W9-BQV-427

Health
in the
Americas

1998 Edition
Volume II

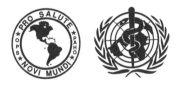

Scientific Publication No. 569

PAN AMERICAN HEALTH ORGANIZATION
Pan American Sanitary Bureau, Regional Office of the
WORLD HEALTH ORGANIZATION
525 Twenty-third Street, N.W.
Washington, D.C. 20037, U.S.A.

1998

Also published in Spanish (1998) with the title:
Las salud en las Américas, Edición de 1998
Publicación Científica de la OPS No. 569
ISBN 92 75 31569 8

PAHO Library Cataloguing in Publication Data

Pan American Health Organization.
  Health in the Americas, 1998 edition.
  Washington, D.C.: PAHO, ©1998—2v.
  (PAHO Scientific Publication; 569)

  ISBN 92 75 11569 9

  I. Title.   II.   (Serie)
  1. HEALTH STATUS   2. HEALTH STATUS INDICATORS
  3. DIAGNOSIS OF HEALTH SITUATION
  4. AMERICAS
  NLM WB141.4

The Pan American Health Organization welcomes requests for permission to reproduce or translate its publications, in part or in full. Applications and inquiries should be addressed to the Publications Program, Pan American Health Organization, Washington, D. C. , U. S. A., which will be glad to provide the latest information on any changes made to the text, plans for new editions, and reprints and translations already available.

© Pan American Health Organization, 1998

CONTENTS

PREFACE

A key function of the Pan American Health Organization (PAHO) is to disseminate information on the health situation and trends in the Region of the Americas. The Organization has performed this function without interruption since 1956, the first year in which an assessment of the health status of the population in the Americas was published. Entitled *Summary of Reports on Health Conditions in the Americas, 1950–1953*, that report was presented to the 15th Pan American Sanitary Conference, held in Santiago, Chile, in 1954. In 1966, the name of the report was changed to *Health Conditions in the Americas*, and from that year on it has been published every four years under that title. Continuing the tradition, the 1998 edition, entitled *Health in the Americas*, becomes the twelfth publication in this series of quadrennial reports. It is being presented to the 25th Pan American Sanitary Conference in September 1998.

Health in the Americas is PAHO's principal vehicle for producing, compiling, analyzing, and disseminating information on the health situation for use by Member Governments. The Organization also produces and distributes other publications that complement the information contained in this one, including *Basic Health Indicators, Health Statistics from the Americas, the Epidemiological Bulletin*, surveillance reports, progress evaluations of progress toward attaining the goal of health for all by the year 2000, and technical documents produced by various specific programs.

Over the years, PAHO has modified the publication's content and format, in order to adapt it to changes in the health profile of the Region's populations, a greater complexity of health systems and services, better and more available information in the countries, characteristics of technical cooperation among countries, and technological advances in the electronic production and processing of data.

The two volumes of this edition of *Health in the Americas* deal mainly with the period between 1993 and 1996. Volume I presents an overview, from PAHO's perspective, of the most relevant aspects of the health situation of the Region's population and analyzes the trends of that situation and the relationship between health and living conditions. It also examines the leading problems that affect special population groups and the manifestations and distribution of diseases and other health impairments. In addition, Volume I looks at the response of health services systems, with special attention to health sector reform and activities in health promotion and environmental protection. The final chapter reviews the trends and characteristics of regional financial assistance and new modalities of technical cooperation among countries. Volume II contains current information on the health situation and trends in each member country and territory of the Organization.

As with previous editions of this report, PAHO hopes that *Health in the Americas* will fulfill the function of keeping the Member Governments informed, and that it also will serve as a reference and source of information for national and international agencies and institutions and for investigators and other professionals working in the health field.

PAHO acknowledges the growing importance of information for decision-making, policy formulation, and evaluation in the countries and in the Secretariat, and it will continue to provide cooperation to strengthen methods, techniques, and procedures for the generation and dissemination of health information. PAHO also is aware that modern technology provides an exceptional opportunity to have universal access to information—thus democratizing it. In so doing, it can enhance and energize the collaboration between the countries and the Organization to achieve better health for the people of the Americas, with equity and sustainable human development.

George A. O. Alleyne
Director

ANGUILLA

GENERAL SITUATION AND TRENDS

Socioeconomic, Political, and Demographic Overview

Anguilla, the northernmost of the Leeward Islands, lies to the north of the island of St. Maarten, and covers an area of 71.3 km². The island is coral limestone formation, with a generally undulating surface; its highest elevation is 738 m above sea level. The climate is tropical, and average annual rainfall is low, ranging from 20 to 50 inches.

It is difficult to distinguish urban from rural settlements in Anguilla, due to the small physical size of the island, its population, and the spatial distribution of development. The Valley is the designated capital. All major settlements are easily accessible by the main road network, which consists of paved and unpaved roads. The island is accessible by sea and air. There are two seaports that accommodate cargo and passenger ferries servicing the St. Maarten/Anguilla route.

In December 1980, Her Majesty Queen Elizabeth signed the "Anguilla Act, 1980," which formally decreed the separation of Anguilla from Saint Kitts and Nevis. The island is a British Dependent Territory. The Governor presides over the Executive Council, which is composed of the Chief Minister, a Cabinet of Ministers, and the Deputy Governor. The Deputy Governor and Governor are representatives of the United Kingdom. The Administration reports to the Legislative Council. General elections are held every five years; the present coalition government was elected in March 1994.

A 1992 review of the Anguilla economy led to the development of the National Development Plan, 1994–1998. The primary goal of the Plan is to ensure sustained and stable economic growth, while minimizing environmental and social losses. Several of the objectives in the Plan have implications for the health sector. These include a planned annual increase in recurrent government revenue of 4.5%; maintained annual growth in recurrent expenditure of 2%; investment of EC$ 22.2 million in the public sector; and promotion of human re- source development through the expansion of education, health, and other social infrastructure in line with population growth and the needs of the economy.

The Anguillan economy registered an annual average growth rate of 7.2% (in constant prices) from 1992 to 1994, but a negative growth rate of 4.4% in 1995 as a result of the devastation caused by Hurricane Luis in September 1995. Gross domestic product in 1990 constant prices was US$ 52.4 million in 1995, compared with US$54.8 million in 1994. Hotels and restaurants, agriculture, and transportation were the sectors that suffered the greatest loss in 1995. Conversely, wholesale and retail, mining and quarrying, and construction registered significant growth, benefiting from post-hurricane reconstruction and rehabilitation. Per capita GDP demonstrated steady growth from US$ 5,128 in 1992 to US$ 5,517 in 1994, with a decline in 1995 to US$ 5,085, in 1990 constant prices.

The tourism industry is the mainstay of the economy, and Government policy advocates investment in large tourism infrastructure projects. According to the 1992 census, the tourism sector employed 21% of the labor force. The offshore financial services sector is being developed as a means of strengthening and diversifying the overall economic base. New legislation governing this sector was passed in 1995. Anguilla has no direct taxes, personal or corporate, and no currency exchange controls.

The 1992 census reported a 7% unemployment rate. The male-female ratio for the employed was 1.2:1, a change from the 1984 ratio of 1.8:1. Increased female employment is related to growth in the tourism sector and increased opportunities for women in the service industries. According to the 1992 census, the distribution of the labor force by occupation group was: 32.3% in production, construction, and transportation; 25.1% in service industries; 20.6% in clerical and sales; 12.5% in professional and technical occupations; 5.6% in agriculture: 3.0% in administration and management; and 0.8% in unspecified occupations. The decline in economic activity following Hurricane Luis in 1995, particularly in the tourism sector, led to contraction in employment, especially for women.

The 1992 census reveals that there were 2,619 housing units in Anguilla in 1992. However, a survey carried out by the Lands and Survey Department in the same year found 4,048 dwelling units, including houses, apartments, and villas. This apparent discrepancy exists because the 1992 census only recorded occupied dwellings. The housing stock improved during the 1992–1995 period, with an increase in speculative building of rental properties by Anguillans. The Land and Survey Department study describes 91% of houses as "constructed from concrete," with 42% of all houses judged to be in good structural condition. Fourteen percent were under construction at the time of the survey.

Sixty-four percent of households have telephones installed, 75% have access to electricity and sewerage, and 90% have water available in their houses. Most households have access to radio and television. Average occupancy is three persons per household.

Anguilla's 71.3 km² of territory is divided into 7,394 parcels, 66% of which are under 1 acre in size. Approximately 95% of the land is privately owned, in small family plots.

Education is compulsory through age 15 in Anguilla. The number of primary and secondary schools has remained constant during the period under review. Primary schools are distributed throughout the island; one secondary school is located in the Valley. Students are provided with transportation to secondary school. There is no screening test for entry into secondary school.

Student enrollment in primary schools from 1992 to 1995 ranged from 1,370 in 1992 to 1,484 in 1995. The teacher-student ratio at this level is 1:20. Secondary school enrollment was 840 in 1992 and 962 in 1995. Females accounted for 51% of students in primary school, and 54% of total enrollment. Government scholarships and loans from the Anguilla Development Board facilitate access to tertiary education.

Over 80% of the labor force received a secondary school education. A further 6% were educated at a technical college, and 7.6% received an university education. The adult literacy rate is 92% (1994), with no reported differential rate by sex.

The estimated population in 1995 was 10,302. The last census, conducted in 1992, established the population as 8,960, of which 49.9% were males. Average annual population growth rate has been 1%. The average annual rate of natural increase for the last 10 years (1986–1995) was 11.4.

Table 1 shows the results of the 1992 census population by age group and sex. According to the Statistical Unit of the Anguilla Ministry of Finance, the total population in 1993 is estimated at 9,248; in 1994, 9,926; and, in 1995, 10,302. Population density is 106 persons per km².

The crude birth rate was 16.7 per 1,000 population for the period 1992–1995. It has shown a decline in the period, with

TABLE 1
Population by age group and sex, Anguilla (1992 census results).

Age group	Total No.	Total %	Male No.	Male %	Female No.	Female %
All ages	8,960	100.0	4,473	49.9	4,487	50.1
0–4 years	986	11.0	494	5.5	492	5.5
5–14	1,749	19.5	867	9.7	882	9.8
15–24	1,558	17.4	796	8.9	762	8.5
25–34	1,668	18.6	848	9.5	820	9.2
35–44	1,098	12.3	560	6.3	538	6.0
45–54	610	6.8	317	3.5	293	3.3
55–64	480	5.4	229	2.6	251	2.8
65 and over	811	9.0	362	4.0	449	5.0

141 live births registered in 1992, 171 in 1993, 163 in 1994, and 167 in 1995. The percentage of births to teenage mothers also declined. Nineteen of the 141 live births in 1992, and 18 of the 163 live births in 1994 were to teenage mothers. The general fertility rate in 1995 was 74.2 per 1,000 women 15–44 years of age.

There has been increasing migration into Anguilla, particularly from neighboring Caribbean islands. In the 1992 census, non-Anguillans accounted for 16% of the population, with even sex distribution. They were mostly of working age and children. No significant trend towards urban migration has been observed.

Mortality Profile

During the1992–1995 period, 237 deaths (124 females and 113 males) were reported. The number of deaths by year was 68 in 1992, 63 in 1993, 52 in 1994, and 54 in 1995. During this period, 64.6% of all deaths were in the 70 and older age group (153 deaths), 12.7% were 60–69 years old (30 deaths), 11.6% were 40–59 years old (25 deaths), 4.2% were 20–39 years old (10 deaths), and 5.1% were less than one year old (12 deaths). Seven deaths occurred in the 1–19-year age group.

The infant mortality rate for the 1992–1995 period was 18.7 per 1,000 live births. There were 12 infant deaths in this period: 4 in 1992, 2 in 1993, 1 in 1994, and 5 in 1995. Infant deaths occurred mostly in the neonatal period. During the 1992–1995 period, 671 deliveries and 8 stillbirths were recorded. One maternal death occurred in the entire 1992–1995 period. A summary of mortality by cause during the 1992–1995 period is shown in Table 2.

Among deaths due to communicable diseases, septicemia was the most common cause of death (44%). No deaths due

TABLE 2
Mortality by cause of death, Anguilla, 1992–1995.

Cause group	Deaths	Percent
Total deaths, all causes	237	100.0
Ill-defined conditions	54	22.8
Total deaths, defined conditions	183	100.0
Communicable diseases	27	14.8
Neoplasms	36	19.7
Diseases of the circulatory system	75	41.0
Conditions originating in the perinatal period	9	4.9
External causes	7	3.8
All other diseases	29	15.8

to tuberculosis were reported. Among deaths caused by neoplasms, 14% were due to cancer of the stomach. In the category of diseases of the circulatory system, cerebrovascular diseases were the predominant cause of death (34.7%). This was followed by deaths due to ischemic heart disease (21.3%) and hypertensive disease (14.6%). Hypoxia and birth asphyxia were the most common causes of death due to conditions originating in the perinatal period (67%). Of the deaths in the "external causes" category, one was due to a motor vehicle accident and one was a homicide.

SPECIFIC HEALTH PROBLEMS

Analysis by Population Group

Perinatal and Child Health

Because many Anguillans seek health services in neighboring islands, these data are not complete.

Over the 1992–1995 period, there were 9 neonatal deaths and 16 perinatal deaths reported. An analysis of perinatal deaths revealed that 67% were due to asphyxia and hypoxia, and occurred during the neonatal period. Twelve deaths under age 1 were recorded in 1992–1995.

There were 76 low-birthweight infants registered from 1992 to 1995. Three deaths in the 1–4-year age group were recorded during 1992–1995.

Acute respiratory tract infection is the leading cause of morbidity in this age group. Gastroenteritis is not reportedly a serious problem. Cases are generally managed in the clinics by district nurses, using oral rehydration salts and referring them to another level as appropriate. There is no defined prevention and control program for diarrheal diseases.

Growth monitoring of all children under 5 years old is performed at district clinics. An informal descriptive study was conducted in 1997, reviewing a sample of infants registered and monitored at the Valley Clinic. Results indicate that obesity in this group (estimated at 10%) is emerging as a problem. Breast-feeding is declining; only 3% of infants were observed to be breast-fed at three months, and 50% of infants were "eating from the family pot" at 6 months of age.

Immunization coverage during the 1992–1996 period was 100% for BCG, MMR, polio, and DTP. Two suspected cases of flaccid paralysis were investigated in 1995, but neither was confirmed as polio. All pregnant women are immunized against tetanus.

The school health service provides screening for children in the 5–9-year age group, including physical examinations and dental, hearing, and vision screening. There is no organized vision referral service, but a visiting specialist offers limited services. Worm infestation was reported in 4% of 5–6 year olds.

Health of Adolescents

The number of births to teenage mothers is declining. During the 1992–1995 period, births to mothers under 19 years old averaged 13.5% of total births. Family planning services are available to adolescents, and a family life education program, which includes peer counseling and skills training, has been implemented in schools. There are no other formally organized health services for this age group.

An increasing number of cases of abuse in children under 16 years old have been referred to the Social Welfare Department. Between 1991 and 1994 there were 122 cases, compared with 51 cases in the 1987–1990 period. Most of the cases were female.

Health of Adults

Prenatal care is provided by midwives in district clinics and by the resident obstetrician/gynecologist. Approximately 80% of pregnant women attending prenatal clinics enroll before the 16th week of pregnancy. Routine supplements of iron, folic acid, and vitamins are distributed. A review of laboratory reports of hemoglobin estimates for pregnant mothers for the period January to June 1995 revealed that 15.6% of these women had hemoglobin levels below 11 mg/dl.

Prenatal referrals to the hospital for complications of pregnancy and other medical reasons comprised 43% of prenatal clinic attendance in 1993, 57% in 1994, and 55% in 1995. Virtually all deliveries (>99%) are performed at the hospital and attended by trained health personnel. No home deliveries are performed. During the 1992–1995 period, 20% to 23% of all deliveries were by cesarean section. No special reason for this high rate can be deduced from the available data. There are no available data on abortions.

Immediate postpartum care begins in the hospital and continued through home visits by district midwives. The communication between hospital and the districts in this area requires strengthening.

Family planning services are delivered at the health centers. Registered clients totaled 560 in 1993, 747 in 1994, and 601 in 1995. New acceptors constituted 10%–15% of current users, but a decrease in the number of new acceptors has been reported (83 in 1993, 86 in 1994, and 63 in 1995). Oral contraceptives and injectables were used by 54% and 31% of clients, respectively, in 1995. No intrauterine device insertions were recorded between 1993 and 1995.

Pap tests are available in the private and public sectors. Coverage is low, with 279 examinations conducted in 1993, 189 in 1994, and 261 in 1995. Of these, abnormalities were reported in 53% of specimens in 1993, 68% in 1994, and 47% in 1995. Two cases of cancer in situ I and cancer in situ II were discovered in 1993 and 1994, and 19 in 1995. Three deaths from cervical cancer were reported during the 1992–1995 period.

Chronic noncommunicable diseases, mainly diabetes and hypertension, contribute significantly to the morbidity and mortality in this group.

Health of the Elderly

The elderly (60 years and over) constitute 12% of the total population as outlined in the 1992 census report. Females comprise 55% of age group. Most elderly persons live at home with extended family, but a growing number live alone. Health care providers, mainly nurses, make periodic home visits to the housebound elderly for routine monitoring and medical care, averaging 329 visits annually (1993–1995).

Chronic noncommunicable diseases are the main contributors to mortality and morbidity in this age group. In 1995, 70% of diabetic admissions to the hospital and 57% of hypertensive admissions were over 60 years old. Other problems affecting the care of this group include social isolation, lack of occupational and recreational facilities, and disabilities.

Family Health

The 1992 census revealed that 25% of households housed single persons; 42%, nuclear families; 12%, extended families; and 2%, composite living arrangements.

Statistics compiled by the Social Welfare Department indicate that during the 1991–1994 period, the average annual number of reported cases concerning child support was 133; child abuse cases averaged 31; an average of 9 cases concerned divorce; 69 related to domestic disputes; and 72 concerned juvenile delinquency.

Family members have access to public and private health services. Public health services at primary and secondary care levels are very accessible, and include maternal and child health services and general medical care. Families can seek exemptions from the nominal charges at the hospital through the Social Welfare Department.

Workers' Health

There is no specific program that addresses occupational health. Both the Environmental Health Department and Labor Division are proposing surveillance and promotion activities in this area.

Analysis by Type of Disease or Health Impairment

Communicable Diseases

Vector-Borne Diseases. No cases of malaria or yellow fever were reported on the island during the 1992–1995 period. Cases of dengue fever occur in Anguilla, but no known case of dengue hemorrhagic fever was identified during the reporting period. The *Aedes aegypti* mosquito is highly prevalent on the island, but no reliable estimate of the household or Breteau index is available.

Vaccine-Preventable Diseases. There were no confirmed cases of poliomyelitis, tetanus, measles, tuberculosis, rubella, or diphtheria reported from 1992 to 1996.

Acute Respiratory Infections. Acute respiratory infections cause significant morbidity in children and adults. Eight deaths in 1995, mainly in the 65 and older age group, were attributed to acute respiratory infections.

Sexually Transmitted Diseases. Sexually transmitted diseases (STDs) are prevalent, but no data are available because many persons go to St. Maarten for treatment. Pap tests from 1993 to 1995 indicated the presence of STDs. There were 312 blood donors for the 1993–1995 period, all of whom were screened. None tested positive for HIV or syphilis, nine were positive for hepatitis B (3% prevalence).

Noncommunicable Diseases and Other Health-Related Problems

Nutritional Diseases and Diseases of Metabolism. Obesity, particularly among women and children, is cited as one of the major health problems facing Anguilla. This is related to lack of physical activity and over-consumption of processed or refined foods. Most of the food eaten in Anguilla is imported.

Anemia was found in an estimated 22% of 5- and 6-year-olds and 7% of 11-year-olds in 1996. In 1992, an estimated 14% of women were anemic.

Accidents and Violence. Data on accidents and violence are inadequate, as are data on morbidity due to domestic violence. From 1992 to 1995, two deaths due to accidents and one from violence were recorded. Police statistics for 1992 to 1994 register 24 reported cases of rape and indecent assault, 3 cases of murder and manslaughter, and 76 serious assaults and wounding. These figures show a moderate increase compared with the 1989–1991 period.

Oral Health. Oral health screening and treatment take place at the Dental Clinic. The ratio of tooth extractions to fillings, while declining, is approximately 1:2, an unacceptably high level. No dental epidemiological survey has been conducted in the last five years, so scores for decayed, missing, and filled teeth (DMFT) are not available. The number of visits to the dental clinic steadily increased from 5,670 visits in 1992, to 6,156 in 1993, and 6,564 in 1994. Visits decreased to 6,009 in 1995. Tooth extractions have consistently declined in this period, from 2,526 in 1992, to 1,788 in 1993, 1,614 in 1994, and 1,508 in 1995. No clear trend is seen in the number of fillings: there were 2,347 in 1992, 3,733 in 1993, 2,935 in 1994, and 3,323 in 1995.

Natural Disasters. Anguilla lies in the tropical storm belt and is at risk from hurricanes and storm surges. In September 1995, the island's infrastructure was damaged by Hurricane Luis, adversely affecting Anguilla's main sources of national and personal income. Thirty-five percent of houses were damaged, and direct damages to the health sector's infrastructure, equipment, and supplies totaled US$ 218,000.

There is a national disaster plan, and a national emergency relief committee coordinates mitigation and response activities. There is a need for operational plans at village and departmental levels.

Risk Factors. There is evidence of degradation of coastal and marine environment due to pollution caused by discharge of sewerage from hotels and restaurants, and discharge of sewerage and oil from visiting yachts and ships. No coastal pollution-monitoring program has been implemented.

There are no rivers in Anguilla, and a significant portion of the water supply is derived from wells. The groundwater is at risk of contamination from direct discharges of effluents, chemicals, and pesticides in areas near the aquifer; intrusion of salt water; and uncontrolled disposal of solid waste. The Environmental Health Department does not monitor water quality.

The septic tank is the most common method of liquid waste disposal in Anguilla (81% of households). Poor design frequently results in malfunction and the release of partially treated effluent into the underground water system, from which the public supply is drawn. The Environmental Health Department lacks expertise in regular monitoring of effluent from package treatment plants.

The high prevalence of the *Aedes aegypti* mosquito, which breeds in water cisterns and rock holes, poses a constant threat for dengue and dengue hemorrhagic fever outbreaks. No estimate of the *Aedes aegypti* index is available.

RESPONSE OF THE HEALTH SYSTEM

National Health Plans and Policies

In September 1995, the Minister of Social Services outlined the key policies and priorities for health development. The stated aim of the Government's health policy is to provide high-quality, accessible primary and secondary health care services to the population of Anguilla and to include provisions for the transfer of patients overseas, thereby maintaining and promoting the health of the population, and supporting the continuing socioeconomic well-being of Anguillans.

The health policy advocates a partnership of private and public health care providers. The Government's top priorities involve improvements in the following areas: quality care; performance of environmental health services; access to health care; and the scope, accessibility, and performance of primary health care services. The policy promotes good physical and mental health and greater service efficiency and cost-effectiveness.

The policy statement acknowledged that the achievement of these priorities is dependent on improved performance in the private and public sector through more consumer-oriented service, better management, improved public/private sector collaboration, and a more proactive approach to planning.

Organization of the Health System

Institutional Organization

The Ministry of Social Services is responsible for the management of health services. The Director of Health Services bears responsibility for the effective functioning of all departments, and delegates responsibility through the Senior Medical Officer of the Hospital, the Primary Health Care Manager, Health Services Administrator, and Principal Nursing Officer. The post of Primary Health Care Coordinator was recently created.

In 1995, a new management structure for health services, which utilizes four teams, was approved by the Executive Council with the objective of making demonstrable and expeditious improvements to health care management. The four teams are described below.

The Health Services Strategy group is responsible to the Ministry of Social Services for health planning, advice on policy issues, financial and budgetary review, and quality assurance in the public and private sector. This group comprises senior technical and administrative staff and a representative of the Ministry of Finance.

The Senior Management group is responsible for the overall management and coordination of publicly provided health services. It is chaired by the Director of Health Services, and is composed of senior technical heads of departments.

The Primary Health Care Management team and the Hospital Management team are each responsible for day-to-day management of services in their respective departments. A Department of Primary Health Care supervises the delivery of services at the community level.

The private health sector in Anguilla is small, limited to primary and selected tertiary care. Anguillans frequently go to Saint Kitts, Puerto Rico, St. Maarten, and elsewhere for medical services, even those available in Anguilla. The Government proposes strengthening the private sector through greater sharing of facilities, information, and joint training. By enhancing the role of the private sector, the Government aims to retain a portion of the scarce private and public funds spent overseas.

The Medical Council certifies and monitors medical practices. There is no mechanism for regulating the practice of other health professionals.

Health Services and Resources

Organization of Services for Care of the Population

Health Promotion and Community Participation. Community participation has been recognized as an essential component of the Anguillan approach to primary health care. The Department of Primary Health Care works to empower communities to take decisions concerning their own health. Health committees have been formed in two health districts. While no formal structure exists presently in support of intersectoral collaboration, several informal intersectoral programs have been established, including programs on water monitoring and solid waste management, a dental mobile unit, and a health/education liaison committee.

Two health educators deliver education programs that focus on the promotion of health and wellness, and emphasize behavior modification and lifestyle changes, targeting schoolchildren, young adults, and community groups. Alliances have been formed with the media, and a weekly radio program disseminates health information.

Epidemiological Surveillance. An epidemiologist was appointed in 1995. The health information system is being improved through the Community Health Information System and Health Sector Adjustment projects. The system aims to improve medical record-keeping and to provide more timely and appropriate information for purposes of quality assurance, epidemiology, resource management, and planning.

The Environmental Health Department is responsible for waste management, food hygiene, vector control, liquid waste management, the monitoring of drinking water, environmental sanitation, beach and roadside cleaning, building better hygiene practices, occupational health and safety, and the provision of low-cost sanitation services. The department is severely constrained by inadequate manpower, limited training, and a lack of technology.

The Department retains responsibility for collection of refuse from government institutions, public roads, and beaches. Domestic solid waste is collected twice weekly, free of charge. No provision is made for the removal of construction waste, old appliances, and derelict vehicles. Hotels and other commercial establishments are required to make their own arrangements for collection of waste. An estimated 12 tons of garbage are disposed of daily at the 10-acre landfill, where waste is placed in pre-excavated trenches and covered with fill.

Potable water supplies encompass rainwater collected in cisterns, groundwater abstraction from wells, and reverse osmosis treatment of salt water: 41% of households receive their water from rainwater collected in cisterns, and 32% from both cisterns and a private piped source. All homes have access to piped water within the home or in the yard. The two main aquifers supplying water are located in the Valley, and contain 70% of the groundwater resources of the island. Over 70% of local demand is supplied by the public water system, with an average daily production of 285,000 gallons; 28% comes from rainwater collected in cisterns. The commercial sector (restaurants, bars, shops, and some hotels) is allegedly the largest consumer of public water. The Government received funding from the British Government and the European Union for a water development project that includes new storage and distribution facilities and upgrading the abstraction system.

The Anguilla Water Authority is responsible for the planning, construction, operation, and maintenance of water supply works. Treatment and testing of groundwater is the responsibility of the Anguilla Water Authority, while the Environmental Health Department carries out inspection and treatment of cisterns. The Environmental Health Department does not conduct water quality surveillance, and monitoring by the Water Authority is not continuous.

There is no sewerage system in Anguilla. All wastewater/ sewerage is treated and disposed of on-site by means of septic tanks (81% of households), soakaways, pit latrines (13%), and package treatment plants, which are used primarily by hotels, some commercial establishments, and government institutions.

Environmental conditions in schools, health facilities, and public buildings are monitored. Routine vector control activities are performed at these compounds.

The 1978 Food Hygiene regulation empowers the health department to conduct periodic inspections of premises where food, drink, and other commodities are sold. The food handlers' program involves the examination, certification, and registration of all food handlers and premises. Education of food handlers is an integral component of the program. In 1996, 180 food establishments and 500 food handlers were registered.

Vector control activities concentrate on the control of the *Aedes aegypti* mosquito and rodents. A national *Aedes aegypti* control program uses a community-based approach. Activities include the stocking of cisterns and water storage facilities with larvicidal fish, house inspections, and treatment. There is significant breeding in the environment. Rodent control is ongoing, with baiting at food premises, schools, and public institutions. Rodenticides are sold to the public.

Organization and Operation of Personal Health Care Services

The health care delivery system consists of a public and private sector. The private sector services include primary and secondary care. The public sector delivers primary care services from five district health centers. Secondary care is delivered at the Princess Alexandra Hospital, a new, 36-bed facility. Hospital services include emergency treatment; outpatient and inpatient care for surgical, medical, pediatric, gynecological, and obstetric cases; laboratory and radiological diagnostic services; and pharmacy service. A nurse or doctor makes referrals to services at the hospital from the primary care level.

For primary health care delivery, the island has been divided into five health districts each with a health center and defined boundaries. Two levels of care—Level III and Level II have been distinguished. Level III comprises the smallest four health clinics, which are staffed by a public health nurse, clinic aide, and environmental health officer. These clinics provide basic core services, including maternal and child health, family planning, immunization, nutrition advice, basic medical clinics conducted twice weekly, care of the elderly, management of chronic diseases, health education, and environmental health. Level II care is provided from the Valley Health Clinic, which serves as a referral center for Level III,

and offers daily medical clinics as well as basic primary care services to its defined catchment population. Support from the nutritionist, health educator, pharmacist, and district medical officer is provided from this level. Referrals are made from Level II to the hospital. Except for puerperal mothers, there is no systematic mechanism for referral of patients from the hospital back to the primary level of care.

Public dental services are located at the central unit in the Valley, and supported by a mobile unit that provides care to the primary schools. Two dental surgeons, three dental auxiliaries, and two dental assistants staff the service.

A 10-bed geriatric care unit provides institutional care for the elderly.

A psychiatric nurse provides community mental health services, and is responsible for maintenance care of all mentally ill patients. A visiting psychiatrist supports the services in diagnosis and treatment review. Emergencies can be referred to a district medical officer. There is no mental health facility. Violent cases are detained at Her Majesty's Prison, and patients requiring specialized hospital care can be referred to neighboring Caribbean islands, at the Government's expense.

The island has no facilities for tertiary care, which is sought from the United Kingdom, St. Maarten, Puerto Rico, and other Caribbean islands.

Inputs for Health

Anguilla has become an active member of the Eastern Caribbean Drug Service (ECDS), a regional procurement scheme for pharmaceutical and medical supplies. The ECDS also gives support in the areas of inventory control and organization. The situation has vastly improved as a result of ECDS cooperation. Prior to this, the drug service experienced high costs, frequent shortages, large quantities of expired drugs, and poor inventory control.

There is no national formulary and purchases are guided by the regional Eastern Caribbean Formulary. Similarly, there is no stipulated list of essential drugs.

Vaccines are obtained from the Expanded Program on Immunization. Inventory control is good, and a reliable service is maintained.

Drug expenditure has remained constant in the 1992–1995 period. During that period, a total of US$ 658,145 was spent. The highest annual expenditure in this period was US$ 168,552 in 1993.

Human Resources

There are no training institutions for health personnel in Anguilla. Depending on health staffing needs, personnel are sent to various Caribbean islands, the United Kingdom, or the United States of America. Increasingly, local training workshops, particularly in primary health care issues, are organized. It is the Government's policy to support training for health personnel in the public and private sectors, and to open all locally organized training to participation by the private sector.

In 1995, there were 9 doctors, 37 trained nurses, 2 dentists, 4 pharmacists, 2 dental auxiliaries, 3 laboratory technicians, 2 radiographers, 4 environmental health officers, 1 nutritionist, and 3 health educators. New categories of workers have been trained to enhance delivery of services at the primary health care level in the fields of nutrition and dietetics, health information, epidemiology, environmental health, and public health nursing. Nursing personnel were redistributed in the primary care sector for improved island coverage.

Expenditures and Sectoral Financing

The Government is the major provider of health services in Anguilla. Recurrent expenditure on health in 1995 was 18% of total Government expenditure, which ranks second after education, and represents 4.5% of the gross domestic product. Approximately 12% of the total recurrent expenditure for health is collected in users' fees for dental, hospital, and pharmacy services. Some 90% of the cost of health services is subsidized through exemption of persons from charges and unrealistic user fees.

The level of private expenditure is not known. However, it was estimated that in 1993, nationals spent at least US$ 1.48 million for private doctor fees and for accessing treatment outside of Anguilla.

The country's decision in 1995 to restructure its health care process has led to greater definition in the health budget, and a separate budget line for primary health care with delegated financial control for expenditure and monitoring.

External Technical and Financial Cooperation

The health services received assistance for capital expenditure from the Dependent Territories Regional Secretariat of the British Foreign Office, totaling US$ 1.3 million from 1992–1995. This was allocated to Princess Alexandra Hospital, the Infirmary, and East End Clinic, which were damaged by Hurricane Luis.

The Overseas Development Agency of the United Kingdom funded the health sector adjustment project, which examined restructuring of the health services with a particular focus on equity, efficiency, effectiveness, quality, and strengthening primary health care.

ANTIGUA AND BARBUDA

GENERAL SITUATION AND TRENDS

Socioeconomic, Political, and Demographic Overview

The nation of Antigua and Barbuda comprises the islands Antigua and Barbuda, and the uninhabited island of Redonda. Located at the center of the Eastern Caribbean's Leeward Islands group, the country is 440 km^2 in area, with Antigua occupying 64% of the land mass and containing 98% of the population.

Antigua has relatively flat topography characterized by central plains and volcanic hills rising in the southwest (reaching altitudes of 400 m), all of which strongly influence the island's hydrology. To the north and east, the soil is mainly calcareous limestone. Annual rainfall is low, averaging 40 inches, and droughts occur every 5 to 10 years. There are no rivers and very few streams. A desalination plant supplies approximately 50% of the water needs of the island.

Antigua and Barbuda became independent in November 1981. It is governed by an elected parliament representing majority and opposition parties, with elections occurring at least every five years. The country is divided into 17 administrative constituencies, which include Barbuda. Executive authority is vested in a cabinet that is headed by a Prime Minister and comprises 10 Ministers.

Population

Table 1 shows results of the most recent national population census conducted in mid-1991 and mid-year estimates for 1995. Life expectancy at birth is 70 years for males and 74 years for females. The 1995 estimated mid-year population was 64,353, representing a 1% increase from the estimated 1988 mid-year population that was recalculated at 63,683. The number of registered live births varied over the past sev-

TABLE 1
Population by age group and sex in 1991 and estimated mid-year population in 1995, Antigua and Barbuda.

Age group	Population by age group and sex, 1991				Estimated mid-year population by age group and sex, 1995			
	Total	Total population (%)	Male	Female	Total	Total population (%)	Male	Female
0–4	6,152	10.4	3,080	3,072	6,670	10.4	3,339	3,321
5–14	11,925	20.1	5,961	5,964	12,929	20.1	6,462	6,467
15–44	28,653	48.3	14,874	13,779	31,066	48.3	14,940	16,126
45–64	7,740	13.0	3,671	4,069	8,391	13.0	3,979	4,412
65+	4,885	8.2	2,121	2,764	5,297	8.2	2,300	2,997
Total	59,355	100	28,612	30,743	64,353	100	31,020	33,333

Source: Population and Housing Census—1991, Antigua and Barbuda Ministry of Health, Health Statistics Department.

eral years, peaking at 1,347 in 1995. The birth rate also peaked in 1995 at 20.93 per 1,000 population.

According to the 1991 census, approximately 91% of the population was of African origin, 3.7% of mixed race, and 2.36% white. There were small groups with Syrian, Lebanese, Chinese, East Indian, and Portuguese ancestry.

Antigua and Barbuda attracts immigrants from many countries. Foreign-born residents came primarily from Dominica, the Dominican Republic, Guyana, Jamaica, Montserrat, Saint Kitts and Nevis, Saint Lucia, and Saint Vincent and the Grenadines. There was a noted increase in Spanish-speaking residents, which had an impact on the delivery of health and education services. In addition, a number of expatriate retirees and their offspring returned from the United Kingdom and the United States of America. The number of work permits granted to foreign workers in 1993 was 2,278 compared to 3,417 in 1994, and 3,657 in 1995. CARICOM citizens accounted for 68.6% of these permits in 1993, 74.7% in 1994, and 77.7% in 1995.

Economy and Education

The country's economy depends primarily on tourism, which, with related services, accounts for 65% of the GDP. Other major contributors were government services, wholesale and retail trade, construction, communications, real estate, and housing. The Government continues to focus on further developing the tourist industry and diversifying the economy through expansion of the financial and information sectors.

There was a steady increase in GDP at factor cost in constant prices from 1992 to 1995, averaging US$ 403 million. In 1995, tourism, finance and information sector activities, and agriculture contributed US$ 59.2 million, US$ 30.5 million, and US$ 13.6 million, respectively. The contribution from tourism declined substantially, dropping from US$ 70.8 million in 1994, in part because of damage caused by Hurricane Luis. Contributions from agriculture showed only slight increases, with an average of US$ 14 million, while banks and financial institutions averaged US$ 28 million over the period. Per capita GDP in constant prices was US$ 2,399.1 in 1994 and US$ 2,288.1 in 1995, compared to US$ 2,192.0 in 1991.

The external debt was approximately US $340 million in 1995, an increase from US$ 270 million in 1992. In 1993, the Government imposed a home-grown structural adjustment program that includes the satisfaction of Government debt obligations and other financial commitments. Debt repayment (domestic and external) totaled 19.2% of actual expenditure in 1995. The inflation rate in 1994 was 3.5% (IMF Interim Index), down from 7.0% in 1990.

Since 1973, Antigua and Barbuda has had a free and compulsory system of education for children 5–16 years old. In 1994–1995, there were 12,059 students enrolled in 30 public and 12 private primary schools; 4,646 children were enrolled in 9 public and 4 private secondary schools. The percentage of males attending decreased at higher education levels in the 1994–1995 period. While male attendance at the primary level was slightly higher than female attendance, at the state college level it was 2% less. A survey done in 1993 by the Antigua Literacy Program found that 15.6% of the adult population was illiterate.

The education system's infrastructure was badly damaged by Hurricane Luis, and intensive effort has been concentrated on repairs. The quality of both academic and technical tertiary level education at the State College continued to improve. The local center for the University of the West Indies (an institution jointly operated by the English-speaking Caribbean Governments) provided continuing education through the distance teaching system that links the University's centers in different Caribbean locations through satellite. Private institutions provided technical and secretarial education courses.

Mortality and Morbidity Profile

Death certificates completed by physicians generate mortality data. The crude death rate remained at approximately 7 per 1,000 population in 1995 compared to 6.3 per 1,000 in 1990.

Malignant neoplasms remained the leading cause of death in Antigua and Barbuda. The other leading causes of death include cerebrovascular and heart diseases, hypertensive diseases, and diabetes mellitus. Unfortunately, "signs, symptoms, and ill-defined conditions" were recorded for almost 6.6% of all deaths, reflecting the lack of attention paid to details of death certification.

Infant mortality rates have declined steadily since 1988. In 1995, the infant mortality rate decreased to 17.1 per 1,000 live births compared to 22.7 in 1991. The yearly average during the period was 20.3 per 1,000 live births, compared to 24.6 for 1988–1991. The most frequent cause of infant mortality is prematurity, reported in 57 of 109 (52.3%) deaths in 1991–1995.

In 1995, the most frequently reported communicable diseases were influenza and respiratory infections, gastroenteritis (notifiable only for children under 5 years old), chickenpox, conjunctivitis, syphilis and other venereal diseases, and foodborne illness.

The leading conditions for which persons sought treatment in the community health centers were hypertension (24.7% in 1994 and 32.9% in 1995, compared with 31.1% in 1992), diabetes mellitus (9.8% in 1994 and 12.2% in 1995), and accidents and injuries (3.5% in 1994 and 4.6% in 1995). Other common conditions included arthritis, heart disease, acute respiratory infections, alcohol and drug abuse, gastroenteritis, bronchial asthma, mental illness, and sexually transmitted diseases.

SPECIFIC HEALTH PROBLEMS

Analysis by Population Group

Health of Children and Adolescents

According to the 1991 census, the age group 0–4 years old accounted for 10.4% of the total population, with a male-female ratio of 1:1. During the period 1992–1995 there were 5,012 live births, an average of 1,275 births annually. The average birth rate was 19.8 per 1,000 population. In 1995, 90% (1,216) of the 1,347 live births took place in Holberton Hospital, Anguilla's main hospital. Seven percent (96) of births occurred at the Adelin Medical Center (a private hospital), and 2.6% (35) took place outside of the secondary care system. There was no clear reason for this trend, as the Government's policy sought to maximize the number of births taking place in institutions. The health sector was well equipped with adequate facilities, including a special care unit for premature and other infants requiring intensive care. Twenty of the 21 stillbirths occurring in 1995 were in Holberton Hospital, with one in the district service.

There were no substantial changes in the percentages of low-birthweight infants based on standards of the Caribbean Food and Nutrition Growth Chart; figures remained at approximately 4.9%. There was a decline in the number of infants considered underweight and overweight in the under-1 year category: a decline from 2.3% to 1.4% in the underweight category and from 9.3% to 8.5% in the overweight category. Similar decreases were seen in the 1–4-year age group.

The most common health problems seen among infants and in the 1–5-year age group attending health clinics are acute respiratory infections, diarrheal diseases, injuries, and skin infections. In the 1988–1991 period, the leading cause of admission to Holberton Hospital among children under 1 year old was gastrointestinal infection; for those 1–4 years old it was respiratory tract infections. In the 1992–1995 period, bronchial asthma replaced gastroenteritis and neonatal jaundice as the leading cause of child hospitalization.

During the 1992–1995 period, there were 103 deaths of infants under 1 year old, with 43% occurring on the day of birth. There was, however, a decline from 27 day-of-birth

deaths in 1991 to only 6 deaths in 1995. In 1995 there were no marked differences between the death rates for male and female infants.

Perinatal deaths declined from 38.4 per 1,000 deliveries in 1991, averaging 28.2 over the 1992–1995 period and 27.8 per 1,000 in 1995. Perinatal mortality seemed related to two factors: birthweight of infant and age of mother. During the 1991–1995 period, 95% of all infants born weighing less than 1,001 g died (49% of those who weighed 1,001–1,500 g and 20% of those 1,500–2,000 g). Only 3% of infants born weighing over 2,500 g died.

In 1995, births to women aged 35 and older represented 11.2% of total births. The percentage of stillbirths to mothers in this age group for the period 1991–1994 was 18.6% while the same age group contributed 9.94% of all live births. Percentage contributions to stillbirths markedly exceed contributions to live births in this age group.

Regular child health sessions screened for developmental and other problems and provided parents with child care guidance and counseling. More than 60% of infants attended clinics at or before the age of 6 weeks in 1994, and over 70% attended in 1995.

Children 5–19 years old comprise 30% of the total population. School-aged children periodically receive screening by family nurse practitioners for vision, hearing, speech, dental health, mental health, hemoglobin levels, weight/height, etc. Family life education was not officially introduced into the school curriculum, but family nurse practitioners and family life educators worked in the schools through invitation from the principals.

Ninety-three percent of school entrants (5 or more years old) had complete immunizations (DTP, DT, polio, and MMR) before beginning school. In 1995, it was estimated that there were 1,733 first visits to clinics by school-aged children and adolescents.

Respiratory illness accounted for 80% of the conditions presented by school-aged children who attended clinics for the first time in 1995. Dental and vision problems were the next two reasons for visits to community clinics in this age group.

Births to women under 20 years of age represented 15.8% of total births in 1995, a figure that has remained constant over the period.

The United Nations Fund for Population Activities (UNFPA) funded a peer counseling and youth health services project that ended in 1996. Part-time staff, including a nurse with training in adolescent health, a family nurse practitioner, and a gynecologist managed the school-based program. They addressed the social and health care needs of adolescents by providing health assessments and ongoing treatment, guidance and counseling, education on AIDS and other sexually transmitted diseases, substance abuse awareness, family life education and family planning, Pap tests, and other services.

Health of Adults

Fifty percent of the estimated mid-year 1995 population was between 20 and 59 years old; 52% was female. In 1994 and 1995, twice as many females as males made first time visits to clinics. Hypertension and diabetes accounted for the majority of cases seen at community health clinics. Persons in this age group also made substantial numbers of visits for accidents and/or injuries, respiratory infections, and heart disease.

The leading causes of death in the age group 15–64 years old in 1995 were diseases of the circulatory system and neoplasms. Males accounted for more than twice as many deaths as females. Women in this age group were targeted for maternal health interventions. In 1995, women in this age group accounted for 84.2% of all births, a figure consistent with the average over the 1991–1994 period. No maternal deaths were recorded.

Community health records indicate that the condom was the preferred contraceptive method among new family planning acceptors. Among active users, however, there appeared to be equal preference for oral contraceptives and injectables. Increasing awareness about AIDS and other sexually transmitted diseases (STDs) among all age groups suggests that the use of contraceptives increased significantly since 1988. Contraceptives were procured primarily through the private sector, so community health clinic figures are not necessarily indicative of the national situation.

Health of the Elderly

The 1995 estimated mid-year population indicated that 7,114 persons were age 60 or older; 4,000 (56%) were female. In 1995, there were 296 deaths in the 65 and older age group, representing 69.5% of all deaths.

Most of the health problems affecting the elderly were due to chronic, noncommunicable diseases. Hypertension and diabetes accounted for the majority of cases seen in clinics. Malignant neoplasms, heart disease, cerebrovascular disease, hypertensive disease, and diabetes mellitus were the main causes of death in this group. The community program for adults and the elderly served 4,164 patients in 1995; 1,759 of them were over 65 years old. Many had risk factors related to obesity, alcoholism, and smoking.

The Citizens Welfare Division of the Ministry of Home Affairs introduced a home help program for the elderly. A number of small private homes for the aged emerged to supplement services provided by the Fiennes Institute, a Government institution.

Family Health

According to a 1991 report, approximately 58% of all households were headed by women, who constituted about 52% of the labor force. There is no specific program for family health. The Citizens Welfare Division provided a variety of services including advice regarding probation and rehabilitation; foster care placement and monitoring; counseling on parenting; and reporting on court investigations.

Issues related to the situation of abused, neglected, and abandoned children are a priority on the national policy agenda. A Sexual Offences Act passed in 1995 provided severe penalties for statutory rape and incest. The Citizens Welfare Division and the Collaborative Committee for the Promotion of Emotional Health in Children works closely with the police to monitor parental neglect and abuse. In the 1991–1995 period, 103 cases of sexual abuse were reported to the police, with 24 occurring in 1994 and 19 in 1995.

Workers' Health

There was no specific workers' health program, but the workman's compensation legislation applies to most workers. All employed persons are required to participate in the medical benefit and social security schemes through monthly contributions of a fixed percentage of salary. The medical benefits scheme provides medication, laboratory, X-ray, and other services to persons diagnosed with certain chronic diseases including hypertension, diabetes, cancer, glaucoma, and mental illness. Social security benefits include grants for disability, maternity, and pension.

Health of the Disabled

The Council for the Handicapped, which coordinates activities for the disabled, was revived in 1995. Special programs for the visually handicapped included general education and technical and craft training, which are organized by nongovernmental organizations with some support from the Government. Hemiplegia and blindness due to cataracts, glaucoma, and diabetes were common causes of disability among the elderly.

Analysis by Type of Disease or Health Impairment

Communicable Diseases

Vector-Borne Diseases. There were no recent outbreaks of vector-borne illnesses. Dengue is endemic in the Caribbean and the *Aedes aegypti* mosquito, vector of dengue and yellow fever, is present in the island. While there is constant surveillance to prevent the importation of malaria, two imported cases were detected in 1995.

Ciguatera poisoning is associated with locally caught barracuda and other fish. There were 322 cases reported in 1995 and 330 in 1994. Many cases go unreported because they are commonly treated with home remedies.

Vaccine-Preventable Diseases. In 1994 and 1995, there was approximately 100% coverage for infants under 15 months for diphtheria, tetanus, and pertussis (DTP) and polio (OPV), and 94% coverage for measles, mumps, and rubella (MMR). Between 1993 and 1995 an average of 40% of pregnant women were immunized against tetanus.

The most recent case of tetanus was recorded in 1993. There have been no cases of diphtheria or pertussis in recent years, and there were no confirmed cases of measles in 1994–1995. No cases of typhoid fever have been reported in the last 10 years. In the first quarter of 1995, meningitis was suspected in one death. Five cases each of hepatitis B were identified in 1994 and 1995.

Cholera and Other Intestinal Infectious Diseases. A cholera plan was prepared and enforced. No cases were identified in Antigua.

Chronic Communicable Diseases: Tuberculosis and Leprosy. There were 10 patients with leprosy on the national register. The Leper Home was closed since the lepers did not require active treatment.

Six cases of tuberculosis (four suspected and two confirmed) were reported in 1995. BCG vaccine was not routinely given as part of the immunization program. The increase in cases of AIDS and its relationship to tuberculosis were causes for concern.

Acute Respiratory Infections. Acute respiratory infections ranked as the leading communicable disease in the last two years, with a sizeable increase from 1994 to 1995. Pneumonia was the sixth leading cause of death in 1994 (19 deaths at a rate of 3 per 10,000 population, or 4% of all deaths).

Rabies and Other Zoonoses. The veterinary authority and the Ministries of Health and of Agriculture are responsible for the inspection of local and imported meat and animal products. There were no problems with rabies or other zoonoses in Antigua and Barbuda.

AIDS and Other Sexually Transmitted Diseases. According to the AIDS Secretariat of the Ministry of Health, since AIDS was first identified in 1985 through 31 December 1995, 70 AIDS cases were reported, including 6 children. Of the 64 adults infected, 55 were male and 9 were female (6:1 ratio). There were 56 deaths.

In the same period, 77 persons tested HIV seropositive (37 adult males, 36 adult females, and 4 children under the age of 13). Heterosexual spread seemed to be the recent pattern of HIV infection. Intravenous drug abuse was uncommon in Antigua and Barbuda. All blood donors are screened for HIV.

Of other STDs, there were 70 cases of gonorrhea and syphilis reported in 1994, and 60 in 1995. Of particular concern is the recurrence of cases of congenital syphilis. Nongonococcal urethritis was the most commonly reported STD; there were 37 cases in 1994 and 62 cases in 1995.

Noncommunicable Diseases and Other Health-Related Problems

Nutritional Diseases and Diseases of Metabolism. In 1995, 24 infants (under 1 year) and 25 1–4-year-olds were diagnosed with mild to moderate protein-calorie malnutrition as determined by weight-for-age on the Caribbean Growth Chart. The national rate for mild/moderate malnutrition was less than 0.87%. Only one child was diagnosed with severe malnutrition in 1995.

In 1993, the Ministry of Health estimated a prevalence of 2.5% for iron deficiency anemia in children under 5 years old. This rate was derived from abnormal hemoglobin test results obtained from public health clinics. A prevalence of 6.3% was estimated among pregnant women.

Approximately 95% of new mothers were breast-feeding on discharge from the hospital. In 1995, the Ministry of Health estimated that 26% of infants were solely breast-fed for six weeks, 68% breast-fed partially for six weeks, and 87% breast-fed continually at three months.

A 1993 Ministry of Health survey identified a national rate for obesity of 4.6%. Sixty percent of women over 40 years were obese; of these, 33% were grossly obese (>140% standard weight). Twenty-five percent of men over 40 years were obese.

Cardiovascular Diseases. Diseases of the circulatory system accounted for 146 (37.7%) of all deaths in 1995, and 164 (38.8%) of all deaths in 1994. This disease category includes heart disease, cerebrovascular disease, and hypertensive disease. In 1995, these three disease groups were among the five leading causes of death in Antigua. There was a relatively high prevalence of hypertension and heart disease among first-time visits to public health clinics.

Malignant Tumors. The leading cause of death in Antigua and Barbuda was malignant neoplasms. In 1995, there were 66 deaths from malignant neoplasms compared to 87 in 1994. Of the 33 deaths in men, 14 (42%) deaths were from prostate cancer. Of 33 cases of malignant neoplasms in women, 7 (21%)

deaths resulted from breast cancer. In 1991, the respective figures for deaths related to prostate cancer were 14 of 37 (38%), and for breast cancer, 5 of 26 (19%).

Accidents and Violence. Deaths caused by traffic accidents averaged 10 per year for the last three years (13 in 1993, 10 in 1994, and 7 in 1995). Many injuries resulted in long periods of hospitalization. There was increased vigilance of drivers by the police traffic department.

Behavioral Disorders. The treatment of behavioral disorders was a priority health initiative during the period. Activities took place through a community mental health program that also provided follow-up care for clients discharged from the Mental Hospital.

Use of crack cocaine, cocaine, and marijuana and alcohol abuse were causes for concern. A rehabilitation program for drug abusers was developed, and services were offered through the Mental Hospital and the community mental health program.

Oral Health. Three dentists, a dental nurse, a hygienist, and two assistants working in a three-chair dental unit in the community health services provided dental care. In 1993, a fluoride rinse program was carried out in public schools, treating an estimated 12,000 students.

Natural Disasters. Hurricane Luis devastated Antigua (along with the neighboring islands St. Maarten and the U.S. Virgin Islands) in September 1995. Two deaths and 165 reported injuries resulted. Ninety percent of homes were damaged (40% sustained major damage); 60% of Government facilities were damaged, including 75% of schools and 50% of Holberton Hospital. Approximately 2,000 persons became unemployed. The Government suffered a shortfall in revenue collection of US$ 10 million to US$ 12 million.

The National Organization of Disaster Services, a body established within the Ministry of Home Affairs to coordinate disaster mitigation, prevention, preparedness, response and recovery, was severely tested by this event. There was a regional call for the development of a "vulnerability index" to be factored into the evaluation of need for preferential aid and trade arrangements for countries like Antigua and Barbuda that lie in the hurricane belt.

RESPONSE OF THE HEALTH SYSTEM

National Health Plans and Policies

A health policy drafted in 1994 committed the Government to understand health as a "human right," adopt the pri-

mary health care approach, and support all national, regional, and international activities necessary to achieve "health for all by the year 2000." Attempts were made to redefine policy and planning goals to meet the aims and objectives of both the Caribbean Cooperation in Health agreement and the Caribbean Charter for Health Promotion.

Strategies and Programs for Health Sector Reform

Reorganization of the health system was a high priority, and several initiatives were undertaken during 1996. A five-year development plan was drafted for the Ministry of Health that included recommendations for the hospital sector. The recommendations address the direction and development of all hospital services, financing, human resources development, community participation in management and evaluation of services, private participation in the delivery of hospital services, and relations with public and private sectors (national and regional). Specific legislation was proposed for governing the organization and management of Holberton Hospital. A training component was devised that complemented the Ministry's main development plan. It details training requirements in management, professional, and technical areas, including training activities for all levels of management (dependent on availability of financing). Finally, proposals were made for alternative health financing mechanisms.

Organization of the Health Sector

Institutional Organization

The Ministry of Health provides leadership in public health care, regulation, and the delivery of services. The system is financed through public taxation or levies in support of the medical benefit scheme. The participation of private insurance in health financing is minimal and will be the subject of further examination during reorganization attempts.

The Minister of Health is a Cabinet member and delegates authority to a Permanent Secretary for management of the Ministry. Technical and administrative staff assists the Permanent Secretary in achieving the Government's health goals and objectives. The Chief Medical Officer is the technical advisor to the Ministry and is responsible for coordinating health services delivered in hospitals and health centers.

Antigua is divided into seven geographically determined medical districts. Each is served by a government-appointed district medical officer responsible for providing medical services to district residents. Primary health care services in the districts include: maternal and child health, health education, management of common health problems, environmental sanitation, community mental health care, nutrition, diabetic and hypertensive care, communicable disease control and surveillance, home visitation, and referral services.

Organization of Health Regulatory Activities

The legislative framework directing public health activities in Antigua and Barbuda was last revised in the mid-1950s, and is now considered inadequate. It was recognized that new regulatory standards are required to meet the expansion of private and public provision of health services. Legislation has been drafted on the administration and management of health institutions, a new Medical Act, and revision of the Pharmacy and Midwifery Acts.

The Medical and Nursing Councils continue to regulate eligibility to practice medicine and nursing.

Health Services and Resources

Organization of Services for Care of the Population

Immunization coverage with DTP and OPV was estimated at approximately 100% for infants under 15 months of age. In 1994 and 1995, coverage for measles, mumps, and rubella was about 94%.

The vector control program focused on the control and eradication of mosquitoes, particularly *Aedes aegypti,* the vector for both dengue fever and yellow fever. The control program consists of fogging, community education, inspection, treatment, and provision of larvae-eating fish for water storage facilities. The house infestation index was 11.1 in 1995, down from 15.3 in 1994.

Efforts to strengthen the Health Statistics Division continued through the provision of equipment, trained staff, and adequate physical facilities.

The responsibility for distributing potable water lies with the Antigua Public Utilities Authority. In 1995, it was estimated that about 60% of households had piped potable water connections; the remaining 40% used standpipes or private collections (drums and cisterns) as their source. Barbuda is supplied from a central well. The Central Board of Health monitored the quality of both drinking water and coastal waters.

The Authority and international consultants developed a project for a central sewerage system for St. John's (the capital city). Because of damage caused by Hurricane Luis, it was estimated that the percentage of homes without sanitary facilities increased from 8% in 1993 to at least 12%. Septic tanks and soakaways served approximately 60%–65% of the population. The majority of the remaining population was served by pit latrines and pail closets that are removed by the night soil

service of the Central Board of Health. Holberton Hospital and coastal hotels have private sewage plants.

The Central Board of Health maintains responsibility for solid waste management. This function will be assumed by a National Solid Waste Management Authority recently established by the Government (November 1995) with responsibility for solid waste storage, collection, treatment, and disposal. Work began in 1996 to engineer the existing dumpsite into a sanitary landfill. All other official dumpsites were closed, although a number of unofficial sites have yet to be shut down.

Efforts to control littering continued through public education and awareness programs. Enforcement of the 1983 Litter Control Act was reviewed.

The Central Board of Health conducted intense inspection of restaurants and other food-shops. No outbreak of food-borne illness occurred in the 1992–1995 period. The proliferation of itinerant roadside food vendors was a matter of increasing concern. Discussions took place between the Ministries of Health and Civil Service Affairs and the Small Vendors Association to address location problems and health concerns. The Central Board of Health embarked on education programs for staff in food establishments as well as for independent operators.

Organization and Operation of Personal Health Care Services

Both Government and private health facilities provided personal health care services. The medical benefits scheme provided pharmacy service to its beneficiaries.

Holberton Hospital is central to the health system, since it is the only public acute care health institution. General and specialist services are provided in medicine, surgery, obstetrics and gynecology, pediatrics, radiology, and pathology. In addition, private sector or foreign specialists provided services in otolaryngology, ophthalmology, orthopedics, neurology, and radiology. In 1995, there were 4,271 discharges from the general hospital; the average length of stay was 8 days. The hospital was damaged by the 1995 hurricane, and its bed component was reduced to 135 beds from 200 beds in 1991. Plans are under way to build a 200-bed acute care hospital to replace Holberton Hospital.

There are two long-stay facilities, the Mental Hospital with 150 beds (average occupancy in 1995 was 85 patients) and the Fiennes Institute, which serves 100 geriatric patients. Springview Hospital in Barbuda serves mainly as an outpatient facility. A private secondary care facility, the 15-bed Adelin Medical Center provides outpatient and inpatient care. There were two group practice medical centers with private physicians and dental offices.

Community health services are provided through a network of nine health centers and 18 satellite clinics or subcenters linked to the health centers. These facilities are evenly distributed across the country. Teams that include the district medical officers (physicians), family nurse practitioners, public health nurses, district nurse-midwives, community health aides, and clinic aides provide services in the health centers. District nurse-midwives and clinic aides provide services at the subcenters with support from health center teams.

The commitment to decentralize health services as a basis for developing local health districts did not yield the expected results. The system is still centrally managed. Patients from rural areas continue to travel to St. John's for X-ray, laboratory, and drug services. In 1994, 82,988 visits were made to all services in the clinics, with approximately 20% for child health services, 17.6% for hypertension, and 9.1% for diabetes.

All resident medical specialists, including the Government consultants and district medical officers, had private practices in the capital city. In addition, there were four private ophthalmology/ophthalmic centers, two private laboratories, and a private physical therapy center. Blood banking is centrally provided in Holberton Hospital and the Adelin Center.

Inputs for Health

All drugs, immunobiologicals, reagents, and equipment were imported.

Human Resources

In general, there was an adequate supply of health personnel; 309 worked in the public sector and 58 in the private sector. In 1995, there were 11 physicians (1.7 per 10,000 population) and 218 trained nurses (34 per 10,000). Specialists among the physicians included two gynecologists, two ophthalmologists, and two pediatricians. Of the 218 nurses, 31 were district nurse-midwives, and 10 were public health nurses. In addition to the local health personnel, Caribbean and other nationals as well as returning residents supplemented the cadre. There were large numbers of staff vacancies in the health establishment and nationals filled many of these positions.

The only certified program for the education of health personnel is the School of Nursing. The Government transferred the School from its hospital base to a community college setting at the Antigua State College, and allocated funding for its first year of operation. Difficulties existed in attracting qualified and motivated entrants to the nursing program. Training for other allied health personnel was accessed through regional training institutions. Continuing education was provided both locally and abroad through the efforts of the Min-

istry of Health, professional organizations, and international and regional agencies.

Research and Technology

Commitments to conduct national health research projects resulted in small retroactive studies on utilization of health services and specific diseases. However, these studies were more reflective of individual interests than program objectives.

Over the last five years there has been a marked increased in the availability of new technology. Holberton Hospital received mammography, fluoroscopy, and CAT scan equipment, and a well-equipped Intensive Care Unit.

Expenditures and Sectoral Financing

Both the actual amounts spent on health care and the percentage of the national budget continue to increase, from US$ 96 million (11.9% of the budget) in 1991 to US$ 141.2 million (13.9% of budget) in 1995. Per capita expenditure on health increased in nominal terms from US$ 186.8 in 1991 to US$ 305.6 in 1995, an increase of about 64%.

In 1995, 45% of the health budget was spent on institutional services that include Holberton Hospital, the Mental Hospital, and Fiennes Institute (the geriatric facility), and approximately 45% on environmental health and community health services. This percentage allocation remained constant over the period.

Sectoral Expenditure

Despite the decline in economic growth in recent years, the health sector maintained high priority in the Government, and garnered 13.9% of the Government's expenditure budget in 1995. In 1996, 13% of the national budget was allocated to the Ministry of Health and Home Affairs (about 12% for health). Financing for the health sector comes from general revenue and the medical benefits scheme.

Improved efforts at recovering costs at Holberton Hospital have resulted in the collection of EC$ 2.96 million in 1993, but this still represents a small percentage of potential revenue from user fees. Improvements in monitoring the accounting system are expected to increase this revenue.

For 1996, EC$ 400,000 has been allocated for capital expenditure on district clinics and EC$ 750,000 for additional equipment for Holberton Hospital. About EC$ 300,000 is earmarked for expenditure on equipment for the solid waste management sector.

The recurrent expenditure estimated for health activities for 1996 is EC$ 40.47 million, with EC$ 12.4 million going to the Central Board of Health and EC$ 17.06 million to Holberton Hospital. EC$ 1.14 million is allocated to the public health, medical, and sanitary services in Barbuda.

External Technical and Financial Cooperation

Antigua and Barbuda participated in regional programs and projects for drug procurement, health service development, information systems improvement, environmental protection, solid waste management, and disaster preparedness. Benefits such as cost savings, training, consultant services, and, in some cases, direct investment were received. Official development assistance from the Development Assistance Committee of the Organization for Economic Cooperation and Development, multilateral organizations, and Arab countries fell in 1993 to US$ 3.0 net million from US$ 7.0 net million in 1991.

ARGENTINA

GENERAL SITUATION AND TRENDS

Socioeconomic, Political, and Demographic Overview

The Argentine Republic is a federal democracy and, accordingly, all powers not expressly vested in the national government are attributed to the provinces. The Constitution—as amended by a constitutional convention in 1993—is the supreme law of the land and all legislation must conform to its precepts.

Argentina has an area of 3,761,274 km² and shares borders with five other countries. It is divided into 23 provinces and a federal district (*Capital Federal*), which are responsible under the constitution for the health and protection of the population. Within the general framework of political, economic, and social reforms that the country has embarked upon, the structure of relationships between the central and provincial governments, and between the State and society in general, is changing.

Since taking office in 1989, the present administration has implemented three economic stabilization plans. The most recent one—the Convertibility Plan—was unveiled in early 1991. It tied the local currency to the United States dollar and set a course for structural adjustment based on export-driven growth. As a result, the Government has been able to shore up the country's fiscal accounts and generate surpluses to pay its financial commitments.

Fiscal adjustment efforts have sought to cut productivity costs by scaling back government spending through such measures as privatizing State-run companies, tax reform, more efficient staffing patterns and levels, a new fiscal pact between the federal and provincial governments, and the updating of labor legislation to allow for more flexibility in civil service. Hand in hand with these changes came a substantial reform of the pension system and a new policy framework for the social security system.

Studies by the UN Economic Commission for Latin America and the Caribbean (ECLAC) have shown that sustained export growth beginning in 1990 led to a trade surplus that—coupled with the abundant supply of external credit and capital inflows—spawned a surge in local demand for goods and services. This, in turn, triggered a boom in imports, especially with the lowering of customs tariffs that had been responsible in part for negative trade balances in preceding years. Demand for goods and services stabilized around 1995, and favorable conditions on international markets led to expansion in the country's exports, bringing trade flows back into balance and boosting economic activity. Although the ratio of foreign debt to exports improved somewhat (dropping from a factor of 5 in 1994 to 4.3 in 1995, while interest as a percentage of exports of goods and services remained stable at 21%–22%), the total foreign debt rose from US$ 58,413 million in 1991 to approximately US$ 96,000 million in 1996 and continues to be a heavy burden for the country.

The prospect of broader regional integration under the economic integration treaty signed by Argentina, Brazil, Paraguay, and Uruguay, MERCOSUR, makes economic stability all the more important. In addition to fostering trade in the subregion, MERCOSUR has been instrumental in forging closer macroeconomic ties among the countries. In 1995, for instance, Argentine exports were able to satisfy a jump in consumer demand in Brazil.

The financial crisis that shook the Mexican economy at the end of 1994 had repercussions throughout the Region, albeit of much lesser magnitude. Despite a fledgling capital market and sparse internal savings, however, Argentina was able to consolidate its monetary and fiscal policy and thereby shore up its economic model. The subsequent contraction of the economy in 1995 was short-lived; progress continues to be made, but it has come at a high social cost.

Economic indicators for the 1991–1996 period confirm the success of the Convertibility Plan and other adjustment efforts in strengthening the country's macroeconomic situation: inflation was reined in and the gross domestic product (GDP), exports, and capital flows all improved. Following a jump of 84.00% in 1991, the consumer price index (CPI) rose only 10.3% in 1992. As inflation continued falling, so did shifts in the CPI, which stood at 3.9% in 1994 and only 1.5% in 1995. By 1996, the CPI rise was only 0.4%, and investment rates had returned to positive figures. GDP growth from 1990 to 1994 showed a cumulative rate of 35.0%.

The Argentine labor market in 1995 was influenced by stable prices and a drop in economic activity—both of which were factors that affected wage and employment trends. For example, even though GDP grew between year-end 1990 and year-end 1994, overall employment decreased. This drop, coupled with the influx of new entrants into the labor market, led unemployment rates to increase, despite the period's economic expansion. The surplus in the supply of labor was further compounded by broad fluctuations in labor market activity and demand.

The recession was already apparent in early 1995, and employment began to drop dramatically. Unemployment surged to 18.4% in April, and underemployment rose to just over 11.0% of the economically active population (EAP). Employment levels continued to fall during the first months of 1996. Although the metropolitan Buenos Aires area was hit hardest, other areas were not immune. In Argentina's major cities, open unemployment (expressed as a percentage of the EAP) soared from 6.0% in October 1991 to 16.4% by October 1996.

In the years following the hyperinflationary period (1989–1990), short-term fluctuations in real wages abated, and the evolution of pay levels was similar in the various sectors and employment categories. In the industrial sector, however, real wages crept downward despite higher productivity levels, falling 7 points between 1991 and early 1995 (using 1991 as a base level of 100). By early 1993, the cost of the basic food basket for an average family had risen 56%, but industrial wages had increased by only 27%. Further adjustment measures were unveiled in 1995: higher-level civil service salaries were pared back, the tax base for income and personal-property taxes was broadened, and payment plans for outstanding taxes were put in place; legislation was passed limiting pension outlays. Employment levels in the industrial sector declined over the course of 1996, while real wages remained virtually unchanged.

The new labor reform package included authorization for small and medium-sized companies to revise their employee-termination policies (e.g., they would now pay fewer associated costs for the termination of recent hires) and redefine job positions. A new kind of apprenticeship contract was created for people under 25, whereby trainees would not be considered full-benefit employees. Accordingly, hiring them would not produce any social-security obligations or any other costs for the company when their contracts expired. Legislation was also passed changing the system of compensation for work-related accidents, replacing employer payments with a compulsory insurance scheme.

The country's vibrant economic activity between 1990 and 1994 did not bring about any change in income distribution. Between 1992 and 1994, income levels rose significantly among the top 10% of Argentina's wealthiest households, but the increase was considerably smaller for the poorest 40% of the population. In other words, the gains secured in terms of better wealth distribution over the first two years were lost.

The shift from inflation to stability and from economic stagnation to economic growth in the first half of the 1990s brought an end to these two factors that had pushed the neediest sectors of society into poverty. The labor market, however, could not offset the accumulated setbacks; on the contrary, it created new sources of vulnerability that, in effect, undermined the progress made thus far. Unemployment continues to accentuate the unequal patterns of growth.

On the Human Development Index (HDI), Argentina was given a value of 0.839 in 1991, placing it among those countries having high human development. The figure in 1993 was slightly higher (0.884). Estimated HDI values for the various provinces point to considerable differences in socioeconomic conditions and are evidence of the complex geography of human development.

The Permanent Household Survey conducted in 1994 by the National Statistics and Census Bureau showed significant variation from one city to another in the percentage of households and persons with unmet basic needs. The incidence of poverty ranged from 32.2% of households in Palpalá (Jujuy province) to 8% in Río Gallegos (Santa Cruz province). For individuals, the highest percentage of unmet basic needs (35.5%) was in Resistencia (Chaco province) and the lowest in two locations in Tierra del Fuego province, Río Gallegos (8.9%) and Ushuaia (8.5%). The discrepancy between these two measures of poverty incidence reflects the fact that households with unmet basic needs are normally larger.

Compared with the October 1995 level, the 1996 Permanent Household Survey showed an increase in the number of people living in poverty in the metropolitan Buenos Aires area. This is a continuation of the trend seen since 1994, and it also is linked to the area's rising unemployment, higher prices for basic staples, and increase in the number of families who are forced to live in substandard dwellings. According to the 1991 census, 30% of the total of 10 million homes had some substandard condition. The emergence of new shantytowns and housing takeovers also are consequences of this situation.

Early in 1996, the Epidemiology Directorate of the Ministry of Health and Social Action began working with PAHO to design a situational-analysis methodology that could generate political and technical criteria to define risk groups, implement geographical targeting, and identify critical problem areas. Such indicators as general living conditions, use of health care services by the population, and the overall health situation would be measured in 524 observation units (or "departments") into which the country had been subdivided.

Data were first stratified by living conditions, taking into account for each department the percentage of homes with unmet basic needs, illiteracy rates, population lacking coverage under an individual health plan or an *obras sociales* employee-benefits plan, population over 60 years of age, and years of potential life lost (YPLL). Summary indicators were constructed and then plotted along a bell curve. After allowing for standard deviation, five categories were identified: atypical, favorable, average, unfavorable, and precarious. Most of the departments (60.9%) fell in the average range and accounted for 61.2% of the total population; 17.8% of the departments were ranked as having unfavorable or average living conditions (5% of the total population). In other words, the groups with the least favorable living conditions were found in the less densely populated departments.

The population's use of health care services was analyzed according to the number of doctor visits and hospital discharges. Data came just from the public subsector, and were presented mainly by service provider rather than by the patients' area of residence. In the departments for which data by patient residence were available (19.3%), those with lower population densities showed a higher rate of hospital discharges than did departments with higher population densities.

In terms of the overall health situation, a study on preventable deaths revealed that—except in the category ranked as having "atypical" living conditions, where preventable deaths were identified exclusively in the age group older than 50 years—preventable deaths occurred in the age group 1–4 years old in every category, although they were highest in the category of "unfavorable" living conditions. The data clearly showed that the number of preventable deaths in the 1–4-year-old age group increased as the quality of life worsened. The data also showed that the more favorable conditions were found in the more heavily populated departments located along or near major national highways, thereby establishing a correlation between geodemographic characteristics and the stratification by living conditions.

The 1991 National Population and Housing Census projected a total population of 35,219,612 for 1996. The average annual growth rate was expected to be 1.261%, lower than in previous periods. The projected male-to-female ratio was 0.96 for 1996 and subsequent years, up to 2005. The total fertility rate continued declining, going from 3.15 children per woman in 1980 to a projected 2.82 for the period 1990–1995 and 2.62 for 1995–2000. The figure varied from one province to another, ranging from 1.58 children per woman in the federal district to 3.58 in Misiones. The birth rate declined very slightly, but steadily, from 19.8 per 1,000 population in 1993, to 19.7 per 1,000 in 1994, and 18.9 per 1,000 in 1995.

Life expectancy at birth for the total population was estimated at 71.93 years for the period 1990–1992 (75.69 years for women and 68.44 years for men) and 75.59 years for the period 1995–2000 (75.75 years for women and 69.55 years for men).

Looking at the country's age distribution, children under 15 years old accounted for less than 30% of the overall population, while persons over 60 years represented 13% of the total. The population's median age in 1985 was 27.6 years, and was projected to rise to 28.4 years by the year 2000. The population over 65 years of age represented 9.0% of the total in 1990, is currently estimated at 9.5%, and is expected to reach 9.8% by the year 2000, with a strong predominance of women. In terms of age structure, the 60-and-older age group (13.9% in 1995) had grown, while the other two cohorts—24 years old and younger (46.0% in 1995) and 25–59 (40.8% in 1995)—had shrunk.

In 1996, the urban population was projected at 88.6% of the total population, concentrated mainly in seven cities of more than 500,000 inhabitants. A full one-third of the country's population lived in the metropolitan Buenos Aires area; elsewhere in the country, residents of suburban and rural areas were moving to provincial capitals. More than one-half of the country's urban population lived in cities of 500,000 or more inhabitants.

Mortality and Morbidity Profile

Argentina's mortality profile improved over the 1990–1995 period. A total of 268,997 deaths were reported in 1995, of which 9,708 (3.6% of the total) were due to ill-defined causes. The total mortality rate was 7.7 per 1,000 population. Maternal mortality, which had risen between 1994 (3.9 per 10,000 live births) and 1995 (4.4 per 10,000 live births), experienced a decrease of close to 14.0% in 1995. Infant mortality fell 15.7% between 1990 and 1995, reaching a level of 22.2 per 1,000 live births. Similar declines were observed in neonatal and postneonatal mortality over the same period, falling by 14.7% and 16.0%, respectively.

In 1995, infant mortality in the city of Buenos Aires stood at 13.1 per 1,000 live births, contrasting with the provinces of Chaco and Formosa, which had levels of above 30 per 1,000 live births. Eleven provinces had infant mortality rates above the national average. The northwest and northeast regions of the country showed the highest levels, but with gradual declines everywhere except in Formosa, San Juan, and Tucumán, where the rates increased. The province of Tierra del

Fuego had the lowest rate of all, with 11.1 deaths of children under 1 year of age per 1,000 live births.

Neonatal mortality was higher than postneonatal mortality in all provinces. Early neonatal was higher (10.8 per 1,000 live births) than in late neonatal mortality (2.8 per 1,000). Nationwide, postneonatal mortality rose by 6.2% between 1994 and 1995, rising from 7.6 per 1,000 live births to 8.1 per 1,000. The increase was seen in all provinces except Chubut, Jujuy, La Rioja, Santa Fe, and Tierra del Fuego. Some 60% of all neonatal deaths could have been prevented by timely diagnosis or treatment during pregnancy and childbirth or for the newborn, and 54.4% of them avoided through prevention, treatment, or both.

Of the 8,570 fetal deaths, 65.2% were classified as late fetal deaths. Fetal mortality in 1995 was calculated at 13.0 per 1,000 live births, although figures varied significantly from one region to another. Low birthweight (<2,500 g) was registered in two-thirds of all fetal deaths. Between 1990 and 1995, the percentage of newborns weighing less than 2,500 g increased from 6.1% to 6.6% nationwide. Underreporting makes it impossible to identify which provinces have greater incidences of low birthweight.

An analysis of mortality by leading cause of death and by sex reveals that the number of deaths attributable to heart disease nationwide fell 10.9% between 1990 (252.6 per 100,000 population) and 1995 (227.7 per 100,000 population). Over the same period, mortality from cerebrovascular diseases and accidents also decreased significantly, by 16.7% (from 80.8 to 69.2 per 100,000 population) and 16.4% (from 32.6 to 28.0 per 100,000), respectively. Deaths from malignant tumors registered a smaller decline, falling from 143.7 per 100,000 population in 1990 to 141.6 per 100,000 in 1996.

Heart disease, malignant tumors, and cerebrovascular diseases were the leading causes of death among both sexes. For men, the death rate from heart disease in 1995 was 244.5 per 100,000 population, while for women it was somewhat lower, 206.4 per 100,000. The male death rate was also higher for malignant tumors (157.6 per 100,000, compared with 124.1 per 100,000 for women) and cerebrovascular diseases (70.4 per 100,000, compared with 66.5 per 100,000 for women). Accidents were the fourth most common cause of death among men, with 6,766 of the total 9,740 accidents ending in death (39.7 per 100,000 population); the specific mortality rate from this cause among women was 16.1 per 100,000 population.

The most striking change in the country's mortality profile has been the increase in the contribution of deaths from pneumonia and influenza since 1994. These diseases ranked fifth as a cause of death in males, displacing conditions originating in the perinatal period. Among women, deaths from pneumonia and influenza rose from the sixth leading cause in 1990 to the fourth in 1995. Also worth mentioning is the increase seen in female mortality from infectious causes as of 1995.

Conditions originating in the perinatal period were the leading cause of infant mortality (7,125 deaths), accounting for 50% of deaths from all causes in children under 1 year old. The specific mortality rate from this cause dropped 17.1% between 1990 and 1995 (from 1,267.2 to 1,081.6 per 100,000 population). Congenital abnormalities were the second most common cause (396.8 per 100,000). Deaths from pneumonia and influenza (690 in 1995) declined 5.7% between 1990 and 1995, and intestinal infectious diseases moved from fourth to sixth place.

Among children 1–4 years old, accidents were the leading cause of death by a wide margin (16.9 per 100,000 population). Although the 1990–1995 period saw a 28.9% drop in mortality from accidents, this cause still claimed 458 lives in 1995 (21.4% of all deaths), of which approximately 45% were traffic accidents or accidents in the home. The risk of dying from pneumonia and influenza dropped nearly 22.0% in 1995, moving this group of causes into fourth place. Mortality from intestinal infectious diseases also declined, and these diseases no longer rank among the five leading causes of death. The relative decrease in deaths from these leading causes is responsible for the relative increase in mortality from congenital anomalies and heart disease.

Accidents were also the leading cause of death in the age group 5–14 years old, with 571 deaths in 1995 (8.6 per 100,000 population). Nevertheless, mortality from this cause dropped 26.7% between 1990 and 1995. Malignant tumors were the second most common cause of death (3.7 per 100,000 population). Mortality from cancer decreased 45.9% (244 deaths).

In the population aged 15 to 49, heart diseases and malignant tumors represented the first and second most common causes of death in 1990, at rates of 33.8 and 33.7 per 100,000 population, respectively. In 1995, there was a decline in mortality from heart diseases (27.9 per 100,000), leaving malignant tumors as the leading cause that year (31.1 per 100,000 population). Accidents continued to be the third most common cause of death in this cohort (25.1 per 100,000).

In the age group 50–64 years old, mortality from heart diseases and malignant tumors exhibited patterns similar to the previous age group. The number of deaths attributable to heart diseases declined considerably between 1990 and 1995, dropping from 340.8 to 289.3 per 100,000 population. Mortality from malignant neoplasms fell slightly, and malignant tumors came to rank as the leading cause of death.

In the population 65 years of age and older, heart disease continued to be the leading cause of death in the 1990–1995 period. Tumors and cerebrovascular diseases ranked second and third; mortality from pneumonia and influenza increased 21.0%.

An analysis of mortality based on years of potential life lost (YPLL) from the leading causes of death revealed that accidents were the number-one cause of death among persons between the ages of 0 and 64 years, followed by conditions originating in the perinatal period and heart diseases, in that order. Accidents and perinatal conditions took the highest toll, since each such death was responsible for the loss of an average of 53.6 and 63.5 years of potential life, respectively. If children under 1 year of age are not included in the calculation, accidents remain as the leading cause, but suicide ranks fifth. Each death from these two external causes represented, on average, 50 and 32 YPLL, respectively.

SPECIFIC HEALTH PROBLEMS

Analysis by Population Group

Morbidity data for this analysis were difficult to collect, because in Argentina records are not generally kept on patient visits, nor are periodic health surveys conducted.

Health of Children

Of the 14,606 deaths among children under 1 year of age reported in 1995, 56.2% were males. Although mortality from conditions originating in the perinatal period declined 17.1%, they continued to be the leading cause of death between 1990 and 1995, accounting for 48.8% of the total. Deaths from pneumonia and influenza rose nearly 6.0%, while those caused by intestinal infections dropped. The apparent increase in deaths attributed to congenital abnormalities may be due to the relative decrease in the other causes. Accidents climbed from the fifth most common cause in 1990 to fourth in 1995. Although accidents were responsible for only 4.0% of all deaths, their risk to children under 1 year of age rose considerably. Data collected from records of discharges from public-sector hospitals give an idea, albeit partial, of morbidity in this age group. Conditions originating in the perinatal period, intestinal infectious diseases, and pneumonia accounted for 60.3% of hospitalizations.

A total of 2,142 deaths were reported in children between 1 and 4 years of age; 54.3% in males. The specific mortality of this cohort fell from 1.2 per 1,000 population in 1990 to 0.8 per 1,000 in 1995. The high number of deaths from preventable causes underscores the need for a more comprehensive approach to health care for this group. Morbidity data based on discharge records from public hospitals show that, in 1992, 43% of hospital visits were due to diseases of the res-

piratory system and intestinal infections. A 1994 survey covering eight major cities found that more than two-thirds of Argentina's children had presented with episodes of upper respiratory infections.

In the age group 5–9 years old, accidents continued to be the leading cause of death, although their actual number was much lower than for other childhood age groups. A significantly higher number of cases occurred among boys. The 251 accidents reported in 1995 accounted for 28.6% of all deaths in this age group; over one-third were from traffic accidents. Malignant neoplasms, especially those of lymphatic and hemopoietic tissue, constituted the second cause of death (147 cases in 1995).

In the northern provinces, moderate chronic malnutrition was detected among children entering first grade. A prevalence of 11.8% was calculated for Jujuy; in the more densely populated provinces, levels were much lower (prevalence of 4% in Córdoba, La Pampa, Rosario, Mendoza, and Río Negro). According to data from public hospitals, diseases of the digestive and respiratory systems accounted for one fourth of all cases of hospitalization. Fractures were the third most common diagnosis and reflect, by inference, morbidity from accidents.

Health of Adolescents (10 to 19 Years Old)

A total of 1,064 adolescents between the ages of 10 and 14 died in 1995. The risk of dying from an accident—especially traffic accidents (130 deaths in 1995)—was much higher in this age group than it was for children. The general profile of mortality and morbidity was similar to that of the 5–9-year-old age group, except that suicides (32 deaths) and homicides (14 deaths) begin to gather importance as causes of death in this age group. Almost two-thirds of all adolescent deaths were males.

The health of young people between the ages of 15 and 19 was closely linked to their greater use of tobacco, alcohol, and psychoactive drugs, and the resulting deaths from accidents, homicides, and suicides. Sexual initiation occurred between the ages of 15 and 19 years for 50% of the population, and this was a factor in sexually transmitted diseases (STDs), AIDS, and unwanted pregnancies.

External causes were the most frequent cause of death among adolescents in 1995. Specific mortality from traffic accidents was 23.8 per 100,000 population; from suicide, 10.3 per 100,000; and from homicide, 8.8 per 100,000. With a male-to-female ratio of 3:1, these three causes accounted for 29.7% of all deaths in this age group. Malignant neoplasms and cardiovascular diseases ranked second and third. Mortality from obstetric causes was less than 3.0 per 10,000 live births.

Hospital admissions of adolescents at public-sector facilities were attributed, in order of importance, to obstetric causes, abortions, and diseases of the digestive system.

Health of Adults (15 to 60 Years)

Cardiovascular diseases, malignant tumors, and accidents were the leading causes of death among adults. Accidents were the most prevalent external cause of death among persons 30 years and younger, followed by suicide (574 deaths in 1995). From age 30 on, the leading cause of death shifted toward cardiovascular diseases and malignant tumors. Males accounted for more than 50% of all deaths.

The scant information available on contraceptive use was based on a survey conducted in Buenos Aires and six other cities. Roughly 60% of Argentine women used some form of family planning. Among adolescents under age 20, that percentage dropped to levels as low as 30% and 50%, and was indirectly proportional to the individual's level of formal education and directly proportional to the level of unmet basic needs. The ratio between normal deliveries and cesarean sections ranged from 1.8 to 4.4 in the areas studied.

Of the 290 maternal deaths reported in 1995, two-thirds were due to direct obstetric causes in which the preventable risk factor was greater than 80%. For indirect obstetric causes, the preventable risk factor was over 50%. However, these figures do not reflect the true seriousness of the situation, since underreporting is estimated in more than half of these cases. Maternal mortality fell from 5.9 per 10,000 live births in 1985 to 4.4 per 10,000 in 1995, a decline of 34.1%. Even so, the level is still considered to be high, bearing in mind that 96.0% of deliveries between 1990 and 1995 occurred in health care facilities. Women from northern and western Argentina were found to bear children at a younger age, and their fertility rates were higher than the national average (total fertility rate of 2.58 for the period 1990–1995). Such regional differences are cause for concern, and the fact that 11 provinces had a maternal mortality rate of over 5.0 per 10,000 live births underscores the seriousness of the problem. The higher rates were attributed to abortions and direct obstetric causes. Seventy percent of the deaths from direct obstetric causes occurred subsequent to a cesarean section, and the most common complication was septicemia. These two causes of death, both of which are avoidable, accounted for 67.3% of all maternal deaths. Risk of maternal death was highest for females below age 15 and over age 35. Nearly three-fourths of these deaths were among women from lower socioeconomic strata.

According to data from public hospital records, morbidity in this group presented a pattern similar to that of the 15-to-24 age group, with a clear predominance of obstetric causes and abortions (20.8% of all diagnoses). The third most common cause of morbidity were diseases of the digestive system, e.g., ulcers of the stomach and duodenum, appendicitis, disorders of the gallbladder, and cirrhosis of the liver.

Health of the Elderly (60 and Older)

Heart diseases, malignant tumors, and cerebrovascular diseases were the three leading causes of death in this age group, although mortality had declined considerably. In 1995, the mortality profile underwent a marked change as deaths from heart disease and cerebrovascular diseases fell 10.9% and 16.9%, respectively, between 1990 and 1995, and malignant tumors became the leading cause of death (922.3 per 100,000 population). That notwithstanding, more than one-half of the deaths in this age group continued to be attributable to heart diseases and malignant tumors.

Mortality from pneumonia and influenza increased significantly in this cohort, rising from the fifth leading cause of death in 1990 to the fourth five years later (208.0 per 100,000 in 1995). Heart diseases, malignant tumors, and cerebrovascular diseases accounted for 63.2% of all deaths in 1995; next in order were pneumonia and influenza (4.0% of the total).

Morbidity data were collected from statistics compiled by the National Social Services Administration for Retirees and Pensioners (INSSJyP) under its Comprehensive Health Care Plan (the PAMI plan). Based on a sample of 500,000 beneficiaries from the three sectors that provide health care (public sector, *obras sociales* plans, and private sector), an examination of the principal diagnoses indicated that diseases of the digestive system, cardiopulmonary diseases, and respiratory diseases accounted for 29% of all hospitalizations. Men showed a greater incidence of genitourinary and respiratory diseases, while endocrine diseases (mainly diabetes mellitus), nutritional deficiencies, and injuries were the main causes of hospitalization among females. In outpatient services, the most common causes of morbidity reported were cardiovascular diseases, followed by diseases of the musculoskeletal system and connective tissue, and endocrine and metabolic diseases. Patient visits from males were mainly for specialized consultations related to the urinary system, while diseases of the musculoskeletal system and connective tissue were the most common cause among women.

Family Health

The National Council on Children and the Family—an agency of the Secretariat for Social Development, which reports directly to the Office of the President of the Republic—provides assistance for teenage mothers nationwide. Between

1985 and 1993, the percentage of children born to mothers under the age of 19 rose from 13.3% to 15.7%. The provinces with the highest percentages of adolescent mothers (>20%) were Catamarca, Chaco, Corrientes, and Misiones. Of these young mothers, 1.1% were illiterate and 11.8% had not finished primary school.

Workers' Health

Data compiled by the Ministry of Labor from a broad sample of companies showed that most work-related accidents between 1991 and 1993 occurred in the food and metallurgical industries. During that period, the accident rate rose 5%. This apparent increase in the risk of accidents in all industries (except textile and nonmetallic mineral) was attributed to better reporting by the companies.

Among the so-called "occupational diseases," psychiatric disorders were especially prevalent in the transportation sector, where workers are exposed to highly stressful conditions; construction workers, on the other hand, suffered mainly from joint-related ailments, respiratory conditions, and alcohol addiction. The food and metallurgical industries accounted for 47.1% of all occupational diseases, and incidence rates were high. It was in the sanitation and basic metal industries, however, that occupational diseases (although lower in absolute numbers) posed the highest risk, followed by the metallurgical, nonmetallic mineral, and construction industries.

The Argentine work force in 1995 included an estimated 200,000 children and adolescents between the ages of 10 and 14; in the country's major cities, an additional 24,000 were engaged in some marginal economic activity such as begging or selling small items or services.

Health of Indigenous People

Since health statistics for Argentina are not broken down by ethnic group, the necessary data are not available to accurately diagnose the health situation of the indigenous population. Nevertheless, the experience of local programs—such as those for the prevention of cholera and Chagas' disease, environmental sanitation, and maternal and child health—points to generally poor health conditions in this population group. In the wake of the cholera epidemic, which hit indigenous communities particularly hard, an agreement was signed by the Ministry of Health and Social Action, the Ministry of Labor, the social security system, the provincial governments, and indigenous organizations, setting up the Health Program for Indigenous Peoples. The program was launched in the northern provinces in January 1994 and has thus far trained and outfitted 250 indigenous health agents who provide pri-

mary health care in their communities; gradually, these agents have been incorporated into the local health teams. Initial coverage efforts focused on communities at risk, for a total of 40,000 persons.

Analysis by Type of Disease or Health Impairment

Communicable Diseases

Vector-Borne Diseases. The risk of infection by *Triatoma infestans* was present across 86% of continental Argentina. Efforts to control transmission of Chagas' disease had significantly reduced household infestation indexes, which were estimated at 4% in many areas. In Santiago del Estero (the province where the disease was most endemic), acute cases had fallen 90% since the 1980s. Serological prevalence among the general population was less than 8%. Thirteen percent of the infected population was under 20 years of age, while persons over age 60 presented the highest rates (>10%). In 1996, the serological prevalence as detected at blood banks stood at 3.7%. The lower infection rate among young people was attributed to the decrease in *Trypanosoma cruzi* transmission after vector-control strategies and serological controls began to be implemented at blood banks in the 1980s. The benefits of these actions were evident in the drop in serological prevalence among 18-year-old males reporting for military service: from 10.3% in the late 1960s to 1.8% in 1993.

The program to control Chagas' disease aims to increase the number of homes sprayed with insecticide while promoting surveillance and control actions toward the ultimate objective of halting vectoral transmission of this disease. The program was able to meet 90% of its target of spraying 685,000 homes in 1996.

The incidence of Argentine hemorrhagic fever, which had been declining since 1988, experienced an increase in 1990, with 727 cases reported (2.2 per 100,000 population). After an initial doubling of reported cases in the provinces of Buenos Aires, Córdoba, and Santa Fe, the level dropped and eventually stabilized in the following years. In 1995, only 65 cases were reported (0.3 per 100,000 population). This dramatic decline in incidence was attributed to the application of Candid#1 vaccine, an attenuated live-virus vaccine that was developed with international cooperation.

The downward trend observed in malaria incidence since 1989 was reversed in 1993, and by 1995 annual case reports had risen to 1,065. Most of these were imported cases, with Jujuy, Misiones, and Salta being the provinces most affected. Given the steady decline in the number of autochthonous cases, the increase in the overall level (incidence of 3.3 per 100,000 population in 1995) was mainly due to imported cases associated with the steady migration into the country from southern Bolivia. In 1996, 2,020 cases were reported, with the proportion of native cases remaining the same (44.0%). Salta—the province with the most cases—continued to display residual endemic conditions. All reported cases of malaria involved *Plasmodium vivax* infection.

No cases of yellow fever were reported; vaccination coverage has been provided for groups at risk since 1946. A total of 98,700 doses of yellow fever vaccine were administered in 1995.

Vaccine-Preventable Diseases. From 1991 on, the highest number of cases of diphtheria reported in any single year was five; no cases were reported in 1996. The incidence of whooping cough declined over the five-year period, with 737 cases reported in 1996 (2.2 per 100,000 population). Twenty-six cases of neonatal tetanus were reported between 1993 and 1996; a program to eradicate this disease was unveiled in July 1994.

A serious measles epidemic swept Argentina in 1991, striking at a rate of 129.1 per 100,000 population. A mass vaccination campaign was launched in 1993, targeting all children under age 15. Nationwide coverage reached 97% among children under 1 year old, and new cases fell back sharply, with only 655 cases reported in 1995 (2.0 per 100,000 population).

The last reported case of wild poliovirus occurred in 1984. In June 1994, the health authorities declared the disease eradicated in Argentina.

In 1992, the country was hit by an epidemic of mumps and rubella, with more than 80,000 cases of each disease reported. Case reports remained within expected levels during the years that followed. At the time, neither disease was part of the Expanded Program on Immunization (EPI), but both have been slated for inclusion as of 1997.

Cholera and Other Intestinal Infectious Diseases. The first cases of cholera in the 1992 epidemic were reported in January among indigenous communities in the province of Salta, along the Bolivian border. The pathogen isolated was *Vibrio cholerae* O1 biotype El Tor. Subsequent epidemic outbreaks of cholera occurred in 1993 and 1994, striking mainly the population over 15 years old (56.5%) and children 1 to 4 years old (23%–25%). Jujuy and especially Salta were the provinces hardest hit, accounting for 94.3% of all cases. The main foci were located in three areas along the Bolivian border in northern Salta: Pilcomayo, Bermejo, and San Martín, in descending order. Incidence peaked in 1993 at 2,080 cases (6.5 per 100,000 population) and a case fatality rate of 1.6%; in 1995, incidence dropped to 188 (0.6 per 100,000 population), only to rise again to 474 cases in 1996 (1.4 per 100,000). The case fatality rate remained stable at 1.1% in 1995 and 1996.

Diarrheal diseases were reported among children in all age groups. In order to provide benchmarks for early detection of cholera cases and to track the increase in cases of diarrhea among older children, in 1992 the reporting categories were changed from under and over 2 years of age to under and over 5 years of age. The steady increase observed in the number of reported cases of diarrheal diseases since 1992 was attributed to better reporting practices.

Typhoid fever registered a slight decline between 1989 (1.1 per 100,000 population) and 1996, when 275 cases were reported (0.8 per 100,000 population). Incidence was highest in the provinces of Buenos Aires, Salta, and Formosa, at rates equal to or greater than 6.0 per 100,000 population.

Acute Respiratory Infections. A total of 561,189 cases of influenza (161.4 per 10,000 population) were reported in 1996. The increase in reported cases during that year was ascribed to a combination of better reporting and a real increase in morbidity in Santa Fe, La Pampa, and the northern provinces. Historically, the city of Buenos Aires has had the lowest rates; in 1996, 9,777 cases were reported (32.3 per 10,000 population). The influenza virus, type A (H3N2) was isolated in 1993, followed later by the influenza B virus, involving a strain similar to B/Panama/90. The incidence of pneumonia was much lower and stood at 91,740 cases in 1996 (26.4 per 10,000 population), although improved reporting had contributed to a general upward trend. Here too, the highest incidence was found in the northern part of the country.

Rabies. Human rabies is now a controlled disease thanks to the success of prevention and animal vaccination programs that have reduced the incidence of animal rabies by 99%. In 1994, a single case of human rabies was reported, the first one since 1985.

AIDS and Other STDs. AIDS was first reported in 1982 and incidence has grown with each passing year. From 720 cases in 1991, the number rose to 1,624 in 1995. Underreporting is thought to be very high, with the actual number of cases estimated to be at least 40% higher than the reported level. The serological prevalence of the human immunodeficiency virus (HIV) was calculated at 0.3% among blood bank donors. Although the disease was present throughout the country, 90% of all cases were reported in the provinces of Buenos Aires, Córdoba, and Santa Fe, which account for over 60% of the total population. A full 75% of the cases reported in the province of Buenos Aires were concentrated in the metropolitan Buenos Aires area; most of the cases in the other two provinces were reported in the cities of Córdoba and Rosario, respectively.

As of 1992, the pattern of distribution by sex began to shift, dropping from 4.1 male cases for each female case that year to 3.5 in 1996. In the province of Buenos Aires, the shift was even more marked, dropping to 3 male cases for each female case; Buenos Aires was also the province with the highest percentage of female and pediatric cases (52% of all cases).

Sixty-one percent of all AIDS patients were between 20 and 34 years of age. Before 1989, though, the age group with the most cases had been the 30–49 age group. This shift toward a younger age group is attributed to an increase in intravenous transmission associated with drug use. The average age was 33 years among males and 28 years among females.

The epidemic's profile has changed not only in terms of the higher number of women infected (rising from 0 cases in 1985 to 21.9% of cases in 1996), but also because of the gradual spread of intravenous drug addiction as a means of transmission. Sexual transmission, which accounted for 100% of cases between 1982 and 1985, dropped to roughly 50% of cases in 1996; 40% to 45% of cases were transmitted by way of blood, and from 5% to 10% were cases of perinatal transmission. For the 1992–1996 period, a full 68.5% of the cases were associated with heterosexual transmission, an HIV-positive mother, or intravenous drug addiction.

Other STDs (including syphilis and gonorrhea) remained relatively stable over the period, although the incidence of syphilis was lower. Widespread underreporting continues to distort the true picture of the health situation with regard to these diseases. Provisional figures on incidence for 1996 indicated 1,339 cases of primary and secondary syphilis, 3,246 cases of unspecified syphilis, and 6,620 cases of gonorrhea. Congenital syphilis was first reported as a separate category in 1994; 275 cases were reported in 1996. This trend is attributed in part to better case reporting. Misiones and Santa Fe were the provinces with the highest incidence.

Emerging and Re-emerging Diseases. Reported cases of meningococcal encephalitis started to show an increase as of 1989. In 1993, incidence was highest in the province of La Pampa with 79 cases (30.4 per 100,000 population), followed by Misiones with 205 cases (26 per 100,000). A total of 3,793 episodes were reported for the country as a whole (11.2 per 100,000 population). Tierra del Fuego, Formosa, Buenos Aires, Tucumán, Chaco, and Santa Fe all reported levels above the average. Children under 5 years old were the age group most severely affected (56.3%).

Bacterial meningitis accounted for most of the cases (roughly 69% of the total), although the viral meningitis was on the rise, accounting for 20% of the total in 1994. In 1991, *Neisseria meningitidis* surpassed *Hemophilus influenzae* as the most prevalent causative agent of meningitis: the former accounted for over 45% of cases in 1993–1994, while the latter was identified in roughly 20% of cases (showing a slight increase in 1994). Pneumococcus infection also was identified in roughly 20% of cases. Meningococcal infections were reported in children between the ages of 0 and 9 years, al-

though they were concentrated in the age group 1–4 years old. *H. influenzae* infection was found mainly among children under 1 year old and in the 1-to-4 age group. Meningococcal meningitis remained constant at around 800 cases a year from 1993 on, while the incidence of meningitis from *H. influenzae* dropped to 300 cases in 1996.

Cuban AB meningococcal vaccine was tested by immunoassay in the province of La Pampa in 1994. A total of 9,339 doses were administered to children between the ages of 2 and 14, with coverage estimated at 82.5%. The results had not yet been evaluated.

Hantavirus pulmonary syndrome was first reported in 1981. Of the 81 cases confirmed as of early 1997, 39 of them (48.1%) occurred in 1996 and presented a case fatality rate of 55%. Six provinces reported cases, with the highest levels being registered in Río Negro and Salta. The causative agent identified in Argentina was the Andes virus, a variant of the USA virus that had triggered an epidemic in the United States. The proven chain of transmission is from reservoir (a wild rodent of the genus *Oligoryzomys flavescens*) to humans; however, person-to-person transmission is thought to be possible as well, and is currently under study.

Hepatitis case reporting has improved since 1993. A diagnostic laboratory network was set up, comprising 14 regional sentinel units for viral hepatitis, and reporting is being monitored more closely, with data broken down by type (A, B, other, and unspecified). The serological prevalence of hepatitis B and C was 0.6% and 0.7%, respectively, based on donors screened at blood banks. In 1993, reported cases of hepatitis A began to show an increase; by 1994, the disease had assumed epidemic proportions, with an incidence of 28,488 cases (87.4 per 100,000 population) that climbed even further to 32,880 cases in 1995 (100.8 per 100,000). With regard to hepatitis B, data from blood banks revealed a serological prevalence of 0.6% in 1996 among the general population; the percentage was higher for at-risk populations (e.g., health workers), however, owing not only to better quality reporting but also to case detection efforts undertaken prior to the hepatitis B vaccination campaign for health workers at high and medium risk. The goal is to vaccinate 95% of these workers; 60% coverage has been attained. Vaccine is also administered to newborns of HBsAg-positive mothers and, since 1996, to personnel of the armed forces and the penitentiary system. The vaccination target for 1997 was to provide coverage for all children 0 to 16 years old who live in at-risk areas.

Chronic Communicable Diseases. A total of 12,185 cases of tuberculosis were reported in 1991, the year with the lowest incidence in the 1991–1995 period (37.3 per 100,000 population). From that year on, reported cases increased and, in 1993, they reached a total of 13,914 (41.3 per 100,000 population). Jujuy and Salta were the only provinces reporting more than 100 cases per 100,000 population. Some 13,450 cases were reported in 1995, representing a decline of 1.7% over 1994 and 3.4% over 1993. Underreporting is suspected to be high. Recent data point to a potentially explosive situation, given the rise in the number of reported cases, the decrease in preventive and bacteriological diagnostic measures, and the increase in drug-resistant forms (primary resistance was reported to be 12.4% and acquired resistance 41.3%). The association between tuberculosis and AIDS continued to grow: tuberculosis was present in 17% of AIDS patients in 1996.

The incidence of leprosy changed very little. Approximately 500 new cases were reported each year (1.5 per 100,000 population), mainly in the provinces of Misiones, Corrientes, Chaco, Formosa, and Santa Fe.

Noncommunicable Diseases and Other Health-Related Problems

Nutritional Diseases and Diseases of Metabolism. The studies conducted in this area present partial or limited data, making it difficult to draw comparisons and estimate indicators at the national level. Iodine deficiency and, even more so, iron deficiency were reported in the age group 1–6 years old. The prevalence of iron deficiency anemia in children ranged from 24% to 47%, depending on the province; there was a strong correlation with socioeconomic level.

The most frequent nutritional disorder among pre-school and school-aged children was growth retardation (i.e., below normal height-for-age) owing to chronic malnutrition. Although the range varied significantly from one region to the next, case reports were concentrated in the northwestern and northeastern provinces and in periurban areas around major cities. In the province of Buenos Aires, 8.5% of schoolchildren were short for their age (below the tenth percentile), compared with 18%–24% in the northwestern region and 16% in the northeastern provinces. According to an anthropometric analysis of data compiled from medical examinations of 18-year-old males reporting for compulsory military service in the 1992–1993 period, recruits from the northern provinces and from Patagonia were found to be up to 8 cm shorter than the average height for Buenos Aires.

The prevalence of chronic malnutrition as measured by body mass index (BMI < 18.5) was calculated at 4.2%, with the highest levels being recorded, once again, in the northwestern and northeastern areas of the country. At the same time, 19.5% of the population was classified as overweight (BMI > 25) and 4.1% as obese (BMI > 30), making this the most widespread type of malnutrition for the country as a whole; figures indicated an upward trend in almost all the provinces.

Cardiovascular Diseases. Aside from nutrition-related factors, arterial hypertension also plays a role in cardiovascular risk. Among adults 18 to 59 years of age, 13% of males and 7% of females suffered from high blood pressure. Smoking—to cite another contributing factor—had a prevalence of 40% among men and 32% among women; and an estimated 75% of the population led sedentary lifestyles. Of the various types of heart diseases classified (ICD-9, 390–429), acute myocardial infarction was the leading cause of morbidity and mortality, with a rate of 44 per 100,000 population in 1995 and a male-to-female ratio of 2:1.

Malignant Tumors. Mortality from malignant tumors remained relatively stable over the 10-year period ending in 1995. The overall rate was 141.6 per 100,000 population in 1995, making malignant tumors the second leading cause of death that year. The absence of a national registry of tumors makes it impossible to identify the exact profile of morbidity from this cause.

The mortality rate from malignant tumors was calculated at 157.6 per 100,000 population among men and 124.1 per 100,000 population among women. Tumors of the trachea, bronchus, and lung were the leading cause among males (accounting for 24.3% of the total), followed by prostate cancer (11.0%). Among females, the most frequent cause was breast cancer (21.2%), followed by cancer of the colon (8.8% of all deaths from malignant tumors).

Stomach cancer was the third most common cause of death in this category among men. Among women, malignant tumors of the respiratory tract and lungs ranked third, surpassing cancer of the uterine cervix and taking the place of stomach cancer among the leading causes of death from malignant neoplasms.

Accidents and Violence. Accidents were the fourth leading cause of death. Despite a drop from 32.6 per 100,000 population in 1990 to 28.0 per 100,000 in 1995, accidents remained a serious health problem and were responsible for the loss of considerable years of life potential lost (estimated total YPLL of 522,966). Their relative weight in the five leading causes of death increased among children under 1 year old, remained relatively stable in the 1–4 age group, decreased considerably in the 5–14 group, and remained constant in the 15-to-49 group. There was a strong predominance of males (4:1) in accident-related deaths (6,766 deaths, representing 69.4% of the total). Among external causes, traffic accidents were responsible for 3,797 deaths (20.8%); suicide, 2,241 (12.4%); and homicides, 1,472 (8.2%). These three causes accounted for 41.4% of all deaths from external causes in 1995. However, the high number of deaths from injuries undetermined whether accidentally or purposely inflicted (4,542 cases) indicates that these percentages may be even higher.

Behavioral Disorders. Information on the prevalence of mental illness is very scant. Data from public-sector establishments are incomplete, but indicate that 2.5% of all hospitalizations were related to this category of diseases. Mental illness was more predominant among males and among the 30-to-55 age group. Mental disorders accounted for an estimated 5% of all hospital admissions nationwide.

Different studies placed the prevalence of smoking at somewhere between 40% and 50% for males and between 25% and 35% for females. An increasing percentage of adolescents were becoming addicted, and teenagers over 15 years of age were estimated to smoke 1,500 cigarettes per capita per year. Of the total number of deaths (268,997 for all age groups in 1995), 20% could be attributed to smoking, given its direct association as a risk factor for cardiovascular and cerebrovascular diseases and cancer of the respiratory tract.

Studies on the prevalence of alcoholism do not provide full data, but they do indicate a high percentage of alcoholics among economically active males (between 30% and 50%). Recently, there has been a trend toward alcohol use at younger ages: in the metropolitan Buenos Aires area, for instance, 70% of adolescents drank beer on a daily basis.

Industrial Accidents and Natural Disasters. Twenty-nine industrial accidents were reported in 1995, resulting in 15 deaths. In 1996, a total of 24 accidents were reported in the chemical industry: 85% were chemical spills, 8.3% involved leaks, and 4.2% were fires. Of these accidents, 62.5% occurred during transport operations and 37.5% at fixed installations, leading to the exposure of 1,035 persons and chemical intoxication of 19.

Periodic flooding is another source of growing concern, given the vulnerability of many residents in at-risk areas. The danger of flooding and the damage it wreaks is exacerbated by improper land use, deforestation, and inappropriate building practices.

RESPONSE OF THE HEALTH SYSTEM

National Health Plans and Policies

The national health policies adopted in July 1992 were designed to ensure the population's right to health on the basis of the principles of equity, solidarity, efficiency, effectiveness, and quality; enhance the accessibility, efficiency, and quality of health care; strengthen health promotion and protection by targeting specific population groups; and redefine the role of the State in line with federalization and decentralization efforts. Steps were taken to revamp the health care system—including reform of the *obras sociales* em-

ployee-benefit plans—and a series of new initiatives were unveiled, such as the National Program for Quality Assurance in Medical Care, the Self-Managing Public Hospitals Program, and the Compulsory Health Plan. Health promotion and disease prevention were given a higher profile through a variety of programs and concerted epidemiological and preventive actions, such as studies on prevalent diseases and vaccination campaigns. Among the relevant strategies adopted in this regard, special mention can be made of the programs to eradicate polio, measles, and tetanus, programs to control and eliminate cholera and Chagas' disease, AIDS control programs, and support for maternal and child health.

These changes in the health sector were preceded by broad-based reform in the country's retirement and pension system, which now combines compulsory and voluntary coverage modalities. The compulsory portion has two components: the government-administered component is financed through tax revenue (on a pay-as-you-go basis) and guarantees a standard minimum benefit according to principles of redistribution and insurance; the private component is geared toward savings and security, and takes the form of individual member-capitalized savings plans or company-managed plans that are funded by joint employee and employer contributions, fully and individually capitalized and regulated by the government (i.e., fully funded plans). The voluntary plans are identical in all respects to the fully funded plans with the exception that they are capitalized exclusively by the beneficiary.

In 1995 and 1996, a new system was devised for managing occupational hazards: private operators were brought in as a way of eliminating one of the inherent weaknesses in the previous system, which assigned full liability to employers. The new system introduced entirely new guidelines and arrangements and allowed for the rapid organization of a structure encompassing 43 specialized insurance companies, 380,000 participating firms, and some 3.5 million workers. Over 24,000 workers receive monthly benefits under this legislation. Overseen by the Superintendency for Occupational Hazards (which is linked organizationally to the Ministry of Labor and the social security system), the new system is looking to extend coverage beyond the formal labor market, while updating the accident information system and broadening the initiative's general objectives of accident prevention and mandatory implementation of plans to improve working conditions and settings.

Health Sector Reform

Current health reforms respond to the macroeconomic objective of paring back the costs of productive activity. Change is also sweeping the health sector at the microeconomic level, as it learns to work with new actors (i.e., insurance companies) and other intermediaries, as well as with new forms of contracting that are redefining its relationship with the private sector.

Until recently, health care costs were managed through a system of egalitarian benefits, fixed-percentage payroll deductions, the Redistribution Fund of the *obras sociales* employee-benefit plans, and additional contributions from employers. Under the *obras sociales* plans, payments were made pursuant to agreements with service-provider groups, i.e., the physicians' association or the association of private clinics and sanatoriums. The main form of contractual relationship was fee-for-service.

The National Health Insurance Administration (ANSSAL) regulates prices (by establishing weighted values for each type of service on the basis of a national fee table), enforces guidelines and regulations, administers subsidies paid out of the Redistribution Fund, and allocates funding for public hospitals (whose services are often used by *obras sociales* plan beneficiaries). In an attempt to circumvent this regulatory structure, service providers have engaged in such practices as billing for services not actually provided, performing unnecessary procedures, and invoicing patients directly for any amounts that exceed the ANSSAL-set fees.

This fee-for-service approach—combined with insufficient management control in the *obras sociales* plans—gave rise to a series of incentives in the system that led to a health care structure based on increasingly expensive curative services and characterized by overbilling, overtreatment, the subcategorization of specialties, and heavier use of technology. Private-sector growth and the steady introduction of technology produced a glut of service providers, making it virtually impossible to financially sustain the burgeoning delivery structure. New sources of financing had to be found. The solution ultimately adopted was to have plan members pay a higher share for the lower-cost and less complex care services; the idea of institutional prepayment was developed by the service providers themselves.

In other words, the system shifted from a fee-for-service basis to a capitation-based system that concentrated the risk in the provider organization. The private subsector took on a greater role in providing health care services, as the role of the *obras sociales* and public subsectors shrank in the face of fiscal constraints, lower wage levels, unemployment, and lower employer contributions.

In 1993, the Government gave approval for plan members to move from one *obras sociales* plan to another. A reform program (known as the PROS program) was launched in 1995 to get the *obras sociales* plans and the INSSJyP's PAMI plan on a solid enough financial footing so they could pay "eligible" debts and come up with new contracting arrangements that

would guarantee their viability, financial soundness, and ability to honor outstanding commitments. Decree 206/97 extended the deadline for *obras sociales* plans to join the PROS program to 30 April 1997, and moved to 30 August 1997 the deadline for members to switch to any prequalified plan that had submitted a proposal for institutional modernization within the PROS framework. According to data from the National Social Security Administration (ANSES), some 150,000 requests to switch plans had been received as of May 1997. The PAMI plan, which provides health care coverage for retirees and their dependents, was transferred to the national budget by executive order in 1995. In March 1997, the Government declared its intervention complete in this area and, from that point on, the plan was to be managed exclusively by its beneficiaries, i.e., the retirees.

Reform of the *obras sociales* plans led to the formulation of the Compulsory Health Plan (PMO). To develop, negotiate, and implement this proposal, a commission was set up that included the Ministry of Health, ANSSAL, and Argentina's largest labor union, the Confederación General del Trabajo. The approved PMO opened the way in late 1996 for full beneficiary mobility in choosing an *obras sociales* plan. In January 1997, Law 24,754 (governing private-sector activity in this area) made it compulsory for voluntary insurance plans to offer PMO coverage as well. This legislation supersedes and overrides all existing agreements; any user may demand the coverage established in the PMO, which encompasses transplants, dental care, services for hemophiliacs, dialysis for chronic patients, and psychological care. The PMO is the cornerstone of compulsory insurance reform, since it defines the product that the *obras sociales* plans will compete with each other to supply.

ANSSAL, the National *Obras Sociales* Board (INOS), and the National *Obras Sociales* Directorate (DINOS) were merged to create the National Heath Services Superintendency, a decentralized agency under the Ministry of Health and Social Action. The agency enjoys administrative, economic, and financial autonomy, and is responsible for supervising, inspecting, and overseeing all the players in the National Health Insurance System. The superintendency will focus its action on monitoring the PMO and the National Program for Quality Assurance in Health Care at service providers throughout the system, enforcing guidelines pertaining to self-managed public hospitals, and ensuring the exercise of people's right to freely select the *obras sociales* plan of their choice.

Organization of the Health Sector

Institutional Organization

The health services system in Argentina is composed of three main subsectors: the public subsector (i.e., government-provided financing and services), the *obras sociales* (employee-benefit plans formerly run by unions and now organized by professional category), and the private subsector (prepaid voluntary insurance plans based on actuarial risk). There is a strong bias toward curative care, with emphasis on hospital services. Although national, provincial, and municipal policies all define primary health care as their basic strategy, most of the jurisdictions that have adopted this strategy approach it in the form of "programs" to be carried out at the primary care level.

The public subsector provides care services through the public network. After a prolonged process, hospitals were decentralized in 1991 and directors were given administrative flexibility. Local authorities outsourced such non-core activities as food services and housekeeping, and the new system of self-management allowed them to charge the *obras sociales* plans for services provided to plan members as well as others with the ability to pay. The Ministry of Health and Social Action transferred the remaining medical care services that were under its jurisdiction to the provinces and *municipios;* from that point on, its sphere of activity has been limited to central planning and evaluation. This reform brought with it significant improvements in terms of planning, statistics, data analysis, data banks, systems automation, and communications between the provincial and the central levels.

In December 1996, the Ministry of Health and Social Action was reorganized into two separate units: the Health Policy and Regulations Secretariat and the Health Programs Secretariat, each with oversight responsibility for several decentralized agencies. The Health Policy and Regulations Secretariat oversees the INSSJyP; the National Food, Drug, and Medical Technology Administration; and the National Health Services Superintendency, while the Health Programs Secretariat oversees the Dr. Carlos Malbrán National Health Institutes and Laboratories Administration, the National Institute for Centralized Coordination of Ablations and Implants (INCUCAI), the National Center for Social Re-education (CENARESO), the National Institute for the Rehabilitation and Support of the Disabled, Baldomero Sommer National Hospital, Professor A. Posadas National Hospital, and Dr. Manuel Montes de Oca National Facility.

The *obras sociales* plans are a system of compulsory social insurance that includes other benefits in addition to health care. Their financing comes from employer and employee contributions; many of them do not provide services directly, but rather subcontract with the private sector. In all, there are currently some 300 such plans (between the union-related plans and those for management-level employees), but the figure is expected to drop to around 80 after the processes of institutional modernization and sector reform have been completed. Roughly 10% of the overall contribution goes into the Redistribution Fund, an ANSSAL-administered equalization fund

that subsidizes plans having lower capitalization levels. In 1994, the amount managed by the *obras sociales* plans came to a total of US$ 2.5 billion. The Government is expediting deregulation of the sector in order to foster competition between the *obras sociales* plans and private (prepaid) health insurance companies, encourage beneficiaries to take an active role in choosing their *obras sociales* plan, and guarantee that all plans afford the basic benefits package of main services, diagnoses, and treatments (PMO) as required by law.

In 1993, the National Tax Directorate (DGI) was charged with levying, collecting, and allocating all social security funds, including contributions to *obras sociales* plans. Late in 1996, the DGI, ANSES, and ANSSAL began working on a beneficiary profile to be used in carrying out this activity.

In the private subsector, the two main subgroups are: professionals who provide independent care services to members of *obras sociales* or private, prepaid plans; and health care facilities that are contracted by *obras sociales* plans. A few non-profit agencies are active in this subsector as well. In recent years, some of the larger service providers have merged, crowding out smaller firms that were unable to attain economies of scale. Most of the private providers are located in the country's major cities. When Argentina privatized its national retirement scheme and set up pension fund administrators, a series of new and related services came into existence linking health, retirement, and life insurance.

There are over 200 private, prepaid medicine companies (the lack of a central registry makes it difficult to know exactly how many). The number of beneficiaries covered is estimated at two million. The October 1996 legislation that deregulated the *obras sociales* plans and established controls for prepaid medicine also authorized private medical companies to function as *obras sociales* plans. Accordingly, they are subject to the same controls, are required to be financially solvent, and must meet specific medical care requirements.

Organization of Health Regulatory Activities

The current reform process called for new legislation on sector organization, regulation, oversight, and control. Statutes, decrees, resolutions, and ordinances were enacted in such areas as health policy approval, organizational changes in the Ministry of Health, the creation of agencies to oversee new programs or perform supervisory, oversight, or control functions, the operation of various health-sector entities (self-managed public hospitals, *obras sociales* plans, the PAMI plan, and the private subsector), food and drug regulations, and environmental protection. In some instances, however, enabling regulations are lacking, enforcement structures are fragmented, and overlapping responsibilities create conflict with other jurisdictional levels. Coordination is still at an incipient stage, bearing in mind that under the country's federal system of government not all subnational jurisdictions have to adopt the norms and procedures generated at the national level.

The State's regulatory role is outlined in the National Program for Quality Assurance in Health Care and in the new procedures instituted to upgrade the certification and recertification of health professionals. A call has been issued to academic, scientific, and professional groups, as well as to health service providers, to take part in preparing regulatory guidelines for diagnosis and treatment procedures and the organization and operation of health services. In this connection, highest priority has been attached to reaching consensus in such areas as the accreditation of specialties, professional certification and recertification, standardization of degrees and titles, and interinstitutional arrangements for redesigning academic curricula and in-service training.

The National Program for Quality Assurance in Health Care oversees the exercise of professional activity in this sector and, accordingly, examines the health team's overall professional performance as well as specializations, registration, certification, and recertification. In this regard, the Ministry of Health has provided crucial input through its work with the Argentine Association of Medical Schools, the National Academy of Medicine, the Argentine Medical Association, the Argentine Medical Federation, the Ministry of Education, medical societies, and scientific associations in order to ensure proper preparation of the human resources that make up the health team.

The Ministry of Health's National Health Resources Commission has updated procedures for medical accreditation, licensing, certification, and recertification. The National Coordination Commission for Human Resources in the Pharmaceutical and Biochemical Professions has analyzed proposed profiles and areas of responsibility for biochemical specialties and has taken up the matter of pharmaceutical certification raised by the Argentine Pharmaceutical Federation.

The National Food, Drug, and Medical Technology Administration (ANMAT) is a decentralized agency that serves as a national reference center and training site for specialized human resources. Its mandate includes quality control, and it is the highest authority for matters pertaining to the control and inspection of the safety and quality of all products likely to have an impact on human health.

Argentina's national surveillance system is linked to the WHO International Drug Monitoring Center, and a national drug surveillance system was inaugurated in 1993. Food quality is monitored through a surveillance strategy based on concerted action by hospitals, other institutions, and the Ministry of Health and Social Action. Work has also begun at ANMAT toward organizing the inspection, control, and surveillance of medical technology.

In 1993, a policy framework for the system of self-managing public hospitals was adopted. The goal was to decentralize public hospitals in operational terms, boost their institutional management capacity, and make them more efficient and financially self-sustaining. Some of the core features of the system are the ability of public hospitals to incorporate at the request of the authorities, the requirement that entities of the National Health Insurance System make immediate payment for services received by their respective beneficiaries, and unrestricted contracting between these entities and self-managing public hospitals. These hospitals must meet a series of general conditions, although individual performance standards can be set by each province. The system also outlines specific functions and responsibilities, including the obligation to provide egalitarian and undifferentiated care to the entire population and to provide care services to those who lack coverage or the means to pay. The policy framework furthermore allows for participation by the provincial governments. Since most public hospitals are not owned by the national government, their inclusion in the national registry has depended on local government decisions.

Argentina is a regular participant at MERCOSUR meetings designed to deepen the process of regional integration with regard to foods, drugs, the environment, and the safety of consumer products. In the health sphere, however, several items of paramount importance remain unaddressed, such as consensus on regional guidelines and the standardization of relevant policy. Argentina is also an active participant in MERCOSUR's cooperation arrangements (information and communications systems, border health, medical technology and care, and technical cooperation).

Health Services and Resources

Organization of Services for Care of the Population

Health Promotion. Reform of the State has led not only to the aforementioned technical and political restructuring of the Ministry of Health and Social Action but also to a reorientation of strategies and programs in several core technical units, such as the Maternal and Child Health Program. In 1994, an initiative entitled "Commitment to Women and Children" was formulated, national strategies and targets were set, and substantial central-government funding was re-allocated for the implementation of provincial programs (whose management responsibilities have increased).

The Ministry of Health stepped up its health promotion and protection efforts by establishing programs for public awareness, health education, and tobacco and health, and encouraging a shift in service networks' care focus. A fledgling movement combining cultural, political, social, economic, and intersectoral interests has been advocating the adoption of public health policies that promote changes in the population's lifestyles.

The Ministry's promotion and protection activities have also addressed air quality, workers' health, pesticides, waste disposal, and basic sanitation, including a special effort to lower arsenic levels in water in areas where high concentrations of arsenic in the water supply is endemic. The evaluation of environmental health risks was another topic of special concern and, accordingly, the Argentine Environmental Waste Management Network (REMAR) was set up, comprising the Ministry of Health, the Secretariat for Natural Resources and Sustainable Development, the Argentine Industrial Union, the General Federation of Industries, Coordinación Ecológica del Área Metropolitana Sociedad del Estado (CEAMSE), and PAHO. At the provincial and municipal level, responsibility for environmental protection is shared by various institutions.

Disease Prevention and Control Programs. Argentina's Program for the Prevention and Control of Communicable Diseases merits special mention. The national vaccination program seeks to increase levels of vaccine coverage and surveillance under the Expanded Program on Immunization and to enhance coordination with provincial programs; as a specific initiative, a campaign to eliminate measles has also been launched. In 1996, coverage stood at 89.7% for polio vaccine, 82.8% for DTP, 100% for BCG, and 100% for measles vaccine. The system for communicable disease surveillance has also been upgraded, resulting in an increase in case reportings. The 1992–1994 period witnessed an intense mobilization effort to deal with the cholera outbreaks; programs were established for public awareness, health education, training for personnel, and outfitting of services. Poliomyelitis was declared eradicated in 1994. At present, campaigns are under way for the eradication or elimination of measles, neonatal tetanus, leprosy, diphtheria, human rabies, and Chagas' disease. The program is currently emphasizing health situation analyses that could be useful in identifying at-risk areas and groups for the principal health problems and establishing an early warning system capable of detecting outbreaks of emerging and re-emerging diseases.

Virtually all the provinces are participating in the National Human Retrovirus and AIDS Control Program, which works to enhance capabilities in diagnostic laboratories and medical care services, the awareness and knowledge of at-risk groups, and epidemiological surveillance. In 1996, a new initiative was launched in Argentina under the Joint United Nations Program on HIV/AIDS (UNAIDS), guiding principles and mandates were defined, and a thematic group was set up.

Epidemiological Surveillance and Public Health Laboratories. The National Epidemiological Surveillance System dates back to the 1950s, when monthly data were already reported for communicable diseases by jurisdiction. The system was reformulated in 1993 under the auspices of the National Epidemiology Directorate of the Ministry of Health and Social Action, and case reportings subsequently increased by around 174% between 1993 and 1996. Almost all data came from the public subsector and referred to morbidity as recorded by outpatient, emergency, and inpatient services. In 1996, the National Network of Argentine Public Health Laboratories (RELAS) was created, linking various networks of laboratories.

Water Supply and Sewerage Systems. The service infrastructure in this subsector presents yawning inequalities. Urban growth over recent decades did not benefit from proper planning and, as a result, the problems of Argentina's major urban centers progressively worsened. Inadequate water supply and excreta disposal generate high-risk conditions that especially endanger the country's poorer areas.

The Undersecretariat for Water Resources Management of the Ministry of Economic Affairs and Public Works and Services concluded a study in late 1996 that presents an updated overview of water supply and sewerage coverage. Data from cities of more than 10,000 inhabitants (84% of the total population) are compared and analyzed. From 1991 to 1995, the study showed that service coverage rose from 71% to 81% for water supply and from 37.3% to 50% for sewerage. An estimated 6.6 million people lacked access to public water supply and nearly 17 million had no sewerage connections. These figures were somewhat lower for the scattered population (around three million) that cannot be served by public service networks. Water supply coverage exceeded 90% in seven provinces, and sewerage coverage reached a level of 84% in the province of Tierra del Fuego. In the metropolitan Buenos Aires area, coverage at year-end 1995 was 78% for water supply and 61% for sewerage (up from 46% in 1991, a reflection of the efforts made).

An estimated 10% of all sewage was treated, creating a situation that undoubtedly contributes to higher levels of environmental pollution. As of the end of 1996, privatized systems covered 65% of the total population served; municipal or provincial systems covered 25%; and the remaining 10% was in a state of transition.

National action in the areas of water supply and sewerage coverage is coordinated by the Public Works and Communications Secretariat and the Water Management Undersecretariat, both under the Ministry of Economic Affairs and Public Works and Services. The country's National Water and Sanitation Agency is part of the Water Management Undersecretariat.

Municipal Solid Waste Disposal (Including Hospital Waste). No reliable data were available on municipal solid waste. In the metropolitan Buenos Aires area, each resident produced around 0.88 kg of solid waste per day; collection coverage stood at 91%, and the sanitary landfill situation was considered good. Elsewhere in the country, solid waste disposal was a serious environmental and public health problem owing to inappropriate siting of landfills. Recycling had not yet been incorporated on a large scale in waste management systems, and reported levels were insignificant. Only 50% of poor homes in the metropolitan Buenos Aires area received regular waste collection services.

A study on hazardous waste carried out by the province of Buenos Aires in late 1991 estimated that the chemical, petrochemical, and oil and gas industries produced roughly 29.9% of all waste. Various sources calculated hazardous waste production at between 50,000 and 100,000 tons a year for the province of Buenos Aires, the country's most highly industrialized province. As of January 1996, the company responsible for solid waste collection had counted 103 garbage dumps in the metropolitan Buenos Aires area alone; these dumps received around one million tons of household and hazardous waste and occupied a total surface area of 557 hectares.

As for hospital waste, data from the Ministry of Health and Social Action indicated a total of 155,749 hospital beds in 1995, with an estimated 1.0 to 1.5 kg of hazardous waste generated per bed per day. Over 50% of this waste was concentrated in the city and province of Buenos Aires.

Prevention and Control of Air Pollution. Environmental quality suffered from a wide range of problems. Generally speaking, though, environmental conditions were poor in marginal urban areas and in regions undergoing rapid economic development. The monitoring system continued to be deficient. Many of the stations included in the Global Environment Monitoring System did not have permanent monitoring systems in place, making it impossible to undertake a specific analysis. Even though maximum contaminant levels had been exceeded on only a few occasions, specific instances of pollution caused by mobile or fixed-point sources had particularly deleterious effects for specific population groups. The privileged geographic situation of the city of Buenos Aires favors the dissipation of ambient contaminants, thus helping to keep pollution levels below international limits. However, certain areas of the city (i.e., the urban core and surrounding areas) commonly have levels of gaseous contaminants and particles that exceed those limits, e.g., the daily carbon monoxide level was between 1.5 and 6 times the legal limit for air quality in Buenos Aires.

In 1991, two new offices were created: the Secretariat for Natural Resources and the Human Environment, linked directly to the Office of the President of the Republic, and the Water Management Undersecretariat, under the Ministry of Economic Affairs and Public Works and Services. The Federal Council on the Environment (COFEMA) was set up in 1992 and provided a central forum for government representatives from all the provinces. In 1994, the Federal Environmental Pact was signed as a further step toward building consensus in the area of environmental policy.

As of the end of 1996, only 43.5% of the provinces had specific structures (and specific assigned responsibilities) in place to address environmental issues at the governmental level. In the other provinces, these responsibilities were fragmented among various areas; a similar situation was observed at the *municipio* level. Fragmentation is not necessarily a problem in and of itself, but such low levels of coordination greatly hinder the planning and implementation of activities. The provinces did not always adopt standards and procedures that were agreed upon at the national level. Furthermore, legislation on pollution control is not compiled into a single compendium, so enforcement is difficult at times. National legislation takes a sector-based approach that sometimes prevents concerted action for dealing with specific environmental problems; in other cases, it limits itself to regulating the management of individual areas.

Food Assistance Programs. Food assistance is one of the specific components of the Social Plan. Revenue share-outs are used to distribute powdered whole milk to at-risk children and pregnant women as a way of preventing malnutrition. This program has been an incentive for health check-up attendance. Beneficiaries are selected on the basis of unmet basic needs.

The Maternal and Child Health and Nutrition Program focuses on nutritional support and food supplements for pregnant women and children under 6 years old. These activities are carried out as part of child health and development actions.

The Children's Food and Nutrition Program of the Social Development Secretariat provides food supplements as part of the actions geared toward improving living conditions and access to appropriate and adequate food for children between the ages of 2 and 14. In 1996, the Maternal and Child Health Directorate of the Ministry of Health and Social Action earmarked US$ 46,299,290 for this program.

Organization and Operation of Personal Health Care Services

Insurance Schemes and Coverage. Given the overlapping of categories and coverage levels, the exact extent of health insurance coverage is hard to estimate. According to the 1991 National Population and Housing Census, 62.2% of the population had some kind of insurance coverage, although specific percentages varied from one region to the next (from 79.5% in

Buenos Aires to 42.1% in Jujuy). The percentage of the population not covered by an *obras sociales* or other kind of health care plan also varied from jurisdiction to jurisdiction, ranging from Formosa (56.39%), Santiago del Estero (54.08%), Chaco (51.23%), Misiones (48.96%), Salta (41.83%), and Corrientes (47.53%), at one extreme, to the federal district (19.49%) and Santa Cruz (22.94%), at the other.

Studies conducted by ANSES in 1992 revealed that nearly 80% of all beneficiaries in the *obras sociales* subsector were covered by the 34 largest plans; the 10 largest *obras sociales* plans covered one half the beneficiary population; the 30 largest plans covered nearly 75%; and the 40 largest plans covered 80%. Based on INDEC figures, ANSES projected that members of ANSSAL-associated *obras sociales* plans would total approximately 8 million by 1997; provincial plans would have a total membership of 6.5 million; the PAMI plan would cover 4.5 million beneficiaries; other *obras sociales* and health care systems (prepaid medicine and *obras sociales* plans for university and armed forces personnel) would cover some 5.5 million; and the population served by the public subsector would total 12.3 million persons.

Outpatient, Hospital, and Emergency Services. Public hospitals provide care services for the poor and, on a reimbursable basis, for members of *obras sociales* plans. They also cover demand from social sectors having greater ability to pay, they provide emergency and accident care, and they perform the functions of a medical school. Free public care services—despite the prevailing crisis—have had to absorb the increase in demand created by the shrinking coverage of many *obras sociales* plans, and in the final analysis have ended up subsidizing the system. For patients who have some kind of insurance coverage, however, self-managed public hospitals are now authorized to bill third-party insurers, be they *obras sociales* plans or some other type of insurer. The public subsector continues to be the principal provider of emergency and psychiatric services and of care for the chronically ill.

In 1995, the Ministry of Health and Social Action conducted a survey of the country's health care facilities and found that they had increased from 9,051 in 1980 to 16,085 in 1995. The largest increase was observed in establishments that did not offer inpatient care (they more than doubled), while those that did offer such care grew by around 10%. Of the total number of establishments, 43.3% were in the public subsector, 1.4% were operated by *obras sociales* plans, 55.2% were privately run, and 0.1% were "mixed." Compared with the structure in 1980, the share of the private subsector had increased (up from 44.6%), with a consequent reduction in the shares of the other two subsectors. At the same time, a new kind of establishment (classified as "mixed") appeared on the scene combining features of the public and private subsectors.

The number of available beds rose from 145,690 in 1980 to 155,749 in 1995, for a 1995 rate of 4.5 beds per 1,000 population. This indicator represented a drop from the 1980 level; in other words, the number of beds increased at a slower rate than the population did. Bed availability in 1995 broke down as follows: 54% in the public subsector (62.5% in 1980), 2.8% in the *obras sociales* subsector (5.5% in 1980), 43.1% in the private subsector (32% in 1980), and 0.1% at mixed-administration establishments (which did not exist in 1980). Two trends came together to create this situation: the number of beds available in the public and *obras sociales* subsectors was dropping just as more beds were rapidly becoming available in the private subsector, outpacing the decrease in the other two subsectors.

A series of new care and service delivery arrangements also surfaced: emergency transport services, which provide in the street and for home emergencies; day hospitals and short-stay facilities, which introduced new formats of inpatient care; and vaccination centers, which apply vaccines as an exclusive service or in combination with other treatments (in 1980, vaccinations were performed at outpatient clinics or, on occasion, at health care facilities with inpatient services). New trends continue to take shape. More and more, establishments operating under a given company name are using differentiated resources to do business at different sites, while other companies are operating under different names at the same site. At least two new forms of care delivery have appeared that mix public and private-subsector modalities. One is the presence of private diagnostic services at public-sector inpatient facilities (an outgrowth of service fragmentation); and the other is the siting of public-sector primary care centers in buildings that belong to community development associations, neighborhood associations, or others. In the provinces, the number of such facilities varies according to the type of unit and the subsector under which they operate.

In 1996, there were 824 self-managing public hospitals, offering a total of 62,402 beds (almost 75.3% of the country's public beds). Under the new arrangements, *obras sociales* and other plans will have to pay for services provided at these hospitals to plan members.

Auxiliary Diagnostic Services and Blood Banks. Plans have been under way since 1996 to institute laboratory control procedures aimed at guaranteeing high-quality diagnoses. Since 1984, the Chagas National Epidemiological Research Institute has overseen quality control of procedures and reagents. Hemotherapy services are coordinated by the Argentine Hemotherapy and Immunohematology Association. The organization of data from serological tests and reagents was performed as an entirely separate activity from quality control until 1992. The initiative launched that year to eliminate *Triatoma infestans* and screen all blood used for transfusions made it possible to build a continuously updated database that covers both public and private institutions. Argentina has 776 registered hemotherapy services and blood banks, some of which serve as compilation points for data from various centers. Included in this number are 536 laboratories that screen blood for transfusions and perform other blood control functions for various institutions. Currently, serological testing is done for hepatitis B and C, *Trypanosoma cruzi*, HIV, and syphilis. All donors in both the public and private subsectors are screened.

Specialized Services. The public subsector has 40 mental health establishments, including 35 residential care facilities for chronic patients. These facilities account for the highest percentage (98%) of the total 15,069 beds available. The private subsector operates 187 establishments, including residential care facilities for cases classified as acute, chronic, acute chronic, or of undetermined duration; these are the most common type of private facility (139) and account for the highest percentage of available beds (80% of the total 9,047 beds for mental health care in the private subsector). From these data it can be seen that virtually all the resources for chronic patient care are located in the public subsector.

Twenty-four establishments with a total of 953 beds provide physical rehabilitation services. Nine of these establishments (532 beds) are in the public subsector and ten (421 beds) are in the private subsector.

Inputs for Health

Drug prices were deregulated near the end of 1991, along with the legal mark-up limits that retail pharmacies may charge. Drug registration procedures were streamlined in 1993, resulting in considerable time savings; drug surveillance and inspections were stepped up as well. The private pharmaceutical sector instituted new drug distribution, administration, and dispensing systems that are used by *obras sociales* plans and prepaid systems for which specific regulations are not yet in place.

Following prolonged parliamentary debate on the issue, the new Patent Act was passed into law in late 1995. The sector was becoming progressively more concentrated as mergers and acquisitions were rapidly negotiated by multinational laboratories. Of the top 20 companies in terms of sales volumes in 1996, 10 were Argentine firms (with 54% of the market) and the other 10 (with 46% of the market) were multinationals.

In the period 1993–1996, the pharmaceuticals market showed a steady downward trend in the number of units sold, for an accumulated drop of 15.8% (from 482 million units in

1992 to 406 million in 1996). Retail sales, however, rose from US$ 2,575,000 to US$ 3,644,000 over the same period, representing point-of-sale price increases of between US$ 5.34 and US$ 8.98 per unit.

Except for those included under special programs, the public subsector does not cover drugs for outpatient care. The public-sector *obras sociales* plans defray a percentage of members' drug costs and fully subsidize all the uncommon, high-cost drugs included in the PMO. Prepaid medicine companies also cover about 50% of beneficiaries' drug costs.

Efforts to contain drug spending began in the 1980s when several price controls were implemented. The controls were based on PAMI-defined treatment modules or on reference prices set by the Medical Care Institute (IOMA); success was limited in both instances. The effective deregulation of prices triggered a jump in spending in 1992 estimated at around US$ 1 billion. Actions to contain spending by promoting more rational use of inputs have not had the intended impact.

Human Resources

Work Force Size. The current size of the health work force cannot be determined accurately in view of the fact that no comprehensive studies have been done since 1980. That year, the health sector employed some 210,000 persons, equivalent to approximately 2.9% of the national work force. Estimates made in 1985 (but based on 1980 data) indicated that some 400,000 persons were employed in the health sector (4% of the economically active population). Argentina's health work force presents an inverted pyramid structure in which the professional categories greatly outweigh the technical and support categories.

Total personnel in the various nursing categories was estimated at 85,000 (on the basis of figures from 1988 and 1994): 1,000 graduate nurses (1.2%), 25,000 tertiary-level nurses (29.4%), 49,000 nursing auxiliaries (57.6%), and 10,000 lay nurses (11.7%). Many lay nurses were receiving training to become nursing auxiliaries as part of a policy that has led to a significant increase in the number of nursing auxiliaries and professional nurses over the past five years: the number of auxiliaries had already doubled, and provincial professionalization programs were expected to train an additional 10,000 tertiary-level nurses by the year 2000.

Training. The training of health human resources exhibits some very specific characteristics owing to the medical model's hegemony over the sector. There are seven public and seven private medical schools, which together form the Argentine Association of Schools of Medical Sciences (AFACIMERA). The country has two other private medical schools that are not members of the association.

Universities train some 3,500 physicians each year. Available data indicate, however, that fewer than 1,000 university residencies are made available each year, a level that could drop even further in light of recent budgetary restrictions. Very few public universities—and none of the private ones—have their own hospital.

Medical residencies in a limited number of specialties are offered at the national universities, and recent graduates are thus able to continue studying and defer their entry into the labor market. According to data from the Ministry of Health and Social Action, a total of 1,700 residencies were available in all of Argentina in 1995. Privately-operated and *obras sociales* establishments offer a wide diversity of residencies and, on occasion, enter into agreements with universities located in their respective catchment areas. Overall, residency prospects are very dim for a high percentage of graduates.

The medical schools—represented by AFACIMERA—have been working with the Ministry of Culture and Education to improve medical training and thereby raise Argentina's health levels. An agreement was signed in 1994 defining mechanisms for self-evaluation of medical curricula and, in December 1996, a second agreement was formalized setting forth the necessary conceptual and methodological bases for moving ahead with the accreditation of medical programs. The two agreements, each with its own specific objectives, created a framework for consultation between the Government and the academic sector aimed at building consensus before setting the new guidelines. Medical schools were called upon not only to incorporate technological and scientific advances, but also to be responsive to changes and needs in the health sector. Under the current reform process, the PMO has increased the demand for a specific professional profile (i.e., general practitioners) and this demand must be met by the system that trains the country's health personnel; changes will also need to be made in working arrangements and in the management of the system that uses these resources.

Schools of dentistry (seven public and two private) are organized under the Argentine Association of Schools of Odontology (AFORA). Self-evaluation and external evaluation processes and accreditation of graduate curricula are at various stages of progress. Advanced training is offered in a variety of formats, ranging from specialization courses, refresher training, and residencies to master's and doctoral programs.

Argentina's medical and dental schools are now facing other challenges as well, as regional economic integration imposes new demands in terms of personnel training, flows of health goods and services, individual health, and the environment.

Continuing Education. A continuing education program is currently under way at several health services in the province of Córdoba, with the stated purpose of strengthening management capacity and adjusting nursing services and hospital administration on the basis of an analysis of specific problems.

Labor Market for Health Professionals. Many areas of the labor market need to be studied in greater detail, data need to be updated, and points of consensus need to be established. In 1992, there was an average of only one physician for every 367 residents, although the level ranged from one physician per 113 people in Buenos Aires to one per 911 in Formosa. At a ratio of 1 nurse for every 4 physicians, and 5.4 nurses per 10,000 population (with broad regional variations), levels in this category, too, were considered insufficient.

Research and Technology

Organization and Financing of Scientific Activity and Training of Human Resources. Reorganization of the science and technology sector began with the transfer of the Science and Technology Secretariat (SCyT) to the Ministry of Culture and Education. The SCyT formulates sector policy, draws up the National Multiyear Plan for Science and Technology, prepares the national budget for the sector, and sets sector priorities.

The Secretariat's current management attaches high priority to regional integration, with special emphasis on MERCOSUR as a forum for promoting scientific and technological research, closer cooperation between research institutions, exchanges, and training. The SCyT plans to launch joint efforts for technology management, applied research, and social issues. The 1997 budget for the science and technology sector was US$ 777.4 million, with 69% of that amount corresponding to payroll costs.

The Ministry of Health operates a multi-city network of national research institutes covering the fields of epidemiology, viral diseases, genetics, nutrition, and health laboratories. Over the course of the past five years, the Ministry has lent support for studies on the effectiveness of vaccines against Argentine hemorrhagic fever and meningitis, diagnosis of Chagas' disease, specific chemotherapy for leishmaniasis, and various research projects on hantavirus, leprosy, tuberculosis, goiter, accidents, nitrite contamination, acute respiratory infections, mental retardation, fibrocystic disease of the pancreas, and AIDS, to name just a few.

Scientific and Technical Documentation: Access, Production, and Dissemination. The dissemination of science and health information enjoys a certain level of importance in the Argentine market. According to data from the Argentine Publishers' Association, approximately 8% of all books published between 1993 and 1996 dealt with subjects related to the health sciences. There are 117 health-related journals: 80% of articles were on clinical research, 11% on biomedicine, and 9% on public health.

A 1996 survey conducted by the National Health Sciences Information Network identified 250 individually-operated health science libraries, most of which lacked appropriate infrastructure, specialized staff, and the necessary resources for proper knowledge dissemination. In this connection, it should be noted that the Ministry of Health and Social Action and many of the provincial ministries lack documentation centers for use by sector services. The main health science libraries are located at universities or in the private sector.

The field of applied information sciences has benefited from the development of the Electronic Network for the Health Sector, which links over 1,500 institutions and serves as a hub for the country's various networking initiatives.

Expenditures and Sectoral Financing

Expenditures. Most of the country's health spending is financed by the State and by the *obras sociales* plans through payroll deductions. Spending by these two subsectors as a percentage of GDP grew between 1980 and 1994 from 3.6% to 4.4%. According to data from the Ministry of Health and Social Action, health spending by these two subsectors in 1994 accounted for 16.49% of all public spending, for a per capita level of US$ 388 in public health expenditure that year.

Total health spending in 1995 was calculated at US$ 20,147 million, broken down as follows: public sector (i.e., national, provincial, and municipal governments) US$ 4,676 million; *obras sociales* plans (national and provincial schemes, and the PAMI plan) US$ 7,055 million; and private sector (prepaid and out-of-pocket) US$ 8,416 million.

Cutbacks in federal funding between 1980 and 1994 were offset by a significant increase in provincial and municipal spending (35.8% increase in 1994–1995). The broader presence of municipal flows was due in part to the decentralization of a number of services by the provincial governments, with municipal expenditures ultimately accounting for US$ 580 million (equivalent to 0.23% of GDP).

Despite some intermediate oscillations, public health spending as a percentage of GDP climbed from 1.24% in 1980 to 1.71% in 1994. Data compiled by the Economic Planning Secretariat, the Finance Secretariat, and INSSJyP indicated the following percentages for public health spending in 1995: national government 4.8%, ANSSAL 2.6%, INSSJyP/PAMI 22.6%, federal transfers to the provinces 0.8%, provinces and municipalities 36.1%, national *obras sociales* plans 20.9%, and provincial *obras sociales* plans 12.2%.

As these figures show, the percent share of the national *obras sociales* plans fell sharply—from 32.7% to 23.5%—be-

tween 1992 and 1995. Also worth noting is the fact that PAMI coverage represented between one fifth and one fourth of all public spending. The expansive trend observed in the national *obras sociales* plans in the 1980s was reversed in the 1990s; the provincial *obras sociales* and PAMI plans, on the other hand, practically doubled their spending levels.

Total health spending by the non-private sectors (i.e., the public sector and *obras sociales* plans) was estimated at US$ 11,073 million in 1994. According to the Economic Planning Secretariat of the Ministry of Economic Affairs, this spending represented 4.44% of GDP in 1994 and 4.70% in 1995. The rise was attributed to increased activity under the PAMI plan.

Private-sector spending as a percentage of GDP declined from 4.5% in 1970 to 2.7% in 1993. The outlook for the future is one of continued restraint in this area, and spending is not expected to outpace the level of overall economic growth. A November 1995 survey revealed that 34% of out-of-pocket spending by families in the metropolitan Buenos Aires area went toward drugs, 18% toward private insurance premiums (the level was 26% for the federal district), 10% for doctor's visits, 17% for visits to other health professionals and dentists, and the remainder for inpatient care and other headings.

Between December 1991 and December 1996, the consumer price index (CPI) for health goods and services grew at more than double the rate of the general CPI (53.25% against 25.5%). Between May 1991 and May 1995, service costs (physicians' and dentists' fees and prepaid medicine premiums) jumped nearly 87%, while drug prices rose a full 59%.

Information from the Economic Planning Secretariat indicates that consolidated public spending represented 18.04% of GDP in 1994 and was distributed thus: education 3.83%; health, social action, and sanitation 5.26%; housing 0.47%; social security 6.84%; labor 0.76%, and other urban services 0.88%. Consolidated public spending in the social sectors as a percentage of GDP in 1995 was 18.41%; expenditure in the health sector as a percentage of GDP was 1.75%.

The trends in spending on health, education, and culture over recent years reveal no clear correlation between the level of wealth generated (GDP) and public outlays for health and education. Such spending remains a function of budgetary constraints.

The Ministry of Health, the provincial health ministries, and the municipal health secretariats spent an estimated US$ 800 million on health prevention and regulatory activities (US$ 2 per capita). Outlays to hospitals and health centers were calculated at US$ 4 billion. Cost-recovery arrangements have become increasingly widespread: in the first six months of 1996, 824 self-managed hospitals billed an estimated US$ 6.8 million through automatic debiting systems. This figure is equivalent to approximately 1.5% of the resources allocated by the public sector. An additional US$ 80 million was paid to public hospitals by the *obras sociales* plans.

Financing. Argentina's health sector is financed through various channels. The national government (the federal administration and its decentralized agencies) earmarks funds from the National Treasury (except for ANSSAL and the PAMI plan); the provincial governments and the city of Buenos Aires allocate resources from the federal tax share-outs they receive and from their own tax revenues and transfers from the federal government; the municipal governments assign a portion of the tax share-outs they receive from the provincial governments as well as their own levies; the national and provincial *obras sociales* plans use funds from employee and employer contributions (and, sometimes in the latter case, from the provincial government); the PAMI plan draws on payments by contributing and noncontributing members and employer contributions; and out-of-pocket family spending is used to defray the costs of voluntary insurance or coinsurance, make copayments, and purchase goods and services directly.

Expressed in terms of percentages, these funding sources break down as follows: public subsector 21.76% (national government 1.94%, provincial governments 16.34%, municipal governments 3.48%), *obras sociales* plans 36.34% (national 15.17%, PAMI plan 12.03%, provincial 7.13%, other 2%); and the private subsector 41.9%, which can be further broken down into indirect (prepaid health care plans) 19.26% and direct (drugs, health care services) 22.64%. Within the public subsector, the national government provides resources for health system financing through various central or decentralized agencies; this source accounts for a very small share of health spending, representing between 0.22% and 0.40% of GDP and between 5.4% and 9.0% of public health spending (over the period 1993–1996).

According to Finance Secretariat data, the national public subsector disbursed a total of US$ 1,197,499,497 in 1996, distributed thus: financing 44.85%, care 31.57%, investment 5.2%, prevention and care 4.42%, administration 3.95%, prevention 2.88%, training 2.47%, research and production 1.97%, regulation, control, and supervision 1.63%, and standardization 0.33%. As can be seen, the bulk of the budgeted amount went to financing and care. The "financing" heading included, in addition to ANSSAL's Redistribution Fund, allocations for the Garrahan Hospital. The funding earmarked for prevention was low. The "investment" category included projects that were funded partly by multilateral lending agencies and were not exclusively physical infrastructure or equipment projects (as can be seen in the structure of spending by economic use), but rather included technical assistance and training components.

Upon analyzing the changes that have occurred in allocation levels over time, it can be seen that funding for medical and other residencies and for investments has risen, although such funding's share in the total remains insignificant. The

jump in the financing level in 1996 was due to the purchase, with a loan from Spain, of medical equipment that was distributed among various jurisdictions.

The national *obras sociales* plans are funded through mandatory employee and employer contributions. Between 1993 and 1995, the exact payroll percentage of these contributions was modified three times with an eye to bringing labor costs down. Pursuant to Decree 492/95, the rate now stands at 5%, nearly 17% below the percentage stipulated in Law 23,660/89 (the National Health Insurance Act).

While it is true that ANSSAL is included in the national public sector budget, its status as regulatory agency for the health insurance industry and coordinator of the Redistribution Fund makes it necessary to analyze it in conjunction with the national *obras sociales* plans. Of the total amount collected by these plans in 1996, US$ 340 million went to ANSSAL and US$ 2,592 million to the plans per se. Between 1993 and 1996, there was a slight decrease in the total amount collected (from US$ 3,400 million to US$ 2,932 million).

The legislation that reformed the *obras sociales* system (Decree 492/95) set a new rate for employer contributions and stipulated that a portion of the Redistribution Fund resources be distributed automatically so as to ensure a minimum coverage of US$ 40 per entitled beneficiary under the national *obras sociales* plans. An estimated US$ 35.9 million was distributed under this arrangement during the last quarter of 1995 (US$ 12 million monthly average) and US$ 180.7 million in 1996 (US$ 15 million per month).

The PAMI plan provides health care and other benefits to the population covered under the National Retirement System; it is financed with payments from contributing and noncontributing subscribers and employer contributions. Data from ANSES indicate that these resources rose from US$ 1,758,150 in 1992 to US$ 2,602,700 in 1995, and then fell to US$ 2,458,800 in 1996. PAMI health care spending followed an upward trend from 1992 to 1994 but then dropped in the following two years, when the plan was transferred to the national budget. By that time, though, these outflows (i.e., health care plus other benefits) had already risen well beyond the level of incoming revenue, and the plan fell deep into debt with government agencies (Banco Nación, ANSES, and ANSSAL) and with service providers. The tensions triggered by the resulting financial imbalance led to the current process of rationalization under way at the INSSJyP/PAMI.

External Technical and Financial Cooperation. According to data from the Ministry of Health and Social Action, the main projects benefiting from external financial cooperation were:

The Maternal and Child Health and Nutrition Program (PROMIN). This program is targeted at the poor population and assigns top priority to the strategies of primary health care, child development centers (as a referral level), food supplements, and institutional strengthening of the sectors responsible for program activities. The program has a budget of US$ 160 million, toward which the International Bank for Reconstruction and Development (IBRD) is providing US$ 100 million; disbursements are scheduled through 1999. The rest of the budget is covered by the federal government (US$ 40 million) and the provincial and municipal governments (US$ 20 million).

The Health Sector Reform Project (PRESAL). The PRESAL project is bolstering reform in the three subsectors (public, private, and *obras sociales*) by redefining implementation arrangements and relationships and promoting cooperative and competitive synergy among them, with an eye to efficient, equitable, and high-quality medical care. The project has three components: countrywide studies, pilot experiments with self-managed hospitals, and nationwide implementation of the reform, including self-managed public hospitals and training. The budget of US$ 144.65 million is funded in part by the IBRD.

The *Obras Sociales* Reform Program. Negotiations have been concluded for an IBRD loan to finance the reform program as well as institutional strengthening. The program will seek to shore up the financial positions of the *obras sociales* and PAMI plans and, as part of a gradual restructuring effort, to adjust staffing levels in line with the profiles best suited to achieving the stated objectives. The program has a total budget of US$ 375 million.

The Health Infrastructure Rehabilitation Program. Financed by the Inter-American Development Bank (IDB), this US$ 64.09-million program will build four highly complex provincial hospitals.

ARUBA

GENERAL SITUATION AND TRENDS

Socioeconomic, Political, and Demographic Overview

Aruba is an island in the Antilles located 24 km from the northern coast of Venezuela. It is the smallest (194 km²) and westernmost of three Dutch islands. Aruba is divided into eight regions: Noord/Tank Leendert, Oranjestad (West), Oranjestad (East), Paradera, Santa Cruz, Savaneta, Sint Nicolaas (North), and Sint Nicolaas (South).

The official language is Dutch, which is used in the school system and civil service. Papiamento, which is spoken on Aruba, Bonaire, and Curaçao, is the language of the Parliament and the mass media. English and Spanish are mandatory languages taught in the upper grades of primary school and are widely spoken.

As an autonomous entity within the Kingdom of the Netherlands since 1 January 1986, Aruba is responsible for its own political affairs and administration, with the exception of defense, foreign affairs, and the Supreme Court. Its constitution provides for free and democratic elections every four years to elect the 21 members of Parliament. The Cabinet, headed by the Prime Minister, consists of a maximum of nine ministers. Officially, the head of state is the Dutch monarch, represented by a Governor.

The service sector—especially tourism—is the mainstay of the economy, although the oil refinery has reopened and several small industries, notably construction, are developing.

The per capita gross national product (GNP) in 1993 was US$ 12,900. In 1994, the gross domestic product (GDP) was US$ 16,630. This index makes Aruba more similar to Western Europe and the United States of America than to other countries of the region; nevertheless, these numbers should be viewed with caution because they were calculated for a relatively short period and are estimates. A study is currently under way to determine the GNP; preliminary data indicate that it probably represents 60% of the GDP. The in-

flation rates in 1990, 1993, and 1994 were 7.1%, 6.0%, and 4.7%, respectively.

Between the census of 1991 and the Labor Force Survey (LFS) of October 1994, the population of the island grew from 66,687 to 79,837, an increase of almost 20%. This growth has affected employment and unemployment in Aruba. Proportionally, in 1994 the number of non-Aruban employees was higher than it was in 1991. According to the LFS, of the 2,722 persons employed in 1994, 28% were not from Aruba. Between 1991 and 1994, employment increased more among women than among men.

After the LAGO refinery was closed, unemployment levels climbed to 28% in 1985. Since then, the Government has adopted a series of measures aimed at improving the national economy. In particular, it has promoted strengthening the tourism industry, whose growth, together with that of parallel activities in the construction and service sectors, has helped to bring down unemployment. The growth of tourism led to a 6.5% increase in the transient population between 1994 and 1995. In the latter year, the number of visitors to the island totaled 618,915, which is 7.3 times the population of Aruba.

According to the 1994 LFS, Aruba's total unemployment rate was 6.4%. Among women the rate was 7.8%, and among men it was 5.3%.

The estimated population in 1995 was 83,652. Of that number, 41,592 (49.7%) are male and 42,060 (50.3%) are female. The population density was 445 inhabitants per km². Oranjestad, with approximately 20,045 inhabitants, is the most densely populated region.

The highest registered population growth rate (9.35%) was in 1993. In 1994 the rate decreased to 3.03%, and in 1995 it was 4.13%. These fluctuations basically are due to migration. Net migration between 1984 and 1987 was negative, with values ranging from −264 in 1984 to −501 in 1987. Net migration became positive in 1989, with a value of 586 for that year, and since then it has risen steadily, reaching a high point in 1993

(5,734). According to the 1991 census, immigrants made up about 23.9% of the resident population of Aruba.

The total fertility rates for the years between 1993 and 1995, respectively, were 6.7, 6.5, and 6.8 per 1,000 women 14–44 years of age. No figures on age-specific fertility are available. The crude birth rate in 1995 was 17.0 per 1,000 people; this rate has remained relatively stable since 1991. In 1991, life expectancy at birth was 77.1 years for females and 71.0 years for males.

The population of Aruba is mainly urban and can be considered predominantly young—55.2% of the inhabitants are under 35 years of age. The population over the age of 65 represents 6.6% of the total.

Mortality Profile

The crude death rate ranged from 5.2 per 1,000 inhabitants in 1993 to 6.0 per 1,000 in 1995.

The five leading causes of death in the period 1987–1993 were diseases of the circulatory system; malignant neoplasms; endocrine, nutritional, metabolic, and immunological disorders; external causes; and diseases of the respiratory system. In 1993, the last year for which figures on causes of death are available, of a total of 402 deaths, 25.6% were attributed to ill-defined causes. Of the deaths from defined causes, 138 (46.1%) were due to diseases of the circulatory system; 47 (15.7%) to malignant neoplasms; 30 (10%) to endocrine, nutritional, metabolic, and immunological disorders; 30 (10%) to external causes; and 12 (4%) to infectious and parasitic diseases.

Conditions that originate in the perinatal period are the leading cause of death among children under 1 year old. Among males aged 1–44 years, external causes are the leading cause of death. Heart disease is the primary cause of death for both sexes over the age of 45.

For the 1991–1993 period, the leading specific causes of death were diseases of pulmonary circulation and other forms of heart disease, ischemic heart disease, diabetes mellitus, cerebrovascular diseases, and malignant neoplasms of the breast and stomach.

SPECIFIC HEALTH PROBLEMS

Analysis by Population Group

Health of Children

The child health service of the Department of Public Health seeks to promote the well-being of and provide care for children and adolescents aged 0–12 years. The physicians employed by the service provide medical care through the Yellow and White Cross Foundation and administer vaccines to schoolchildren.

Mortality among children under 1 year old has decreased since 1991, when 10 deaths were certified. Between 1993 and 1995, four, five, and one infant deaths, respectively, were registered. All four deaths in 1993 were attributed to conditions that originated in the perinatal period; two (50%) were due to intrauterine hypoxia and birth asphyxia.

In the 1–4 age group, in 1991 one male child died of a malignant neoplasm, no children died in 1992, and one died in 1993 due to an unspecified accident. In the group aged 5–14 years old, four deaths were certified in 1991—three from diseases of the respiratory system and one from an accident. No deaths occurred in this age group in 1992, and in 1993 there was only one death, which was due to infectious disease.

Health of Adults

The Family Planning Foundation, created in 1970, aims to promote parental responsibility, bearing in mind the cultural and religious traditions of the population. The Foundation provides contraceptive services through the Aruban Family Planning Clinic. According to data from 1994, the most widely used methods were oral contraceptives (41.7%), condoms (41.1%), sterilization (5.7%), injectable contraceptives (5.2%), intrauterine devices (4.8%), and others (1.4%). Although there are no data on coverage, it is known that the number of women coming to the Foundation is on the rise: 5,005 visits in 1988 and 7,178 in 1994, an increase of 43%.

Aruban women can opt to receive care during pregnancy and childbirth from a general practitioner, a midwife, or an obstetrician/gynecologist, but in practice this choice is somewhat limited. Women who have private health insurance and those who are employed in the public or private sector have the greatest freedom of choice. Those who have PPK ("pro-paupere kaart"), a special card for persons of limited economic means, are required to use the services of a midwife. To prepare for the birth, women may take a prenatal exercise course. The Yellow and White Cross (community nursing service) also offers a full range of parenting courses for future mothers and fathers, teaching them about diet and nutrition for mother and baby, growth and development of the fetus, hygiene, nursing, labor and delivery, and postnatal care. Delivery usually takes place at the General Hospital, although women may elect to give birth at home.

Premature births are relatively rare, but when it is suspected that one may occur, the mother is transferred to Curaçao (Netherlands Antilles), where the necessary services are available. If a premature birth does occur on Aruba, the infant is transferred to Curaçao as soon as his/her medical condition permits.

Abortion is a crime prosecutable under the Aruban Penal Code. No data on abortion are available.

No maternity deaths were recorded for the period 1991–1993.

Health of the Elderly

The most frequent causes of death in the group 65 years old and older are diseases of the circulatory system and malignant neoplasms, which account for 51% and 15% of all deaths, respectively. Sixty-five percent of the deaths attributed to ill-defined causes occur in this age group, which has grown considerably as a proportion of the total population over the past three decades: in 1960, persons 65 and older made up 3.1% of the population; in 1991, 7%; and in 1995, 6.6%.

According to the 1991 census, the employed population who were older than age 60 years decreased from 1,187 (5% of the employed population) to 887 (3%). At the time the census was conducted, 13% of the population aged 60 and over was working. This proportion is considerably less than the numbers registered in the 1981 census (20.5%). One possible explanation is the recent decision (1 July 1992) to reduce the age at which persons are eligible to begin collecting their pensions, from 62 to 60 years. Aruba has an officially regulated old-age pension program designed to ensure a minimum income for the elderly.

Stichting Algemene Bejaardenzorg Aruba (SABA), an organization that provides services for adults aged 60 and over, manages three residences for the elderly with a total capacity of 236 beds, which is insufficient. The Government subsidizes the personnel costs of foundations that provide social assistance services to elderly persons in the community.

The Yellow and White Cross Foundation at the district level offers home care for the elderly. There are also two day-care centers that provide services only in the mornings; their programs are mainly recreational.

Workers' Health

A public-sector service provides pre-employment medical examinations for workers as well as monitoring and following up on sick workers. This service also is responsible for prevention and control of occupational risks, health education for workers, and management of data on occupational accidents and illnesses.

In 1995, 40% of all workers in the public sector were women, and this percentage has been increasing. Participation in the labor market by people under the age of 20 has de-

clined dramatically as the number of years spent in school has increased, and currently the percentage of employed young people under 20 is quite small. In the group aged 20–24 years, the rate of participation is considerably higher (70.2% for males, 62.7% for females).

Studies of the years 1994 and 1995 reveal that the causes of morbidity that lead to the greatest absenteeism among workers are colds and flu, digestive disorders, and headaches.

Health of the Disabled

According to data from the 1991 census, the prevalence of disability (including both physical and mental disability) was 5.5% (3,700). The most frequent form of disability was impairment of a limb (28.7%), followed by motor and visual impairments (18.3% and 13.2%, respectively). Disabilities were slightly more frequent in males (5.7%) than in females (5.4%).

Analysis by Type of Disease or Health Impairment

Communicable Diseases

In May 1995 the first case in an eight-month dengue outbreak was reported. A total of 67 suspected cases were reported (57 in 1995 and 10 in 1996) and 45 were confirmed through serological testing, in which serotype 2 was isolated. No deaths or cases of hemorrhagic dengue were reported. This dengue epidemic is the second that has occurred in Aruba; the first occurred in 1984–1985 and affected 24,000 persons. There were two deaths. Serotype 1 was isolated in that epidemic. No other cases of vector-borne disease have been reported.

Aruba has had no reported cases of poliomyelitis or acute flaccid paralysis, diphtheria, whooping cough, or tetanus. Four cases of measles were reported in 1994, none in 1995, and four suspected cases in 1996; serological studies of the latter four cases revealed that three were rubella, and measles was ruled out in the fourth case. Another five cases of rubella were reported during 1996. One case of mumps was reported in 1994, two in 1995, and none in 1996.

There are no consolidated data on vaccination coverage, but estimates indicate 80% coverage with vaccines against diphtheria, tetanus, and pertussis, (DTP), and against poliomyelitis for 1.5-year-old children and 100% coverage for 6-year-olds.

Three cases of hepatitis B were reported in 1994, one in 1995, and one in 1996.

The island has had no cases of cholera. Between 1981 and 1996, the number of cases of shigellosis ranged from 10

(1981) to 89 (1990). During the past three years the numbers have fallen from 24 (0.3 per 1,000 inhabitants) to 20 (0.2 per 1,000 inhabitants) to 13 (0.1 per 1,000 inhabitants), but this reduction is attributed to underreporting. During the same period, the number of reported cases of intestinal infectious diseases caused by other salmonella organisms ranged from 23 (1985) to 116 (1989).

Data from the period 1981–1996 indicate that the highest incidences of tuberculosis were registered in 1992, when seven cases occurred, and in 1995, when eight cases were reported, and most of those were foreigners. No drug resistance has been detected, and no association with AIDS has been found. Aruba had only one case of leprosy, which was diagnosed in 1994.

Although there is no information on the number of medical visits for acute respiratory infections (ARIs), it is estimated that they are a major cause of morbidity; a review of hospital discharge records for 1994 reveals that the likelihood of being hospitalized for a clinical picture consistent with ARI was 2.9 per 1,000 inhabitants. Children aged 1–4 years and adults aged 65 and over were three times more likely than other age groups to be hospitalized for ARI.

During the 1987–1996 period, 25 cases of AIDS were reported, 18 in males and 7 in females; 22 people have died. Epidemiological studies indicate that 94.4% of the males were infected through sexual transmission and 5.6% (one case) through blood that was probably infected (as a result of intravenous drug use). All HIV-positive individuals who report to the Division of Infectious Diseases receive medical and psychological counseling following detection. In addition to counseling and clinical care for HIV-infected patients, control measures include education and screening, especially of prostitutes, patients with sexually transmitted diseases, and blood donors. During the 1986–1995 period, blood testing for HIV detected one seropositive case in 1986, three in 1987, and one in 1995. There were no positive tests in the other years. Approximately 50% of the seropositive individuals were immigrants who had applied for work permits. Most returned to their native countries, which made it impossible to determine how many later developed or died from AIDS.

The number of physician-reported syphilis cases ranged from 14 (the highest number reported) in 1990 to 7 in 1995. In 1996, it was decided that laboratories would be asked to submit information on seropositive cases directly and 86 cases were thus detected, which suggests that the previous numbers reflect a significant degree of underreporting.

There is also underreporting in the case of gonorrhea; the highest number (53 cases) was reported in 1990. In 1996 only three cases were detected.

No cases of rabies or any other zoonoses were reported.

Noncommunicable Diseases and Other Health-Related Problems

A nutritional survey conducted in 1991–1992 (Kappel/Kock) indicated that 67% of the Aruban population was overweight, with a body mass index (BMI) of 25 or more, and 52% of the population had a BMI of more than 27. The mean BMI found among persons aged 22–64 was 27.8. Overweight affects both sexes equally. Significantly higher BMIs were found in low-income than in upper-income groups. The BMI among persons aged 50 and over was 28.5, while among younger adults aged 21–34 it was 27.

In 1995–1996, first- and fifth-graders were screened for overweight and the results were compared with screening results obtained in 1994–1995. It was found that the percentage of overweight among first-grade children had declined from 13.4% to 12.0%. Among fifth graders, an increase from 26.1% to 29.4% was observed. No data are available on protein-energy malnutrition among children under the age of 5.

Aruban authorities have not established an official policy on promotion of breast-feeding. In practice, many mothers do breast-feed their children, although they generally use bottle-feeding as a supplement.

The 1990 National Health Survey was a descriptive study of the general population aimed at obtaining information on health status, alcohol consumption, demand for medical services, and degree of satisfaction with those services. The results of the survey indicated that 66% of the population felt healthy and that hypertension and diabetes were the most prevalent diseases (affecting 9.8% and 4.3%, respectively, of the population).

Hospital admissions for diabetes mellitus were more frequent among females than males, which may indicate that the disease is more prevalent among females. The risk of requiring hospitalization for this cause increases with age and is three times higher in the group aged 65 and over than in the 45–64 age group. Diabetes mellitus was the fourth leading cause of death during the 1987–1993 period, and the rate has tended to remain stable. In 1993, the risk of dying from this cause was twice as high among females.

Ischemic heart disease ranked first or second as a cause of death in the 1991–1993 period.

In 1989, a study of a sample of the population aged 15–74 yielded information on the prevalence of coronary risk factors. The prevalence of arterial hypertension was found to be 17% with no significant differences associated with sex, nor were cholesterol levels significantly different in the two sexes (12% of males and 11% of females showed seriously high cholesterol levels, and 23% of males and 28% of females had moderately high levels of 5.2–6.4 mmol/l). The study showed the prevalence of diabetes to be 6% and that of smoking to be 32% among males and 13% among females. Overweight was detected in 60% of the sample; 35% were moderately overweight and 23% were severely overweight. Significantly more females than males were overweight.

Malignant neoplasms were the second leading cause of death during the period 1987–1993. The most frequent tumor sites were the stomach and breast. A decline in mortality from this cause was noted between 1991 and 1993, which may be due to the fact that a high percentage of deaths was attributed to ill-defined causes in the latter year. According to anatomopathology reports for 1995 and 1996, in 100% of the cases of cervical cancer diagnosed, the carcinoma was in situ, but of 49 cases of breast cancer, 45 (92%) had progressed to an invasive stage at the time of diagnosis.

During the 1987–1993 period, accidents ranked third as a cause of death. In 1993, the only death in the 1–4 age group was attributable to this cause. Among males aged 15–44, accidents (specifically, motor vehicle accidents) were the leading cause of death. The only death among females aged 15–24 years was due to a violent cause (homicide). According to hospital discharge records, at least 8 of every 1,000 persons required hospitalization each year as a result of an accident, a number 2.8 times higher than the rate of hospitalization for acute respiratory infections.

With regard to behavioral disorders, during the 1995–1996 school year, the Drug Abuse Foundation carried out a survey among secondary school students. Of a sample of 625 students, a response rate of 98% was obtained. Of those who responded, 25% admitted using legal or illegal drugs. Of those who admitted to drug use, 19.3% indicated they drank beer, 16.5% drank wine, 12.2% drank rum or whiskey, 9.1% smoked cigarettes, 5.6% used marijuana, and 0.4% used cocaine. The students were more aware of the harmful effects of legal than of illegal drugs. The latter most often were obtained on the street, in discotheques, and at friends' houses.

With respect to oral health, in 1990 the School Oral Health Division of the Department of Public Health conducted a study of oral health among schoolchildren aged 4, 6, 9, and 12 and found that 66% had dental caries, while 34% were caries-free. The average DMFT (decayed, missing, filled teeth) index for the sample was 2.9. Dental caries were the most frequent oral health problem found, followed by extractions. Of the 37 schools surveyed, 17 had a DMFT index below 2.9, 6 had an index of 2.9, and 14 had an index above 2.9. Both the extent and the seriousness of caries were greater in Santa Cruz and Sabaneta than in other parts of the country. Oranjestad, the capital, was where the dental caries problem was least severe. The DMFT index was lower among females than males. Higher percentages of deficient oral hygiene were found in Sabaneta.

As for emerging and re-emerging diseases, no cases of meningococcal meningitis, hantavirus, or Venezuelan equine encephalitis have been reported.

No natural disasters or industrial accidents have been reported.

RESPONSE OF THE HEALTH SYSTEM

National Health Plans and Policies

The current Government is committed to reorganizing public health services, ensuring efficient and coordinated management of health activities, distributing financial resources appropriately, providing information to the population about the importance of preventive medicine, and maintaining and improving medical and paramedical care.

Reorganizing the public health sector means revising existing laws; applying the general insurance law, the aim of which is to reduce and control medical costs; inventorying and coordinating the areas related to public health; promoting good health and accentuating health education, including primary, secondary, and tertiary prevention; and introducing a system of inspection of public health services.

The Public Health Law (1952) comprises a set of general laws—also known as organizational regulations, which deal with matters relating to organization and supervision of health services as well as promotion of health—and specific laws, grouped according to whether they concern the health professions—mental health, sanitation, diseases, health inspection of animals and plants, meat inspection, livestock and marketing of meat products, and burials and cemeteries. The specific laws were enacted between 1917 and 1969.

Health Services and Resources

Organization of Services for Care of the Population

The Department of Public Health of Aruba is responsible for promotion of public health, mental health, and psychiatric care; administration of the public laboratory; and application and enforcement of laws relating to public health.

Health Promotion. The Department of Public Health makes information available to the population via radio and television. Its Public Relations and Health Promotion Section distributes informational materials (posters, pamphlets, brochures, and stickers). Other services within the Department provide information to the general public, including schools, about various health-related topics.

Disease Prevention and Control. The Youth Health Service performs physical examinations of all first- to fifth-grade students each year, and also provides vaccinations.

Vector control is the responsibility of the Department's Vector Control Division, which monitors all dwellings on the island for *Aedes aegypti.*

The Animal Health and Veterinary Public Health Division of the Department of Public Health conducts research and analysis in the field and in the veterinary laboratory. These activities are regulated by veterinary law.

The Communicable Diseases Division ensures epidemiological surveillance of communicable diseases through a reporting system in which the health services participate. This service regularly provides consolidated information to the Division of Epidemiology and Research. Reporting of communicable diseases is required by law. Nurses from the Communicable Diseases Division are responsible for patient monitoring and follow-up. This division also monitors and counsels patients with HIV.

Aruba has a public health laboratory, which makes diagnoses for surveillance purposes. Internal and external controls ensure the quality of laboratory tests.

Water Supply and Sewerage Systems. Drinking water is supplied on Aruba by the Water and Energy Company (WEB), which serves some 26,000 homes. Average per capita consumption of water in 1995 was 9 metric tons a month. Drinking water is produced by desalinization of sea water. WEB Aruba obtains more than 31,000 metric tons of desalinated water per day, which represents a total of about 11 million metric tons per year. On the basis of the water-quality standards of the World Health Organization, Aruba's water is one of the best in the world; chemical and bacteriological tests are performed monthly at 20 sites on the island to ensure water quality.

Wastewater is treated through both individual systems—including cesspits, septic tanks, and direct drainage into the ocean—and the collective system, which may be by central cesspit, purification of wastewater, and drainage into the ocean.

Municipal Services for Management of Solid Waste, Including Hospital Waste. For disposal of solid waste, there is a 12.5-hectare refuse dump located in Parkietenbos. Different types of waste are taken to this site (refuse from homes, offices, industry, hotels, restaurants and cafes, construction and demolition sites), but no documentation is available regarding the exact amounts. Hospital waste also is transported and disposed of in the municipal dump. Infectious waste is burned in an incinerator, which may pose operation and maintenance problems.

Food Safety. The Communicable Diseases Division tests food-handlers every six months for shigella, salmonella, and tuberculosis. Food samples are collected regularly and sent to the laboratory for testing.

Organization and Operation of Personal Health Care Services

Everyone who legally resides on the island has access to medical care. Individuals may obtain insurance privately or through their employers. The unemployed, the elderly, and the disabled are eligible to receive a PPK card, which entitles them to receive care from government physicians. The Government also furnishes any drugs that PPK cardholders require.

The main hospital on Aruba is the Doctor Horacio Oduber Hospital, which is a private, nonprofit institution managed by a foundation. It has 253 beds for inpatients and 26 beds for psychiatric care. In 1994 the hospital had 9,970 admissions, with an occupancy rate of 87.2%. The hospital possesses radiology equipment and performs 2,000 imaging studies and 40,000 X-ray studies annually. Other services provided include internal medicine, surgery, urology, gynecology and obstetrics, pediatrics, otorhinolaryngology, ophthalmology, neurology, psychiatry, and rehabilitation. The emergency room operates 24 hours a day and in 1994 attended 25,293 patients, of whom 2,516 (9.9%) were tourists.

The Dr. Rudy Engelbrecht Medical Center is centrally located in Sint Nicolaas to provide medical care for the city's residents as well as those from Savaneta, Pos Chiquito, Brasil, and Cura Cabay and the inmates of the Correctional Institute. The Center provides mainly primary care. It has an emergency room that operates 24 hours a day under the supervision of a general practitioner. Except for pregnant women in labor, who may be admitted by their general practitioners, only patients referred by a specialist are admitted.

As of 31 December 1996, Aruba had 32 general practitioners, 50 specialists, 20 dentists, 15 pharmacists, 4 veterinarians, 4 psychologists, and 3 midwives.

Human Resources

Most physicians receive their training in recognized institutions in the Netherlands or, to a lesser extent, in Colombia, Costa Rica, the United States, or Venezuela. The Hospital has a school of nursing, which trains practical nurses. Nursing degrees are usually obtained from schools on Curaçao or in the Netherlands.

Health research is considered an important activity for the development of public health. In 1996, the Public Health Department budget allocation for research development was US$ 29,000.

Investments

Equitable and sustained economic growth is clearly an objective of Aruba's public spending policy. For example, a specific objective of the Sasaki Development Plan and many other public investment projects is to promote sustained and equitable economic development. Public investment plays an important role in the formation of both human and physical capital. Public investment in basic infrastructure is also an essential requirement for the accumulation of wealth in the private sector.

Investment is one of the factors that has allowed Aruba to experience rapid growth. Total investment increased from around US$ 95.3 million, or 20% of GDP, in 1986 to US$ 436 million, or 31% of GDP, in 1991; however, it fell to around 24% of GDP in 1993, but subsequently rose again to approximately 27% of GDP in 1994–1995, a level consistent with the macroeconomic policy objective of 5% real growth in the GDP.

Three distinct trends can be identified in the period 1980–1995. Between 1980 and 1985, there was a decline in investment and in related economic growth, coupled with a significant rise in unemployment; during the period 1985–1990 investment increased to an annual average rate of 31.5%, with the highest rate (32.2%) occurring in private investment, which provided a strong impetus for the economy and, more importantly, fueled a recovery of economic growth, which had stagnated during the crisis years. In the period 1990–1995, investment increased only slightly, with slow economic growth.

Analysis of available statistical data shows that the contribution of private investment to overall growth of the GDP has been considerable and that there has been an increase in capital formation efforts in the past 10 years. In January 1991, average private investment as a percentage of GDP reached a high of 27%, subsequently declined to 20.8% in 1993, and then recovered in 1994, rising to 24.4% of GDP in 1995. Throughout the period, private investment exceeded public investment. Access to foreign capital was a key factor in the increase of the gross investment rate. The Government stimulated investment through a combination of fiscal incentives. These measures had a significant impact on private investment, which became the principal motor of economic growth.

During the period 1986–1995, average public investment reached 3.8% of the GDP and 12.8% of total government spending. Both, however, began to decline in 1987, which affected public investment in the social sectors, especially education and health. The drop in public investment was linked to two main factors: a salary increase in the public sector and relatively low tax revenues. Public investment—including foreign aid provided through the Dutch Development Cooperation Program, administered by the Cabinet of the Netherlands Antilles and Aruba—which decreased to a relatively lesser extent than private investment, underwent significant changes in terms of prioritization. These changes favored state-run companies, especially in the energy sector. The negative effects included a decrease in capital outlays, spending on operations and maintenance, and investment in social programs (education and health, in particular).

Investment began to rise in 1995 and continued to do so into the first half of 1996. Public investment is expected to increase considerably during the period 1996–2000, especially as a result of early application of the Sasaki Development Plan.

With regard to planned investment in health for the next period, the Ministry has assigned high priority to the construction of a psychiatric hospital with 60–80 beds by the end of 1996. The objective is to link the psychiatric hospital to a small general hospital (70 beds) so that they can share services such as laundry, laboratory, technical maintenance, and food service.

Under the present plan, the general insurance system will be implemented in phases. During the first two years, health expenditures will probably increase, but then they are expected to decline. It is also expected that the reorganization of health services, with an emphasis on prevention, will lead to a reduction in health care spending. In this connection, the activities of the Yellow and White Cross Foundation are seen as very important, and it is considered necessary to enhance and intensify them. Home health care, which is becoming increasingly prevalent, should also be expanded so that it becomes a truly viable option.

BAHAMAS

GENERAL SITUATION AND TRENDS

Socioeconomic, Political, and Demographic Overview

The Commonwealth of the Bahamas is an archipelago of some 700 islands with a total land mass of 5,382 mi^2 scattered over 80,000 mi^2 of the Atlantic Ocean. Over 95% of the population lives on just seven islands. The two major population centers are Nassau, the capital, located on New Providence, and Freeport, located on Grand Bahama. The other populated islands and cays are called Family Islands. New Providence is the most densely populated island, with 2340.4 persons per mi^2. Only three other islands/island groups have population densities greater than 100 per mi^2. As of the 1990 census, New Providence accounted for 67.4% and Grand Bahama 16% of the population. The 1990 census showed an average household size of 3.8, with 3.9 in New Providence and 3.6 in Grand Bahama. Although there are areas where crowding is known to exist, this problem has not been quantified.

The Government's commitment to social development is evidenced by the fact that approximately 30% of the national recurrent budget is allocated to social sectors, with special attention given to education, health, and housing. The people enjoy universal access to health care, and basic services are available regardless of ability to pay.

Education is available to all segments of the Bahamian population and is compulsory to age 14 years. There are 213 schools in the country, 163 of which are in the public sector; total enrollment at the primary and secondary levels is about 61,500 and the teacher-to-student ratio is 1:18.

Tertiary education is provided at the Government-owned College of the Bahamas, which offers both associate's and bachelor's degrees in the arts and sciences. There are also a number of privately run institutions that also offer associate degrees and are affiliated with tertiary educational institutions in the United States of America. Technical and voca-tional training is also available at the Bahamas Technical and Vocational Institute.

In the 1996–1997 recurrent budget, US$ 102,021,118 (13.3% of the total budget) was allocated to the Ministry of Health, representing a per capita expenditure of approximately US$ 359.[1] Although expenditure in the health sector has increased steadily between 1986 and 1995–1996, it has decreased as a percentage of the national budget from 15.6% to 13.6%.

As an independent unitary state within the British Commonwealth of Nations since July 1973, the Bahamas is governed as a parliamentary democracy based on the Westminster/Whitehall model, with a Governor General who represents Her Majesty the Queen, a bicameral legislature including an elected House of Representatives, and an independent judiciary. The Cabinet of Ministers is headed by a Prime Minister who is also a member of the legislature. Government business is carried out by ministries, headed by a minister (political) and permanent secretary (administrative), and by quasi-governmental institutions. The 1992 elections brought the first change of government in 25 years, and this same government was returned to power in 1997.

The wide geographic dispersion of the islands presents the Government with many logistical problems for the organization and delivery of services, including health care services. In response, a system of local government, which gives Family Islands/Districts greater control over the administration of governmental business in their communities, has been established. The Ministry of Health has also embarked on an initiative to bring management of the health services closer to the people by development of local health systems on three Family Islands—Andros, Eleuthera, and Long Island. If successful, this initiative will be extended to other islands on a phased basis.

Tourism, including tourism-related commerce, constitutes by far the major economic activity, accounting for over 50% of

---

[1] Since 1972 the exchange rate with the US$ has been 1:1.

the gross domestic product (GDP) and 60% of employment. Service industries (such as government services, tourism, banking, and insurance), fishing, and agriculture employ approximately 80% of the eligible labor force. Some 30.4% of workers are employed in community, social, and personal services, 13.5% in hotels and restaurants, 13.2% in wholesale and retail trading, and 7.4% in financial, insurance, real estate, and business services.

According to data received from the Department of Statistics, the overall unemployment rate in 1996 was estimated at 11.5%, down from a high of 14.8% in 1992. New Providence, with a 1996 rate of 11.9%, has the largest number of unemployed persons; in Grand Bahama the rate is 10.6%.

Economic recovery from the 1991–1992 recession began in 1993 and has continued. Output grew by 1% in 1995. That year, GDP was estimated at US$ 3,053 million (in 1990 dollars), having increased steadily since 1993 after declining between 1990 and 1992. The average growth rate in the period 1990–1995 was –0.5%. During the same period, GDP per capita fell from $12,291 to $11,059, for an average annual rate of change of –2.1%. With respect to health expenditure, in 1990 public expenditure was estimated at 2.63% of GDP, while private expenditure was approximately 2.20%.

The main objectives of underlying monetary and fiscal policies pursued by the authorities remain the maintenance of macroeconomic stability, improvement in all aspects of competitiveness, and stimulation of sustainable development by the private sector in the short and medium term. A key issue in the Bahamas is diversification of the economy, which is to be accomplished by improving intersectoral linkages between the tourism sector and the rest of the economy and by improving infrastructure in the Family Islands to promote their economic development. This initiative, which started in 1994—particularly with regard to roads, airports, the water and sewerage systems, and electricity—has started to pay dividends, as evidenced by increased foreign investment outside of New Providence and Grand Bahama.

The budget for 1996–1997 reaffirmed the Government's commitment toward consolidating the improvements achieved in economic and social conditions, implementing necessary institutional reforms, and maintaining a climate conducive to domestic and international investment.

Demographic Situation

The 1996 midyear population of the Bahamas was estimated at 284,000. About one-third of the population is under 15 years of age and about 5% is over 65. Annual population growth was estimated at 1.97% between 1980 and 1990, while urban growth was 2.35%. The crude rate of natural increase rose from 18.1 per 1,000 population in 1988 to 20.4 in 1992,

then dropped steadily to 16.2 in 1995. At the time of the 1990 census the dependency ratio was 58.5; youths (under 15 years) accounted for 51.0 of that number and the elderly (65 and over), 7.5.

Life expectancy at birth has increased steadily, rising from about 60 years in the period 1950–1955 to approximately 73 years in 1990–1995 (76 years for females and 69 years for males).

From 1988 to 1992 the crude birth rate fluctuated between 22.7 and 25.6 per 1,000 population. Thereafter, the rate fell steadily to 22.4 in 1995. The pattern of fertility has remained similar in the years between 1976 and 1995, with fertility being highest in the 20–24 and 25–29 age groups. There has been a marked decrease in fertility rates in these age groups in the last decade. However, in the 15–19 age group, which has the third highest fertility, and in the 40+ age group, there has been no change. The only group showing an increase is the 35–39 age group, probably because some women are opting to delay pregnancy in order to pursue a career.

Reliability of Vital Statistics Data

The registration of births, deaths, and marriages in the Bahamas is required by law. By statutory requirement, births must be registered within 21 days of the event. For deaths, a medical certificate of death giving details of direct and underlying causes must be provided by a physician (or, on rare occasions and in remote areas, a nurse) and submitted to the Registrar of Deaths before burial can take place. This officer registers the death and issues a death certificate.

An ongoing assessment of the coverage of the birth registration system is possible because the birthing facilities throughout the country, including private and public hospitals and clinics, routinely provide the Ministry of Health with reports of all births occurring in their establishments. These reports serve as the basis for an estimate of the actual number of births. This assessment revealed an underregistration percentage that has steadily increased to a high of 33% in 1995. It also allowed the necessary adjustments to be made to the basic health indicators derived from data on births, such as neonatal and infant mortality rates. The validity of this procedure is supported by studies that have shown that no more than 1% of the births in the country occur outside a health facility or without the knowledge and probable attendance of trained health personnel, who file their statistics on all known births with the Ministry of Health.

The data on stillbirths, particularly for 1991 and 1993, suggest that the registration system has less-than-satisfactory coverage, probably because of failures in documentation and in adherence to definitions.

In the Bahamas, current practices allow duplicate cause of death coding for all deaths occurring in government hospitals: first by medical records staff, and second by the staff of the Department of Statistics, the agency officially responsible for the publication of death statistics. For coding purposes, the Department of Statistics uses copies of the medical certificates of death obtained from the Department of the Registrar General, whereas the hospital staff have access to the medical records in addition to the certificates. Coding at these institutions is completely independent, with no cross-checking. National cause of death statistics are based on the coding of the Department of Statistics.

A study to assess the quality of mortality data was conducted in 1996 using 1994 data from the Princess Margaret Hospital, where upward of 80% of all medical certificates of death originate. Results indicated that underregistration, estimated at less than 5%, was not a major problem. However, the system for coding and processing death data needs to be improved. When the International Classification of Diseases (ICD) codes assigned to deaths occurring in or passing through the Princess Margaret Hospital were compared to the codes applied by the Department of Statistics, the agreement was only 65.7% for three-digit codes and much lower for the more precise four-digit codes. As a result of this study, it was recommended that workshops for physicians and other staff on the proper completion of the medical certificates of death be held (such a workshop was conducted in the first quarter of 1997), and that the institutions cross-check their coding and resolve discrepancies through bilateral discussions.

Less than 2% of the deaths recorded in 1995 were classified as due to ill-defined conditions.

Mortality Profile

In 1995, 1,604 deaths were recorded, for a crude death rate of 5.75 per 1,000 population. The 10 leading causes accounted for 86.3% of the deaths from defined causes. The crude death rate has been below 6.0 for at least the past two decades, but between 1990 and 1995 it increased from 5.3 to 5.7 per 1,000—the highest rate since 1989, when it was 5.9.

Diseases such as hypertension, diabetes, myocardial infarction, stroke, and cancers are major concerns for the population of the Bahamas. These diseases are among the leading causes of mortality and account for nearly 45% of all deaths in the country. These diseases also cause more morbidity than any other group of problems.

The top five causes of death are lifestyle-related, and three of those are nutrition-related. In 1995 the leading cause of death in the general population was diseases of the heart (102.9 per 100,000 population), which accounted for 18.2% of deaths. It was followed by AIDS (97.1 per 100,000 and 17.2%),

malignant neoplasms (85.3 per 100,000 and 15.1%), cerebrovascular diseases (46.6 per 100,000 and 8.2%), and accidents, violence, and poisonings (39.8 per 100,000 and 7.0%).

Over the past decade or so, diseases included among the leading causes of mortality have remained relatively stable with the exception of AIDS and its related disorders. Since 1985, when testing for HIV was instituted in the Bahamas, the proportion of deaths attributable to AIDS has grown steadily, and in 1994 it replaced malignant neoplasms as the second leading cause of death. Also in that year, accidents, violence, and poisonings switched rank order with cerebrovascular diseases to become the fourth and fifth leading causes of death, respectively. In 1986—the first complete year for which data are available on HIV infection and AIDS—the proportion of all registered deaths attributable to AIDS was approximately 2%. By 1995 this proportion had increased to 17.2%. Prior to the appearance of AIDS, the only infectious disease appearing among the leading causes of death was pneumonia.

There are significant differences in the mortality levels and the ordering of the principal causes of death between males and females. In 1995 the death rate for men was 635.5 per 100,000 males, while the rate for women was 515.6 per 100,000 females. Since 1991 there has been a rise in the death rate of both sexes. But whereas the rate among men remained fairly constant between 1993 and 1995, that for women rose steadily from 441 in 1991 to 515.6 in 1995. Nevertheless, despite the increase in death rate among women in general, the death rate among the 15–44-year age group decreased from 195.1 to 132.4 between 1993 and 1995.

The three most significant causes of death among men were AIDS (a rate of 130.4 per 100,000 male population, 20.9% of deaths from defined causes), diseases of the heart (102.9 per 100,000 and 16.5%), and malignant neoplasms (91.3 per 100,000 and 14.6%). Accidents, violence, and poisonings, the second leading cause in 1994 at 113.6 per 100,000, fell to fourth place (66.7 per 100,000, 10.7%). When men 15–44 are examined as a group, by far the two most common causes are AIDS (171.0 per 100,000 population, 46.5%) and accidents, violence, and poisonings (85.5 per 100,000, 23.3%). They are followed by diseases of the heart and malignant neoplasms (both with rates of 18.5 per 100,000 and accounting for 5% of deaths each).

Among females the most frequent causes of death were diseases of the heart (102.8 per 100,000 female population, 20.3%), malignant neoplasms (79.4 per 100,000, 15.7%), and AIDS (64.5 per 100,000, 12.7%). Cerebrovascular diseases, the fourth most common cause of death, accounted for 10.6% of all female deaths, with a rate of 53.9 per 100,000. The biggest difference among leading causes between men and women is in accidents, violence, and poisonings, which ranked ninth in females, with a rate of 13.5 per 100,000. The order of the top three causes is reversed in the 15–44-year-old age group, with

AIDS being the most common (83.3 per 100,000 women in that age group, accounting for 41.1% of deaths), followed by malignant neoplasms (29.2 per 100,000, 14.4%) and diseases of the heart and accidents, violence, and poisonings (both at 12.5 per 100,000 and 6.2%). The top 10 causes of death in this age group account for 87.7% of deaths from defined causes.

According to 1995 data, cerebrovascular diseases and diabetes mellitus are the only two causes that pose a greater risk to the lives of the general female population than they do to males in the Bahamas. Diabetes, which seemed to be posing less risk of death to women in recent years (moving from third to sixth rank and with rates falling from 39 per 100,000 female population in 1991 to 27.7 in 1993), increased its toll again in 1994 and then moved to a ranking of fifth in 1995, with a rate of 42.6 per 100,000 and proportional mortality of 8.4% of deaths from defined causes. The death rate among men from this disease, already lower than that in women, had also fallen from 20 per 100,000 in 1991 to 16.7 in 1993, when it ranked 10th as a cause of death. But in 1994 diabetes moved up to seventh place and, as in females, the rate further increased to 29.7 per 100,000 in 1995, when it ranked sixth.

Accidents and acts of violence rank high on the list of causes of deaths in the overall population. Thirty-one percent of injury-related deaths in 1994 were due to violence. The problem is most significant among men 15–44 years of age and children under age 15 years. In 1994, about 37% of all deaths among men 15–44 were due to accidental events or acts of violence.

Between 1984 and 1995 maternal deaths were very few (between one and four per year) and therefore the rate fluctuated widely—from 1.5 to 6.4 per 10,000 live births, where it peaked in 1995. There were only two years between 1988 and 1995 when more than one death occurred: 1989 (two deaths) and 1995 (four deaths).

SPECIFIC HEALTH PROBLEMS

The main sources of the data in this section are the discharge diagnoses records from the Princess Margaret Hospital (PMH), which accounts for approximately 75% of all acute inpatient discharges in the public sector, and the Rand Memorial Hospital, which accounts for the rest. Data from the monthly reports of the community health clinics and the notifiable disease surveillance system are also used.

Analysis by Population Group

Health of Children

In 1994 the under-5 years age group had the highest number of admissions to the Princess Margaret Hospital per 1,000 population. Diseases of the respiratory tract were responsible for more than 75% of all admissions of children under 5; asthma, bronchitis, and pneumonia were the main causes within that group of diseases.

At the community clinic level, upper respiratory tract infection (URTI)—excluding the common cold—was the most common illness seen in children under 5 years between 1992 and 1995. This held true when the data were disaggregated for New Providence, Grand Bahama, and the Family Islands. In Grand Bahama and the Family Islands, injuries were the second most frequent problem seen in this age group, while in New Providence it was ear diseases. This may be a reflection of the health care choices available in New Providence, as children with injuries are probably taken directly to the Princess Margaret Hospital. Acute bronchitis was also among the top five causes of illness in the under-5 age group in Grand Bahama and New Providence, but not in the Family Islands. Acute gastroenteritis was among the top three causes in New Providence and the Family Islands, but was not among the top five causes in Grand Bahama. Thrush was among the top five causes in Grand Bahama and appeared as number five in New Providence in 1995, but was not among the most common causes in the Family Islands.

Children under 1 Year of Age. There has been a decline in infant mortality from the 1986 level of 30.2 per 1,000 live births to 19.0 in 1995. For the past two decades "certain conditions originating in the perinatal period" has been the principal cause of infant deaths. Between 1984 and 1994 the rate for this cause increased steadily from 10.4 to 16.8 per 1,000 live births. In 1995 it dropped to 8.8 deaths per 1,000 live births. Since 1989 "congenital anomalies" has been the second most frequent cause of death, with a rate between 2.4 and 3.9 per 1,000. Between 1989 and 1995 AIDS moved from the fifth to the third-ranked cause of death in infants; the rate increased from 1.2 in 1989 to 2.8 in 1994 and then dropped to 1.1 per 1,000 live births in 1995. This rate was expected to drop even further in 1996 because of the introduction of a program for treatment of HIV-positive pregnant women with AZT. The same three causes are responsible for both neonatal and post-neonatal deaths. Rounding out the picture, there were an estimated 79 stillbirths (10.7 per 1,000 total births, and perinatal and neonatal mortality rates were 19.4 and 11.5 per 1,000 total births and live births, respectively. The trend in both of these rates has been downward since the late 1970s.

In 1993 it was estimated that approximately 10.2% of infants were born with a low birthweight (defined as less than 2,500 grams). Records for 1995 show that 9.8% of newborns at the Princess Margaret Hospital in New Providence had low birthweights. At the Rand Memorial Hospital in Grand Bahama, 9.1% of newborns were so defined, and in the Family Islands this figure was 5.1%.

In 1991 (the most recent year for which data are available) there were 1,563 admissions to Princess Margaret Hospital of children under 1 year of age. The leading cause, accounting for 18.9%, was pneumonia and influenza, followed by intestinal infectious diseases (12.7%), certain causes of perinatal morbidity (12.5%), diseases of the upper respiratory tract (9.0%), and other diseases of the respiratory tract (5.4%). The most frequently reported infectious disease was gastroenteritis. In male infants it accounted for more cases than the other four leading causes combined: amebiasis, dysentery, influenza, and chickenpox, in that order. In females the order was reversed.

No data are available on the nutritional status of children in this age group. For information on the diseases included in the Expanded Program on Immunization (EPI), see the section "Vaccine-Preventable Diseases."

Children 1–4 Years of Age. In 1995 the age-specific mortality rate in the 1–4-year age group was 4.1 per 10,000 population. There was a dramatic reduction in the number of deaths in this age group between 1994 and 1995, from 28 to 10. This was mainly due to the reduction in deaths from accidents, violence, and poisonings and from AIDS, the two most common causes of death in this age group between 1991 and 1994. Almost half (46.4%) of the 28 recorded deaths in 1994 resulted from accidents, violence, and poisonings, while AIDS was responsible for 21.4%. In 1995 AIDS was replaced by congenital anomalies as the second leading cause of death (two deaths, 20%). Accidents, violence, and poisonings, with three deaths and a rate of 12.0 per 100,000 age-specific population, accounted for 30% of deaths. The other causes of death accounted for one death each.

Children 5–14 Years of Age. In the 5–14 age group, 5 of the 20 deaths (25%) in 1995 were due to AIDS (9 per 100,000), and 3 (15%) each to pneumonia and to accidents, violence, and poisonings (5 per 100,000). Two deaths each (10%, 4 per 100,000) were due to malignant neoplasms and diseases of the heart. In recent years deaths in this age group have fluctuated between 10 (1993) and 20 (1991, 1994, 1995). The most common cause of death was accidents, violence, and poisonings until 1995, when it was replaced by AIDS.

Of the deaths in 1995, 11 were in the 5–9 age group and 9 in the 10–14 age group. In both groups AIDS was the leading cause, and other causes were pneumonia; accidents, violence, and poisonings; and diseases of the heart.

Health of Adolescents and Young Adults (15–44 Years)

Although there has been a steady downward trend in the birth rate among women under 20 years of age, teenage pregnancy continues to be a matter of concern in the country. In 1994 approximately 15% of births were to women in the 15–19-years age group. One disturbing development is the re-

cent increase in registered births to girls under 15 years of age—a jump from 7 and 5 births in 1991 and 1992, respectively, to 34 and 20 births in 1993 and 1994, respectively. The number of births occurring to females in this age group in 1993 was the highest since 1987.

For the most part, birth rates among teenagers were highest in New Providence and Grand Bahama until 1990. Then there was a dramatic reduction in the rate in Grand Bahama, approaching the consistently lower levels found in the other Family Islands. This phenomenon may reflect the migration of persons in the reproductive age group to New Providence, even from Grand Bahama.

Only six deaths occurred in the 15–19 age group in 1995, two of which were classified in the category accidents, violence, and poisonings and one each in other categories.

The five leading causes of death in the 15–44-year age group in 1995 were the same for both males and females, but the rank order differed. In both sexes the leading cause was AIDS and AIDS-related complex. In males the age-specific rate was 170.5 per 100,000 population, up from 120.0 in 1993. AIDS replaced accidents as the highest ranking cause between 1991 and 1993 and has continued in that position. The other leading causes in males in 1995 were accidents, violence, and poisonings, at 85.5 per 100,000 (down from 97.6 in 1993), and diseases of the heart and malignant neoplasms (both at 18.5 per 100,000). The latter two causes have tended to increase. "Other diseases of the respiratory system" ranked number five in 1995 (17.1 per 100,000). There was an increase in the total number of deaths of males in this age group from 180 in 1991 to 260 in 1995.

The number of deaths among women in the 15–44 age group increased from 103 in 1991 to 147 in 1995. The age-specific mortality rate for AIDS in women was 83.3 per 100,000 population in 1995. The second most common cause of death among women was malignant neoplasms (29.2 per 100,000), followed by diseases of the heart and accidents, violence, and poisonings (both at 12.5 per 100,000). It should be noted that AIDS has by far the greatest impact of any cause on women in this age group, while for men AIDS and injuries are both important.

The total fertility rate of women in the Bahamas was estimated at 2.43 for 1995. A comparison of recent age-specific fertility rates with those in the 1970s and 1980s indicates that fertility is declining among all age groups except women 35–39 years, in which it has been increasing since the mid-1980s. Although women of this cohort are having more babies than women of the same age group in the 1980s, they are having fewer than those in the 1970s. The highest fertility rates are found in women 20–24 years of age (129.6 per 1,000 women), followed closely by the 25–29 age group. Women are choosing to postpone starting a family and are having babies for the first time at an older age, and the National Health and Nutrition Survey (1988–1989) found that older women pregnant for the first time had a higher level of education.

Between 1992 and 1994 the number of new prenatal clients attending community clinics decreased from 5,427 to 4,805. This pattern held true in New Providence, Grand Bahama, and the Family Islands. Women in the Family Islands and Grand Bahama tended to attend clinics earlier than those in New Providence, as evidenced by the percentage of those registering before the 16th week of pregnancy (38%, 31%, and 24%, respectively). The average number of visits per client during this time period remained fairly constant at about 7.1 in New Providence, 5.6 in Grand Bahama, and 5.5 in the Family Islands—the inverse of the order for early first-time registration at the clinics.

Health of Adults Aged 45–64 Years

Current data on morbidity in this age group are not readily available because incomplete computer software changes have delayed processing. The most recent morbidity data refer to leading causes of inpatient morbidity at the Princess Margaret Hospital in 1991. These were diseases of the heart, "other diseases of the digestive system," and diabetes. These data were not disaggregated by sex. The changes in ranking between the younger age group and this group mainly reflects the increased prevalence of chronic diseases.

In 1995 the three leading causes of mortality, together accounting for 57% of deaths, were malignant neoplasms (21.0%, with an age-specific rate of 2,136 per 100,000 population), diseases of the heart (19.7%, 2,004 per 100,000), and AIDS (16.6%, 1,688 per 100,000).

Health of the Elderly (65 Years of Age and Over)

Mortality in persons 65 years and over is dominated by the chronic diseases. In 1995 the four leading causes of death accounted for 72% of mortality. The most common cause was diseases of the heart (28.4%), with an age-specific rate of 1,376.5 per 100,000 population. It was followed by malignant neoplasms (18.6%, with a rate of 900.3 per 100,000), cerebrovascular disease (14.3%, 692.0 per 100,000), and diabetes mellitus (10.7%, 520.8 per 100,000). Although the rates for all of these diseases increased in the three years prior to 1995, that for diabetes mellitus almost doubled: from 283 to 521. Diseases of the respiratory and circulatory systems are also among the most frequent causes of death in this age group.

Between 1984 and 1995 the death rate from diseases of the heart remained much the same, although it rose slightly in 1989 and again, but to a lesser extent, in 1995. Up to 1993 the rates from malignant neoplasms and diabetes mellitus were falling, then they increased again. On the other hand, the death rate from cerebrovascular disease has been increasing steadily since 1984. Pneumonia deaths, which peaked in 1979, fell consistently thereafter.

In 1991 (the most recent year for which such data are available) ischemic heart disease and hypertensive disease were the major causes of death from heart disease in this age group. Malignant neoplasms of the digestive organs and the peritoneum, and the prostate were the leading causes of cancer deaths.

Family Health

The rate of marriages (number of marriages during a given year per 1,000 population) was fairly constant between 1988 and 1995 at between 8.6 and 9.7. In 1994, the most recent year for which such information is available, the majority (55%) of women getting married were between the ages of 25 to 30, while 52% of men got married between the ages of 30 and 39. During the same period the divorce rate (number of divorces during a given year per 1,000 marriages in the same year) fluctuated, showing no clear tendency. It peaked in 1994 at 18.7 (474 divorces granted). Divorces were more prevalent among couples who had no children (30%) and those who had only one child (26%). In contrast, couples who had five or more children accounted for only 4% of the divorces.

Just over half (53.3%) of all registered births were outside of wedlock in 1995. Of these births, 525 (23.1%) were to teenagers, 1,578 (69.3%) were to women aged 20–34 years, and 173 (7.6%) were to women aged 35 years and over.

According to the 1990 population census, 25.3% of private households were headed by single parents. The majority of these household heads (57.1%) were females.

Although it is known that domestic violence is a problem in the Bahamas, very few data are currently available upon which to estimate its extent. In 1993, of the 1,226 cases of assault against women seen at the Accident and Emergency Department of the Princes Margaret Hospital, the perpetrators were known in 245 cases, but their relationship to the victims was not documented. The Crisis Center (a nongovernmental organization), in cooperation with the Ministry of Health, operates a counseling and education service aimed at helping persons cope with violent home situations. In 1993 only 66 victims of domestic violence sought the assistance of the Center.

Workers' Health

Currently, medical care and compensation to workers injured on the job remains the responsibility of the National Insurance Board (NIB). Through this institution, workers with job-related injuries receive full coverage of all medical bills, both locally and abroad, if the correct referral procedures are followed.

Data from claims processed by the National Insurance Board suggest that in 1996 the five most common causes of absenteeism in the workplace were "female disorders," musculoskeletal problems, fractures, sprains/strains/dislocations, and infections, including AIDS. For invalidity, the five most frequent causes were AIDS, psychiatric disorders, cardiovascular diseases, arthritis/fractures/skin problems, and neurological disorders.

As would be expected from their proportional representation in the work force, hotel workers were the category of employees most frequently injured on the job, followed by government workers. The third highest frequency of injuries was found among construction workers.

Health of the Disabled

In 1993 the Bahamas was included in the Caribbean Cooperation in Health (CCH) initiative's Program on Community-based Rehabilitation. In preparation for the development of the project proposal, several islands were surveyed to identify prevalence and types of disability, so that pilot areas for this project could be established. An additional assessment was made from the National Insurance Board register. Out of a population of approximately 8,000, Eleuthera had 371 (4.6%) registered persons with disabilities. Of these, 108 (29.1%) had lower limb disabilities, 69 (18.6%) had impaired vision, 29 (7.8%) had a hearing deficit or were slow learners, 28 (7.5%) had speech problems, and 26 (7.0%) were mentally retarded. In Abaco 492 (4.8%) of the approximately 10,100 inhabitants were registered as disabled. As in Eleuthera, the most common disabilities were related to the lower limbs (130, 26.4%), with the second most frequent being sight-related (66, 13.4%), followed by hearing and speech deficits (43, 8.7%), upper limb problems (40, 8.1%), and mental retardation (39, 7.9%). In Long Island (north), 305 (16.0%) of the approximately 1,900 persons were registered as having disabilities. This was the site chosen to initiate the Community-based Rehabilitation Project. Subsequent evaluations have shown the project to be quite successful, and efforts are under way to extend it to Eleuthera and Abaco.

Analysis by Type of Disease

Communicable Diseases

The prevention and control of infectious diseases is one of the concerns of the Ministry of Health and Environment.

Vector-Borne Diseases. Malaria is not endemic to the Bahamas. However, the large number of illegal immigrants from countries where malaria is endemic, along with the presence of the *Anopheles* mosquito, increases the risk of this disease being reintroduced. Between 1993 and 1995 there were from 1 to 3 imported cases each year. No cases were reported in 1996. Although there has not been a case of yellow fever in the Bahamas for over three decades, the *Aedes aegypti* mosquito is indigenous to the islands and the threat is ever-present. The risk of an outbreak of dengue fever is high. There was one confirmed case of dengue in 1995. Prior to that, the last reported cases (numbering 87) were in 1989. The Vector Control Unit of the Department of Environmental Health Services carried out an *A. aegypti* survey in 1993 in Yellow Elder Gardens, a section of an urban area on the island of New Providence. It documented excesses in all the indices used to determine the extent of the problem. A second survey of the same area in 1996 showed a reduction in all the indices except the potential container index. The house index fell from 30.4 to 17.7, while the Breteau index fell from 43.1 to 21.1. This area was included in a pilot vector control project as part of the Caribbean Cooperation in Health initiative.

Vaccine-Preventable Diseases. Immunization of children against diphtheria, tetanus, whooping cough, poliomyelitis, measles, mumps, and rubella is available free of charge through the community health clinic system. As a result, immunization coverage against these diseases has been fairly high. In 1995, 87% of children under 1 year of age were fully immunized with three doses of DTP and OPV, and 90% with MMR. BCG is not included in the country's EPI protocol.

Like the rest of the Region, the Bahamas was declared free of poliomyelitis, the last cases having been recorded in the 1960s. The country's participation in the subregional initiative to eradicate measles has resulted in no confirmed case of measles being recorded since 1990. Diphtheria and whooping cough are no longer problems in the Bahamas. There have been no cases of diphtheria since prior to 1988, and the last three indigenous cases of whooping cough were recorded in 1993, with one imported case each in 1994 and 1995. Mumps continues to occur at low levels; the number of cases fell from 11 in 1993 to 2 in 1994 and 1 in 1995, then rose again to 6 in 1996. There have been no reported cases of neonatal tetanus since 1988, but in 1996 one case of tetanus was reported in an adult. Since an outbreak of rubella in 1990 (which caused 121 cases) there have been only sporadic cases, two or fewer per year between 1992 and 1996. No cases of congenital rubella syndrome have been reported since the 1970s.

The numbers of *Haemophilus influenzae* infections have been small, with decreases observed between 1993 (15 cases) and 1996 (10).

There was a sharp increase in hepatitis B cases between 1993 (92 cases) and 1994 (246). Since then, case numbers have declined steadily to 137 in 1996. As of that year, the policy was to provide hepatitis B immunization to medical personnel and all members of the uniformed services. Donated blood is routinely tested for hepatitis core antibody, as well as hepatitis B and C.

Intestinal Infectious Diseases. The threat of cholera to the Region in 1992 put the Bahamas on full alert. Active public and environmental health teams were put in place for the prevention and control of this problem.

During May and June of 1991, a localized outbreak of seafood-related illness occurred in New Providence. Upward of 380 cases were reported during the peak week of the outbreak. This illness was primarily associated with (1) the consumption of raw conch obtained from wet storage sites in the waters of Nassau Harbor; and (2) contamination resulting from the food-handling practices of the vendors in that area, combined with the sanitation conditions in the area itself. The immediate response was to suspend all food sales in or around the suspected area and to launch a mass campaign to educate the public about the problem. Once its source was identified, the problem was rectified. In an effort to avoid future outbreaks of this type, the Department of Environmental Health has stepped up its campaign to eliminate illegal roadside sales of seafood and other products.

In spite of these efforts, intermittent outbreaks of foodborne illness due to the ingestion of raw conch continue. The identified pathogen was *Vibrio parahaemolyticus* in all outbreaks. The number of reported cases of foodborne diseases in 1996 was 1,061.

The occurrence of diarrheal diseases among children under 5 years of age continues at a high level. From 1988 to 1994 the number of reported cases fluctuated between 1,095 and 2,705, but showed a tendency to increase. In the over-5-year age group, the number of diarrheal diseases was low in 1993 and 1994, more than doubled in 1995, and increased another fivefold in 1996.

Intestinal infectious diseases are not a common cause of admission to hospital. In 1995 they ranked 10th at the Princess Margaret Hospital, accounting for 2% of admissions, and 15th at the Rand Memorial Hospital, where they accounted for 1%, although at the latter institution they had represented 3.1% of admissions the previous year. In terms of outpatient contacts, intestinal infectious diseases were the fifth most common reason for attendance at the general practice clinic of the PMH (1,390 cases, 3.5% of visits).

Chronic Communicable Diseases. The number of tuberculosis cases, which had been constant at about 50 per year, peaked at 63 in 1992 and then fell again in 1993. This reduction continued up to 1996, when only 32 cases were reported. Bahamas has been using the multidose regimen of rifampin,

ethambutol, pyrazinamide, and isoniazid supplemented with vitamin B_6. A drug compliance methodology is utilized, whereby nurses visit patients on a periodic basis to confirm that they have been taking their medication as prescribed. As the human resource situation improves, this practice will be converted into the full "directly observed treatment, short course" (DOTS) method. Given the association between AIDS and tuberculosis and the high incidence of HIV infection in the Bahamas, a careful watch must be kept on the situation.

HIV-positive persons accounted for over 60% of all tuberculosis cases in 1996 (40 out of 59). A recent study of the incarcerated population demonstrated a positivity rate for tuberculosis of 20%. An alarming developing situation is the occurrence of an unknown multidrug-resistant strain of the bacillus in New Providence and the Family Islands. Its existence has been confirmed by the government research laboratory in Canada. Moreover, active tuberculosis has recently been identified in staff working in several acute care institutions.

Leprosy is not endemic in the Bahamas, but a case was diagnosed in 1996. The last known indigenous case was diagnosed in 1982.

Acute Respiratory Infections. This group is represented by diseases of the upper respiratory system, pneumonia and influenza, and bronchitis and asthma. Inpatient data from the PMH and the Rand Hospital between 1990 and 1995 were analyzed. Discounting normal delivery, acute respiratory infections (ARI) were the second most common reason for admission to hospital, after complications of pregnancy. Between 1991 and 1995, numbers fluctuated at the PMH, peaking in 1994 (1,764), when ARI was the leading cause of admission, then falling to below the 1991 figure. At the Rand Hospital, ARI was the third most common reason for admission, but cases have been declining since 1990.

Preliminary analysis of available inpatient data indicates that by far the most commonly affected age group is children under 5 years old, who account for more than 50% of the cases. More male children than females were affected.

In terms of outpatient attendance at the Princess Margaret Hospital in 1995, diseases of the respiratory system constituted the second leading reason for consultation (7,074 or 18.3%). Within this disease group, diseases of the upper respiratory tract (3,440 or 8.6%) and bronchitis and asthma (3,255 or 8.1%) were the most frequent causes of outpatient visits.

AIDS and Other Sexually Transmitted Diseases. Estimates of the prevalence of chlamydia were obtained from a study conducted in Grand Bahama in 1995. Results indicated that approximately 13% of all prenatal patients were infected. The percentage was the same among all clients with a suspected STD.

The incidence rates of syphilis and gonococcal infection have been decreasing since 1986 and 1987, respectively. Case numbers of the latter fell from 1,804 in 1987 to 92 in 1995, while the former decreased from 837 cases in 1987 to 115 in 1995. During the second half of 1985 the Ministry of Health and Environment started its campaign against AIDS, promoting abstinence and safe sex through the use of condoms. The decline observed in the reported incidence of these two STDs may well be a secondary effect of that campaign. If this is true, then one can expect a leveling off of the annual incidence rate of HIV infection in a few years, although the number of AIDS cases will continue to rise for some years to come.

The problem of AIDS and HIV infection has had a significant impact on the health services of the Bahamas ever since reporting of the disease began in 1985. It is now the second most frequent cause of death in the general population. Furthermore, it has become the leading cause of death among all males and among males and females 15–44 years of age. As of 31 December 1996, a total of 2,481 cases had been reported, of which 63% had died. A further 3,941 individuals were known to be HIV-positive, without symptoms of the disease. A geographic breakdown shows that 12 of the 22 inhabited islands have reported HIV infection; 86% of the cases have occurred on New Providence, 6% on Grand Bahama, 3% each on Eleuthera and Abaco, and the rest on the other Family Islands.

The disease occurs primarily among heterosexuals (87%), with a male-to-female ratio of 1.6 to 1. Homosexual and bisexual transmission accounts for approximately 4% of infections. At the start of the epidemic in the country, as many as 70% of the persons identified as HIV-positive were non-Bahamians (mostly illegal immigrants). The increasing spread of the virus has changed the percent distribution for Bahamians and non-Bahamians. Immigrants now constitute only 14% of the cases and known carriers. Freebase/crack cocaine addicts represent approximately one-third of individuals with HIV infection and AIDS. There has been a steady increase in the number of new cases of AIDS each year since 1985; however, the rate of increase has been declining since 1994.

A successful, voluntary, confidential contact-tracing program for HIV and other STDs has been in place since 1985. This program is well established and is probably one reason for the level of surveillance and completeness of data on HIV in the Bahamas.

Because of the mode of transmission, AIDS affects predominantly those in the sexually active age groups, with 75% of all reported cases since 1985 occurring in persons 20–49 years of age. Data indicate that most people are becoming infected between the ages of 15 and 25. The rapid increase in the death rate from this disease among women aged 15–44 indicates that young women are at particular risk. The fastest growing group of HIV-positive persons is teenage girls. Pre-

natal clients are now routinely tested for HIV (with informed consent).

A seroprevalence study carried out in 1990–1991 indicated that about 2.9% of prenatal clients were HIV-positive; in 1996 this figure was estimated at 3.2%. The study included approximately 95% of pregnant women attending prenatal clinics in New Providence and approximately 65% of all delivered pregnancies in that period. Bahamians constituted 79.2% of the women tested and Haitian-born women 17.7%. The rate of infection in the former was 2.5%, as compared with 4.5% in women of Haitian origin included in the study, a significant difference. None of the women included in the study who had been born in other countries were infected. The highest incidence was in women aged 25–34, and the prevalence of infection increased with increasing numbers of pregnancies, from 1.9% among women in their first pregnancy to 7.9% among women who had been pregnant seven or more times.

HIV prevalence figures for STD clinic patients were 10% and 5.2% in 1992 and 1996, respectively. Among male prison inmates the prevalence was 10.4%, and among female inmates, 19.6%. A 1993 study of inmates upon admission showed an even higher rate of HIV (up to 18%). These high rates are related to the fact that the majority of inmates have had a close association with the drug culture.

As evidenced by the sex ratio, AIDS affects women almost as frequently as men. There will therefore be an increase in deaths in a population—young women—that, prior to the emergence of this disease, was not at any increased risk of death from lifestyle-related causes.

Given the estimated lag period of eight or more years between infection and appearance of the disease, it is clear that young people in the 15–19 age group are at great risk. Among young people in this age group the rate of HIV infections per 10,000 population increased from 6.7 in 1990 to 14.0 in 1993, then fell slightly to 12.2 in 1994. In the general population, HIV infections steadily increased from 20.6 per 10,000 population in 1990 to 28.8 in 1994, and over the next two years the rate declined to 19.0 in 1996.

As of the end of December 1996, 339 children had tested positive for HIV since the beginning of the epidemic, of whom 173 had developed AIDS and 125 had died. Between 1990 and 1995, the transmission rate between mother and infant was about 30%. In 1995 a program providing AZT to selected pregnant women was introduced. In 1996 the transmission rate had been reduced to 7%.

There have been no cases of HIV linked to blood transfusion since HIV testing began in 1985 in the Bahamas. Screening revealed that the prevalence of HIV-positive potential blood donors was 0.4% in 1996.

The campaign against AIDS has focused on reducing sexual transmission by stressing condom use and partner reduction and by targeting young people and women.

Noncommunicable Diseases and Other Health-Related Problems

Nutritional Diseases. The diet-related noncommunicable disorders—such as obesity, cardiovascular disease, type II diabetes, hypertension and stroke, and various forms of cancer—are the leading causes of morbidity and mortality among adults. The problem of anemia in children and pregnant and lactating women is also an area of concern. Reports generated throughout the Bahamas by the Government's community health clinics indicate that approximately 19% of the prenatal clients screened in 1994 had hemoglobin levels <10g/dL. This proportion remained at 18.5% to 19% between 1992 and 1995. The problem is most prevalent in New Providence and least prevalent in the Family Islands. Severe anemia was diagnosed in less than 1% of the prenatal population.

Protein-energy malnutrition among children 0–5 years of age is not a serious public health problem, nor are deficiencies of micronutrients. The National Health and Nutrition Survey (NHNS), 1988–1989, revealed a general adequacy to a slight excess (15%) of energy, a large excess (83%) of protein, and an even larger excess (87.4%) of fat supply (based on average intake in relation to daily dietary allowance). These excesses are largely due to the high consumption of animal products, cereals, sweeteners, and fats and oils. Such dietary habits have implications for the progression of chronic noncommunicable diseases.

The survey also revealed that 6.7% of children 5–14 years of age were obese (based on NCHS standard weight-for-age). Overall, 48.6% of the population was obese (body mass index >25), with more females (53.6%) being affected than males (43%).

Findings from a 1988–1989 survey of preschool children indicated that a very small number of infants were exclusively breast-fed up to 4 months of age. Furthermore, 80% of the infants were introduced to bottle-feeding as early as the first week of life—90% of that group while in hospital—although 63% of mothers attempted to breast-feed.

In 1993 a Lactation Management Project was initiated to strengthen the breast-feeding promotion programs in the country. The project involved the training of more than 300 persons in government and private hospitals and clinics, as well as community health workers and health personnel from nongovernmental institutions. At the time of discharge from the Princess Margaret Hospital, where 72% of births take place, 34.6% of women were exclusively breast-feeding. Reports from clinics in New Providence indicate that three months after giving birth, 7.4% of women were exclusively breast-feeding, 8.6% were predominantly breast-feeding, and 40% were partially breast-feeding. However, since 1993 the percentage of women exclusively breast-feeding at three months fell steadily to 4.9% in 1995. In terms of differences between islands, the largest percentage of such women was in the Family Islands, followed by New Providence, and the lowest in Grand Bahama.

Cardiovascular Diseases. Based on results from the National Health and Nutrition Survey, it was estimated that 13% of the population 15–64 years of age of the Bahamas could be classified as hypertensive in 1989. The percentage was slightly higher for males (15%) than for females (12%). Another 17% could be considered borderline. Among the elderly (65 and over), 38% were hypertensive. The prevalence of hypertension was fairly equal in New Providence, Grand Bahama, and the Family Islands.

These results are in contrast to the figures reported from hospitals, which clearly show more females being treated than males. Given that the hospital figures are representative of other branches of the health care delivery system, this difference is a clear indication of the failure of the health service to detect and treat many male hypertensive cases. This observation is supported by the fact that in all three areas investigated in the NHNS (New Providence, Grand Bahama, the Family Islands), the proportion of persons in the community with hypertension who did not know that they had the disease was consistently higher for men than for women.

During 1991, there were 404 hypertensive patients admitted to the Princess Margaret Hospital, and in 126 (31.2%) of them, hypertension was the primary diagnosis. Almost two-thirds (62.1%) of all hypertensive admissions were female, a trend consistently observed over the last five years. For those cases with a primary diagnosis of hypertension, the total number of days spent in hospital in 1991 was 2,058, for an average length of stay of 16.3 days. In those cases where hypertension was accompanied by diseases of either the heart or kidney, the average length of stay was much longer. Approximately 83% of admissions diagnosed with hypertension were persons aged 45 and older.

Data available for the same period from the Rand Memorial Hospital indicated a total of 120 admissions, 29 (28.4%) of which had a primary diagnosis of hypertension. Of these, 62.5% were female.

The total number of new cases of hypertension reported from the community clinics in 1993 was 1,141. A total of 23,163 visits were made to these clinics by new and old hypertensive patients seeking care for their disease.

Diseases of the heart is the most common cause of death in the overall population and the leading cause in females. It was also the leading cause in males up until 1994, when it was replaced by AIDS. In the over-65 age group it is the leading cause of death, and between 1993 and 1995 the age-specific death rate slowly increased, from 125.8 to 137.7 per 100,000 population.

Between 1979 and 1989 the overall death rate from diseases of the heart increased from 78.8 per 100,000 to 104.8; thereafter it fell to 90.7 in 1993 and climbed again to 102.9 in 1995. This pattern was seen among both women and men.

Malignant Tumors. Between 1991 and 1993 malignant neoplasms were the second most common cause of death for all ages and both sexes. In 1994 and 1995 this cause moved to third place. Between 1970 and 1984 the rate per 100,000 population almost doubled, from 57.1 to 102.2. Thereafter, it slowly declined to 85.3 in 1995. This trend was found in both sexes: among men the rate went from 51.4 per 100,000 to 122.9 to 91.3, while among women it changed from 63.4 per 100,000 in 1970 to 87.5 in 1989 to 79.4 in 1995.

Between 1992 and 1995 the two most common sites of fatal cancer in males were the prostate and the trachea, bronchus, and lung. In 1995 cancer of the prostate caused 22.2% of all cancer deaths in males, while cancer of the trachea, bronchus, and lung accounted for 17.5%.

The two most common causes of cancer deaths in women are cancers of the breast and the cervix uteri. Deaths due to breast cancer comprised 23.2% of total female cancer deaths in 1995 and 3.6% of all deaths in females. Cervical cancer accounted for 9.8% of female cancer deaths and 1.5% of all female deaths.

Accidents, Violence, and Poisonings. In 1995 accidents, violence, and poisonings ranked as the fourth leading cause of death. This cause group is a leading reason for emergency room visits and admissions to both major hospitals, exceeded only by childbirth and complications of pregnancy, childbirth, and the puerperium, and respiratory infections. About 25% of these injury-related hospital admissions were due to violence, the main cause being homicide and injuries purposely inflicted by others. Motor vehicle traffic accidents, as a group, constituted the second leading cause of injury-related hospital admissions. In 1995 accidents, violence, and poisonings were also the leading cause of attendance at the General Practice Clinic of Princess Margaret Hospital, accounting for 34.1% of the 13,645 visits.

The problem is most significant among men, particularly those in the 15–44 age group, and among children 5–14 years of age, especially for accidents. In 1995 approximately 23% of all deaths of men 15–44 years old were due to accidents and violence. In women of that same age group, although accidents and violence ranked fourth as a cause of death, it accounted for only 6.2% of deaths.

In general, deaths from accidents, violence, and poisonings have been decreasing. Between 1990 and 1992 the rate of such deaths fell from 60.6 per 100,000 population to 43.6. It increased to 65.2 in 1994, and fell again to 39.8 in 1995. Be-

tween 1990 and 1994 homicide deaths increased from 24 to 56, then declined slightly in 1995 to 44. The weapon most commonly used was a handgun (44%) followed by a knife or sharp instrument (20%). During the 1990–1995 period, the number of deaths from motor vehicle accidents declined from 39 to 20, although it spiked to 36 in 1994.

Based on data from all three acute care hospitals (including a private one), in 1993 assaults (4,596) accounted for 4.5% of the 102,657 emergency room visits, and gunshot wounds (161) accounted for 3.5% of all trauma due to assaults. With respect to motor vehicle accident trauma presenting at the Princess Margaret Hospital, the numbers were fairly constant at about 2,200 between 1990 and 1992, then fell to 2,088 in 1994. The latter represented 11.5% of all trauma cases seen at the hospital. This percentage held true for the first half of 1994.

Behavioral Disorders. Alcoholism and other substance abuse, particularly cocaine addiction, are major health problems that remain at unacceptably high levels. This is of particular concern because of the positive correlation between cocaine abuse and HIV infection.

The number of new cases of cocaine abuse presenting for treatment at the Community Mental Health Clinic (the principal outpatient treatment facility in the country) jumped from 69 in 1993 to 102 in 1994; in 1995 the number of new cases was down to 52, but it rose again to 82 in 1996. The number of persons presenting with alcohol abuse tended to decline between 1990 (134) and 1996 (68), while the number of marijuana abusers who were treated rose from 8 between 1990 and 1992 to 47 in 1996.

The number of patients hospitalized for cocaine abuse at the Sandilands Rehabilitation Center had declined from the 1987 level, but not consistently. Indeed, there was no change in the annual number of new cases (109) during the three year period 1993–1995. A sharp drop to 53 followed in 1996.

In terms of the total picture of mental disorders seen at the Community Mental Health Clinic, there was a steady decline in numbers of new clients registered between 1988 (677 clients) and 1993 (476). Thereafter, numbers increased to 704 and 705 in 1994 and 1995. The trend was the same among both males and females. Between 1988 and 1994 the three most common disorders presenting at the clinic were drug abuse, alcohol abuse, and depression. Psychotic and psychosocial disorders rounded out the top five. In 1995 the number of psychosocial disorders doubled, making this problem second to drug abuse and more frequent than depression.

Oral Health. Data provided for 1995 from the school dental clinic in New Providence show that there was a 50.6% increase over 1994 in the number of procedures performed. Of the 3,971 procedures done in 1995, 15.8% were restorations of permanent or deciduous teeth; almost three-quarters of the restorations involving fillings were done on deciduous teeth. Extractions accounted for 14.5% of all procedures; 9.5% of extractions involved permanent teeth, and 90.5% deciduous teeth.

In addition to the above-mentioned clinic there are three community dental clinics on the island of New Providence that serve the general population. Although the number of patients seen decreased between 1994 and 1995, the number of procedures increased. Extractions accounted for 27.5% of all procedures performed, and fillings and restorations 17.4%. Of the 994 extractions done, 68.2% were of permanent teeth.

According to data available from the Community Health Clinics, the most common problem noted among 5–14-year-olds in the school system is dental caries. This problem is most severe in New Providence, and least in Grand Bahama. Between 1993 and 1995 the percentage of children with caries in New Providence schools increased from 24.1% to 39.4%, while that in the Family Islands rose from 20.5% to 34.0%. On the other hand, in Grand Bahama the rate fell from 14.7% in 1993 to zero in 1995.

Natural Disasters. The Bahamas was hit in 1996 by two hurricanes, Bertha and Lili, but they were less powerful than the severely destructive Hurricane Andrew in 1992. The 1996 hurricanes caused infrastructural damage (power outages and disrupted telephone communications) and property damage in several Family Islands, but no deaths and few personal injuries. Several cases of post-traumatic stress syndrome were reported. Concerted efforts were made to reinstall services, remove debris, control insect proliferation, provide bottled water, and advise the public to boil drinking water.

Industrial Accidents. No major industrial accidents have been recorded in the Bahamas, but an emission of noxious gas in Freeport, Grand Bahama, resulted in the relocation of a school that was near the industrial site. During 1996 a fire in an old oil holding tank of the Bahamas Oil Refinery in Grand Bahama caused some concern. Although the fire itself was contained, residents worried about the potential for air pollution.

RESPONSE OF THE HEALTH SYSTEM

National Health Plans and Policies

The Government of the Bahamas subscribes to the internationally accepted principle that health is a fundamental human right, not a privilege, and to the view that quality health care must be universal in its application. There is full commitment to the global goal of "health for all," and community participation is accepted as a vital element of the health strategy.

The Ministry of Health's Policy Document, which was originally drafted in 1980 and most recently revised in 1988, is due for review and revision. In the meantime, the manifesto of the ruling party provides guidance in the form of politically directed emphases for the health services.

The people of the Bahamas already enjoy universal access to health care. However, the production of health services is inconsistent with the level of per capita government expenditure on health. The monitoring, evaluation, coordination, and planning of services need to be improved. Therefore, current emphasis is on upgrading managerial capacity, quality of care, and intersectoral coordination for development of local health systems. In this context, much attention is being paid to the development of human resources, establishment of norms and standards, and the strengthening of not only information systems but also the capacity to make effective use of them for planning, evaluation, and monitoring. In addition, a Planning Unit has been established within the Ministry with responsibility for coordinating and facilitating the internal planning process. It functions as the administrative and executive arm of: (1) the core planning group at Ministry Headquarters, comprising the chief administrative and technical officials, and (2) the extended planning committee, which includes the chairpersons of the executive management committees of each of the institutions/departments. The development and implementation of health projects of national priority are also facilitated through the Planning Unit.

The Government has indicated its intention to improve and expand services available at the Princess Margaret Hospital and to transform the hospital into a state-of-the-art diagnostic and therapeutic inpatient facility. Given that high technology demands the highest technical skills for maintenance of medical equipment, the Ministry is actively involved in strengthening the equipment maintenance program through pursuing the strategy of technical cooperation between countries. In addition, the availability of competent clinical and technical staff is being ensured through training in critical areas.

The Bahamas is experiencing a shift in its epidemiologic patterns away from deaths due to communicable diseases and toward those caused by chronic noncommunicable diseases, AIDS and AIDS-related complex, and accidents, violence, and poisonings. These changes, coupled with increasing health care costs, have served to highlight the importance of health education and promotion as a vital component of the health care system. The Ministry of Health and Environment is therefore putting in place the mechanism for development of a healthy public policy.

Health promotion and community participation are recognized as strategies to reduce health risk through mobilizing the populace to develop appropriate healthy lifestyles. Considerable effort is needed to educate the community as to its role in this regard, as it is only through the involvement of all social, political, and economic sectors that the state of wellness of a community can be enhanced. These strategies will be incorporated in all program plans, which will emphasize the need for proper food and nutrition, exercise, and smoking cessation, and pay particular attention to the areas of chronic diseases, STD/AIDS, and maternal and adolescent health.

In 1991–1992, the Ministry of Education implemented a comprehensive Family Life Education Program in primary and secondary schools. The Program is an important health promotion strategy that promises to have significant impact with time. A three-year National Plan of Action for Nutrition has already been developed, and its implementation will be the primary focus of the Nutrition Unit.

Maternal and child health concerns remain high on the health agenda. Within the context of the regional goal of health for all, the Bahamas has already achieved two of the three goals directed toward these at-risk groups. The regional goal for infant mortality at the end of the century is 30 or fewer deaths per 1,000 live births, while for children 1–4 years old it is 2.4 or fewer deaths per 1,000 population in the age group. In 1995 these two child health indicators were 19.0 and 0.41, respectively, for the Bahamas.

It is clear from the available data that in order to reduce the infant mortality figures further, special attention has to be paid to improving prenatal and perinatal care. In 1993 an Infant Mortality Reduction Project was developed. This project deals with three aspects:

- improving the quality of care during the prenatal period through the development and implementation of protocols for the management and referral of women with risk conditions;
- improving monitoring during the labor, delivery, and early neonatal periods; and
- providing special care for pregnant teenagers.

An important adjunct to the maternal and child health program is the establishment of an adolescent health care program. This program involves intersectoral collaboration between the several ministries. As an initial phase, a clinic for adolescents has been established at one of the comprehensive clinics on New Providence. The purpose is to promote healthy lifestyles in boys and girls, to reduce teenage pregnancy, and to encourage community-based services for adolescents.

A special group of youths will be targeted for specific family and community-based interventions. This will include any teenager who is sexually active and those who have been ad-judicated by the courts for any criminal offense. The integration of this program will be greatly facilitated by the new ministerial portfolios, in place since April 1995, when Education and Youth became the responsibility of the same Minister. There is now a Minister of State for Youth, Sport, and Culture to give continued emphasis to youth issues.

Interventions aimed at promoting healthy choices among adolescents have been developed. Also, in collaboration with the ministries of Education and Social Services, the needs of pregnant teenagers are being addressed by coordinating reproductive health services with health promotion and continuing education.

The Ministry of Health has formulated a National Family Planning Policy, which was mandated by the Cabinet following the Caribbean subregional follow-up meeting (hosted by the Bahamas) to the UN International Conference on Population and Development (ICPD). This policy is seen as a priority within the overall health policy, which aims "to improve the quality of, and provide the opportunity for a productive life for every Bahamian . . . ." The policy stipulates that all members within a family should have access to information and services that empower them to enrich their quality of life.

Access to information will be provided through the family life education program offered by the Ministry of Education, and through parenting, peer counseling, and other programs integrated with existing programs in the workplace, places of worship, social clubs, and sporting and recreational environments. Services will be provided through community clinics, where all clients within the childbearing age group attending any designated health care facility for the first time each year will be offered counseling, education, and physical assessment, including cervical smear, breast examination, urine testing, and screening for specific STDs, including HIV. Prostate examination will be offered to males over 30 years of age. A full range of contraceptive methods will also be available to clients. These services will be provided on a cost-recovery basis, but no one will be denied service because of inability to pay. All providers of family planning services will be certified in family planning and STD counseling, contraceptive technology, and related screening techniques.

Client education will be provided through a comprehensive health education and promotion program, making full use of the mass media. In recognition that a national program requires the full involvement of many sectors of the community, an effort will be made to strengthen government agencies' collaborative ties with each other and with nongovernmental organizations, through the establishment of a National Family Planning Committee comprising representatives of related government programs and private-sector organizations.

Substance abuse, including the abuse of alcohol, is a high-priority public health problem in the country. The efforts of the National Drug Council (NDC) are geared toward providing public education, fostering national awareness and serving as a catalyst, and facilitating and coordinating multisectoral, NGO, and community involvement and interventions.

A major NDC program aimed at demand reduction is well under way. Substantial support for this program was obtained under a special project funded by the United Nations International Drug Control Program. This project emphasizes the following demand reduction plans over the next three years:

- community prevention, which includes the development or strengthening of community organizations dealing with the antecedents to drug abuse and the establishment of alternative economic activities for young people in order to reduce the likelihood of them engaging in drug trafficking;
- prevention education, including ongoing support for the family life education curriculum, training for teachers and other persons responsible for the care of children who are at special risk for drug abuse, an aggressive public education campaign, and the training for youth in the techniques of peer counseling and the establishment of such activities in schools and communities; and
- treatment and rehabilitation, including ongoing evaluation of programs and the establishment of quality standards for treatment and rehabilitation activities, training of treatment and rehabilitation personnel, development of community-based outpatient rehabilitation and aftercare services, and rehabilitation services specifically designed to satisfy the needs of women, youth, and incarcerated persons.

There has been general agreement for many years now on the need to develop a comprehensive mental health program, integrated at all levels of the health system on all islands. The operationalization of this concept has been slow. The Ministry's recent decision to undertake a National Family Health Care Initiative, which will incorporate a mental wellness component (with emphasis on preventing family violence and coping with stress), will help solidify a comprehensive mental health program.

The Ministry of Health's dental health program is largely palliative in the public sector, with most of the preventive and restorative work carried out in the private sector. The ratio of dentists (public and private) to population was 3.0 to 10,000 in 1994. Continued expansion of the school dental program is warranted, as is greater emphasis on dental education and preventive care.

Disease surveillance and programs for the control of communicable diseases have a long history of development in the Bahamas. Prevention programs include immunization against vaccine-preventable diseases such as diphtheria, whooping cough, poliomyelitis, measles, mumps, and rubella; management of acute diarrhea; and screening programs for STDs including HIV/AIDS.

The HIV/STD 1993–1996 Medium-Term Plan II (MTP II) fostered a supportive social environment for the effective implementation of risk reduction and behavioral interventions directed toward vulnerable populations: young people between the ages of 10 and 19 years, females of childbearing ages, persons with multiple partners, pregnant women, incarcerated populations (past and present), and blood donors. All of the aforementioned groups include persons from the Creole community.

The National Disaster Preparedness Program focuses the Ministry's attention on the continued development and refinement of its Health Disaster Plan through training and disaster simulation exercises.

In response to growing dissatisfaction with the erratic availability and the high cost of pharmaceuticals to the public sector, the Ministry put in place a system of procurement and distribution of pharmaceuticals to ensure the population's access to essential drugs. The Bahamas Drug Agency was established in 1994 to address these issues as well as the development and maintenance of the pharmaceutical formulary for the country.

The Ministry has extended basic laboratory services to selected Family Islands, including services to facilitate the diagnosis of STDs. The laboratories at the Princess Margaret and the Rand hospitals participate in several WHO quality control programs and make full use of the facilities of the Caribbean Epidemiology Center for monitoring of blood bank and transfusion services. Within the hospital setting, a quality assurance program is being strengthened through participation in the Regional Hospital Accreditation Program and in a Ministry of Health initiative that began in 1996.

The Government proposes to privatize the collection of both commercial and domestic wastes. To this end, a comprehensive waste classification study (completed in 1992) was used as the basis for developing the privatization plan. A preinvestment study on solid waste and hazardous materials management was carried out through an agreement with the Inter-American Development Bank (IDB). It resulted in a Solid Waste Master Plan, developed in 1996. The Plan recommends, *inter alia,* waste reduction, rationalization of the collection system, and sanitary landfilling (in combination with composting in New Providence). Studies have indicated that total solid waste generation is 2.6 kg per person per day. Implementation of the Plan has commenced in several Family Islands.

Several air pollution monitoring stations have been installed in New Providence and in Freeport, Grand Bahama, as part of the Air Pollution Prevention and Control Strategy.

These monitoring stations are operated by the Department of Environmental Health Services, an agency of the Ministry of Consumer Affairs and Aviation, and measure suspended particulate matter, nitrogen oxides, and sulfur oxides.

Most fuel stations in the Bahamas now sell unleaded gasoline, with one company providing only unleaded gasoline. It is anticipated that a significant reduction of lead in the environment will result from this development.

The 1995 data on water supply indicated that 88% of houses in urban areas were connected to the drinking water supply system, while another 8% of urban houses had reasonable access to water. The situation was reversed in rural areas, where 86% of houses had reasonable access to water but no indoor connections. In contrast to the water supply situation, only 16% of houses in urban areas are connected to a public sewer, but the remaining 84% have adequate on-site excreta disposal. In the rural areas, 100% of the houses have an adequate on-site excreta disposal system. In addition, regular collection of solid waste is provided to nearly all (99%) of the houses in urban areas, but to none in rural areas.

A major concern with regard to drinking water quality is the proliferation of private shallow-water wells. Especially in residential and commercial areas with on-site sanitation, groundwater quality is compromised by nitrates, pathogens, and substances used in commercial activity. Although this well water is mostly used for washing, cross-connections have been reported, which could allow this polluted water to be pumped into the public distribution system and thus affect the potable supply.

Use of private wells is discouraged. Those who use them are urged to have their water tested periodically. Switching between public and private supply is also discouraged in order to reduce the risk of contamination.

In terms of human resource development, particular attention is being paid to the areas of maternal and child health, the health inspectorate, disease surveillance/epidemiology, hospital administration, program management, and project design and management. The Ministry recognizes that adequate human resource planning, coupled with development for health professionals and staff at all levels and in all areas, is a key to success.

Other Ministry programs include strengthening of the health information system and infrastructural development of hospitals and community clinics.

Health Sector Reform

In keeping with Region-wide developments related to changing national health systems, and as a part of the overall public sector reform efforts, the Bahamas' focus for health sector reform is on issues of modernization and decentralization; the organization and operation of services; complementarity with the private sector; and rationalization of human and financial resources.

Specific reform efforts under way in the Bahamas include (but are not limited to) the following:

- preparations for the devolution of management of the three public hospitals from the centralized Ministry to an autonomous, quasi-governmental hospital services board/authority;
- privatization of selected diagnostic health services in the public sector;
- the adoption of policies for the purchase, financing, and distribution of pharmaceuticals;
- selective privatization of decentralized financing/capital funding and decentralized management policies and practices; and
- the development of local health systems in the Family Islands.

Devolution of Hospitals. The decision to devolve the management of hospitals resulted from a determination that highly centralized government bureaucracy militates against the efficient and effective operation of the hospitals. The long-range goal is the establishment of a hospital corporation, directed by a board that will be responsible for the executive management and direction of the corporation. Some services within the hospital have already been privatized and the decision taken to contract out selected services.

Selective Privatization. Selective privatization grew out of the need and desire of Bahamian physicians to deliver quality health care to all residents of the Bahamas, in both the private and public facilities. Selective privatization was initiated within the context of availability of first-world health care providers, the existence of patients with first-world expectations, and the reality of limited budgets within the public health sector.

The central feature of selective privatization is the relationship between the management of the Princess Margaret Hospital and a private entity, the Physicians Alliance. Through this partnership, the Physicians Alliance provides capital for the purchase of equipment and for the renovation of the facilities and is responsible for equipment selection, transport, installation, maintenance, and replacement. In addition, the Physicians Alliance is responsible for employing the clerical and administrative staff, managing the service, and paying the technical and medical personnel. The Princess Margaret Hospital contributes the physical plant, staff for renovation of facilities, housekeeping and security staff, and funds for utilities payments and customs duties on imported equipment and supplies.

The other feature of the partnership is the equal sharing of any profits between the Physicians Alliance and the Princess Margaret Hospital. The policy of the Alliance is that indigent patients are not denied service. Fees for public patients are much lower than those charged in the private sector; fees for private patients, while higher, are set at competitive rates and are still significantly lower than the fees charged in the private sector.

On a smaller scale, radiology services, once provided to community clinic clients by the Princess Margaret Hospital, have been privatized.

Development of Local Health Systems. The concept of a local health system was first realized on Grand Bahama in 1985, when all the health services on the island were brought under one administrative umbrella. This arrangement afforded the maximum utilization of hospital-based skills, to the advantage of the entire system, and allowed for a two-way sharing of resources. During 1993–1994 this system was evaluated and a study was done to assess the feasibility of implementing a similar system in the Family Islands. As a result, a modified form of the system was introduced on the islands of Andros, Eleuthera, and Long Island. These islands are divided into health districts, each with its own health team. This system has not only brought the management of the services closer to the population being served, but has also facilitated the sharing of resources between districts. With the establishment of local government during 1996, it has become necessary to find ways to manage the health system within the mandates of local government to the benefit of the population. The phased extension of the system to other major Family Islands is proposed.

Within the context of local health systems, innovative ways will be sought to involve clients in determining the extent of the services provided and in setting priorities.

Organization of the Health System

Government Sector

In April 1997, following elections, responsibilities within the public sector of the health system were reordered. The Ministry of Health has overall responsibility for ensuring the health of the nation. It discharges this responsibility through establishing national policies and strategic plans for personal health; providing public services and facilities to support these interventions; and ensuring that public health regulations and activities for disease control and health promotion are maintained.

The Ministry is headed by the Minister of Health, who is assisted by a Parliamentary Secretary with specific responsibility for updating health legislation. The administrative structure is managed by the Permanent Secretary, and the technical head is the Chief Medical Officer. The senior technical directorate is completed by the Chief Hospital Administrator and the Director of Nursing.

The service areas and programs of the Ministry that fall directly under the purview of headquarters management include the Health Education Division, the AIDS Secretariat, the National Drug Council, Materials Management, the National Drug (Pharmaceutical) Agency, the Human Resources Development Unit, the Health Information Coordinating Unit, and the Health Planning Unit.

Hospital Services. The public sector operates three hospitals, the two largest of which are located on New Providence. The Princess Margaret Hospital, with 436 beds, provides general acute and specialized services including intensive care, hemodialysis, cardiology, and urology. The Sandilands Rehabilitation Center provides both psychiatric/mental health care on an inpatient and outpatient basis (352 beds) and geriatric care (130 beds). The third institution, the Rand Memorial Hospital, is in the nation's second largest city, Freeport, on Grand Bahama. It provides general acute care as well as basic levels of specialized services, and has a bed complement of 82.

Between 1992 and 1994 the occupancy rate of the Princess Margaret Hospital was around 90%, but in 1995 it dropped to 82%. High occupancy rates were also recorded at the Sandilands Rehabilitation Center in both the Psychiatric Unit (84%–88%) and the Geriatric Unit (93%–95% in 1992–1994, falling to 88% in 1995). At the Rand, however, occupancy rates were between 52.8% (1992) and 54.0% (1994).

The Executive Management Committee of each hospital consists of the Hospital Administrator, the Medical Staff Coordinator, and the Principal Nursing Officer; at the Princess Margaret Hospital it also includes the Financial Controller and the Chief Hospital Administrator. In 1996 a new category of staff was introduced: the Resident Specialist. These persons are full-time clinical managers who are responsible for managing their respective units and who sit on the Hospital Planning and Development Committee.

Laboratory, X-ray, and Pharmacy. These facilities are available within both the public and private sectors. The laboratory of the Princess Margaret Hospital serves the hospital and the Community Health Clinics. It also functions as the public health and referral laboratory and manages the blood bank. The Rand Hospital performs similar functions on Grand Bahama. These services are also available at the Doctor's Hospital, a private institution, and stand-alone facilities exist in the private sector.

The pharmaceutical services within the public sector are managed by the National Drug Agency, which was established in 1994. It is responsible for the procurement and distribution of pharmaceuticals and biologicals to hospitals and community health services. In 1993 a technical cooperation project was instituted between the Ministry of Health and the Barbados Drug Agency to streamline the procurement and distribution of pharmaceuticals to government health facilities. This project is ongoing.

Purchasing of equipment and materials for the Ministry is carried out by the Materials Management Department. Requests are forwarded to it by the respective institutions following careful review by an in-house purchasing committee.

Public Health Services. These services are delivered through a network of 57 community clinics and 54 satellite clinics in New Providence and the Family Islands. They also encompass community-based programs such as home and district nursing, disease surveillance, and home-based rehabilitation. The management team in this area consists of an Administrator, Medical Staff Coordinator, Principal Nursing Officer, and Medical Officer of Health. There is a unit specifically responsible for coordinating service delivery to the Family Islands. Public health services include general practice, maternal and child health, and dental health. They are provided at the following types of health facilities:

(1) Comprehensive clinics (available only in Nassau), which are staffed by general practitioners, public health nurses, and other registered nurses. They have X-ray, pharmacy, dental, and limited laboratory services.

(2) District health centers, which have a resident doctor, nurse-in-charge, and administrative/clerical officer. These centers are the focal medical facilities in defined health districts and are equipped with most of the standard life-sustaining equipment.

(3) Community clinics, which take care of the needs of a specified community. A resident nurse is stationed at each clinic, and the district doctor makes weekly visits.

(4) Satellite clinics, which have no resident staff and are visited at intervals ranging from twice monthly to every six weeks by a doctor or nurse-in-charge.

Environmental Health Services. The environmental concerns of the Ministry are managed by the Department of Environmental Health Services (DEHS), whose functions are conducted through three divisions: the Health Directorate, Environmental Monitoring and Risk Assessment, and Solid Waste Collection and Disposal. The management team comprises a Director, Deputy Director, and the Assistant Directors responsible for the three divisions. In April 1997 this department was transferred from the Ministry of Health to the Ministry of Consumer Affairs and Aviation.

DEHS activities include monitoring the quality of groundwater, drinking water (including bottled water), and air; man-

agement of solid waste, chemical safety, and hazardous waste; inspection of ports for compliance with sanitation rules; monitoring of food quality; inspection of premises; and control of vector proliferation.

Most solid waste is disposed of in a landfill. In New Providence 28% of the total waste delivered to the landfill is hauled by DEHS (residential trash and waste from small businesses), and 72% by private haulers and waste management companies (from hotels and industrial and commercial enterprises). Infectious waste from hospitals is incinerated on-site, while the other waste is transported to the landfill.

The supply of drinking water is the responsibility of the Water and Sewerage Corporation (WSC). It is legally responsible for water resource management, water supply, and the provision of adequate facilities for the drainage and safe disposal of sewage and industrial effluent in the Bahamas, except on Grand Bahama, where a separate utility has been established for water supply and wastewater management.

The primary source of drinking water is shallow groundwater. The groundwater has a detectable saline taste, and many people use bottled drinking water (locally produced in reverse osmosis plants). Desalination plants have also been constructed at major hotel developments. A reverse osmosis plant was scheduled to be operational by the end of 1997 to augment public supply and reduce overall salinity levels. Rainwater collected in tanks and cisterns supplies less than 3% of the water consumed. Drinking water is also brought by barge from Andros to New Providence, the most populous island.

Since the Bahamas is heavily dependent on the tourism sector for its economic survival, sustained tourism development is vital. The Government has established the Bahamas Environment, Science, and Technology Commission (BEST) within the Office of the Prime Minister to address the issue of sustainable development. Commission membership is drawn from ministries, departments, corporations and private sector organizations, and individuals responsible for or involved in matters related to the environment, science, or technology.

The responsibilities of BEST are, *inter alia:*

- To serve as the Bahamas' national focal point for contact with all international organizations on matters relating to the environment, science, and technology.
- To coordinate work pertaining to international environmental conventions, treaties, protocols, and agreements to which the Bahamas is or will become a signatory.
- To coordinate national efforts to (i) protect, conserve, and responsibly manage the environmental resources of the Bahamas; (ii) develop a National Conservation and Sustainable Development Strategy Plan; (iii) identify suitable scientific and technological advances that can

contribute to the development of the Bahamas; (iv) draft legislation to enforce the provisions of the National Conservation Plan and other environmental policies; and (v) identify and apply for technical assistance and financial grants to meet the Commission's responsibilities.

Areas of environmental concern include pollution from automobiles, solid waste management, protection of the natural environment, coastal zone pollution, drinking water supply, and sewage disposal.

Legislation. Health legislation has not kept pace with the health care industry, technological advances, or the many environmental concerns that currently confront the country. New categories of staff and new types of facilities, especially within the private sector, need to be accommodated. Current legislation only covers the registration of doctors, nurses (including midwives), and dentists. Top priority is being given to laws governing the registration of pharmacists and laboratory technologists, and work has begun on laws pertaining to such disciplines as X-ray technology, optometry, podiatry, chiropractic, and physiotherapy.

Another legislative priority is the regulation of health facilities, including private hospitals, walk-in clinics, laboratories, and X-ray facilities.

Work has been ongoing in environmental health legislation, but much remains to be done. No legislation exists to control smoking in most public places, but the national airline and, as of 1 August 1997, national airports are smoke-free.

No legislation is currently in force regulating the use of seat belts or car seats for children, but active consideration is being given to such legislation. In the interim, the driving public is being encouraged to use seat belts.

Private Sector

Services. The private sector provides primary care services, emergency services, secondary inpatient care, and specialized clinical, diagnostic, and treatment services in both the medical and dental fields. There are two private hospitals providing secondary care. Doctor's Hospital has 72 beds and its services include emergency care, specialized medical care (including rheumatology and nephrology), surgery (including cardiovascular and neurosurgery), obstetrics, and diagnostic services (including nuclear medicine). The other private hospital, Lyford Cay, has 12 beds. It provides specialty services in cardiology, plastic surgery, urology, and podiatry. In addition, a number of private practices have birthing facilities but are not classified as hospitals.

Specialized ambulatory services are available in the areas of cardiology and nephrology. The Bahamas Heart Center offers a full range of cardiac evaluation techniques, including nuclear stress testing and cardiac catheterization. Pacemaker implantation is also available. Renal House offers kidney dialysis.

Health Insurance. There is no national health insurance scheme, but the National Insurance Board provides medical benefits for job-related injuries and illness. Partial salary replacement is provided during illness, as well as paid medical care for industrial injuries. Other benefit types include maternity, disability, and death. In addition, provision is made for invalidity, retirement, and survivor's benefits. Several options for health and dental insurance are available through the private insurance system.

Health Resources

Human Resources

The Bahamas is well supplied with physicians and dentists. Doctors increased from 373 (14.13 per 10,000 population) in 1992 to 417 (14.98) in 1995, and dentists from 58 (2.2 per 10,000 population) in 1992 to 80 (2.9) in 1995. In terms of distribution, 235 physicians were in government service and 182 (excluding consultants) were in the private sector. Consultants work in both the private and government sectors.

Within the government sector, 152 doctors (including 25 consultants) are attached to the Princess Margaret Hospital, 32 (including 7 consultants) to the Rand Hospital, 13 (including 5 consultants) to the Sandilands Rehabilitation Center, and 37 to the Community Health Services. It is noteworthy that in 1994, 15 of the Community Health Services doctors were based in New Providence, while 20 were in the Family Islands. In 1995, however, this situation was reversed, with 21 in New Providence and 16 in the Family Islands.

Of the 80 dentists in the country, 21 are in government service and 59 in private practice. Of the government service dentists, 13 are attached to the Princess Margaret Hospital, 1 to the Rand, 1 to the Sandilands Rehabilitation Center, and 6 to the Community Health Services.

The number of registered nurses in the government service increased only slightly between 1989 and 1995 (from 623 to 653). Thus the rate per 10,000 population decreased from 25.0 to 24.1. Between 1989 and 1993 the number of trained clinical nurses (TCNs) decreased from 467 to 416; it then recovered to 464 in 1995—still below the 1989 level. During that period the rate per 10,000 population dropped from 18.8 to 16.6. In terms of distribution, 362 registered nurses and 249 TCNs are attached to the PMH, 56 registered nurses and 53 TCNs to the Rand, 104 registered nurses and 88 TCNs to the Sandilands Rehabilitation Center, and 131 registered nurses and 74 TCNs to the Community Health Services.

With respect to other categories of staff, the Princess Margaret Hospital has 16 pharmacists and 16 pharmacy aides, 32 laboratory technologists, 7 physiotherapists and 5 aides, and 1 occupational therapist. The Rand Memorial Hospital has 7 laboratory technologists, 4 lab technicians, and 1 cytotechnologist.

There is no medical or dental school in the Bahamas. Most national doctors and dentists are trained at the University of the West Indies or in North America. As of April 1997 the Bahamas Government entered into an agreement with the University of the West Indies, whereby the Princess Margaret Hospital and community health facilities will provide clinical experience to medical students from the University.

Nursing training is carried out at the College of the Bahamas. The nursing department offers a program in midwifery, an associate of science degree in nursing, a continuing education program, and, since 1995, a bachelor of science degree nursing program for registered nurses. While there were 199 students registered in the associate of science degree program in 1995, the number of graduates had been relatively small in the period 1992–1995 (64), with only 7 graduating in 1995. There was only one graduating class of midwives during that time (15 in 1994). These numbers cannot satisfy the demands of the health sector, and nurses are still recruited from overseas from time to time.

The Health Sciences Department of the College of the Bahamas offers an associate's degree in environmental health. An associate of science degree in health sciences, with options in medical technology, pharmacy, occupational health, and physiotherapy is presently being developed.

Expenditures and Sectoral Financing

The national health expenditure by the Government has shown a steady increase since 1970, mirroring the increase in the total national recurrent expenditure. The percentage of the total government expenditure devoted to health increased from 10.8% in 1970 to 15.6% in 1986. Since that time, the proportion has fluctuated and has tended to fall; in the 1995–1996 budget it amounted to 13.6%. Nevertheless, because of the strengthening of the national economy, the actual amount spent has increased. The distribution of expenditure between the different divisions of the Ministry has remained fairly constant, with approximately 15% going to administration, 65.5% to hospitals, 8% to environmental health, and 11% to community health services. It is not possible to determine how much is spent on preventive as opposed to curative services, since both types of services are provided through the public health system.

The financial resources for health provided by the central government come from the consolidated fund. In addition, limited amounts are obtained from inpatient charges and fees for clinical and diagnostic services.

In addition to medical benefits, the National Insurance Board has provided funding for the construction of 11 health facilities on New Providence and five of the Family Islands, and another 5 are under construction.

The out-of-pocket expenditures of families for physician's fees, medications, diagnostic services, and private health insurance contribute to private sector resources. The IDB has estimated that private health expenditure amounts to 2.2% of GDP and 45.6% of the total health expenditure in the country.

Several nongovernmental organizations provide health services of one kind or another. Some of these organizations take an active part in government-sponsored health programs. Notable among these are the Cancer Society, Crippled Children's Committee, AIDS Foundation, Family Planning Association, Crisis Center, and Diabetic Association. Other organizations exist in the areas of drug abuse and care for persons living with AIDS.

BARBADOS

GENERAL SITUATION AND TRENDS

Socioeconomic, Political, and Demographic Overview

Barbados, the easternmost Caribbean island, extends over 430 km², over mostly flat terrain. Given the country's small size, it is difficult to define areas as urban or rural, but the most densely populated areas are found along the western, southwestern, and southern coasts.

The country has a good network of roads, and the international airport has several daily flights to major cities around the world. The population also is well served by a system of private and public transportation. Because the island lies within the hurricane belt, each year there is increased vigilance from June through November. The Central Emergency Relief Organisation is responsible for disaster preparedness and response.

Barbados has a democratic system of government with parliamentary elections held every five years. The parliament consists of a nominated 21-member Senate and an elected House of Assembly of 28 members.

During 1992–1995, Barbados's economy recovered from the recession that began in 1989, showing growth in real output and in international reserves, as well as improvements in the balance of payments. In fiscal year 1991–1992, the Government introduced an 18-month stabilization program, designed to restore balance to the country's finances and external accounts.

Real gross domestic product in 1992 had fallen to US$ 395.5 million, due to the recession in 1989. In 1993, however, real output had risen to US$ 401.9 million, reaching US$ 428.4 million by 1995. The main sectors of the economy that contributed to this growth were tourism, manufacturing, wholesale and retail trade, and business and general services.

Tourism recorded real growth during the period, with annual revenues from this sector rising from US$ 56.8 million to US$ 65.4 million between 1992 and 1995 and with indicators such as average length of stay and hotel and bed occupancy rates showing increases. Growth in cruise passenger arrivals outstripped the long-stay arrivals.

The first surplus in three years on the current balance of payments was recorded in 1992; it was sustained during 1993–1995, largely through the performance of manufacturing for the export market and tourism.

The rate of inflation, recorded at 6.2% in 1992, dropped to 0.1% in 1994, but rose again 1.9% in 1995. Increases in the prices of food and beverages and housing in 1995 were partially offset by declines in the price of transportation and household operation and supplies.

In April 1993, the Government, trade unions, and social partners negotiated the first protocol on prices and incomes, which froze public- and private-sector wages and contained the price of goods and services.

Government current expenditure increased from US$ 543.1 million in 1992/1993 to $616.2 million in 1995/1996. Current revenues increased from $502.2 million to $574.5 million in the same period. Capital expenditure each year from 1992–1993 to 1994–1995 was about $22 million and rose to $58.5 million in 1995–1996. Government expenditure as a percentage of GDP, however, had declined from 26% in 1993 to 23% in 1995. The fiscal deficit net of amortization, which was $25.9 million in 1992/1993, had declined to $10.6 million in 1995/1996.

The labor force increased from 132,100 in 1992 to 136,800 by 1995. The unemployment rate reached its highest rate (24.3%) in 1993, during the implementation of the structural adjustment program; by 1995, unemployment had fallen to 19.7%.

The literacy rate in Barbados, estimated at 95%, is one of the highest in the Caribbean. Education at the primary and secondary levels is compulsory until age 16.

In 1990, there were approximately 75,170 households in Barbados and 70,693 (94%) of them had piped water. The other 6% had easy access to public water-supply facilities.

More than 75% of households have telephones, and telecommunication services are readily available, and more than 90% of households have electricity. According to the Statistical Service's Continuous Household Survey, in 1996 the average household size was 3.5 persons; the 1990 census revealed that women headed 44% of households.

During 1992–1995, the population grew at an annual rate of less than 1%. For the last decade, the population's demographic profile has changed, with an increasing proportion of elderly persons. In 1995, approximately 12% of the population was older than 65 years old, and 23% was under 15 years. By 1995, the mid-year population was estimated at 265,173: 47.9% were males and 52.1% females; however, there were 19.4% more females than males in the age group 65 years and older. Life expectancy at birth is 72.9 years for males and 77.4 years for females. Birth registration is complete—more than 98% of babies are delivered in hospital, and births are required to be recorded immediately.

Mortality Profile

The crude death rate has remained fairly constant over the past four years, around 9 per 1,000. During the 1992–1995 period, the total number of deaths was 9,692. In 1995, the five leading causes of death were as follows, in descending order of importance: cardiovascular disease (393–398; 410–429), 18.8% of deaths; malignant neoplasms (140–208), 17.2%; cerebrovascular disease (430–438), 13.7%; diabetes mellitus (250), 10.0%; and other diseases of circulatory system (440–459), 3.9%. In 1995, the five leading causes of death in children under 5 years old represented 3% of all deaths. In the age group over 45 years old, 905 deaths (41%) were attributed to heart related causes and 373 (13.3%) to neoplasms of the genitourinary tract and digestive organs. Remaining deaths were attributed to various other causes. These data are in keeping with an aging population with a lifespan over 75 years.

SPECIFIC HEALTH PROBLEMS

Analysis by Population Group

Health of Children

In 1995, the infant mortality rate was 15.2 per 1,000 live births and the neonatal death rate was 11.3 per 1,000 live births. Infant and neonatal death rates varied little between 1992 and 1995.

Neonatal deaths account for 75% of all infant deaths and 54% of neonatal deaths are in the age group under 1 day old.

The leading causes of death in children under 5 years of age were certain conditions originating in the perinatal period, followed by congenital anomalies, pneumonia, and AIDS.

The number of children under 1 year old who die from AIDS has remained relatively constant, but since AZT is now being given to pregnant women who are HIV-positive, this number may decrease. Even though diseases of the respiratory system were not a leading cause of death, they were the second most common cause of hospitalization among children under 5 years old; prominent in this group of diseases is asthma, reflecting the increasing prevalence of this disease, which is estimated at 12% among the general population.

Over the last four years, the percentage of newborns with low birthweight (<2,500 g) fluctuated between 9% and 11%, signaling a need for the health system to target mothers who give birth to underweight babies for follow-up services. Malnutrition in childhood is uncommon and so is an infrequent cause for hospital admission.

For 1992–1995, the mortality rate for children 1–4 years old was 0.4 per 1,000 children of this age; for the age group 5–14 years old, it was 0.2 per 1,000.

Health of Adolescents

Health services for adolescents (age group 10–19 years old) are provided at the government-operated polyclinics; clinic-based family life education and school outreach programs also are provided. These programs aim to improve family life and reduce teenage pregnancy and child abuse.

Data from the Government Statistical Department indicate that there was a consistent reduction in births to adolescent mothers. During the period under review, births to adolescent mothers were 13.9% of all births in 1995, down from the 1977 high of 23%. This decline coincided with a strengthened adolescent health program, the implementation of family life education programs in schools, and an expansion of the adolescent peer-counseling program run by the Barbados Family Planning Association.

Substance abuse is an issue of much concern in this age group. Marijuana and cocaine are the substances most abused. In 1994 and 1995, between fifteen and twenty 20-year-old men received treatment for simultaneous use of both drugs. It is believed that, owing to the stigma attached to attendance at the Psychiatric Hospital's Rehabilitation Unit, the services were underused. No intravenous drug use was reported.

In the period under review, several programs were geared to improving family health. In the 1990 census there were 70,460 persons in the 15–29 age group, representing 27% of the total population. Increased violence and deviant behavior in this age group have been causes of concern. Reports indicate that most people who participate in drug rehabilitation programs conducted by the Ministry of Health started using illegal drugs between the ages of 13 and 16.

Health of Adults

Lifestyle is critical to the health of adults (20–60 years old). The population's disease profile shows an increase in the incidence of noncommunicable diseases from age 45 years on.

Much attention was given to women in this age group. For the last 40 years, the birth rate has significantly dropped, going from 34 per 1,000 in 1955 to 13.4 per 1,000 in 1995. Family planning clinics were established in all public clinics between 1993 and 1995.

Legal abortions represented 2.8% of the leading causes for hospitalization in 1995, compared with 3.9% in 1992. There were five maternal deaths in the 1992–1995 period (3.3 per 10,000 live births), as compared with 14 in the 1988–1991 period (8.4 per 10,000 live births).

Health of the Elderly

Coping with problems among the elderly (age group 60 years old and older) is one of the health care system's major challenges. Noncommunicable diseases such as arthritis, hypertension, and diabetes mellitus continue to be the main health disorders among the elderly. The leading causes of death in this age group were heart disease and cardiovascular disease. The most common disabilities affecting the older adult were blindness and impaired vision.

In Barbados, the elderly have unrestricted access to primary health care, which is available at the polyclinics, and to secondary care that is available at Queen Elizabeth Hospital and the psychiatric hospital. Five Geriatric/District Hospitals mainly provide inpatient care for the elderly; they have a combined bed capacity of 744 and an annual average occupancy rate of 95.5%. Excessive demand for geriatric care in public institutions forces these hospitals to operate at maximum capacity. According to statistics from Queen Elizabeth Hospital's Social Services Department, in August 1996 there were 604 persons on the waiting list for admission to the Geriatric Hospital. As a way to solve the problem of insufficient beds in public geriatric institutions, in 1995 the Government allocated several beds at the Queen Elizabeth Hospital to elderly persons who did not need acute medical or nursing care. An expansion of care for the elderly is one of the components of the IDB-funded health rationalization study.

The Government is committed to allowing the elderly to continue to live within their communities. Attempts to deinstitutionalize the elderly and return them to their own homes,

however, have not always been successful because not enough support systems and programs have been available in the country. The Government also is exploring ways to provide domiciliary care for the elderly.

Workers' Health

There is no evidence of child labor in Barbados because the Compulsory Education Act that requires children ages 5–16 years to attend school is strictly enforced; Student Attendance Officers investigate reports of children who are absent from school for two weeks.

Information on informal sector employment was not available, but the Ministry of Labour, Community Development, and Sports is currently conducting a study of that sector.

Women represented an increasing proportion of the economically active population, accounting for 48.2% of the labor force in 1992 and 49.3% in 1995. In 1992, 80% of employed women worked in service industries. The effects of the work environment on women's health need to be investigated, particularly in those establishments where chemical substances are used and where adequate lighting is required; the agricultural sector also should be studied.

In May 1996 at a Regional Multipartite Conference on Workers' Health, held in Barbados, a draft Regional Workers' Health Plan was presented and discussed. Its components included: health and human development, health systems and services development, health promotion and protection, environmental protection, and disease prevention and control.

The Government is currently considering legislation on health and safety in the workplace, which will replace the 1982 Factories Act. The Barbados Employers Confederation encourages its members to promote workers' health by making workplaces healthy, through such measures as establishing smoke-free offices, measuring air quality, providing exercise facilities, and sponsoring seminars on health issues at the workplace; employee assistance programs also are available at some work sites.

Health of the Disabled

The Children's Development Centre is a unit within the Ministry of Health that provides physical, psychological, and emotional support for disabled persons, offering such services as occupational therapy, physiotherapy, behavioral therapy, speech therapy, audiological testing, and counseling.

There are currently 1,417 persons with disabilities registered with the Centre, 924 men and 493 women. The age group 1–12 years old was most affected with mental retardation and development delays, accounting for greater percentages of the classified diagnoses.

In 1992, the Barbados Council for the Disabled, working with the Barbados Chapter of Partners in Appropriate Technology for the Handicapped (PATH), developed a long-range project designed to bring about more and better services for children and young adults with disabilities by involving parents. Since then, the Council established education programs to sensitize the general public regarding the disabled and has helped to advance the process of national planning for physical and mental disabilities. A national policy for persons with disabilities began to be formulated in 1994, and a task force commissioned by the Ministry of Labour, Community Development, and Sports was established to propose legislation to facilitate the integration of the disabled into national life. The Ministry of Health was a member of the task force, and the proposals are currently under consideration by the Ministry of Labour, Community Development, and Sports.

Analysis by Type of Disease or Health Impairment

Communicable Diseases

Vector-Borne Diseases: Dengue Fever. In an epidemic in 1995, 2,076 cases of dengue fever were reported, 870 of which were laboratory-confirmed. The outbreak was concentrated in the country's south and southwest, and the group most affected were women 15 to 39 years old, who are more economically active and make up almost half of the country's labor force. There were two cases of dengue hemorrhagic fever and one death. Type 2 and Type 4 were the circulating serotypes during this epidemic. Dengue fever appears to be endemic, as cases are being reported throughout the year.

Vaccine-Preventable Diseases. Barbados was declared free of poliomyelitis in 1994; no cases of polio have been notified in more than 10 years. The last case of diphtheria was reported in 1980. One case of whooping cough was reported in 1993 and one in 1995. Two cases of tetanus were reported in 1993, two in 1994, and none in 1995. All of the cases of tetanus occurred in elderly persons.

The last case of measles was reported in 1991. In 1996, there was an outbreak of rubella, with 229 suspected cases notified; 3 cases of rubella were notified in 1993 and 16 in 1995. No cases were reported in 1994. Of the suspected cases, 83 were laboratory-confirmed, 15 of which occurred in pregnant females. A surveillance system for congenital rubella was implemented to track the outcome of these pregnancies and plan any necessary intervention strategies for dealing with the babies. The cost-effectiveness of an immunization program for at-risk mothers is being examined.

Two cases of *Haemophilus* meningitis were reported in 1993, five cases in 1994, and one case in 1995. *Haemophilus influenzae* is being considered for inclusion among the EPI diseases for which vaccination would be made available.

In 1993, one case of meningococcal meningitis was reported; it was believed to be imported but the epidemiological linkage was not clearly demonstrated. Immediate contacts were treated with Rifampicin.

Cholera and Other Intestinal Diseases. No cases of cholera have been reported in Barbados. The diarrheal disease surveillance system reported 1,606 cases of diarrhea in 1993, 1,549 cases in 1994, and 2,099 cases in 1995. Fifty-three cases of gastroenteritis were reported in 1993; the corresponding figures for 1994 and 1995 were 37 and 102, respectively. An increase in circulation of viral pathogens and the improved active surveillance systems are factors in the rise of reported cases of diarrheal diseases in the last year.

In 1993, the Public Health Laboratory reported 8 cases of hookworm infestation on stool samples submitted for analysis; the corresponding figures for 1994 and 1995 were 15 and 10, respectively. In 1993, 15 cases of *Trichuris* infestation were reported; 14 were reported in 1994 and 8 in 1995. Two cases of Ascariasis were reported in 1993 and no cases were reported in 1994 or 1995.

Chronic Communicable Diseases: Tuberculosis and Leprosy. In 1993, two cases and two deaths of tuberculosis were reported; eight cases and six deaths were reported in 1994 and six cases in 1995. One case of leprosy was reported in 1993; no cases were reported in 1994 or 1995.

Acute Respiratory Infections. In 1993, 21 cases of bronchopneumonia were reported in the age group under 5 years old; there were 12 and 13 cases reported in 1994 and 1995, respectively.

Asthma is a significant cause of morbidity, with a prevalence rate of 12%. The Accident and Emergency Department of Queen Elizabeth Hospital records an average of 8,000 to 10,000 attendances every year.

Rabies and Other Zoonoses. No cases of rabies were reported in the 1993–1995 period. Of the 31 leptospirosis cases reported in 1993, 6 died. In 1994 there were 17 cases and 4 deaths, and in 1995, there were 34 cases and 8 deaths. Barbados has the only leptospirosis laboratory in the subregion, which performs diagnostic work for other Caribbean territories; the laboratory also provides training for these other territories.

AIDS and Other STDs. Although sexually transmitted diseases are not notifiable by law, basic figures obtained from government clinics show a decline in syphilis and gonorrhea between 1992 and 1995.

Sexual contact is the predominant mode of HIV transmission, accounting for approximately 98.9% of total cases in the adult population. Perinatal transmission accounted for 4.2% in 1995. Of the 95 cases diagnosed in 1995, two occurred in the age group under 5 years old; 5 occurred in this age group in 1994.

In 1993, 59 males and 29 females were diagnosed as having AIDS; in 1994, the figures were 92 males and 27 females; and in 1995, there were 76 males and 19 females.

Of 3,053 blood donors tested for HIV in 1993, 10 were positive. The figures for 1994 and 1995 were 9 out of 2,830 and 9 out of 2,824, respectively. Of 2,904 blood donations tested in 1996, 6 (0.2%) were positive for syphilis (VDRL): 13 (0.4%), positive for hepatitis B; 8 (0.3%), positive for hepatitis C; and 22 (0.8%), positive for HTLV1.

Noncommunicable Diseases and Other Health-Related Problems

Cardiovascular Disease. In 1993, there were 593 (3.9%) hospital admissions for heart disease, out of a total of 16,980. Diabetes mellitus accounted for 422 of admissions to the Queen Elizabeth Hospital in 1993. For both diseases and for the same year, the age group over 45 years old accounted for more discharges from the Queen Elizabeth Hospital than any other age group.

Malignant Tumors. In 1993 there were 804 hospital admissions for malignant neoplasms, distributed in the following sites: 47 stomach; 41 colon; 128 prostate; 46 cervix; 103 female breast; and 43 trachea, bronchus, and lung. Benign neoplasms of the uterus accounted for 493 admissions and hyperplasia of prostate, 81.

The most common cancer site in women 15 years old and older was breast, followed by the cervix. About 10,000 Pap smears are performed every year. A 1995 KAP survey showed that 90% of the at-risk population had been screened in the preceding five years; the survey also showed that those at greatest risk (women aged 55–70) were not being adequately screened. In men, cancer of prostate is the most frequent cancer site, accounting for 82 deaths in men 45 years and older.

Accidents and Violence. Accidents and violence accounted for 3,131 admissions (16.8% of total) in 1993. From 1992–1995, admissions due to accidents, falls, and motor vehicle accidents accounted for most admissions to Queen Elizabeth Hospital. There were fewer admissions for accidents caused by fire.

Certain highly vulnerable groups such as women, young men, children, and the elderly, suffer disproportionately from violence. The 1982 Family Law Act continues to provide protection for women and children. Studies of child abuse in Barbados confirm that sexual violence against children, especially incest, is increasing and dealt with as a priority.

Many young men suffer serious physical injury from armed confrontations (stabbing, gunshot, and cutlass wounds). Use of guns and cutlasses is a serious problem, and recent statistics show that it costs Queen Elizabeth Hospital $1,500 per day to treat a person suffering from such wounds. Armed confrontation has become a public health epidemic that is putting a strain on the health budget and has become a high public health priority. The Ministry is currently developing strategies to deal with violence.

Behavioral Disorders. In 1995, there were 1,107 admissions to the Psychiatric Hospital; in 1991, there were 1,181. The mental health care system provides outpatient services, day care programs, specialized professional services (social work, psychology, psychotherapy, occupational therapy, and workshops), and consultation services at Queen Elizabeth Hospital and at the medical clinic at Her Majesty's Prison.

RESPONSE OF THE HEALTH SYSTEM

National Health Plans and Policies

The Government of Barbados views health care as a fundamental right of all Barbadians. It is responsible for ensuring that basic conditions for healthy living exist and for creating an atmosphere that fosters healthy choices. To this end, the Government aims to provide comprehensive health care to all its citizens at an affordable cost to the country and to ensure that environmental concerns are considered in all aspects of national development. Further, the Government is committed to ensuring that all citizens have access to clean drinking water, proper sanitation, and a safe environment free from health hazards.

The Ministry of Health, through its Environmental Engineering Division, regulates and monitors the environmental impact of development projects with respect to water quality, solid and liquid waste disposal, air quality, noise pollution, and the control and disposal of hazardous chemicals. The Ministry of Health's Sanitation Service Authority is responsible for the collection and disposal of domestic household garbage.

The Public Health Inspectorate—staffed by environmental health officers—is the main mechanism for monitoring domestic environmental quality. Food safety and the control of communicable diseases fall under this division.

The Government has begun to implement a solid waste management plan that will encompass waste minimization, waste recycling, and waste reuse. Inadequate financing continues to significantly constrain environmental quality programs; maintaining environmental quality will incur increasing recurring costs, and new programs will require significant additional capital.

In keeping with the Declaration of Alma Ata, emphasizing "health for all by the year 2000," primary health care has remained an integral part of the country's health care delivery system and of the community's overall social and economic development. A community approach to primary health care and better utilization of governmental and nongovernmental organizations are being emphasized.

Services at government facilities are free of cost at the point of delivery. Private health services also are offered and are mainly used by those who can afford to pay.

The Ministry's priority programs, which are in keeping with the goals and targets of the Caribbean Cooperation in Health initiative, are committed to improving the conditions of vulnerable, high-risk population groups such as the elderly, the disabled, women of childbearing age, children, adolescents, the physically challenged, and the mentally ill.

Nutrition programs geared at improving the nutritional status of the Barbadian population have continued in the polyclinics, at the community level, and within the schools. The family planning and family life education programs have been strengthened and are now in place at all of the polyclinics.

The Ministry of Health continues to view health promotion and education as a critical component of its primary health care strategy and to collaborate with NGOs to promote healthy lifestyles. Health promotion programs such as those operated by the Barbados Youth Service and the Juvenile Liaison Scheme address illegal drug use among youth. Some NGOs, such as the Barbados Family Planning Association, the Barbados Cancer Society, the Heart Foundation of Barbados, the Kidney Association, the Association for Disabled Persons, and the Diabetic Association, are actively involved in providing services.

The Ministry of Health, insofar as its financial resources have permitted, has continued to arrange for personnel training both domestically and abroad.

The Government's policy regarding drugs and related items is to provide them free of cost at the point of services to clients seen by a government doctor. Under the Special Benefit Service, listed in the Barbados Drug Formulary also are free at the point of service to persons 65 years of age and over; children under 16 years of age; and persons being treated for hypertension, diabetes, cancer, asthma, and epilepsy. In 1995, the Government adopted a policy to distribute Zidovudine (AZT) to all pregnant women who were HIV-positive; a protocol was set out for mother and child.

Given the fact that the Government accounts for the larger share of spending in health, restrictions in government revenues have a significant and direct effect on health sector activity.

Data indicate that for the most recent seven years the Government of Barbados has committed an average of 18% of its revenues to the Ministry of Health. This level was maintained even during the difficult economic period between 1988 and 1993, when the country's GDP fell from 3.5% to 0.04%, after a brief spike to 5.6% in 1992, and its fiscal deficit ballooned from 4% of GDP in 1988 to 7.2% in 1990, before falling back to 2% by 1993.

Health Sector Reform

As a way to improve health care quality, enhance delivery efficiency, contain costs, increase equity in access, and strengthen public/private collaboration, the Government commissioned a study on the rationalization of the health sector as a whole. The results of this IDB-funded study, which is near completion, will be used to improve existing services so they can better meet the needs of the community. Although the study will examine all areas of the health sector and recommend strategies for effective and efficient allocation of programs and facilities, it will focus on three major areas.

First, chronic care, rehabilitation, and health promotion will be assessed, with a view to rationalizing care for the elderly, the disabled, and persons with chronic diseases and conditions and psychiatric care. A review of current health promotion and education efforts will lay the foundation for addressing lifestyle health choices and changes into the 21st century. Second, primary, secondary, and tertiary care will be studied to evaluate how these health services might function in the future, in light of a greater demand for high-cost technology, an aging population, an increase in chronic health problems, and constraints on public financial resources. Finally, the health sector's efficiency will be analyzed as a way to provide cost and service information for developing or modifying health care policies and ensuring their financial sustainability.

The Government also is contemplating reforms of other sectors that provide health-related services. A Green Paper on Housing is expected to become national policy for ensuring the provision of adequate shelter and financing home ownership for all.

Organization of the Health Sector

Institutional Organization

The Government operates Queen Elizabeth Hospital (a large secondary and tertiary care facility), a network of four district hospitals for geriatric care, a main geriatric institution, a mental health hospital and a half-way house, two small rehabilitation institutions for the physically and mentally handicapped, an AIDS hostel, a development center for disabled children and adolescents, and a nutrition center.

A nationwide network of eight polyclinics provides a wide range of preventive and curative services, as well as limited rehabilitative services. These polyclinics and four satellite stations provide traditional public health services such as maternal and child health, family life development, communicable disease control, community mental health, chronic disease programs; dental health, nutrition, and general practice. These services also cover environmental health, which includes food hygiene, mosquito and rodent control, building development control, atmospheric and chemical pollution monitoring and control, monitoring and control of water quality, monitoring and control of sewage disposal, solid waste disposal, the maintenance of cemeteries, and the licensing and control of stray dogs.

The Government also operates the Barbados Drug Service, a WHO Collaborating Center that controls the importation and distribution of essential drugs in the country, thus ensuring that Barbadians receive affordable quality drugs and pharmaceuticals.

The private sector is well developed, with about 100 general practitioners operating singly or in multiple practice; consultants (senior doctors working in government hospitals or polyclinics) also have private practices. There is only one small private hospital in the country—Bayview Hospital—with fewer than 30 beds, representing under 4% of the country's total acute bed capacity. Private sector health services and facilities also include 18 homes for long-term care, as well as pharmaceutical, laboratory, diagnostic, dental, psychiatric, and physical therapy services.

Staff at all levels are well trained and continue to receive regular updates. All of the polyclinics are supplied with the necessary equipment for the delivery of quality health care. There is a referral system between clinic, hospital, and other support services.

The Ministry maintains autonomy over the health services. The decision on how money is to be spent lies within the Ministry, but the Ministry of Finance appropriates the overall budgetary allocation. And while the Government exercises some independent control over health professionals with regard to health service legislation, physicians and nurses maintain involvement in health policy dialogue through their own trade union.

In order to improve health, the health sector must work with other public sector agencies, the private sector, civic organizations, community groups, and citizens. The Ministry of Health, the private sector, and other government ministries collaborate on several activities, such as the vector control ed-

ucation program, "World Health Day," "World Environmental Day," and "World AIDS Day."

Health Services Delivery. Health service delivery falls into the following seven program areas: primary health care; 24-hour acute, secondary, tertiary and emergency care; mental health care; care for the elderly including rehabilitation services; drug service; assessment services and rehabilitative care; and health promotion. Primary health care services encompass maternal and child health; family life development, including family planning and ophthalmic and dental care for schoolchildren; care for the disabled, pregnant women, and the elderly; general medical care with clinics for hypertension, diabetes, and sexually transmitted diseases; nutrition; pharmaceutical services; and community mental health and environmental health care.

The Chief Medical Officer is responsible for all matters affecting public health and medical services on the island, advising the Minister of Health and Environment on these matters; the Chief Medical Officer also plays an integral role in health planning and health infrastructure development. Two Senior Medical Officers support the work of the Chief Medical Officer, and a team approach is applied for each program area.

Each polyclinic is managed by a Medical Officer, who functions as a clinician and an administrator, heads a team of clinical medical officers and public health nurses, and works closely with the Public Health Inspectorate. Additional staff comprises pharmacists, community nutrition officers, dental officers, and other ancillary personnel. An administrator, a clinician, support medical staff, and other ancillary staff similarly run other institutions.

The major problem at the primary health care level is the shortage of staff resources, especially at the clinical level. This results in longer waiting periods and the inability to offer services at some of the polyclinics after 4:30 p.m. and on weekends.

At the secondary care level, the Government operates the Queen Elizabeth Hospital, a 547-bed facility that offers 24-hour acute, secondary, tertiary, and emergency care. The hospital houses more than 90% of the country's acute care beds; clinical services include accident emergency and outpatient and inpatient care in surgery, medicine, pediatrics, obstetrics and gynecology, pathology, radiology, radiotherapy, rehabilitation therapy, ophthalmology, and ear, nose, and throat. The hospital's diagnostic equipment includes a CAT scan and ultrasound and modern radiotherapy equipment. A cardiac catherization unit was established in 1993, and by the end of 1996 had performed 50 open-heart surgeries and 242 cardiac catherizations.

Mental health care is provided by the government owned psychiatric hospital, which has 627 beds, and at the 8-bed unit at Queen Elizabeth Hospital. The Psychiatric Hospital offers the following services: acute psychiatric care, including child and adolescent care; long-stay psycho-geriatric care; forensic psychiatric care; care for the subnormal; and addiction services. Community mental health services include a district nursing service that follows up persons who have been discharged from the hospital, and a primary community mental health program offered from the polyclinics.

Organization of Health Regulatory Activities

The country has a comprehensive health legislation. The Health Services Act and its regulations, which were enacted in the late 1960s and early 1970s, cover all areas that fall under the jurisdiction of the Ministry of Health and the Environment. The Ministry has undertaken to improve the legislation for effective administration of the health services, the regulation of related public activity, and the services given to the public. Among laws to be reviewed and amended are: the Dental Registration Act; regulations regarding alternative medicine; food hygiene and restaurant regulations as they relate to street vending operations, random testing of food-handlers for foodborne illnesses, and mandatory training of food-handlers; the Mental Health Act and all related legislative instruments that affect mental health, such as housing; and the General Nursing Council Act, regarding the enforcement of the regional examination and registration for nurses. In addition, the solid waste management plan, the regulation of private hospitals and nursing homes, regulation of organ donation and organ transplant, the development of a national oil spill contingency plan, registration of medical specialists, and the establishment of criteria for general fitness to practice medicine will all be part of the review and reform process.

Certification and Practice of Health Professions. Several pieces of legislation regulate the registration, licensing, and governance of health professionals through the establishment of councils. There are councils for medical, dental, general nursing, pharmacy, and paramedical professions. The last one, which encompasses such professions as physiotherapists, occupational therapists, chiropractors, and laboratory technologists, may be amended to include nutritionists, acupuncturists, and osteopaths.

Food Safety. Barbados has specific health regulations designed to control food safety, and public health inspectors who issue licenses to all food establishments enforce these regulations. Currently, these regulations are under review, so that food handlers will only be issued their annual licenses after undergoing several training sessions. Legislation dealing with the licensing and control of the increasing number of itinerant vendors also is being reviewed.

Health Services and Resources

Organization of Services for Care of the Population

Health Promotion, Health Settings and Environments, Social Communication. Health promotion is viewed as a strategy for protecting and improving public health through the encouragement of individual and collective initiatives and actions. Barbados regards health promotion as key in achieving "health for all by the year 2000" by promoting healthy lifestyles; involving community residents in the delivery of their own health care, especially preventive care; and creating an environment that makes it possible to live a healthy life.

The country has no formal health promotion program. Various groups working in advocacy and support activities emphasize different components, but the links among these groups are often weak, resulting in poor communication and duplication of efforts. The Government acknowledges the need for better links and for strengthening the role of the Ministry of Health and the Environment as coordinator and facilitator.

In October 1993, Barbados participated in a PAHO-sponsored subregional workshop on health promotion designed to develop a cadre of health educators who could help integrate health promotion principles and strategies into health programs and projects. As an outgrowth of this workshop, in 1997 a national consultation on health promotion will bring together multisectoral private- and public-sector groups to develop a common framework for understanding and advancing health promotion in Barbados.

The Ministry of Health sees public relations, information, and communications as important aspects of policy and strategy, and attaches importance to ensuring that the public is informed about the principles, policies, and achievements of the Ministry, as well as the Ministry's position on any issue. The Government Information Service assists the Ministry in maintaining effective channels of communication with all identifiable public within the nation as a whole.

Programs for Disease Prevention and Control. Special clinics have been established at the polyclinics for diabetes mellitus, hypertension, and STDs.

A national AIDS Program was established in 1988 to implement projects aimed at reducing HIV transmission and providing care and support to persons who were HIV-infected or affected by the disease. The program uses a multisectoral approach. To date, the program has organized workshops to sensitize public and private sector policymakers; identified community members who are working in AIDS education and care, as a way to establish a national network; trained doctors to deliver lectures/presentation on HIV/AIDS; established a 9-bed residential care facility for homeless persons with AIDS; and trained primary and secondary school teachers to educate students about HIV.

The Ministry of Health's Vector Control Division routinely conducts mosquito surveillance throughout the country, targeting high risk areas; *Aedes aegypti* indices, which help to identify target areas for intervention, are reported weekly. The services of the Vector Control Division integrate central strategies with those of the Public Health Inspectorate services. Identified foci are treated with larvicides and insecticides where indicated; in addition, thermal fogging of areas for greater coverage is ongoing, and areas where greatest mosquito activity or dengue fever occurrence is reported are targeted.

The Rodent Control Unit in the Vector Control Division distributes rat bait free of charge to all residents through the polyclinics. The Ministry of Agriculture and the Barbados Agricultural Society also supply rodenticide to the business sector, plantations, and estates. Government facilities including the seaport and airport are included in the Rodent Control Unit's programs and are baited at regular intervals.

Dengue fever is a notifiable disease and is passively reported. Since 1995, an active surveillance program was put in place to facilitate the early detection of an outbreak. The public health inspectorate's efforts included education programs, surveillance of the disease by geographic mapping of cases (suspected and confirmed), and surveillance of the mosquito index within the various catchment areas. In addition, in March 1995, a national clean-up campaign was launched to reduce potential breeding sites for *Aedes aegypti*. The campaign covered the private and public sectors, and removed more than 1,500 truckloads of solid waste from various locations throughout the country.

The country's Expanded Program of Immunization includes vaccination for polio, diphtheria, pertussis, tetanus, measles, mumps, and rubella. The program has attained a coverage of 93% of the eligible population (i.e., infants reaching their first birthday). In order to ensure adequate immunization coverage for EPI target diseases, the need for immunization was publicized to all the population, immunizations were made a legal requirement for school entry, and a computerized tracking system for all births was set up.

Epidemiological Surveillance Systems and Public Health Laboratories. Barbados has no physical epidemiological unit, but one of the Senior Medical Officers has been designated national epidemiologist; he is assisted by five deputies who are public health inspectors trained to investigate diseases at the community level.

The country has developed and implemented an active surveillance program for diarrheal disease, acute flaccid paralysis, acute febrile rash illness, and, more recently, congenital rubella syndrome. There is one public health laboratory located at the largest polyclinic, which performs tests in bacteriology, parasitology, and urinalysis.

Between 80% and 90% of essential drugs are available on location at most facilities, and the remainder can be made available at the Barbados Drug Service.

Drinking Water Services and Sewerage. The Barbados Water Authority (BWA) is the statutory corporation responsible for providing potable water to the citizens of Barbados. BWA conducts water quality monitoring (surveillance) programs for groundwater supply in conjunction with the Public Health Inspectorate. In 1995, the Authority commissioned a study on water loss that identified leaks throughout the island and recommended ways to minimize water losses. It is estimated that 90% of the groundwater resources are already committed, and are being utilized for public and private abstractions.

The Government acknowledges the importance of preserving the country's ecosystem, by improving sewage disposal along the densely populated tourist service areas on the south and west coasts and in Greater Bridgetown. The Bridgetown Sewerage Project was completed, and the contract for the construction of the sewage treatment plant for the south coast sewerage project was awarded in August 1995; several million Barbados dollars are expected to be spent in the construction. The sewerage project for the west coast is in its final design stage.

Management of Municipal Solid Waste Services. Concern over the increase in the generation of solid waste and the subsequent high incidence of illegal dumping practices has led the Ministry of Health and the Environment to give high priority to integrated solid waste management. In 1997, the Ministry was expected to complete the construction of a modern landfill that is destined to have a life-span of 10 to 15 years. In addition, the Government will also increase its monitoring of these dumps and prosecute anyone disposing of waste illegally.

Environmental Quality. The Environmental Engineering Division of the Ministry of Health and Environment is responsible for environmental protection. Its main functions include ensuring that buildings conform to public health standards; monitoring and controlling freshwater and marine water quality; monitoring and controlling noise pollution; recognizing, evaluating, and controlling air pollutants; managing disposal sites for derelict vehicles, blood, grease, asbestos, and night soil; monitoring and controlling derelict buildings and vehicles; monitoring the operations license regulations of public swimming pools; evaluating and carrying out corrective measures for dealing with workers' health; monitoring and controlling waste disposal, including hazardous waste; conducting public education programs on environmental matters; advising and assisting the Ministry of Health in all environmental engineering matters; and applying relevant provisions of the Health Services Regulations.

Food Protection and Control. The Ministry provides food handling courses for its institutions and for the hotel industry. Since 1995, food handling training has been structured as programs or clinics organized for certain health institutions and several hotels.

Food Assistance Program. The school-meals program for primary school students is heavily subsidized so as to make daily meals affordable to almost all children. The Welfare Board, the Barbados Red Cross Society, church-based organizations, and other NGOs provide food assistance to the needy. In the public sector, the National Assistance Board assigns home helpers to prepare meals and take care of the elderly who live alone. The National Advisory Committee on AIDS facilitates a food bank program by soliciting donations for persons with AIDS.

Organization and Operation of Personal Health Care Services

Ambulatory Services, Hospitals, and Emergency Services. Ambulatory visits are made to a variety of public sector facilities and programs, including primary and specialist care, outpatient clinics and services offered weekly at Queen Elizabeth Hospital, the polyclinics and their associated outpatient clinics and district outreach activities, outpatient clinics and district activities at the Psychiatric Hospital, two general practice clinics associated with the University of the West Indies, and the clinics at the Barbados Defence Force and Glendairy Prisons.

More than one-half of medical visits to public ambulatory care facilities were made at polyclinics and their satellite outpatient clinics, and the overwhelming majority of dental visits for children, pregnant women, and the elderly (95%) were made there as well. These findings are consistent with the Government's continuing emphasis on general access to primary care through strategically located clinics. During 1995, there were 596,571 ambulatory visits, of which 60% were to polyclinics. In the same year, oral health visits accounted for 620,808 outpatients, 95% of them in polyclinics.

The private sector supplies most of the ambulatory services each year, although trend data on private sector utilization of ambulatory services are not available. The private sector surpasses public clinics as a provider of medical/surgical ambulatory services only by a modest margin (55% vs. 45%,

respectively, in 1995), and it overwhelmingly outdistances them as a provider of dental services, because free dental care is available at the polyclinics only on a limited scale—to children under the age of 18, pregnant women, and elderly persons under certain circumstances. In short, the adult population is financially responsible for its own dental care.

Visits for medical services (740,647) in the private sector are largely made up of visits to private practice physicians (97%). However, some nongovernmental organizations also provide services: for example, the Family Planning Association provides clinical services, the Heart Foundation offers cardiac rehabilitation services, and the Cancer Society and the Diabetic Association offer disease screening and management services.

The two largest components of outpatient service at Queen Elizabeth Hospital are the specialist clinics and the Accident and Emergency Department. While utilization of the department has remained relatively stable since 1988 (between 50,000 and 57,000 attendances), utilization of the specialist clinics has increased to 63% since that year. This increase could be due to the expansion of the population in Queen Elizabeth Hospital's catchment area. However, utilization of the Sir Winston Scott Polyclinic, which is in the same catchment area, has actually decreased. The previously mentioned study on the health sector's rationalization is expected to explain the discrepancy.

Auxiliary Services for Diagnosis and Blood Banks. More than 1.25 million individual laboratory tests were completed in Barbados in 1995, amounting to approximately 5 tests per person per year; 81% of all tests were performed at the two public laboratories at Sir Winston Scott Polyclinic and Queen Elizabeth Hospital. Four private laboratories on the island together account for one-fifth of the national laboratory testing. The blood bank routinely screens donor blood for HIV, hepatitis B, hepatitis C, HLTV1, and syphilis.

As a way to renew the strategy for health in diagnostics, laboratory capacity is being strengthened to facilitate dengue testing, more health promotion and education materials are being produced, the collaboration of NGOs, churches, and other community groups is being enlisted, and the infrastructure to deliver the support services for individuals in need is being further developed.

Specialized Services. Specialized services in obstetrics and gynecology; ears, nose, and throat; ophthalmology; invasive cardiology; renal dialysis; gerontology; radiotherapy; radiology; mental and physical rehabilitation; and oral and maxillofacial surgery are available in both the public and private sectors. Other specialist services include an AIDS hostel, a Soroptomist Village for the elderly, and the privately run substance abuse foundation.

Inputs for Health

Drugs. The drug supply service has been generally successful in maintaining a continuous supply of formulary drugs and related items in the country. The Barbados Drug Service procures its drugs from the one local drug manufacturer, and more extensively from market sources in the U.S.A, Canada, South America, and Europe.

Immunobiologicals and Reagents. Vaccines are bought through the PAHO Revolving Fund. Reagents for use in the laboratory and diagnostic procedures are readily available; most are imported.

Human Resources

According to the Ministry of Health's Statistical Records, in 1994, Barbados had the following numbers of health personnel, by category: 355 doctors, 48 dentists, 898 nurses, 2 sanitary engineers, 9 veterinarians, and 970 technologists and assistants.

Continuing education is promoted as an integral part of personnel development and as a means of keeping the various disciplines updated. In 1988, the Ministry of Health prepared a five-year development training plan to meet its requirements. Much emphasis has been placed on in-service and local training, especially in priority areas such as geriatric nursing, radiography, orthopedics, environmental impact assessment, health planning, and hospital management.

Queen Elizabeth Hospital is a teaching hospital and is used by the University of the West Indies Faculty of Clinical Medicine and Research for preclinical training or internships for medical graduates. The internship is a carefully supervised and monitored system of continuing medical education.

The Barbados Community College School of Nursing provides similar apprenticeships for nurses. A wide range of allied health professionals such as public health inspectors, medical records clerks, medical laboratory technicians, pharmacists, and occupational therapy assistants receive training at the College.

In general, the numbers in medical and nursing professions have reached an equilibrium, in that enough are produced to meet the needs of the country; this is particularly true in the medical arena. The Government is being forced to revisit the issue of medical student sponsorship because of the rapid growth in Barbadians seeking to enter the medical profession and Queen Elizabeth Hospital's strained finances. However, in light of the growing need for social support and rehabilitative services, some of the paramedical professionals such as nutritionists, physiotherapists, chiropodists, and x-ray technicians are still needed.

Research and Technology

Health research and technology development both within and outside the Ministry, particularly at the University of the West Indies, have been undertaken in chronic noncommunicable diseases such as obesity, hypertension, and diabetes and their complications. Other research projects that have been undertaken by the Ministry within the period dealt with major causes of morbidity and mortality such as AIDS and cancer, including the risk factor survey and a knowledge attitude and practice (KAP) study relating to a cervical cancer control project. The Faculty of Medical Sciences at the University of the West Indies has already undertaken extensive research in the areas of hypertension and diabetes. Collaboration between the Ministry and the University has led to the setting up of a diabetes model clinic and the preparation of guidelines for the clinical management of diabetes. Funding for research remains the main constraint to improving health research and technology, but government initiatives such as the Chronic Disease Research Centre, should lessen the impact of financial constraints. Donations for this center are expected from private sector enterprises.

BELIZE

GENERAL SITUATION AND TRENDS

Socioeconomic, Political, and Demographic Overview

Belize is bordered by Mexico on the north, Guatemala on the west and south, and the Caribbean Sea on the east. Its land area is 22,700 km². The northern and southern coasts are plains, with mangrove swamps. The Maya Mountains are in south central Belize and occupy much of the country. Some 65% of the country is classified as forest, 36% of which is set aside as reserves and protected areas. The climate is subtropical, with temperatures ranging from 10°C to 35°C; annual mean rainfall ranges from 150 mm to 2,650 mm. Belize is the only English-speaking country in Central America, although Spanish is also widely spoken; it is more similar to Caribbean countries in culture, politics, and economy.

Belize is a sovereign state governed by a parliamentary democracy based on the British system. The Head of State is Queen Elizabeth II, who is represented by a Governor General. The Prime Minister and Cabinet constitute the executive branch, and a 29-member elected House of Representatives and an 8-member appointed Senate form the bicameral legislature. The Cabinet members are appointed by the Governor General on the advice of the Prime Minister.

The country is divided into six administrative districts: Corozal, Orange Walk, Belize, Cayo, Stann Creek, and Toledo. Each district is administered by a locally elected board, and a mayor and village council govern at the village level. Although the capital was moved to Belmopan in 1981, Belize City remains the commercial center with almost a quarter of the population.

Population

The 1991 census put Belize's population at 189,392, while the estimate for 1996 was 222,000. Over 42% of residents were under the age of 15, and 61% are under 25 years of age, with similar proportions of women and men. In 1991, the rural population surpassed the urban due to an influx of immigrants. According to reports from the Office of the United Nations High Commissioner for Refugees, the migrant population was approximately 30,000, or 14% of the total; the 1995 National Survey conducted by the Central Statistics Office indicated that immigrants comprised 12% of the population.

According to the census, the Mestizo ethnic group (persons of mixed heritage descended from Spanish colonists and indigenous peoples) represented 44% and the Creole (of mixed African and European heritage) represented 30% of the population. Other ethnic groups include the Maya (12%), Garífuna (7%), East Indian (4%), and other smaller groups. Between 1984 and 1996 the Government promoted immigration, mainly targeted at Asian immigrants. In 1996, Belizeans of Asian origin comprised 2.5% of the population.

The annual population growth rate in 1996 was 2.5% compared to 2.6% in 1991. The total fertility rate was estimated at 4.6 children per woman, showing a steady downward trend from 7 children per woman in the 1960s. In 1991, estimated life expectancy at birth was 69.9 years for males and 74.1 years for females. A 1996 estimate showed the crude death rate to be 4.3 deaths per 1,000 population.

Economic Situation

The country has an economy primarily based on agriculture and services. A stable currency is one of the attractions for foreign investment. The 1996 per capita income was US$ 2,308 compared to US$ 1,664 in 1989, a growth of 39%. The gross domestic product (GDP) increased by 67% from US$ 306 million in 1989 to US$ 512 million in 1996, while the population grew by 21%. The GDP had a real growth rate of 1.5% in 1996, compared to 3.8% in 1995. Although inflation is low, it increased in 1996. The consumer price index was 2.8% in 1995 and 6.4% in 1996, averaging 3.2% the previous five years.

The economy is dominated by agricultural exports including sugar cane, citrus concentrate, bananas, and marine products, which made up 77% of exports in 1996. Belize also relies on forestry, fishing, and mining, which, combined with agriculture, account for 22% of the GDP.

Recent trends have increased the trade deficit, putting pressure on net foreign reserves. A lack of public savings, expansion of fixed investments, declining foreign assistance, and rising levels of external debt increased government deficits. Although the Government reduced expenditure, it has not succeeded in generating the resources needed to expand the infrastructure base. Reduced Government spending has resulted in cuts in health services for rural communities and curtailed services in health posts and mobile clinics. The Government is reorganizing its tax structure, which will affect the poor. The Social Investment Fund, containing US$ 10 million, was created to promote productive and social interventions in highly underprivileged population groups, and should help to alleviate poverty.

Social Situation

A 1995 Poverty Assessment Report by the Caribbean Development Bank, the Ministry of Economic Development, and the Central Statistics Office concluded that 33% of Belizeans were poor (unable to meet expenditures on basic food and non-food items), while 13% were very poor (unable to meet expenses on basic food items). Of heads of households, 24% of males and 31% of females were considered poor. In Toledo district, where a majority of the Maya live, 58% of the population was poor; 41% in Cayo District, and 25% of Orange Walk, Corozal, Belize, and Stann Creek Districts were classified as poor.

The 1991 census indicated that the majority of households consist of five or more persons. The 1996 Labour Force Survey showed a drop to 4.5 persons per household. Over 20% of households in the country comprise less than two persons. Average household size in the rural areas was larger than in urban areas. Nationwide, 22% of households were headed by females, except in Belize District, where the figure was as high as 33%. The census also indicated that 63% of houses had two or fewer bedrooms. Approximately 66% of all houses were either owned or being bought, while over 20% were rented. Houses were more often owned in the rural than in urban areas.

Of the estimated 1996 population, the survey indicated that 65,025 persons were employed and 10,425 unemployed, which gives an unemployment rate of 13.8%, a 1.3% increase

from 1995. Unemployment was highest in Belize District (18.4%), followed by Stann Creek (15.4%), Cayo (15.2%), Toledo (14.3%), Orange Walk (6.6%), and Corozal (5.8%). Unskilled labor occupied 63% of the workers in 1996. Of the employed force, 22% had not completed primary school, 47% had a primary school education, and 15% had completed high school. Mennonites had the highest employment rate (99.3%) and the Garífuna had the lowest (75.7%). The Creole and Mestizo comprised 75% of the unemployed force. Around 71% of the employed were males. In the 14–19-year-old age group, 32.2% of males and 45.5% of females were unemployed.

It is estimated that 100% of the urban and 69% of the rural population had a safe and adequate water supply. Belize District had the highest coverage levels (91%) and Toledo, the lowest (71%). The other districts have coverage levels between 82% and 85%. Nationwide, 39% of the population had adequate sanitation facilities; the figures were 59% in urban and 22% in rural areas. Solid waste management is a problem throughout Belize; this is exacerbated by drainage problems in Belize District.

Primary school attendance is free and compulsory up to age 14, but approximately 36% of children do not complete it. Census data were used to assess the basic literacy rate, considering those who completed up to standard five or beyond of the formal education system to be literate. Using this definition, the basic literacy rate was 70%. In 1996, the Central Statistics Office added a literacy survey module to the Labour Force Survey in order to assess functional literacy (measured by specific reading and comprehension skills) as well as basic literacy nationwide. The survey showed basic literacy to be 75.1%, although only 42.4% of the population 10–65 years old were functionally literate. According to the census, 48.6% of primary schoolteachers were fully trained; these figures were 81% in Belize District, compared to only 27% in Toledo.

Although few statistics are available by sex, some provide a profile of the status of women in the society. Women are classified as poorer than men. One of 29 seats in the House of Representatives is held by a woman. Only 2.4% of females complete pre-university education. Senior management positions are held by 1.9% of women; 22% are employed in unskilled jobs, and 18% are unemployed. Over half of pregnant women (51.7%) suffer from iron deficiency anemia. Since the passage of the Domestic Violence Act in 1993, the number of protection orders granted has increased by over 300%.

Mortality Profile

Life expectancy at birth increased from 68.4 years in 1980 to 71.8 years in 1991. In 1980, females had 2.2 more years of life expectancy than males (69.8 vs. 67.6), a gap that widened to 4.8 years by 1991 (74.7 vs. 69.9). The infant mortality rate showed a decreasing trend, from 31.5 deaths per 1,000 live births in 1993 to 26.0 in 1996. Maternal mortality fluctuated from 16.1 in 1993 (10 deaths) to 8.2 (5 deaths) in 1995, increasing to 13.9 (9 deaths) in 1996. The leading causes of maternal deaths were hemorrhage, pulmonary embolism, eclampsia, and abortion.

The crude mortality rate remained around 4 deaths per 1,000 population from 1993 to 1996 (4.0, 3.6, 4.3, and 4.0 for those years, respectively). The mean mortality rate among males (4.6) was 40% higher than that of females (3.4). Belize District reported the highest rate (6.0), while Cayo had the lowest (2.5).

Mortality was dominated by noncommunicable and chronic causes during the 1992–1996 period. Heart diseases were the leading cause for both males and females. An average of 20% of deaths were due to heart diseases, with a decreasing trend from 22% in 1993 to 16% in 1996. Respiratory diseases were the second most frequent cause (10%–14% of deaths), except in 1994 when it ranked fourth (7%). Cerebrovascular diseases and malignant neoplasms accounted for 7%–9% of deaths, but neoplasms were more frequent as a cause of death among females (8%–11%). The assessment of neoplasms is limited by the lack of oncological services in Belize. External causes (excluding road traffic accidents, homicides, and suicides) accounted for 4%–5% of deaths, ranking fifth. Among males, road traffic accidents were an increasing cause of death, while among females it did not figure in the leading causes. Suicides increased from 1 case in 1994 to 11 cases in 1995, totaling 20 cases over the period. Nineteen of the suicides were males.

The leading causes of morbidity, as measured by the number of hospitalizations, were respiratory diseases, particularly in males. The second cause of morbidity in males was intestinal disease. Among females, complications of pregnancy ranked first, respiratory diseases, second, and abortion, third. The high prevalence of anemia in pregnant women (51.7% at prenatal clinics) aggravates the outcome of pregnancy complications. Orange Walk, Stann Creek, and Toledo districts reported respiratory diseases as leading causes of hospital morbidity during the period. In contrast, Cayo District reported complications of pregnancy as the leading cause, followed by respiratory diseases. In Orange Walk District, "other injuries" was the second cause of morbidity among males, while complications of pregnancy ranked second among females. In Belize District, abortion was the second cause of hospital morbidity among females, while "other injuries" ranked second among males for the years 1993 and 1996. Malaria ranked among the five leading causes of hospital morbidity in Stann Creek District.

SPECIFIC HEALTH PROBLEMS

Analysis by Population Group

Health of Children

Infant Health. In children under 1 year old, mortality rate decreased by 20% from 31.5 deaths per 1,000 live births in 1993 to 26 in 1996. Corozal and Cayo Districts had the lowest rates (13.8 and 17.9), while Orange Walk, Stann Creek, and Toledo Districts had the highest (32.6, 33.2, and 30.1, respectively). The decreasing trend observed nationally was seen in Corozal, Cayo, and Stann Creek Districts. The rate increased in Toledo from 29.4 in 1993 to 52.1 in 1994, and decreased to 30.1 in 1996 (no known explanation exists for this change). It increased in Belize District in 1995 and 1996. More males (62.1%) than females died during this period.

The main cause of infant mortality during the 1993–1996 period was "conditions originating during the perinatal period" (36% of deaths), increasing from 29% in 1993 to 39% in 1996. Asphyxia was the most important cause of death among conditions originating in the perinatal period (32%), followed by low birthweight (28%), and infections (11%). Nearly 62% of perinatal deaths occurred in males; 68% of asphyxia cases were males. The second cause of infant mortality was infectious diseases (24% of deaths); respiratory diseases were responsible for 12% of deaths. The frequency decreased from 25% in 1993 to 19% in 1995, but increased again to 31% in 1996. Congenital diseases caused 10% of deaths in the 1993–1996 period, decreasing from 16% in 1994 to 9% in 1996.

Infectious diseases prevailed in the morbidity pattern among infants, accounting for 50% of hospitalizations in the 1993–1996 period; 57% were males. Admissions due to infectious diseases decreased from 64% in 1993 to 40% in 1996. Respiratory and intestinal diseases were responsible for 63% and 32% of admissions, respectively. Nationally, hospitalizations per 1,000 live births increased from 104 in 1993 to 216 in 1994, and remained stable thereafter. Hospitalizations were most frequent in Toledo (289), followed by Belize District (261); Corozal had the lowest number (74).

A low proportion of babies, approximately 46%, were exclusively breast-fed to four months of age, with no change in trend. This rate reflects the fact that hospitals are not complying with the requirements for "baby-friendly hospital" certification.

While infant mortality declined during the 1992–1996 period, morbidity remains associated with quality of care, in particular in terms of basic health services and prevention of infections.

Health in Early Childhood. Among children in the 1–4-year age group, mortality rates increased from 9.0 deaths per 10,000 persons in 1993 to 12.1 in 1996. External causes, including road traffic accidents, accounted for the highest proportion of deaths (24%). This figure increased from 21% in 1993 to 33% in 1996. The second leading cause was infectious diseases, accounting for 22% of deaths; respiratory diseases accounted for 65% of these deaths. No differences were found in rates between males and females.

Morbidity based on hospitalizations showed that 35% were due to respiratory diseases, followed by intestinal diseases (18%), and external causes (12%). There were no differences found between males and females in hospitalization due to these causes.

Undernutrition measured by weight-for-age deficit (Z score −2.0) occurred in 6% of children attending health clinics in 1992 at the national level, more than twice the number expected. In Toledo, a survey showed that 16% of children were undernourished in 1992 and 18% in 1994. The study suggested that while breast-feeding practice and duration were appropriate, undernutrition was caused by poor weaning practices related to food quality and quantity. Also associated with undernutrition were the poor quality of drinking water, household sanitation, and hygiene practices.

Health in Late Childhood. Children in the 5–9-year-old group had the lowest mortality rates of all age groups at 3.3 deaths per 10,000 persons over the 1993–1995 period, with an increase to 5.5 in 1996. Mortality rates were higher in males (4.4) than in females (3.0). External causes accounted for 43% of deaths. More males (62%) died from these causes than females.

Respiratory diseases were the leading cause of morbidity in this period for both males and females, accounting for 21% of all hospitalizations. Second in rank were external causes (12%). Hospitalizations due to fractures were more frequent in males (67%) than females.

Data from a national census showed that the prevalence of growth retardation (low height-for-age) in schoolchildren in 1996 was 15%–18% in males and 13% in females. This prevalence was much higher in rural areas (23%) than in urban areas (7%) and in Mayan children (45%) than in Mestizo and other ethnic groups (18%). With the exception of Belize District (4% prevalence), the districts with the highest levels of poverty also had the highest level of growth retardation (Toledo District had a prevalence of 39%). The ethnic group most affected was the Maya (45%), and the least affected, the Creole (4%). Maya children had four times more growth retardation in Toledo District (52%) than in Belize District (12%).

Health of Adolescents

The mortality rate among adolescents (10 to 19 years old) over the period averaged 6.2 deaths per 10,000 persons. Mor-

tality among males was twice as high (8.7) as females (3.6), males accounting for 72% of all deaths. External causes were the leading cause of death (37%); 80% of these deaths were in males. Belize District had the highest number of deaths due to external causes, followed by Orange Walk; Toledo District had the lowest percentage (6%).

Complications of pregnancy were the leading cause of hospitalization for adolescents in the 1993–1996 period (17%), followed by injuries and poisoning (16%). Females represented 60% of all admissions. Complications of pregnancy accounted for 42% of female admissions, while injuries and poisoning accounted for 31% among males. Fractures accounted for 37% of all injuries and poisoning, with males hospitalized in 78% of cases. Among complications of pregnancies, abortion and early labor were each responsible for 19% of the admissions; cesarean section represented 7%.

Health of Adults

Among adults 20–49 years old, mortality was stable over the period, with an average rate of 2.3 deaths per 10,000 persons of this group. Mortality rates among males were higher (2.7) than for females (1.4). External causes were the leading cause, accounting for 24% of deaths, followed by heart and respiratory diseases (12% and 7%, respectively). Males represented 69% of all deaths in the age group. Road traffic accidents were responsible for 51% of externally caused deaths; 88% involved males. The highest frequency of deaths due to external causes occurred in Orange Walk, 94% in males. The frequency of deaths due to heart diseases was higher in females (17%) than males (9%).

Complications of pregnancy were the leading cause of hospitalization in this age group (29%) in the 1993–1996 period, followed by digestive disorders (8%). Females in this age group comprised 69% of hospital admissions. Complications of pregnancy were responsible for 42% of female admissions of all ages, and 37% of these cases were related to abortion. Injuries and poisoning were the leading causes of hospitalization for males (29%). Within this category, "other injuries" was the leading cause (61%), 81% occurring in males. Fractures were the second leading cause of morbidity in the injuries and poisoning group, accounting for 35% of hospitalizations.

In 1995, 51.7% of pregnant women attending health clinics were found to be anemic (hemoglobin levels below 11.0 g/dl).

Adults 50 years old and older had a mortality rate in the 1993–1996 period of 20 deaths per 10,000 persons. Rates were higher in males (20.8) than females (18.4). Heart, respiratory, cerebrovascular diseases, and neoplasms were the leading causes, accounting for more than 50% of all deaths.

Respiratory, heart, and digestive system diseases and diabetes were the leading causes of hospitalization in this age group. Other causes for hospitalization were hypertension, cerebrovascular disease, and neoplasms. No difference was observed between male and female hospitalization patterns.

Workers' Health

Approximately 29% of the total population of the country was employed in 1996, and a total of 1,522 benefit claims were filed. The majority of claims were for sickness (37%), followed by injury (19%). The leading morbidity conditions were respiratory diseases, followed by back pain and fever. Of all injury claims, 42% were due to open wounds and injuries. The highest numbers of injury claims were in Orange Walk (29%), Corozal (26%), and Stann Creek Districts (25%), districts where agro-industry is more developed. The 20–39-year age group filed 65% of all claims.

Analysis by Type of Disease or Health Impairment

Communicable Diseases

Vector-Borne Diseases. Malaria continued to be a major public health problem in Belize. The number of cases, the rise in the number of positive localities, the number of cases due to *Plasmodium falciparum,* and the percentage of cases occurring among children increased during the 1992–1994 period. A study in 1995 on the distribution of malaria showed that, in Toledo, 56% of cases occurred among children under 14 years of age. In other districts, most cases occurred in young adult males.

Although the situation improved during 1995, the malaria incidence rate continued to be high. There were 9,413 cases diagnosed in 1995, a decrease of 10% compared to 1994. Cases decreased by approximately 50% in Orange Walk and Corozal Districts. Almost 95% of cases in 1995 were due to *P. vivax.* Of the *P. falciparum* cases, 86% occurred in Stann Creek and Cayo. Cayo was the most affected district, with 40% of all cases, while Toledo reported 23% and Stann Creek, 18%. In 1996, there were 6,605 reported cases, a reduction of 30% with respect to 1995.

There were no reported cases of dengue between 1991 and 1993. In 1994, 14 cases were detected and in 1995, 107 suspected cases were registered, 9 being confirmed by laboratory. Belize does not have the capacity to conduct serological testing, but sends samples abroad for confirmation. No cases were reported for 1996.

Cholera and Other Intestinal Diseases. Cholera appeared in Belize in January 1992; 159 cases were reported in 1992 (mainly in Toledo District), 135 in 1993, and 26 in 1996.

Four deaths occurred during the first year of the epidemic, followed by two deaths in 1993 and two in 1996. Hospitalizations due to intestinal diseases decreased from 913 in 1994 to 593 in 1996, particularly in children 1–4 years old.

Tuberculosis. Mortality rates due to tuberculosis were 2.0 per 10,000 persons in 1993, 4.3 in 1994, 2.8 in 1995, and 5.4 in 1996. During the period, 232 new cases of tuberculosis were diagnosed.

Respiratory Infections. Respiratory diseases were the major cause of hospitalization in the 1993–1996 period, accounting for 12% of all admissions. The most common diagnoses were chronic obstructive lung disease (45%), which includes asthma, followed by pneumonia and influenza (29%). There were no differences in hospitalization between males and females. The highest morbidity rate occurred in Stann Creek (3.2 per 1,000 inhabitants), followed by Toledo (2.8), with the lowest in Corozal (1.0).

Respiratory disease was the second leading cause of death (11%). Pneumonia was the diagnosis in 69% of these deaths.

AIDS. Since the detection of the first AIDS case in 1986, 195 cases were reported through December 1996. There were 18 cases of AIDS in 1994, 28 in 1995, and 38 in 1996. The majority (80%) were in the 20–44-year age group. AIDS mortality was over 90%; life expectancy after developing the disease is between 18 and 24 months.

Through the end of 1996, 486 cases of HIV infection were reported by the Central Medical Laboratory, the number increasing from 60 in 1994 to 78 in 1996. The male-to-female ratio of reported HIV cases declined from 13:1 in 1989 to 1.6:1 in 1996. Transmission occurs mostly through heterosexual contact, although 27 persons with AIDS reported homosexual and bisexual activities. Eight pediatric cases have been reported, five attributed to perinatal transmission and three to blood transfusion. In 1995, the Sentinel Surveillance project showed 0.96% HIV prevalence in women attending prenatal clinics, and 0.8% prevalence in cord blood. Although the epidemic affected the entire country, Belize and Stann Creek districts reported 78% of the cases (61% and 17%, respectively). The number of HIV cases also diagnosed with tuberculosis increased to nine in 1996, compared to an average of three cases per year in the preceding period.

Noncommunicable Diseases and Other Health-Related Problems

Nutritional Diseases and Diseases of Metabolism. Nutritional problems range from deficiency to obesity. Deficiencies in weight- and height-for-age, as well as in serum iron and vitamin A in preschool children were present in all ethnic groups in Toledo, and in rural populations of the Maya and Mestizo in the other districts. Anemia was found among pregnant women. Data from a study conducted among adults in 1995 indicated that obesity was a problem.

Food supply in Belize is highly dependent on imports, and it is necessary to monitor imported food for iodized and fluorinated salt. The Government policy is to promote self-sufficiency in food production.

Cardiovascular Diseases. Cardiovascular diseases accounted for 30% of reported deaths in the 1993–1996 period. Mortality rates varied from 125.8 per 100,000 inhabitants in 1993 to 113.5 in 1996. Heart diseases were the leading cause of death for males and females, accounting for 67% of cardiovascular deaths. The highest death rate occurred in Belize District (183.0), followed by Stann Creek District (141.3); the lowest death rate was in Toledo (64.0).

Heart disease was a major cause of hospitalization among adults 50 years or older, accounting for 10% of all hospitalizations in this group. However, it did not appear among the leading causes of hospitalization in other groups. There were no sex differences in hospitalization due to heart disease. The districts with the highest hospitalization frequency due to heart diseases were Corozal and Belize, each with 13%, and the lowest was Cayo (6%).

Malignant Tumors. Malignant neoplasms were among the leading causes of mortality during the period, particularly in the 50 and older age group. Mortality remained stable at 34.7 deaths per 100,000 persons. No sex differences were observed. The districts with the highest number of deaths due to neoplasms in the 50 and older age group were Cayo and Orange Walk, each registering 17%; the lowest was in Toledo (7%). Neoplasms were also a leading cause of hospitalization for the age group 50 years old and older, accounting for 5% of all hospitalizations. There were no differences by sex.

Diabetes. Diabetes appeared among the 10 leading causes of mortality only in the 50 and older age group (88% of all diabetes deaths). The annual average number of diabetes-related deaths per year was less than 25, accounting for 2% of reported deaths in this age group. The annual average number of females (28) that died from diabetes was slightly higher than that of males (21) in this age group. Hospitalizations due to diabetes decreased from 308 in 1993 to 235 in 1996, with women accounting for 67% of admissions. Five out of six amputations in Belize are due to diabetes, and 9% of cases of blindness were related to diabetic retinopathy.

Accidents and Violence. External causes were among the leading causes of mortality, accounting for 9% of reported

deaths in the general population in 1993–1996; males accounted for 79% of these deaths. Road traffic accidents caused 41% of deaths in this category. The mortality rate for motor vehicle accidents increased from 10.7 per 100,000 population in 1993 to 16.7 in 1996. In men, the rate increased from 14.4 to 26.1 per 100,000 between 1993 and 1996, while in females it increased from 6.9 to 7.2.

Although suicide did not appear among the leading external causes of mortality, its frequency increased from 1 death in 1994, to 11 in 1995, and 8 in 1996; almost all suicides were males. Nearly half occurred in Corozal; 75% were in the age group 20–49 years old. Forty-two percent of suicides were by shotgun, 21% by hanging, and 15.9% by paraquat ingestion.

The Domestic Violence Act has been in effect since 1993, but documentation on domestic violence is almost nonexistent and information is not channeled to the Medical Statistics Office or other information systems. The Department of Women's Affairs is presently coordinating the development of a national five-year plan of action on domestic violence, and the Ministry of Health and Sports is coordinating the development of a national registration form for domestic violence through its Epidemiology Unit.

A 1996 study in Orange Walk identified important issues relating to domestic violence, including compromised medical response; weak networking; increased utilization and demands on the legal system; increased awareness of domestic violence coupled with stereotypical attitudes; and the need for support services (counseling, data registration, and management protocols).

Abortion. Although abortion did not figure among the leading causes of mortality, it is probable that some deaths due to abortion were reported as complications of pregnancy. There were 2,603 abortions reported. While hospitalizations due to abortion decreased from 7% in 1993 to 5% in 1996, abortion ranked fourth in causes of hospitalization. Twenty percent of hospitalizations related to abortion occurred in the 10–19-year age group, decreasing from 21% in 1993 to 17% in 1996.

Mental Health. Information on mental health is based on hospitalization at the national psychiatric hospital. Neurotic disorders and alcoholic syndrome are included in the five leading causes of hospitalization; schizophrenia and other psychoses are not.

A recent psychiatric nurse practitioners' study cited "stress and inadequate coping skills" as the leading contributing factor for psychiatric illness, followed by chemical abuse.

Oral Health. Oral health improved among schoolchildren, with a reduction in dental decay and gum disease. However, a recent study of 3–4-year-olds showed that 43% had dental caries and 15% had rampant caries. The risk of caries in 4-years-old was 1.5 times higher than in 3-year-olds. Increased fluoride use by children from 1993 to 1995 was associated with a decrease in the demand of dental services. The index for decayed, missing, and filled teeth (DMFT) in 1989 ranged 3.4 in Orange Walk to 4.7 in Cayo in schoolchildren from 6 to 12 years of age. For 12-year-olds, the index was 4.3 for the districts included in the study. There were no differences by sex. Among adults, an increased request for dental fillings, prophylaxis, and bacterial plaque removal was noted.

Ocular Health. Information on ocular health is limited, most of it coming from Government clinics (in Cayo, Belmopan, and Belize Districts) and the Belize Council for the Visually Impaired, a nongovernmental organization that maintains a national registry on blind persons. As of December 1996, there were 806 recorded cases of blindness, a rate of 3.6 per 1,000 inhabitants. This is below the rate of 8 per 1,000 expected in developing countries according to WHO estimates. Stann Creek and Belize districts had the highest rates (5.2 and 4.6, respectively); the other district rates ranged from 2.4 to 2.8. The most common diagnoses among blind persons were cataracts (39%), glaucoma (23%), diabetic retinopathy (9%), congenital blindness (5%), retinal blindness (5%), and others (15%). Persons age 60 and older represented 25% of all those registered as blind; by district, this age group comprised 41% of the blind in Belize, 15% in Cayo, 14% in Stann Creek, 13% in Orange Walk, 10% in Corozal, and 7% in Toledo. Hospitalizations due to eye diseases decreased from 125 in 1993 to 43 in 1996.

Natural Disasters. The most important natural hazards in Belize are hurricanes, fires, and floods. During 1995, a flood in the north required the evacuation of several villages, an event that reduced immunization coverage. To minimize the impact that natural or man-made disasters have on health services, simulation exercises, training, dissemination of information, and intersectoral cooperation have been carried out. Constraints in this area include the coordination and allocation of funds for disaster mitigation measures.

RESPONSE OF THE HEALTH SYSTEM

National Health Plans and Policies

In November 1996, the Prime Minister launched the National Health Plan 1996–2000 and the Ministry of Health started reorganization to implement the plan, focusing on the development of new programs and approaches, and decentralization. Areas of concern include information systems, health financing, health service administration, equipment maintenance, human resource development, and institutional development and planning. The Ministry has received support from PAHO and the Inter-American Development Bank in the reform process. The policy reform project of 1993 provides policy options for implementing the National Health Plan and consolidating equity and efficiency in the health sector.

The National Health Plan provides a framework to guide the Ministry of Health and others in efforts to ensure universal access to a set of comprehensive health services of acceptable quality, through primary health care. The development of the National Health Plan has been a participatory process, promoting active involvement of different sectors in identifying priority areas and proposing solutions and desired outcomes at central and local levels.

The National Health Plan defined five programmatic areas for achieving its goals: environmental health; early childhood; late childhood and adolescence; early and late adulthood; and sports. Support services include information systems and epidemiology, health education and community participation, nutrition, development of a health facilities network (including a referral system, maintenance, laboratory, and drug supplies), physical education, and administration.

While State reform is under way, and consultative and participatory processes have won new supporters in recent years, change depends on the pace and direction of the reform. Decentralization is not uniformly accepted, and will require changes in culture and attitude. An environment conducive to democracy and community decision-making is necessary to ensure community participation.

Organization of the Health Sector

Institutional Organization

The Government has provided health services at practically no charge over the years, including the provision of pharmaceuticals. Cost recovery mechanisms are gradually being instituted, particularly for curative care.

Health care management, centralized until recently, now allows more district autonomy in the decision-making process. In April 1997, finances were decentralized to the district level, but guidelines for budget distribution and management had not yet been established. There was progress in cooperation and coordination between the preventive community-based programs and the District Medical Officers (who usually administer the hospital and are responsible for overall health care management), but there were problems due to lack of management training at the community level.

While both public and private sectors contribute to health care, there is no clear definition of their roles or coordination.

The Ministry of Health is responsible for the design of policies and arrangements between institutions and providers, including the utilization of public hospitals by physicians and dentists for private practice.

Intersectoral cooperation is recognized as a sound approach to health and development. Multisectoral bodies such as the National Commission for Families and Children, the National Women's Commission, the Appraisal Environmental Committee, among others, exist, but their impact is compromised by a lack of effective mechanisms for intersectoral coordination and cooperation at the national level.

The Ministry of Health has embraced primary health care, and has created an infrastructure of district health teams that work toward health related goals. The teams were established to promote intersectoral and community participation in health development, but are composed mainly of health care providers. The teams have no legal authority or assigned budget with which to operate.

Organization of Health Regulatory Activities

Although specific statutes have been approved, there have been no major changes in health legislation for nearly three decades. The laws of Belize refer to medical services and institutions, public health, food and drugs, and certification and practice of health professionals. Revision of existing health legislation is an expected outcome of the health policy reform. There are no effective regulatory mechanisms, norms, or standards to enforce legislation.

The Ministry of Health is responsible for making regulations on health related issues. The Chief Medical Officer (Director of Health Services), appointed by the Governor, is responsible for executing ordinances and recommending necessary regulations to the Minister, and in cases such as control of communicable diseases has the authority to make regulations. Regulatory bodies such as the Medical Board, the Nurses and Midwives Council, and Board of Examiners of Chemist and Druggists are responsible for registering professionals in specific areas and advising the Minister on regulations concerning those categories.

Authority to prevent and control environmental pollution is contained in provisions of the Public Health Act, the Pesticide Control Act, and the Solid Waste Management Authority Act. The Environmental Protection Act of 1992 established a Department of the Environment, which is charged with enforcing provisions of the Act. Over the past five years, legislation was developed for the control of pollutants in land and water. Air quality standards for industry, traffic, and exposure to environmental tobacco smoke in public buildings are still required. The Housing Department set standards for housing ventilation.

Legislation on food safety and security is under development. Food standards and regulations based on regional references exist for most processed food, whether for internal or external markets.

The Factories Act, governing occupational health and safety in factories, no longer meets the needs of most workers. The Workers' Health Plan replaced it in the form of the Occupational Health and Safety Act, relevant to diverse working environments.

Health Services and Resources

Organization of Services for Care of the Population

Health Promotion and Education. Belize ratified the 1994 Caribbean Charter for Health Promotion. Health education was incorporated into vertical programs, but inclusion of health promotion as a strategy was not achieved. The utilization of the mass media and community mobilization was a countrywide strategy. The establishment of local health promotion coordinators contributed significantly to the decentralization of health education and promotion. Health sector reform should ensure that the strategy continues to influence health. Major constraints are the emphasis of the budget on curative care, and the limited availability of training institutions for health educators.

Programs for Disease Prevention and Control. The Ministry of Health developed vertical programs in response to major communicable diseases such as vaccine-preventable diseases, malaria, dengue, rabies, tuberculosis, and AIDS and other sexually transmitted diseases. As part of the Maternal and Child Health Program, the Expanded Program on Immunization increased its coverage for targeted diseases. Between 1993 and 1995, there were major achievements in this area: the elimination of measles and the introduction of the measles, mumps and rubella vaccine. In addition, congenital rubella syndrome surveillance was initiated in 1997, and a pilot project for hepatitis-B vaccination was implemented in the Stann Creek District. The Government assumed the purchase of vaccines. To ensure coverage for targeted diseases, emphasis is given to surveillance, ongoing training, maintenance of cold chains, and regular mobile clinic outreach. The constraints are individual refusals, a vulnerable outreach program, and deficient equipment maintenance.

The vector control program of the Ministry of Health carried out systematic spraying of houses (particularly in rural areas), identified areas of infestation, and applied treatments when required. The Public Health Bureau conducted rabies vaccination and health education campaigns to encourage individuals to vaccinate domestic animals. The tuberculosis program runs a chest clinic for the prevention and control of tuberculosis cases. The productivity of the clinic decreased between 1992, when 409 patients were seen (20% with tuberculosis), and 1995 when 129 patients were seen (47% with tuberculosis).

A National AIDS Program has been in place since 1987, and it has implemented two middle-term plans within the framework of the Global Program on AIDS. Activities included public awareness campaigns, targeted outreach programs, blood safety measures, counseling, HIV testing, and the development of policies and standards. Since 1987, 100% of blood for transfusion has been screened for HIV, and its cost is assumed by the Government. Despite these efforts, attitude changes on sexual behavior are limited, stigma and discrimination persist, access to care and support is limited, and there are no defined policies and regulations for the prevention and control of HIV/AIDS. In 1996, a group of organizations and individuals from the public and private sectors established a task force to develop a national strategic plan within the framework of the new AIDS program. Building on previous experiences, the intersectoral group has focused its efforts to meet the needs of the population and those directly affected by the epidemic.

There are no programs for prevention and control of non-communicable diseases, although special services are available for priority diseases such as diabetes and hypertension. It is important to mention the contribution of certain non-governmental organizations that provide complementary care in this area, such as the Belize Council for the Visually Impaired, Belize Diabetes Association, Belize Cancer Society, the Red Cross, and the Lions Club, among others.

Despite many successes, the disease-oriented and vertical approach being used for the organization of health services delivery compromises an efficient response. The life cycle/gender approach seeks to ensure an integral focus on health for all ages, male and female. The challenge is to develop an efficient health model that is sensitive to local needs and cultural diversity.

Workers' Health. The largest program providing benefits to workers is the Belize Social Security Scheme, covering approximately 89% of the working population. Those not covered include people employed for less than 24 hours per week and the self-employed. The scheme does not target workers' health; rather, it provides for medical care for injuries suffered on the job only. The Social Security Sickness Benefit consists of cash payments for wages lost during illness; health care services are mainly provided by the Ministry of Health.

Food Protection and Control. Government policy has aimed at self-sufficiency in food production. Recent reforms include tax exemptions for local food production and allowing producers a more competitive position in the market.

Responsibility for food safety is shared by the ministries of Health, of Agriculture and Fisheries, and of Trade and Industry. Efforts to establish a coordinating body have not yet succeeded, but steps to establish a Codex Alimentarius Commission by the public and private sectors are under way. The public sector is represented by the Ministries mentioned above, and the private sector, by the Chamber of Commerce and Better Belize Bureau. Laboratory facilities for a food safety program are limited and devoted mainly to water quality control. Food testing is done outside of the country.

Drinking Water Services, Sewerage Systems, and Solid Waste Management. Responsibilities for management of water sources are not clearly defined nor coordinated. Five Government Ministries and the Water and Sewerage Authority are involved in the water and sanitation sector, each undertaking partial control and managing fragmented resources with only minor regard for overall planning criteria. The Ministry of Health, through its Public Health Bureau, monitors water quality and implements rural sanitation programs. The Water and Sewerage Authority operates water systems in urban centers and sewerage systems in Belize City, Belmopan, and San Pedro Ambergris Key. Although water supply and sanitation coverage increased between 1990 and 1995, and had a positive impact on the control of waterborne diseases, there is still a shortfall of facilities in rural and urban areas. In 1995, the Government discontinued the Rural Water Supply and Sanitation Unit to streamline public service and to improve efficiency, but this affected the monitoring of rural water systems and their maintenance.

In urban communities, refuse disposal is the responsibility of the local governments. In rural communities, refuse disposal is not organized at the community level; each household is responsible for the disposal of its solid waste. When disposal methods are inadequate and cause health concerns, the Ministry of Health may intervene to ensure corrective actions. There is one hospital solid waste management system functioning in the national referral hospital; the rest of the hospitals do not have a standardized system, and bury and burn their waste in open sites.

Epidemiological Surveillance Systems and Public Health Laboratories. Surveillance systems exist for poliomyelitis and measles, and to control HIV and AIDS, malaria, cholera, tuberculosis, typhoid fever, and congenital rubella syndrome. These systems do not always coordinate with the Medical Statistics Unit of the Ministry of Health, and are more responsive to the vertical nature of existing programs.

Public Health Laboratory activities are supported by the Central Medical Laboratory and the Water Quality Laboratory, which both need further development.

Organization and Operation of Personal Health Care Services

The Government, through the Ministry of Health, is the main provider of health services. There are eight public hospitals, one in each district, with the exception of Cayo and Belize Districts, which each have two. Karl Heusner Memorial Hospital is the national referral hospital and serves the Belize District population with general and specialized services for primary, secondary, and some tertiary care. Rockview Hospital, located 22 miles from Belize City, is the national psychiatric hospital.

District hospitals function as primary level care facilities and provide some secondary care. There are no studies on the response capability of the health services facilities network, but Ministry of Health personnel recognize that this is an area needing improvement. Referrals are made to neighboring countries, but no standardized protocols are in place.

There are 75 public facilities functioning as health centers (40) and rural health posts (35). Health centers provide pre- and postnatal care, immunization services, growth monitoring of children under age 5, treatment for diarrhea and minor ailments, and general health education. Some specialized clinics offer services for hypertension, diabetes, tuberculosis, sexually transmitted diseases, and AIDS, also providing referrals and follow-up. There are no standardized protocols and mechanisms for referrals to district hospitals or to the national referral hospital. Each center serves 2,000 to 4,000 persons, and most also provide a mobile clinic that visits smaller and more remote villages every six weeks, accounting for 40% of the centers' service delivery.

Specialized services in mental health, maternal and child health, and dental health are provided through this public facility network. Mental health care follows a psychiatric service delivery model based on incarceration, although an outpatient clinic and psychiatric social welfare services were established and extended to the districts through monthly clinics. In 1992, a psychiatrist was hired for the Government program. Today there are two psychiatrists and nine trained psychiatric nurses providing mental health care. A community-based project was initiated in 1997 to strengthen mental health care outreach services.

The Dental Health Program has been successful through specialized clinics and school-based services.

The Maternal and Child Health Program is one of the more structured programs. Clinic attendance records from children's services show that follow-up visits manifest an increasing trend for preschoolers and a decreasing trend for children 1–4 years of age; the first visit remained stable for both age

groups. More than one-fourth of hospitalization services were for normal deliveries. The Ministry of Health does not provide contraceptives, and family planning is limited to health education during pre- and postnatal services. Belize Family Life Association, a nongovernmental organization, is the main provider of contraceptives.

The private medical sector is limited in number of providers and range of services. Only two private hospitals exist, one nonprofit hospital in Cayo District (20 beds) and a for-profit facility in Belize District (4 beds). In addition, there are 54 private clinics, 27 of which are in Belize City; Toledo District has one private clinic. The private sector is mostly limited to outpatient services. Secondary care is provided for maternity cases and simple surgeries.

Private health insurance is limited but increased rapidly during the 1990s. Many insurance companies are affiliates of large international firms and benefit packages are fashioned to cover expenses for medical care outside of Belize. Premium levels are high and out of reach for the average worker. Family coverage can cost as much as US$ 100 monthly for a group medical policy.

Regulations that restrict the number of physicians authorized to practice privately, the proximity of higher-quality services in Mexico, low population coverage of group medical insurance, the absence of linkages between financiers and providers of health care, and the use of public hospitals by government-contracted and independent specialists to treat private inpatients are some of the structural problems influencing the underdevelopment of private practice.

Although the number of health professionals increased, particularly specialist physicians, the services provided, coverage, and productivity decreased in the public health sector in the 1993–1996 period. There are no data available on private sector productivity. According to the Medical Statistics Office, the total number of hospital discharges decreased from 19,480 in 1993 to 16,557 in 1996. Hospital occupancy rates decreased from 44% in 1993 to 37% in 1996. The total number of consultations decreased from 218,993 in 1993 to 178,016, while specialist consultations went from 19,364 in 1993 to 14, 115 in 1996. Productivity indicators were as follows: 0.60 discharges/physician/day; 0.23 C-sections/obstetrician/day; 13.9 general consultations/general practitioner/day; 0.94 specialist consultations/specialist/day; 0.78 major surgeries/surgeon/day, and 0.04 emergencies/physician/day. Productivity was lower in the Karl Heusner Memorial Hospital than the average for the rest of the district hospitals.

Inputs for Health

The Central Medical Laboratory is the hub of the public laboratory network. Except for Cayo, all district hospitals have a laboratory that is administered from the central level. Quality control of private laboratories is the responsibility of the Central Medical Laboratory. The quality of services in public laboratories is compromised by staff shortages, low budgetary allocation, and waste of supplies.

Private diagnostic facilities consist of one laboratory in Belize and a radiology unit; neither is affiliated with a patient facility. Regulation of private sector diagnostic facilities does not exist. Although the Ministry of Health has radio-image diagnosis equipment, it is underutilized due to a shortage of trained personnel.

There are three main problems regarding drug management and supply in the public sector: the annual budget is too low to cover needs; procurement is ineffective, with many purchases occurring at unnecessarily high prices; the distribution system is dysfunctional and items are frequently out of stock for prolonged periods. Drug supply is a priority area being addressed by the health policy reform project. The Ministry of Health developed a Drug Formulary in 1994.

Routine maintenance of facilities is compromised because of limited budget.

The health information system suffers from limited standards for routine reporting, late reporting, lack of feedback, and shortage of staff trained in data processing and analysis. There are various vertical information systems but there is minimal coordination among them. A large amount of data is compiled and made available but not properly used for decision-making.

Human Resources

The number of health personnel increased by 57% from 1976 to 1994. The 1994 health personnel survey counted 500 health workers, 465 of whom were active. Physicians, dentists and professional nurses accounted for 58% of the personnel; 33% were professional nurses, 21% were physicians, and 3% were dentists. Almost 75% of health personnel work in the public sector, the largest group being nurses (84%). The majority working in the private sector are physicians and dentists (58%). Approximately 14% of health personnel work in both the public and private sectors. Fifty-five percent of physicians working in the public sector also held jobs in the private sector. Most dentists (67%) work exclusively in private service. Community health personnel include 117 midwives and 135 traditional birth attendants; 110 have undergone some training. Other Ministry of Health staff include 14 supply clerks and a supply officer, 16 public health inspectors, 68 vector control staff, 7 health educators (two with health education training), and a network of 171 community health workers.

Belize allocates financial resources to staff the health sector at a level that is comparable to that of other countries, but it has one of the lowest coverage of physicians and only an average coverage of nurses. Health personnel are concentrated in the metropolitan district of Belize, where more than half of the health staff is employed (60% of physicians, 54% of practical nurses, and 63.3% of professionals work at the central level), most in the Karl Heusner Memorial Hospital. Lack of infrastructure and available specialists result in low utilization of district inpatient facilities and a high level of referral to the Karl Heusner Memorial Hospital. The distribution is unequal in all districts for both physicians and nurses in rural and urban areas. Although Belize has the highest distribution rates for all categories of personnel, it has no physicians in rural areas.

Expenditures and Sectoral Financing

The budget for health increased from US$ 862,950 in 1992 to US$ 11,035,500 in 1995. However, the health sector's share of the national budget decreased from 9% in 1992 to 8% in 1995. The relative allocation of resources showed an emphasis on curative services (74% allocated to hospitals), and within curative services, an emphasis on secondary care (28%). Only 17% of the budget was allocated to public health programs. The budget structure remained the same over the 1993–1996 period. Personnel costs consume over two-thirds of Ministry of Health expenditures (75%) and increased in recent years, while drugs and medical supplies consume 17%. Over 60% of Ministry of Health capital expenditure is covered by foreign aid, and little funding is available for routine maintenance. Inadequate resources and inefficiencies in allocation and use contribute to the deterioration of the quality and quantity of services provided by the Ministry of Health.

External Technical and Financial Cooperation

International partnership contributed to health sector development and the multisectoral process, positively affecting the health status of the population. The Government emphasized building and strengthening bilateral, regional, and global relations and commitments. Since the last "Health for All" evaluation, the Ministry of Health strengthened its technical cooperation efforts within the framework of the Caribbean Cooperation in Health, the Central America Health Initiative (CAHI-III), the Binational Cooperation in Health Mexico/Belize, and the Trinational Cooperation in Health Mexico/Guatemala/Belize. Belize cooperated with nontraditional partners in health, such as the Inter-American Development Bank involvement in the health reform project.

Although legal agreements exist between agencies and the Government through the Ministry of Foreign Affairs, there are no formal arrangements for the coordination and execution of international donor-funded technical cooperation in health and development. Coordination of international cooperation and health assistance is done on an ad-hoc basis by the Ministry of Health.

The Ministry of Health set up a planning unit in 1996 to coordinate international assistance for health. A technical cooperation manual was developed in 1996 as part of a Ministry of Health and PAHO/WHO initiative to streamline their joint planning, execution, monitoring, and evaluation in health. UNICEF is also strengthening inter-ministerial coordination within its new program of work.

BERMUDA

GENERAL SITUATION AND TRENDS

Socioeconomic, Political, and Demographic Overview

Bermuda comprises a small group of islands that cover an area of approximately 20.5 mi^2, located 586 miles east, southeast of Cape Hatteras, North Carolina. It has a population of 59,807, of which 51.6% is female, with a density of 3,160 persons per mi^2.

Bermuda has virtually no natural resources, and it imports all of its consumer goods. The economy is based almost entirely on tourism and international company business. About one-third of the work force is engaged in wholesale and/or retail trade; one-third, in restaurants and hotels; and the other third, in community, social, and personal services. The country usually has a small balance of payments surplus, the Bermuda dollar (BD$) is pegged to the US dollar on an equal basis, and inflation is estimated to be at around 2.6% per annum. Hotel occupancy rates have slowly improved over the past few years, reaching 64% in 1995.

Education is free in public schools and compulsory up to age 16 years. In 1995, 10,056 students were enrolled in government and private primary and secondary schools and in Bermuda College. In 1994, the literacy rate was estimated at 97%.

Living standards are high, with good housing and well developed communications systems. Roads are good, and public transportation (buses, taxis, and ferries) is well-developed. All the population has safe drinking water at home, as well as sanitary waste disposal.

In 1991, the median household income was US$ 48,588, an increase of 16.4% since 1988, when it was last measured, and women represented 50% of the work force.

The country's per capita health expenditure was US$ 943 in 1995, representing approximately 5% of the GDP.

In 1991, the census reported a population of 58, 460 inhabitants in Bermuda. The yearly population growth has been approximately 0.7% in recent years, yielding a population of 59, 807 in 1995. Between 1991 and 1995 the average number of births per year was 902, but births have declined steadily during the period, with numbers in the latter years falling by more than 10% to 840, compared to the 959 at the beginning of the period. Crude birth rates declined from 16.4 per 1,000 population in 1991 to 14.0 in 1995. The racial composition of the population is 58% black and 42% white and other races. According to the 1991 census, the island had 22,430 households. Over time, multiple family-member households have given way to smaller units, with the average number of persons per household dropping to 2.61.

The population is gradually aging. It was estimated that in 1995 only 6.8% was under 5 years old, 12.9% between 5 and 14 years of age, and 9.8% 65 years old and older. That same year, life expectancy was 63.4 years for males and 78 years for females.

The average infant mortality rate for the 1992 to 1995 period has been approximately 13 per 1,000 live births. The crude death rate has hovered around 8 per 1,000 in the same period (Table 1).

Mortality Profile

A total of 2,388 deaths were recorded in Bermuda between 1991 and 1995, an annual mean of 478 events.

Overall, the average percentage of deaths according to broad groups of causes in the 1991–1995 period showed that diseases of the circulatory system were the most frequent ones, with 40.9% of the cases, followed by neoplasms, with 26.1%. Among the diseases of the circulatory system, the most frequent causes of death were ischemic heart disease (23.7%) and cerebrovascular disease (9.9%). Among neoplasms, lung, colon cancer, and female breast were the most frequent sites. External causes accounted for 4.5%; communicable diseases, for 4.3%; and conditions originating in the perinatal period, for 2.2%. The distribution pattern of deaths by sex was similar, except for external causes, where the frequency was almost four times higher among males, and for communicable diseases, where the frequency was twice as high among females.

SPECIFIC HEALTH PROBLEMS

Analysis by Population Group

Health of Children and Adolescents

The infant mortality rate in Bermuda is low (an average of 11 deaths per 1,000 live births in 1991–1995), and practically all deaths in this age group are due to conditions originating in the perinatal period. There were no recorded deaths in infants due to communicable diseases during this period. Only three deaths were registered during this period among children aged 1–4 years old and none for the age group 5–14 years old. Seven percent of newborns weighed 2,500 grams or less at birth.

Respiratory infections were the leading cause of hospitalization for infants, and respiratory infections and accidents were the leading hospitalization causes for children from 1 to 14 years of age.

Obesity is a public health concern in the age group 5–9 years old. Because immunization coverage has been consistently high, the incidence of vaccine preventable diseases is low or nonexistent. In 1995, coverage was 80.5% for measles vaccination, 90.7% for OPV3, and 93.7% for DTP3 in the age group under 1 year of age.

Dental decay has decreased over the past decade and oral health in children is generally excellent. This is largely attributed to a preventive dental care program for children that provides free fluoride rinses. The voluntary, school-based program has maintained high participation rates.

In youths 15 to 19 years old, accidents were the leading cause of death and one of the major causes of hospital admissions, along with pregnancy and respiratory diseases.

Health of Adults

Approximately 57% of the total population was between 25 and 64 years old in 1995. The most important causes of mortality and morbidity in these population groups were chronic diseases, accidents and violence, and AIDS. Mortality in these age groups has increased in the past 10 years due to AIDS and HIV infection, particularly in males. AIDS was the main cause of death in the group aged 35 to 44 years. For those aged 50 to 64 years, the leading causes of death are diseases of the circulatory system, cancers, and diseases of the digestive system.

Maternal health indicators are good. In 1995, more than 95% of pregnant women received prenatal care, 99% were fully immunized against tetanus, and all births took place in a hospital.

Health of the Elderly

The population group 60 years old and older are the most rapidly growing segment of the country's population. The leading causes of death and hospitalization in this group are diseases of the circulatory system, cancer, diseases of the digestive system, and diseases of the respiratory system. Social security benefits to persons in the age group 65 and older include health insurance. Special programs are in place to enable the aged to remain independent and active as long as possible.

Workers' Health and Health of the Disabled

Regulations related to workers' health are enforced under the Public Health Act, which is designed to ensure safety in the workplace. Many women occupy professional positions, and there is no evidence of child labor.

The Government has special programs to enable the disabled to remain active, independent, and employed as much as possible.

Analysis by Type of Disease

Communicable Diseases

Communicable diseases are not an important health problem. In 1990, three imported cases of malaria were recorded, but none has been recorded since 1992. Dengue and yellow fever have never been reported, and the last registered cases of rubella (4 cases) occurred in 1992.

AIDS is an important health problem. Since Bermuda's first case was reported in 1982, 339 cases and 269 deaths have been recorded.

In 1991 there were three reported cases of tuberculosis and seven in 1992.

Noncommunicable Diseases and Other Health-Related Problems

Chronic noncommunicable diseases are the most important health problems. Both circulatory system diseases and cancers are leading causes of hospitalization and death. Ischemic heart disease and cerebrovascular disease are the most important causes of death among diseases of the circulatory system. The most frequent types of cancer include: female breast, lung, colon, and stomach.

Accidents are a major cause of death in the age group 15–34 years old, and motor vehicle accidents are the most important in this category; males are disproportionately affected.

RESPONSE OF THE HEALTH SYSTEM

National Health Plans and Policies

The Government's health policy emphasizes maternal and child health, health of schoolchildren, community nursing for the elderly, dental health, control of communicable diseases, mental health, and alcohol and drug abuse. Public health policy rests on the following principles: the Government should be the provider of last resort and should serve as the guarantor of public health; all residents should be able to participate in determining health care system priorities; and individuals, the community, and the Government share responsibility for maintaining the public health and assuring conditions whereby individuals can maintain and improve their health status.

In response to community concerns about escalating health care costs and the quality of health care on the islands, in 1993 the Government undertook an in-depth review of health care that brought together providers, consumers, the Government, and the insurance industry to examine health care costs, financing, quality, and needs assessment.

The general practitioner will likely continue to function as a "gatekeeper," controlling access to specialized care; the Government, in an effort to cope with rising health care costs, will develop more formal arrangements with preferred providers abroad (USA and Canada) for providing tertiary and some secondary care. Insurers are facing increased pressure to expand coverage and increase benefits, particularly for the treatment of addictions and for preventive services.

Both the Public Health Service and the Bermuda Hospitals Board have explored the development of additional ambulatory services and a greater integration of existing community services, particularly those geared at the elderly.

Organization of the Health Sector

Bermuda's health care system comprises a public and a private sector. The Ministry of Health, Social Services, and Housing is responsible for health matters in the country. The Ministry is mandated to promote and protect the health and well-being of the island's residents and is charged with assuring the provision of health care services, setting standards, and providing coordination within the health care system.

The Minister of Health sets public policy and reports to the Cabinet. The Ministry has responsibility for health planning and evaluation. There is no central planning agency.

The Ministry comprises several departments and agencies, including Ministry Headquarters, the Department of Health, the Department of Child and Family Services, the Prisons Department, the Department of Financial Assistance, and the Housing Corporation. Ministry Headquarters coordinates and controls the Ministry's departments; each department is responsible for its own operation, under the direction of the department head or director and the authority of the Permanent Secretary.

The Ministry also is responsible for the island's hospitals. These are administered by the Bermuda Hospitals Board, a statutory body appointed by the Ministers. Public health services are provided by the Ministry through the Department of Health.

Primary health care services are delivered from private physicians' offices, government centers, and hospital outpatient clinics. The private sector delivers a significant proportion of primary health care. Additional ambulatory care services are provided through specialty clinics and the hospital's emergency room.

Responsibility for providing public health services rests with the Department of Health, which includes a mandate to provide disease prevention and control and health promotion services. The Department also serves as a regulatory agency; monitors food safety and water and air quality; and provides various public health services, including personal health, dental health, and environmental health.

The public health service administers several public health programs, including maternal and child health, school health, immunization, and communicable disease control. It also manages home care, including health visiting and district nursing, and selected specialized care, such as care for AIDS patients, rehabilitation, health education, and health promotion programs. The country is divided into three health regions, and the department operates a health center in each. These centers offer prenatal care, family planning services, immunizations, child health and other primary care services, and dental clinics for children.

Private voluntary agencies, assisted by the Government, provide some specialized services such as community based oncology nursing and personal services for HIV-infected persons.

Health Services and Resources

Organization and Operation of Health Care Services

Bermuda has two hospitals: the King Edward VII Memorial Hospital, a general hospital with 234 beds, plus an additional

90 geriatric and rehabilitation beds, and Saint Brendan's Hospital, a psychiatric hospital with 166 beds. An executive director is responsible for the management of each hospital; he or she is assisted by several senior managers and by a medical staff committee that represents the physicians. There are no private hospitals in the country.

King Edward VII Memorial Hospital provides diagnostic and treatment services, including medicine, surgery, pediatrics, obstetrics and gynecology, rehabilitation, and geriatrics. The hospital also provides some specialized and intensive services, including oncology, medical and surgical intensive care, and renal dialysis. In addition to its specialty and ambulatory care clinics, the hospital operates a primary care clinic for indigent patients. A neonatal care unit is being developed. Both hospitals undergo periodic accreditation reviews by the Canadian Council on Hospital Accreditation.

The average length of stay at the general hospital was 8.7 days in 1993, and this figure has remained stable for several years. The average occupancy for that same year was 75%, and there were 63,905 patient-days.

There are no secondary or tertiary referral hospitals on Bermuda, although there are links for the provision of tertiary care with the United States, the United Kingdom, and Canada.

Mental health services are provided through psychiatrists, psychologists, a psychiatric social worker, and mental welfare officers attached to Saint Brendan's Hospital. This hospital provides treatment for both mentally ill and mentally handicapped persons. The hospital operates a day hospital and an outpatient clinic, provides community-based services, and functions as a halfway house. There is only one psychiatrist in private practice; all others are employed by the Hospital Board.

Long-term care facilities are operated by the Hospital Board and the Government. Skilled nursing care facilities include Lefroy House, with 57 beds, and the extended care unit at the general hospital, with 90 beds. A hospice facility for the terminally ill that opened in 1991 provides care for AIDS patients and other terminally ill persons. It is operated by the Hospital Board and partially subsidized by public funds. There are 11 residential care facilities for the elderly, including nursing homes that provide room and board and limited assistance with personal services. Most of these facilities are partially funded through public monies.

Human Resources

There were 94 physicians in active practice in the country in 1995, which represents one physician per 637 inhabitants: 25 of those are general practitioners, 6 work in public health and preventive medicine, and the remainder are specialists.

There are 27 dentists, including specialists in periodontics, orthodontics, and others; 5 of the general dentists work in the public health service. This represents 2,174 inhabitants per dentist.

In 1995, the number of licensed nurses was 689, including registered nurses, enrolled nurses, and psychiatric nurses. More than 75% are registered nurses, and most are based in hospitals.

There is a variety of other health personnel, including 15 physiotherapists, 40 medical laboratory technologists, 23 radiographers, 15 occupational therapists, 9 nutritionists and dietitians, and 7 speech-language pathologists.

Most physicians and dentists work as independent, private practitioners. Most other health care providers are employed on a salaried basis by the hospitals, the public health service, or private physicians. There is a small number of multi-specialty practices and a few partnerships among specialists.

There are 38 pharmacists who provide services ranging from retail pharmacy to clinical pharmacology. Most pharmacists are employed on a salaried basis.

Health Care Financing

The health care system is financed through a variety of mechanisms. Health services are either paid through an insurer, by a government agency, or by consumers. Funding for the hospitals includes insurance payments and government subsidies. There is no universal, publicly funded health insurance, although hospitalization insurance is mandatory for all employed or self-employed persons. Insurance coverage is nearly universal, and some persons are insured by more than one provider. Both employers and employees contribute an equal share of insurance premiums. The administration of Hospital Insurance is provided through the Hospital Insurance Commission, which regulates insurance sold both by private companies and public agencies. All policies must provide a minimum set of benefits, known as the Standard Hospital Benefit.

Government employees are insured through the Government Employees Health Insurance Scheme, and several major employers operate "approved schemes" to cover their employees. The Hospital Insurance Commission also operates a health insurance plan, which has an annual open enrollment period designed to ensure access to health (hospitalization) insurance for all Bermuda residents.

A Mutual Reinsurance Fund covers dialysis, kidney transplants, diabetes education and counseling, drugs to prevent graft rejection, hospice care, and extended-stay (inhospital) patients. It is funded through a compulsory levy on all health insurance premiums collected and was introduced to spread the cost of high risks claims among all insurers. The fund also is administered by the Insurance Commission. Hospitalization is provided free-of-charge to children and the aged, and it is covered through a government subsidy to the Bermuda Hospital Board.

Public health services are generally free or provided at modest cost; they are funded through general revenues.

The prevailing method of payment for doctors and dentists is fee-for-service. There are no restrictions on direct payments to providers by consumers, and physicians may bill patients for charges in excess of standard insurance reimbursement or agreed fee schedules. For hospital-based physician services there is a fee schedule, established on an annual basis by agreement between the Bermuda Medical Society and the Health Insurance Association of Bermuda. The Government determines overall increases in hospital fees and regulates the acquisition of major equipment and services.

BOLIVIA

GENERAL SITUATION AND TRENDS

Socioeconomic, Political, and Demographic Overview

Bolivia has a land surface of 1,098,581 km², spread over three distinct topographies: highland plateaus (*altiplano*) and Andean mountain slopes (25%), valley area (15%), and plains (60%). In terms of population distribution, 45% of Bolivians live in the highland plateaus, 30% in valley areas, and 25% in the country's eastern plains. Social organization, access to goods and services, and morbidity and mortality profiles vary considerably among the three regions. Although the country is officially divided into nine departments (*departamentos*), regional autonomy is still at an incipient stage.

In 1995, the gross domestic product (GDP) posted growth of 3.7%, the fiscal deficit was cut by 2% of GDP, and the currency issue rate dropped from 36.7% to 20.8%—all in a year. At the same time, however, annual inflation rose from 8.5% to 12.6%, owing mainly to higher international prices for imported staples and local market shortages triggered by the severe drought and its impact on farm output that year. These two factors also had repercussions for the country's trade balance, because imports grew at a faster rate (19.9%) than exports (5.7%). The burden of reform and structural adjustment fell most heavily on Bolivia's poor, and it pushed more people into poverty and out of the socioeconomic mainstream; furthermore, as the peasant farming and mining sectors shrank, activity in the informal sector of the economy expanded.

According to the 1992 National Population and Housing Census, Bolivia had a total population of 6,420,792 that year, estimated to rise to 7,413,834 by 1995. In the period since the previous census (1976), the population had grown at an average annual rate of 2.11% (compared with 2.05% over the 1950–1976 period). The highest rates were observed in Santa Cruz (4.16%), Beni (3.16%), and Tarija (2.82%); Potosí, however, posted a negative rate, with its population shrinking

0.12% annually. People were moving away from the highland plateaus and into the country's central and eastern regions. Overall population density averaged 5.84 inhabitants per km², ranging from 0.6 in Pando to 19.9 in Cochabamba. Life expectancy at birth in 1992 was 61 years for women and 58 years for men. That same year, 57.5% of the population was classified as urban (i.e., living in towns of more than 2,000 inhabitants): three metropolitan areas (La Paz, Santa Cruz, and Cochabamba) were home to 36.2% of Bolivia's population, with 21.3% living in 112 other cities. Children under 15 years of age accounted for 42% of the population, and people over 64, approximately 4%; for urban areas, these figures were 39% and 4%, rising to 44% and 6% in rural areas. Women represented 50.6% of the total population. The total fertility rate was 5 children per woman, more than 1 child less than in the previous decade; the rate ranged from 4.2 children per woman in urban areas to 6.3 for rural women. The indigenous population, estimated at over 3.6 million, encompasses 35 ethnic groups; the Quechua and Aymará are the largest groups, especially in the cities of Potosí, Oruro, Sucre, El Alto, La Paz, and Cochabamba.

In 1992, 70% of Bolivia's 1,322,512 homes lacked adequate access to basic education, health, and housing and were classified as poor (51% of urban homes and 94% of rural homes). Thirty-seven percent of these families lived in conditions of extreme poverty (32% were considered indigent and 5% lived in abject poverty); 13% lived at the poverty threshold, with a minimum level of satisfaction of their basic needs; and only 17% were able to properly meet their basic needs. At the department level, the percentage of poor households ranged from 58% in Santa Cruz to 81% in Pando. The highest poverty levels were found among monolingual indigenous populations and households headed by individuals working in the informal sector. Over 70% of poor households were headed by someone who had not completed primary school. Roughly 70% of children under 9 years of age lived in extremely poor homes and did not attend school. Studies on the determining factors of poverty indicate that indigenous populations are 40% more likely to be poor; each additional child increases this probability by 6.5% and an unemployed head of household increases it by a further 14%; each additional year of schooling, however, reduces the likelihood of poverty.

According to 1992 census data, 19.8% of the population aged 15 or over was illiterate (11.8% among males and 27.7% among females); this represents a 50% drop with respect to the 1976 census. In rural Bolivia, over one-third of the population (23% of males and 50% of females) was illiterate, with school attendance calculated at 74.3% for children between the ages of 6 and 19 (76.5% for boys and 72.1% for girls); at the primary education level (children aged 6 to 14 years), the rate was 83.9%. Women are gradually assuming a broader role in the country's political and economic life. In the 1993–1997 legislative assembly, women held 3.7% of the seats in the Senate and 7.7% in the Chamber of Deputies. Only 31.6% of university graduates were women. Although their overall participation in the economy reached 39.9%, women earned on average 30% less than men at the same level of employment. Of every five rural landowners, only one was a woman.

Morbidity and Mortality Profile

In 1993, the 10 principal causes of general morbidity were diseases of the respiratory system (22%), intestinal infectious diseases (16%), other infectious and parasitic diseases and delayed effects of parasitic diseases (3%), diseases of the musculoskeletal system and connective tissue (1.6%), diseases of the skin and subcutaneous tissue (1.4%), diseases of the female genital organs (1.4%), diseases of the oral cavity (1.2%), tuberculosis (0.7%), direct obstetric causes (0.4%), and fractures (0.2%). Only 20% of deaths were certified by a health professional.

The principal causes of hospital mortality in 1993 were diseases of the circulatory system (27%), diseases of the digestive system (14%), diseases of the respiratory system (7%), cerebrovascular disease (4%), diseases of the urinary system (3.5%), certain conditions originating in the perinatal period (3%), injuries (2.5%), malignant neoplasms (1.5%), tuberculosis (0.6%), and endocrine and metabolic diseases and disorders of the immune system (0.6%).

Infant mortality decreased from 151 per 1,000 live births in 1976 to 75 per 1,000 in 1992 (based on census data for the two years), a trend that was confirmed by the 1994 National Survey of Population and Health (ENDSA 94). However, the rate in rural areas (94 per 1,000 live births) was approximately 40% higher than in urban areas (58 per 1,000 live births). Diarrhea and acute respiratory infections were the two leading causes of infant mortality. A differential analysis

of infant mortality underscores the gap between rich and poor departments. The rich departments comprise the so-called central corridor (La Paz-Cochabamba-Santa Cruz), and it is here that the country's population and economic activity are concentrated. Tarija and, to a certain extent, Chuquisaca are included in this group, although the latter's socioeconomic situation is more precarious. The mining departments of Oruro and Potosí and the departments of Beni and Pando, located in the Bolivian Amazon, are not included in the group. In the period 1976–1992, the gap between these two groups in terms of infant mortality grew even wider.

SPECIFIC HEALTH PROBLEMS

Analysis by Population Group

Health of Children

According to the ENDSA 94 survey, infant mortality stood at 75 per 1,000 for the period 1990–1994, down from 99 per 1,000 live births in the period 1984–1989. For rural areas, the rate was 92 per 1,000 live births, compared with 60 per 1,000 in urban areas; the rates for the period 1984–1989 were 120 and 80 per 1,000, respectively. Infant mortality was highest in the country's valley regions (101 per 1,000 live births), compared with 96 per 1,000 in the highland plateaus and 53 per 1,000 in the plains. Neonatal mortality was calculated at 41 per 1,000 live births, with a postneonatal rate of 34 per 1,000. Mortality in the group aged 1 to 4 dropped from 57 to 44 per 1,000 over the period in question. Child mortality for the period 1990–1994 stood at 116 per 1,000.

Data from ENDSA 94 indicated that 28% of children under 3 years of age suffered from chronic malnutrition (low height-for-age), a figure 10% lower than that reported in ENDSA 89. One of every three rural children and one of every five urban children suffered from chronic malnutrition, which was more prevalent in the highland plateaus (32%) and valley regions (30%) than in the plains (18%). According to the same source, 15% of children whose mothers had completed an intermediate or higher level of education showed stunted growth, compared with 46% of children whose mothers had no formal education. Acute malnutrition (low weight-for-height) was reported among 4.4% of children under 3, higher than the level recorded by ENDSA 89 (1.6%). The high rates of acute malnutrition in Chuquisaca (14.6%) and Potosí (10%) resulted in a higher national average for 1994.

ENDSA 94 data on prevalence and duration of breast-feeding showed that 22% of children were breast-fed within the first hour after birth and 62% within the first day. Three departments reported low levels of breast-feeding 24 hours after birth: Beni (44%), Pando (44%), and Chuquisaca (51%). A total of 61% of infants under 2 months of age were exclusively breast-fed; at 4 months of age, that figure was only 25%. At the same time, 80% of children aged 10 to 11 months were still being breast-fed (although not exclusively), and 30% were still being breast-fed at 24 months.

Health of Adolescents

The median age for a woman's first childbirth is 21.2 years. Eighteen percent of all Bolivian females between the ages of 15 and 19 were either pregnant or had already borne a child (the average age at the time of a woman's first delivery is 21.2 years). By age 19, some 37% of Bolivian women are mothers and 9% already have two or more children. Specific fertility rates have declined over the past 30 years for all age groups except the 15-to-19 group (rate unchanged), which, because of its size, has caused the total fertility rate to increase; indeed, it is estimated that, by the year 2000, 13% of all births will occur among adolescents. There is a trend toward initiating sexual activity in early adolescence (currently 2.7% of sexual activity is among people under the age of 15) as well as early initiation of sexual activity (91% of individuals before age 18 in rural areas and 84% in urban areas). Very few female adolescents used family planning methods (5.7%). Adolescent health care—sexual and reproductive health in particular—is very unsatisfactory; as a result of the country's educational reform, however, sexual education is now part of the curriculum.

Health of Adults and the Elderly

According to ENDSA 94, fertility dropped 26% during the previous five years; reproduction rates indicated that women had 4.8 children on average, compared with 6.5 in the early 1970s. Some 62% of women aged 15 to 49 lived in a conjugal relationship, and four-fifths of them were married (matrimony is the most common way of starting life as a couple). Familiarity with contraceptive methods was rather limited, although the situation is improving. In 1994, three of every four women had heard of modern methods of birth control, compared with two of three women in 1989; moreover, 64% said they knew about the pill and intrauterine devices (IUDs), compared with 54% in 1989. Knowledge about sterilization remained unchanged from the 1989 level (54%), although one-half of the women who lived with their partners knew about condoms, compared with 29% in 1989. IUDs were the modern contraceptive method most used in 1994. The use of contraceptives is more prevalent among urban women with higher levels of formal education, especially in the departments of Tarija and Santa Cruz, where roughly

55% of women used contraceptive methods (60% of the methods were modern).

The ENDSA 94 survey data indicated that maternal mortality had remained relatively unchanged: 416 deaths per 100,000 live births in the 1984–1989 period, compared with 390 in the 1990–1994 period. For the highland plateaus, the rate was estimated at 602 per 100,000 live births, more than twice that of the valley regions (293) and almost six times the figure for the plains areas (110). Urban maternal mortality was calculated at 274 per 100,000 live births; the rate among rural mothers was 524 per 100,000, although it reached 887 per 100,000 in the rural highland plateaus. Only one-half of all pregnant women received prenatal care from trained personnel (physician, nurse, nursing auxiliary); 47% received no prenatal care whatsoever. Only 50% of women had been vaccinated against tetanus; in departments in the plains, the area where coverage is highest, the level was only 60%. A high percentage of babies are delivered at home (57%), often without professional care (only 40% of cases). The principal causes of maternal death are, by order of frequency, hemorrhage, toxemia, infection, and obstructed labor; abortions account for an estimated 27% to 35% of maternal deaths.

Persons over age 60 represented 6.1% of the population in 1992, and many of them still worked. The estimated mortality rate among persons over 65 years of age was 7.8 per 100,000 population (8.2 among men and 7.4 among women). There is no explicit government policy on care for the elderly, and health plans and programs for this age group are not assigned priority.

Workers' Health

In 1994, the economically active population (EAP)—defined as all people 10 years of age or older—represented 59% (3,921,236) of the total population; 42% of them worked in the agricultural sector. Women have been increasing their participation in the work force and in 1992 they accounted for 39% of the EAP. An estimated 8% of the EAP is between the ages of 7 and 14. Unemployment oscillates between 9% and 24% of the EAP. Employment activity is not limited to the formal sector; Bolivia's National Statistics Bureau estimates that 1,366,060 people work in the informal sector of the economy. Of the 125,853 economic units identified by the second National Survey of Businesses (1992), 81% had fewer than five employees.

Reliable data on work-related accidents are limited. Of the country's eight existing insurance funds, only the National Health Insurance (which covers approximately 80% of all insured workers) reported data: 1,085 cases of work-related disabilities each year. Among the 15,000 workers exposed to occupational diseases, the most prevalent ones were silicosis

(7.6%) and silicotuberculosis (1.4%). Until the 1980s, when traditional mining activities began to drop off, the reported prevalence among 67,000 exposed workers was around 24%. The occupational hazards of mining and other extractive activities have now been compounded by those of agroindustry and the machine tool, metallurgical, and refining industries (the gas industry, in particular). Specific-risk studies have recorded blood lead levels over the maximum allowable limit among 48.5% of foundry workers and 11.5% of workers at volatile chemical plants; unacceptable urine mercury levels were found among 70.0% of foundry workers; and excessive urine arsenic levels were found among 53.2% of foundry workers and 2.7% of workers at volatile chemical plants. Research conducted between 1989 and 1993 on agricultural workers directly exposed to organophosphorus-containing pesticides revealed blood levels of cholinesterase that were 2.9% below normal in the highland plateaus, 7.0% below normal in valley areas, and 8.8% below normal in the plains.

Only 0.5% of workers in the agricultural subsector of hunting and fishing have health insurance, compared with 30% in the transportation subsector, 55% in construction, 86% to 90% in manufacturing and trade, 90% to 100% in the health and education sectors, and 100% in the banking and financial sector. In economic terms, it has been estimated that the country is losing up to 9.4% of its GDP in direct and indirect costs deriving from work-related injuries. The Labor Act of 1938, which addresses occupational hazards, officially established the principle of worker safety, and Law 16,998 of 1979 assigned responsibilities to the various government agencies and defined the rights and obligations of employers and employees. The Social Security Code outlines standards and socioeconomic arrangements for worker disabilities and mandates the payment of a pension to disabled workers or, in the event of death, to their lawful heirs. The workers' health subsector has undergone a major upheaval since 1997, when the newly created pension fund administrators were charged with managing professional risk up to the year 2001, at which time the law stipulates that specific pension funds are to be in place to provide such management.

Health of Indigenous People

In 1994, a census was carried out in Bolivia's lowlands (i.e., the Oriente, Chaco, and Amazonia regions) aimed at identifying the country's indigenous groups on the basis of language, territory, and self-identity. Three major linguistic groups were identified—the Aymará, the Quechua, and the Guaraní—which are further subdivided into 35 ethnic groups, each with its own cultural identity. It is estimated that nine ethnic groups have died out since the beginning of the twentieth century.

The Aymará group represents 23.5% of the population and is located in the departments of La Paz, Oruro, and Potosí. Infant mortality in La Paz was 106 per 1,000 live births; in the Aymará provinces of the departments of Oruro and Potosí, however, it fluctuated between 120 and 135 per 1,000 live births. Serious to moderate malnutrition among children under 5 years old was higher than the national average in the provinces of Inquisivi, Tamayo, and Omasuyos (department of La Paz). The highest fertility rates (more than seven children per woman) were reported in Tamayo and Villarroel. With the exception of Murillo (La Paz) and Cercado (Oruro), over 10% of the Aymará population used traditional medicine, with that percentage rising to over 30% in the provinces of Tamayo, Camacho, Muñecas, and Aroma in La Paz and in the provinces of San Pedro de Totora, Litoral, and Nor Carangas in Oruro. The proportion of the population with access to Western medicine ranged from 11% to 65%, with the lowest figures being registered in northern La Paz. The areas with the highest percentage of people lacking access to any type of service (over 30%) were situated in the provinces of Los Andes, Pacajes, and Pando in La Paz. Self-medication was found to be most prevalent among the inhabitants of Tamayo, Nor Yungas, and Larecaja (La Paz).

The Quechua account for 34% of the population and they are the group whose health situation is the most precarious: 9 of Bolivia's 10 poorest provinces are located in predominantly Quechua areas; the most seriously disadvantaged groups are found in northern Potosí, western and southern Cochabamba, and in some provinces in Chuquisaca. Of the 36 provinces having Quechua residents, 23 have over 20% monolinguals, a percentage that rises to 60% in Arque (Cochabamba) and 89% in Charcas (Chuquisaca). In 20 of the provinces, the illiteracy rate exceeds 40%, and in 12 provinces over 90% of the population lacks at least one basic service. Child mortality is above the average for rural areas in Iturralde (La Paz); Zudáñez and Azurduy (Chuquisaca); Charcas and Ibáñez (Potosí); and Ayopaya, Bolívar, and Arque (Cochabamba). In some places, child malnutrition is twice the national average. Access to health care services displays patterns similar to the Aymará areas, ranging from 70% in the provinces of Oropeza and Tomás Frías to 11% in Tapacarí. There is a strong preference for traditional medicine, especially in the provinces of northern Potosí (where it is used by 85% of the population in Charcas, 70% in Ibáñez, 69% in Bilbao, and 52% in Chayanta). A similar situation is observed in southern Cochabamba (provinces of Bolívar and Arque), where over 55% of the population opts for traditional medicine; these two provinces also have the highest percentage of people who have no access whatsoever to any type of health service (14% and 20%, respectively).

The Guaraní group comprises 33 different ethnic subgroups spread across the Chaco and Oriente regions, for a total population of 150,483. The main subgroups are the Chiquitano (47,000), Guaraní (36,900), Mojeño (6,600), and Movima (7,200). Their annual population growth of 1.9% was higher than the 0.1% reported for the general rural population. The fertility rate was 8.5 children per woman, higher than the average for rural areas (6.3 children). Maternal mortality stood at 395 per 100,000 live births, which is lower than the average for rural areas (458). A full 90.5% of the lowland population lacked electricity, 51.2% lacked basic sanitation services, and only 9% had access to drinking water. The overall illiteracy rate was 23%, rising to 30% among females and 37% in rural areas. In the Oriente region, 46.3% of families did not have title to their property, compared with 42.4% in the Chaco and 50% in the Amazonia regions.

These groups are not only highly exposed to communicable diseases, they are also more vulnerable to them. The incidence of tuberculosis was five to eight times greater than the national average, and cholera took a particularly high toll among the Weenhayek (Mataco) and Guaraní communities. Gastrointestinal diseases (acute diarrhea in particular) are the leading cause of death among infants and children under 5 years of age; although these diseases strike with greater frequency and more virulence, they are not deemed a medical priority. Vaccine-preventable diseases (especially neonatal tetanus and measles) are also more prevalent among indigenous children, whose vaccination coverage is lower than for children living in urban areas. Indigenous women, too, are at a significantly greater risk of death, because they start bearing children at a younger age, they have larger families, the intervals between their pregnancies are shorter, they are breastfeeding during a large part of their reproductive lives, they receive inadequate care during delivery, and they have limited access to family-planning services. Furthermore, indigenous women are more submissive and more dependent on men (for cultural reasons) and this leads to higher levels of physical and sexual violence. Such factors, coupled with their greater reproductive risk, place these women in a group that is at high biological and social risk.

Analysis by Type of Disease or Health Impairment

Communicable Diseases

Vector-Borne Diseases. In 1996, a total of 64,012 cases of malaria were reported in eight of Bolivia's nine departments, six of them located in areas at high risk of uninterrupted transmission. Between 1991 and 1996, the annual parasite index rose from 7.0 per 1,000 population (19,031 cases) to 19.4 per 1,000. The number of localities at high risk jumped from 746 in 1993 to 2,124 in 1996, showing increases of between 8.9% and 667%. The departments of Tarija and Beni accounted for 68% of the cases reported. *Plasmodium vivax* was involved in 92% of the cases and *Plasmodium falciparum* in 8%. Cases involving *P. falciparum* had increased significantly, from 1,110 in 1991 to 4,164 in 1996. Chloroquine resistance was encountered in 15% to 45% of cases, mainly in Riberalta and Guayaramerín (Beni) and in certain areas of Pando. Fourteen hospital deaths involving malaria were reported in 1996.

With respect to Chagas' disease, the main vector—*Triatoma infestans*—was present in 60% of the country (six of Bolivia's nine departments). General seroprevalence was estimated at 40%, although it may run as high as 70% in some areas. Infestation indexes for this vector were 70% to 100% in rural areas, 40% to 60% in periurban areas, and 20% to 40% in urban areas. Chagas' disease is estimated to have a mortality rate of 13% among the general population, 29% among men aged 24 to 44, 22% among women aged 24 to 44, and 26% to 46% among children, with 32% of the latter cases attributable to the congenital form of the disease. In 1993, the National Laboratory Institute detected seroprevalences of 5% and 51% at blood banks in La Paz and Santa Cruz, respectively. A seroprevalence of 20.2% was found the following year among 14,200 donors screened by blood banks; in 1995, the level stood at 13.7% for 14,579 blood samples. Among seropositive individuals, 15% to 28% presented with Chagasic myocardiopathy and 16% suffered from gastrointestinal disorders. Chagas' disease is estimated to have cut the country's labor capacity by 25%, equivalent to 105,000 years of productive life lost and an economic cost to the country of US$ 39 million. Bolivia is an active participant in the Southern Cone initiative to eliminate vectoral transmission of *Trypanosoma cruzi* by spraying with residual-action insecticides. Of the 90,000 homes sprayed over the course of the 1990s, 35,000 were sprayed in 1996.

Leishmaniasis is found in tropical and subtropical areas of La Paz, Beni, Pando, Santa Cruz, and Cochabamba. A total of 5,780 cases were reported between 1989 and 1996; of those, 40% (2,310) were reported in 1996: 93.2% were the cutaneous form and 6.8% were the mucous form (the only cases of visceral leishmaniasis were reported in 1993, and even then only in certain valley areas). Men accounted for 65% of all cases, and 75% of those cases occurred in males aged 15 and older. In 1996, only 55.2% of diagnosed patients were treated with a full regimen and proper dosages.

No cases of Bolivian hemorrhagic fever were reported between 1975—the year when seven cases and two deaths were reported in San Joaquín—and 1993, when a case was reported in the province of Mamoré. In 1994, nine cases were reported in the province of Iténez; six of them ended in death. In 1996, there were three nonfatal cases, all in the department of Beni.

Laboratory tests conducted in January 1996 detected the presence of dengue fever in Santa Cruz de la Sierra. The serotypes I and II were in circulation, and a total of 66 cases had been reported as of January 1997. Women accounted for

66% of all cases, with 90% of those cases occurring in females aged 15 and older. No cases of dengue hemorrhagic fever were reported. The infestation index for the *Aedes* mosquito was calculated at 18% in 1996.

Jungle yellow fever continues to be a problem. Starting in 1984, when 12 cases were reported, the disease followed an upward trend that reached 107 cases in 1989, 50 in 1990, and 91 in 1991, only to drop off sharply to 8 cases in 1994. Subsequently, in 1996, 30 cases were reported, pointing to a new upswing in transmission of this disease. The cases occurred in the departments of La Paz, Santa Cruz, Beni, and, in particular, Cochabamba. The disease struck adult males the hardest, producing a 70% case fatality rate. Vaccination campaigns are conducted in areas at risk, usually in response to reports of an outbreak, and protection is provided to military troops stationed in at-risk areas.

In December 1996, there was an outbreak of plague (27 cases) in the town of San Pedro (Apolo, La Paz), with an attack rate of 11%, a case fatality rate of 15%, and general mortality of 2%. Cases were concentrated in the 15-to-49 age group (73%). A blood sample tested positive for *Yersinia pestis*. Actions to control the outbreak included treating individuals with streptomycin and spraying homes with deltamethrin.

Vaccine-Preventable Diseases. The last case of clinically confirmed poliomyelitis in Bolivia was in 1988. In 1994, the last case considered as polio-compatible was seen. Flaccid paralysis in children under 15 years of age was reported at a rate of 2.2 per 100,000 population in 1993, falling to 1.7 in 1994, 1995, and 1996.

Vaccination coverage stood at 81% in 1993, 82% in 1994, 86% in 1995, and 82% in 1996. In 1992, there was a major outbreak of measles, the largest Bolivia had seen in 10 years (4,937 cases). An elimination program was launched and succeeded in raising vaccination coverage to 90% in 1997, ultimately bringing down the number of cases to 16 in 1995 and 4 in 1996 (based on clinical diagnosis).

Neonatal tetanus had declined since the 1992 level of 42 reported cases, with only 14 cases reported in 1996 (0.1 per 1,000 births); between 1992 and 1996, vaccination coverage rose from 52% to 55% among women of child-bearing age and from 77% to 82% among infants under 1 year of age.

Diphtheria dropped from 20 cases in 1992 to 1 case in 1996, and whooping cough fell from 284 cases in 1992 to only 14 in 1996; vaccination coverage now exceeds 80%. A seroprevalence of 1.1% was detected for hepatitis B among 13,276 donors screened at blood banks in 1994, rising to 1.5% based on 13,295 samples screened in 1995.

Cholera and Other Intestinal Infectious Diseases. In 1992, there were 23,862 reported cases of cholera (349 per 100,000 inhabitants), with a case fatality rate of 1.7%; in

1993, 10,290 cases were reported (150 per 100,000 inhabitants), with a case fatality rate of 2,5%; in 1994, 2,718 cases were reported; in 1995, 3,136 cases were reported; and in 1996, 2,632 cases were reported, with a case fatality rate of 2.4%. The highest case fatality rates were observed in remote, rural areas of La Paz and Potosí that lacked easy access to health services. Cholera cases were concentrated in the 15-to-59 age group, with a slightly higher prevalence among males.

The prevalence of diarrheal diseases in children under 3 years of age declined from 36% (ENDSA 89) to 30% (ENDSA 94). An average of five diarrheal episodes were calculated per child per year, and an estimated 7,900 deaths among children under 5 were attributed each year to this cause. The hospital fatality rate for cases involving diarrhea in this age group was 5% in 1992 and 4.8% in 1995.

Chronic Communicable Diseases. Tuberculosis-related care services increased sixfold between 1993 and 1995 and are evidence of the high priority accorded to this disease by the country's health authorities. The number of health care facilities with control programs in place rose from 214 to 1,269 (with government-run services providing 71% of overall coverage). The network of diagnostic laboratories grew from 127 in 1987 to 302 in 1995; the number of diagnostic bacilloscopies performed between 1983 and 1995 quadrupled, going from 18,528 (0.2 per symptomatic patient) to 81,252 (1.3 per symptomatic patient) and, ultimately, in 1996, to a level of 2.8 bacilloscopies per symptomatic patient. Reported cases of tuberculosis (all forms) dropped from 165 to 129 per 100,000 population between 1990 and 1995, with the incidence in 1995 calculated at 116 per 100,000 males and 73 per 100,000 females. Case reports were highest in La Paz, Santa Cruz, and Cochabamba. In the cohort of pulmonary tuberculosis cases treated with directly observed treatment strategy (DOTS), a cure rate of 76% was recorded. Primary resistance was found to be 5.8% for isoniazid, 1.8% for rifampicin, and 4.4% for streptomycin; acquired resistance was reported at 14.7%, 12.6%, and 11.5%, respectively. The case fatality rate of 4.5% had remained stable since 1988.

Leprosy is present in rural areas of Beni, Pando, Santa Cruz, Cochabamba, Chuquisaca, Tarija, and La Paz. Between 1989 and 1996, a total of 3,793 cases were reported (71% were the multibacillary form and 29% were paucibacillary). Eighty-six new cases were detected in 1995, and there were an additional 32 in 1996. All the reported cases involved persons over 15 years of age (60% were males). The case detection rate in 1996 stood at 5 cases per 100,000 population, with a prevalence of 110 per 100,000 population. The country has adopted the use of multidrug therapy.

Acute Respiratory Infections. Acute respiratory infections (ARIs) continue to be the leading cause of morbidity and the second most common cause of mortality among children. The ratio of ARI mortality to mortality from pneumonia decreased 30% between 1989 and 1994 (dropping from 28% to 20%). According to ENDSA 94 data, 18% of children under 3 years of age had symptoms of ARIs in the two weeks preceding the survey; this percentage was 25% among infants 6 to 11 months old, and 13% for infants under 6 months. The departments of Beni and Pando accounted for 33% of all cases. Estimates from the National Office for the Health and Nutrition of Women and Children indicate that each year some 5,600 children under 5 years of age die from causes attributable to ARIs. The hospital fatality rate from pneumonia in this age group, based on information from the National Health Information System, was 10% in 1992 and 7.2% in 1995.

Rabies and Other Zoonoses. Between 1977 and 1994, a total of 269 cases of human rabies were reported, 71% of them in Santa Cruz and Cochabamba. Eight cases were reported in 1995, and an additional three cases in 1996. Sixty-five percent of the patients were males; 55% were persons under the age of 20. The predominant form of transmission was by dogs (91%). As for animal rabies, 92% of the cases occurred in dogs, 2% in cats, and 6% in other domestic and wild animals.

Tomography studies on teniasis conducted in 1990 at neurological centers in Cochabamba detected 107 cases of neurocysticercosis. In 1995, research on teniasis and cysticercosis in 25 high-risk localities found seroprevalence levels of 12% and 16.4% in Chuquisaca, 7% and 4.7% in Potosí, 1% and 2.5% in Santa Cruz, 8.2% and 3.7% in Tarija, 7% and 7% in Cochabamba, 8% and 3% in La Paz, and 0% (teniasis) and 5.1% to 5.8% (cysticercosis) in Oruro, Cobija, and Trinidad. Parasite disinfestation campaigns (with praziquantel) were carried out. Cases of other zoonoses (e.g., fasciolasis and foot-and-mouth disease) were also reported.

AIDS and Other STDs. The first case of AIDS was reported in 1985; as of 1996, a total of 123 cases had been detected in addition to 111 cases of asymptomatic infection with the human immunodeficiency virus (HIV). Ninety-two percent of the cases were in the 15-to-49 age group, and 75% of the patients were males. The means of transmission were sexual contact (92%), blood transfusions (6%), and perinatal transmission (2%). Cases of HIV/AIDS infection were reported in eight of the country's nine departments, although most were concentrated in Santa Cruz, La Paz, and Cochabamba. Blood banks screened 16,093 donors in 1994, detecting a seroprevalence of 0.02%, and 14,227 donors in 1995, detecting a seroprevalence of 0.03%.

The number of reported cases of syphilis (all forms) is on the rise; the rate of incidence per 100,000 population increased from 44 in 1992 to 55 in 1995. In the 20-to-29 age group, 48% of the cases were among women. Blood banks screened 13,334 donors in 1994 and 14,092 in 1995, detecting seroprevalences of 2.4% and 1.3%, respectively. Gonorrhea was observed at a rate of 73 cases per 100,000 population in 1995, compared with 30 per 100,000 in 1992. The age group most affected was 20-to-29-year-olds, with 65% of the cases occurring among males.

Noncommunicable Diseases and Other Health-Related Problems

Nutritional Diseases and Diseases of Metabolism. According to information from the International Fund for Agricultural Development (IFAD), the daily per capita availability of calories showed a gradual downward trend between the periods 1979–1981 and 1986–1988 (dropping from 2,082 to 1,987 kcal per day). Data for 1994 showed a level of 2,115 kcal per person per day. Studies undertaken in 1994 and 1996 by a committee of experts (the International Council for the Control of Iodine Deficiency Disorders) revealed a level of iodized salt consumption calculated at 91.6%, average levels of urinary iodine among the general population at 25.02 µg/dl, and 4.5% prevalence of goiter in schoolchildren. With regard to vitamin A deficiency, a 1991 study of 979 children between the ages of 12 and 71 months found serum retinol levels to be below 20 µg/dl in 11.3% of the cases (19.5% in rural areas of the highland plateaus and 16.5% in the plains area) and below 30 µg/dl in 48.3% of the cases (marginal or subclinical deficiency). Vitamin A deficiency has been targeted under the Expanded Programme on Immunization (EPI) by means of campaigns promoting the administration of capsules containing 200,000 international units of this vitamin. A 1992 study by the Bolivian Institute for High-Altitude Biology focusing on highland children between the ages of 6 months and 9 years showed a prevalence of iron deficiency (as manifested by the presence of nutritional anemia) ranging from 14.6% to 42.6% at an altitude of 3,600 m above sea level and from 23.3% to 67.2% at 4,800 m above sea level; the prevalence of anemia was found to decrease with age.

Domestic Violence. In one 12-month period (1992–1993), Bolivia's four largest cities recorded 21,500 official reports of violence against women, 73% of which involved domestic violence. In almost all cases, the aggressor was a male (a companion or former companion of the woman); the forms of violence were classified as physical (48% of cases), psychological and other (42%), and sexual (10%). Since 1994, the Undersecretariat for Gender Affairs has been overseeing implementation of the National Plan for the Prevention and Eradication of Violence against Women, and in December 1995 the National

Congress passed the Domestic Violence Act. A network of legal support and family protection services has been set up in the country's main cities. The fact that the number of reported cases of family violence has increased since 1996 is attributable to greater public awareness and mobilization in this area. Given the delicate nature of the issue of sexual abuse, available data do not always reflect the true situation of sexual abuse of children and adolescents. According to the Undersecretariat for Gender Affairs, of every 10 women who were victims of violence in Santa Cruz, at least 2 of them had been raped; in Cochabamba, at least 1 had been a victim of rape.

Oral Health. In June 1995, the then National Health Secretariat conducted a study of 2,666 children between the ages of 6 and 15 in 128 periurban and rural schools; the study revealed an overall index of decayed, missing, or filled teeth (the DMFT index) of 7.6 (9.5 for 6-to-9-year olds and 6.9 for 6-to-15-year olds). The DMFT index for children from families considered to be moderately poor was 4.5 in valley areas, 7.3 in the highland plateaus, and 10.9 in the plains. The average fluoride content of the water supply—at 0.29 ppm—was below the recommended level. A ministerial resolution was subsequently signed attaching high priority to this issue and launching a salt fluoridation program.

RESPONSE OF THE HEALTH SYSTEM

National Health Plans and Policies

The Government of Bolivia has responded to the country's health situation by passing the Community Involvement Act (*Ley de Participación Popular,* April 1994). The act transfers ownership of all local service infrastructure to the *municipios,* allocates funding for this purpose (which would now be apportioned on a population or per capita basis rather than discretionally), and delegates to them all responsibility for the operation, maintenance, and administration of that infrastructure. Under the legislation, the *municipios* are granted full title to all revenue generated by the sale of such services; they are also required to formulate social and economic development plans (for health actions as well) under a participatory approach that involves the user population. Lastly, the act created a supervisory committee that would be responsible for overseeing activities and the appropriate use of funds. Human resources and countrywide programs would continue to be financed out of the national budget. Subsequent legislation (the Administrative Decentralization Act) transferred human resource administration to the local government level (*prefectura*) of each department, although funding would continue to come from the national budget.

The then National Health Secretariat that had become part of the Ministry of Human Development devised a national health model that was intended to help the health sector adapt to the recent legislative developments. Approved in 1996, this new model provided the legal framework for restructuring the health sector. It defined the public health system as a decentralized, participatory structure that served as both the sector's response to and its instrument for policy and for technical, administrative, and citizens' concerns in the face of the current situation of poverty and health. At the conceptual level, the model framed health policies and plans against the broader backdrop of human development and called for greater coordination between health and education actions, giving due consideration to variables such as gender, ethnic heritage, age, degree of urban development, and the fight against poverty. At an operational level, the model outlined a structure and organization for the national health system, sector management arrangements, and the responsibilities of the various social participants in the production of health.

Organization of the Health Sector

Institutional Organization

Under the model described above, the national health system comprised all public and private services that are engaged in health-related activities under the aegis of the then National Health Secretariat; these include the public health system, the social security system, private for-profit and not-for-profit entities, religious groups, and traditional medicine.

In 1998, the Ministry of Health and Social Welfare designed a new health model that defines the Bolivian Health System as a universal access system based on primary care and embracing gender and intercultural approaches. In terms of operations, the new model establishes care, management, and financial modalities. The Bolivian Health System is defined as accessible, efficient, and solidary and having sustainable quality and multiple providers.

Public Health System. The public health system is a decentralized, participatory system that is funded out of the national budget. Its mission is to provide health care and respond to the population's health needs while observing criteria of universal access, solidarity, and efficiency. The system is essentially a network of services that are administered locally and jointly by the community and by the department and *municipio* governments. This network is organized into three care levels. The first level is formed by the country's 896 health centers and 1,210 health posts, which provide a total of 2,276 beds for attending to normal deliveries and emergency hospitalization;

traditional medicine is included in this level. Basic hospitalization services and specialized consultations make up the second level, represented by 63 district hospitals (a total of 1,717 beds). The third level—highly specialized consultations and hospital care—is made up of the country's 81 general hospitals (5,277 beds), 29 specialized hospitals (including social security facilities and psychiatric hospitals, for a total of 2,071 beds), and national reference and technical support centers.

Health promotion, preventive and curative care, and rehabilitation services are provided throughout the network and at all levels, in accordance with each level's ability to respond to the community's health care needs and the programs and strategies defined locally as part of the participatory planning and programming process.

The system basically has two kinds of management arrangements: management by sector institutions and management that is exercised jointly with the local community. Management by sector institutions refers to the administration of all actions involved in the definition and administration of policies, plans, and programs for the delivery of health care services. Jointly exercised management refers to the responsibilities assumed in cooperation with the local community to administer health care services in a given *municipio*. This kind of management is performed through the local health boards, which provide a locus for consensus building, negotiation, and coordination with an eye to the smooth development and operation of the municipal health system. The health boards are overseen by the local level of government (which provides infrastructure and operational support) and are made up of a sector representative (from the office of the *prefecto*, which provides the human resources) and a representative of the users or the organized community (who provide community monitoring and contribute to the overall financing of the local health system through payment of fees, whence the need for shared management).

Nongovernmental organizations (NGOs) and the churches in the country play a significant role in health care delivery. At the national level, a broad-based agreement has been signed by the Ministry of Finance and the National Health Secretariat; at the local level, specific agreements are signed with each local health board allowing NGOs to work directly with local governments.

Traditional-medicine practitioners are allowed to practice at health care establishments or at the *municipio* level; they also are authorized to set up practice independently in the private sector. There are no legal restrictions on the practice of traditional medicine, and the local health boards are permitted to use these practitioners in the public care network, which in fact occurs in the case of midwives. This notwithstanding, their integration into the public network has not been smooth. Surveys reveal that the public sector provides health care for about 40% of the national population.

Health Insurance. Aside from the coverage provided by the public sector per se, Bolivia has an additional health insurance scheme that covers hourly workers. These "insurance funds" (*cajas de salud*), however, are separate from the pension plans, even though they are tied in to conventional social security financing arrangements. The funds currently provide coverage to 20% of the population, but their growth has been very slow or even negative in recent years. There are eight health insurance funds and two special, comprehensive insurance funds; benefits and quality of care vary from one to the next. The largest of these funds is the National Health Insurance, which provides 85% of the country's social security coverage and whose principal guarantor is the Republic of Bolivia. These health insurance schemes do not cover informal, self-employed, or migrant workers, nor do they cover peasant farmers, operators of for-hire vehicles, housewives, domestic workers, miners who are members of cooperatives, or employees of small businesses; all these people must be covered by the public subsector. Ambulatory care is provided at the outpatient services of hospitals and clinics run by the various funds. This subsector is essentially self-governing, although its activity is coordinated by a unit of the National Health Secretariat and by the National Health Insurance Institute, which performs oversight and policy-setting functions. It has an extensive service network of some 9,300 employees and possesses suitable technological capacity. The subsector focuses on hospital care and on the urban population (only 4% of the rural population is covered), it is relatively inactive in the area of health promotion, and it lacks arrangements for user participation in management and planning.

Private Subsector. This subsector is made up of for-profit and nonprofit, privately run companies and organizations that have their own funding. It is regulated by the National Health Secretariat and other government authorities and agencies, who make sure that services are safe and efficient and that qualified personnel are employed. The private subsector comprises:

• Private firms, such as health care providers and suppliers of inputs, diagnostic support services, and drugs. Although the private subsector is perceived to operate efficiently, only 10% of the population is thought to use its services regularly. The subsector is experiencing significant growth in urban areas and is able to respond well to the socioeconomic conditions of the neighborhoods where it operates. Even so, private medicine has yet to be taken into account in the planning and organization of the health system, and oversight of the subsector continues to be weak. Some of these services are consumed by the health insurance funds, although a large portion are, in essence, subsidized by the public sector, because private care providers use the public sector's infrastructure.

• Nonprofit organizations. NGOs are the main participants in this category; there are many of them in Bolivia and their presence locally depends on the area and poverty level of the *municipio*, as well as on the churches' activity. Many conduct health promotion activities, and some provide health care services directly, under agreements with the *municipios*; yet others focus on helping the *municipios* and existing services to strengthen their management capacity and organization (e.g., Medicus Mundi, Doctors Without Borders, and Plan Internacional). An association of health-related NGOs has been set up to coordinate the work of local and international NGOs in this sphere. Most receive international funding, with very few benefiting from local financing. The majority of these NGOs work in depressed urban areas; a few, mainly those with international financing, are active in extremely poor *municipios*. NGOs are gradually being incorporated into the public health insurance system and into the revamped structure of the new health model. An estimated 10% of the national population uses these services, chiefly at the primary care level; for health promotion activities, the figure is much higher.

Churches provide important services to the community, especially in areas of extreme poverty and in marginal urban areas. In most cases, work is organized around government-sponsored human resources, the churches' infrastructure, and partial financing by users. The churches' work in some departments has helped to set up service networks that include all three care levels, usually in combination with health promotion activities. In some *municipios* and communities, the churches are the sole service providers.

• Traditional medicine is practiced widely, and almost every rural or marginal urban community has some kind of practitioner (e.g., midwives, traditional healers, etc.). The health system is gradually moving to incorporate traditional midwives into local care networks. Demand for these services is high and they are often used in conjunction with other public and private services. Some of the Western-style care providers who also practice traditional medicine have formed an association (SOBOMETRA), and their establishments have been gaining acceptance around the country. An estimated 20% to 30% of the population has serious difficulties in accessing formal public and private health care services, because of either a shortage of such services or their inaccessibility for cultural, economic, geographic, or functional reasons. These are the people who turn to self-treatment and traditional medicine. Against such a backdrop, the inauguration of national insurance for mothers and children in July 1996 was a major milestone; coverage is provided for ambulatory care; medical, surgical, and pharmaceutical assistance; basic laboratory services; hospital care during pregnancy, delivery, and puerperium; obstetric emergencies; and medical,

pharmaceutical, and hospital care in cases of acute diarrheal diseases or ARIs, including pneumonia in newborns and children under 5 years old. The plan is funded out of the 3% transferred to the municipal governments under the country's revenue-sharing arrangements. Another milestone was establishment of the national old-age insurance scheme (financed with earnings from the national charity lottery), which provides access to care at no cost to persons aged 65 and older.

Health Services and Resources

Organization of Services for Care of the Population

Water Supply and Sewerage Systems. Services in this sector fall within the sphere of the National Basic Sanitation Directorate, which is the agency in charge of coordinating the supply of basic sanitation services with the local governments and service providers. Between 1993 and 1995, water supply coverage rose 6.4% and sewerage coverage 2.8%; in 1996, the levels stood at 58.2% and 44.5% respectively, dropping to 24% and 17% in rural areas. The Basic Rural Environmental Sanitation Program, with support from the World Bank, the United Nations, and PAHO/WHO, hopes to close these gaps by promoting community participation at the municipal level.

Hospital and Municipal Solid-Waste Management. Considerable progress has been made in this area since 1992. As of 1996, seven of the nine major cities had effective solid waste collection and disposal services; coverage at the national level was 60%. In 1997, a second phase of activity was launched in seven medium-sized cities, which brought coverage up to 70%; service coverage for the scattered rural population is the principal challenge remaining. Plans are to greatly expand coverage by the year 2010 by means of self-sustaining microenterprises that have been trained in solid waste management. With regard to hospital waste, a pilot project has been implemented at a number of tertiary-level hospitals with support from international technical cooperation; the project is now slated for upscaling to the national level.

Prevention and Control of Air Pollution. Programs to control fixed-point and mobile-source emissions have been launched with a view to bettering air quality in two major cities. In 1994, Bolivia enacted Law 1,484, which adhered to international agreements for protecting the ozone layer; in 1996 the Governmental Ozone-Protection Commission was created, and a nationwide calendar was adopted for mandatory phasing-out of chlorofluorocarbon use.

Environmental Risks

Water. Several major watersheds continue to register high pollution levels, and only four major cities have wastewater treatment plants (in the past four years, only one new treatment plant was opened). Industries—mining concerns in particular—do not exercise adequate control over the materials they discharge into waterways and, accordingly, there is a high risk of chemical contamination, especially with heavy metals and especially in the departments of La Paz, Oruro, and Potosí. The Porco incident—240,000 tons of mining waste that spilled into the Pilcomayo River when a dike broke—is a dramatic example of the risk that water contamination poses to the population's health and the ecological damage that can be wrought. Panning for gold has led to mercury contamination in rivers throughout most of Pando, Beni, and La Paz, and it could affect the health of area residents who eat contaminated fish. Similarly, the waste dumped from sugar mills in Santa Cruz has been polluting rivers and destroying local flora and fauna.

Air. Fixed-point emissions of metallic dusts and gases contribute to high air pollution indexes in mining areas, especially around foundries in Potosí, Oruro, and La Paz (El Alto). Studies of children in Oruro and El Alto have found blood arsenic and lead levels three to four times higher than the allowable limit. Significant amounts of lead are emitted by mobile sources (e.g., from gasoline) and contribute to the problem of air pollution in urban areas.

Soil. Commercial logging activities in the warm valleys of La Paz and the *chapare* area of Cochabamba have left extensive tracts of former forestland bare, and other forest areas have been burned down to clear land for agricultural use. These practices have triggered a serious ecological imbalance that threatens the survival of various species of local flora and fauna. In the department of Tarija, deforestation coupled with drought and strong winds has led to soil erosion and destroyed a unique ecosystem, converting it into desert. A similar phenomenon is being observed in the warm valleys as a consequence of intensive coca cultivation, a practice that depletes the soil's nutrients and reduces its productive capacity. The heavy rains that flooded several areas of the country in 1997 resulted in a national emergency that had repercussions for some 77,330 persons.

Housing. According to the National Fund for Low-Income Housing, 40% of the Bolivian population lacks access to housing. Approximately US$ 80 million is being invested in the construction of 35,000 homes in different areas of the country, especially in medium-sized cities and department seats. To solve the quantitative housing deficit, though, some 200,000 homes would need to be built each year, and an estimated half a million existing homes are in need of qualitative improvements. Electricity is available in 87% of urban dwellings (68% in Beni, 90% in Potosí and Oruro) but only 15% of rural dwellings (6% in Chuquisaca, 23% in Cochabamba).

Chemical Safety. Bolivia is drawing up a national profile of chemical substances and preparing a project entitled "*Sustancias Químicas Bolivia*" (Chemicals Bolivia). Consideration is being given to legislation that would control the importation, transport, storage, and use of chemicals, and negotiations are under way for Bolivia to join the International Network of Chemical Substances.

Food Protection and Control. Food surveillance and control is performed at the production, handling, transportation, and storage stages. Any foodstuff that is made available to the public is subject to monitoring by the local Municipal Sanitation Directorate and by the National Health Secretariat's Food Control Directorate. The central level maintains a national registry of foods processed in the country and a registry of authorized food importers, and it grants authorization for the sale of imported processed foodstuffs.

Surveillance of Foodborne Diseases. The VETA project has been providing stepped-up epidemiological surveillance of foodborne diseases since January 1996 in the departments of Santa Cruz, Cochabamba, Potosí, and La Paz. As the policy-setting body in this sphere, the Office for Food Control is represented on the Technical Standards Committee of the National Industry Secretariat and the Bolivian *Codex Alimentarius* Committee; it is also the focal point for the subcommittee on food safety. As of 1996, the National Registry contained 3,855 listed food products and 850 controlled products (importation, registry, and follow-up).

Organization and Operation of Personal Health Care Services

As of 1996, Bolivia had 2,279 registered health care establishments (2,007 of them operated by the National Health Secretariat, NGOs, or the churches, and 272 operated by the social security system) and a total of 11,939 beds (8,503 and 3,436 respectively), averaging out to 3,291 persons per establishment and 1.6 beds per 1,000 population. The occupancy rate of 41.1% is a clear indicator that hospital services (i.e., the ones that use the most resources) are underutilized. According to 1995 data from the National Health Information System, 56.1% of the total of 4,764,742 outpatient consultations were performed by the public subsector, 24.3% by the social security system, 10.8% by health NGOs, 6.9% by church-affiliated services, and 2.0% by the private sector that reports. In terms of sector output, this comes to 0.63 consultation per person per year. Deliveries attended by qualified personnel had a coverage level of 35.5%. Prenatal care coverage (i.e., a series of four checkups) was calculated at 26.9%; the average was 1.97 consultations per pregnancy. Of the 434,546 prenatal checkups performed, 63.0% were done at public sector facilities, 16.8% at social security establishments, 11.8% by NGOs, 6.5% by church-affiliated services, and 1.9% by private sector providers. According to the same source, only 46% of the population had first-time contact with the public health system during the year. As for hospital discharges, in 1995 the National Health Information System recorded 2.8 discharges per 100 population nationwide (ranging from 1.5 in Cochabamba to 5.4 in Beni), an average stay of 5.8 days per bed, and an occupancy rate of 46%.

The public sector's emergency services are in need of greater operating capacity and more modern and expeditious systems for communications and transportation. La Paz and Santa Cruz are the only two cities to have implemented the Dial-118 emergency telephone line, which has been handling calls and transportation for medical emergencies since 1996. A similar service is run by the police department (Dial 110).

Diagnostic and therapeutic support services are present at most secondary and tertiary level hospitals, but they are relatively rare in rural areas. According to the National Health Secretariat, Bolivia had 224 working laboratories in 1997. In 1995, a total of 1,322,096 laboratory tests were performed; 40 public sector and 20 private hemotherapy services were registered, bringing donor totals to 15,743 public sector and 6,403 private donors; and 20,451 blood transfusions were performed (compared with 18,991 in 1994).

Regarding oral health, there were 355,971 first-time consultations and 220,390 follow-up visits in 1996, with 266,339 extractions and 158,127 fillings performed. A total of 5,735 children under 5 years of age received follow-up fluoride applications; and 47,486 dental surgical procedures were performed.

Inputs for Health

Essential Drugs and Medications. There is inequitable access and inefficient use of essential drugs and medications, which has led to the marketing of drugs that are not only more costly but are of doubtful efficacy and safety. With total annual sales of roughly US$ 70 million (US$ 10 per capita), the pharmaceutical market is supplied by 26 local manufacturers (40%) and by importers (60%). The market is very concentrated: three large laboratories cover about 40% of the domestic market. The National Program for Essential Drugs was launched in 1990, and efforts are under way to strengthen the regulatory framework, shore up the supply of low-cost essential drugs, enhance quality, and promote the rational use of drugs. In the service network, drugs are purchased directly by patients and health establishments.

Bolivia is an active participant in the Expanded Program on Immunization and, accordingly, is able to purchase vaccines of proven effectiveness at stable, affordable prices. The national budget has made the necessary allocations for the purchase of EPI inputs since 1995. Several vaccines, such as those for rabies and malaria, are supplied by friendly governments at low prices or, in some cases, at no cost. EPI vaccinations are administered free of charge throughout the public health services network. Most medical and surgical inputs are procured directly by health establishments from private sources or from NGOs; financing for such purchases comes directly from cost-recovery measures (fees) or local government allocations.

Human Resources

According to 1992 census data, the allied health professions had an economically active population of 25,229 (10,287 men and 14,942 women); 24,872 persons were employed and 357 were unemployed. Of the total staff employed in the public health subsector (21,373), 12,056 worked in the decentralized public subsector and 9,317 in the autonomous public subsector, distributed as follows: 4,011 physicians (1,976 under the National Health Secretariat and 2,035 in the social security system), 1,894 nurses (1,003 and 891), 4,792 nursing auxiliaries (3,134 and 1,658), and 10,541 administrative and support staff (5,808 and 4,733). These resources were concentrated in the country's economic development corridor (La Paz, Cochabamba, and Santa Cruz); roughly 80% of the country's specialists worked in tertiary-level facilities located in cities. With the passage of the 1996 Administrative Decentralization Act, staff was transferred to the local government level (*prefecturas*), and guidelines were drafted for the reorganization of personnel departments and chains of command; however, municipal health service networks are only now being reorganized and staff reassigned. Twenty percent of Bolivia's 311 *municipios* lack qualified health personnel; in those *municipios*, health care is provided by lay staff. Training has been provided to midwives, health promoters, and other community resources over the past 20 years with an eye to meeting the population's health demands; over 5,000 of these trained midwives and health promoters are thought to be active in the health system.

Training opportunities for health personnel have expanded dramatically with the founding of private universities. The supply of undergraduate courses in medicine has tripled over the past six years; for nursing and dentistry it has doubled.

Rural areas continue to be at a disadvantage, not only because of the lack of permanent positions, but because of the dire shortage of basic and intermediate-level technical staff; indeed, there are no human resource management systems or policies in place to boost productivity and keep health care personnel in areas where they are needed, nor are there any arrangements for in-service training. Between 1991 and 1995, 766 new positions were created for physicians, compared with only 111 new positions for professional nurses; this phenomenon is especially noticeable in the social security sphere. The system's bias toward medical care is evident in the supply of training: most undergraduate programs tend to focus on hospital practice, with public health programs receiving considerably less attention. The Government has sought to address this issue by means of the health care teaching committees that it set up in 1993. High levels of staff turnover, however, have resulted in more than 50% of the trained personnel being lost in less than two years.

Expenditures and Sectoral Financing

The main sources of funding for Bolivia's health sector are:

• The National Treasury. The National Health Secretariat executed a budget of US$ 99 million in 1995. Of that amount, US$ 57 million went directly to health care services (equivalent to 4.1% of the national budget), with the remaining US$ 42 million going toward transfers, pensions, and retirement fund payments. The National Treasury allocated an additional US$ 83,000 to health spending for the purchase of drugs under the Ministry of Defense's *Sanidad Operativa* initiative. Funds earmarked for payroll were transferred to the local departmental governments (*prefecturas*) in June 1995 as part of government decentralization. Despite a series of constraints stemming from recent structural adjustments (revenue sharing, foreign debt service, transfers to projects), the national budget's share in financing personnel costs actually increased 18% between 1993 and 1996.

• The *municipios*. As of 1994, the Community Involvement Act transferred ownership of all physical infrastructure for health, education, culture, sports, irrigation, microenterprise irrigation arrangements, and rural roads to the *municipios*, along with the responsibility to administer and maintain them, outfit them with the necessary installations and supplies, build new infrastructure as required, and oversee the respective service providers. Of Bolivia's 311 *municipios*, 219 have qualified to receive funds under national revenue-sharing arrangements; the other 92, which have populations smaller than the requisite 5,000, have joined together to form 47 legally recognized pairings or groupings of municipalities in order to receive revenue-sharing entitlements. In 1994, the

municipios' revenue share outs came to US$ 74 million. Starting in 1995, these funds have been allocated according to strictly population-based criteria; in that year, the budget allocation came to US$ 141 million. Of the total funds transferred under the revenue-sharing arrangement, the amount earmarked for health in 1994 was US$ 2 million (2.7%), rising to US$ 8 million in 1995 (5.7%); for 1996 the amount was estimated at between 6% and 10%. Some *municipios,* such as Capinota and Tupiza, have invested up to 30% of their revenue in the health sector. All income from service fees and other cost-recovery measures belongs to the *municipio* and is ploughed back into supporting the operation of the services. This contribution is considered under the heading of private family health spending: families pay a fee to the decentralized public sector, which pays for drugs and inputs for diagnosis, treatment, or maintenance of the services.

• Companies. Health sector financing from this source is limited to legally established public and private companies that contribute to the social security system (short-term benefits). Applicable legislation stipulates that this contribution (calculated at 10% of payroll) is to be borne exclusively by the employer. In 1995, the amount furnished under this category came to an aggregated US$ 107 million (including the resources from the military's separate social security fund), equivalent to an annual average contribution of US$ 312 per premium-paying insured individual and US$ 69 per covered beneficiary. The total sum available for covering health care needs was around US$ 6 million, equivalent to US$ 106 per beneficiary.

• Families. Data on the health spending of Bolivian families are very limited. According to a 1990 survey of family budgets conducted in the cities of La Paz, Cochabamba, Santa Cruz, and El Alto, health spending (for all subsectors of service providers) represented 4% of the household's overall expenditures, ranging from 2.4% in the poorest quintile to 4.9% in the richest one. Forty percent of health spending went toward the purchase of drugs, and service fees accounted for the other 60%. This category was estimated at a total of US$ 105 million.

• External cooperation. Available data on external financing indicate that the total contribution from this source stood at around US$ 312 million for the period 1989–1995; budget execution averaged US$ 28 million per year, or 63% of the overall amount committed to the health sector. As a rule, external cooperation has focused on infrastructure, equipment, development of national programs, and support for municipal health development efforts, and it has thus helped to enhance equity in the system.

• NGOs. There are 141 NGOs working in the Bolivian health sector according to the country's consolidated registry of NGOs. A 1994 survey of 63 of these NGOs revealed a combined investment of US$ 9 million from outside sources. The aggregate amount invested by this category is estimated at US$ 20 million.

Factoring together all the contributions from the various subsectors, the country's total health sector expenditure was reckoned at US$ 323 million for 1995 (4.7% of GDP), equivalent to an annual per capita spending of US$ 44. The main source of financing for national health spending was social security (35%), followed by family contributions (32%), the National Treasury (15%), external cooperation (15%), and, lastly, the *municipios* (3%). If external cooperation is removed from the equation, the total comes to US$ 275 million per year (4% of GDP), equivalent to US$ 37.50 per capita. The public sector's spending on health (from the National Treasury, *municipios,* and company contributions to social security) came to US$ 170 million (2.5% of GDP), equivalent to US$ 23 per capita.

As can be seen, financing for the health sector has been relatively stable. The prospects for any substantial increase in this area are directly proportional to the funding sources' ability to increase their contributions, be it from families, companies, or the government (at both the national and *municipio* levels). That said, there are some yawning inequities in the current financing situation; social security spending, for instance, accounts for 35% of the total although it covers less than 20% of the population. Steps to close these gaps will need to include a redistribution of sector financing and broadened coverage of the social security system.

External Technical and Financial Cooperation

The past four years have seen a marked increase in technical cooperation between countries, not just in the Andean Subregion and Southern Cone but with other countries in the Region as well. Technical and scientific exchanges were carried out with Argentina, Brazil, Colombia, Costa Rica, Cuba, the Dominican Republic, Mexico, and Peru. The countries pooled efforts in a vast array of fields: epidemiology, traditional medicine, food control, vector control, blood banks, hospital administration, health service maintenance, disaster prevention and mitigation, salt fluoridation, organization of oncology services, plastic surgery and burn treatment, exchanges between pediatric associations, improvement of housing, basic sanitation and water supply, actions at the *municipio* level, health development activities in border areas, and exchanges among traditional midwives. Technical cooperation activities were carried out with the participation of the National Health Secretariat, the academic community, the National Oil-and-Gas and Health Funds, and the Agriculture Secretariat.

Funding from external cooperation sources falls into two broad categories—official (both multilateral and bilateral) and nongovernmental. In the health sector, this cooperation is provided under one of two formats: grants or loans. Bolivia has extensive bilateral cooperation arrangements with partners such as the European Economic Community, the United States of America, Japan, and the Scandinavian countries, and it also receives significant cooperation from the United Nations System (PAHO, UNICEF, the World Food Programme, the United Nations Population Fund, United Nations Volunteers) and other agencies. The multilateral development banks (the World Bank and the Inter-American Development Bank) also are lending support to crucial projects to strengthen the country's service network and health care programs. This category breaks down as follows: 65% in bilateral aid, 20% in technical multilateral aid from the United Nations System, and 15% in aid from development banks. International NGOs, it should be noted, account for a sizable share of technical and financial cooperation in some *municipios.*

BRAZIL

GENERAL SITUATION AND TRENDS

Socioeconomic, Political, and Demographic Overview

Brazil has an area of 8.5 million km² and shares borders with all the countries of South America except Ecuador and Chile. The Federative Republic of Brazil is currently governed by the Federal Constitution of 1988. Its political and administrative organization includes the three branches of government—executive, legislative, and judicial—as well as 26 states, 5,508 *municipios,* and the Federal District (the seat of government).

The country is divided into five major regions. The North, the largest region, occupies 45% of the national territory, but has only 7% of the population; the Southeast occupies 11% of the territory and has 43% of the population. The South is the smallest region, with 7% of the territory and 15% of the population. Each of the other two regions occupies approximately 18% of the territory, but the Northeast has 29% of the population, and the Central-West has only 6%.

In 1991 and 1994, based on the human development index (HDI) of the United Nations Development Program, Brazil ranked very close to the point at which countries are considered to have attained a high level of human development. However, the global HDI figure masks tremendous internal disparities. The HDI in the South, Southeast, and Central-West regions places them in the upper ranges of human development, whereas the North and Northeast regions are at an intermediate level, with the latter region bordering on lower levels of the index. The nine states in the Northeast have the lowest socioeconomic indicators in the country.

Brazil is one of the countries with the most pronounced socioeconomic inequalities in the world. In recent years growth of the economy has raised the median income in all strata of the population, but the unequal distribution has exacerbated existing differences. The median income of the wealthiest 10% of the population is almost 30 times greater than that of the poorest 40%, whereas in other countries with comparable levels of development it is only 10 times greater. Between 1960 and 1990, the share of national income of the poorest half of the population fell from 18% to 12%, and that of the richest 20% increased from 54% to 65%.

The proportion of women in the economically active population (EAP) has increased from 31% to 35% in the past decade. Nevertheless, the median wage of women is 63% that of men. Ethnic disparities are evident in the lower wages received by blacks and *pardos* (other dark-skinned groups), who make up 44% of the country's total population and in 1990 earned, on average, 68% of the amount earned by whites. In the Northeast, an estimated 46% of the population lives in poverty. This percentage is 43% in the North, 25% in the Central-West, 23% in the Southeast, and 20% in the South. Whereas the poverty in the Northeast is typical of traditional societies that have been largely left out of urban-industrial growth, poverty in the metropolises in the Southeast, especially the peripheral areas surrounding the cities of São Paulo and Rio de Janeiro, is associated socially and economically with this region's role as the dynamic center of the national economy.

Educational levels have improved significantly in recent decades, with a reduction in illiteracy, an increase in school enrollment, and a rise in the average number of years of schooling of the population. In 1991, the average school enrollment rate among children aged 5–17 years was 73%, with rates ranging from 81% in families earning more than two times the monthly minimum wage per capita to 37% among the poor. Between 1991 and 1995, the proportion of children aged 7–14 years who did not regularly attend school decreased from 16% to 10% for the country as a whole, although the rate was higher in the states of the Northeast (15%). In 1991, among groups earning less than half the per capita minimum wage, 15% of children aged 10–14 years worked while attending school and 12% worked but did not attend school. Among adolescents aged 15–17 years, these percentages were 39% and 15%, respectively. Blacks and *pardos* have greater difficulty enrolling and remaining in school. The rate of illiteracy in the population over 25 years old in 1991 was approximately 35% among blacks and *pardos,* whereas among whites it was 15%.

In 1995, the proportion of the EAP that was employed was 58% of the total population aged 10 years and over (5% in the group aged 10–14 years, 11% in the group aged 15–19, 59% in the group aged 20–39, 28% in the group aged 40–59, and 6% in the group aged 60 and over). Data from 1990 indicate that, among poor families, 23% of children aged 10–14 years worked. These children generally work in adverse conditions, are not protected by labor laws, and often work more than 40 hours per week, earning less than the minimum wage.

According to the Brazilian Geography and Statistics Institute, the unemployment rate remained at about 5% for the period 1990–1995. However, the quality of jobs has deteriorated, with a decline in industrial jobs and absorption of the unemployed into the service sector. In addition, the proportion of workers with a formal employment contract has fallen from 60% to 50%, and the proportion of "self-employed" workers who are excluded from the benefits and protections of labor legislation has increased.

Economic Growth and Stability

During the 1980s and the early 1990s the Brazilian economy was characterized by extreme instability and inconsistent growth, with inflation rising to extremely high rates. Reflecting external imbalances (the debt crisis), as well as the internal instability (persistent public deficit and hyperinflation), the period saw the demise of the industrial development strategy initiated in Brazil during the 1950s, which was based on import substitution and extensive state intervention in productive activities. The poor economic results of the 1980s and successive frustrated attempts at stabilization can be attributed to an inability to effect the structural changes necessitated by the new development model. Although there were some isolated successes, the Brazilian economy grew scarcely 1.2% per year between 1980 and 1992; at the same time, per capita income fell by 7.5% and the living conditions of the population deteriorated sharply, as did the prospects for overcoming the inherent problems associated with poverty and social inequality.

In 1994, the "Real Plan" (named for the country's new currency unit, the *real*) was launched, ushering in a period of growth in per capita income and the beginnings of a redistribution of the wealth. The poorest half of the population saw its share of national revenues increase by 1.2%, and that of the richest 20% decreased by 2.3%. The gross domestic product (GDP) grew 7.4% between 1994 and 1996 (at 1996 prices), rising from US$ 662,000 million to US$ 711,000 million, with an increase in per capita GDP from US$ 4,305 to US$ 4,503.

In 1995 per capita income reached its highest level since 1990, with an increase of 30% over the 1993 level if all sources of income of persons aged 10 years and over are taken into account. Wages for persons with formal employment contracts have grown at a slower rate (18.5%). In 1996 the annual inflation rate was 9.8%, compared with rates of as much as 45% per month at the time the stabilization plan was initiated.

The MERCOSUR Treaty (1991) laid the foundations for the establishment of a common market comprising Argentina, Brazil, Paraguay, and Uruguay. In addition to the immediate objective of promoting subregional economic integration, the MERCOSUR modernization process is aimed at improving living conditions for the population. The new economic programs adapted by the MERCOSUR countries favor economic liberalization, promoting competition, and increasing the efficiency and competitiveness of their economies in the global market. The ultimate objective is sustained long-term growth.

Population

According to the national census of 1991, Brazil has a total of 146.8 million inhabitants, with a ratio of 97.5 males for every 100 females. There are 17.2 inhabitants per km^2, and 75.6% of the total population is urban. Only the state of Maranhão continues to have a predominantly rural population. Mean population growth declined from 2.4% per year during the 1970s to slightly less than 1.9% in the 1980s, and it is expected that it will fall to 1.36% by the year 2000. Projections put the total Brazilian population in 1998 at 161.8 million.

During the 1980s urban population growth slowed significantly. Cities with more than 20,000 inhabitants grew at a rate of 2.6% annually, compared with 4.9% annually in the previous decade. The population of the nine metropolitan regions grew at an annual rate of 2%, considerably less than the 3.8% of the preceding decade. As a result of the exodus of the population from the Northeast in search of better living conditions in other regions of the country, the Northeast has the smallest proportion of nonnative inhabitants.

The fertility rate has decreased rapidly in recent decades. The rate dropped from 2.57 children per woman in 1991 to 2.52 in 1995. The crude birth rate fell from 31.2 live births per 1,000 inhabitants in 1980 to 23.6 in 1990, and it is estimated that the rate will be 18.2 per 1,000 in the year 2000. Total mortality followed the same trend, with a rate of 7.2 deaths per 1,000 inhabitants in 1990. It is estimated that the death rate will be 6.7 per 1,000 in the year 2000. Life expectancy at birth increased 3.9 years (6.3%) between 1980 and 1990. In 1999 it is expected to be 64.8 years for males and 71.2 for females.

The age structure of the Brazilian population has also changed in recent decades. The oldest generations, born before fertility began to decline rapidly, form a broad-based pyramid, while the age structure of younger generations is much less regular and unlike the distribution of the older generations. In 1991 there were fewer children under 5 years old than between 5 and 10 years old. Between 1970 and 1991 the proportion of children under 15 years of age decreased from 42% to 35% of the total population, while the group aged 15–64 years increased from 54% to 60% and the group aged 65 and over grew from 3% to 5%.

Around 1970 the economically dependent population (persons under 15 or over 64 years of age) made up almost 50% of the total population, and of every 20 dependents, fewer than 2 were elderly. By the turn of the century, it is estimated that dependents will make up only 33% of the total population and that of every 20 dependents, 3 will be elderly. The total dependency rate has declined notably as a result of the rapid reduction in the proportion of the population under 15 years of age and the still slow growth of the elderly component. This situation creates a special opportunity for significantly improving the quality of nutrition, health, and education policies aimed at children and young people.

Mortality Profile

Given the difference between the number of deaths estimated on the basis of population projections of the Brazilian Geography and Statistics Institute and the number of deaths registered by the mortality information system of the Ministry of Health, it is estimated that the mean number of unreported deaths for the country as a whole in the period 1990–1994 was approximately 20% of the total number. The figure exceeded 50% in some parts of the North and the Northeast. In most of the South and the Southeast, underreporting was less than 10%, and it was close to 0% in urban areas. Among the reported deaths, ill-defined causes accounted for 17.8% in the period 1990–1994. The North and the Northeast have the highest proportion of deaths due to ill-defined causes (28.6% and 42.1%, respectively, in 1990), which calls for caution in analyzing the distribution of deaths due to defined causes in these regions. A more accurate picture of the evolution of total and age-specific mortality rates for the country as a whole will probably be obtained by using population projections as indicators, reserving data from death records for the analysis of causes of death.

Demographic data indicate that mortality levels in the Brazilian population have declined significantly in recent decades. This reduction has resulted mainly from the decline in mortality in the population under 5 years of age; deaths in that age group as a proportion of total mortality between 1980 and 1994 decreased from 24.0% to 9.8% for the subgroup of children aged under 1 year and from 4.6% to 1.7% in

the group aged 1–4 years. Consequently, proportional mortality in the group aged 50 and over rose from 48.4% to 62.4% during the same period.

Part of the reduction in mortality during the last decade was canceled out by an increase in male mortality from external causes in the group aged 15–29 years. A comparison of mortality curves for both sexes reveals a clear difference between the ages of 15 and 44 years; the patterns are similar for the other age groups. The reduction in mortality from complications of childbirth and the puerperium among females and the increase in deaths due to homicide and suicide among males explain the increase in the difference between the sexes in life expectancy at birth. For every female between the ages of 15 and 19 who died in 1991, there were 2.8 deaths of males in the same age group, 3.2 in the group aged 20–29 years, and 2.6 in the group aged 30–39.

Analysis by cause of death according to the categories used by PAHO shows that in the period 1990–1994, excluding ill-defined causes, diseases of the circulatory system constitute the leading cause of death, accounting for 33.9% of the total. In the North and Northeast, where communicable diseases continue to be an important cause of death, cardiovascular disease also ranked first, although it accounts for a smaller proportion of deaths than in the South and Southeast. Within this group of illnesses, ischemic heart disease is the predominant one among males and cerebrovascular disease is the leading cardiovascular disease among females.

The second leading cause of death is composed of external causes, which includes injuries and poisoning. This group accounts for 14.8% of all deaths in the country, with higher proportions in the North (19%) and Central-West (20%). Within this group, homicide is a major cause of death, especially in large urban centers.

The third leading cause of death is malignant neoplasms, which between 1990 and 1994 accounted for 13.0% of all deaths from defined causes. The most common malignant neoplasms among males are stomach cancer and lung cancer. Prostate cancer ranked third as a cause of male mortality from malignant neoplasms in virtually all regions. Among females, breast cancer is most frequent, followed by cervical cancer, which is the leading cause of death from malignant neoplasms in the North and the Northeast.

Communicable diseases (including all those listed in Section I of the Ninth Revision of the *International Classification of Diseases*, as well as meningitis, acute respiratory infections, pneumonia, and influenza) ranked fourth as a cause of death in the Brazilian population, accounting for 11% of all deaths from defined causes with no significant annual variations during the 1990–1994 period.

The maternal mortality rate dropped during the 1982–1991 period from 156.0 to 114.2 deaths per 100,000 live births. According to data for 1989, the rate was 380 per

100,000 live births in the North, 153 per 100,000 in the Northeast, 134 in the Central-West, 97 in the Southeast, and 96 in the South. The national average was 124 per 100,000 live births.

The most frequent direct cause of maternal mortality is toxemia of pregnancy (30% of all maternal deaths). Hemorrhage during pregnancy, childbirth, or the puerperium constitutes the second leading cause, accounting for 18% of all deaths, followed by puerperal infection, which accounts for 15%. Abortions cause 12% of all maternal deaths; the remaining 25% are due to other causes.

A study conducted in 1996 showed a clear decline in mortality in all the age subgroups of children under 5. During the 10 years preceding the study, infant mortality fell from 56 to 39 per 1,000 live births, with significant variations according to region, social class, and other characteristics. In urban populations, infant mortality decreased from 51 to 32 deaths per 1,000 live births in children less than 1 year old. In rural areas, the reduction was only from 69 to 61 per 1,000. There are also marked interregional disparities. Infant mortality in the Northeast (64 per 1,000 live births) is 2.5 times higher than in the South (25 per 1,000). Infant mortality rates tend to decline as the educational level of the mother rises, with rates of 93, 42, 38, 28, and 9 deaths per 1,000 live births in groups of mothers with less than 1 year, 4 years, 5–8 years, 9–11 years, and 12 or more years of schooling, respectively. In urban areas, postneonatal mortality is declining significantly, while in rural areas it continues to account for two-thirds of infant mortality.

Among children under the age of 5 years, mortality patterns are similar to those described above for infant mortality. During the same 10-year period, the overall rate fell from 64 to 49 per 1,000 live births; however, the rate in the Northeast (89 per 1,000) is more than triple the rate in the South (29 per 1,000). With respect to maternal levels of education, the mortality rate of children under 5 decreases from 119 per 1,000 in the group whose mothers have less than 1 year of schooling, to 48 in the group whose mothers have 4 years, and 9 in the group whose mothers have 12 years or more of schooling.

Morbidity Profile

In Brazil general morbidity data are generated by the hospital information system, which encompasses institutions within the public health system. It is estimated that these hospitals provide close to 80% of all hospital care, with a monthly total of approximately 1.2 million hospitalizations. According to data for the period 1991–1994 on principal diagnosis by groups of causes according to the Ninth Revision of the *International Classification of Diseases,* 22.8% of all hospitaliza-

tions were related to pregnancy, childbirth, and the puerperium; the vast majority were for childbirth. The leading causes of the remainder of hospitalizations were respiratory disorders (15.9%), circulatory disorders (10.6%), infectious and parasitic diseases (9.4%), genitourinary disorders (8.4%), digestive disorders (7.5%), and external causes (6.0%). During this period—excluding hospitalization for causes related to pregnancy, childbirth, and the puerperium—no significant variations according to sex were observed in the distribution of morbidity.

SPECIFIC HEALTH PROBLEMS

Analysis by Population Group

Health of Preschool Children

Recent improvements in the evolution of morbidity and mortality indicators among children stem from the interaction of various demographic, economic, and social factors. Specific health-sector interventions, such as immunization, use of oral rehydration therapy, and promotion of breast-feeding, were key to the eradication of poliomyelitis, the virtual elimination of deaths from measles, the dramatic decline in neonatal tetanus, the reduction by half of deaths from diarrhea, and the reduction of malnutrition, especially the severe forms. The sustained decline in infant mortality can be attributed to a reduction in the most frequent causes of death in the postneonatal and late neonatal periods. At present, causes originating in the perinatal period account for more than half of all infant deaths from defined causes.

The mean values of national indicators tend to mask large disparities between urban and rural areas, among regions, among states in the same region, and among *municipios* within the same state. Of all deaths of children under age 1, half occur in the Northeast, where 29% of the country's population resides. In that same region, 39% of the reported deaths of children under the age of 1 year in 1993 were attributed to ill-defined causes, whereas in the Southeast the proportion was only 6%. The qualitative deficiency of the data in the poorest areas is associated with high rates of underreporting of deaths, which makes analysis of mortality by cause difficult. The lack of data is most noticeable in the case of diseases typical of underdevelopment, such as diarrhea and acute respiratory infections.

With regard to morbidity, 22% of hospital discharges in the public health care system in 1995 were of children under the age of 1 year; and the principal causes of hospitalization were pneumonia (30%), diarrheal diseases (25%), and conditions originating in the perinatal period (13%). Of the hospital deaths occurring in this age group, 32% were due to conditions originating in the perinatal period, 11% were due to pneumonia, and 8% were due to diarrheal diseases. Prematurity and low birthweight accounted for 69% of all perinatal deaths. Considering that the coverage level of care during the prenatal period and at childbirth is high, even in rural areas, these data demonstrate the need to focus efforts on improving the quality of the care provided.

Overall malnutrition among children under 5, according to anthropometric indicators, has declined significantly since the 1970s, particularly in urban areas. Even in the Northeast, the region with the largest proportion of malnourished children in the country, it will be possible to attain the target proposed for the year 2000 (6.4%) if the current rate of reduction of malnutrition is maintained. The incidence of low birthweight decreased from 10% in 1989 to 9.2% in 1996, a very slight reduction compared with the decrease in prevalence of malnutrition and infant mortality.

In 1990 a system of information on live births (SINASC) was implemented in virtually the entire country. Data for the system are supplied directly by hospitals. SINASC will provide a better basis for calculating infant morbidity and mortality rates at the municipal level in addition to supplying information for the development of a profile of live births by birthweight and other variables.

Health of Schoolchildren

Only 0.7% of the deaths reported in the country in 1994 occurred in the 5–9-year age group. External causes were responsible for 45% of the deaths in this group, followed by malignant neoplasms (12%) and diseases of the respiratory system (10%). Close to 60% of deaths from all causes occurred among male children; the proportion rises to 66% when only external causes are considered.

Information on health care for the school-age population is not consolidated at the national level. In 1996, the Ministry of Education launched an integrated health care project (PAISE) aimed at carrying out health education and preventive and curative activities for elementary school students residing in impoverished areas of capital cities in Brazil.

Health of Adolescents

External causes are responsible for the largest proportion of deaths in the group aged 10–19 years. According to data from 1993, this group of causes accounts for 53% of all deaths from defined causes in the group aged 10–14 years and for 70% of deaths in the group aged 15–19 years. Homicide and injury from traffic accidents accounted for a total of 63% of the deaths due to external causes in the group aged 15–19;

the vast majority occurred among males (93% of the homicide deaths and 74% of the deaths from traffic accidents). The second leading cause of death in the groups aged 10–14 and 15–19 is malignant neoplasms, which accounted for 10% and 5% of total deaths, respectively.

The specific fertility rate among women aged 15–19 years increased from 75 to 87 children per 1,000 women between 1965 and 1991. The increase was most evident in urban areas, where fertility rose from 54 to 80 per 1,000. Although the data from 1996 suggest a change in this trend, they also indicate that 14% of the women in the 15–19 age group had already given birth to a child.

Another problem of growing importance in this age group is drug use. Surveys conducted in 1987, 1989, and 1993 in primary and secondary schools in 10 capital cities showed that the six most frequently used drugs are alcohol, tobacco, solvents, tranquilizers, amphetamines, and marijuana, in that order. Of a sample of 24,634 students surveyed in 1993, 23% had used drugs at least once and 19% drank alcohol frequently.

Health of Adults

Unintentional injuries and violence constitute the leading cause of death in the group aged 15–60 years. This cause accounted for 30% of all deaths from defined causes in this age group in 1994. The next most frequent causes of death are diseases of the circulatory system (24%) and malignant neoplasms (13%). The distribution of deaths by age subgroups shows a strong predominance of external causes in the groups aged 15–19 and 20–29 years (71% and 62%, respectively). This group of causes also ranks first as a cause of death in the group aged 30–39 years (38%); diseases of the circulatory system (16%) and endocrine and metabolic disorders (12%) also account for a significant proportion of deaths in this age group. In the groups aged 40–49 and 50–59 years, the leading causes of death are diseases of the circulatory system (30% and 39%, respectively), followed by malignant neoplasms (16% and 21%) and external causes (20% and 9%). Close to 70% of all deaths in adults aged 15–60 years occur in males. Excess female mortality has been noted only in the case of malignant neoplasms (breast and cervical cancers) in the group aged 30–49 years. Mortality from malignant neoplasms in persons aged 20–59 years in 1997 was estimated at 36,000 deaths, 53% of which occurred in the oldest quartile (50–59 years).

The information available on the health conditions of women relates mainly to reproductive health. Data from a national study conducted in 1996 show that 96% of births in urban areas took place in health care institutions (78% in rural areas) and 86% of the mothers had received prenatal care. The percentage of cesarean births remains quite high, having increased from 32% in 1986 to 36% in 1996 for the country as a whole. By region, the highest rate of cesarean deliveries (52%) occurs in the state of São Paulo. Of the women of childbearing age living with a male partner, 79% of those in urban areas use some method of contraception (69% in rural areas). The most frequently used methods are female sterilization by tubal ligation (40%) and oral contraceptives (21%). Surgical sterilization is being performed on increasingly younger women, with a consequent rise in the incidence of complications. Hospital data indicate that of approximately 3 million discharges of patients hospitalized for obstetric causes in 1996, about 246,000 (8%) were due to postabortion curettage.

Maternal mortality remains high. The rate in 1991 was estimated at 114 deaths per 100,000 live births. The high maternal death rates are associated with a large proportion of high-risk pregnancies (45%), which are more frequent in rural areas (59%), where the population has less access to health services.

Health of the Elderly

Diseases of the circulatory system caused 47% of reported deaths among Brazilians aged 60 and over in 1994. The second leading cause of death was malignant neoplasms (16%), followed by diseases of the respiratory system (14%). Of the deaths from cardiovascular disease, cerebrovascular disease accounted for 34% and ischemic heart disease accounted for 28%.

In 1997 an estimated 60% of all deaths in Brazil from malignant neoplasms occurred in the group aged 60 and over. Bronchopulmonary, gastric, and prostate cancers were the most frequent forms (13.6%, 13.0%, and 7.3%, respectively).

Steady growth of the elderly population, in both absolute and relative terms, has led to higher spending for the care of chronic and degenerative diseases and has resulted in reorganization of the health care system to meet the needs of this age group. Studies conducted in the state of Rio Grande do Sul have shown that elderly patients who are hospitalized do not receive adequate medical and psychosocial care. A large proportion of these patients have problems typical of old age—such as incontinence, balance and mobility problems, dementia, delirium, and depression—which these studies found were often not diagnosed or were treated improperly.

Of the total 12.7 million hospitalizations in 1995, almost 17% were persons 60 years or over, among whom the hospital discharge rate is 197 per 1,000. This figure contrasts with the rates found in the groups aged 0–14 and 15–59 years, which were 53 and 93 per 1,000, respectively. The average hospital stay for patients aged 60 and over was 7.1 days, whereas for those aged 15–59 it was only 5 days and for those under 15 it was 5.5 days.

Workers' Health

Information on accidents in the workplace comes from claims submitted to the social insurance system. The system does not provide the type of data necessary for constructing an epidemiologic profile that shows the distribution of these accidents. In 1994 a total of 338,304 work-related accidents were reported in the country. Analysis of these records indicates that close to 90% of the accidents occurred in the Southeast and South regions, and approximately half occurred in the industrial sector. Among male workers, those employed in the construction industry have the most accidents. Almost 60% of the accidents reported involved workers between 18 and 35 years of age; this age group also accounted for a similar percentage of total mortality from work-related accidents. Male workers have three times as many accidents as female workers, and deaths from work-related accidents are 26 times more frequent among males.

Health of the Disabled

There are no data at the national level to indicate the magnitude of the problem of disability. A study conducted in 1985 in the municipality of Salvador, Bahía, found the prevalence of disability to be 5.3%. This statistic suggests that the mean prevalence nationally could exceed 1%, based on census data from 1991. Between 1993 and 1996 studies of the prevalence of disability were carried out in various cities and states utilizing a research protocol developed by PAHO. The findings indicated rates ranging from 2.8% in Brasília to 9.6% in Feira de Santana, Bahía. Disorders of the nervous system and sense organs were found to be the most frequent causes of disability, followed by mental disorders and diseases of the osteomuscular system, connective tissue, and circulatory system. These studies also showed that disability was generally associated with lack of steady income, low educational levels, substandard housing, and limited access to health care.

Health of Indigenous People

The indigenous population has been reduced to about 300,000 persons (0.2% of the Brazilian population), grouped in 206 ethnic groups, which occupy 554 "indigenous territories" distributed across 24 states. Approximately 50% of the indigenous population lives in the North region. The state of Amazonas is home to 25% of the country's indigenous population (3.2% of the population of the state). Roraima is the state with the largest proportion of indigenous people (10.4% of the total). The living and health conditions of indigenous communities are generally poor, owing in large part to the aggressive economic exploitation to which they have been subjected and which has steadily reduced their territories and caused environmental deterioration and loss of their cultural identity.

Since the early 1990s, efforts have been under way to coordinate intersectoral health care activities for indigenous peoples, and two national conferences on the subject have been held, one in 1986 and the other in 1983. In the state of Roraima, the Yanomami Health District has been created. However, current legislation assigns responsibility for indigenous health care to a variety of governmental entities. The Ministry of Health is responsible for preventive activities, control of communicable diseases, and basic sanitation.

In the absence of a national policy that would ensure comprehensive care for the indigenous population, the information available is disparate and does not lend itself to comparison or provide a complete picture of the health of these population groups. Among the most common problems detected in 1996 were acute respiratory infections and diarrheal diseases. Malnutrition, parasitic diseases, anemia, tuberculosis, and skin disorders, especially scabies, are also common. As a result of changes in lifestyle, an increase in alcoholism and in accidental and violent injuries has also been observed. In the Amazon region, malaria, cutaneous leishmaniasis, and hepatitis B are common. In the Yanomami territory, which occupies 9.4 million hectares, with 7,882 inhabitants organized in 169 communities, 17% of deaths are due to acute respiratory infections and 10% are due to malaria. The leading cause of death in the Yanomami population is malaria (2,142 cases in 1996, 753 caused by *Plasmodium falciparum*). Onchocerciasis is endemic throughout the region.

In 1996, investments in basic sanitation benefited 39,000 indigenous persons and financed the construction or upgrading of 481 simplified water supply systems. Various institutions trained personnel in health care for the indigenous population. A total of 2,306 persons received such training, and 1,322 of them were members of the indigenous community.

Health of the Black Population

The black population in Brazil shows some unique characteristics from the genetic standpoint, having resulted from the mixture of individuals of diverse ethnicity from several regions in sub-Saharan Africa. In 1993, the black or *pardo* population was estimated at 66.7 million, or 45% of the total population. Among the genetic diseases that affect the black population, the most prominent is sickle cell anemia. Other common diseases, such as high blood pressure, diabetes mellitus, and glucose-6-phosphate dehydrogenase deficiency, are aggravated by the poor socioeconomic conditions in which most of the black population lives. Sickle cell anemia is the

most common monogenic hereditary disease, with 8,000 cases and 2 million carriers of the hemoglobin S gene. The implementation of a sick cell anemia control program and other governmental initiatives have been aimed specifically at improving health care for the black population. The inclusion of race on death certificates beginning in 1997 will provide mortality data for this population group.

Analysis by Type of Disease

Communicable Diseases

Vector-Borne Diseases. Approximately 19 million persons (12% of the Brazilian population) live in areas at risk for malaria. These areas are located in the Amazon region, where more than 99% of the 444,049 cases of the disease reported in 1996 occurred. The annual parasite index (API) was 29.6 per 1,000 in 1995. Ninety-five municipalities in the Amazon region have an API of more than 50 per 1,000, which puts them at high risk for malaria. The three states that reported the largest number of cases in 1996 were Pará (33% of the total number of cases), Rondônia (2%), and Amazonas (16%). Few outbreaks of malaria occurred outside the high-risk areas. Of the cases reported in 1996, 128,418 (29%) were caused by *P. falciparum,* a reduction of 51% with respect to the number reported in 1988. *Plasmodium vivax* and *Plasmodium malariae* were responsible for 71% and less than 1%, respectively, of the cases reported in 1996. Virtually all *P. falciparum* cases are believed to be chloroquine resistant to some degree. Malaria mortality decreased 67% between 1988 and 1995. The persistence of malaria in Brazil is due mainly to low coverage of integrated control activities; unregulated emigration to urban, agricultural, and mining areas; and delays in the process of decentralizing services in the highest-risk areas.

No cases of yellow fever have been reported in urban areas in Brazil since 1942, although *Aedes aegypti,* the urban vector of the disease, is abundant. The reasons for this are not clear, given that the level of vaccination being carried out is probably not sufficient to prevent transmission. Cases of jungle yellow fever continue to occur every year. Between 1993 and 1996 a total of 102 cases were reported in the states of Amazonas, Goiás, Maranhão, Minas Gerais, Mato Grosso do Sul, Pará, and Roraima. In 1996, 14 cases and 12 deaths from jungle yellow fever were reported, all in the state of Amazonas. The high case fatality rate probably indicates a high rate of underreporting. The principal measure for prevention of yellow fever is vaccination. In the past two years more than 3.6 million persons were vaccinated, almost all of them were either residents of the states where jungle transmission occurs or persons who travel in those areas.

The incidence of dengue is increasing in the country. More than 175,000 cases were reported in 1996. Despite the high number of cases reported annually, which exceeds the number reported in any other country on the continent, there are few cases of hemorrhagic dengue. In the past four years 127 cases have been reported, with 14 deaths, and in 1996 there were only 6 cases and 1 death. Indigenous cases of dengue have been reported in 20 Brazilian states. In 14 of those states two serotypes of the virus, dengue-1 and dengue-2, are circulating. Sequential infection by two different serotypes is the most important risk factor for hemorrhagic dengue, which suggests that there is high risk of a major epidemic. Given the potential seriousness of hemorrhagic dengue and urban yellow fever, the Government has implemented a plan to eradicate *Aedes aegypti,* under which it proposes to spend US$ 4,300 million over the next 3-year period in 2,000 infested *municipios* located in 26 of the 27 states.

Of the five triatomid species that are vectors of Chagas' disease, the most important is *Triatoma infestans.* The area infested by this vector has been reduced from 711 municipalities in 1992 to 83 in 1993. The success of the national control program was fundamental for the launching, in 1991, of the initiative of the Southern Cone countries to eradicate *T. infestans* and interrupt transmission of *Trypanosoma cruzi* through blood transfusions. In 1996 insecticide spraying was carried out in 104,500 dwellings, mainly in residual foci that persist in the northern portion of the state of Rio Grande do Sul, in the western portion of Bahía, in the southeastern portion of Tocantins, and in the northeastern region of Goiás. In studies conducted between 1989 and 1996 among schoolchildren aged 7–14, in which some 180,000 samples from 18 states and 662 municipalities were analyzed, a seroprevalence level of 0.2% was found. In 1996 almost 2 million blood samples were processed in blood banks, yielding a seropositivity rate of 0.8%. The continuity of the activities and the attainment of the eradication goals makes it possible to anticipate that transmission of the disease by *T. infestans* will have been stopped by the year 2000.

Schistosomiasis is endemic in almost all the states of the Northeast and in two states in the Southeast (Minas Gerais and Espírito Santo). In addition, there are foci in all other regions of the country: North (northeastern Pará), Central-West (Federal District), and South (Paraná and Santa Catarina). Despite numerous systematic activities for the diagnosis of stool samples and treatment of cases (2.7 million examinations in 1995), it has not yet been possible to extend the control activities—which include improvements in household sanitation and environmental management—to all the endemic areas. In some areas the prevalence continues to exceed 25%, which poses a serious risk for the development of the more severe forms of the disease. Generally speaking, however, the trend is toward reduction of the prevalence and clinical severity of the disease.

Visceral leishmaniasis (kala-azar) is concentrated in the Northeast region, which accounts for more than 90% of the 2,000 cases reported annually. There are also major foci in the North, Southeast, and Central-West. Since the 1970s the disease has tended to become endemic in urban areas, a trend associated with poor living and nutrition conditions among the affected population. Epidemics in the capital cities of the states in the Northeast during the period 1981–1985 and 1993–1994 necessitated emergency control measures. The incidence of cutaneous and mucocutaneous leishmaniasis increased from 10 to 23 cases per 100,000 inhabitants between 1985 and 1995. This form of the disease is most common in the North and Northeast regions. The increase is associated with two distinct epidemiologic phenomena: one is the expansion of the agricultural frontier and the other is growth in outlying urban regions, with a possible adaptation of the parasites to reservoirs outside the jungle.

The remaining foci of plague in Brazil—almost all of them located in mountain and plateau regions in the Northeast—are controlled. Nine human cases were reported in 1995 and one case was reported in 1996.

The principal focus of lymphatic filariasis is in the metropolitan area of Recife, Pernambuco, where more than 1,500 cases were reported in 1995. Efforts are under way to implement a national plan to eliminate the disease through mass application of new treatments.

Onchocerciasis affects mainly the indigenous Yanomami population living along the border with Venezuela. Cases have been reported in nearby tribes and also in white individuals who were visiting the region, which poses a potential risk for spread of the endemic to other parts of the country.

Vaccine-Preventable Diseases. The last cases of poliomyelitis in Brazil were reported in 1989, and interruption of the indigenous transmission of wild poliovirus was certified in 1994. The incidence of acute flaccid paralysis in children under the age of 15 years—the indicator used by the epidemiologic surveillance system to monitor the disease— has remained at a mean annual rate of 0.9 cases per 100,000 inhabitants.

The incidence of measles has declined dramatically throughout the country since 1992, when measles vaccine was administered to more than 90% of the under-16 population. Since then, epidemiologic surveillance and outbreak control activities have been intensified, with a view to eliminating the disease. Measles was ruled out in more than 70% of the 4,000 suspected cases reported and investigated annually since 1994. In 1995 there were 19 laboratory-confirmed cases and 887 cases were clinically consistent with measles. No measles deaths were reported in the country in 1995 and 1996. Two outbreaks in 1996, in the states of Santa Catarina and São Paulo, represented a setback in the plan to eliminate the illness. In June 1997, the São Paulo outbreak continued to worsen, with 383 laboratory-confirmed cases since the beginning of the year, more than half of which were in persons aged 20–29 years.

Neonatal tetanus continues to occur sporadically in Brazil. More than half the cases are concentrated in small municipalities in the North and the Northeast. In 1995, 127 cases were reported, about half the number reported in 1992. The other forms of tetanus occur mainly in adults. Between 1992 and 1994 a total of 1,238 deaths from tetanus were reported, with the highest rates occurring among persons over the age of 40. In 1995, 900 cases were reported (0.6 per 100,000 inhabitants).

The incidence of diphtheria has declined steadily. Two hundred cases were reported in 1995 (0.1 per 100,000), with 62 deaths during the 1992–1994 period. The highest rates occur in the South and in the 1–4-year age group.

Whooping cough was the reported cause of 124 deaths during the 1992–1994 period, and almost all (118) were infants. In 1995, 3,236 cases were reported (rate of 2.1 per 100,000), with the lowest rates occurring in the Southeast region.

Cholera and Other Intestinal Infectious Diseases. From the beginning of the cholera epidemic in 1991 up to 1994, a total of 150,000 cases were reported nationwide, with 1,700 deaths. In 1995, 5,000 cases were reported, approximately 10 times less than in the preceding year. In 1996, there were only about 900 confirmed cases. Throughout the period, the transmission area of the disease has expanded steadily, and it now encompasses 1,226 Brazilian municipalities (22% of the total), almost all of them in the North and the Northeast. In the past two years the disease has continued to spread in practically all the vulnerable areas, where poor sanitation conditions are favorable for endemicity.

The use of oral rehydration therapy increased 35% in the Northeast region between 1991 and 1996, which helped to significantly reduce mortality from diarrhea. Nevertheless, in 1995 and 1996, 25% of hospital discharges of children less than 1 year old reported this as the cause of hospitalization.

Chronic Communicable Diseases. The downward trend of tuberculosis observed during the 1980s has slowed in recent years, and the incidence of the disease has begun to increase in some major cities, including Rio de Janeiro. Some 6,000 deaths annually are attributed to tuberculosis. In 1995, a total of 91,013 cases of all clinical forms of the disease were reported, making the incidence 29 per 100,000 inhabitants. Approximately half these cases were the pulmonary form. Of the 258,616 patients with respiratory symptoms examined in 1995, 10% had positive sputum smears. The North region has shown the highest incidence of laboratory-confirmed pulmonary cases, followed by the Northeast. The state of Rio de Janeiro, in the Southeast, had the highest reported rates in 1995 for all types of tuberculosis (127 per 100,000) as well as for the pulmonary form (56 per 100,000). Recent data indicate worrisome levels of multidrug resistance. A nationwide epidemiologic study to more accurately determine the magnitude of the problem is currently under way. Tuberculosis occurs as an opportunistic infection in 15% of AIDS cases.

Leprosy remains a significant problem. As of late 1996 there were 105,744 known cases, which makes the prevalence 6.8 per 10,000. In the same year, 39,792 new cases were diagnosed (detection rate of 2.5 cases per 10,000). The most affected regions continue to be the North and the Central-West. However, as a result of the activities of the national control program, especially multidrug therapy, notable progress has been made toward eliminating the disease as a public health problem, which means achieving a prevalence of less than 1 per 10,000. During the 1991–1996 period the number of reported cases decreased from 278,692 to 105,744, a reduction of 172,948 cases. During the same period, the prevalence fell from 18.2 to 6.8 per 10,000 inhabitants.

Acute Respiratory Infections. Acute respiratory infections are one of the three leading causes of illness and death among Brazilian children. Data from a national study carried out in 1996 indicate that in the 15 days preceding the household survey, 47% of children under the age of 10 years had suffered cough accompanied by difficult breathing, 25% had suffered fever, and 18% had been seen in health services for symptoms of respiratory infection. Children aged 6–23 months are most frequently affected.

Rabies and Other Zoonoses. The incidence of human and canine rabies has been reduced enormously since the national control program was instituted in the 1970s. A priority activity under the program has been annual canine vaccination campaigns in urban areas. In 1995, 31 human cases and 712 canine cases were reported. In 1996 there were 25 human cases. The canine vaccination rate in 1996 was 89%. The disease was eliminated in the southern states of the country during the 1980s. Over the 1980–1996 period a total of 76 cases of human rabies transmitted by vampire bats were reported, almost all of them in rural settlements in the Amazon region. Prophylactic antirabies treatment for humans has been standardized and adopted nationally.

Human leptospirosis is endemic in the principal urban centers and seasonal outbreaks occur during periods of flooding. Between 1986 and 1995, a total of 25,482 cases and 2,966 deaths were reported. Since then, an increase in the incidence of the disease has been observed.

The seriousness of the problem of taeniasis-cysticercosis is evident from the fact that some 100 deaths from neurocysticercosis are reported every year in the states of the Southeast and the South, where the best conditions for diagnosis of the disease exist. Human hydatidosis continues to be an important problem, mainly in the southernmost region of the country.

Tuberculosis and brucellosis in animals are considered diseases of low prevalence, although the incidence may be medium to high in cattle in some dairy regions. Reporting of human cases of brucellosis is not required in Brazil.

In the period 1990–1993 there were 81,611 reports of snake bites, with 355 deaths. Some 8,000 scorpion stings are reported annually, mainly in children under 14, with a case fatality rate of 1%. The incidence of spider bites is 1.5 per 100,000 inhabitants; most cases occur in the South and Southeast regions. Eighteen deaths from this cause were reported during the period 1990–1993.

AIDS. The AIDS epidemic began in 1980 in the cities of São Paulo and Rio de Janeiro and has since spread to all the other states in the country. As of February 1997, 103,262 cases had been reported, and 74% of them were in the Southeast region. For the entire period, the mean cumulative incidence for the country as a whole was 74 cases per 100,000 inhabitants. By region, incidence ranges from 125 per 100,000 in the Southeast to only 21 in the Northeast. The human immunodeficiency virus (HIV) has not tended to spread rapidly in the interior of the country, especially in rural areas. At least one case has been reported in 1,740 of the 5,508 municipalities in Brazil, but only 427 municipalities have reported five or more cases. Preliminary estimates indicate that between 338,000 and 448,000 adults aged 15–49 years may be infected with HIV. Serologic surveys show high HIV-positive levels among the prison population. Nationwide, AIDS continues to spread fairly slowly, especially in comparison with what is happening in the areas where the epidemic started and has affected large segments of the population.

Significant changes in the epidemiologic profile of the disease have been observed in recent years. Sexual transmission continues to predominate (66% of all cases for which the route of transmission is known), but around 1990 the initial concentration of cases in homosexual and bisexual males began to decline steadily and the number of cases detected in heterosexual males and females began to increase. As for acquisition of the virus through exposure to infected blood (31% of cases for which the route of transmission is known), intravenous drug use has become the primary risk factor (87.4% of reported cases in 1995), replacing blood transfusion, which accounted for 40% of cases in 1986 but only 11% in the 1993–1996 period. The latter reduction stems from the implementation of blood donor screening throughout the country. An HIV seroprevalence rate of 0.49% was found among blood donors in 1995. There has been a gradual rise in perinatal transmission, which was responsible for 3.8% of the cases reported in 1995 (86% of pediatric cases).

A steady increase in cases among patients with low levels of education is being observed. In 1994, 70% of the cases reported were in patients who had only an elementary education or were illiterate. In females, the proportion was 78%.

There has been a steady decline in the excess incidence of the disease among males. The male-to-female ratio decreased from 28:1 in 1985 to 3:1 in 1993, which may indicate an increase in heterosexual transmission by bisexual males and heterosexual drug users. Among women, 27% of the cases reported up to 1995 occurred among drug users and 12% occurred among partners of bisexual men.

Other STDs. Between 1987 and 1996, a total of 504,219 cases of sexually transmitted disease (STD) were reported in Brazil. In descending order of magnitude they were distributed among the following categories: nongonococcal urethritis (28.5%), venereal syphilis (28.3%), gonorrhea (27.7%), condyloma acuminata (11.3%), chancroid (1.8%), lymphogranuloma venereum (1.0%), congenital syphilis (0.9%), granuloma inguinale (0.3%), and gonococcal conjunctivitis (0.2%). The majority of cases occur in the South (40.9%), but the available data are believed to reflect large variations in the reporting systems of each state, which mask the true epidemiologic situation. According to data from public blood banks, 1% of blood samples collected from blood donors in 1995 tested positive for syphilis; by region, the seropositivity rate was 0.5% in the South and 2% in the North.

Emerging Diseases. About 28,000 cases of meningitis are reported annually, and 15%–20% of them are considered to be meningococcal meningitis. Since 1985 *Neisseria meningitidis* serogroup B has been the most common causal agent, although since 1987 a progressive increase in the frequency of serogroup C has been observed, especially in the South and the Southeast, where in some states these two serogroups occur with about the same frequency. The most commonly affected age group has been children under the age of 4 years. The overall case fatality rate for meningococcal meningitis in the country was approximately 20% in 1995–1996. Other important causes of meningitis are pneumococcal infections (responsible for 6% of all meningitis cases), *Haemophilus influenzae* type B (5%), *Mycobacterium tuberculosis* (2%), and viral infections (30%). Of the 1,500 cases of *H. influenzae* meningitis reported annually, more than 90% occur in children under 5 years old.

Viral hepatitis is very common in Brazil and in 1995 and was responsible for 16,851 hospitalizations and close to 800 deaths. Various studies have demonstrated the enormous impact that hepatitis B and hepatitis delta have on the population of the western Amazon region. Both types of hepatitis have also recently been found to be highly endemic in states in the Southeast (Espírito Santo) and the South (Santa Catarina). Data from public blood banks in 1995 showed sero-prevalence rates of 1.2% and 0.6% for hepatitis C and B, respectively, among blood donors.

Like other countries, Brazil is seeing a worrisome emergence of diseases caused by previously unknown agents. During the 1970s, the Rocio virus, a new arbovirus, caused about a thousand cases of encephalitis in the state of São Paulo. In the 1980s, Brazilian purpuric fever caused by *Haemophilus aegypti* led to outbreaks of septicemia among children in the states of São Paulo and Paraná. In 1993 a family outbreak of Hantavirus infection was detected serologically. This and other episodes demonstrate the need to pay greater attention to new infectious diseases. In 1995 a project of scientific and technological training in emerging and re-emerging diseases was launched, with special emphasis on biosafety.

Noncommunicable Diseases and Other Health-Related Problems

Nutritional Diseases and Diseases of Metabolism. Data on malnutrition among children under 5 in Brazil in 1996 show that 10.5% had height-for-age deficits, 2.3% had low weight-for-height, and 5.7% had low weight-for-age. During the past two decades, a steady decline in malnutrition has been registered among children under 5 years old (malnutrition is defined as weight-for-age two standard deviations or more below the expected mean value), with a reduction of 60% between 1975 and 1989 and 20% between 1989 and 1996. The mean height of Brazilian children born during the 5-year period 1980–1984 is significantly greater (3.3–4.6 cm) than during the 1960s, with a larger increase among girls. The reduction in malnutrition during the period 1975–1989 has changed the ratio between malnutrition and obesity, which was more than four malnourished children for each obese child and is now two malnourished children for each obese child. During the same period, the proportion of obese adults almost doubled, rising from 5.7% to 9.6%. In 1989 the proportion of obese women exceeded the proportion of malnourished women in all income groups; among men, this occurred only in the middle- and high-income groups.

The most important micronutrient deficiencies are vitamin A, iodine, and iron deficiencies. Vitamin A deficiency is common in the Northeast, where more than 40% of children have serum retinol concentrations under 20 (μg/dl. This deficiency is also considered to be endemic in the Jequitinhonha Valley in Minas Gerais and in the Ribeira Valley in São Paulo. In these areas, 6.5 million children between 6 and 59 months of age are given food that has been fortified with vitamin A.

In 1975, a national survey of the prevalence of endemic goiter in the school population found rates ranging from 1% to 33.5% in different states. Subsequent studies carried out in 1984, 1989, and 1990 in municipalities selected to participate in the activities of the national endemic goiter control program showed a general downward trend in the prevalence in these areas, although increases were reported in some municipalities.

Iron deficiency anemia is a major problem, especially among pregnant women and children under the age of 2 years. Among pregnant women receiving prenatal care, the prevalence of iron deficiency anemia has been found to range from 25% to 44%, with an extremely high value of 65% in the state of Pará. Among children under 5, published studies show a prevalence that ranges from 59% in São Paulo to 70% in Pará. In the state of Pernambuco, 85% of children aged 6–11 months, 82% of those aged 12–23 months, and 17% of those aged 5 to 6 years were found to be anemic. The only national study on iron consumption in the Brazilian population, conducted 20 years ago, showed adequate mean values, with marked deficiencies in the low-income population.

The practice of breast-feeding has increased steadily in recent years as a result of concerted action by government agencies, professional health associations, scientific institutions, and other organizations. Between 1989 and 1996 the mean duration of breast-feeding increased from 5 to 7.5 months, and the frequency of exclusive breast-feeding increased 11-fold in infants up to 3 months of age and 25-fold in infants 4–6 months of age. In 1996 the general prevalence of breast-feeding for infants aged 0–3 months and 4–6 months was estimated at 85.4% and 63.7%, respectively; the prevalence of breast-feeding as the predominant form of feeding was estimated at 43.5% and 18.4%, respectively; and that of exclusive breast-feeding was estimated at 0.3% and 12.8%, respectively. These prevalence rates are considered very unsatisfactory, given that more than 95% of Brazilian children are breast-fed at birth. However, exclusive breast-feeding is being discontinued very early and weaning is taking place long before it should.

A multicenter study on diabetes mellitus conducted in nine Brazilian capital cities between 1986 and 1988 showed a mean prevalence of 7.6% in the urban population aged 30–69 years, with higher values in São Paulo (9.7%) and Porto Alegre (8.9%). Between 5% and 10% of the cases were insulin-dependent. The prevalence of diabetes was found to rise steadily with age, from 2.7% in the group aged 30–39 years to 17.4% in the group aged 60–69, with no significant variations according to sex.

Cardiovascular Diseases. In recent decades diseases of the circulatory system have been responsible for an increasing proportion of total mortality. Between 1930 and 1980 mortality due to these causes rose from 11.8% to 30.8% in the capital cities. More recent analyses of all deaths reported in Brazil in the period 1990–1994 indicate that 33.9% were due to cardiovascular diseases, which are the leading cause of death in all regions of the country. Mortality from this cause is proportionally higher among women (36.2% of the deaths in 1986 compared with 29.0% among men). This difference is explained by the greater frequency of external causes of death in males. In 1991 the most frequent specific causes of death from diseases of the circulatory system in the capital cities were cerebrovascular disease (11.6%), ischemic heart disease (9.8%), and hypertension (2.3%).

In 1991 health system spending for the care of patients with cardiovascular diseases was estimated at about US$ 500 million for hospital care alone. When the costs of outpatient care, prostheses, and special materials are added to this sum, the figure rises to US$ 1,000 million. Diseases of the circulatory system are responsible for 25% of all hospitalizations according to hospital discharge records and they consume 13% of total health care resources.

Malignant Tumors. With decreasing birth and infant mortality rates and the consequent increase in life expectancy, malignant neoplasms have assumed a more important role in the morbidity and mortality profile in Brazil. According to estimates of morbidity for 1997, the six principal cancer sites, in decreasing order of frequency, were breast (28,310 new cases), uterine cervix (22,500), stomach (19,820), lung (19,015), colon and rectum (17,630), and prostate (14,020). The female population suffers a disproportionate cancer burden, especially in the younger age groups, because the two most frequent forms of cancer occur exclusively in women. The overall incidence of all types of cancer is 176 cases per 100,000 females and 162 per 100,000 males. Among males, lung cancer is the most frequent form, with an incidence of 20.1 per 100,000, which far exceeds the estimated rate in females (5.9 per 100,000), among whom lung cancer is the sixth most frequent malignant neoplasm. The next most frequent cancer sites in males are the prostate and the stomach. Gastric cancer is much more frequent in males (18.6 per 100,000) than in females (8.5 per 100,000), among whom it is the fourth most frequent type. Colon and rectal cancer is the fourth most frequent type in males and the third in females, with similar incidence rates in both sexes (12.4 and 11.6 per 100,000).

It is estimated that in 1997 deaths from malignant neoplasms in all sites totaled 97,700. The largest number were due to lung cancer (11,950 deaths) and stomach cancer (11,150), followed by deaths due to breast cancer (6,780), cervical cancer (5,760), colon and rectal cancer (5,440), and prostate cancer (4,690). Unlike morbidity, mortality from cancer is higher among males (72.5 deaths per 100,000, compared with 60.7 per 100,000 in females).

The cancer morbidity and mortality profile varies somewhat from region to region. Among males, prostate cancer ranks first in the Southeast and Central-West regions, whereas in the North and Northeast cancer of the stomach is the leading cause and in the South lung cancer predominates. Among females, breast and cervical cancer are the two most frequent types in all regions, but the third most frequent type in the North and Northeast regions is stomach cancer, whereas in other regions of the country colon and rectal cancer ranks third.

Accidents and Violence. Accidents and violence (external causes) have ranked second as a cause of death in Brazil throughout the present decade. They account for close to 15% of all deaths from defined causes, with a rate of 70 deaths per 100,000 inhabitants. In the group aged 5–39 years they are the leading cause, and in the group aged 15–19 they are responsible for almost 80% of all deaths. Homicide ranks first among all external causes of death, accounting for close to 30% of deaths attributable to this group. Between 1977 and 1994 the specific death rate due to homicide increased 160% nationwide. The principal victims are young adult males, particularly those between the ages of 20 and 29. Among all the external causes, one of the most important is traffic accidents, which increased rapidly until the mid-1980s and began to decrease slightly in 1990. Mortality from this cause is greater among males than females, with a ratio of 3:1.

Morbidity from external causes account for 6% of hospitalizations. However, because hospital discharges are not classified by the nature of the injury, no data are available on morbidity from specific causes within this group.

According to national statistics on traffic accidents, in 1995 there were 255,000 accidents with injuries; a total of 321,000 people were injured and there were 25,513 deaths, of which 80% were males and 70% were in the 15–59 age group. The total cost of these accidents is estimated at US$ 966 million. Since 1992 there has been a slight decrease in the mortality rate from traffic accidents, which was 9.6 deaths per 10,000 vehicles in 1995. A large proportion of the deaths were pedestrians who were struck by automobiles. In 1995 such pedestrian accidents made up 28% of all reported accidents. In 1997 a national transportation safety program was implemented with a view to reducing accident rates, deaths, and the severity of injuries. Over a 5-year period US$ 400 million in resources from the Inter-American Development Bank (IDB) will be used for this program.

Behavioral Disorders. The most recent data on the distribution of mental disorders in the Brazilian population come from a study conducted in 1990–1991 in three metropolitan regions. Neurotic disorders, especially anxiety and phobia, were found to be most frequent, with prevalence rates ranging from 7.6% in São Paulo to 17.6% in Brasília. Nonpsychotic depression was detected in 14.5% of women in Porto Alegre.

The prevalence of various forms of alcoholism point to a significant potential demand for psychiatric care in the population over the age of 15, with rates ranging from 4.5% to 8.7% and up to 15% among males in some cities.

Drug use is a growing problem, especially among young people; illegal drugs are the most frequently used type of drug in this population group. Alcoholism and drug use together account for close to 20% of all hospitalizations for mental disorders in Brazil. The proportion is as high as 28% in the South, according to data for 1995. Alcoholism was the underlying cause of 3,621 deaths (only 10.8% of those were women), 35.5% of which were of persons under the age of 40. A study conducted in the five state capitals found the proportion of street children who use drugs—excluding alcohol and tobacco—to be 82.5% in São Paulo and 90.5% in Recife. Intravenous drug use is an increasingly important factor in the transmission of AIDS, accounting for 20.7% of all cases reported up to 1996. Use of illegal drugs is also associated with an increase in violence and prostitution, problems that impact in various ways on the health situation in urban areas.

It is estimated that some 30 million Brazilians smoke and that 80,000 deaths each year are due to causes related to tobacco use. Control activities have prioritized the dissemination of educational materials in schools and workplaces, restriction of advertising, and prohibition of smoking in public places.

Oral Health. The prevalence of dental caries in the Brazilian population has declined markedly in recent years. Surveys by the Ministry of Health in state capitals show that the index for decayed, missing, and filled teeth (DMFT) index among 12-year-olds fell from 6.67 in 1986 to 3.06 in 1996 as a result of various educational and preventive activities implemented with the participation of the public sector and dentistry entities. In 1996, 42% of the population had access to fluoridated water through public water supply systems.

Natural Disasters and Industrial Accidents. The most frequent types of disasters in Brazil are floods, landslides, cave-ins, and droughts, which have the heaviest impact on low-income populations in urban slum areas. Data on the state of São Paulo indicate a progressive increase in the number of technological accidents since 1978, with 215 recorded in 1995 and 398 in 1996. The majority of the accidents reported between 1978 and 1996 involved modes of surface transport (39%) or maritime transport (12%), or they occurred at fuel storage sites (8%), households (8%), and industrial areas (6%). The chemical products most frequently involved in these accidents were flammable liquids (41%), corrosives (14%), and gases (11%). In 1995, the explosion in a shopping center in the municipality of Osasco, São Paulo, caused 45 deaths; and in 1996, a plane crash in a residential neighborhood close to the São Paulo airport caused some 100 deaths.

The national civil defense system is responsible for disaster preparedness and response activities. Created by law in 1993 and coordinated by the Special Secretariat for Regional Policies within the Ministry of Planning and Budget, the system encompasses state and municipal subsystems. Its priorities are training human resources to respond to chemical disasters, to practice radiation safety in hospitals, and to care for the population affected by floods and droughts. Most companies in the chemical and petrochemical sector—whether private or state-run—have accident prevention programs and procedures for emergency situations.

RESPONSE OF THE HEALTH SYSTEM

National Health Plans and Policies

The social policies of the Government of Brazil that provide the framework for the health policy are coordinated by the Social Policy Committee, which is composed of the ministers of the social sectors with the participation of the Ministries of Finance and Planning, under the direction of the President of the Republic. This committee establishes strategies for coordinated action by the various agencies responsible for carrying out social programs.

During the 1980–1990 period, public spending on health as a proportion of GDP peaked in 1989 at 3.3%. This percentage decreased dramatically over the next several years and then began to rise again in 1994, reaching 2.7% in 1995. If private spending by individuals—estimated at 34% of all health spending in 1990—is included, total health spending in 1995 was about 4.1% of GDP. This may be an underestimate, because the tremendous reduction in public spending on health between 1990 and 1993 led to an increase in direct out-of-pocket spending by individuals to pay for private services. Federal spending on health activities carried out by the Ministry of Health in 1996 represented approximately 10% of tax revenues, compared with 19% in 1989.

Government action in the area of health is geared toward the achievement of two basic objectives: improvement of the health situation, especially reduction of child mortality, and political and institutional reorganization of the sector aimed at modernizing and enhancing the operating capacity of the health system. To achieve the first objective, activities are being carried out with regard to communicable disease control, prevention and treatment of malnutrition, integrated management of maternal and child health, and improvement of basic sanitation. Joint effort by the health and sanitation sectors seeks to reduce infant mortality to 22.6 deaths per 1,000 live births in 1999. The political-institutional reorganization will entail broad reform of the health care model. The priority strategy in this effort will be intensification of the decentralization process. These objectives are specified in the plan of priority goals and activities for the 1997–1998 biennium, implemented in March 1997 by the Ministry of Health. The plan stresses prevention, with emphasis on primary care, as well as improving the quality of services and interaction of the health system with society through strengthening of the health councils. A basic instrument for implementing the activities and achieving the goals of the plan is a financial agreement signed by the Ministry of Health with the IDB and the World Bank for the execution, beginning in 1997, of the Unified Health System Reorganization and Strengthening (RE-FORSUS) project. The project's specific objectives are to strengthen the physical and technological infrastructure of the health services system and develop the system's management capacity at its various levels. The project prioritizes maternal health care and emergency care in large urban centers, hemotherapy and public health laboratory networks, and family health activities. It also encourages innovations in sector management, information and evaluation in the health field, formulation of policies on health system decentralization, managerial training for personnel in management units, and quality assurance in health systems and services. The project will run for three years with a total budget of US$ 650 million; it will cost US$ 195 million for the first year.

Health Sector Reform

Health reform efforts in Brazil grew out of the Eighth National Health Conference, held in 1986, and are aimed at bringing about broad financial, organizational, and institutional restructuring of the public health sector, with three main objectives: (a) to transfer responsibility for the provision of health care benefits from the national government to the local governments; (b) to consolidate the financing and delivery of public health services, seeking to achieve equity and comprehensive care; and (c) to facilitate the effective participation of the community in planning and control of the health system. The legal and institutional foundation for the reform is provided by the Federal Constitution of 1988 and subsequent legislation.

The Federal Constitution of 1988 deals specifically with health in the chapter on social security. The Constitution makes health a right of all and a responsibility of the State, which it should fulfill through economic and social policies aimed at reducing the risks of illness and other health impairments, as well as through universal and equitable access to activities and services for the promotion, protection, and recovery of health within a Unified Health System (UHS) that is public, federal, decentralized, and participatory in nature

and provides comprehensive care. The constitutional framework that allows for the development of the UHS has been complemented by subsequent legislation, including organic health laws (8.080/90 and 8.142/90), decree 99.438/90, and the basic operational guidelines of 1991, 1993, and 1996. Law 8.080/90 regulates the UHS, which is responsible, though not exclusively, for giving concrete expression to the constitutional principles regarding the right to health. The UHS encompasses all public services (at the federal, state, and municipal levels) as well as private services that have been duly accredited by contract or agreement.

The changes sought through health sector reform are not intended to be "quick fixes" or compensatory measures but rather are part of a process of structural change that includes (a) a cultural change and affirmation of the rights of citizens, in which the right to health is considered a determinant of the quality of life; (b) the consolidation of a national public system in which the federal, state, and local levels work in a complementary and harmonious fashion and have the necessary instruments of power; (c) the organization and regulation of a private health care system, with specific objectives that are consonant with the constitutional precepts of universal, comprehensive, and equitable health care; (d) competitive functioning of the public and private subsystems, as a means of promoting quality and reducing costs; (e) the adoption of innovative technical and operational models aimed at providing care that is comprehensive, personalized, appropriate, and accessible to all; (f) the implementation of a system of monitoring, control, and evaluation that will help to effectively reduce unnecessary spending; and (g) the introduction of decentralized management practices that will prevent inefficient and unfair duplication of effort.

In the framework of MERCOSUR, studies are being conducted with a view to harmonizing national legislation applicable to the health sector, a process that will be intensified in the next four years to meet the requirements of specific trade and production agreements. Pursuant to recommendations of the third meeting of ministers of health of MERCOSUR, a working subgroup on health was established for the general purpose of harmonizing quality parameters for health-sector goods, services, and production factors and health regulatory mechanisms.

Organization of the Health Sector

Institutional Organization

The Brazilian health services system comprises a complex network of health care providers and financers in the public and private sectors. The public segment of the system consists of public providers at various levels of government, including the federal level—the Ministry of Health—which oversees national management of the UHS; university hospitals operated by the Ministry of Education; and the Armed Forces health services. The state and municipal levels include a network of establishments operated by entities at those levels. The public health services, complemented by private services that work under contract with the Government in the framework of the UHS, cover 75% of the population. The exclusively private segment consists of for-profit services paid for directly by individuals and private institutions that provide care under private health insurance plans. Most inpatient hospital services are provided under a system of public reimbursement for services provided by private entities (80% of hospitals that provide services within the UHS are private). In contrast, 75% of outpatient care within the UHS is provided by public establishments.

Private health insurance plans fall into four main categories: (a) group practices, a prepayment modality that represents 47% of the private health care market; (b) medical cooperatives, a prepayment modality that represents 25% of the market; (c) company health care plans, which combine self-managed services and services purchased from third parties in various modalities and represent 20% of the market; and (d) traditional indemnity insurance, through which benefits are paid to the insured or to third parties, which represent 8% of the market. In 1995, 20% of the Brazilian population, some 34 million persons, were covered under private health insurance plans, at a total cost of US$ 6,400 million.

Management, Regulation, and Delivery of Services

Basic operational guidelines (BOG) for the UHS were approved under the organic health legislation. At present BOG 01/96 is being implemented. This BOG defined the managerial responsibility of each level of government within the UHS. In addition to strengthening managerial functions and the capacity of the municipal governments and the Federal District to deliver services to the population, BOG 01/96 promotes the process of decentralization through mechanisms for the automatic transfer of federal resources to the states and municipalities. It also strengthens processes of shared management between the Federal Government and the state and municipal governments through tripartite and bipartite joint management commissions, which serve as permanent forums for negotiation and consensus-building. The municipal UHS card is an instrument that helps to ensure citizen access to the health care system. It is a document that is valid nationwide, entitles the UHS user to receive services outside his or her area of residence, and insures reimbursement of the costs to the system that provided the services.

BOG 01/96 establishes a mechanism for joint integrated programming and defines responsibilities, requirements, and prerogatives for health management at the municipal and state levels. Municipalities are entitled to take over full management of basic health care or of the entire municipal system; those that do not opt to do so continue to be service providers within the state system. Similarly, the states are entitled to take over full management of the state system.

The joint management commissions are intended to facilitate coordination between the municipal, state, and federal governments and ensure unified management of the system at each level, without duplication or omission of activities. The tripartite joint management commission is composed of equal numbers of representatives of the Ministry of Health, the National Council of State Secretaries of Health, and the National Council of Municipal Secretaries of Health. It is a forum for negotiation and agreement between managers of the three levels of public health administration for the implementation of national policies and guidelines. The bipartite joint commissions are made up of equal numbers of representatives of the state secretariat of health and the representative entities of the municipal secretaries of health within the state.

The health councils are permanent advisory bodies established at each level of government. Their principal functions are to formulate strategies for the implementation of sectoral policies and to oversee the execution of health policies and activities, including their economic and financial aspects. They consist of equal numbers of representatives of the various groups of users (labor unions; neighborhood associations; associations of retired persons, patients, and disabled persons; and other groups of society) and representatives of the various segments of the health sector (governments, service providers, and health professionals). At the federal level, the National Health Council was created pursuant to legislation enacted in 1990 and has been functioning regularly and systematically since its creation. Health councils are now operating in all 26 states, the Federal District, and almost 3,000 municipalities.

Health conferences are held regularly as a means of encouraging social participation in the development of the health system. They are convened every four years to assess the health situation and propose guidelines for the formulation of health policies. In preparation for the national conference—the most recent one was held in September 1996—health conferences are held at the municipal and state levels.

Organization of Health Regulatory Activities

Delivery of Health Services: Health Care Facilities and Standards of Care. The construction and upgrading of health care establishments is regulated by technical standards set by the Ministry of Health for physical infrastructure projects, taking into account cost-related criteria and the needs of the health care system. The training program in health facility architecture includes two specialized courses at the federal universities of Brasília and Bahia.

Evaluation and certification of health services is one of four strategic projects being carried out under the Brazilian quality and productivity program for the 1996–1998 period. The Ministry of Health also has several initiatives aimed at enhancing quality management in health services, with emphasis on hospital management. Another line of action in this area is the process of health service accreditation. Two institutions were recently created for this purpose: the Brazilian Institute of Hospital Accreditation (1995) and the Pará Institute of Hospital Accreditation (1996).

Special mechanisms have been instituted to monitor and evaluate procedures that are considered highly complex and costly for the UHS. For example, technical regulations have been established for the operation of renal therapy services, which set specific standards for units that perform kidney dialysis and transplants. In addition, a specific federal law regulates the extraction of human organs, tissues, and body parts for transplant and treatment purposes and lays the foundation for the creation of a national transplant system.

Certification and Practice of Health Professionals. Authorization to practice the various health professions is granted by the respective professional boards to candidates who hold a degree from a university or technical school. These boards are autonomous public entities created by law and entrusted with regulating and monitoring the practice of professionals in their respective areas of specialization throughout the country.

Basic Health Markets: Technologies, Drugs, and Other Inputs. Technology assessment has been a constant feature of health reform in Brazil and is seen as a means of establishing appropriate criteria for the use of technological resources. The general basis for action in this area is provided by the Organic Health Law and the conclusions of the First National Conference on Health Science and Technology. A set of proposed policy guidelines on health technology is currently under discussion within the Ministry of Health.

The health regulations on drugs, equipment, and cosmetic and hygiene products are enforced by the Health Surveillance Secretariat within the Ministry of Health. Federal legislation regulates the manufacture of these products and requires market authorization before they can be sold. Within the framework provided by the Constitution of 1988 and the legal instruments adopted subsequently, in particular those that created the UHS and the consumer protection code, a national health surveillance system has been established. This system facilitates intersectoral coordination and defines the responsibilities of the three levels of government within the health system. The National Health Quality Control Institute serves as a national reference and quality control laboratory for an integrated network of state and university institutions. A technical and administrative structure for the national health surveillance system, which will enable it to fulfill its assigned responsibilities, is still being developed.

Environmental Quality: Water, Air, Soil, Housing, and Chemical Safety. The foundations for Brazilian environmental policy are established by the Constitution and by Law 6.938/81, which created the national environmental system. Decentralization of the execution of environmental policy to the state and municipal levels is currently a priority. Guidelines have been formulated for the establishment of a national health and environment plan oriented toward ensuring sustainable development, with broad multisectoral participation.

Several World Bank-financed projects for the cleanup of rivers, bays, and watersheds in major Brazilian cities are currently under way. Recent federal legislation created the national system for the management of water resources, which regulates the use of watersheds through specific interinstitutional committees. To alleviate the housing shortage (there are 5.1 million housing units that lack adequate infrastructure or are located in extremely overcrowded areas), the national housing system invested US$ 2.83 million in 1995–1996, benefiting 393,000 families.

Air pollution is a major problem in large urban areas, especially the São Paulo metropolitan region. In every month of the year this region registers pollution levels that exceed the limits considered tolerable, especially particulate matter and carbon monoxide, mainly from automobile exhaust.

Control of agricultural toxins is regulated by intersectoral legislation and involves the Ministries of Health, Agriculture, and Environment. The health sector is responsible for toxicology assessments. Eleven Brazilian states are currently participating in the system that monitors the health effects of agricultural toxins.

Food Control. Food control is a component of the national health surveillance system. Specific legislation establishes basic regulations for the registration, control, and labeling of food products as well as product identification and quality standards, monitoring, and related administrative procedures. The state secretariats of health participate in technical analysis for product registration processes, and health inspection activities are decentralized to state or municipal agencies. The Ministry of Agriculture, through the Secretariat for the Protection of Agriculture and Livestock, is responsible for registration and inspection of products of animal origin, beverages, pesticides, and pharmaceutical products for veterinary use. In the case of agricultural products intended for export, regulatory activities are carried out directly at the federal level. The National Codex Alimentarius Committee and the Technical Advisory Commission on Food are currently operating. The National Health Quality Control Institute coordinates regulatory activities relating to laboratories.

Health Services and Resources

Organization of Services for Care of the Population

The UHS encompasses the diverse activities carried out at the three levels of government to meet health care and environmental health needs. Health care services for individuals or groups are provided through outpatient facilities, hospitals, or home health care services. Environmental health activities focus on control of vectors and hosts, operation of environmental sanitation systems, and health conditions in the home and work environment. Policies outside the health sector deal with the social determinants of the health-disease process.

The establishments that make up the municipal level of the UHS need not necessarily be owned by the municipality or located within its territory. The important thing is that they organize and coordinate among themselves so that the municipal government can ensure the population's access to health services and the availability of comprehensive care.

Health Promotion. Since 1994 the Ministry of Health has been carrying out a program of family health as a strategy for reorganizing primary health care. The program seeks to incorporate health promotion into traditional medical care through reorganized health units that focus on families and their social relations within a given area. As of December 1996 the program had been extended to 228 municipalities. The community health agents program is also being expanded. The objective of this program is to develop community-based health care and organize basic activities at the local level. As of December 1996, there were some 45,000 health agents working in the program.

Several programs at the national level are aimed at ensuring comprehensive care for the health of women, children, and adolescents. They emphasize education and prevention, identification of risk groups, and early detection of health problems. Maternal and child health care also include specific activities carried out under the programs on immunization, breastfeeding, care for children with physical and mental disabilities, control of specific nutritional deficiencies, care for malnourished children and pregnant women at nutritional risk, and control of AIDS and other STDs. Since 1995 the project on reduction of infant mortality has been coordinating specific maternal and child health and basic sanitation activities in the 913 municipalities with the highest levels of poverty.

The national policy on aging includes guidelines on health of the elderly, which seek to ensure prevention and health promotion activities for this population group as well as care for the recovery of health at the various levels of the UHS. The policy also encourages the participation of the elderly in social management of the health care system.

Some of the muncipalities that have made the most progress in decentralization have succeeded in mobilizing the local community and initiating intersectoral health promotion activities in the framework of the healthy communities strategy. A pioneering experience launched in 1993, in Campinas, São Paulo, highlighted the importance of formulating policies aimed at improving the living conditions of the poor population through public programs and projects on public housing, sanitation and public services in low-income housing developments, food processing, assurance of a minimum family income, creation of jobs, etc. As a result of this experience, in 1996 Campinas received the Latin American "Healthy Community" award, granted by PAHO. Similar activities were carried out in the state of Paraná under a project in the municipality of Palmeira. These initiatives have served as models for other districts in the country.

Health promotion efforts receive an important boost from the national mass communication campaigns carried out by the Federal Government to focus attention on priority areas of action. The Government spends some US$ 50 million annually on these campaigns, which are developed by advertising agencies and broadcast on television and radio. AIDS prevention is one of the major campaigns.

The press is also devoting increasing attention to health issues in response to concerns revealed by public opinion surveys.

Disease Prevention and Control Programs. Communicable disease control activities are carried out through specific programs and initiatives overseen by the National Health Foundation, with variable degrees of interinstitutional articulation and coordination. The creation of the UHS and the general process of sector restructuring have necessitated the development of new models for the management of these activities, with managerial decentralization to the municipal level and organization of statewide and nationwide technical support systems in strategic areas (information and research).

In the area of vector-borne disease control, similar efforts are under way to replace the traditional model of intervention, based on short-term centrally managed campaigns, with ongoing intersectoral activities managed at the local level. These efforts have stressed training of personnel in decentralized services in the application of control instruments whose use was previously very limited. Interaction with the academic sector and scientific associations, such as the Brazilian Society of Tropical Medicine, provides technical support for government actions and is a source of crucial input in specific areas. Among the most noteworthy of the programmatic initiatives carried out thus far are the integrated malaria control project, the plan for the eradication of *Aedes aegypti*, the extension of training in entomology, and joint projects with states and municipalities for the control of schistosomiasis, filariasis, and onchocerciasis. An important element of support of the process of decentralization is the program for the development of zoonoses control centers to monitor animal populations that serve as reservoirs and vectors of disease. Eighty-five of these centers are currently operating in large and medium-sized Brazilian cities.

National programs for the control of lung diseases and skin diseases of public health importance have been decentralized for many years and are carried out by the general health services system with technical support from the Ministry of Health. In the case of tuberculosis and other lung diseases, support is provided by a national reference center and by macroregional technical units in close coordination with the Brazilian Society for the Study of Lung Disease and Tuberculosis. One of the activities planned for the future is the implementation of an emergency plan for tuberculosis control in 250 municipalities in which 70% of the country's tuberculosis patients reside. With regard to leprosy and other skin diseases of public health importance, there are three national reference centers and a plan for the elimination of leprosy as a public health problem by the year 2000. State control programs have been strengthened and epidemiologic stratification of the problem to the municipal level has been undertaken with a view to developing differentiated interventions in some 400 municipalities where 85% of all leprosy patients are concentrated. Projects for the detection of cases in areas surrounding the principal Brazilian capitals are also under way.

Control of vaccine-preventable diseases is routinely carried out by the health services system. Special strategies are adopted for certain types of vaccines or specific areas, in accordance with the programming established jointly by national, state, and municipal managers of the UHS. Data on coverage and doses of vaccine administered have been available in all municipalities of the country since 1995. The oral polio vaccine continues to be given annually on two national immunization days, when 90% of children under the age of 5 are vaccinated. Other vaccines are also administered on these immunization days, selectively and according to local needs. To prevent a buildup of susceptible people after the mass measles vaccination campaign carried out in 1992, a new campaign was conducted in 1995. As a result of these campaigns, 86% coverage has been achieved among children under age 4. Mean annual coverage levels among children less than 1 year old for the routinely administered vaccines are approximately 95% for BCG, 75% for DTP, and 80% for the measles vaccine. The percentage of children who fail to com-

plete the three-dose DTP series is about 15%; the North and Northeast regions have the lowest coverage rates. Vaccination against groups A, B, and C meningococci is carried out sporadically in response to epidemic situations. In areas with a high prevalence of hepatitis B, children under the age of 1 are routinely vaccinated. The governments of six states in the South and Southeast have utilized their own resources to implement routine administration of the triple measles-rubella-mumps vaccine. Some municipal health programs have also begun to use the *H. influenzae* type B vaccine.

Under a national program for the control of cervical cancer launched by the National Cancer Institute in 1996, pilot projects are to be implemented in five state capitals.

Epidemiologic Surveillance Systems and Public Health Laboratories. The national epidemiologic surveillance system comprises a set of technical norms and procedures applicable at all levels of the health system to make relevant and timely information available to guide activities for the control of specific diseases and health impairments. At the national level, the Ministry of Health determines which diseases are reportable and establishes the corresponding requirements. The state and municipal secretariats of health are responsible for carrying out the activities in their respective territories, complementing the regulatory guidelines, and adding to the national list other diseases of regional or local importance. When necessary, the technical agencies of the Ministry of Health provide additional support to the states, including investigation of epidemics. Currently, there are 25 diseases that are required to be reported at the national level in Brazil. The list includes communicable diseases targeted by national control programs. Food and nutrition surveillance is carried out by a specific system, which is currently operating in 1,050 municipalities.

In recent years the Ministry of Health has been working to ensure better coordination of the activities of its various technical agencies. The creation of the National Epidemiology Center in 1990 was an important step in this direction. This center provides standardized instruments for the collection of data and disseminates information regularly by means of a national epidemiologic bulletin. The system is currently in the process of adapting to the changes in the sector through the establishment of local structures, which implies decentralization of activities that have traditionally been carried out by national health agencies and training of central-level personnel to support the state and municipal systems.

Laboratory support for disease control activities is coordinated nationally through a network of specialized services composed of reference centers and macroregional laboratories that provide technical support for state and municipal epidemiologic surveillance systems. As of 1994 the network included reference laboratories for meningitis, diphtheria, tuberculosis, leprosy, leptospirosis, cholera and other bacterial infections, hepatitis, arboviruses, enteroviruses, measles, rubella, rabies, Chagas' disease, and leishmaniasis. With financial support from the Ministry of Health, this network produces technical manuals, trains human resources, provides technical assistance and supervision, and produces some diagnostic reagents.

Drinking Water and Sewerage Services. Constitutional provisions specify that municipal governments are responsible for the management of basic sanitation services. Available information indicates that approximately 15% of Brazilian municipalities are managing these services directly and 75% have services managed by state-run sanitation companies. No information is available for the remaining 10%. Funding for the national sanitation policy is provided out of the national budget and user contributions. The Ministry of Health manages part of these resources directly through the National Health Foundation.

Data from 1995 indicate that 76% of households nationwide are connected to a water supply system. In urban areas the proportion is 90%, and in rural areas it is about 17%. By region, coverage levels are highest in the Southeast (96%), followed by the South (93%), the Northeast (84%), the Central-West (82%), and the North (70%).

Of the households included in the national survey carried out in 1995, 60% overall were connected to a sewer system or had a septic tank, but the coverage was much higher in urban areas (71%) than in rural areas (14%). By region, the highest coverage is in the Southeast (87%), followed by the South (72%), the Northeast (47%), the North (46%), and the Central-West (42%). Septic tanks are used in 20% of households (23% in urban areas and 45% in rural areas), while 29% of households (25% in urban areas and 45% in rural areas) have rudimentary cesspits or dispose of their waste in rivers or irrigation trenches. In comparison with the 1991 census, there has been a reduction of 4.3% in the number of households that lack any sanitation facilities or any system of waste elimination. Of the total amount of wastewater collected, only 20% is treated at a water purification plant, stabilization or aerobic-anaerobic lagoon, oxidation pond, or by some other method.

Management of Municipal Solid Waste. In 1995, 72% of Brazilian *municipios* had regular refuse collection by public or private sanitation services. In urban areas, 87% of households have refuse collection services, but the proportion is only 10% in rural areas. In the other municipalities (28%) refuse is burned, buried, or simply dumped in vacant lots, lakes, rivers, or the ocean. In urban areas, data from 1989 indicate that of all the waste collected daily, 49% is disposed of in open-air dumps, 22% is disposed of in controlled landfills, 23% is dumped in sanitary landfills, and only 6% is composted, recycled, or incinerated.

Prevention and Control of Air Pollution. Resolutions of the National Council on the Environment (CONAMA) have established national air quality standards and have also established air pollution standards for the development of an emergency plan to be applied in critical situations. A program to control air pollution produced by motor vehicles has been in operation since 1986 and has established maximum emission levels. As of 1997, all new cars are required to meet maximum emission levels similar to those in developed countries. Almost one-third of the national vehicle fleet runs on hydrated alcohol fuel, and all gasoline must be blended with alcohol. Air pollution from fixed sources, especially industry, is regulated in the case of new industries through the establishment of emissions standards for combustion processes.

Food Protection and Control. A national system for epidemiologic surveillance of foodborne diseases is currently being organized. In 1996, 349 outbreaks were registered in seven states, with 11,341 cases. Investigation of the outbreaks revealed *Staphylococcus aureus*, *Salmonella* sp., and *Clostridium perfringens* as the causal agents. The principal determining factors were faulty raw materials; lack of hygiene; incorrect food-handling, cooking, or reheating practices; and storage at improper temperatures. New food-processing technologies are being introduced, and risk analysis as well as analysis of critical control points is being applied. A total of 1,040 professionals have been trained in this area in the past five years.

Food Aid Programs. To combat vitamin A deficiency, close to 5.8 million children received vitamin A supplements during the immunization campaigns carried out in the Northeast region between 1983 and 1991. In 1994 the program was extended to other endemic areas, and a coverage level of more than 80% was achieved.

In 1995 new legislation relating to iodine deficiency disorders was enacted. The Ministry of Health is responsible for ensuring the supply of iodine to salt distributors. Regulation of this supplement and establishment of a higher standard for salt iodization (from 40 to 60 mg/kg) have been important steps toward reducing this problem in the country.

Activities at the national level aimed at controlling iron deficiency anemia are limited to ensuring the availability of ferrous sulfate supplements through health services within the health care system.

Organization and Operation of Personal Health Care Services

According to the most recent data on current capacity of the health sector, in 1992 there were 49,676 health care establishments: 27,092 (55%) in the public sector and 22,584 (45%) in the private sector. There were 24,016 outpatient care facilities (65% public); 7,415 hospitals (28% public); 8,440 emergency care facilities (38% public); 16,400 specialized diagnostic centers (25% public); 1,078 blood banks (28% public); 7,050 specialized treatment centers—radiation therapy, chemotherapy, etc. (28% public); and 429 psychiatric care facilities (20% public). Eight percent of public establishments and 24% of private establishments provide inpatient care. The country has 544,357 hospital beds, or 3.6 per 1,000 inhabitants, 25% in the public sector and 75% in the private sector. The vast majority of psychiatric hospital beds (100,749, of which 30% are in public-sector facilities) are concentrated in the Southeast (63%), compared with the North (less than 1%), and the Northeast (18%). The Southeast and South regions of the country possessed about 60% of the total installed capacity in terms of establishments and available beds.

The implementation of the REFORSUS plan is expected to enhance the current capacity of the UHS. The objectives are to upgrade the physical facilities and technological capabilities of the health system—especially in the areas of obstetric, perinatal, and emergency care in large urban areas—as well as to expand the family health program and improve the capacity and quality of the hematology and hemotherapy system and the public health laboratories.

In some states intermunicipal health consortia are being formed. These are civil associations established by the governments of several municipalities. The consortia pool institutional resources of the municipalities and ensure referral to public facilities that provide hospital and specialized care for the entire population living in the intermunicipal area, thus reducing dependence on health care facilities in the large urban centers.

Inputs for Health

Drugs. Brazil is one of the world's 10 largest consumer markets for drugs, with a 1.5%–2.0% share of the world market. Gross receipts in the domestic drug market totaled US$ 9,700 million in 1995, a 15% increase with respect to the previous year. The pharmaceutical industry directly generated 47,100 jobs in 1996, with overall investments of US$ 200 million in that year. The sector comprises some 500 companies, including drug producers, chemical-pharmaceutical industries, and importers. There are 45,000 pharmacies that sell 5,200 products in 9,200 different forms. The population segment whose income is more than 20 times the minimum wage—which comprises 15% of the total population—accounts for 48% of all spending on drugs, with a mean annual expenditure of US$ 193 per capita. The segment whose income is 4–10 times the minimum wage makes up 34% of the population and accounts for 36% of spending on drugs, with

a mean annual expenditure of US$ 64 per capita. Another 51% of the population accounts for 16% of spending on drugs, with a mean annual expenditure of US$ 19 per capita.

The government drug program is administered by the central drug exchange (CEME). This is an agency linked to the Ministry of Health, which is responsible for the procurement and distribution of drugs for 23 specific programs coordinated by the Ministry, with an approximate value of US$ 1,000 million in 1997. Of the resources allocated by the CEME to meet this demand, 47% are from public-sector laboratories, which supply 38% of the products procured.

In 1995, pursuant to MERCOSUR agreements, the Secretariat for Health Surveillance officially adopted the good manufacturing practices recommended by WHO. The same year, a national program for the inspection of the pharmaceutical and pharmacochemical industries was established and several courses on good manufacturing practices were offered. Inspection activities have been stepped up considerably during the past few years.

Immunobiological Products. Since 1985 the country has had a program for national self-sufficiency in immunobiological products, aimed at ensuring the availability of the vaccines and sera used in public health programs. The program has strengthened national institutions, mainly in the public sector, which have gained experience in the development of immunobiological products. In its 11 years of existence, some US$ 100 million in federal funds have been invested for the construction and improvement of laboratories, purchase of equipment, and training of human resources. To ensure the quality of the products supplied to health services, whether or not they are manufactured in Brazil, the program sends each production lot to the national quality control institute for analysis.

In 1996, the national immunization program used 196 million doses of 26 different types of vaccines and sera worth a total of around US$ 84 million. Of this amount, close to 76 million doses were manufactured in the country, which was sufficient to meet the total demand for BCG, tetanus toxoid, double antigen, yellow fever, and human and canine rabies vaccines as well as antivenom, antitetanic, antipertussis, and antirabies sera. If all the production facilities currently under construction are completed, by the year 2000 Brazil will be in a position to supply other South American countries with DTP vaccine and its components, BCG, antitoxins, and antivenins.

Equipment. The total national stock of medical and hospital equipment in the public sector has an estimated worth of US$ 7,000 million. However, 20%–40% of this equipment is inoperative because of procurement-related problems, poor quality, improper use, deficient management and maintenance, and lack of regular programs to finance investment in modernization. This situation is related to the shortage of equipment management and maintenance units, which exist in only 1% of hospitals with more than 120 beds, and also to the shortage of specialized professionals (maintenance engineers and technicians). Consumption of medical and hospital equipment and materials in Brazil in 1995 totaled close to US$ 2,000 million, which represents 1.7% of the world market for these products. Domestic industries met about 60% of internal demand, with equal participation by the public and private sectors.

Since 1991 the Ministry of Health has been promoting the establishment of equipment management and maintenance systems, training of specialized human resources, institution of quality assurance systems, and development of proposals for technology assessment. These initiatives, though not yet consolidated, have produced notable results in the institutionalization of professional training programs, assessment and establishment of regulations relating to equipment, and projects for investments in the health services system, especially projects financed with external resources, such as REFORSUS.

Human Resources

Brazil has 513,338 health professionals, of which 40.1% are physicians, 26.8% are dentists, 13.2% are professional nurses, 10.1% are pharmacists, and 9.8% are veterinarians. There are 757 inhabitants per physician, 1,132 per dentist, 2,330 per nurse, and 2,981 per pharmacist. Increasing numbers of women are entering the medical profession. In 1996, 31.9% of all practicing physicians in the country were women.

The distribution of health services and health professionals in the country is characterized by a heavy concentration of human resources in the most developed regions and in the state capitals. Fifty-nine percent of all physicians, 51% of nurses, 50% of pharmacists, 63% of dentists, and 44% of veterinarians reside in the Southeast. The region with the smallest proportion of medical professionals is the North, which has only 5.3% of the human resources in all categories.

The number of graduates in the medical profession during the 1992–1994 period remained relatively stable, with a slight upward trend in the fields of dentistry and pharmacy and a reduction in the area of physical therapy. Data from 1992 indicate that there were some 300,000 health professionals who had not completed a degree or certification program. These professionals make up 56% of the total health work force in Brazil and 52% are employed in the public sector.

The health sector accounts for about 8% of all jobs in the formal economy of the country. One-third of these health sector jobs are in public administration at one of the three levels of government.

Research and Technology

In recent decades, activity in the area of health science and technology in Brazil has come to depend on extrasectoral support, mainly from federal development agencies, which have allocated 25%–35% of all the funds they invest to health. This support has strengthened the infrastructure for research, especially in the biological sciences. Nevertheless, in the sectoral sphere, institutional research has been weakened and has become increasingly less responsive to the needs of the health system.

With regard to Brazilian scientific output, records from the LILACS (Latin American and Caribbean Literature on Health Sciences) database for the 1981–1992 period show that more than half the indexed publications were Brazilian. According to the database of the Institute for Scientific Information, the number of citations with one or more Brazilian authors increased from 1,317 in 1981 to 2,841 in 1992, totaling 23,975 publications for the period in 1,429 specialized journals; only nine of these journals were published in Brazil.

The need for guidelines for the development of science and technology in the country led to the organization of the First National Conference on Health Science and Technology, which brought together representatives of institutions from all concerned segments of society. This conference approved a set of basic principles for the development of a national policy in this area. One of the most important outcomes of this process was the adoption by the National Health Council—in 1996, after a broad process of social consultation—of guidelines and standards to regulate research on human subjects.

Expenditures and Sectoral Financing

According to the Constitution, the funding allocated for the UHS includes financing for the social security system, which is organized by the Government and encompasses health, social insurance, and social welfare services. The resources come from public budgets at the three levels and from direct taxes on wages, billing, benefits, and financial transactions. In the framework of the REFORSUS project, external resources will be invested in the service delivery infrastructure, in managerial training for personnel in the state and municipal health secretariats, and in the family health program.

Public spending on health at the three levels of government, which in 1989 was US$ 13,200 (US$ 96 per capita), declined enormously in subsequent years, dropping to US$ 8,700 million (US$ 63 per capita) in 1992. This sharp reduction paralleled a reduction in federal spending, which historically has accounted for three-fourths of total public spending, and was 42% lower in 1992 than in 1989. In 1993, federal public spending began to rise again gradually, reaching US$

14,000 million in 1996, approximately 25% more than in 1989.

In January 1997 the country instituted a temporary tax on financial transactions, aimed at raising funds to address the urgent needs of the health sector. The tax, which was to remain in effect until February 1998, was expected to generate some US$ 4,800 million, making it possible to increase the federal health budget by approximately 30%. After the tax is discontinued, the higher level of health spending is to be financed through alternative sources of funding created as a result of a constitutional amendment formulated by the National Congress and in negotiation with the Federal Government.

In 1995, private insurance plans mobilized resources totaling US$ 6,400 million. The median per capita value of the resources managed by private insurers ranges from US$ 83 to US$ 150 monthly.

External Technical and Financial Cooperation

Brazil receives international technical cooperation for health from a broad range of sources, most of it aimed at meeting needs relating to management and quality control in connection with the establishment of the UHS. This cooperation is formalized through projects with an average duration of three to five years.

Scientific cooperation is provided in response to the needs of Brazilian and foreign investigators, generally on a sporadic and short-term basis without formal agreements between the parties involved.

Currently, Brazil is participating in bilateral technical cooperation initiatives with Canada, China, France, Germany, India, Italy, Japan, Russia, Spain, the United Kingdom, and the United States. The characteristics of this cooperation differ with each country. Some involve single, long-term projects and a large volume of resources (the United Kingdom); in other cases the projects are smaller and are renewable every two years (France). Diversified cooperation is not the norm, except as in cases where training programs are linked to the projects (Japan). Brazil offers attractive conditions for foreign projects in the field of clinical research, but before allowing such research projects to be carried out the country has had to establish agreements on technology transfer, intellectual property rights, internationalization of production, and compliance with legal provisions concerning research on human subjects.

Brazil cooperates bilaterally on health matters with various developing countries, including Bolivia, Colombia, Cuba, El Salvador, Paraguay, Venezuela, and Palestine. There are also official cooperation arrangements with several foreign non-governmental organizations, which are mainly interested in health of the indigenous population.

With regard to multilateral cooperation, the Brazilian health sector participates in technical commissions in various spheres: MERCOSUR, the Treaty for Amazonian Cooperation, entities that regulate medical care on the country's southern border, and the Community of Portuguese-Speaking Countries. PAHO cooperation with Brazil is based on strategic and programmatic orientations validated in the country by means of a joint evaluation process that establishes biennial priorities and regular programming instruments.

Two major sources of international financial cooperation in the area of health are the United Nations Population Fund, which contributes significantly to the program on women's health, and the World Bank, which has supported large-scale projects, such as those for control of endemic diseases in the Northeast and control of malaria in the Amazon region. The REFORSUS project, as noted above, is being financed by the IDB and the World Bank. Also under way are two projects for the prevention and control of drug use, which are receiving support totaling US$ 2.4 million from the United Nations International Drug Control Program.

BRITISH VIRGIN ISLANDS

GENERAL SITUATION AND TRENDS

Socioeconomic, Political, and Demographic Overview

The British Virgin Islands is a Dependent Territory of the United Kingdom. It has full internal self-government through a democratically elected Legislative Council. The Government is formed by an Executive Council consisting of a Chief Minister and three other Ministers. The Governor exercises reserve powers on behalf of the Crown. There is no local government machinery or town councils. District Officers with administrative functions have been appointed for the smaller inhabited islands—Virgin Gorda, Jost van Dyke, and Anegada.

Offshore financial services and tourism are the two main activities of the economy. The offshore financial sector is characterized by international business company registration; there are approximately 200,000 companies registered in the territory. Recently proposed legislation expanded the offshore sector to cover mutual funds, shipping registration, captive insurance companies, and limited partnerships. There are 100 mutual fund companies registered as international business companies, and they manage more than 1,500 funds with assets exceeding US$ 55 billion, including offshore trusts. In 1996 the financial services sector accounted for US$ 55 million, or 49.1% of total government revenue receipts.

The growth of tourism, government infrastructure projects, and house building has fueled activity in the construction industry. Economic activity in these sectors also has led to the importation of labor, mainly from other Eastern Caribbean countries. Unemployment was estimated at approximately 3.6% in 1991.

The Government relies on locally generated revenue and loans for most of its recurrent and capital spending. It also receives grants-in-aid from the British Government, mainly for internal security and foreign affairs, the areas covered by the Governor's reserve powers, and to support "good governance."

The standard of housing is good, with an average of four occupants per dwelling. There are small pockets of poverty in the two main urban areas, Road Town and East End/Long Look. In 1994, it was estimated that 17.7% of the population was living in poverty. Zoning laws and development controls have not yet been introduced, so residential, commercial, and industrial land use coexist in the same area.

A compulsory social security scheme covers all paid employees, and both employees and employers make contributions. Self-employed workers also are required to enroll in the plan. The social security plan provides a wide range of benefits, including maternity, employment injury, unemployment, old-age pension, sickness, and survivor's benefit, as well as providing a funeral grant.

Literacy rates are approximately 98.7% for females and 97.8% for males. School attendance is compulsory up to age 15. The average school attendance is 9.4 years per person. An increasing number of preschools have been established. The University of the West Indies has an active center in the territory. The British Virgin Islands Community College has been renamed the H. Lavity Stout Community College, and it occupies a new campus at Paraquita Bay. There are plans to extend the College, including relocating the University of the West Indies center to the Paraquita Bay Campus.

Much of the population growth in the territory has been the result of incoming migrant laborers and their families from other parts of the Eastern Caribbean. In 1995, the population was 18,314 (51.5% male), with 287 births.

Mortality and Morbidity Profile

A medical practitioner certifies all deaths. Those that occur in a hospital are reported directly to the National Registration

Office; deaths that occur at home are reported to the Office by district registrars.

Between 1992 and 1995, an average of 84 deaths were registered annually in the British Virgin Islands. About 6% of them were coded as ill-defined conditions. Diseases of the circulatory system accounted for 36% and malignant neoplasms for 18% of all deaths. External causes accounted for 7%, conditions originating in the perinatal period for 8%, and communicable diseases for less than 5% of the total. There were no maternal deaths in the period under review, and, with 34 infant deaths, the infant mortality rate for 1992–1995 was 28.7 per 1,000 live births.

More than 60% of all primary care contacts occur in the private sector. The remaining 40% occur at district clinics and at the emergency department of Peebles Hospital. An unknown number of persons also seek primary care in the neighboring United States Virgin Islands. The local health information system does not capture routine data from the private sector, apart from that for communicable diseases. As a result, the only general source of reliable morbidity data is that which can be derived from the pattern of hospital admissions.

Between 1992 and 1995, aside from normal births, diabetes mellitus was the first cause of hospitalization in the Islands, with an average of 62 admissions per year. Alcoholism (in males), hypertension (mostly in females), cholelithiasis (in females), abortions, asthma, and injuries were some of the other important causes of hospitalization. In 1992 there were important outbreaks of fish and shellfish food poisoning cases.

SPECIFIC HEALTH PROBLEMS

Analysis by Population Group

Health of Children

There are very few hospital admissions among children under 5 years old. The leading causes in 1994 were tonsillitis (3 cases), respiratory tract infection (3 cases), bronchopneumonia (5 cases), asthma (6 cases), and hernias (3 cases). The leading illnesses in children 12 years old and younger who attended government district clinics were diarrheal diseases, acute respiratory infections, skin conditions, and intestinal parasites. Between 1992 and 1994, immunization coverage for DTP, polio, MMR, and BCG was 100%.

Health of Adolescents and Adults

There are no specific services for adolescents, although they are recognized as a group with particular needs. Births to teenagers accounted for about 10% of births between 1992 and 1995; in 1% of births mothers were under 15 years old.

Injuries and accidents primarily affect the adult population, particularly young males. Chronic noncommunicable diseases were the characteristic health problems of adults. The leading causes of hospitalization throughout the period were mental disorders, diabetes, and hypertension. For women, pregnancy complications and gynecological disorders were the main causes of hospitalization. Among older men, alcohol abuse was associated with traffic injuries, domestic violence, and workplace injuries.

Health of the Elderly

Cardiovascular and cerebrovascular diseases continue to be the main causes of mortality and morbidity among the elderly. Arthritic conditions also are significant problems. District nursing reports show that in the 1993–1995 period the leading reasons for home visits, in descending order, were diabetes, hypertension, arthritis, accidents and injuries, dressings, and respiratory tract infections.

Analysis by Type of Disease or Health Impairment

In 1995 there were 34 confirmed cases of dengue. There were no cases in 1994 and three confirmed cases in 1993. The recorded increase is probably the result of better reporting as well as an increase in the mosquito population following a very active hurricane season.

Between 1992 and 1995 there were 22 reported HIV cases (13 were males, 7 females, and in 2 cases the sex was not recorded). Over the same period there were 8 cases of AIDS (4 males and 4 females), and 7 deaths as a result of AIDS (4 males and 3 females). Reported cases peaked in 1993 (9 cases), and decreased to 4 cases in 1994 and 5 cases in 1995. Heterosexual contact is the main mode of transmission; those at highest risk for transmission are in the 20–44-year age group.

Among adults alcoholism is a contributing factor to mental disorder. With younger persons the use of illegal drugs is highly correlated with psychiatric problems.

RESPONSE OF THE HEALTH SYSTEM

National Health Plans and Policies

The Government's policy ensures that the public and private health sector provide services that are as comprehensive as possible using available resources. Government services focus on providing care for children, the elderly, the mentally ill, and the disabled. The Government is the main provider of acute medical and surgical services. Health activities and policies emphasize health promotion. The British Virgin Islands has not formulated a health plan; however, Government health priorities are to improve hospital services, strengthen public primary health care services, and enhance all aspects of environmental health, including solid waste management.

In accordance with the 1976 Public Health Act, which provides the statutory framework for protecting and promoting the population's health, government health services are provided free at the point of use to certain groups, including full-time schoolchildren, nursing mothers, the elderly, the mentally ill, health workers, firefighters, the police, prisoners, and prison officers.

Health Sector Reform

The Government of the United Kingdom funded a health sector adjustment project in the 1990s covering four British Dependent Territories in the Caribbean, including the British Virgin Islands. The Project was managed by Keele University in the United Kingdom, which provided two full-time health sector development advisers, based in the Caribbean. In addition, the Project hired consultants to assess issues such as health information, solid waste management plan, mental health services, and services for the terminally and chronically ill. Proposals for restructuring the management in the Ministry and in the Public Health Department were accepted by the Government in 1995 and are in the process of implementation.

Organization of the Health Sector

Institutional Organization

The Ministry of Health and Welfare is responsible for providing public health and social services, as well as for monitoring and regulating private sector providers. Policy decisions are made by the Minister in consultation with the Director of Health Services and the Permanent Secretary. The Director of Health Services is charged with the day-to-day management and planning of health services. The Permanent Secretary is responsible for the administration of the Ministry headquarters and for supporting the Minister in his policy role.

The Public Health Department is responsible for managing government health services. The Department is organized into hospital and primary health care services; each is headed by a senior manager who reports to the Director of Health Services. Budgetary responsibility is devolved to the heads of the respective units.

The Medical Act, which currently is under revision, provides for the registration of doctors and certain allied professionals. There is a separate Nursing Act that provides for certification of nursing professionals.

The territory has a vigorous private health sector, encompassing both inpatient and ambulatory care. Many residents also go off-island for health care, mainly to the United States Virgin Islands or Puerto Rico, either through choice or because they require specialized care unavailable locally. British Virgin Islands residents also have access to specialist care in the United Kingdom, which is arranged through the International Division of the United Kingdom's Department of Health.

Health Services and Resources

Organization of Services for Care of the Population

Maternal and Child Health Services. The Health Department has the following objectives regarding prenatal care: to initiate prenatal care for 90% of pregnant women by the 16th week of pregnancy; attain 90% coverage of all pregnant women, with a minimum of 10 prenatal visits; have 95% of deliveries take place at the hospital; ensure that every woman with complications or known health risks receives the care her condition warrants; and attain 90% tetanus toxoid coverage of all pregnant women.

Pregnant women are encouraged to seek prenatal care from district clinics or private doctors. All pregnant women are referred to the hospital clinic by the 12th week of pregnancy, where an obstetrician conducts comprehensive assessments to identify high-risk cases. Hemoglobin levels are appraised, anemia treated, VDRL tests performed, and tetanus toxoid is administered. All pregnant women are referred to Peebles Hospital for delivery. Between 1992 and 1995 there were 1,208 hospital deliveries, an average of 302 annually.

District clinics provide a full range of child health services, including growth and nutritional monitoring, development assessment, treatment of common illnesses, counseling, school health, vision and hearing screening, and screening for anemia, including sickle cell anemia. All school students undergo a complete physical examination prior to entering high school.

Fort Charlotte School is a 12-slot facility for children with special needs run by the Department of Education. Attendees include children with Down's syndrome, cerebral palsy, physical disability, autism, and attention deficit disorder. The school had an average of 10 attendees during the review period.

Family Planning. There have been wide fluctuations in enrollment in family planning services. In 1991, there were 1,764 acceptors, increasing to 3,606 in 1992, falling to 2,542 in 1993, and dropping further to 1,431 in 1994. Condoms are available from many shops and stores in the territory; about 1,500 condoms were dispensed through health clinics. In 1994, 56% of acceptors chose oral contraceptives, 40% chose injections, and 1.5% chose the IUD. The diaphragm and tubal ligations were chosen by fewer than 0.5% of acceptors.

AIDS Prevention. The British Virgin Islands has an intersectoral National AIDS Committee. All blood for transfusion is screened for HIV. Community education is a key national strategy for combating AIDS, and there have been numerous campaigns and a consistent media strategy to maintain AIDS awareness.

Control of Noncommunicable Chronic Diseases. Diabetes and hypertension rank among the top five causes of death and reasons for hospital admission, district clinic attendance, and home visits by nurses. The Ministry of Health, in conjunction with the Diabetic Association, has undertaken major initiatives to control these diseases, including public education and improved clinical advice for diabetics and their families. There are protocols for the management of persons with diabetes and hypertension, and hypertension and diabetic clinics are conducted on Tortola at Road Town, East End, Capoons, and Carrot Bay. On Virgin Gorda there are hypertension and diabetic clinics at North Sound and the Valley. In 1993 there were some 1,800 clinic visits and 1,978 visits in 1994 for both conditions territory-wide.

Mental Health. Mental disorders, including alcoholism, drug-induced psychoses, non-specific psychoses, and schizophrenia have been the leading causes of hospitalization for the past 10 years. The community mental health center located in Road Town provides most of the ambulatory care for the territory. Its approach emphasizes treating individuals in their community, including monitoring and administering medication, providing family counseling, and promoting self-care. Mental health center staff visit the hospital, the prison, and the geriatric home as necessary. In 1991, there were about 1,873 patient contacts, 1,001 in 1993, and 1,566 in 1994. Most were seen at weekly clinics, including drop-in sessions. Since 1993, the male-to-female ratio for mental health services has been 2:1.

Psychiatric patients are admitted to the medical ward of Peebles Hospital, an arrangement that is less than satisfactory from a clinical point of view. There are only two secured rooms on the medical ward and non-disruptive patients are admitted on the general medical ward. There are no psychiatric nurses on staff and quarters are cramped.

In 1995, a drug rehabilitation facility was opened within walking distance of the community mental health center. The drug treatment center saw 90 persons during 500 contacts in 1995–1996. Once it began to operate, the center's mandate was expanded to cover all substance abuse, domestic violence, and child abuse problems.

Environmental Health. The Environmental Health Division is part of the Health Department. The Solid Waste Department is directly responsible to the Permanent Secretary of the Ministry of Health and Welfare. Several other ministries and departments also are involved in environmental health matters, including the Conservation and Fisheries Department, the Department of Agriculture under the Ministry of Natural Resources and Labor, and the Water and Sewerage Department under the Ministry of Communications and Works. Consideration is being given to transferring responsibility for water supply to the Electricity Corporation, which now produces a substantial amount of potable water and sells it directly to the public.

The Environmental Health Division is responsible for food hygiene, vector control, water quality surveillance, institutional hygiene, the maintenance of public conveniences on Tortola and Virgin Gorda, and the investigation of nuisance complaints such as septic tank problems, rodents, and abandoned vehicles. The bulk of the Division's non-salary budget is allocated to vector control activities, which mainly involve efforts to reduce the *Aedes aegypti* mosquito population to a level where the risks of transmission of dengue are reduced to a minimum. The usual control measures are fogging, oiling, and the supply of larvivorous fish. During 1995, four cycles of treatment and inspection took place. The house index was 5.4%, which is comparable to the 5% figure seen in 1992. There has been increasing demand for rat baiting, but the Government has not allocated funds for this purpose. An estimated US$ 6.40 per capita was spent on vector control activities in 1995.

Food Safety. The food hygiene program inspects food-handling premises and provides training for staff involved in food handling. All food handlers are required to have physical examinations, laboratory tests, including tests for tuberculosis and VDRL, and stool examinations for ova and parasites. In 1995, 90% of establishments met food hygiene requirements.

Drinking Water. All households have access to potable water, which is mainly supplied through rainwater collected in household cisterns. Piped water is supplied by the Water and Sewerage Department, and is obtained from several groundwater sources and from a desalination plant. Tortola's main water supply only reaches Road Town and its environs; pipes are being laid to extend the supply eastward along

Ridge Road, and plans are under way for further expansion of the system.

The Water and Sewerage Department monitors the quality of the water it produces, as does the Environmental Health Division. The Division's water quality and institutional hygiene programs deal with the surveillance of water supplies and ensuring the maintenance of a basic level of sanitation in public institutions such as schools, preschools, day-care centers, and clinics. The bacteriological quality of the public water supply is monitored at least once every two months, cistern water is examined, and employees of water bottling companies are certified. In late 1995, the Division received a portable testing laboratory that enables it to undertake its own fecal coliform testing. The Conservation and Fisheries Department, in association with the Water and Sewerage Department, monitors water in recreational areas.

Pollution. Land and sea pollution continues to be a problem. The leading pollution sources are used motor oil, effluent from septic tanks, garbage, surface run-off, old batteries, and household and commercial chemicals. Untreated sewage continues to be discharged into the sea by some yachts, marinas, seafront hotels, businesses, and residences. The increase in the number of cruise ships poses an additional threat of water contamination and added demand for solid waste services.

Only about 7% of households (400) are connected to the sewerage system, and most households rely on septic tanks; some 4% have no approved toilet facilities. Malfunctioning soakaways resulting from poor soil permeability continue to pose serious problems, particularly in communities where large apartment buildings have been constructed.

Solid Waste Disposal. The Solid Waste Department is responsible for the collection and disposal of solid waste, operation of the Pockwood Pond incinerator on Tortola, street and road cleaning, roadside trimming, gully cleaning, and beautification. The Department is no longer responsible for liquid waste disposal, but the transfer of this responsibility is still under consideration. The Department now controls an annual budget of US$ 2 million and has 8 salaried personnel and 55 daily paid personnel.

A combination of landfill and open burning is used on all major inhabited islands, except Tortola. Solid waste is collected by private contractors and by staff directly employed by the Solid Waste Department. The Government covers the cost of solid waste collection and disposal, although some owners contract and pay private collectors. There are no dumping fees or taxes levied. Although services are considered to be good, glass recycling may become necessary in the future to avoid incinerator capacity limitations and to extend landfill life. Hazardous and special waste is disposed of at the incinerator on Tortola.

There is a need for a long-term landfill site for Tortola, and alternative management practices to reduce the bulk of waste and to increase recycling need to be considered. More guidelines must be developed and a better system established for the collection and disposal of hazardous or special waste.

Health Promotion. The Health Education Division of the Public Health Department is responsible for most of the formal health promotion undertaken in the British Virgin Islands. It carries out health education, public relations, and communications activities pertaining to health matters, and also provides technical support to other parts of the Health Department and to certain NGOs. It relies on radio programming, advertising, video presentations, printed material, press releases, press contacts, and audiovisual presentations to conduct programs aimed at the public at large and at target groups. A senior health educator, a health educator, a communications specialist, and an audiovisual technician staff the Division. Priorities for the Division are the prevention and control of AIDS and other sexually transmitted diseases, cancer, heart disease, and diabetes. Health promotion activities regarding drug demand reduction are undertaken by the National Drug Advisory Council and its service arm. The Solid Waste Department also undertakes health promotion activities related to its area of responsibility.

Organization and Operation of Personal Health Care Services

The first level of public health care is the district clinic. District clinics are supported by Road Town Health Center and Peebles Hospital, located in the same compound in Road Town. Catchment populations for district clinics range from 141 persons at the Jost van Dyke Clinic to 9,106 persons at the Road Town Health Center on Tortola, numbers augmented by tourists and temporary residents, such as yacht dwellers. The Road Town Health Center serves as a referral point for the district clinics and includes a family planning service. Public health nurses are being trained to take on family planning duties at the district level. Other primary care facilities available include a drug-treatment center, a community mental health center, and a dental unit, all of which provide services that are not routinely available at district clinics. The drug-treatment center and mental health center are based in Road Town.

The island of Virgin Gorda has two clinics. The clinic in The Valley may expand the scope of its services. The clinic in North Sound has a catchment population of 582; it has one bed and a resident nurse. A full-time physician serves Virgin Gorda, in addition to a public health nurse, midwife, environmental health officer, and several junior nurses. The clinics on Jost van Dyke and Anegada both have resident nurses and a physician who makes weekly and bi-weekly visits, respectively, to the two islands. Private medical practitioners based in Tortola also visit Virgin Gorda, Jost van Dyke, and Anegada.

Doctor clinics are held at all health clinics. In 1994 these accounted for 293 clinic sessions, 3,984 total attendances, or an average of 14 patients per session. Doctor clinics mainly served the elderly and other persons who are exempt from fees. The leading causes of clinic visits by adults, in rank order, were diabetes, hypertension, arthritis, accidents/injuries, dressings, and respiratory tract infections.

The 50-bed Peebles Hospital in Tortola (44 beds in operation) is the main provider of secondary care and is administered by the Government. It offers surgical, obstetric, medical, pediatric, and psychiatric care on an inpatient basis. All service areas are covered by local doctors, except for psychiatry, which is served by a part-time consultant psychiatrist based in Barbados. Hospital ambulatory care includes emergency care and several outpatient clinics, including pediatrics, surgery, medicine, ophthalmology, dermatology, and obstetrics. Clinical support includes physiotherapy, x-ray, and laboratory services. In 1995 there were 1,918 outpatient visits; 17,168 emergency department visits, and 1,423 inpatient admissions. The occupancy rate (based on 44 beds) was 51% and the average length of stay was five days.

The Community Mental Health Center provides psychiatric service on an outpatient basis. The Adina Donovan Home, which is adjacent to Peebles Hospital, is a residential facility for the elderly run by the Ministry of Health and Welfare.

One dentist, two dental nurses, and one dental hygienist staff the Government's three-chair dental unit in Road Town. There is one dental chair in Virgin Gorda and one in Anegada, where services are provided one day per week and one day per month, respectively. Government oral health services mainly treat children; the dental officer treats adults in private clinics part-time on a split-fee basis with the Ministry. In 1994, US$ 112,000 was spent on public dental services. No index for decayed, filled, or missing teeth (DMFT) is available for the territory.

There is an active and well-established private health sector. An eight-bed clinic performs reconstructive, general, and hand surgery, and had an annual average of 354 patients during the review period. There are two private dental clinics in Road Town. The dental workload in the private sector was an estimated 18,000 courses of treatment per year, compared with the public sector dental workload of 2,182 in 1991, which rose to 5,000 in 1993. The vision center conducted 1,500 consultations in 1992 and 2,500 in 1993. In addition, there are several private medical practices; the two largest are located in Road Town, and one has a branch in Virgin Gorda. Both centers have a pharmacy and mammography, ultrasound, and x-ray diagnostic equipment. They also provide a broad range of family practice services, including extended hours for walk-in treatment. There are at least two private physicians working in individual practices on a part-time basis. One full-time chiropractor and 8 to 12 traditional practitioners work on a fee-for-service basis.

During the 1991–1993 period it was estimated that between 55% and 60% of primary health care contacts were in the private sector, and for some specialties such as ophthalmology and gastroenterology, around 90% of the care is in the private sector. The distribution of laboratory tests, prescriptions, and imaging also follows this pattern.

Specialized services are provided through referrals to institutions abroad (the U.S. Virgin Islands, Puerto Rico, and the United States mainland). The individual usually pays for this care, but, in some cases, employment-based health insurance, personal health insurance policies, or the industrial injury provision within the social security scheme cover the costs. The Social Security Board has consistently made grants to the Health Department to widen the scope of local services, so that a larger number of those experiencing work-related injuries can receive treatment locally, rather than being sent off-island.

Human Resources

Nursing assistants are trained locally. In 1994, a degree level program for nursing began at the Community College, in association with Hocking College of Ohio (United States). Further professional training is done in other Caribbean countries, the United States, or the United Kingdom. Health personnel also participate in local staff development programs organized by the Health Department and the Government's Training Division. They also take advantage of programs provided through the University of the West Indies' distance education facilities.

Overall reliance on foreign-born and trained nurses and doctors remains high. Nurses tend to come from within the Caribbean, doctors from further afield. Non-nationals usually receive two-year contracts, and there is high turnover of foreign staff.

Expenditures and Sectoral Financing

Public health services are almost wholly financed by the Government. User fees generally raise only 5% of the operating costs of hospital, primary health care, and solid waste services. In 1991, expenditures on public health services stood at US$ 5.96 million with hospital services accounting for 58% of expenses, primary health care for 22%, and solid waste management for 18%. By 1994 the total figure had increased to US$ 10 million, with hospital services accounting for 64%, primary health care for 18%, and solid waste management for

16.8% of expenditures. Financial analysis of the health sector estimated that in 1993 the public sector accounted for approximately 51% of health care expenditure in the territory. There was no significant capital expenditure in the health sector during the review period.

In the private sector, health insurance premiums paid by employers, including the Government, parastatals, and private sector employers accounted for an estimated 21% of expenditures. Direct payments to practitioners represented 9%; medicines, dental, and optical appliances, 12%; fees paid to traditional practitioners, 1%; and fees paid to government providers accounted for 2% of private sector health outlays. No estimates were made of the amount spent by the population for health care services purchased off-island.

Health insurance premiums have been a growing area of expenditure in the territory. All government and parastatal employees are now eligible to join group schemes. Many private companies also offer this as a benefit. The premium-to-claim ratio for Government and parastatal schemes are 4:1 or worse. In other words, 25% or less in claims are met from the premiums paid. These payments now represent a large financial outflow, while offering little enhancement of local services.

CANADA

GENERAL SITUATION AND TRENDS

Socioeconomic, Political, and Demographic Overview

Canada is the largest country in the Western Hemisphere, with a land area of 10 million km². It is a confederation governed by 1 national, 10 provincial, and 2 territorial governments. Canadians enjoy one of the highest standards of living in the world. This is evident in the fact that Canada has ranked first in the United Nations Human Development Index each year between 1994 and 1997.

In 1994, it was determined that the majority of Canadians between ages 16 and 69 have the literacy and numeracy abilities to meet everyday living requirements. Overall, 99% of the population is considered literate. Educational levels also continue to rise. The number of First Nations students living on reserves has increased from less than half to 75% in the past six years.[1]

Since 1992, the Canadian economy has expanded at a moderate pace. The 1995 gross domestic product (GDP) per capita was Can$ 26,184. Health expenditures for 1996 reached Can$ 2,510 per capita. This represented 9.5% of the GDP, down from the 1992 peak level of 10.2%.

As of 1 July 1996, there were 29,963,000 people living in Canada, a 9.7% increase since 1991. The 1995–1996 increases in population yielded a growth rate of 1.2%, lower than the 1.7% average annual rate for the 1991–1995 period. Census figures for 1991 revealed the self-identified Aboriginal population to be 1,002,675, or 3.6% of the total Canadian population. There were nearly 602,700 registered Indians, of whom 346,291 lived on-reserve and 256,400 lived off-reserve. According to the 1991 census, 60.5% of the population reported English as their mother tongue, 23.8% reported French, and 13% reported a mother tongue other than English or French.

There are more women than men in the oldest age groups (65–74 years and 75 and older), but in all other age groups, there are virtually equal numbers of women and men. The number of young Canadians (age 0–19) decreased from 8.6 million in 1970 to a low of 7.5 million in 1985. Since then, the absolute number has grown slightly to 7.9 million in 1993. Still, the proportion of Canadians under age 19 has decreased from approximately 40% in 1970 to 26.6% in 1996, largely due to the aging of the "baby boom" generation.

Canadians 20–64 years of age now make up 61% of the population. The number of Canadians age 65 and older has doubled from 1.7 to 3.5 million since 1970, and account for 12.2% of the population. This proportion is expected to increase to 14% by 2011. As the "baby boomer" population approaches retirement, health services consumption will likely increase.

The majority of the Canadian population is concentrated in two provinces: Ontario (37%) and Quebec (25%). Twenty-nine percent lives in Alberta, Saskatchewan, Manitoba, and British Columbia, compared with 9% in New Brunswick, Nova Scotia, Prince Edward Island, and Newfoundland. The vast differences in provincial population size are illustrated by the ratio of the largest (Ontario) to the smallest (Prince Edward Island), which is 81:1. The territorial populations are even less than that of the smallest province.

Canada's population is highly urbanized. From 1991 to 1995, the percentage of the population residing in rural areas declined from 23% to slightly less than 20% and by 1995, over 80% of the population was urban. At present, metropolitan areas account for 61% of the population, with the balance living in smaller urban places.

Immigration has diversified the ethnic and cultural makeup of the Canadian population. In 1996, there were 209,000 international migrants, down slightly from 255,740

---

[1] The term "First Nations" refers to those persons who are registered as Indians under the terms of the Indian Act, and whose names appear in the Indian Register maintained by the Department of Indian Affairs and Northern Development. The term "Aboriginal" refers to all indigenous persons of Canada, specifically those of North American Indian, Inuit, or Metis ancestry.

in 1993. The majority of immigrants were from Asia (136,982), followed by Europe (40,735). Since immigrants tend to settle primarily in urban areas, immigration has the greatest impact on urban centers.

The Canadian population has grown substantially since 1970, the two principal reasons being immigration and new births. More than 383,000 babies were born in Canada in 1995, a rate of 12.9 per 1,000. The 1995 crude birth rate is the lowest since 1972. The birth rate for First Nations peoples was 27.5 per 1,000 in 1993, approximately twice that of the general Canadian population, whose crude birth rate was 13.4 in the same year.

For 1995, the fertility rate varied dramatically by age group. Women in the 25–29-year age group account for 109 births per 1,000 women, followed by those in the 30–34-year age group (86.8 per 1,000); almost two-thirds of all babies were born to women within this 10-year range. Less than 1% of babies were born to mothers aged 10–14 and only 1.3% to women age 45 or older. There is a wide range of fertility rates by geographic area, from a low of 1,250 per 10,000 women in Newfoundland, to a high of 2,778 per 10,000 women in the Northwest Territories.

Mortality Profile

Overall mortality rates have declined significantly since the early 20th century. As Canada moved into public insurance coverage of health care services, specific causes of mortality showed further declines.

In 1995, the crude death rate for the general Canadian population was 7.1 per 1,000. The crude death rate for First Nations peoples in 1993 was 5.52 per 1,000. This rate was slightly lower than that of the general Canadian population, whose crude death rate in 1993 was 7.08 per 1,000. It is plausible that the favorable difference is attributable to the larger proportion of youth in the First Nations population rather than to better health.

Average life expectancy (1995) at birth for a male is 75.4 years while the average life expectancy for a female is 81.3 years. Total life expectancy decreased marginally from 1992 to 1993 due to an influenza epidemic; nevertheless, the gains since 1971 are impressive for both sexes. Improvements in living conditions, infectious disease control, and health care have contributed to increases in longevity.

At all ages, females have a greater total life expectancy than males, although the 6-year advantage that exists at birth declines to a 3-year advantage upon reaching age 75. To some extent, the female advantage with respect to length of life is offset by a lower quality of life, as the additional years lived by a woman are frequently accompanied by an increasing degree of poor health.

TABLE 1
Vital statistics summary, Canada, 1993 and 1995.

Indicator	General Canadian population (1995)	First Nations population (1993)
Live births[a]	12.8	27.5
Deaths[a]	7.1	5.5
Infant deaths[b]	6.1	10.9
Neonatal deaths[b]	4.2	4.0
Post-neonatal deaths[b]	1.9	6.9
Perinatal deaths[b]	7.0	11.8
Maternal deaths[c]	4.0	...
Stillbirths[b] (20+ weeks)	6.2	7.0

[a] Rate per 1,000 population.
[b] Rate per 1,000 live births.
[c] Rate per 100,000 population.

With respect to First Nations people, between 1980 and 1990, the life expectancy of the population increased by six years for both sexes. In 1992, the life expectancy of First Nations females was estimated at 74.9 years, or 6 years less than females in the general Canadian population. Life expectancy for First Nations in 1992 was estimated at 67.8 years or 6.8 years less than the general Canadian population.

A major reason for the overall increase in life expectancy in the general Canadian and First Nations population is the drop in infant mortality, largely due to better pre- and postnatal health care and improved nutrition. Infant mortality rates declined about 83% between 1951 and 1991, and reached 6.1 per 1,000 live births in 1995 (see Table 1). Infant mortality rates for the First Nations population have declined from 27.6 per 1,000 live births in 1979 to 10.9 per 1,000 in 1993. The First Nations post-neonatal death rate (defined as deaths of infants from the 28th day to 1 year of age) dropped 60% from 14.5 per 1,000 live births in 1979 to 6.9 in 1993. By comparison, the post-neonatal mortality rate for the general population was 3.7 in 1979 and declined to 2.1 in 1993.

Since the 1970s, death rates from most major causes have declined, particularly deaths due to heart disease and injuries. Diseases of the circulatory system (including ischemic heart disease and stroke) are the leading causes of death in Canada, accounting for 36.3% of deaths among men and 39.7% among women. Although there were an estimated 54,671 deaths from cardiovascular disease in 1995, this represents a decrease in absolute terms. The decline has been due to a combination of factors: reduced smoking among men, less consumption of dietary fat, improved control of hypertension, and improvements in medical and surgical care. Exceptions to the positive trend are the fairly stable death rates due to suicide, and deaths from all types of cancer combined. Other major causes of death in Canada, for both men and

TABLE 2
Nine leading causes of death, Canada, 1991–1993 and 1995.

Leading causes of death	General Canadian population (1995)[a]	First Nations population (1991–1993)[a]
Circulatory disease	267	350
Neoplasm	199	182
Injury and poisoning	46	174
Respiratory disease	59	108
Digestive disease	26	56
Endocrine and immune system disorders	23	45
Infectious and parasitic diseases	12	17
Congenital anomalies	4	6
Perinatal condition	3	4

[a] Rates per 100,000 population.

Sources: Health Canada. *Trends in First Nations Mortality: 1979–1993;* 1996. Statistics Canada, *Mortality Summary, List of Causes,* 1995.

women, include respiratory diseases, and adverse effects and diseases of the digestive system (see Table 2).

Deaths due to injury have declined as a result of several factors, including increased safety consciousness and safer behaviors. Legislation and programs aimed at such issues as improved roads and vehicles, impaired driving, and seatbelt and helmet use have also contributed to the improving trend.

In the First Nations population, the four leading causes of death have not changed significantly since 1979, although three of the four causes (injury and poisoning and diseases of the circulatory and respiratory systems) have seen significant decreases in their crude mortality rates. Injury and poisoning remains among the leading causes of death. This category has seen a 36.6% improvement in mortality rates, from an average of 243 deaths per 100,000 in the 1979–1981 period to an average of 174 deaths per 100,000 in the 1991–1993 period. Diseases of the circulatory and respiratory systems, the second and fourth leading causes of death in First Nations people, have had lesser decreases in crude mortality rates over this period: 11.1% and 6.5%, respectively. The third leading cause of death among First Nations peoples is neoplasms, which have continued to rise from 55 deaths per 100,000 in 1979–1981 to 76 in 1991–1993, an increase of 38.2%.

Among the Canadian population as a whole, obesity is an emerging health problem. Data indicate that there has been a significant increase in obesity since the mid-1980s, particularly among women. In 1994–1995, almost one third of Canadians aged 18–74 were overweight, to the point of probable health risk. Other chronic health problems for Canadians apart from those that result in death include arthritis and rheumatism; disorders of the back, limbs, and joints; mental disorders; allergies; and dental trouble.

SPECIFIC HEALTH PROBLEMS

Analysis by Population Group

Health of Children

Children in Canada generally have a healthy start in terms of their mothers' health, access to prenatal care, and limited exposure to drugs and alcohol during pregnancy, and the health conditions surrounding their birth. Nevertheless, despite significant health gains since the 1970s, the majority of childhood health indicators for the First Nations population are worse than the Canadian average.

The infant mortality rate for the general Canadian population has declined significantly, reaching 6.0 per 1,000 live births in 1996. The First Nations infant mortality rate has also fallen from 27.6 per 1,000 live births in 1979 to 10.9 per 1,000 in 1993, but it still remains 1.7 times higher than the national average. Although the First Nations neonatal mortality rate was 61.7% higher than the Canadian rate from 1979–1981, it has declined more sharply than the Canadian rate, and by 1991–1993, rates reached an average of 4.7 deaths per 1,000 live births, a rate that was 14.6% higher than the Canadian rate for the same period.

The First Nations perinatal mortality rate has shown substantial improvement from 21.8 deaths per 1,000 births in 1979–1981 to 11.8 deaths per 1,000 births in 1993. Even so, the First Nations perinatal death rate continues to be well above that of the general Canadian population (7.1 in 1994).

Infant mortality and perinatal morality rates are higher for boys than girls, the most pronounced ratio being for early neonatal death at 1.25:1. Provincial and territorial variations in these rates are quite striking. Infant mortality is lowest in Quebec and British Columbia (5.7 per 1,000) and highest in Prince Edward Island (9.1 per 1,000) and the Northwest Territories (9.6 per 1,000). By contrast, Prince Edward Island has the lowest rate of perinatal mortality (5.7 per 1,000), while the highest is in Yukon (11.7 per 1,000).

While the majority of Canadian babies are born healthy, the rate of low birthweight babies has not declined since the early 1980s. Between 1991 and 1995, almost 6.0% of all newborns had low (1,500–2,499 g) or very low (500–1,500 g) birthweight. Women who live in the poorest urban neighborhoods have 1.4 times as many low birthweight babies as women in higher-income areas. A mother's age or racial background did not seem to contribute significantly to low birthweight.

Breast-feeding initiation and continuation varies widely across Canada; the average is 75% initiation and only 30% continuation at 4–6 months. Among those of lower socioeconomic status, the rate of breast-feeding initiation is lower.

Since the mid-1980s, all provinces have stressed infectious

disease elimination through immunization and education programs. Between 85% and 90% of 2-year-olds in the general Canadian population have been fully immunized against diphtheria, tetanus, pertussis, *Hemophilius influenzae* type b (Hib), polio, mumps, rubella, and measles. Ninety-six percent of 2-year-olds have been immunized against measles, 85% have been immunized against DPT, and 90% against polio. Unfortunately, statistics are not as positive for First Nations children. The highest rate of coverage for this population in 1993 was for measles, mumps, and rubella at 73.6%, and the lowest was for pertussis at 45.8%. Nevertheless, figures from 1993 reveal that deaths from infectious and parasitic diseases have become less frequent among the general population of Canadian and First Nations infants.

In 1996, the mortality rate for children of both sexes under age 5 was 8 per 1,000. This represents a 4.3% decline in males and a 1.7% decline for females under age 5 since 1980. Along with premature birth, conditions such as sudden infant death syndrome and congenital anomalies are among the main contributors to infant death.

Injuries also pose a national threat to the health and well-being of children. Unintentional injuries are the leading cause of death for children over 1 year of age and account for more child deaths in Canada than the next six causes combined. The leading causes of injury-related deaths in Canadian children from infancy through early adolescence are suffocation, burns, drownings, falls, and motor-vehicle–related accidents. Injuries during play are typical of the 5–9-year age group. Males are at two to four times greater risk of injury than females, and the severity of injuries is also greater for males.

The prevalence of obesity in children has increased in the past decade from 14% to 24% among girls and from 18% to 26% among boys. At the same time, there are approximately 2.4 million Canadians, of whom 900,000 are children, who rely on government food banks to supplement their diets.

Injuries in the 10–14-year and 15–19-year age groups are more likely to occur at school, a playground, or a sports facility. Poisoning is also common among youth in the 15–24-year age group.

Health of Adolescents and Adults

Lifestyle choices such as alcohol and tobacco use affect the health of young Canadians. Alcohol-attributable mortality remains a major cause of death, particularly among youth in Canada. This is especially true when drinking is combined with driving.

In 1994–1995, 55% of Canadians age 12 and over reported drinking at least one drink per month in the previous year. The proportion of drinkers rose steadily with age. Twelve percent reported never drinking. Nearly 20% of teens aged 15–19 and 30% of youths aged 20–24 reported regular heavy drinking. With the exception of the 12–14-year-old age group, males were significantly more likely than females to have reported being drinkers. There is also a relationship between drinking and education. University graduates were almost twice as likely as those with less than high school education to report drinking at least once a month (71% and 47%, respectively).

While overall tobacco consumption declined by 27% from 1970 to 1990, it has remained steady since 1990. In 1994–1995, 29% of Canadians age 12 and over smoked. Among those in the 15–19-year age group, 29% (261,000) of girls and 26% (244,000) of boys were regular or occasional smokers. While smoking by teens in the 15–19-year age group is not as prevalent as among those 20–44 years old, teen smoking is distinctive in a number of ways. Most significantly, the rate of current teen smokers increased substantially between 1991 and 1995, from 21% to 29%. Teenage females were more likely than males to smoke. For example, in the 12–14-year age group, 15% of girls are current smokers—three times the rate of boys the same age.

Sexual health has become an increasingly important part of healthy living. In 1990, approximately 63% of Canadians age 15 and over reported having their first sexual intercourse before the age of 20. Relatively few (9%) reported their first sexual intercourse as occurring before the age of 15. Differences between genders, age groups, and education levels all characterize variations in sexual practices. The gender variation regarding number of sex partners is most pronounced among 15–19-year-olds: 83% of females report having had only one sex partner in the previous year compared with 64% of males.

Educational and provincial differences in sexual practice are less pronounced than gender and age differences, but some are notable. For instance, the population with a high school education are slightly more likely to have had sex before the age of 20 than are university graduates (69% and 50%, respectively).

The prevalence of sexually transmitted diseases (STDs) other than AIDS, in particular chlamydia, gonorrhea, and syphilis, is highest among youth and young adults in 15–29-year age group. Chlamydia and gonorrhea infection rates are highest among female teens (1,358.7 and 124.9 per 100,000, respectively). Syphilis infection rates among 20–24-year-old males and females are 1.3 and 1.6 per 100,000, respectively.

Low socioeconomic status also continues to be associated with poorer sexual and reproductive adolescent health. Between 1987 and 1994, the rate of teenage pregnancy rose by more than 20%. The teenage pregnancy rate in the poorest neighborhoods was nearly five times that of teenagers living in affluent areas.

Among Canadian women age 15–44, 86% report using contraception. The vast majority of Canadian women also consult with trained personnel at some point during their pregnancy. Women who do not receive prenatal care are more likely to live in isolated communities, are new to Canada, or experience other marginalized circumstances. Prenatal care is universally available, usually from a doctor (92.4%), nurse (2.9%), or midwife (1.4%). In 1992–1993, physicians performed 98% of deliveries.

Studies indicate that a disproportionate number of low-income women live in areas, both rural and urban, where there are few facilities for sexual and reproductive health services, including abortion services and STD clinics. Lower-income women are also more likely not to have had, or to have delayed preventive procedures such as mammograms and Pap tests.

Health of the Elderly

The population age 65 and over experience activity limitations that are almost three times that of younger age groups. The poorest segments of the senior population tend to experience the highest rates of activity limitation. However, this pattern is most evident among younger seniors (age 65–69). Close to 20% of low-income seniors age 65–69 reported a health-related activity limitation as compared to 12% for middle- and upper-income seniors in the same age bracket. This is particularly pronounced for seniors from First Nations, Inuit, and other minority groups, and for seniors with disabilities, who tend to experience a lifetime of low income, sporadic employment if any, or little opportunity to acquire savings.

Twenty-nine percent of seniors 65–69 years old experience chronic pain. The number increases to 35% for those 75 years and over. The severity of pain increases with age, being 17% for those 65–74 years old and 20% for those 75 and over. Sources of chronic pain include migraine headaches, arthritis, rheumatism, angina, and vascular disease. Among both age groups, women were more likely to report chronic pain than men (34% and 27%, respectively).

Falls and home injuries also impact the health of seniors. For both genders, the injury and mortality rates from accidental falls increase with age. Of deaths resulting from accidental falls in 1993, 35.7% occurred among men and 51.6% among women age 65 and over. Visual impairment affects 9% of the population age 65 and over. Women tend to experience the onset of these and other health-related activity limitations earlier than men. In every age group of the senior population, the rates of activity limitation are higher for women than for men, though the difference is pronounced only in those 75 years and older.

A problem that has only recently come to public attention is elder abuse, a term generally used for the physical, psychosocial, or financial mistreatment of seniors. Approximately 4% of non-institutionalized seniors reported being abused. Financial abuse is the most prevalent type of abuse, affecting 60,000 Canadian elders. Chronic verbal aggression affects approximately 34,000 seniors, and 12,000 seniors experience physical abuse. In the majority of physical abuse cases, the abusers are spouses of the victim.

Health of the Family

In Canada, as in almost all other parts of the industrialized world, marriage rates are declining. The number of marriages peaked in 1972 at around 200,500. Subsequent brief upturns merely moderated the downward trend, which resulted in fewer marriages being registered in 1994 (159,959) than 25 years earlier, although the population had increased by almost 30% during this time. The number of divorces in 1994 was 78,880, with small annual variation since 1989.

In 1994, 80% of the population or 23.5 million Canadians were living in families. While more families are being formed, fewer births are occurring; in 1995, average family size was 3.0. Thirteen percent were single-parent families. Although this percentage has remained steady since 1986, it represents an increase of 4% since 1971. Men headed only 17% of all single-parent families.

Family violence, particularly wife and child abuse, has become a major social issue. In 1993, 10% of women age 18 and older had experienced violence in the preceding year. Women in the 18–24-year age group were significantly more likely to have reported experiencing violence than any other age group.

One-half of Canadian women (51%) have experienced at least one incident of physical or sexual violence since the age of 16. There are some striking geographical variations in the occurrence of violence against women. Women in Newfoundland were significantly less likely than average to have been victims of violence (33%), while women in Alberta and British Columbia were the most likely to have experienced violence (58% and 59%, respectively).

The presumed child abuse mortality rate for infants less than 1 year old between 1985 and 1990 was 2.7 per 100,000 live births. In 1992, 40,000 children were removed from their homes and taken into protective custody by the state. While children of all ages are at risk of child abuse, those 3 years old or younger are most likely to suffer from neglect, and children 12–15 years old from physical abuse. Child abuse is not confined to any one social class or sector of the population, but economic disadvantage is a major contributor to child neglect.

Workers' Health

Substantial proportions of Canadians are in the labor force (63.8%). Unemployment rates are higher for men in all age groups than they are for women. Female labor force participation increased from 36% in 1970, peaking at 59% in 1992, and declining to 57% in 1995. The overall increase in female participation has important health implications, given that women are entering the labor market at unprecedented rates but often maintain the majority of child-rearing responsibilities. A 1991 survey found that 19% of employed mothers in Canada with children under 13 years of age reported experiencing a great deal of tension on a daily basis balancing work, family, and child-care responsibilities. Thirty-two percent of women in dual-income households reported high work–family conflict, compared with 23% of men. Single mothers are more likely to report high levels of work–family tension: 27% of employed single mothers with children under age 13 experience severe work–family tension on a day-to-day basis, compared with 18% of employed married mothers.

The vast majority of men and women in the paid labor force report experiencing considerable satisfaction with their work, even though this figure has declined since 1991. At the individual level, the pace and volume of work, the sense of control, the repetitiveness of tasks, and the range of skills used are all related to health outcomes. Organizational factors such as level and method of remuneration, the quality of benefits, the degree of worker participation in decision-making, and the overall management philosophy toward workers and workers' well-being have all been found to be related to health in the workplace.

Health of the Disabled

The functional health status of Canadians in general age 12 years and over has been assessed based on self reported data on vision, hearing, speech, mobility, use of hands and fingers, memory and thinking, feelings, and pain and discomfort. Data from 1994–1995 indicate that most Canadians either are in perfect health or have fully correctable minor problems, for example, nearsightedness and slight hearing loss.

Close to 5 million Canadians age 12 and over report a disability or limitations on a continuing basis because of a health problem. Conditions causing these limitations include non-arthritic back problems (17%), vision or hearing difficulties (17%), respiratory or digestive conditions (9%), and heart conditions other than coronary heart disease (7%). Thirteen percent are limited in home activities, 5% of students are limited in school activities, and 8% of working persons are limited on the job.

In all age groups, females are somewhat more likely to report an activity limitation at home or at school, while males are more likely to report work limitations. With the exception of school, the rate of limitations decreases sharply with age, until age 65. Over 36% of older seniors report some limitation of activity at home. Among working Canadians, those in the 45–64-year age group are most likely to report work limitations.

Health of the Indigenous People

Unlike the general Canadian population, 1991 data indicate that 31% of First Nations people have some form of disability. Forty-five percent reported problems with mobility, 35% with agility, 35% with hearing difficulties, and 25% with vision. Sixty-five percent of these disabilities were classified as mild and 12% as severe. Among Inuit people, 29% report a disability. Forty-four percent suffer from hearing impairment (a higher proportion than found in other subgroups or in the general Canadian population), 36% report problems with mobility, 26% with agility, and 24% with vision. The literature suggests that the major causes of disabilities in First Nations and Inuit peoples are high accident rates, poor housing and community conditions, alcohol and substance abuse, and chronic conditions such as diabetes.

First Nations and Inuit peoples continue to be among the country's most socially and economically disadvantaged groups. Despite ongoing problems, however, over the past three decades significant improvements have been made in many aspects of First Nations and Inuit health. These advances are due mainly to improved living conditions, better access to good health care, and greater involvement by indigenous communities in the health care system. In 1994–1995, 6% of First Nations dwellings lacked an adequate water supply, and 12% were without adequate sewage disposal, compared with 1986 when over 25% were without adequate water and 33% without adequate sewage disposal.

Analysis by Type of Disease

Communicable Diseases

In Canada, communicable diseases considered to be of particular public health importance are Creutzfeldt-Jacob disease, blood-borne pathogens such as hepatitis B and C, influenza and respiratory syncytial virus, antimicrobial-resistant *Streptococcus pneumoniae,* nosocomial infections, vancomycin-resistant enterococci, methicillin-resistant *Staphylococcus aureus,* waterborne enteric diseases, measles, hantavirus, acute flaccid paralysis, congenital rubella syndrome, and HIV/AIDS.

Vector-Borne Diseases. Data from 1996 indicate that there were 744 new cases of malaria, up from 637 in 1995. All cases of malaria were contracted overseas. There were no reported cases of yellow fever or plague in 1996. There have been no reported cases of yellow fever in Canada for a few decades.

Vaccine-Preventable Diseases. In 1995, there was one vaccine-associated case of polio. In 1996, there was an importation of the wild poliovirus, but no reported cases. There were two reported cases of diphtheria in 1994 (non-travel related) and no cases in 1996. There were six reported cases of tetanus in 1995 and two reported in 1996. In 1996, there were 280 new cases of the mumps and 237 incidents of rubella. The number of new cases of hepatitis B for 1996 was 2,774, down slightly from 3,034 in 1995. It is estimated that 85%–95% of the eligible population in each province or territory has been fully immunized against hepatitis B.

In 1995, there were 2,362 reported cases of measles compared with 503 in 1994. In 1996, the reported number of new measles cases was only 322. In 1996, 11 provinces and territories introduced a routine two-dose measles vaccination program to replace the one-dose strategy. Combined with a massive campaign, the two-dose vaccination programs have resulted in 97% coverage. This has significantly decreased the transmission and incidence of measles.

The introduction in 1992 of *Haemophilias influenzae* type b (Hib) conjugate vaccines for routine immunization of infants has led to a reduction of more than 85% in the reported incidence of Hib disease in Canada. In 1996, there were only 56 reported cases of invasive Hib.

Immunization coverage in First Nations and Inuit communities is below average. Several factors inhibit coverage: the absence of families from their communities for hunting, fishing, berry-picking, or other seasonal employment; the failure of authorities to enforce immunization standards; religious beliefs or philosophical positions; and negative media coverage, particularly regarding pertussis vaccinations.

Cholera. In 1996, there were four reported cases of cholera.

Acute Respiratory Infections. Bacteria and viruses that are carried in or infect the human respiratory tract cause substantial morbidity and mortality among adults and children in Canada. Between April and November, the influenza virus causes an estimated 70,000 hospitalizations and 6,700 deaths per year, especially among the elderly and those with underlying illnesses. Respiratory syncytial virus, a common childhood infection, causes approximately 34 hospitalizations per 1,000 children annually. Recent studies done at Health Canada's Laboratory Center for Disease Control suggest that *Streptococcus pneumoniae,* the most common bacterial cause of pneumonia, affects approximately 15 Canadians per 100,000 per year, especially the very young and the elderly. Similar research has identified rates of disease due to other respiratory tract pathogens, such as group A streptococci (approximately 3.5 cases per 100,000 people per year) and *Neisseria meningitidis,* a common cause of meningitis (approximately one case per 100,000 people per year).

Rabies. There have been no reported cases of human rabies for at least a decade.

AIDS and Other STDs. Since the first diagnosed case of AIDS in 1979, the total number of cases has risen steadily, cumulating in a total of 10,689 cases in 1994. In 1996, there were only 558 new cases of AIDS, representing a decrease from 1,266 in 1995. In 1995, Canada's rate of AIDS cases was 4.0 per 100,000.

In Canada, most persons with AIDS have been exposed to the human immunodeficiency virus (HIV) through sexual contact with infected individuals; the remainder have been infected from using contaminated needles or through the use of blood products and blood transfusions from donors infected with the virus. Only 6% of all reported AIDS cases are among women, and 99% of AIDS cases are in the adult population. The majority of reported cases (77%) occur in homosexual and bisexual men.

The highest rate of infection is in the age group 30–39 years old, followed by the age groups 40–49 years old, and 20–29 years old. These age differences are not believed to reflect current sexual practices, but rather the lengthy incubation period for HIV. Ontario, Quebec, and British Columbia have the largest number of AIDS cases and deaths. The concentration of AIDS in these provinces exceeds their respective proportion of the population.

As of 1996, chlamydia was the most common STD, whereas five years earlier gonococcal infection was the most frequently reported STD. In 1996, there were 24,476 reported cases of chlamydia, down from 37,061 in 1995. In 1996, there were 3,914 gonococcal infections, which represents over a 10-fold drop in the number of cases reported since 1981. In 1996, there was one reported case of congenital syphilis, 14 reported cases of early latent syphilis, 45 reported cases of early symptomatic syphilis, and 248 cases of other syphilis. Across all ages, men are more likely than women to be infected with gonorrhea or syphilis, but women are three times more likely than men to contract chlamydia.

Tuberculosis and Leprosy. In 1994, there were 2,074 reported cases of tuberculosis. In children under 4 years of age, there were 91 reported cases of tuberculosis. For the population as a whole, there were 110 reported deaths attributable to tuberculosis (69 male and 41 female). In 1995, the incidence of tuberculosis decreased to 1,930. The majority of cases of active tuberculosis now being reported in Canada occur among those who have come from other countries where the disease is more prevalent.

The total number of reported cases of active tuberculosis among First Nations Canadians has remained constant in the recent past. In 1980 there were 390 reported cases, while in 1995 there were 343 reported cases. These totals constituted 14% and 18% of all reported cases in Canada for 1980 and 1995, respectively.

In 1996, there were five reported cases of leprosy.

Noncommunicable Diseases and Other Health-Related Problems

Nutritional Diseases and Diseases of Metabolism. Protein-energy malnutrition in children under 5 years old is not generally considered to be a problem in Canada. All salt marketed for table or general household use must be iodized and less than 5% of school-age children have goiter. As a result of fortification programs, the general Canadian population does not suffer from vitamin A deficiency. However, food intake studies since 1991 have identified segments of the First Nations population as being at risk for low intake of vitamin A. Calcium intake is inadequate in some population groups. In addition, folic acid is a micronutrient for which intakes, particularly in women, may not always meet requirements when standard Canadian diets are consumed. Recently, steps have been taken to increase the fortification of flour and other grain products with folic acid to assist in reducing the risk of neural tube birth defects, such as spina bifida.

Iron deficiency anemia and its impact on growth and development remains a problem, especially in certain subgroups of women. Data indicate that iron intakes are low in women 18–49 years of age in Nova Scotia and Quebec. Also, infants in some regions of Canada and among some low-income families are at risk for iron deficiency in later life due to the use of whole cow's milk in infant feeding. Breast-feeding, an important part of infant nutrition, is quite high in mothers of children under 2 years old; 75.3% of children have been or are being breast-fed.

Being overweight is generally more prevalent in Canada's eastern provinces, ranging from 61% in Newfoundland to 44% in British Columbia. Men are more likely to be overweight than women: 57% of Canadian men are at increased risk of cardiovascular disease due to being overweight, compared to 40% of women.

While one out of every two Canadians age 20–69 is at a healthy weight, approximately 48% of Canadians have a body mass index of 25 or more, which puts them at risk of cardiovascular disease and other conditions such as high blood pressure and diabetes. A significant proportion of the population was overweight to the point of possible health risk (17%) and probable health risk (32%). At the other end of the spectrum, close to one-tenth (9%) of the population is underweight. More women (15%) than men (5%) are likely to experience health problems associated with being underweight.

Diabetes has been diagnosed in 1.5 million Canadians. Approximately 60,000 Canadians are diagnosed with diabetes every year. Ten percent of all people with diabetes have Type I diabetes and the remaining 90% are diagnosed with Type 2 diabetes. Eighty percent of people with Type 2 diabetes are overweight, and 5% of women will develop diabetes during pregnancy. Canadian men and women are about equally likely to report having diabetes and the overall prevalence is generally low (4% for women, and 5% for men). Diabetes is at least two to three times higher among First Nations Canadians than the rest of the population.

Cardiovascular Diseases. Death rates from all major categories of cardiovascular diseases have been declining at a rate of about 2% per year in Canada since the mid-1960s. Nevertheless, cardiovascular disease remains a major cause of death, disability, and illness in the country. In 1994, cardiovascular disease accounted for 38% of all deaths. Men experience almost twice the death rates of women in all categories of cardiovascular disease, except stroke, for which the death rates are approximately equal for all ages.

First Nations populations in Canada had, until recent decades, experienced much lower cardiovascular disease death rates than the general population. Yet during the past decade, First Nations men have experienced a death rate for ischemic heart disease similar to that of the general male Canadian population. The age-standardized death rate from stroke for the First Nations population is decreasing as is the relative difference between their death rates and those of the general Canadian population. First Nations women experience higher death rates than the general Canadian female population for both ischemic heart disease and stroke. During the past decade, the difference between First Nations women and the general population with respect to stroke has decreased noticeably, whereas that for ischemic heart disease has remained the same. The higher prevalence of risk factors for cardiovascular diseases such as high blood pressure, diabetes, obesity, and smoking may partially account for this trend.

The prevalence of one or more major modifiable risk factors for cardiovascular disease is uniformly high among men and women ages 18–74 (66% and 62%, respectively). There are no marked gender differences in the overall prevalence of regular smoking. About one-quarter of Canadian men and women age 18–74 smoke on a regular basis. High blood pressure is more prevalent among Canadian men than women; 19% of men have high blood pressure and 13% of women. More than 20% of adults are at increased risk of cardiovascular disease due to elevated blood cholesterol; differences in levels between men and women are not significant. Education level is strongly linked to risk-factor prevalence. Canadians with 11 years of education or less are much more likely to have at least one of the major risk factors for cardiovascular disease than those with more than 11 years of education (76% as compared with 59%).

Malignant Tumors. Trends in the incidence and mortality for all forms of cancer combined have been relatively stable since the mid-1980s, although the number of new cases and deaths continues to rise because of the aging population. In

1995, 125,400 new cases of cancer were diagnosed and an estimated 61,500 Canadians died from cancer in that year. Rising rates of lung cancer and the aging of the population have offset reductions in death rates for many types of cancer, such as leukemia and colorectal cancer. Cancer in its many forms was the second leading cause of death in 1994 and accounted for over 891,000 years of potential life lost. Cancers, including lung and prostate cancer, account for 28.3% of total deaths in men and 27% in women. In 1997, there will be an estimated 60,700 deaths from cancer, an increase of 25% since 1987.

Accidents and Violence. In 1993, accidents, poisoning, and violence accounted for 8% of hospitalizations. The death rate from injuries is higher among First Nations people than in the general Canadian population. However, injury death rates have decreased substantially since 1979, particularly among men. Over the 1990–1994 period, the main causes of death from injury among First Nations people, were, in order of importance, motor vehicle accidents, suicide, homicide, and drowning.

Traffic accidents are one of the leading causes of death among Canadian youth. Teenagers and 20–24-year-olds are twice as likely to be injured or killed in accidents than any other age group. Although traffic accidents are caused by many factors, including driver error, recklessness, and poor road conditions, the combination of drinking and driving is one of the key causes in many serious car accidents each year.

Years of potential life lost as a result of traffic accidents are approximately three times greater for males than for females. There are some important geographical variations in traffic accident casualties. Although Ontario and Quebec account for the most deaths and injuries due to motor vehicle accidents, Quebec is underrepresented in injuries in terms of its current proportion of the population, and Ontario is underrepresented in deaths. In contrast, there is an overrepresentation of traffic accident deaths in Prince Edward Island, Alberta, and British Columbia. British Columbia also has a disproportionate number of injuries due to road user collisions. Quebec and Alberta are distinguished from other provinces by the high proportion of motor vehicle collisions that result in death.

Alcohol, Tobacco, and Drug Use. Aside from caffeine, the most commonly consumed psychoactive drug is alcohol. Nevertheless, alcohol consumption continues to decline: 72.3% of Canadians reported drinking (defined as the consumption of at least one drink each month) in 1994 compared to 79% in 1990. A survey on alcohol and other drugs found that only 5% of Canadians drank on a daily basis. Groups considered to be at particular risk from harm associated with alcohol and other drugs include women, youth, seniors, First Nations and Inuit peoples, and driving-while-impaired offenders. First Nations youths are at two to six times greater risk for alcohol-related problems than their counterparts in other segments of the Canadian population.

There are large geographic variations in alcohol consumption, with Prince Edward Island and New Brunswick both well below the average in terms of current drinking prevalence, and Quebec and British Columbia above average.

Nicotine is the third most commonly used psychoactive drug. In 1995, 27% of Canadians age 15 and older reported smoking on a regular basis, a decrease of close to 5% since 1989 (31.9%). The average Canadian smoker age 15 and over smoked an average of 20.5 cigarettes per day. In general, more males than females smoke (28.4% and 25.6%, respectively). Rates of use are highest among 20–24-year-olds (37%) and lowest for adults over 65 (14%). There are wide variations between the provinces in the prevalence of regular smoking, ranging from a high of 33.6% in Quebec to a low of 22.4% in Ontario. The majority of First Nations Canadians (57%) smoke; half of those who smoke do so daily.

One in five First Nations youth has used solvents. One-third of all users are under 15 and more than half began to use solvents before the age of 11.

Oral Health. In 1990, 75% of Canadians had visited a dentist in the previous 12 months. From 1993 to 1995, the decayed, filled, missing teeth (DFMT) index was 2.1 for 12-year-olds in the general population. The DFMT index for First Nations children was 4.4.

Approximately 40% of the population receives fluoridated drinking water. Since 1986, there has been little change in the number of cities in Canada who have implemented programs to fluoridate their water. Nearly 72% of the population is served by treated water supplies, and, of that population, 53.7% receives artificially fluoridated water. Fluoride levels in municipal water supply are controlled and monitored by provincial, territorial, and municipal governments.

Natural Disasters. In May 1997, severe flooding caused the evacuation of 28,000 residents in the province of Manitoba. Although the waters damaged 2,500 homes and the cost of the flood is estimated to be close to Can$ 200 million, well-coordinated disaster relief efforts prevented the loss of life.

RESPONSE OF THE HEALTH SYSTEM

The national principles of the health care system are set out in the Canada Health Act. These principles include public administration on a nonprofit basis, comprehensive service, universal population coverage, accessibility to services, and portability of benefits. Canada's taxpayer-financed, comprehensive health insurance system covers medically necessary hospital, inpatient, outpatient, and physician services for all residents. No resident may be discriminated against on the basis of such factors as income, age, geographic location, or health status.

National Health Plans and Policies

What has come to be known as "Medicare" comprises 12 interlinked health plans administered by the provinces and territories, which have constitutional authority for health care. Medicare's two major components are the Hospital Insurance Program and the Medical Care Program. The Hospital Insurance and Diagnostic Services Act of 1957 led to all provinces and territories providing their residents with comprehensive coverage for hospital care by 1961. This was followed by the federal Medical Care Act in 1968, and by 1972, all provincial and territorial health care plans insured physician services. The 1984 Canada Health Act consolidated the previous legislation on hospital and medical care insurance and clarified the broad national standards that provincial plans must meet to qualify for federal funding.

Since the release of the Lalonde report ("A New Perspective on the Health of Canadians") in 1974, followed by the Ottawa Charter in 1986, Canada has broadened its understanding of the factors that contribute to health and has taken action on a number of fronts. Government policies focus on lifestyle choices (e.g., diet, exercise, and smoking) as well as on public policy (e.g., seat-belt legislation). In addition, there is an awareness of the social dimension of health, beyond factors that are within the immediate control of individuals, professionals, and communities.

In October 1994, the federal government launched the National Forum on Health. The Forum's mandate was to advise the federal government on ways to improve the health system and the health of Canada's people. In 1997, after numerous public consultations, the Forum released its final report, "Canada Health Action: Building on the Legacy." The Forum emphasized that strategies to improve population health status must address a broad range of health determinants: social and economic environments, physical environments, personal health practices, individual capacities and coping skills, as well as the availability of health services.

In 1997, the government announced several initiatives to improve population health. These include the creation of a Health Transition Fund, which will provide Can$ 150 million over three years to support provincial and territorial projects and innovative approaches to modernize the health care system. The Fund will consider specific projects such as nationally insured pharmaceutical and home care services, primary care, preventive health, and evidence-based decision-making. The Canadian Health Information System aims to strengthen Canada's health surveillance network and establish a popula-

tion health information database and a First Nations health information system. The Community Action Plan for Children and the Canada Prenatal Nutrition Program build on constructive partnerships with provinces, territories, and stakeholders to provide community-based support that families at risk need to help ensure the health of their children. The Canada Foundation for Innovation will help generate funding for innovative and progressive research in various sectors, including health. Six Networks of Centers of Excellence oriented toward health science (i.e., the Canadian Bacterial Diseases Network, the Canadian Genetic Diseases Network, the Health Evidence Application and Linkage Network, the Respiratory Health Network, the NeuroScience Network, and the Protein Engineering Network) will receive annual funding of close to Can$ 50 million to support the work of health researchers.

In August 1995, the federal government announced a new policy on the inherent right of self-government of First Nations and Inuit peoples. Under this policy, First Nations and Inuit governments and institutions will acquire the jurisdiction or authority to act in a number of areas, including health. At present, consensus between the federal government and First Nations peoples has not been reached with respect to substance of the policy or the implementation process.

Organization of the Health Sector

Institutional Organization

Canada's health care system relies extensively on primary care physicians (e.g., family physicians and general practitioners), who account for about 60% of all active physicians in Canada. They are usually the initial points of contact with the formal health care system and control access to most specialists, many allied health providers, hospital admission, diagnostic testing, and prescription drug therapy.

Doctors are not employed by the government. Rather, most physicians are private practitioners who work in independent or group practices and enjoy a high degree of autonomy. Some doctors work in community health centers, hospital-based group practices or work in affiliation with hospital outpatient departments. Private practitioners are generally paid on a fee-for-service basis and submit their service claims directly to the provincial insurance plan for payment.

In most instances, when Canadians need medical care they go to a physician or clinic of their choice and present the health insurance card issued to all eligible residents of a province. Canadians do not pay directly for insured hospital and physician services, nor are they required to fill out forms for insured services. There are no deductibles, copayments, or dollar limits on coverage for insured services.

A number of allied health care professionals are also involved in primary health care. Dentists work independently of the health care system, except where in-hospital dental surgery is required. While nurses are generally employed in the hospital sector, they also provide support for primary services, typically in conjunction with private practices. Pharmacists dispense prescribed medicines and drug preparations as well as providing information on prescribed drugs or assisting in the purchase of non-prescription drugs.

Specialized ambulatory physician care is provided on much the same basis as general practitioner care. Specialists control access to other physicians and allied providers, admissions to hospitals, and prescribe necessary diagnostic testing, treatment, and prescription drug therapy.

Over 95% of Canadian hospitals are operated as nonprofit entities run by community boards of trustees, voluntary organizations, or municipalities. Hospitals have control of day-to-day resources provided that they stay within the operating budgets established by regional or provincial health authorities. Hospitals are primarily accountable to the communities they serve, not to the provincial bureaucracy. For-profit hospital operations account for less than 5% of the total number of hospitals and are predominantly long-term care facilities or specialized services such as addiction centers.

In addition to insured hospital and physician services, provinces and territories also provide coverage for health services that remain outside the national health insurance framework for certain groups of the population. These supplementary health benefits often include prescription drugs, dental and vision care, services of allied health professionals such as podiatrists and chiropractors, and aids to independent living.

Although the provinces and territories do provide some additional benefits, supplementary health services are largely privately financed. The individual's out-of-pocket expenses may depend on income or ability to pay. Individuals and families can acquire private insurance or may benefit from an employment-based group insurance plan to offset some portion of the expense of supplementary health services. Under most provincial laws, private insurers are restricted from offering coverage that duplicates governmental programs, but they can compete in the supplementary benefits market.

Since the federal, provincial, and territorial governments share responsibility for health, a structure that allows for consultation and collaboration among them has been established. It comprises the Conference of Ministers of Health, the Conference of Deputy Ministers of Health, several federal/provincial/territorial advisory committees, and numerous subcommittees and working groups established to deal with subjects requiring more detailed study. An example is the "Report on the Health of Canadians" prepared in 1996 by the Federal, Provincial, and Territorial Advisory Committee

on Population Health. The Report helped policymakers to measure Canada's progress in achieving better population health and to identify actions that can be taken to make continued improvements.

In most provinces and territories, the administration and payment for health services operate either from within the Ministry of Health or through a separate agency closely linked to the Ministry. These health insurance plans administer payment to service providers on behalf of provincial residents. The operation of these plans must respect the principles of the Canada Health Act in order for the province to qualify for full federal health funding transfers. The Minister of Health in each province or territory is politically accountable for the operation of the health care system in his or her jurisdiction.

The provinces and territories are responsible for providing hospital and physician services to all residents, including First Nations peoples, through provincial insurance plans. The federal government provides treatment and public health services in remote First Nations communities and public services to other First Nations people though the Medical Services Branch of the federal Department of Health. The Medical Services Branch also provides or pays for non-insured health benefits for on- and off-reserve First Nations and Inuit peoples. The Medical Services Branch spends close to Can$ 976 million annually on the development and delivery of health services to First Nations and Inuit peoples. At present, the federal government is working in partnership with First Nations communities to promote good health and to assist them in assuming control of their own health programs.

Provincial, regional, and municipal health authorities also manage other health services such as safe water provision and sewage treatment, operate public health programs such as communicable disease surveillance and health education, provide inspection of food-service establishments, offer home and hospital services to mothers and newborns, and provide school health services such as immunization clinics and preventive care dental clinics.

At the federal level, the Department of Health is the principal agency concerned with health matters. The Department undertakes a broad leadership role in fostering essential national relationships by establishing active health system partnerships with the provinces and territories, supporting initiatives to redress health inequalities, improving knowledge management and research dissemination, and creating innovative and effective health programs to advance the health of Canadians.

The federal Minister of Health is politically responsible for ensuring that provinces abide by the criteria contained in the Canada Health Act. In this respect, the Department of Health regulates monetary transfers to the provinces, which assist in the financing of insured health services.

Organization of Health Regulatory Activities

The Department of Health provides occupational health, environmental health, and emergency health services within its areas of jurisdiction. It is also responsible for regulatory functions to safeguard the quality and safety of foods, cosmetics, pesticides, drinking water, and air quality, as well as the safety and effectiveness of drugs and medical devices. The Department is charged with monitoring disease incidence, assessing risks, providing disease control services, providing national epidemiological and laboratory surveillance of HIV/AIDS, and identifying and assessing environmental hazards.

Monitoring of hospitals is undertaken at many levels. Provinces typically control facilities by monitoring budgets and expenditures. The Royal College of Physicians and Surgeons regularly evaluates hospitals for inclusion in residency training programs. Allied professions, such as physiotherapists, assess individual hospital programs and departments as candidates for internships. The quality of Canadian hospitals is monitored by the Canadian Council for Health Facility Accreditation. The accreditation process requires hospitals to meet minimum standards to maintain their status. Failure to meet these standards may lead to a ratings change, loss of teaching hospital status, or in some cases, a reduction in funding.

In March 1996, the federal government separated responsibility for food inspection activities from food safety initiatives by creating the Canadian Food Inspection Agency. Although the traditional inspection and compliance activities performed by the Health Protection Branch of the Department of Health have been transferred to the Inspection Agency, the Department of Health retains its jurisdiction over food safety and nutritional value of the Canadian food supply. In particular, the Health Protection Branch continues to direct research, risk assessment, and standards setting in the area of food safety. It also evaluates the safety of industry submissions in regard to the use of food and food-related products, for example, veterinary drugs, food additives, and foods derived from biotechnology. Coordinating bodies at the federal level include intersectoral committees on food regulation, food inspection, and food safety in addition to committees of the Canadian Agricultural Research Council.

In Canada, only physicians and dentists can prescribe drugs. Pharmacists who work in private pharmacies dispense prescription medicines. The Health Protection Branch of the Department of Health, which ensures that drugs are safe and efficacious before they are allowed on the Canadian market, conducts the drug approval process at the federal level. All therapeutic products are regulated under the Food and Drugs Act and Narcotics Control Act, which prohibit the importation for sale of any drug that would be in violation of provisions of the Act. As of 1997, the Department of Health requires that an establishment license be issued annually to reflect that a manufacturer or distributor meets the appropriate standard, thereby ensuring uniform requirements for fabricating, packaging, import, distribution, or testing drugs in Canada.

The manufacturer prices of patented medicines are regulated by the Patented Medicine Pricing Review Board, a federal agency established in 1987 when the length of effective patent protection for pharmaceuticals was extended to 20 years. In 1997, the federal government announced its intention to consider broadening the mandate of the Review Board to include non-patented drugs.

The Health Protection Branch of the Department of Health concerns itself with chemical and radiological hazards in the environment, the safety and effectiveness of medical devices, and radiation hazards associated with drugs and devices sold in Canada.

The Canadian Environmental Assessment Act was approved in 1995 and is administered by the Canadian Environmental Assessment Agency. The Act requires federal departments and agencies to assess the environmental implications of all their projects. Intersectoral aspects of the Act provide the means to integrate environmental, health, and economic factors as well as public concerns into the government decision-making process. Jointly administered at the federal level by the Departments of Health and the Environment, the Act evaluates the potential health risks of environmental contaminants, regulates the entry into Canada of new materials that may damage health and the environment, and assesses the health risks of new substances, including those created through biotechnology.

Overall, purchases of expensive technologies such as diagnostic tools are regulated through provincial control of capital expenditures. Assessments to ensure the quality and effectiveness of these technologies are undertaken at the federal level by the Canadian Coordinating Office for Health Technology Assessment and at the provincial level by several similar assessment agencies.

Health Services and Resources

Organization of Services for Care of the Population

Health Promotion. As part of its national mandate, the Department of Health focuses on the promotion of public health through a variety of programs. The Child Development Initiative (formerly Brighter Futures) aims to improve the well-being of Canada's children. Activities have included work to control solvent abuse in First Nations and Inuit communities and the development of a national childhood cancer information system. Aboriginal Head Start is an early intervention initiative to address the needs of First Nations children living in urban centers and large northern communities.

Early intervention typically includes parental involvement, early childhood education, nutrition education, and social services for children and families. The Canada Prenatal Nutrition Program enables community groups to develop and deliver comprehensive prenatal programs to pregnant women who are at risk of having an unhealthy baby due to poor health and nutrition of the mother.

The Student Leadership Development program focuses on developing leadership skills of youth at the elementary and secondary school levels, through their participation in planning and running of intramural physical activities. The Canadian Active Living Challenge is primarily a school-based program that supports more participation in physical activity and a developmental learning process for active living. Canada's "Guide to Healthy Physical Activity" is being developed to provide standard recommendations on physical activity and will complement Canada's "Food Guide." A Guide supplement is also being developed that will highlight special considerations for older Canadians on integrating physical activity into their daily lives.

Violence in families is a serious social problem that negatively impacts mostly women, children, and seniors. The Department of Health, through the Family Violence Prevention Division leads multi-departmental federal efforts to address the problem.

There are 12 federal agencies addressing HIV/AIDS issues. Eleven of these are within the Department of Health. Federal action in the areas of education and prevention, research, community action, care, treatment and support, coordination, and international initiatives are conducted in an environment that encourages partnerships, creates supportive social environments and enhances the ability of persons infected and affected by HIV/AIDS to participate in health care decisions.

The Tobacco Demand Reduction Strategy aims at reducing the incidence of smoking. Funded by a health promotion surtax on tobacco manufacturing profits, the strategy includes a comprehensive public education and awareness component as well as community action initiatives. The Health in Perspective program focuses on smoking prevention and cessation for adolescent females aged 12–15 years of age.

Food Consumption Surveys are carried out in order to assess the potential risks to health resulting from the presence of chemical contaminants or inadequate quantities of nutrients in food.

The St. Lawrence Vision 2000 Knowledge Development Fund, jointly funded by the Department of Health and the Fonds de la Recherche en Santé du Québec, finances research projects to study the direct impacts on human health of contamination in the St. Lawrence River, Canada's major waterway.

Housing. In 1996, the government introduced a new housing policy that provides additional resources and emphasizes community control and flexibility in design, labor requirements, and partnerships with the private sector. The federal government's First Nations and Inuit housing policy is aimed at improving living conditions on reserve by addressing the basic shelter needs of residents. The government provides capital subsidies and loan guarantees to First Nations communities and individuals to help build, buy, and renovate houses on reserves, and allocates operating funds for housing-related administration, training, and technical assistance. First Nations peoples themselves directly administer this program.

Water Supply and Sanitation. In Canada, approximately 99% of the population has safe water. The majority (86%) is served by central systems and 14% by individual systems. Approximately 95% of the population also has satisfactory excreta disposal facilities. The federal and provincial governments recently completed a $Can 6 billion infrastructure upgrading program and are updating drinking water, recreational water, and ambient water quality guidelines.

The federal government provides funding for First Nations and Inuit peoples to acquire, construct, operate, and maintain such basic community facilities as water, electrical and sewage services, schools, roads, community buildings, and fire protection facilities. Over 90% of the capital program budget is managed directly by communities themselves. In 1995 and 1996, 95% of dwellings in First Nations and Inuit communities had water service and 90% had sewage services as compared to 75% and 67%, respectively, in 1985 and 1986.

Organization and Operation of Personal Health Care Services

Canada's hospitals, which are primarily nonprofit and run by community boards or trustees, are highly autonomous of the federal and provincial governments, with the provincial role limited to broad planning functions, funding, and capital budgeting. Currently, the only hospitals directly run by provinces tend to be psychiatric institutions; however, many of the provinces are in the process of divesting themselves of these institutions. The federal government operates a number of hospitals for the military, provides some facilities for First Nations and Inuit peoples, and until recently administered a number of veterans' hospitals.

Hospitals are typically organized as general or acute care facilities, community or secondary care, and long-term or chronic care. Depending on affiliation with a medical school, any of these hospitals may also be classified as a teaching hospital. In the largest cities, some institutions have become highly specialized, with hospitals focused on arthritis care, orthopedics, and children's and women's health. As part of the restructuring of the health system, many highly specialized services are being consolidated into single urban centers that serve an entire province or region.

Public health services are typically funded and provided separately from the main components of health care, and are administered through local or regional health units. They range from broad immunization programs, such as the provision of second-dose measles immunizations, to health programs that educate identified at-risk groups. They provide child and maternal health counseling programs, reproductive health services, and are at the forefront of the effort to control the spread of AIDS. In addition, most public health services coordinate or directly provide personal and home care services such as home nursing care. As such, public health services are an integral part of community care.

Community care services are organized at two levels: institutional-based care and home-based care. Community institutional care is largely focused on the provision of long-term and chronic care, ranging from residential care facilities that provide only limited health services, to intensive chronic care facilities. Increasingly, the majority of patients in these institutions are the frail elderly. Institutional long-term care health services are typically paid for by the provincial government, while accommodation costs (room and board) are largely the responsibility of the individual.

Inputs for Health

Pharmaceuticals are a key component of the Canadian health care system. Drugs include prescription medicines, non-prescription medicines, and personal health supplies. Prescription medicines are usually prescribed by physicians, dispensed by pharmacists, and are received either in a hospital or in the community. Non-prescription medicines, such as cough and cold remedies, are available without prescription through retail outlets. Personal health supplies include items such as oral hygiene products and home diagnostics kits and are also available through retail outlets.

Except for medicines received while in institutional care, drugs are not covered by the Canada Health Act. In 1995, it is estimated that 88% of Canadians had coverage for prescription medicines: 62% were covered under private plans, 19% under provincial plans, and 7% were covered under both. Of the 12% of the population without any coverage, more than half were employees and their dependents whose employers did not provide a supplementary drug benefit plan. For the most part, the consumer pays for non-prescription medicines and personal health supplies out-of-pocket.

Drug expenditure estimates indicate that in 1996, Canada spent Can\$ 10.8 billion on drugs. This estimate encompasses all drug spending in the health care system, including drugs in hospitals and other institutions, drugs in the offices of private practitioners, and public health spending on drugs such as vaccines. Without the controls of a single-payer system, pharmaceuticals have become the fastest growing component of national health care expenditures.

Both public and private sector payers are implementing measures to contain the costs of pharmaceutical benefits. These measures include the use of restrictive formularies with emphasis on the use of generic products and use of pharmaco-economic studies to demonstrate the cost-effectiveness of products as a prerequisite for listing on the formulary. Other measures include increasing deductibles and copayments, restricting eligibility for coverage, capping benefits, and improving information to guide appropriate prescribing. The federal and provincial governments are exploring the possibility of a single-payer pharmaceutical program.

Medical equipment is provided both on a public and private basis. While some equipment is available through hospital or community-based programs, a large proportion of medical equipment is funded by the private sector, either out-of-pocket or through private insurance. Expensive personal equipment such as wheelchairs are often subsidized by service organizations.

Human Resources

Employment in health services represents an increasing portion of total employment in Canada. In 1995, health services employment (723,000 employees in health and medicine, or 244.21 per 10,000) represented close to 5.5% of total employment. From 1975 to 1995, total health personnel employment increased by over 16.4%. Nurses account for almost half of all health personnel (232,869 or 78.66 nurses per 10,000). The number of physicians has also increased significantly from 44,200 in 1975 to 55,006 or 18.58 physicians per 10,000 in 1995. In 1995, there were 22,197 pharmacists (7.50 per 10,000 population) and 15,636 dentists (5.28 per 10,000 population).

Today, there is a general over-supply of physicians in Canada, particularly in urban areas. At the same time, there is a chronic shortage of physicians in rural and remote areas. Some jurisdictions have also found that the ratio of general practitioners to specialists is unacceptable. The problems encountered with physician supply led to the development of a national action plan on physician resources. Provinces have introduced human resource plans to control medical school enrollment, the number of practicing physicians, and the number of foreign medical students and doctors. In addition, many provinces are developing programs to induce physicians to work in under-serviced areas or sectors.

The distribution of nurses is almost entirely dependent on the dispersion of hospitals and clinics. As such, there is a reasonably adequate distribution of nurses in most of the country, although many remote areas remain under-serviced. The supply of nurses is also tempered by downsizing in the acute care sector.

The majority of health care professionals in Canada require some degree of university training. Physicians typically have the longest training programs, which include undergraduate and graduate training, as well as several years of practical instruction. Individuals who specialize undergo even longer periods of formal training. Nurses, physiotherapists, pharmacists, chiropractors, and other allied health professionals require university degrees.

Nurse practitioner and midwifery programs have found renewed support across the country. Two new programs to prepare nurse practitioners were established, and in 1993 a baccalaureate midwifery program was introduced in the province of Ontario. Training for rehabilitation assistants, who work under the supervision of occupation and physical therapists, is available in most provinces.

Utilization of multi-skilled workers in health services has increased as has the general trend toward recognition of alternative health providers. In this regard, in May 1997, the Minister of Health announced that an advisory panel will be established to provide a regulatory framework for herbal remedies, including product licensing, establishment licensing, cost recovery, and international harmonization.

Research and Technology

The Department of Health offers coordination and policy advice on health and health care delivery based on research. The National Health Research and Development Program funds strategic, population-based, applied health research to support departmental policy and program needs.

During 1996, significant developments occurred in the area of health research in Canada. An endowment of Can$ 65 million was made to support health services research, and the Canadian Health Services Research Foundation was created to administer the endowment and to raise additional funds. The Foundation supports peer-reviewed research into health services and is responsible for supporting the dissemination and uptake of the resulting research evidence.

The Medical Research Council of Canada has pursued several private and publicly financed endeavors to facilitate technology transfer. The Council was instrumental in creating the Canadian Medical Discoveries Fund, a labor-sponsored venture capital fund that has raised Can$ 200 million to commercialize promising medical science developments. The Council also administers the health component of the Networks of Centers of Excellence Program, which encourages technology transfer by linking researchers and the busi-

ness community. The program has succeeded in attracting private sector capital to support the development of research in the health sector, such as, for example, the NeuroScience Partners Funds.

The Canadian Coordinating Office for Health Technology Assessment was created by the federal, provincial, and territorial governments in 1989 to provide information on emerging and existing health care technologies to decision-makers and to facilitate the exchange and coordination of information on health technologies. The Office has developed a library that assists in the identification, collection, and dissemination of information on medical technologies, and publishes and disseminates health technology assessment information. Two areas of focus are drug assessment (therapeutic effectiveness and economic impact) and assistive or home-use devices.

Expenditures and Sectoral Financing

In 1996, Canada spent an estimated Can$ 75,224 million on health care, representing 9.5% of the gross domestic product and a real per capita total health expenditure of Can$ 2,510. Public expenditures accounted for about 70% of total national health care spending. Federal transfers accounted for 22% of the expenditures; disbursements by the federal government for health care services for special groups such as First Nations and Inuit peoples, Armed Forces personnel and veterans, and expenditures for health research, health promotion, and health protection accounted for 4%; provincial expenditures made for those insured accounted for 44%; and private funds accounted for 30%. One of the components that contributes heavily to the cost of health care is the aging of the population. In 1996, health expenditures for the population 65 years and older represented almost 40% of the total spent.

Until 1995–1996, federal transfers to provinces and territories included both cash and tax transfers for the health portion of the Established Programs Financing and cash payments under the Canada Assistance Plan, as well as payments made by the Department of Indian and Northern Affairs for medical and hospital insurance plans of First Nations people. Beginning in April 1996, federal transfers to provincial and territorial governments for their health, post-secondary education, and social assistance/social services programs were combined into the Canada Health and Social Transfer, which is a single block transfer of cash and tax points. The need to contain costs in the health system has resulted in an increase of 13% in total health expenditures between 1991 and 1996, compared with a 26% increase between 1988 and 1991. Table 3 provides a breakdown of national and private sector health expenditures by category.

TABLE 3
Total national and private sector health expenditures by category, Canada, 1994 and 1996 (in billions of Canadian dollars).

Category	Total national health expenditure (1996)	Private sector health expenditure (1994)
Institutional and related services		
Hospitals	25.7	2.8
Other institutions[a]	7.5	2.1
Professional services		
Physicians	10.9	0.1
Other professionals	6.6	5.3
Drugs	10.8	6.2
Other health expenditures	13.7[b]	3.8[c]

[a] "Other institutions" refers to residential care facilities and includes homes for the aged, physically and mentally disabled, psychiatrically disabled, and clients with alcohol and drug problems.

[b] Includes public health expenditures, for example, public measures to prevent the spread of communicable diseases, food and drug safety, health inspections and health promotion activities (Can$ 3.8 billion), and capital expenditures (Can$ 1.9 billion).

[c] Includes capital expenditures (Can$ 0.5 billion).

External Technical and Financial Cooperation

Canada's external technical and financial cooperation in health includes ongoing cooperation with other countries through institutions such as the World Bank, the World Health Organization, the Pan American Health Organization, and the Organization for Economic Cooperation and Development. Canadian health regulators have initiated efforts to encourage harmonization of regulations, standards, and labeling requirements related to foods, pharmaceuticals, and medical devices within trading blocs and between countries.

The Canadian International Development Agency (CIDA) is a federal agency responsible for managing approximately 80% of Canada's Official Development Assistance (ODA). CIDA pursues the following programming priorities: basic human needs; women in development; infrastructure services; human rights; democracy and good governance; private sector development; and environment.

CIDA's "Strategy for Health" was launched in 1996. This document presents a comprehensive and integrated approach to health and development. Top priorities are to strengthen national health systems and improve women's health and reproductive health. Other priority objectives include improving children's health; decreasing malnutrition and eliminating micronutrient deficiencies; prevention and control of major pandemics that cause more than 1 million deaths per year (HIV/AIDS, tuberculosis, tobacco use, malaria, trauma, and violence); and support for the introduction of appropriate technologies and special initiatives.

CIDA's development activities in Latin America and the Caribbean are provided through three main delivery channels: (1) the partnership program, which enables CIDA to provide funding in support of health projects in developing countries undertaken by Canadian nongovernmental organizations, institutions such as universities and colleges, professional associations, and private firms; (2) the multilateral program, which supports multilateral development approaches through international organizations such as United Nations agencies, the Commonwealth, and international financial institutions; and (3) the bilateral program, which enables Canada to support projects through consultation and cooperation with recipient country partners.

The bilateral program in the Americas underscores CIDA's principles of equity for sustainable development. CIDA's Americas branch is active in supporting programming in health and supports efforts through various mechanisms. In Bolivia, for example, a small contribution is helping UNICEF to eliminate iodine deficiency disorders. Through UNICEF's Safe Motherhood and Reproductive Health project, CIDA funds supported government establishment of a maternity and childhood insurance program that has increased access to public health services. The "Support to Health Sector Reform in Bolivia" project was developed with Canadian partners to enhance national health policy formulation and implementation, to strengthen health management capacities at the municipal level in selected pilot areas, and to improve information systems. Counterpart funds in Bolivia are used to support a Chagas' disease control program. In Peru, CIDA supports UNICEF's program in primary health care.

In the Caribbean, CIDA supports the Caribbean Epidemiology Center (CAREC), which provides technical support and collaboration among its Member Countries. The aim of this project is to strengthen the capacity of the national ministries of health and community-based organizations in the provision of services for the prevention and control of HIV/AIDS and other STDs, and the care of infected persons in their communities. In Haiti, CIDA funding is being used to reinforce reproductive health care services through support to UNFPA.

In addition to core funding to the UN system, CIDA contributes to various PAHO projects. These include a project to improve perinatal health services and increase community participation through a regional safe motherhood program in Bolivia, Honduras, Nicaragua, and Peru. CIDA has financed PAHO's Regional Program of Surveillance and Epidemiology Strengthening in nine countries in the Region. The aim of this intervention is to enhance the human resource expertise and institutional capacity in epidemiology and surveillance of some of the major causes of early childhood respiratory diseases.

Canada contributes to the World Bank's Energy Sector Management Assistance Program for the elimination of lead from gasoline throughout the Americas.

Areas where future programming is actively being pursued include support to reproductive health initiatives; a regional tuberculosis prevention and control project; and health-related projects through the transfer of technology funds in certain Southern Cone countries and Brazil.

With its limited resources, Canada focuses its interventions on strategic areas where leverage and impact can be achieved and where development efforts reflect both the needs of developing countries and Canada's ability to meet those needs.

CAYMAN ISLANDS

GENERAL SITUATION AND TRENDS

Socioeconomic, Political, and Demographic Overview

The Cayman Islands is a British Dependent Territory comprising three islands: Grand Cayman, Cayman Brac, and Little Cayman. The islands cover an area of about 250 km^2 in the western Caribbean Sea, about 240 km south of Cuba and 290 km west of Jamaica. George Town, the capital city, is located on Grand Cayman, the largest and most populous island. The islands are generally low-lying, with the exception of a massive limestone bluff rising on Cayman Brac. Cayman Brac and Little Cayman are located about 145 km northeast of Grand Cayman. At the end of 1995, the population of the Cayman islands was estimated to be 33,600, an increase of 5% over the previous year.

A Governor, who represents the Queen and presides over the Executive Council, heads the territorial Government. The elected Legislative Assembly designates Ministers to sit on the Executive Council. A 1993 amendment to the Constitution established a new Ministry of Health, Drug Abuse Prevention, and Rehabilitation. Ministers delegate policy implementation and department administration to Permanent Secretaries.

Political stability and a strong economy characterize the Cayman Islands. The exchange rate remained constant over the past two decades at CI$ 0.80 to US$ 1.00. The gross domestic product almost doubled between 1988 and 1994, when it was estimated to be $US 906 million. Average per capita GDP was an estimated at US$ 28,900. The revenue almost doubled in seven years: it was US$ 101.2 million in 1988, US$ 130.4 million in 1991, and US$181 million in 1995. Overall economic growth for 1995 was an estimated 5%, and both inflation and unemployment recorded historically low levels. Inflation averaged about 5% annually in recent years, but stood at 2.3% in 1995. The average unemployment rate during the 1992–1995 period was 6.1%, and in

1995 was 4%, the lowest rate since the 1989 census. The labor force was about 16,830 in 1994, of whom 6,821 (40.5%) were foreign work permit holders. Growth in the economy was fueled largely by successes in finance and tourism, the two main sectors of the economy. In the financial sector, the mutual funds industry achieved remarkable growth. In the tourism sector, visitor arrivals amounted to over 1 million in 1995.

The annual recurring Government expenditure nearly quadrupled in the last decade. In 1986 it was US$ 58.9 million and in 1995 it reached US $211.9 million. In 1995, education was allocated 10.7% of the budget; health, 9.6%; tourism, 9.6%; and social services, 3.6%.

Population

In 1995, the estimated mid-year and year-end populations for the Cayman Islands were 32,500 and 33,600, respectively. According to the 1989 census, 22.7% of the population was under 15 years of age and 6.3% was 65 years and older. A 1993 survey estimated these figures to be 24.9% and 8.6%, respectively. The dependency ratio was 33.5 in 1993.

The annual average crude birth rate has remained almost static during the last decade at 17.6 per 1,000 population; the lowest rate was 14.9 in 1995. The annual average death rate over that period was 4.7 per 1,000 population; the lowest rate was 3.4, also in 1995. The average annual growth rate was 4.6%, with variations from 2.1% to 6.7%. In 1994, 63% of the population was Caymanian, a reduction from 69% in 1988. This is attributed to the rapid increase in the number of foreign work permit holders and their dependents (10,017 in 1995) living in the Cayman Islands.

Births totaled 520 in 1992, 531 in 1994, and 485 in 1995. There was a small increase in live births to mothers 35 years and older (9.5% in the 1988–1991 period and 10.7% in the 1992–1995 period). There were no live births to mothers 45 years old and older during these periods. There has been a slight increase in the percentage of unmarried mothers (37.8% in the 1988–1991 period, and 39.3% in the 1992–1995 period).

According to national sources, life expectancy at birth in 1989 was 77.1 years. Estimates for 1995 were 77.5 years, 75.0 years for males and 79.0 years for females. The average age at death during 1994 and 1995 for both sexes was 71 years, 66 years for males and 76 years for females.

School is free and compulsory for all children between 5 and 16 years old. Health care is provided free of charge to all school children. Adult literacy rate is about 98%.

Mortality Profile

The registration of deaths occurring in the Cayman Islands is 100% complete. Mortality data reported here exclude deaths of visitors (approximately 10% of total deaths) whenever possible to avoid bias. Data are not available on residents who die overseas. As comparisons can be misleading due to the small population size, data were grouped for the 1988–1991 and 1992–1995 periods.

Deaths of residents average approximately 100 per year. During the 1992–1995 period, 469 deaths were recorded, compared with 460 deaths from 1988 to 1991 (14 visitors' deaths were included in the 1991 data). The average annual crude death rate for the 1988–1991 period was 4.6 per 1,000 population, and 4.3 during the 1992–1995 period. The number of infant deaths varied from 2 to 7 per year over the 1988–1995 period. The average infant mortality rate during the 1989–1991 period was 8.8 per 1,000 live births, and 8.6 per 1,000 in the 1992–1995 period. The neonatal mortality rate was 7.3 per 1,000 live births during the 1992–1995 period, and 7.7 during the 1988–1991 period. The average stillbirth rate was 12.0 per 1,000 births from 1988 to 1991, compared with 4.3 per 1,000 births during the 1992–1995 period. There was only one maternal death between 1984 and 1995.

Symptoms and ill-defined conditions accounted for 1.5% of deaths during the 1988–1991 period, while 3.2% of registered deaths were due to ill-defined conditions during the 1992–1995 period. The leading causes of death in the 1988–1991 period were diseases of the circulatory system (39.5%, or 179 deaths), malignant neoplasms (22.3%, or 101 deaths), and external causes, about 11% (50 deaths). During the 1992–1995 period, diseases of the circulatory system comprised 41.9% of total deaths, followed by malignant neoplasms (20.9%). During the same period, external causes were responsible for 7.9% of the deaths. The decline in this category is attributed to a recent decline in deaths due to motor vehicle accidents.

SPECIFIC HEALTH PROBLEMS

Because the Cayman Islands are small territories with similar demographic and socioeconomic profiles, there is no significant variation in health problems due to geographical location. Mortality data during the 1992–1995 period, Georgetown Hospital discharge data for 1995, and data from notifiable disease records were used to describe specific health problems in the Cayman Islands. Data for Georgetown Hospital, which serves 95% of the population, indicated that there were a total of 3,417 discharges in 1995 (105 per 1,000 population). The major causes for admission were: diseases of the digestive system (404 cases, or 11.8%); diseases of the genitourinary system (336 cases, or 9.9%); injuries (305 cases, or 8.9 %); diseases of the respiratory system (265 cases, or 7.8%); and diseases of the cardiovascular system (254 cases, or 7.4%). Normal deliveries accounted for 421 admissions (12.3%).

Analysis by Population Group

Health of Children

The number of infant deaths varied from 1 to 7 per annum during the past 10 years, with 2.8 deaths per 1,000 live births being the lowest rate, and 14.0 per 1,000, the highest. The annual average infant mortality rate during the 1991–1995 period was 8.7; nearly 85% of infant deaths were neonatal deaths. Of the 18 infant deaths occurring during the 1991–1995 period, 9 were attributed to prematurity, and 4 to congenital heart disease. Hypoplastic left heart syndrome was responsible for three infant deaths during this period. Fifteen of the infant deaths were among females (83%), and nine of these deaths were due to prematurity. The stillbirth rate declined from 12.0 per 1,000 births in the 1988–1991 period to 4.3 per 1,000 births in the 1992–1995 period. In 1990 and 1991, 11.2% of infants had low birthweights. This figure decreased to 4.5% in 1995; the average during the 1992–1995 period was 6.4%.

In 1995, 86 admissions to the Georgetown Hospital were for children under 1 year of age (excluding 421 healthy liveborn infants), an admission rate of 156 per 1,000 children under 1 year old. This is the second highest age-specific rate after that of the 65 and older age group. The leading causes of admission among this age group were diseases of the respiratory system (27 cases) and diseases of the digestive system (19 cases). There were 9 cases of bronchitis (10.5%), 8 of gastroenteritis (9.3%), and 6 of asthma (6.8%).

There were no deaths among children 1 to 4 years of age during the 1992–1995 period. Three occurred during the 1988–1991 period, two due to accidental drowning and one from accidental poisoning. There were 259 admissions to the Georgetown Hospital for this age group, for a rate of 106 per 1,000 population. The leading specific causes for admission were gastroenteritis (31 cases), asthma (28 cases), and convulsions (17 cases). These represent 11.4%, 10.2%, and 6.2%, respectively, of all admissions in this age group.

One death occurred in the 5–9-year-old age group during the 1992–1995 period due to a traffic accident. A total of 112 children in this age group were admitted to the hospital in 1995, for a rate of 52 per 1,000 population. The most common causes for admission were diseases of the respiratory system (26 cases) and diseases of the digestive system (25 cases, or 12 per 1,000).

Health of Adolescents

During the past decade, there were between 1 and 2 live births to females under 15 years of age, a rate of 2.2 per 1,000 births during 1988–1991, and 2.5 in 1992–1994. No births were recorded in 1991 and 1992 for this group. One death due to Sanfilippo syndrome occurred among 10–14-year-olds during the 1992–1995 period. In 1995, 68 children in this age group were admitted to the hospital, or 35 per 1,000 population. The main causes for admission were injuries (19 cases, or 28%), diseases of the respiratory system (10 cases, or 15%), and diseases of the digestive system (10 cases, or 15%).

During 1992–1994, 12.9% of births (204 of 1,578) were to mothers between 15 and 19 years old, compared with 17.5% during the 1988–1991 period. From 1992 to 1995, three deaths occurred among the 15–19-year-old age group, two due to motor vehicle accidents and one to homicidal injury. A total of 155 hospital admissions were recorded in 1995, a rate of 82 per 1,000 population in this age group. Females accounted for 121 admissions (78%). The most common causes for admission among females were normal delivery (40 admissions, or 33%); obstetric causes (22 cases, or 18.2%), genitourinary diseases (9 cases, or 7.4%), and diseases of the digestive system (10 cases, or 8.3%). Thirty-four males were admitted in this age group in 1995, accounting for 11 admissions due to injuries (32.4%) and 7 due to diseases of the digestive system (20.6%). Of the 244 clients seeking drug counseling, 21% were under 19 years of age.

Health of Adults

The total fertility rate declined from 381 in 1990 to 335 in 1994. There were no births to women above 50 years of age between 1986 and 1995. Between 1992 and 1994, 89% of live births were to mothers between the ages of 20 and 44, compared with 79% in the 1988–1991 period. In 1995, 98.8% of

pregnant women saw trained personnel during the prenatal period, and trained personnel attended all deliveries. The average number of prenatal visits per pregnancy was 11.8. A survey revealed that 27% of mothers were solely breast-feeding at four months, and 12% were solely breast-feeding at six months. Forty-nine percent of babies were partially breast-fed at six months.

There were 96 deaths among the 25–64-year-old age group (25% of total deaths) in the 1992–1995 period. The most common causes for death were diseases of the circulatory system and malignant neoplasms. In 1995, 61.3% (1,801 of 2,936) of hospital admissions were in the 20–64-year-old age group, a rate of 84 per 1,000 population. Seventy percent (1,258) were females. The main causes for admission for women were normal delivery (208, or 16.5%), obstetric causes (214, or 17%), genitourinary diseases (151, or 12.0%), and diseases of the digestive system (109, or 8.7%). Among males the main causes for admission were injuries (117 admissions, or 21.5%), diseases of the digestive system (91, or 16.8%), diseases of the circulatory system (56, or 10.3%), and mental disorders (49, or 9%).

Health of the Elderly

In 1993, it was estimated that 6.6% of the population was 65 years old and older, a slight increase over 1989, when it was 6.3%. A recent survey revealed that 29% of the elderly are employed. About 36% indicated that they do not have any fears or problems related to aging, while 32% are concerned about their health. The Social Services Department assists those in need, and the Government offers free medical care for elderly who cannot afford treatment.

During the 1992–1995 period, 345 of all deaths (73.5%) occurred in this age group; the most common causes were diseases of the circulatory system and malignant neoplasms. In 1995, 455 (15.5%) of hospital admissions were for persons 65 years and older, representing the highest age-specific rate (212 admissions per 1,000 population). Females accounted for 57% of admissions in this age group. The main causes for hospital admission among females were diseases of the circulatory system (68 cases, or 26%), diseases of the digestive system (33 cases, or 13%), diseases of the musculoskeletal system (23 cases, or 9%), and endocrine and metabolic disorders (18 cases, or 7%). Among males, the main causes were diseases of the circulatory system (48 cases, or 25%), diseases of the digestive system (31 cases, or 16%), diseases of the respiratory system (19 cases, or 10%), and diseases of the genitourinary system (19 cases, or 10%). Of the diseases of the circulatory system, ischemic heart disease accounts for 40% of male admissions, followed by diseases of the pulmonary system (27%), and cerebrovascular diseases (21%).

Family Health

The marriage rate has declined from 10.7 per 1,000 population in 1988, to 7.6 in 1994. The divorce rate declined from 5.56 per 1,000 in 1991, to 2.20 in 1994. During the 1992–1995 period, 39.3% of live births were to unmarried mothers, compared with 37.8% during the 1988–1991 period. A program for young parents was started in 1995 to help develop skills in young mothers. All deliveries are conducted in health facilities.

Workers' Health

All Government employees are offered free health care. While many businesses provide health insurance coverage to their employees, a recently approved National Health Insurance Law will enable all employees and their dependents to have health insurance. Drug and smoking policies are in place in many organizations. Compulsory schooling precludes employment of children under 16 years old.

Health of the Disabled

Special education facilities are available for handicapped and impaired children. More than 60 children attend the Lighthouse School, which caters to the special education needs of disabled children. Data on blindness are not available. In 1992, the prevalence of mental retardation was estimated at 0.08%.

Analysis by Type of Disease or Health Impairment

Communicable Diseases

Vector-Borne Diseases. Vector-borne diseases such as dengue, yellow fever, and malaria are not endemic in the Cayman Islands. *Aedes aegypti* mosquitoes were eradicated from the islands about 20 years ago. Sporadic re-infestations are dealt with immediately by the Mosquito Research and Control Unit.

There have been between two and four cases of imported malaria cases per year, reaching eight in 1995; most malaria cases were imported from Honduras. During 1995, four dengue cases were imported. Whenever malaria or other vector-borne illnesses are detected, the Mosquito Research and Control Unit is notified for appropriate measures.

Vaccine-Preventable Diseases. There were no reported cases of polio, diphtheria, whooping cough, or tetanus during the 1986–1995 period. The last cases of polio occurred in

1957, and there was one case of diphtheria in 1966. During the 1986–1989 period, there were from 1 to 3 cases of measles reported annually. In 1990, 27 cases were reported. Since 1991 there have been no cases of measles. Presently a two-dose schedule of measles, mumps, and rubella vaccine (MMR) is in effect. A national campaign was organized to immunize school-aged children with the second MMR dose. Mumps is estimated to be underreported. On average, 2 to 4 cases are reported each year; in 1991, 8 cases were reported. All blood for transfusions is screened for HIV, venereal disease, and hepatitis B and C.

Cholera and Other Intestinal Diseases. The threat of cholera in the Region in 1991 and 1992 put the Cayman Islands on alert for cholera prevention and control. Reported cases of gastroenteritis among children under 5 years of age have been less than 100 per year, but have fluctuated widely. There have been sporadic cases of food poisoning, especially due to ciguatera poisoning. The incidence of ciguatera fluctuated widely: there were 10 cases in 1990, 18 in 1993, and 2 cases in 1995. A few cases of trichuriasis and ascariasis were identified. Hookworm and amebiasis are not endemic in the Cayman Islands.

Chronic Communicable Diseases. The incidence of tuberculosis varied from 0 to 3 cases per year during the past decade, with 6 cases during the 1988–1991 period, and 8 cases during the 1992–1995 period. Leprosy is not endemic in the Cayman Islands, and there have been no reported cases in the past 15 years.

Acute Respiratory Infections. During the 1988–1991 period, 29 of 460 deaths (6.3%) were due to acute respiratory tract infections. Twenty-five of these deaths (86%) were among persons 75 years and older. During the 1992–1995 period, only 4% (19 of 469) deaths were due to these conditions; 95% (18 of 19) occurred in the age group 75 years old and older. In 1995, 7.8% of hospital admissions were due to diseases of the respiratory system. Of 265 admissions for this condition, 108 were for children under the age of 5; 74 admissions were for persons between 20 and 64 years old; and 39 admissions were for those 65 years and over.

Rabies and Other Zoonoses. Rabies and other zoonoses are not prevalent in the Cayman Islands.

AIDS and Other Sexually Transmitted Diseases. While cases of HIV infection may be underreported, there is little or no underreporting of overt AIDS cases. The first case of AIDS in the Cayman Islands was reported in 1985. One case was detected each year between 1985 and 1989. Four new cases were reported annually in 1991, 1992, and 1994, but there were no new cases in 1993 or 1995. These variations in incidence are attributed to the return of residents from abroad after having tested HIV-positive. Through December 1995, there had been 19 persons identified with AIDS, 16 of whom died. These figures are not consistent with mortality data, since some deaths occurred overseas. At the end of 1995, there were 3 persons living with AIDS, and 18 known HIV-positive cases. Initially, most HIV-infected persons were homosexual, but in 1995, 57% (21 of 37) were heterosexual. Sixty percent of persons infected with HIV (22 of 37 cases) were in the 25–34-year age group; 20 were males (54%). There were two cases of perinatal transmission of HIV, representing 5.4% of all cases.

Sexually transmitted diseases are underreported. Data on the incidence of gonococcal diseases shows a decline from 164 cases in 1992 (57 per 10,000 population), to 81 cases in 1995 (25 per 10,000 population). The incidence of syphilis shows a similar trend: from 249 cases in 1990 (95 per 10,000 population) to 146 cases in 1995 (45 per 10,000 population).

Noncommunicable Diseases and Other Health-Related Problems

Nutritional Diseases. The percentage of newborns weighing less than 2,500 g at birth declined from 11.2% in 1990 and 1991 to 4.5% in 1995. There is not a significant presence of moderate or severe protein-energy malnutrition levels in children. Obesity among children and adults is starting to cause concern, but there are no current data on its prevalence. There have been no cases showing evidence of iodine deficiency disorders.

Most foods are imported from the United States, so Caymanians benefit from food fortification applied in that country. Vitamin supplements are routinely provided to pregnant women and preschool children. A campaign promoting nutrition guidelines is under way, and the Agriculture Department promotes local food production.

Cardiovascular Diseases. During the 1992–1995 period, diseases of the circulatory system were responsible for 41.9% of deaths (190 of 454), for a death rate of 15.4 per 10,000 population. In the 1988–1991 period, these conditions accounted for 39.5% of deaths (179 of 453), a death rate of 17.5 per 10,000 population. They constitute 39.5% of deaths among males, and 43.9% among females. Ischemic heart disease caused 42.6% of these deaths, and cerebrovascular disease 23.7%. In 1995, 8.5% of hospital admissions (254 of 2,996) were related to these conditions (55 per 10,000 population). Most of the cases (191, or 75%) were among people 50 years old and older. Of 455 hospital admissions for persons over the age of 65, 106 (23.2%) were related to diseases of the circulatory system. Of the total admissions, 55.5% (141 of 254) were

females. Prevalence data on hypertension in the Cayman Islands are not available.

Malignant Tumors. During the 1988–1991 period, malignant neoplasms caused 101 deaths, for a mortality rate of 9.8 per 10,000 population. This rate declined to 7.7 per 10,000 in the 1992–1995 period. Malignant tumors comprised 25% of all deaths among males, and 16% among females. Neoplasms accounted for only 2.6% of hospital admissions in 1995, probably because much of the care was conducted through outpatient departments. Of the 86 admissions relating to tumors, 47 were for management of malignant tumors, and 39 for benign tumors. In the 1988–1991 period, malignant neoplasms of digestive organs and peritoneum (excluding stomach and colon) accounted for 19 deaths; trachea, bronchus, and lung cancers for 18 deaths; female breast cancer for 16 deaths; and prostate cancer, 10 deaths. Malignant neoplasms of the trachea, bronchus, or lung accounted for 18 deaths, female breast cancer for 13 deaths, and prostate cancer for 12 deaths in the 1992–1995 period.

Accidents and Violence. There were 17,427 vehicles registered in 1995, or nearly 1 for every 2 people, an increase of 23% over 1990. However, the traffic accident rate per 1,000 vehicles decreased from 33 in 1990, to 23 in 1995. There was also a decline in traffic fatalities (1.4 per 1,000 vehicles in 1990 and 0.5 in 1995) and serious injuries (3.7 per 1,000 vehicles in 1990, and 2.9 in 1995). Accidents not involving vehicles decreased from 61 per 1,000 population in 1990, to 43 in 1995. The incidence of assaults stood at 6.9 per 1,000 population in 1990, compared with 4.2 in 1995. The improvement in these rates are concurrent with public education efforts of the Health Services and Police Department, as well as enhanced enforcement measures.

External causes were responsible for 11% of deaths among residents during the 1988–1991 period, compared with 7.9 % in the 1992–1995 period. While the proportions of deaths due to external causes among males were similar during 1988–1991 (14.7%) and 1992–1995 (13.0%), there has been a more dramatic decline, from 7.0% to 3.3%, among females. In 1995, 10.2% of hospital admissions (305 of 2,996) were due to external causes (injuries, poisoning, and burns). One-third (102 cases) were among those under 19 years of age, and one-half (154 cases) among persons between 20 and 59 years of age. Intracranial and internal injuries accounted for 68 of hospital admissions (22.3%); 45 of these cases were among males. Poisoning and toxic effects accounted for 50 hospital admissions; 37 of these cases were females (74%).

Behavioral Disorders. Based on data on hospital patients and a survey done by district public health nurses, the prevalence of mental illness in the population was estimated to be

5.5% in 1992. The prevalence of schizophrenia was estimated to be 0.61%; depression, 0.17%; and manic depression, 0.19%. Almost all persons suffering from schizophrenia, depression, and manic depression have been in contact with the Mental Health Services.

Oral Health. In November 1995, at the request of the Cayman Islands Government, the Pan American Health Organization carried out a comprehensive survey of oral health and dental disease in the territory. Over 1,000 people were examined, a sample that corresponded to about 11.6% of all schoolchildren and 7% of adults.

Dental health was measured using indices for decayed, missing, or filled teeth (DMFT). The 1989–1990 survey indicated a DMFT rate of 4.6 for 12-year olds. The 1995 DMFT for the same age group was 1.7, a very significant improvement. Ninety-seven percent had no fluorosis; 3% had questionable, mild, or very mild scores. There was no severe fluorosis. Slightly over half of those surveyed needed no dental treatment, and approximately one-third needed routine, non-urgent treatment. Eight percent had decay, and required prompt attention. Areas of high treatment urgency included Cayman Brac and children in Government schools in Georgetown. Only 3.7% of 6- and 7-year-olds needed fillings, but the need was greater in middle-aged adults. A relatively low number of adults needed crowns. Approximately 20% of younger children needed sealants. In 1981, 28% of children in primary schools, 39% in middle school, and 46% in high schools were decay-free. In 1995, the figures had improved significantly: 66.8% of 5-year-olds, 60% of 12-year-olds, and 60% of 16-year-olds were decay-free.

Results from the survey among children are encouraging, but there is room for improvement in the adult population, particularly regarding gum disease and preventive care. With the limited resources available, the strategy would be to target children and reinforce preventive measures.

Other Emerging and Re-emerging Diseases. Emerging and re-emerging diseases such as meningococcal meningitis, hantavirus, and Venezuelan equine encephalitis are not endemic in the Cayman Islands.

Natural Disasters and Industrial Accidents. There are no major industries using heavy equipment in the Cayman Islands, and there have been no major accidents in the construction industry. The last natural disaster to threaten the Cayman Islands was Hurricane Gilbert in 1988. An Emergency Medical Relief Plan is in place in the event of a hurricane or other natural disaster. A National Health Coordinator ensures that the plan is updated each year, that essential supplies are available, and staff is allocated. An Intersectional Committee oversees the Emergency Medical Relief Plan, which forms part of the National Hurricane Plan.

RESPONSE OF THE HEALTH SYSTEM

National Health Plans and Policies

It is the Government's policy to provide community-based health care services with advanced and effective central support. The development of new health centers in all districts was initiated in 1993, and all districts will have new health centers in operation by August 1997. An 18-bed hospital was commissioned in Cayman Brac in 1993, and a 128-bed hospital construction project in Grand Cayman began in 1994, with construction to be completed by the end of 1998. The Government recognizes that it is neither cost-effective nor efficient to provide tertiary care in the Cayman Islands, and maintains a formal contract for such care with the Baptist Hospital in Miami, Florida (USA), as well as arrangements with other institutions in Miami and with the University of the West Indies.

To lessen the burden of escalating health care costs, the Government enacted legislation in June 1997, making it mandatory for all employers to provide health insurance coverage for employees and their dependents. The Government will regulate the provision of health insurance by private carriers.

Strategic Plan for Health Services

There have been significant developments in defining the strategies for health care delivery in the Cayman Islands. A planning committee consisting of 25 members drawn from the health professions, the community at large, nongovernmental organizations, and Members of Parliament was established in 1994 to develop the Strategic Plan for the Health Services. The Plan consists of eight strategies that address the following: development of community-based services; staff participation in decision-making; community involvement in health promotion; maintenance of legislative support and accountability of Ministry departments; alternative approaches to health financing; collaboration between public and private sectors in providing health services; establishment of standards to facilitate health staff development; and assurance that quality of health facilities, equipment, supplies, personnel, and procedures meet international standards.

Institutional Organization

In 1992, the Health Services Authority was established to oversee the day-to-day management of health services. In 1994, it was instituted as a department within the Ministry of Health and Human Services. In March 1994, the new Ministry of Health, Drug Abuse Prevention, and Rehabilitation was established with overall responsibility for health care in the

Cayman Islands. The Health Services Department is responsible for all Government health care services, including public health services. The Health Practitioners Board licenses and disciplines health professionals in the Cayman Islands.

The Director of Health Services reports to the Permanent Secretary of the Ministry of Health, Drug Abuse Prevention, and Rehabilitation and is assisted by the Chief Medical Officer, Medical Officer of Health, Chief Nursing Officer, Senior Dental Officer, Health Service Accountant, and Manager of Ancillary and Support Services.

The primary health care system provides primary care services through the district health centers. When Georgetown Hospital is completed in 1998, it will provide emergency care, specialist services, and inpatient care. While the referral system is in place, specialist services are sought directly, due to the small size of the Cayman Islands.

Constraints to decentralizing responsibility exist because of central Government control of financial and administrative procedures. These issues are being addressed.

The Government operates the 59-bed Georgetown Hospital in Grand Cayman, and the 18-bed Faith Hospital in Cayman Brac, the only two inpatient facilities. In 1995, there were 24 public sector doctors, including two based on Cayman Brac. There were 24 doctors in full-time private practice, providing family health or specialized treatment on a regular basis. Private physicians use hospital services as needed.

Organization of Health Regulatory Activities

There is no specific legislation providing for regulation of health care or facilities. There are, however, regulations in place that allow health practitioners to use only medical equipment or drugs approved for use in the United States and United Kingdom. The Environmental Health Department monitors the food safety program and controls nuisances under public health law.

Health Services and Resources

Organization of Services for Care of the Population

Health Promotion. The national Strategic Plan for Health empowers the community to take responsibility in maintaining personal and community health. Recognizing the importance of health promotion as part of this strategy, the Government created a full-time position for a Health Promotion Officer in 1994. Health promotion activities target disease prevention, healthy lifestyle, health skills, and the environment, and are conducted with intersectoral cooperation. Public education programs are disseminated using radio, television, and newspapers; the recent availability of cable

television has assisted efforts to raise awareness about health among the public. Churches and businesses are other conduits for public awareness programs. Educational materials are produced and widely distributed. Public education programs are organized around special efforts such as the colon cancer screening program, health programs carried out during the Batabano Carnival and Pirates' Week, and the National Trust Fair, as well as the observance of such events as "Health Week," "Choose To Be Drug-Free Week," "World No-Tobacco Day," and "Breast-feeding Week."

Disease Prevention and Control. The Cayman Islands Government offers free immunization program to all resident children. High coverage (above 90%) of polio immunization has been maintained over the years, and consequently, no special campaigns are conducted. The Acute Flaccid Paralysis surveillance is 100% complete, and is effective because of the small population. Ninety-eight percent of infants reaching their first birthday were fully immunized with polio and DPT vaccines.

There were no cases of adult or neonatal tetanus in the 1986–1995 period. Tetanus toxoid is offered to all pregnant women attending public health facilities, and it is estimated that 90% of infants are protected from neonatal tetanus at birth.

There have been no reported cases of measles since 1991. Even though there have been fluctuations, vaccination coverage has been maintained above 90%, sometimes reaching 95%–99% during the past decade, due to small population size.

There have been a few significant changes in the immunization policies and activities during the last five years. *Haemophilus influenzae* B vaccine was introduced into the national immunization schedule in 1992. BCG vaccine was given at the age of 1 year until 1992, when it was changed to 6 weeks (postnatal visit). BCG coverage at times has been low because foreign parents, particularly those from the United States, Canada, and the United Kingdom, decline the vaccine when it is not given nationally to infants in their countries of origin. High-risk groups such as health care workers, police, prison officers, and fire service officers receive hepatitis B vaccine.

Epidemiological Surveillance. The Health Information System has an early warning system to detect communicable diseases of public health importance. The hospital laboratory serves as a public health laboratory and is equipped to diagnose common infectious diseases. An overseas referral system is used for specialized diagnosis. Qualified staff is available to unusual disease occurrences.

Environmental Health Services. Development in the Cayman Islands has proceeded rapidly in the last two decades, with attendant effects on the environment. Growth in the urban and suburban population has been greater than the infrastructure can comfortably support. The results are increased traffic with accompanying air pollution; increased demand for potable water and sewage treatment and disposal; pollution of groundwater (now unfit for human consumption in most urban areas); and increasing noise pollution.

In 1996, the Department of Environmental Health was given departmental status in the Ministry of Agriculture, Environment, Communications and Works. A priority of the newly formed department was to draft legislation, standards, and guidelines on environmental health. The Department of Environment Health is responsible for water quality surveillance, meat and food inspection, monitoring food handling establishments, oversight of solid waste management, and review of building plans.

Certain requirements must be satisfied before licensing is granted to food vendors. Such licenses are renewed on an annual basis. Food is inspected at the port of entry and may be condemned by the food inspector because of improper storage or handling conditions, appearance, or faulty temperature control. All food inspectors are trained in hazard analysis critical control points (HACCP) evaluation.

There are two piped water supply systems in Grand Cayman, both fed by desalinated water, which provide water to approximately 70% of the island's population and all its major hotels. Apart from these systems, rainwater is typically collected from roofs and cisterns, or water is pumped from groundwater sources for drinking and domestic use. Private water trucks transport water from the Water Authority Works to supplement individual rain- and groundwater supplies. Within the next three to five years, the entire population is expected to have access to piped water supply.

The quality of drinking water is routinely monitored throughout the Cayman Islands, with emphasis on public water supplies, public facilities, day-care centers, retirement homes, schools, health care facilities, restaurants, and tourist accommodations.

Solid waste is collected at a minimum of three days per week on Grand Cayman. There are sanitary landfills on all three islands for solid waste disposal. These government-managed landfills are the only legal disposal sites in the Cayman Islands. A major achievement in 1995 was a 10% reduction in the solid waste processed at landfills, achieved through the introduction of a number of recycling strategies. Cardboard, aluminum, and automotive batteries are the main recyclable items being exported to suitable markets. There is great potential for further development of these and other recycling programs, and these will be the subject of increased promotion.

A central sewerage treatment plant serves the main tourist hotel area of Georgetown. All other sewage treatment and disposal is carried out on a site-by-site basis, utilizing septic tanks with deep well injection or soakway fields. Larger apartments, office buildings, and hotels outside the public sewerage service area operate private treatment plants. Adequate excreta disposal facilities are available to 99.5% of the population.

Organization and Operation of Personal Health Care Services

The Government operates the 59-bed Georgetown Hospital, which includes 7 nursery beds in the maternity ward, and a 7-bed extended care unit at the Pines Retirement Home on Grand Cayman. On Cayman Brac, health care is dispensed from Faith Hospital, an 18-bed facility. Primary health care is also provided through four district health centers in Grand Cayman.

Specialist services are available locally in the fields of surgery, gynecology and obstetrics, pediatrics, internal medicine, anesthesiology, public health, orthopedics, ophthalmology, otolaryngology, and periodontology. Visiting specialists provide services in dermatology, cosmetic surgery, maxillofacial surgery, and urology. The surgeon from Faith Hospital (Cayman Brac) conducts an outpatient clinic in urology on Grand Cayman every two weeks. Baptist Hospital, in Miami, Florida (USA), provides tertiary care. A visiting team of orthopedic surgeons from Canada provides care through the Cayman Medical Center and has provided coverage at Georgetown Hospital. Dental care is available through three government dental officers, and privately from six dentists, two orthodontists, and one resident and one visiting periodontist. Oral surgery services are available once weekly from a visiting dental consultant. The ambulance service had a staff of 18, including 3 paramedics in 1995. Emergency and non-emergency calls totaled 1,508 and 743 respectively, a 14% increase over 1994.

In 1995, Georgetown Hospital admissions totaled 3,622, a 2% increase over 1994. Outpatient and casualty visits increased 4.3%, totaling 48,265 in 1995. Faith Hospital had 391 admissions and 6,645 outpatient visits. District health centers accounted for 33,115 visits, an increase of 8.9% over the previous year. Public health nurses made 8,163 home visits in 1995, a 2% increase over 1994. A decompression chamber for diving emergencies is located at the Hospital and is operated by a volunteer group. Eighty-four treatments were given to 43 patients in 1995.

Mental health services are provided in a comprehensive, community-based fashion. Services are delivered via visits to homes, prison, geriatric and day-care facilities, and district health centers. A psychiatrist, psychiatric social worker, and two community mental health nurses comprise the staff.

Health centers in Grand Cayman are located in West Bay, Bodden Town, East End, and North Side. The district health centers offer both preventive and curative services, functioning as an extension of the hospital's outpatient department and public health service. With only a few exceptions, the centers provide all of the services offered by the Public Health

Department in Georgetown. In addition to full-time staff at the health centers, visiting staff include physicians, a public health officer, psychiatric social worker, social worker, medical social worker, nutritionist, health educator, pharmacy technician/pharmacist, community mental health nurse, and counseling center staff. Services offered through district health centers include daily treatment by nurses, and clinics by doctors on specified days in the areas of general practice, psychiatry, nutrition counseling, child welfare, health education, and drug counseling.

The public health services on Cayman Brac and Little Cayman are provided by a public health nurse. All services offered on Grand Cayman are available on these two islands, but on a smaller scale. The Cayman Brac Health Services serve few Cayman Island residents.

Inputs for Health

There is no local production of drugs, vaccines, reagents, or equipment. These are imported from approved companies, mainly from the United States. Vaccines are obtained through the Pan American Health Organization's Expanded Program on Immunization Revolving Fund.

All essential drugs are available at public health care facilities. There are no "remote facilities" in a country the size of the Cayman Islands, but formulary drugs, essential and nonessential, are requisitioned from the central pharmacy storeroom by the appropriate section of the health services department. The formulary contains all drugs deemed essential by WHO guidelines, in addition to other pharmaceuticals.

The primary action being taken to ensure access of all to essential drugs is the expansion of district clinics into health centers. The considerable increases in size and quality of the facilities, as well as extended hours, have been of significant benefit to patients residing in the districts. The addition of pharmacists to the staff of health centers during 1997 will increase the level of pharmaceutical care available in the districts, resulting in improved utilization of essential and other drugs. There are no constraints currently affecting accessibility of essential drugs.

Human Resources

The Health Practitioners Board is responsible for registration of health practitioners for the private sector. Government workers are registered automatically and are subject to Civil Service General Orders.

While there has been an increase in the number of health professionals during the last decade, the rapid increase in population caused a decline in the ratio of health workers to population. Among all health professionals, the rate was 8.4 per 1,000 population in 1988, declining to 7.9 in 1995. There were 4.9 nurses per 1,000 population in 1988 compared with 4.3 in 1995. The physician/population ratio also has declined: from 1.6 per 1,000 in 1988 to 1.4 in 1995. According to 1995 data, human health resources available in the Cayman Islands per 10,000 population are: 14.3 physicians; 4.5 midwives; 38.4 nurses (excluding midwives); 3.9 pharmacists; 3.6 dentists; and 18.2 other health care providers (including community health workers).

Approximately 95% of physicians and 70% of other health care professionals (nurses, pharmacists, etc.) are contracted officers from overseas. Although the Government supports the training of Caymanians as health professionals, there is a shortage of available personnel.

Research and Technology

Health research is not routinely undertaken in the Cayman Islands. Projects in cooperation with the Mailman Center for Child Development in Miami organized research on gene localization of non-progressive cerebella ataxia and Usher Syndrome. An oral health survey was conducted in 1995 with the help of PAHO. Even though the territory's small population and budgetary and staffing constraints limit the scope of research, efforts are being made to strengthen this component.

Expenditures and Sectoral Financing

Due to the small population size of the Cayman Islands, it is not feasible to describe expenditures according to regions and social groups. Data on private sector financing and expenditure on health are not available. While there has been a steady increase in the Government budget for health care services over the last decade (US$ 6.8 million in 1986, US$ 12.7 million in 1990, and US$ 20.2 million in 1995), recurrent expenditures out of total Government expenditures for health care dropped from 11.5% to 9.5% during the same period. Per capita Government health expenditure in 1995 was US$ 623. Data on total national health expenditure as a percentage of GNP and percentage of national health expenditure devoted to local health care are not available.

External Technical and Financial Cooperation

Technical and financial assistance from international agencies is limited to that provided by PAHO/CAREC in the form of fellowships and workshops. This amounts to approximately US$ 25,000.

CHILE

GENERAL SITUATION AND TRENDS

Socioeconomic, Political, and Demographic Overview

Chile has a surface area of 756,626 km². The most recent census, conducted in 1992, showed the population to be 13,348,401, with an intercensus growth rate of 1.64%. The projected population in June 1996 was 14,418,864. The urban population makes up 84.7% of the total. The largest concentrations of population are found in the Santiago metropolitan area (39.8%), followed, in terms of population density, by the Biobío region (12.8%), Valparaíso (10.3%), and the region of Los Lagos (7.1%). The country comprises 13 regions and 341 communes.

Chile's economy has been largely positive in recent years. The gross domestic product (GDP) has grown steadily since 1960, with a significant rise in the past five years and an average annual growth rate of 7.4% in the 1990–1995 period and of 7.2% in 1996. Per capita income, estimated at US$ 2,450 in 1990, increased to US$ 4,987 in 1996. In 1996, Chile ranked 33rd according to the human development index of the United Nations Development Program, up from 38th place in 1994.

The rise in the GDP, together with the improvement in other indicators—including the total investment rate (28.0%), the annual median gross domestic rate (9.8%), exports of goods and services (9.1%), imports of goods and services (11.9%), and prepayment of the foreign debt and a lower inflation rate (6.6% in 1996)—have strengthened the country's economy. The balance of payments was positive throughout the 1991–1996 period, ranging from US$ 577 million in 1993 to US$ 3,194 million in 1994, with an average of US$ 1,294 million. The consumer price index, which is used as a gauge of inflation, fell from 27.3 in December 1990 to 12.2 in December 1993, and then it leveled off at between 8 and 9 in 1994, 1995, and 1996. There was also growth in the construction industry. In 1991 the built-up area totaled 8,633,855 m². Of that area, 64.4% consisted of housing units,

29.0% were industrial or commercial buildings, and 6.7% were service sector buildings. In 1995, the total built-up area increased to 13,101,655 m², of which housing accounted for 62.7%, industrial or commercial facilities for 31.6%, and the service sector for 5.8%.

In the area of education, according to the 1992 census, the literacy rate in the population over the age of 15 years was 91.2% and it was estimated at 94.5% in 1995. The educational system comprises the primary level (primary school attendance is compulsory) and the secondary and higher levels. In 1995, a total of 3,533,047 students were enrolled at all levels—7.5% in preschools, 62.3% in primary schools, 20.9% in secondary schools, and 9.3% in higher learning institutions. These figures indicate enrollment rates of 95.7% at the primary level and 79.3% at the secondary level. The average amount of schooling in 1995 was 9.57 years. A program of educational reform currently under way will increase the number of required hours of school attendance at the primary and secondary levels.

According to the New National Employment Survey, the economically active population increased from 4,550,000 in 1988 to 5,500,000 during the four-month period from January to April 1996. Female participation in the labor force has increased slightly, from 31.8% in 1990 to 33.7% in 1996 for the country as a whole. The biggest increases were registered in Tarapacá (40.4%) and the Santiago metropolitan area (39.4%) and the smallest were in the regions of Araucanía (22.4%) and Coquimbo (26.0%). A comparison of the figures from the survey conducted in the October–December period each year reveals that the unemployment rate has decreased gradually over the past several years, dropping from 5.69% in 1990 to 4.7% in 1995. The four-month unemployment survey for 1996 shows that the rate rose again to 5.4%. This increase can be attributed to the adjustment measures that were adopted for the purpose of curbing the growth rate and thus forestalling inflationary pressures. These measures caused the job market to decline but also reduced consumption and helped keep inflation below double-digit rates for several years running. Annual rates (averages of the rates for 12 months) reveal positive changes, with the unemployment rate dropping from 8.2% in 1991 to 6.4% in 1996, the lowest of the decade. The unemployment rate was higher among women (7.9%) than among men (5.6%), with regional variations ranging from a low of 1.6% in Aysén to a high of 7.9% in Biobío.

In April 1996 the hourly wage index reached a nominal value of 153.28 (April 1993 = 100), which represented an increase of 0.8% with respect to the index for March 1996 and 5.3% with respect to December 1995. The cumulative increase over the 12 months from April 1995 to April 1996 was 14.6%. The sectors of economic activity that posted the greatest cumulative increases over 12 months were transportation and communications (18.0%) and public services (16.1%); the smallest increase was in construction (8.1%). By occupational category, the largest increases were reported in the operation and assembly of tools and machinery (20.3%) and professional services (18.2%); the smallest increases occurred among personal service workers (10.9%) and skilled workers (11.6%). Real wages showed an annual positive trend (4.1% increase, on average, for the most recent period). Negotiations among the Government, business owners, and labor organizations have resulted in a slow but steady rise in the monthly minimum wage, which increased from US$ 92 in 1989 to US$ 157 in 1996.

As for the structure of the labor force by sector of economic activity, the service sector employed the largest percentage of workers (25.16%), followed by commerce (18.1%), and industry and manufacturing (16.16%).

With regard to poverty rates, the results of the socioeconomic surveys (CASEN) conducted by the Ministry of Planning indicate that poverty decreased, although the rates varied from region to region. In 1984, it was estimated that 44.6% of the population could be classified as poor; the proportion fell to 32.7% in 1992 and to 25.0% in 1996. According to the 1994 CASEN survey, the regions with the highest levels of poverty were Maule (VI), with 40.5%, and Biobío (VIII), with 40.3%. The regions with the lowest levels of poverty were Magallanes (XII), with 14.8%, and the Santiago metropolitan region, with 20.9%. In rural areas, the highest level of poverty, 43.5%, was found in the Tarapacá region (I). In urban areas, Biobío (VIII) was the poorest region (40.9%). The distribution of poverty by sex shows that females are at a slight disadvantage compared to males (28.9% versus 28.0%, respectively). The proportion of indigence also was higher among females than among males (8.2% versus 7.8%).

The birth rate has shown a marked decline, especially during the 1960s. This trend has been associated with a decrease in the fertility rate, which was only 2.65 in the 1985–1990 period. In 1945 the birth rate was 35.5 per 1,000, and it remained at that level until the 1960s (36.3 per 1,000 in 1965), after which the rate dropped substantially as a result of programs that were implemented to encourage responsible parenthood. In 1975, the birth rate was estimated at 24.2 per 1,000 population; by 1995, it had dropped to 19.7 per 1,000. That same year, the fertility rate was 2.5 children per woman, which represents a large reduction compared with the rate of 3.2 reported in 1975.

Mortality and Morbidity Profile

After a sharp decline, mortality has leveled off in recent years. In 1995, the rate was 5.5 per 1,000 population. Total mortality in 1945 was around 19.1 per 1,000, a figure that fell by two-thirds during the 1970s (7.2 per 1,000 in 1975). In 1995, mortality among children aged 1 to 4 years was 0.6 per 1,000 population, maternal mortality was 0.3 per 10,000 live births, and mortality in the group aged 15 to 44 was 1.3 per 1,000 population. In the group aged 45 to 54, the mortality rate was 7.5 per 1,000 population, and among those aged 65 and over the rate was 51.4 per 1,000 population.

The leading causes of death in 1995 were diseases of the circulatory system, with a specific rate of 149.5 per 100,000 population (27.8% of all deaths that year); followed by malignant neoplasms, with a rate of 115.7 per 100,000 (20.7% of all deaths that year); injuries and poisoning, with a rate of 63.6 per 100,000 (11.8% of all deaths that year); and diseases of the respiratory system, with a rate of 61.2 per 100,000 (11.4% of all deaths that year).

With the changes in the above-mentioned indicators, life expectancy at birth in 1996 increased to 78.3 years for women, 72.3 for men, and 75.21 for both sexes. For the census interval 1920–1992, the change in these indicators represents an increase of 40.47 years in life expectancy at birth for females over the period (0.62 year per year during the interval), and 45.06 years for males (0.55 year per year during the interval).

There were sex differentials in the causes of death, notably the excess male mortality from injuries and poisoning (almost four times greater). Male mortality from diseases of the digestive system also was greater (1.60 times). Excess male mortality of 1.28-fold for conditions originating in the perinatal period and 1.26-fold for diseases of the central nervous system and sense organs is also observed. Excess female mortality exists in the case of diseases of the musculoskeletal system (3.22 times greater) and diseases of the skin and cellular and subcutaneous tissue (1.86 times greater). An analysis of the leading causes of death in 1960 by the National Statistics Institute reveals that, in that year, 26.2% of all deaths were due to enteritis, colitis, and pneumonia (ICD-7, A89, A104, A132). In 1995, these causes accounted for only 9.15% of all deaths (ICD-9, 008, 009, 480). In 1960, the group comprising arteriosclerosis and other heart diseases (ICD-7, A81 and A82) accounted for 5.69% of all deaths; that percentage rose to 14.43% in 1995 (ICD-9, 410–414, 415, and 416). In 1990 and 1995 no cases of measles were reported, whereas in 1960 measles still accounted for 2.15% of all deaths. Also in 1960, 3.9% of all deaths were caused by pulmonary tuberculosis (ICD-7, A1), whereas in 1995 only 0.5% of deaths were attributed to this cause (ICD-9, 010–012).

Mortality has decreased in all age groups, but the largest reductions have occurred among women and among children under the age of 5 years. In 1980, the latter group accounted for 12.7% of all deaths, and in 1994 it accounted for only 5.4%. The decline in mortality rates in the group aged 55 and older has been comparatively small, which increases the relative importance of older adults in total mortality figures for the country as a whole. Excess male mortality in 1994 was 1.25. For the period 1995–2005, life expectancy at birth was estimated at 75.2 years for both sexes: 78.3 years for females, and 72.3 years for males.

Analysis of mortality by cause in 1995 reveals that the four most frequent causes of death were acute myocardial infarction (ICD-9, 410), which accounted for 7.3% of all deaths that year; followed by bronchopneumonia (ICD-9, 485), which accounted for 5.9%; acute cerebrovascular disease (ICD-9, 436), which accounted for 4.4%; and cirrhosis and other chronic liver diseases (ICD-9, 571), which accounted for 4.2%.

Based on a study of the burden of disease conducted by the Ministry of Health, in which disability-adjusted life years (DALYs) were calculated, the five leading causes of death were congenital anomalies (7.53 per 1,000 population), acute lower respiratory infections (5.23 per 1,000 population), ischemic heart disease (4.9 per 1,000 population), hypertensive disease (4.37 per 1,000 population), and cerebrovascular disease (4.19 per 1,000 population).

A total of 1,404,478 hospitalizations were registered in both public and private institutions in 1996; most were for causes related to pregnancy, childbirth, and the puerperium. In 1995, the occupancy rate in public hospitals was 69.7, with an average hospital stay of 7.10 days and 33.7 discharges per bed. In private-sector establishments, a total of 370,811 discharges were reported, with an average stay of 5.7 days, an occupancy rate of 57.5, and 32.1 discharges per bed.

The leading reason for outpatient consultations is high blood pressure. By groups of causes, diseases of the respiratory system account for the largest proportion of health service visits (24.0%) and are the reason for about 40% of all visits at the primary care level.

The consultation rate per person, which in 1985 was 1.28, decreased to 1.07 in 1996. Of the total number of consultations and routine visits in 1996, almost one-third (30.6%) were children, and of them about 10% were routine well-child visits. Another 10% of the consultations took place in the

framework of the Women's Health Program, and 55% were adult medical visits.

The ratio of nurses to doctors attending children at well-child visits has shown a sustained decline since 1981. In that year, nurses were performing 8.8 well-child examinations for every examination performed by a physician; in 1996, the ratio was 6.03, which is a reflection of the shortage of nurses in the country, especially at the primary care level. The ratio for health service visits for reasons other than well-child care was 0.03 in 1996.

SPECIFIC HEALTH PROBLEMS

Analysis by Population Group

Health of Children

Infant mortality has shown a marked decline, which has continued in recent years, as a result of the sharp reduction in birth rates and high rates of prenatal care and professional care at childbirth. In 1995, 99.50% of births were attended by trained birth attendants. Other factors contributing to the reduction in infant mortality include the extensive coverage of child growth and development monitoring programs, vaccination programs, and supplementary feeding programs; rising educational levels, especially among women; improvements in basic sanitation; and use of perinatal treatment technologies. In 1945, the infant mortality rate was estimated at 165 per 1,000 live births, whereas in 1995 it was only 11.1 per 1,000 live births. The neonatal mortality rate was 6.1 per 1,000 live births in 1995, the late infant mortality rate was 5.0 per 1,000, and the early neonatal rate was 4.5 per 1,000. In 1975, infant deaths accounted for more than one-third of total mortality, and in 1995 they accounted for only 3.96%. Neonatal deaths in 1995 accounted for 57.1% of all deaths in the age group under 1 year old.

With regard to the distribution of mortality in the country, regional disparities in infant mortality were noted in 1995, with rates ranging from a low of 9.6 per 1,000 in Magallanes to a high of 14.6 per 1,000 in Antofagasta. The regions with the highest infant mortality rates, after Antofagasta, are Araucanía (14.3 per 1,000 live births) and Biobío (14.1 per 1,000 live births).

With regard to differences in mortality by living conditions, infant mortality in 1994 in the Western Santiago Health Service, which serves the rural and most impoverished population, was 11.4 per 1,000; in the Eastern Metropolitan Health Service, which serves a higher-income population, the rate was 7.6 per 1,000 live births.

Better nationwide coverage of the Expanded Program on Immunization (EPI) and the cold chain resulted in fewer deaths from vaccine-preventable diseases in the past decade. The coverage of BCG vaccine in 1996 reached 97.99 per 100 newborns. In the same year, the coverage with three doses of DTP (diphtheria, tetanus, and pertussis) was 94.16 per 100 newborns, and coverage with three doses of polio vaccine was 94.26 per 100 newborns. Mortality from diphtheria fell to 0 in 1992. The last death from this cause occurred in 1991. The measles mortality rate decreased from 0.2 in 1989 to 0 in 1990, and since then no deaths from this cause have been reported.

Mortality among children aged 1 to 4 has fallen to 0.6 per 100,000 population in this age group in 1995. This reduction has been associated with the expansion in coverage of primary health care in urban and rural areas and in coverage of EPI, as well as the decrease in morbidity and mortality from vaccine-preventable infectious diseases—in particular, mortality from diarrheal diseases and acute respiratory infections.

Since 1975, the maternal and child health program in Chile has been applying a high-risk approach in obstetric and perinatal care. One of the results of this approach has been a steady decline in the percentage of low-birthweight infants, which fell from 5.7% in 1991 to 5.0% in 1995.

Some improvement also has been noted in nutritional deficiency indicators among children under the age of 6 years participating in regular growth monitoring programs in public health establishments, with slight but sustained decreases in nutritional disorders. At the same time, however, there has been a slight increase in the prevalence of overweight.

In 1996, 60% of hospital discharges of children under the age of 2 years were associated with respiratory causes.

With respect to outpatient consultations, the country has no nationwide tracking system. Data are available only for 1990, when 57% of medical visits by children under the age of 15 were for acute respiratory infections, 18% were for infectious and parasitic diseases, and 9% were for skin diseases.

In studies conducted in 1990 among children enrolled in preschools operated by the National School Assistance and Scholarship Board, 11 episodes of acute illness per child were recorded in children observed over a period of 100 months, 57% of which were due to respiratory infections, 13.9% to skin diseases, and 10.5% to diarrheal diseases. The comprehensive school health system of the Ministry of Health, which covers children aged 6 to 10 who attend municipal and publicly subsidized private schools, reports that 5.8% of all schoolchildren have visual deficiencies, 8.2% have posture problems, and 2.2% have hearing problems. Programs have been implemented to refer schoolchildren with these types of problems to medical specialists in the public and private sectors.

With regard to hospital discharges, the available data indicate that for 1993 the principal cause associated with hospital discharge in the group aged 10 to 14 was injury and poisoning, which was associated with 704.9 discharges per 100,000 population. The next most frequent causes were diseases of the digestive system (569.28 discharges per 100,000 population) and diseases of the respiratory system (404.68 discharges per 100,000 population). As for sex differentials, among males aged 10 to 14, the most frequent causes associated with hospital discharge were injuries (955.99 per 100,000 population) and diseases of the digestive system (625.60 per 100,000 population); among females in the same age group, the most frequent causes were diseases of the digestive system (511.4 per 100,000 population) and injury (445.40 per 100,000 population).

Health of Adolescents

Adolescents in Santiago suffer 2.8 episodes of illness per year, with a medical consultation rate of 1.58 per person in 1995. Based on studies carried out in 1990, ill-defined causes account for the largest proportion of these episodes, followed by acute respiratory infections and digestive disorders. Of the patients referred to the secondary care level, 40% were psychiatric patients, 18% were ophthalmology patients, 11% were dermatology patients, and 5% were trauma patients.

The most frequent cause associated with hospital discharges in the group aged 15 to 19 years is childbirth (2,272 per 100,000 population), followed by injuries and poisoning (823.65 per 100,000 population). In this age group, addiction is a serious problem, to which the Government has assigned high priority. The National Drug Abuse Control Council (CONACE) has implemented a national drug information system. In 1994, CONACE surveyed 8,271 persons age 12 to 64, who represented 80% of the population in the country's urban areas and five geographic regions (Norte Grande, Norte Chico, Santiago metropolitan region, Zona Sur, and Zona Austral). The survey found a lifetime prevalence of drug use (i.e., use of at least one of three illicit drugs—marijuana, cocaine paste, and cocaine hydrochloride—at least once in a lifetime) of 9.43% among those aged 12 to 18 for the country as a whole. By region, the highest lifetime prevalence rates were found in Norte Grande (the Tarapacá and Antofagasta regions), where the rate was 9.7%, and the Santiago metropolitan region, where the rate was 12.4%. Lower rates occurred in Zona Sur (Libertador B. O'Higgins, Maule, and Biobío), where the lifetime prevalence was 6.4%. The lowest rate was found in Zona Austral (Araucanía, Los Lagos, Aysén, and Magallanes), with a prevalence of 5.0%. Norte Chico (Atacama, Coquimbo, Valparaíso) had a prevalence of 7.1%. With regard to the types of drugs used among young people aged 12 to 18, the CONACE study showed that the lifetime prevalence by drug used was 9.03% for marijuana, 1.92% for cocaine paste, and 1.57% for cocaine. For all those surveyed, use of cocaine paste was found to be most frequent among those in the lower socioeconomic strata (lifetime prevalence of 3.16%), and cocaine use was most frequent among those in the upper-middle and upper income groups (lifetime prevalence of 3.24% and 3.59%, respectively). By region, the lifetime prevalence is 3.9% in Norte Grande, 1.0% in Norte Chico, 2.6% in the Santiago metropolitan region, 1.1% in Zona Sur, and 0% in Zona Austral.

The prevalence of tobacco use in the month immediately preceding the survey was 24.27% among young people aged 12 to 18. In the same age group, the prevalence of alcohol use in the month immediately preceding the survey was 24.04% and that of tranquilizer use was 1.08%.

Health of Adults

In 1994, mortality in the group aged 15 to 59 was 2.21 per 1,000 population; male mortality was double female mortality, with little variation in rates by region. Sex differentials were noted mainly in relation to accidents and violence (118.05 per 100,000 population among males versus 18.80 per 100,000 among females) and in diseases of the circulatory system (43.84 per 100,000 population among males and 25.01 per 100,000 among females).

Mortality in the group aged 15 to 44 decreased slightly, dropping from 12.6% in 1984 to 11% in 1995, and the rate in the group aged 45 to 64 decreased to 7.6 per 100,000 persons in this age group. By groups of causes, proportional mortality from infectious diseases decreased for both sexes (from 3.6% of all deaths in 1984 to 2.7% in 1995), as did the rate for external causes (from 12.4% in 1984 to 11.3% in 1995) and that of diseases of the circulatory system (from 28.4% in 1984 to 26.9% in 1995). The proportion of deaths due to malignant neoplasms increased (from 16.6% of all deaths in 1984 to 21.7% in 1995), as did the proportion due to endocrine and metabolic disorders (from 2.3% in 1984 to 3.6% in 1995).

Health of the Elderly

Adults over the age of 60 make up 9.71% of the country's population. Deaths in this age group in 1995 totaled 54,527 (69.4% of all deaths that year), yielding a mortality rate of 39.1 per 1,000. By cause, in 1994 diseases of the circulatory system and malignant neoplasms together accounted for 57.1% of all deaths; the next most frequent groups of causes were respiratory diseases (13.5%) and digestive diseases (6.1%). With regard to hospital discharges, the rate in 1993 was 174.8 discharges per 1,000 population in the over-65 age group. The most frequent causes of hospitalization were diseases of the circulatory system, which generated 35,418 discharges, for a rate of 41.19 discharges per 1,000 population, followed by diseases of the respiratory, digestive, and genitourinary systems; injuries; and malignant neoplasms.

According to data from the only existing study on the needs of the elderly in urban areas, which was conducted in 1984 in a population sample of 1,500 older adults, 71.9% indicated that they suffered from some disease. Of that percentage, 17.7% had a disease of the circulatory system and 14.9% had a disease of the musculoskeletal system (14.9%).

According to the results of the 1992 CASEN, 65.2% of the elderly persons surveyed said they had suffered no episodes of acute illness or accidents during the preceding three months, and most of those who indicated they had been ill (close to 90%) had received medical attention. Around 70% required medication; 57% of them were able to acquire drugs they needed (31.8% purchased them and 18% received them free of charge). The survey also showed that 75% of the population over 65 years of age is covered by the public health care system, 11% go to private physicians, 5% receive care through private health insurance institutions (ISAPREs), and 4% are covered under the Armed Forces health care system.

Health of Women and Families

Maternal mortality, which increased to 30 per 100,000 live births in 1995, has shown a leveling-off trend. In 1960, the rate was estimated at 300 per 100,000 live births, and one-third of the deaths were attributed to abortion. The Responsible Parenthood Program has helped to substantially reduce maternal deaths.

With respect to domestic violence, in 1993 it was estimated that one of every four women, regardless of socioeconomic level, had been the victim of physical or psychological abuse. One-third of women acknowledged having been a victim of psychological abuse. Surveys conducted by UNICEF in 1995 reveal that only 22% of minors interviewed had never suffered any type of abuse, and 34% had suffered severe physical abuse. In response to these high rates, initiatives have been mounted to provide prevention and/or assistance services to victims, and legal changes have been promoted with a view to increasing protection for minors who are victims of violence.

The marriage rate has fallen from 7.5 per 1,000 population in 1990 to 6.1 per 1,000 in 1995. A total of 87,205 marriages took place in the latter year.

Workers' Health

In 1993, an estimated 68% of the employed labor force had some kind of protection against occupational health problems, generally in the form of insurance covering occupational risks (work-related accidents and diseases). This insurance is administered by one of three authorized institutions—the workers' compensation fund, which covers 24% of the employed labor force; employers' mutual insurance, which covers 74% of the employed labor force; and authorized insurance administration companies, which cover the remaining 2%. Oversight functions are carried out by the health services.

Available data indicate that the accident rate in 1993 for workers covered by mutual insurance was 12.5 per 100 covered workers, with significant variations by region and sector of activity (for example, the accident rate is higher in the construction, industry, mining, and agriculture sectors). The accident rate is inversely correlated with the size of the company, which is explained by the fact that all companies with more than 100 employees are required to have a department of risk prevention.

A large proportion of work-related health problems are not reported to the National Health Services System (SNSS). The most frequent claims are for diseases of the skin, hearing disorders, and musculoskeletal system diseases. Based on available information, in 1992 the most frequent work-related health problems were dermatitis, hearing loss, and tendinitis.

Health of the Disabled

Data from the 1992 census indicate that there were 283,888 persons in Chile with some kind of disability (total blindness, total deafness, muteness, paralysis, or mental impairment), which is 2.12% of the total population. Disability is slightly more common among males (male/female ratio, 1.16). The most frequent disability is paralysis (36.2%), followed by mental impairment (30.4%), deafness (21.1%), blindness (14.5%), and muteness (4.8%). Blindness is the only disability that is more frequent among females.

According to available data, in 1955 the pension administration system paid 4,131 disability pensions; 82% were for total disability. The most frequent reasons are psychiatric disorders, followed by neurological disorders, heart problems, and cancer, with significant variations according to age and sex.

Health of Indigenous People

Available epidemiological information, although incomplete, shows that the communes with the largest concentrations of indigenous populations have lower health indicators than the rest of the country. One recent study yields an epidemiological profile based on information from 39 communes where 20% or more of the population is indigenous. The infant mortality rate in the period 1988–1992 varied among different indigenous groups: among the Aymará the rate was 40 per 1,000 live births; among the Atacameños, 57 per 1,000; among the Rapa Nui, 32 per 1,000; and among the Mapuche, 34 per

1,000. Health conditions among the indigenous population appear to have deteriorated more in urban areas than in rural ones. The conclusions of the aforementioned study constitute a first step toward characterizing the health situation of indigenous communities throughout Chile.

Analysis by Type of Disease

Communicable Diseases

Vector-Borne Diseases. *Triatoma infestans* is present in Chile between the 18°30′ and 38°35′ parallels, an area that encompasses regions I (Tarapacá), II (Antofagasta), III (Atacama), and IV (Coquimbo). The population exposed to Chagas' disease numbers 500,000 persons, distributed among 43 communes. Based on serological studies, 19% of the population is seropositive. In the endemic areas, blood is regularly screened in the blood banks of the 57 hospitals that serve 75.7% of the donors in the country. The most recent data available on the incidence of the disease, which date from 1994, indicate a rate of 3.3 per 100,000 population. It is estimated that in 1996 there were a total of 11,721 infested households in regions I and IV. Control programs applied in these regions in 1995 reduced the percentage of infested households from 51% to 2%.

Mortality from hydatidosis decreased from 0.5 per 100,000 population in 1981 to 0.24 per 100,000 in 1994 (34 cases). In 1994 an incidence rate of 2.4 per 100,000 population was reported (332 cases). The prevalence of hydatidosis in slaughterhouses has remained stable at about 10% of slaughtered animals.

There are no known cases of yellow fever. Eight cases of malaria were reported in 1994. No up-to-date studies exist on *Aedes aegypti* infestation in urban areas.

Vaccine-Preventable Diseases. The incidence of diphtheria in 1995 was 0.01 per 100,000 (two cases). The rate has decreased slowly but steadily, with periodic variations. Between 1991 and 1995, 25, 12, 8, 4, and 3 cases, respectively, were reported. Fewer than five deaths have been reported every year since 1987, and no diphtheria deaths have been reported since 1991 (one case).

The number of cases of whooping cough reported in the past five years has varied, because the disease tends to occur in cyclical outbreaks. In 1990, 59 cases were reported, with two deaths; in 1991, 61 cases and two deaths; in 1992, 264 cases and four deaths; in 1992, 59 cases and two deaths; in 1993, 517 cases; in 1994, 10 cases; and in 1995, 361 cases, with no deaths. Two outbreaks were reported during the period 1992–1997. The first occurred in 1993, when the incidence rate was 4.3 per 100,000 population (517 cases and five deaths), and the second occurred in 1996, when the rate was 5.0 per 100,000 population (600 cases and two deaths).

Measles also tends to occur in epidemic cycles of approximately four years' duration. The last outbreak was in 1988, when 45,079 cases were reported, with a morbidity rate of 351 per 100,000. In 1989, there were 13,008 cases. In 1990, the number decreased to 1,958, with no deaths. In 1991 the number of cases rose again to 2,098, but in 1992 it dropped to 397 cases, two of which were fatal. Since 1993, no measles deaths have occurred. Morbidity has been successfully controlled thanks to two national vaccination campaigns conducted in 1992 and 1996 and subsequent active epidemiological surveillance. Between 1993 and 1996, the country had only two cases, both imported; the last case occurred in 1993.

No cases of poliomyelitis were reported during the 1976–1996 period.

Tetanus has been controlled in the country. Incidence rates have remained very low: 0.4 per 100,000 population in 1971 (41 cases) and 0.1 per 100,000 population in 1994 (11 cases, no deaths). No cases of neonatal tetanus occurred in 1995, and in 1994 only 1 of the 11 cases reported was neonatal.

The incidence of rubella has shown a downward trend, with noncyclical outbreaks; the last occurred in 1988. The rate fell from 54.9 per 100,000 population in 1990 to 16.5 per 100,000 in 1994.

Cholera and Other Intestinal Infectious Diseases. Since the outbreak of cholera in 1991—in which there were 41 confirmed cases, with a case fatality rate of 4.8%—the disease has been under control. The last reported case was in 1994.

The number of cases of typhoid and paratyphoid fever decreased by more than 50% between 1980 and 1990. In 1990 the incidence rate was 39.3 per 100,000 (5,172 cases). The reported death rate for that same period was 0.22 per 100,000. However, two distinct phases can be identified in the trend of the disease during the period: between 1980 and 1983, the rate rose from 97.6 to 119.8 per 100,000 and then began to fall again until 1990. The cholera outbreak in 1991 led to the application of a series of control measures, which also brought about a spectacular reduction in typhoid fever as well as hepatitis. In 1994, the morbidity rate for the latter disease was the lowest in Chile's history: 11.2 per 100,000 population (1,565 cases).

Hepatitis A is the most frequently reported sanitation-related enteric disease in the country. The incidence rate between 1980 and 1984 increased from 36.7 to 107.6 per 100,000, subsequently falling to 66.5 per 100,000 in 1990 (11,400 cases). Since the start of the cholera epidemic, the incidence of hepatitis A has declined dramatically from 66.6 in 1991 (8,909 cases) to 38.9 per 100,000 in 1992 (5,291 cases). However, after that year, the rate began to climb again, and in 1994 it reached 90.8 per 100,000 population (12,732 cases).

The rates in these years were higher in regions outside the Santiago metropolitan area. As for hepatitis B, 125 cases were reported in 1994, for a rate of 0.9 per 100,000 population. That same year, three deaths were attributed to the disease (0.02 per 100,000 population). With regard to hepatitis C, it is estimated that <1% of the Chilean population is infected. Studies of blood banks in the country indicate antibody prevalence rates of between 0.15% and 0.35%.

Chronic Communicable Diseases. Mortality from tuberculosis in 1994 was 2.84 per 100,000 population. The rate has been reduced by one-third compared with the rate observed 10 years ago (12.2 in 1980). The prevalence has also decreased from 55.0 per 100,000 in 1985 to 41.1 in 1991 and to 29.5 in 1994 (4,138 cases). In 1994, 6,636 persons were hospitalized for tuberculosis; 81% had the pulmonary form. The median age of the patients was 42.5 years. The incidence rates currently being reported by health services show significant changes, and cases are being reported in children under the age of 15. During the 1989–1996 period, 40,000 cases and 3,800 deaths were reported. In 1994, new cases of tuberculosis totaled 3,646 (60% in males), and 4% of these new cases were in children under the age of 15. Of all the cases reported in 1994, 75% were pulmonary tuberculosis; of these, 62% were smear-positive.

Leprosy cases exist only in Region V, Easter Island. No new cases were reported during the 10-year period between 1984 and 1993, and six new cases were reported between 1994 and 1996.

Acute Respiratory Infections. Acute respiratory infections were the third leading cause of death in the general population in 1990 and the second leading cause in 1994 (5.2% of the total number of deaths). Among children under 1 year of age, acute respiratory infections accounted for 9.3% of all deaths in 1994. The infant mortality rate from pneumonia (ICD-9, 480–486) decreased from 3.04 per 1,000 live births in 1985 to 1.27 in 1994 as a result of the application of specific intervention strategies during the periods of highest incidence. According to hospital discharges associated with this cause, bronchopneumonia accounted for 60% of hospitalizations among children under 1 and for 46% among children aged 1 to 4. This cause is associated with 9.4% of all discharges in all age groups. Respiratory infections are also an important cause of pediatric medical visits in primary care centers and pediatric emergency services (generally, they are responsible for between 40% and 50% of all such visits). Among children under 2, respiratory infections are associated with 60% of all hospital discharges. Hospital discharge rates associated with this cause are very high among children under the age of 15 (2,000 per 100,000 discharges) and among adults over the age of 60 (4,000 per 100,000 discharges).

Rabies and Other Zoonoses. One case of human rabies was diagnosed in Chile in 1972. In 1996, one case occurred in a child in Region VI, following a bite by a vampire bat.

AIDS and Other STDs. The first AIDS cases were detected among males in Chile in 1984; the first female cases were detected the following year. As of March 1996, a total of 1,456 cases (92% in males and 8% in females), 909 deaths, and 2,203 carriers of the human immunodeficiency virus (HIV) had been reported. The male/female ratio was 10:1 for the 1992–1996 period, down from the ratio of 15:1 reported in 1984–1991. As of 31 December 1994, Chile had a cumulative rate of 8.8 cases per 100,000 population, which places it among the South American countries with moderate incidence of the disease. Sexual contact is the most common route of transmission (91%), especially in males. An increase in the incidence rate among the youngest members of the population has been observed over time. The most affected regions are the Santiago metropolitan region, Region V, and Region II. Sixty percent of the cases acquired through contact with infected blood are associated with intravenous drug use. AIDS surveillance in the country is carried out by sentinel centers that monitor specific population groups: blood donors, pregnant women, and patients in STD clinics. The results of this surveillance indicate that in the case of STD patients, who began to be monitored in 1992, the prevalence of HIV-positive individuals has remained stable (1% in 1992, 1% in 1993, and 0.66% in 1994 for all sentinel centers). With regard to the prevalence of HIV infection among pregnant women, an increase has been observed for all sentinel centers, with the rate rising from 0% in 1992 to 0.05% in 1993 and 0.1% in 1994. For blood donors, systematic screening was begun in 1987, and a slow but steady increase in prevalence has been noted (from 0.12 per 1,000 donations in 1988 to 0.31 per 1,000 donations in 1994).

In 1994 the most frequently reported STDs in Chile were syphilis (33.5 per 100,000 population), gonorrhea (26.1 per 100,000), and nongonococcal urethritis (5.9 per 100,000). Rates of syphilis have changed little in recent years, following a period of decline that ended in 1989. In 1994 a total of 4,705 cases were reported, with an incidence of 33.5 per 100,000 population. The incidence of gonorrhea has decreased in recent years, from a rate of 114 cases per 100,000 population in 1981 to 26.1 in 1994. It is known that the disease is underreported, although the number of cases that go unreported has not been determined. The majority of case reports come from public health establishments, and even in these establishments, it is believed that some cases are not reported.

Emerging and Re-emerging Diseases. The incidence of meningitis caused by *Neisseria meningitidis* has increased slightly in recent years, especially in the country's northern region. The rate increased from 0.6 per 100,000 population in 1971 to 3.38 per 100,000 in 1995. The disease affects mainly children under the age of 5 (55% of all cases), and there has been a relative increase in the number of cases in the group aged 5 to 9 years. Children between the ages of 0 and 9 years account for 70% of all cases.

The vaccine against *Haemophilus influenzae* type B was incorporated into the EPI in 1996 and is being administered to all children born after 1 May 1996. It is expected that 973,000 doses will be given in 1997.

In 1995 and 1996, two and three cases, respectively, of laboratory-confirmed Hantavirus infection were reported in Region X, in southern Chile. Three of these cases proved fatal. In 1995, two cases of hemolytic-uremic syndrome were reported after consumption of meat contaminated with enterohemorrhagic *Escherichia coli*.

Noncommunicable Diseases and Other Health-Related Problems

Nutritional Diseases and Diseases of Metabolism. The incidence of child malnutrition, as measured by weight-for-age, was 15% in 1975 and 5% in 1993. In June 1996 the Ministry of Health reported that only 0.6% of children under the age of 6 fell more than 2 standard deviations below the reference values established by the United States National Center for Health Statistics (NCHS). Integrated nutritional assessments, measured at similar points in time, show that 74.4% of children under 6 are classified as normal. Among pregnant women, the prevalence of underweight decreased from 26% in 1987 to 17% in 1996, and the proportion of overweight increased to 46% in 1994. The most recent available study of nutritional status in the child population whose growth was regularly monitored in public health establishments shows that, based on the aforementioned integrated nutritional assessment, 3.1% of children are at risk of malnutrition and 0.7% are malnourished. The majority of children (73.7%) have normal nutritional status, and 22% are overweight or obese. The reduction in child malnutrition is associated with the activities of the National Supplementary Feeding Program, increased coverage of child services, and improvements in the educational levels of mothers.

With regard to micronutrient deficiencies, a national study conducted in 1975 concluded that vitamin A deficiency does not exist in Chile. The incidence of anemia, according to studies by the Food Technology and Nutrition Institute (INTA), is 20% among children aged 6 to 24 months and 20% among pregnant women. Mandatory iodization of salt (in Chile 97% of salt is iodized) has contributed to the control of goiter. Nevertheless, studies of localized school populations in 1995 found a 9% prevalence of goiter.

Studies by the National Breast-Feeding Commission, created by the Ministry of Health to promote breast-feeding, reveal that 87% of children are breast-fed during the first month of life. By the fourth month, the percentage drops to 59%, and by the sixth month, to 25%. Other studies conducted in pediatric care services found that 57.1% of the population surveyed was exclusively breast-fed at 120 days of age.

Based on various studies, obesity is more prevalent among females (between 22.7% and 25.0%) than males (between 13.0% and 17.6%). Differences occur between men and women in different socioeconomic strata; for example, obesity is more frequent among females in lower socioeconomic strata and among males at higher socioeconomic levels.

The prevalence of diabetes ranges from 3.0% to 5.6%, according to various studies of the general population. Diabetes is the primary cause in a rising number of hospital admissions and is also frequently an associated cause. In 1990, 11,650 patients were hospitalized for diabetes mellitus, making the hospitalization rate 8.84 per 10,000 population and 35.8 per 10,000 population in the group aged 45 and over. Diabetes was associated with 70% of hospital discharges for endocrine causes. The increased prevalence of diabetes could be attributable to unhealthy lifestyles as well as to lower mortality from the disease because of better therapeutic management. At the primary care level, this diagnosis accounts for an estimated 2.9% of all visits.

Cardiovascular Diseases. For the past several years, this group of diseases has accounted for the largest proportion of mortality among Chileans, especially adults. More than one-fourth of all deaths are caused by cardiovascular diseases (20,922 in 1994, or 27.7% of all deaths that year, with a specific rate of 149.5 per 100,000 population). Within this group, ischemic heart disease, hypertensive disease, and cerebrovascular disease occur most frequently. According to information on hospitalized patients, cardiovascular diseases generated a hospitalization rate of 5.2 per 1,000 population in the general population in 1991, a 35% increase with respect to 1975. Ischemic heart disease (ICD-9, 410–414) accounts for the largest percentage of deaths. Myocardial infarction (ICD-9, 410) alone accounts for 25.9% of all deaths attributed to this group of causes.

Malignant Tumors. The trend of general mortality from this cause has been upward over the past decade. In 1980 mortality from malignant neoplasms was 101.6 per 100,000. The rate increased to 104.3 per 100,000 in 1987 and to 115.7 in 1994. In 1995, malignant neoplasms were the second leading cause of death in the country, accounting for 16,429 deaths (20.7%). The five most frequent cancer sites are the stomach (16.7%); trachea, bronchus, and lung (10.4%); gallbladder and bile ducts (10%); prostate (6.4%); breast (5.7%); and uterine cervix (4.5%).

In 1994 a total of 10,293 cases of cancer were reported (73.4 per 100,000 population). The most frequent types in females are cancer of the cervix (25.6% of all female cancer cases), breast (15.8%), and skin (8.7%). Among males, the most frequent types are cancer of the stomach (20.5% of all male cancer cases), prostate (12.2%), and lung (10.1%). The male/female case ratio is 0.68.

Accidents and Violence. In 1991 the mortality rate from injuries, poisoning, and violence was 69.1 per 100,000 population, and in 1994 it was 63.6 per 100,000. Accidents and violence have become increasingly prominent as causes of both mortality and morbidity. Persons under the age of 65 account for 84.8% of all deaths from this group of causes (compared with 44.5% for other causes) and persons under the age of 15 account for 16.5%. The latter group's share of mortality from violent causes has ranged between 11% and 12% over the past decade (11.8% in 1994). Thirty-eight percent of the deaths from this group of causes are due to accidents of all types; of these, almost one-fourth are motor vehicle accidents.

According to police records, the number of persons injured or killed annually in traffic accidents increased between 1980 and 1995 from 25,176 to 41,582, an average rise of 9.4% per year. The number of deaths went up from 1,191 to 1,747 over the same period, a 7.4% yearly increase. In 1996, police statistics show 1,925 traffic accident fatalities and a total of 60,093 accidents. In economic terms, private expenditures due to vehicle accidents totaled an estimated US$ 274 million in 1993, including the cost of injury to persons and damage to vehicles. The social cost of these accidents in 1993 is estimated at US$ 321 million, taking into account damage to vehicles, injuries, and deaths. A study of motor vehicle accidents in 1989 conducted by the Ministry of Health and the World Bank in 1993 revealed that about 5.8% of the vehicles in the country had been involved in some kind of accident, with figures ranging from 2.0% of the vehicle fleet in the regions of Coquimbo and O'Higgins up to 12.2% in the Aysén region. The percentage of public transportation vehicles involved in accidents, according to the aforementioned study, was 44.8%—almost half of all the vehicles were involved in some type of accident in 1989. When the information was classified by commune, it was found that this percentage was 63% in the case of public transportation vehicles in the Valparaíso region. This situation prompted the Government to create an interministerial commission on transportation safety, which has established the basic framework for public policy on this issue.

Behavioral Disorders. The prevalence of mental health problems has increased significantly in recent years. Several studies—most of them of small groups, specific groups, or both—provide indirect indicators. Of the medical leave certificates issued by the National Health Fund, 5.6% were for neuroses. In the case of certificates issued to ISAPRE beneficiaries, this percentage was 7.48% in 1994.

With regard to alcoholism, it is estimated that at present 20% of persons can be classified as problem drinkers; 15% of them are not dependent on alcohol, and 5% are dependent on alcohol. Alcoholism is more frequent among males and among persons who are unemployed or irregularly employed. It is the eighth leading cause of disability adjusted life years (DALY: 53,498, with 3.02%). Alcoholism is associated with 38% of hospital discharges. It is the primary cause reported in 4.5% of hospital discharges and in 7% of deaths, and it is an associated cause in 25% of deaths. Alcohol use is a factor in 48.6% of homicides, 38.6% of suicides, and 50% of traffic accidents.

According to information obtained from the CONACE survey, the prevalence of alcohol consumption during the month before the survey, without regard to the amount consumed, was 39.97% (50.23% among males and 31.03% among females). No major differences by age group were found; the lowest values were observed in the group aged 12 to 18 (24.04%), and the highest values were reported in the group aged 19 to 25 (49.74%). By socioeconomic level, higher prevalence was found in the upper and upper-middle strata (56.95% and 47.18%, respectively) than in the lower-middle (35.25%) and low-income (38.52%) groups. The study design included administration of the "Short Survey of Drinking Habits" to determine the percentage of alcohol drinkers who can be classified as problem drinkers. The results showed that 24% of the persons who said they had consumed alcohol in the past year fall into the category of problem drinkers (35.6% of the males and 11.1% of the females surveyed), with higher percentages in the lower socioeconomic groups: 41% in the low-income group and 32% in the lower-middle group, compared with 13.1% in the upper-income group and 11.5% in the upper-middle group. Most of those surveyed had started drinking before the age of 18 (71.35% of the males and 57.07% of the females). Drinking at an early age (before age 12) was more common in the lower socioeconomic strata (11.41%).

Specific mortality from cirrhosis of the liver was 20.8 per 100,000 population in 1994, one of the highest rates in the Region. Liver disease remains an important cause of death, especially cirrhosis, which is responsible for a significant proportion of alcohol- and tobacco-related mortality. The death rates from cirrhosis were 27.4 per 100,000 population in 1989, 28.5 in 1990, and 20.8 in 1994.

According to the CONACE drug addiction survey, among all the individuals aged 12 to 64 surveyed, the lifetime prevalence of illicit drug use (i.e., use of at least one of three illicit drugs: marijuana, cocaine paste, and cocaine) was 13.42%. The rate was 20.63% for males and 7.14% for females. This means that one of every eight Chileans between the ages of 12 and 64 has used one of these substances at some time. The lifetime prevalence is greater for all three drugs considered in the survey in the groups aged 19 to 25 years (22.23%) and 26

to 34 years (20.84%). The lifetime prevalence is also higher in the upper and upper-middle socioeconomic strata (21.11% and 15.35%, respectively) and lower in the lower socioeconomic stratum (11.73%). The most frequently used drug is marijuana (12.85%), followed by cocaine (2.35%) and cocaine paste (1.97%). The only major sex difference occurs in the case of cocaine use, which is six times more frequent among males (4.4%) than females (0.7%).

According to data from the 1994 CASEN, the prevalence of tobacco use is 38% in the male population and 25% in the female population. A slight decrease in prevalence has been noted among males (from 47% to 44%), and the prevalence among females has increased (from 36% to 41%). These data are similar to those generated by the 1995 CONACE, which found a prevalence of 45.43% among males and 36.25% among females. Tobacco use begins before the age of 12 in 8.15% of males and 4.21% of females. The prevalence of tobacco use in the month prior to the survey ranged from a high of 50.82% in the group aged 19 to 25 to a low of 24.27% in the group aged 12 to 18. The prevalence is higher in the upper socioeconomic stratum (42.31%) than in lower socioeconomic levels (31.78%).

The prevalence of use of legal drugs such as tranquilizers (especially benzodiazepines) in the month preceding the survey was 6.2% and was higher among females (8.37%) than males (3.71%). The differences by age range from a low of 1.08% in the group aged 12 to 18 to a high of 11.28% in the group aged 45 to 64. Use of this type of drug is much more frequent in the upper socioeconomic strata (10.77%) than in low-income groups (3.67%).

Oral Health. The estimated prevalence of dental caries in the population exceeds 90% and the average number of damaged teeth is 12 per person. Thirty-four percent of preschool children have dental caries. In the Santiago metropolitan region, the DMFT index (decayed, missing, filled teeth) in children with permanent dentition seen in outpatient services (6 to 18 years of age) was 6.27. Nevertheless, a slight improvement has been observed in these indexes, thanks to the large-scale application of various preventive interventions (education, fluoride rinses, and application of sealants), although the prevalence remains high in the adult and adolescent populations. Another problem is gingivitis, the prevalence of which is estimated at 37.7% in the population aged 6 to 12, and the rate increases with age. Studies conducted to date indicate a correlation between oral health problems and low educational and socioeconomic levels, which are considered risk factors for poor oral health. With regard to coverage of oral health services within the SNSS, it was estimated that in 1995 only 1.97% of the population had received such services. The population aged 0 to 9 had a coverage of 3.91%; the population aged 10 to 19, 2.46%; pregnant women, 0.85%; and the population over the age of 20 had a coverage rate of only 0.85%.

Natural Disasters and Industrial Accidents. Because of its geography, Chile is exposed to various types of natural phenomena that may endanger the population's health. These include earthquakes, landslides, and floods, which in the past decade have affected the population. In 1996, a drought in at least four regions of the country, including the metropolitan region, affected the agricultural sector and also reduced the water reservoirs used to generate electricity. At the same time, water supplies were insufficient for distribution of drinking water in certain sectors of the metropolitan region, which led to the implementation of various strategies aimed at reducing unnecessary consumption. Once this problem had been partially overcome, a new problem emerged due to the opposite climatic phenomenon—excessive rainfall, which produced a state of emergency, especially in the northern part of the country in the regions of Atacama and Coquimbo, both of which normally have a desert climate and so lack the necessary road and drainage infrastructure to deal with such a situation. Many families with limited resources lost their homes or possessions, and several deaths occurred in connection with the rescue operations mounted by social organizations in the most heavily damaged sectors.

In 1992, the city of Antofagasta was flooded by rainfall that saturated the ground around drinking water storage reservoirs, which affected a large segment of the city. In 1993, a similar phenomenon affected the area known as the Macul gorge in the Santiago metropolitan region as a result of rainfall in the mountains, which created a mass of mud and rock that buried a vast sector of the city, claiming more than 100 victims, who either died or disappeared.

Because the country is naturally prone to seismic activity, especially the area extending from the metropolitan region to the North, the population is subjected to earthquakes fairly often. The last one, which was of medium intensity, occurred in 1996 and affected Chile's central area.

Industrial accidents are a recent phenomenon. Their occurrence has led to the formation of teams responsible for prevention and for planning disaster response activities.

RESPONSE OF THE HEALTH SYSTEM

National Health Plans and Policies

Under the Constitution of 1980, health is considered a basic human right and it is the State's duty to ensure that all citizens are able to exercise their right to protect their health and to live in an unpolluted environment. The Constitution recognizes a dual system of health care, in that it guarantees each person's right to choose whether to receive care in the public or the private health care system. The function of the Ministry of Health is to ensure free and equal access to services for the promotion, protection, and recovery of health as well as rehabilitation services following illness. The Ministry also is responsible for coordinating, overseeing, and, where appropriate, executing activities in these areas.

The policies of the country's second democratically elected government are aimed, in broad terms, at bringing about reform of the State and eliminating extreme poverty. In the area of health, the Government is committed to improving the quality of life for all Chileans. In 1996, the Government undertook the modernization of the social sectors through greater efficiency in the use of resources and in the sector's organization, which is considered as fundamental for socioeconomic development and for improving the quality of life. Health planning in Chile is essentially decentralized. The Ministry formulates strategic lines of action and national goals, and the regional health services develop detailed plans and programs. The principal issues confronting the sector are the lack of equity among various regions and communes in the country and between the public and private sectors with respect to the distribution of resources and activities; limitations in the availability of resources and in the organization and management of the public subsector; and the need to ensure that health service users are treated with dignity and are viewed as the primary focus of health sector activities.

The Plan for Strengthening and Modernizing the Public Health Sector, which was carried out in 1994 and 1995, sought to improve efficiency and quality of care, particularly the care provided to the poorest segments of the population. The strategic lines of action under the plan were to transfer to the population the benefits of the modernization process that had been the focus of the government's attention during the first few years and to develop an integrated Social Security system to cover the entire population through a set of individual and collective benefits with mutual financing.

Health reform efforts in Chile are aimed mainly at reducing waiting lists, helping to overcome extreme poverty, humanizing health care and improving the treatment of users, strengthening and modernizing the public health care system, increasing social control and involvement in the health sector, improving coverage and quality of care for the elderly, enhancing health care for adolescents, and strengthening oversight of the ISAPREs.

Organization of the Health Sector

Institutional Organization

The unified public health care system that Chile adopted in 1952, which provided coverage for the entire population, has undergone significant change since 1980, particularly in establishing the ISAPREs and in transferring responsibility for management of primary health care establishments to the municipal level. These changes have been accompanied by decentralization of the management of the regional health services (of which there were 28 as of early 1997).

The public subsector comprises the agencies that make up SNSS: the Ministry of Health, the 28 regional health services distributed throughout the country, the National Health Fund (FONASA), the Public Health Institute, the Central Supply Clearinghouse, and the ISAPRE Authority. All of them have been decentralized. The sector also includes governmental institutions and enterprises that provide health care for their personnel.

In each region, the Ministry of Health is represented by a regional secretariat. The 28 health services and one specialized service (the Metropolitan Environmental Health Service) provide medical attention and health care services for the population in a specific geographic area through their health care establishments and units. Public sector health care personnel include 68,400 SNSS employees and 16,500 primary health care providers at the municipal level.

FONASA is the agency responsible for collecting, administering, and distributing state funds for health. Its main functions relate to financing health activities and to the capital investments required by the system. The agency has a central office and 13 regional offices for managing the free-choice modality, a health care scheme similar to the ISAPRE model in the private sector.

The Public Health Institute serves as the national reference laboratory and is responsible for regulating and supervising the public health laboratories designated by the Ministry of Health in the fields of microbiology, immunology, food science, pharmacology, clinical laboratory, environmental pollution, and occupational health.

The Central Supply Clearinghouse is responsible for centralized procurement and supply of drugs, laboratory and pharmaceutical products, surgical equipment, instruments, and other supplies needed by all agencies, entities, and individuals employed in or affiliated with the system.

The health services system comprises three levels of care (primary, secondary, tertiary), and each service carries out health promotion and protection functions, curative care, and rehabilitation in accordance with its respective level of complexity.

Decree N 1/3063, enacted in 1980, permits the transfer of responsibility for administration of primary health care establishments to the municipal level. The process, which was initiated in 1981, was intended to achieve greater administrative decentralization of the establishments and, at the same time, extend coverage, tailoring it to the needs of each community. It culminated in 1988, by which time responsibility for most primary health care facilities in urban and rural areas, as well as rural health posts and stations, had been transferred to the *municipios*.

The ISAPREs are private entities that withhold 7% of the salaries of workers who voluntarily and individually decide to become members of their health plans. Depending on the plan selected, the worker may be required to pay an additional premium. Generally, a copayment is also required when services are received; the amount varies depending on the plan selected and the time and point of service. When workers do not voluntarily join an ISAPRE, their 7% contribution goes to FONASA, which becomes responsible for their health insurance coverage. This institution also receives tax funds to finance care for the indigent and for the uninsured (self-employed workers, for example).

Health Legislation

Health sector reforms have required that existing legislation be modified extensively. The principal legal reforms currently under consideration are the draft law on professional remuneration and incentives, which reflects an agreement between the Ministry and health professionals; a series of proposed laws aimed at advancing the legislative effort at decentralization; a new law regulating the working conditions and compensation of physicians, dentists, and pharmacists; and draft legislation on bioethical issues such as transplants (this legislation has already been approved), artificial life support, assisted fertilization, and genetic manipulation. The major legislative matters remaining to be addressed include environmental legislation that would clearly define the role of the health sector in environmental issues and expansion of the scope of the law governing production and marketing of drugs.

In the framework of regional integration processes—specifically the Hipólito Unanue agreement (Andean Pact) and MERCOSUR and the Southern Cone Initiative—the country also is engaged in a process of harmonizing national health legislation in the subregion. To date, however, no viable proposals have been advanced for health legislation that would respond to present and future needs associated with regional integration.

The Chilean Congress is bicameral and each legislative chamber has a health commission. These commissions have become forums for debating health sector reform and other sectoral issues, especially the conflicts between the Government and associations of health professionals.

Management of the Health Sector

The legal framework for the process of health service decentralization is provided by the reforms of 1980. The population is covered by 28 regional health services, which enjoy autonomy of action, financing, and budgeting. These services form the core of the Chilean health system. Responsibility for primary health care is delegated to the *municipios,* which coordinate their activities with those of the regional services. The regional as well as municipal health services have financial autonomy and they are financed by either FONASA or ISAPRE, to whom they sell services. One of the fundamental aspects of health reform is separation of institutional functions. The Ministry of Health, historically the provider of basic health services in the country, has progressively adopted a governing and regulatory role; FONASA performs insurance and financial functions; and the regional health entities are responsible for providing service.

In the private sector, health insurance is provided by the 21 open ISAPREs and 15 restricted ISAPREs operating around the country. The open ISAPREs recruit their members from among the working population in general, while the restricted institutions cover workers only in certain companies, generally large businesses, such as mining, petroleum, and railroad companies. Services are provided to members in private clinics and public hospitals (about 10% of beds in public hospitals are available to ISAPRE members). Some ISAPREs have their own outpatient primary care services, but they generally do not provide hospital care.

From a financing standpoint, private participation in the Chilean health care system takes place through the ISAPREs and, in terms of service delivery, through outpatient care facilities and the 11,549 hospital beds available to this subsector, which represent 26.78% of all the hospital beds in the country, with an occupancy index of 57.5. For many years, the number of beds available in SNSS was around 33,000, but it began to decline in 1980, dropping to 31,579 in 1995. There are currently 3.5 beds per 1,000 beneficiaries in the public subsector and 3.0 beds per 1,000 population in the public and private subsectors combined.

Of the 35.3% of the population that receives care in the private sector, 23.7% are covered by ISAPREs, 2.7% by the Armed Forces health care system, 0.9% by other systems, and 8.0% cover their own health care expenses.

Beneficiaries of the public system (FONASA) make up 64.47% of the total population, while beneficiaries of ISAPREs constitute 27%, including the 1.3% who are members of restricted ISAPREs. The rest of the population (9.05%) receives health care from the Armed Forces and police systems or from private or alternative health care providers.

Insurance and Coverage

In 1995 SNSS provided 2.53 consultations per beneficiary; open ISAPREs, 2.9; and restricted ISAPREs, 4.9. In the case of SNSS, if services provided by nonphysicians (nurses, mid-wives, and auxiliary personnel) are taken into account, the proportion rises to 4.04 visits per beneficiary.

In 1995 a total of 1.4 million patients were discharged from all inpatient care facilities in the country. SNSS registered 1,064,000 discharges, with a yield of 33.7 discharges per bed. In the private sector, the proportion was 32.1 discharges per bed. In 1996, the SNSS had 116.2 discharges per 1,000 beneficiaries; the open ISAPREs, 86.4; and the restricted ISAPREs, 139.8. The hospitalization rate (the discharge/consultation ratio) was 4.58% in the SNSS, 2.50% in the restricted ISAPREs, and 2.76% in the open ISAPREs. In the public sector, if consultations provided by nonphysician personnel are considered, the rate is 2.86%.

In public and private establishments, a rate of 2.18 laboratory exams per person was reported in 1996. In the case of imaging studies, the rate was 0.21 per person, and for pathological anatomy studies it was 0.05. The ratio of clinical laboratory exams to consultations was 2.04. The ratio of imaging studies to consultations was 0.20, and that of pathological anatomy studies to consultations was 0.05.

The rate of major surgeries per 100 population in 1996 was 2.67, and the rate of minor surgical procedures per 100 population was 4.82, for a total of 7.49 surgical procedures of all types per 100 population.

Organization of Health Regulatory Activities

The construction of new private health care facilities is regulated by the General Construction and Building Ordinance, which contains a specific chapter on hospital buildings and health care establishments. The regional health services are responsible for authorizing the construction of such establishments.

In 1981 the military government modified the 1948 law on professional associations—which made the College of Physicians responsible for ethical oversight of the profession—and eliminated mandatory physician membership in the College. This has had serious ethical ramifications, as well as consequences for the control over the practice of medicine, because an estimated 20% to 30% of practicing physicians are not members of the College. Currently there are four proposed laws before the National Congress that seek to correct this situation.

The Chilean drug market generates close to US$ 400 million annually. About half the drugs sold are produced in national laboratories and the other half are imported. Under recently updated legislation (March 1997), drug registration falls under the responsibility of the Public Health Institute. Inspections are carried out by the regional health services, and the necessary tests and analyses are conducted by the Public Health Institute.

Health Services and Resources

Organization of Services for Care of the Population

Environmental Protection. The environmental regulatory system was strengthened through the enactment in 1994 of the Basic Law on the Environment and the adoption in April 1997 of regulations for environmental impact assessment in development projects. The implementation of this system has made it possible to disseminate information on levels of pollution in the capital on a daily basis and to declare environmental alerts and emergencies when pollution levels exceed 300 mg/m³, in which case strict restrictions are imposed on motor vehicle traffic and a large number of industries that are fixed sources of pollution are temporarily shut down.

In the Santiago metropolitan region, the Metropolitan Health Service is responsible for monitoring air quality and levels of pollution emitted by fixed sources. The Metropolitan Transport Service monitors mobile sources of pollution.

Monitoring of water quality is done by the General Water Division of the Ministry of Public Works. Marine waters are monitored by Directemar, an agency of the Ministry of the Navy. The regulations on water use are being updated by the National Commission on the Environment (CONAMA).

Food Safety. The Public Health Institute is responsible for controlling the quality of foods, but actual food quality control activities are carried out by the Ministry of Health through the regional health services, which monitor food quality through sampling, authorize the marketing of foods, monitor food-handling practices, and inspect the sanitary conditions in food establishments. The network of public health laboratories carries out analysis of food samples. The country's food legislation is currently being updated to bring it into line with international codes and standards.

Health Promotion. Chile is engaged in a major effort to increase health promotion activities. One of the principal activities is the organization of development councils (community participation councils) at the level of primary care services and establishments and in hospitals. In 1995, 40 development councils were operating, and by late 1996 the number had increased to 111.

Disease Prevention and Control Programs. Disease prevention and control activities are carried out by the municipally administered primary care services and the regional health services. The result of these activities can be seen in the figures: more than 95% immunization coverage, 99.5% attended births, and infant mortality of 12.0 per 1,000.

Epidemiological Surveillance Systems and Public Health Laboratories. The regional health services carry out epidemiological surveillance of communicable diseases through various intervention strategies that involve epidemiologists to control and monitor outbreaks. Traditional epidemiological surveillance models are being enhanced through the incorporation of data processing and transfer technology. One of the best experiences in this process is being carried out within the Atacama health service, which is using the Epivigil system and has adapted the NETSS surveillance model of the United States of America Centers for Disease Control and Prevention to the characteristics of the country's health services.

The national network of public health laboratories is coordinated and controlled by the Public Health Institute through the Program for External Evaluation of Clinical Laboratory Quality (PEEC), which includes eight clinical laboratory sections (clinical chemistry, hematology, parasitology, syphilis serology, bacteriology, immunology, virology, and mycobacteria). All the sections have subprograms for the specialties they evaluate. The organization and administration of PEEC, which is the responsibility of the Public Health Institute, calls for a minimum of two and a maximum of four evaluations per year by each subprogram for each of the establishments affiliated with the program. In March 1997 a total of 886 clinical laboratories were affiliated: 201 public; 77 municipal; 56 within the health systems of the Armed Forces, universities, or religious entities; and 552 private laboratories. In addition to these laboratories, there are 128 blood banks, 75 public and 53 private. All blood banks are required to screen for HIV, hepatitis B, syphilis, and, in endemic zones, Chagas' disease. The PEEC makes it possible to monitor compliance with established quality standards. During 1996, a total of 883 laboratories and 57 blood banks took part in the program, a participation level of 88%.

Drinking Water and Sewerage Services. Ninety-eight percent of the urban population and 67.3% of the rural population has access to safe drinking water. The coverage of sewerage systems is 84.7% in urban areas, although 97% of wastewater is disposed of in waterways without prior treatment.

Water use is 184 liters per person per day in urban areas and 50 liters per person per day in rural areas. One hundred percent of the population that has drinking water service receives chlorinated water.

Solid Waste Disposal. Solid waste collection coverage is 98% in urban areas; 74.2% of the waste collected is disposed of in sanitary landfills. Of the industrial waste generated in 1995 in the metropolitan region, 3.0% was classified as hazardous.

Food Aid Programs. Since the 1920s, Chile has been carrying out supplementary feeding activities. In 1952 these activities were consolidated under the National Supplementary Feeding Program (PNAC). This program, which has demonstrated remarkable stability over the years, largely explains the improvement in the country's infant mortality and immunization indicators (vaccination is carried out in conjunction with supplementary feeding). In 1994, PNAC accounted for 9.12% of total public spending on health.

Organization and Operation of Personal Health Care Services

Outpatient, Hospital, and Emergency Services. The health care establishments affiliated with the regional health services are organized in a network. The municipally administered primary care services also are linked to the regional services and are coordinated by the services through their primary care division, program division, or integrated care divisions.

In 1995, the public health system included 187 hospitals, 15 urban outpatient clinics administered by the SNSS, 215 municipally administered urban outpatient clinics, 146 rural outpatient clinics, and 1,102 rural health posts (without a permanent staff physician). Of the hospitals, 20 (11,855 beds) are high-complexity institutions; 30 are type-2 hospitals, or hospitals with several specialized departments (8,019 beds); 23 are type-3 hospitals, or hospitals that provide care in several basic specialties (4,114 beds); and 105 are operated by general practitioners (5,332 beds).

A network of emergency and prehospital care units operates within several health services in the Santiago metropolitan region, Valparaíso, and Viña del Mar. The prehospital care services are staffed by auxiliary personnel in some cases and by a physician (French SAMU model) in others, which has improved the quality of care in these units.

Auxiliary Diagnostic Services and Blood Banks. With a view to improving the quality of care at the secondary level, since 1994 autonomous diagnostic units (laboratory services and imaging) have been established, especially in the metropolitan region, as well as diagnostic and treatment centers annexed to hospitals and referral centers.

Of the 160 blood banks that existed in the country in 1993, 118 (73.7%) were public, 31 (19.3%) were private, and the rest were associated with the Armed Forces health services (4.4%), universities (1.3%), and independent private establishments (1.3%). In 1996, the Public Health Institute reported that the country had 128 blood banks (58.5% public and 41.4% private).

Specialized Services. In 1994, SNSS had 37 psychiatric establishments with 1,334 beds. The National Mental Health Plan, a comprehensive normative effort, is currently being implemented with the support of multidisciplinary units in the 28 regional health services. The plan seeks to integrate mental health patients into the community through group homes, sheltered workshops, and night hospital services, in addition to delegating responsibility for the care of these patients to primary health care services. The mental health units in the 28 regional health services are concerned mainly with promotion and prevention activities and with the identification of problems that require urgent attention, such as health and violence, alcohol and drug use, child and adolescent mental health, emotional disability, and rehabilitation.

Since 1990 the country has had an oral health program oriented toward health promotion and prevention of oral health problems. Thirty-eight percent of the population receives fluoridated water, and in the regions where this does not occur schoolchildren receive fluoride rinses through programs that currently cover 900,000 of the almost 2 million schoolchildren in the country. In addition, an oral health education program is carried out jointly by the Ministry of Education and the *municipios,* and the decayed, missing, filled teeth (DMFT) index and fluorosis problems are monitored. With regard to oral health care, there is an active effort to introduce new technology, with intensive use of auxiliary personnel. The number of required hours of study has been increased (from 350 to 1,200 hours) in training programs for dental assistants, and practical training is being incorporated into the education programs for oral health professionals. In 1992 one school of dentistry (Temuco) introduced a curriculum that emphasizes the use of new technology.

Inputs for Health

Drugs. Under recently updated legislation (March 1997), the Public Health Institute is responsible for registration and quality control of drugs, foods for medicinal use, cosmetics, and pesticides used for health and domestic purposes. The Public Health Institute also is responsible for the control, authorization, and inspection of establishments that manufacture pharmaceutical products, cosmetics, and pesticides throughout the country. Inspection of warehouses, drugstores, and distributors of these products is carried out by the regional health services; testing and analysis is done by the Public Health Institute.

Immunobiologicals. Chile's Public Health Institute is the official producer of biologicals for the country. The Institute manufactures rabies vaccine from suckling mouse brain for human and canine use. The volume of production is sufficient to fully meet domestic demand; it is also exported to seven countries in the Region. The quality of the manufacturing process for this product has helped to reduce the incidence of rabies and has enabled the Public Health Institute to collaborate in quality control of rabies vaccine produced by other centers in the region. The Institute is also the sole producer in the country of the triple (DTP) and mixed (DT) vaccines, which are prepared with standard strains and by established procedures in sufficient quantities to meet domestic demand with a product of acceptable potency and efficacy. Another product made by the Public Health Institute is the whole-cell typhoid vaccine, which is administered mainly to food-handlers and military personnel. The Public Health Institute also produces purified protein derivative (PPD) for detection of tuberculosis, Rotagel for diagnosis of rotavirus, and standard antigen for diagnosis of rabies. The other vaccines are imported and the Public Health Institute is responsible for quality control.

Reagents. A recently modified law, which introduced changes in the Health Code, regulates quality control activities for a series of products with a view to ensuring their safety and efficacy. The Public Health Institute is currently drafting regulations that will define its inspection functions. Among the products subject to inspection are instruments, equipment, diagnostic reagents, and articles or elements used in the prevention, diagnosis, and treatment of human diseases, as well as prostheses used for anatomical replacement or modification.

Quality control will be carried out in establishments expressly authorized by the Public Health Institute in accordance with technical specifications established by the Ministry of Health based on proposals by the Public Health Institute. No product will be marketed unless it has been subjected to quality control procedures or received a quality certificate issued by an authorized entity.

Human Resources

Of the 13,857 physicians practicing in the country in 1966, 66.2% worked in the public sector and 7,831 were affiliated with SNSS; 11.7% of them practiced at the municipal level. Of the 5,817 dentists, 26.1% worked in the public sector and 8.75% at the municipal level. Of the 6,738 nurses, 59.0% worked in the public sector and 14.5% at the municipal level. As for midwives (5,369), 54.6% worked in the public sector, 17.1% at the municipal level. Of the 1,830 chemists and pharmacists in the country, 15.9% worked in the public sector and 1.5% at the municipal level. With regard to paramedical personnel, 26,972 practiced in the public sector, 19.5% of them at the municipal level. In 1996 the country had 0.54 physicians, 0.07 dentists, 0.22 nurses, 0.14 midwives, and 1.54 auxiliary personnel per 1,000 population.

Training. Undergraduate training programs for health personnel are offered by public and private universities throughout the country. Specialized training became available in 1954 with the creation of the Graduate School within the College of Medicine of the University of Chile. A national certification board (CONACEM) certifies medical specialists on the basis of validation of their credentials or competency exams. The certification board has been operating since 1985 and is composed of representatives from the College of Physicians of Chile, schools of medicine, the Academy of Medicine of the Institute of Chile, and several scientific societies. Its objective is to certify the qualifications of medical specialists and help regulate the practice of medicine. As of December 1995, CONACEM had certified 5,127 medical specialists; the majority were in the fields of pediatrics (735), internal medicine (683), general surgery (561), and obstetrics and gynecology (506). The University of Chile and the Catholic University train about 94% of the specialists who graduate from university programs.

As of December 1995, 8,654 graduates had completed university specialization programs in 1975, 1980, 1985, 1990, and 1995, the majority in internal medicine (1,199). Information provided in November 1995 by the College of Physicians of Chile indicates that 10,988 physicians were members of that association. Of that number, only 10.47% were registered as general practitioners working in urban or rural areas.

Continuing Education for Health Personnel. The legal provisions relating to primary care are innovative in the sense that they explicitly recognize the need for continuing education for health personnel. Continuing education is also a requirement for those employed by the municipal government. The health services are responsible for approving and supervising the annual training programs developed by each municipal government.

In a study of continuing education in a sample of health services in 1996, officials at all levels of the system indicated that since 1994 there has been a marked change in the intensity of training and in the training model, which is now more comprehensive and encompasses a wider range of professionals and auxiliary personnel. This process has responded to the organizational development initiatives of the services.

Job Markets for Health Professionals. In 1996 the Ministry of Health commissioned a study on the job market for health professionals that looked at supply, demand, structure, compensation, motivational factors, and trends. The study revealed that the country has sufficient numbers of medical professionals, except in some specialties such as anesthesiology, procedure-related specialties, oncology, and child neuropsychiatry, by order of relative shortage. In the Santiago metropolitan region there is a relative surplus (of approximately 1,300 professionals, according to the study), and there are shortages of professionals in regions VIII, X, IX, and IV (between 570 and 340). The country has an insufficient supply of nurses, and most of these professionals are concentrated in the metropolitan region. Only one of every four nurses worked at the least complex levels of the system. Of the 5,817 practicing dentists, about 65% work in the metropolitan region, 30% in the SNSS; of these, 45% are specialists.

Research and Technology

Research and development in Chile increased ninefold in real terms between 1965 and 1993, although this sector of activity continues to account for only a small proportion (0.75%) of the GDP. Of the resources distributed by the National Board for the Development of Science and Technology (FONDECYT), the principal official source of funding in the area of technology, 13.4% went to the health sciences.

The main source of financing for research is FONDECYT. In the area of health, two national institutions receive a large share of this funding, which is awarded on a competitive basis: the University of Chile (Santiago), which accounted for close to 50% of all projects in the period 1988–1995, and the Catholic University of Chile (Santiago), which accounted for about 30% in the same period.

Of the 1,796 projects financed through various sources in the country during the period 1985–1994, 12% involved specialized training in medicine. Unfortunately, the other health professions were included under basic and applied sciences (15%), with no breakdown of the figures.

Technical and Scientific Documentation. In 1997, 75 regular publications were identified in the area of health, of which 55 are listed in the LILACS database. In Chile there is an extensive network of entities devoted to consulting and research in the health field, some affiliated with the university system; this network produces many publications. The Ministry of Health/PAHO Documentation Center registers close to 800 titles of this type each year.

Expenditures and Sectoral Financing

Total spending on health in 1997 was estimated at US$ 3,600 million, of which the public subsector accounted for some US$ 2,020 million. Total spending as a proportion of GDP for that year was estimated at 5.02%, of which 2.13% was private spending. Of the public spending, 10.2% was direct expenditures by municipal governments. In the past five years the proportion of the GDP devoted to health grew by 15.1% (from 4.36% in 1993). The public component increased 5.7% during the period (from 2.96% in 1993) and the private component, by 36.5% (from 1.56% in 1993). In 1994, 46.8% of public spending on health was financed by tax revenues and the remainder was financed by the 7% withholding on workers' earnings.

Analysts believe that the growth in private participation in the sector will slow in coming years because of saturation of the ISAPRE market. Moreover, the Government clearly has shown a clear willingness to continue increasing social spending on health and education.

With respect to public and private spending on preventive services, in 1995 SNSS spent a total of US$ 183.17 per beneficiary. In the private sector, the amount spent was US$ 212.69 in the case of the open ISAPREs and US$ 431.88 in the case of the restricted ISAPREs. Of the total institutional spending in the public subsector, 11.99% was for primary care.

With regard to public and private spending on outpatient and hospital care, FONASA spent 33.6% of its resources on inpatient care, 19.3% on diagnostic examinations, 17.1% on outpatient care, 13.9% on surgical procedures, 5.03% on gynecology and obstetrics procedures, 4.8% on oral health care, 1.3% hemodialysis and other benefits, 0.82% on specific protection activities, and 2.31% on environmental activities. In the ISAPRE subsystem, 46.15% of the resources were spent on outpatient care and related diagnostic services, 48.3% for medical programs, including hospital care, 2.18% on dental care (not covered by all health plans), and 0.35% on preventive activities. Of the FONASA expenditures, 13.9% occurred under the free-choice modality, a health care scheme that is similar to the ISAPRE model in the private sector. Beneficiaries may opt for this modality at the time they receive services.

As for the regional distribution of public resources among the 28 regional health services, in 1994 per capita revenues for health ranged from a low of US$ 78.55 (Biobío) to US$ 249.17 (Iquique). The median was US$ 114.67 (Antofagasta); the upper quartile was US$ 162.50 (Valparaíso-San Antonio) and the lower was US$ 94.14 (Viña del Mar-Quillota and the South-East metropolitan region); the semi-interquartile range/median quotient (nonparametric coefficient of variation) was 29.81%.

The public budget for health in 1997 was funded by worker contributions (33%), fiscal revenues (48%), operating income (8%), other income (9%), and borrowing (2%). Of the public resources for health, 10.2% came from municipal fiscal revenues. In 1996 investment in the sector totaled US$ 112 million, which represented 6.3% of total public spending in the sector. Investment increased 651% over the five years prior to 1995.

External Technical and Financial Cooperation

The health development situation in Chile is such that financial cooperation is less important than the joint activities made possible by cooperative projects. Chile participates in a significant amount of cooperation among countries, especially with countries of Central America and the Caribbean, as is the case with Nicaragua and Haiti.

During the 1994–1995 period, Chile received extrasectoral resources in the form of loans from the World Bank for US$ 3.3 million for hospital rehabilitation and upgrading projects; US$ 23.9 million for emergency units in the metropolitan region; US$ 3.5 million for institutional development projects; and US$ 86.5 million for investment in eight regional health services. The Inter-American Development Bank (IDB) extended a loan of US$ 70 million for a project to improve the physical and functional efficiency of the regional services.

The Government of Germany granted a loan of US$ 31.75 million for hospital restoration.

As for bilateral cooperation, during the same period Chile received US$ 894,000 from Germany for a project in the field of rehabilitation; US$ 10.8 million from the United States for primary care in needy communities; US$ 348,000 from the Kingdom of the Netherlands for AIDS prevention; US$ 10.34 million from Italy for health care in socially high-risk areas; US$ 42,000 from France for AIDS control efforts; US$ 700,000 from Japan for the development of health care units at the secondary level; and US$ 416,000 from Sweden, also for AIDS control. With regard to multilateral cooperation, the European Union provided US$ 986,440 for the prevention of drug addiction.

COLOMBIA

GENERAL SITUATION AND TRENDS

Socioeconomic, Political, and Demographic Overview

Colombia has a land area of 1,141,748 km²; its relief map is dominated by three branches of the Andean range (western, central, and eastern) separated by valleys and plains. The population in 1997 was estimated at 40,072,328 inhabitants: 49.5% males and 50.5% females. The population growth rate is 2.05% per year and the demographic density is 32.4 inhabitants per km². The urban population represents 71% and the rural population represents 29% of the total.

Internal migration flows mainly toward the Andean region. One of every four Colombians lives outside his or her native region. External migration is primarily to Ecuador, the United States of America, and Venezuela. According to the 1993 census, emigration exceeded half a million persons. However, this number represents only part of the exodus, because much of the migration is done clandestinely. The volume of immigrants from other countries represents 0.33% of the total population.

Colombia is a multiethnic and multicultural country, with diverse traditions and different languages. There are 81 indigenous groups (1.7% of all inhabitants) as well as a sizable population of African ancestry (25%) and of mixed race. This diversity produces not only cultural differences but also wide variations in living conditions and hence different types of diseases.

In general, the demographic indicators show steady improvement from 1970–1975 to 1990–1995. However, the statistics for the country as a whole obscure large differences among regions, between urban and rural areas, and among social levels. For example, in the period 1990–1995 the Pacific region, where the Colombian population of African ancestry predominates, had the worst indicators: life expectancy at birth was less than the national average by 2 years (64 years for men and 73 years for women), and infant mortality, at 37 per 1,000 live births, exceeded the national average by 20%.

There were also differences between the urban and rural populations: in the former, the overall fertility rate was 2.65 children per woman, whereas in the latter it was 4.41 children per woman. Mortality from communicable diseases was three times greater for the population with an index of unmet basic needs between 90 and 100 than for those with an index lower than 20.

The improvement of living conditions for the general population in the municipal seats (urban areas) has apparently had a positive influence on the demographic indicators. However, despite the encouraging trend observed between 1973 and 1993, the poverty gap between the municipal seats and the rest of the municipalities actually widened. In 1973 the number of people living in poverty (i.e., with at least one unmet basic needs indicator) was 1.5% higher in the municipalities as a whole (excluding inhabitants of municipal seats) than in the municipal seats. By 1993 that number had nearly doubled to 2.9%. The ratio of the population living in abject poverty (presence of two or more unmet basic needs indicators) in rural areas relative to those in the municipal seats increased from 2.2 to 5.0.

In the past 30 years the Colombian Government has taken great interest in extending the coverage of primary and secondary education, but the country's education deficits are still immense. In 1994, 2 of every 10 children between the ages of 6 and 11 were not attending primary school, and 5 of every 10 youths 12 to 17 years of age were not in secondary school. Of every 100 children enrolled in primary school, only 30 completed the ninth grade and only 7 managed to reach that level without having to repeat a year. In urban as well as rural areas, poor people receive the least education. In 1973, illiteracy in rural areas (22.8%) was more than three times higher than in urban areas (6.0%); variations within the country ranged from 3.0% in Bogotá to 25.11% in Tolima to 25.3% in Córdoba. As for number of years of schooling, in the urban population the figure (7 years) was double that in the rural population (3.2 years). The number varies widely from one part of the country to another—4.2 and 4.3 years in Cauca and Sucre, respectively, and 8.1 years in Bogotá. In 1993 the rates of school attendance according to educational level were 36.9% at the preschool level (children aged 3 to 5 years), 79.1% at the primary school level (6 to 11 years old), and 54.1% at the secondary school level (12 to 17 years old); 8.7% of 18- to 24-year-olds pursued a higher education.

In addition to the deficits in educational coverage, there are also problems with the quality of education, especially in the public primary and secondary schools. In rural primary schools the children cover less than half the material prescribed in the curriculum; 25% of secondary school children in seventh grade rank at the lowest level in the language tests, and fewer than 20% in grades seven through nine manage to achieve the highest level.

Public expenditure on education as a percentage of gross domestic product (GDP) has remained almost unchanged: 2.85% in the 1970s, 2.99% in the 1980s, and 3.03% in the 1990s. As for the allocation of this spending, in 1994 the proportion allocated for primary schools was 33%; secondary schools, 29%; and higher education, 17%. Moreover, the distribution of these monies was unbalanced: at the primary level the poorest 40% of the population received 67% of the funds and at the secondary level the poorest 40% received 46% of the total; in higher education, the poorest 40% received only 15% of funds.

Coverage for basic services in the home increased significantly between 1985 and 1993, from 70.5% to 82.1% for water supply and from 59.4% to 69.0% for sewerage connections. Nevertheless, there are still between 6 and 10 million people who lack one or the other of these services. The situation is more critical in rural areas, where between 5 and 8 million people lack at least one of these services. The gaps are even greater when it comes to water quality. Only 62% of the urban population receives water that is fit for human consumption, and in rural areas the proportion is only 10%. The most significant advances in water supply and sewerage services have taken place in the 1990s. Investments made between 1991 and 1994 came to 25% of total spending in this area in the past 30 years. Even so, this expenditure represented only 0.3% of GDP and 2.7% of total spending on social services, which shows how little importance was given to this sector in the past.

The Colombian economy has experienced enormous changes in recent decades, constantly growing and diversifying. In the early 1990s it began to open up dramatically, with protectionist customs barriers falling in almost all sectors. However, in the past six years the economy's performance has been uneven and some sectors have benefited more than others. The GDP grew steadily from 1991 (2%) until 1994 (5.6%), but then it dropped to 4.5% in 1996. Inflation continued to decline until it reached 19% in 1995, but then it reversed and reached 23% in 1996.

Direct foreign investments went from US$ 2,100 million in 1985 to US$ 7,342 million in 1995, not including the mining and petroleum sectors. The foreign debt rose from US$ 17,000 million in 1992 to US$ 20,000 million in 1994, which corresponds to 34.5% and 30.7%, respectively, of the GDP.

Although the GDP increased at rates of 7.5% and 4.7%, respectively, in the first two quarters of 1995, during the same period in 1996 the growth rates were only 3.9% and 2.2%. This net loss is attributable to the liquidation of businesses, temporary shutdowns, and massive layoffs in the large cities, which produced an unemployed work force that for the most part could not be absorbed by other sectors of the economy, which were also affected by the extended recession. The loss of jobs was especially rapid in construction and in the manufacturing industry. On the other hand, jobs increased in the mining and quarrying sector, possibly because of activity in the petroleum industry.

As a result of these trends, the situation in the urban labor market deteriorated seriously and rapidly. In September 1996 the unemployment rate reached 12.1%, its highest level in 10 years. The situation was similar in almost all the large cities in Colombia: Pasto, 15.5%; Cali, 15.1%; Medellín, 13.6%; Manizales, 13.1%; Barranquilla, 12.2%; Bucaramanga, 10.8%; Bogotá, 10.4%. The rise in unemployment was matched by a sharp and almost equal drop in employment (–2.36%) between 1995 and 1996, the largest decline since 1990.

According to a 1994 report by the National Administrative Department of Statistics, informal employment represented 54.9% of total employment and had not changed since 1984. Small businesses accounted for most of this figure, and microbusinesses of five or fewer workers generated more employment than businesses with six workers or more.

There is a large informal subsistence economy in Colombia, and this situation constitutes a hindrance to the country's economic development. The goods and services produced by the informal sector are for domestic consumption. Three-fourths of the informal activities are concentrated in the trade and service sectors.

The recent opening up of the economy has added to the uncertainty of the market and to fluctuations in demand. In 1997 Colombian businesses were threatened by economic instability and had to face increased international competition, which forced them to lower costs and accelerate technological changes. This situation affected labor relations, because businesses had been forced to adopt more flexible working arrangements and to resort to different types of contracting agreements in order to lower costs (temporary and part-time employment, working at home, agreements with subcontractors). New businesses as well as those in crisis tended to rely increasingly on temporary labor.

Women with temporary jobs have much lower incomes than those with permanent jobs, and the gap between the two groups tends to widen with higher levels of qualification: temporary laborers earn 2% less, temporary administrative employees earn 13% less, and temporary professionals earn 22% less than their permanent counterparts. The situation is different among men: temporary laborers earn 10% less and temporary professionals earn 5% less, but temporary administrative employees receive average salaries 10% greater than their permanent counterparts. Thus, the salary patterns are inconsistent.

Contrary to the unfavorable situation with regard to jobs, average earnings of those who are employed have increased in real terms since 1991, especially in the financial sector, while the wages of people working in the industrial and commercial sectors have remained within the national average, which indicates that although employment declined the productivity of workers improved. Although the Government's budget for social spending increased from 9.07% of GDP in 1990 to 15.14% in 1995, there were disparities between urban and rural areas in terms of education, basic services, and employment. This situation necessarily has direct or indirect repercussions on the health of the people because it affects living conditions and the accessibility of services, including health services. Health conditions are currently in a state of transition characterized by progressive but unequal improvements and the concurrence of communicable, chronic, and degenerative diseases, which particularly affect the poor (with notable differences according to sex). On the other hand, there has been an unusual preponderance of injuries and homicide in the overall epidemiological picture.

Mortality Profile

The crude general mortality rate during 1990–1995 was 6.57 deaths per 1,000 inhabitants. Underreporting of deaths in municipal seats was estimated at 15%, compared with 65% in the rest of the municipalities. Underreporting in the population as a whole was 34.0%, with rates of 46.6% for infants under 1 year old and 29.8% in the population aged 70 and over. With regard to men and women, underreporting was 34.8% for males and 32.5% for females. No major changes were noted during the period for either sex- or age-specific rates.

In 1994, circulatory diseases were the leading cause of deaths (168,568), followed by external causes, tumors, communicable diseases, and certain conditions that originated in the perinatal period. In terms of age distribution, 79.5% of deaths due to diseases of the circulatory system were in the population aged 45 and over, whereas 71% of mortality due to external causes was in the group 15 to 44 years of age, and communicable diseases occurred mostly in children under 5 years old. This situation is evidence of a mosaic of causes of age-specific death in the population.

Differences between the sexes were notable. Among women, chronic degenerative diseases were the most frequent cause of death; 35.3% of all deaths were due to diseases of the circulatory system and 17.7% of deaths were due to tumors. Among males, however, 36.8% of all deaths were due to external causes—in other words, males are at greater risk of dying from violent causes.

SPECIFIC HEALTH PROBLEMS

Analysis by Population Group

Health of Children

The main health problems in childhood are infectious diseases. In infants under 1 year of age, 43.5% of all deaths in 1994 were attributable to conditions that originated in the perinatal period, and 61.9% of the deaths in that age group were due to hypoxia. Thus the main cause of death is related to care during and shortly after birth.

In children under 5 years old, acute respiratory infections and diarrheal diseases are the leading reasons for consulting a health professional. In 1995, these reasons accounted for 37.4% and 14.0%, respectively, of all consultations. In addition to the specific health problems of children, there are other problems in Colombia that have not yet been quantified, such as orphanhood as a result of armed conflicts, participation of children in those conflicts, and child labor. On the other hand, at the root of the social problems and major inequities that exist among regions are the difficulties with access to education, especially for children in rural areas. In areas where there is armed conflict, the school dropout rate is nearly 100%.

Health of Adolescents

Colombia has made great strides toward the eradication of illiteracy, especially in the past decade. However, only 1 of 10 youths who begin a bachelor's degree program will graduate. According to data from the National Planning Department, 2.4 million youths (30% of the total adolescent population) neither work nor attend school. Thus, dropping out of school is one of the risk factors to which this population is exposed. Moreover, sexual activity begins between the ages of 11 and 18, and it is more common at younger ages among the population in the lower social strata in large cities. As a result, more than 10% of girls between the ages of 15 and 19 are already mothers. Statistics show that adolescents who are parents before the age of 19 are one-third as likely to graduate from a university.

The foregoing situation has led to the problem of juvenile delinquency. In 1994, 19,250 youths in Colombia between the ages of 12 and 17 had been sentenced and were incarcerated in correctional institutions. Recidivism in this group is nearly 85%, which has led to overcrowding in the correctional system. At the same time, the use of psychoactive substances is widespread among adolescents under the age of 18 in the upper and middle social strata; youths under 18 account for 15.2% of the population that consumes alcohol, and 6.8% of all cigarette smokers are young. Cocaine is used by 3.8% of the general population; 15.2% of the users are between 11 and 15 years old and 30.4% are between 16 and 18 years old. These factors contribute to the fact that external causes, especially homicides and traffic accidents, constitute the principal cause of death among adolescents.

Health of Adults

The main problems in the adult population are unemployment and underemployment, which create and reinforce precarious living conditions and hence exposure to social and environmental factors that affect health.

Rural poverty, among other factors, has been a factor in the displacement of large population groups to the outskirts of large cities. The effect of this migratory flow on the social life and mental health of the Colombian population is not yet fully known. However, it is worth pointing out that one-third of the households are headed by women.

In addition to the foregoing problems, 12.6% of the population over the age of 15 has high blood pressure, and an estimated 7% of the population over the age 30 has non-insulin-dependent diabetes mellitus, 30% and 40% of whom are unaware that they are ill. Second to traumatic injuries, the leading cause of morbidity and mortality in this age group is chronic degenerative diseases, and among women there is a high rate of illnesses associated with reproductive health.

Health of the Elderly

In studies conducted before 1993, it was found that 87.5% of the elderly were not beneficiaries of social security; 42.0% did not have a formal, regular income; 41.93% were living in a state of abject poverty in marginal areas; 11.0% were living in slums; 32.5% were illiterate; 8.7% had the benefit of some form of pension; 30.85% were engaged in remunerative work; and 39.05% worked at various trades in order to subsist. This age group accounted for about 50% of all deaths in Colombia, and cardiovascular disease caused about half of those deaths.

The Ministry of Health has launched the Health Program for the Elderly, which embodies the objectives of the national social security policy—namely, comprehensive coverage of the needs of this group; reinforcement of the identity, self-esteem, and self-recognition of older persons; prevention and treatment of diseases; and improvement of health services.

Health of Women

In 1995, institutional coverage of pregnant women was 80%, each with an average of four checkups, 30% of which took place in the first trimester. In that same year, the coverage rate for institutional delivery was 77%, which means that about one-fifth of pregnant women did not receive any type of medical care. This situation was reflected in the coverage attained by health care programs for women of reproductive age. Of all women, 27% were of reproductive age, and 55% of these were married. Although there is widespread knowledge about contraceptive methods, only 72% of the women who were married or living in established unions used contraceptives; 29.4% of them were supplied by the public sector. Of all pregnancies, 24% were terminated by abortion and 26% resulted in unwanted births.

Abortion is the second leading cause of maternal death, accounting for 15% of all deaths associated with maternity, with the highest incidence in women from 20 to 29 years of age. This situation coincides with the unmet demand for contraceptives in the at-risk population. Of all pregnancies that ended in abortion in 1995, 24% were due to contraceptive failures and the rest were due to lack of access to contraceptives. Because abortion is illegal in Colombia, many women use unsanitary procedures to terminate unwanted pregnancies, which greatly endangers their life and health.

Analysis by Type of Disease or Health Impairment

Violence

The number one health problem in the Colombian population is injury due to external causes, the result of violence, which affects all of society. In 1994 the National Institute of Legal and Forensic Medicine created the National Reference Center on Violence under the directorate of Forensic Services to support social outreach activities for individuals and groups. The Center is responsible for planning and executing interventions against violence. In 1995 there were a total of 213,341 investigations of nonfatal injuries and 11,970 reports of sexual offenses in Colombia. These figures represent a 15% increase in the rate of nonfatal injuries (527 per 100,000 inhabitants in 1994 and 608 in 1995) and a 7.6% increase in the rate of sexual offenses (31.6 per 100,000 inhabitants in 1994 and 34.0 in 1995). The rate of nonfatal injuries in 1995, compared with the previous year, reflects increases in public violence, family violence, sexual offenses, and traffic as well as other accidents.

Of nonfatal injuries, 163,230 (76.5% of all injuries) were personal injuries intentionally inflicted by others; 65.8% came under the heading of public violence (quarrels, holdups, settling of accounts, revenge, social purges, etc.), which represents a rate of 306 per 100,000 inhabitants; 26.3% were attributable to family violence (122 per 100,000); 0.5% to public disturbances; and 7.3% to sexual offenses (34 per 100,000). Most of the injuries were inflicted with blunt instruments (63.7%), followed by stabbing (18.5%). The highest injury rates were in San Andrés, Amazonas, Arauca, and Santa Fe de Bogotá. The areas with the highest rates of public violence are not the same as the regions that have the highest rates of homicide, which suggests that the two have different causes.

In 1995 the Institute reported 42,963 cases of family violence (child abuse, conjugal violence, and aggression among other family members), which represents 20.1% of all personal injuries investigated and is equivalent to a national rate of 122 cases per 100,000 inhabitants. The groups that suffered the highest rates of family violence were females 25 to 34 years of age and males 5 to 14 years old. Santa Fe de Bogotá, San Andrés, Arauca, Meta, Risaralda, Quindío, and Tolima had the highest rates of all forms of family abuse.

In 1995 there were 11,970 reports of sexual offenses, 87.8% of which were perpetrated against women, for a rate of 34 per 100,000 inhabitants; 55.3% of the victims were from 5 to 14 years of age, and in 77.4% of the cases the aggressor was a person known to the victim (9% were the father, 8.5% the stepfather, 11.3% another family member, and 48.6% an acquaintance). In 35.5% of the victims under 14 years of age, physical examination provided positive evidence. When there is no physical proof of a sexual offense, which is usually the case with abusive acts against minors, it is more difficult to conduct a judicial examination, to identify and charge the aggressors, and therefore to punish them.

Fatal and nonfatal injuries from traffic accidents have increased in the large cities. In 1995 a total of 7,874 autopsies were performed on persons who died in traffic accidents, which corresponds to a rate of 22 per 100,000 inhabitants. For every person who died, seven persons were injured in traffic accidents. Examinations were performed on a total of 52,527 victims of nonfatal injuries incurred in traffic accidents, or 150 per 100,000 inhabitants. Males, especially those between 25 and 34 years of age, were at greatest risk for nonfatal injuries (in which the pedestrian is usually the principal victim), whereas mortal injuries were most common in the population aged 60 and over. Various factors may be influencing the increase in traffic accidents, among them the larger number of vehicles on the road, the long distances being traveled, the high percentage of drivers under the age of 25 and their easy access to alcohol, the lack of speed limits, and inadequate procedures for inspecting vehicles.

It is estimated that in 1995 there were a total of 1,450,845 years of potential life lost (YPLL) because of violent deaths, 67.4% (977,725) of which were due to homicide, 18.5% (268,303) to traffic accidents, 10.1% (145,988) to other accidents, and 4.1% (58,830) to suicide.

In 1995 the National Institute of Legal Medical and Forensic Sciences performed 43,800 autopsies in the entire country, 87.9% (38,483) of which were attributable to violent deaths. This is equivalent to a rate of 110 per 100,000 inhabitants, or a decline of 2% with respect to the previous year, when the rate was 112 per 100,000. Of all mortal injuries due to external causes, 65.7% were homicides, followed by traffic accidents, which represented 20.5%.

An analysis of the data by age and sex revealed especially significant differences between the sexes. The ratio for violent deaths in general is 7.7 males for every female; by type of violence, the figures are 14:1 for homicide, 3.3:1 for suicide, and 3.9:1 for each type of accident. In terms of age, 59.7% (22,977) of the violent deaths were in young persons 15 to 34 years old. In this age group the sex ratio (male/female) was 10:1 for violent deaths in general and 15.3:1 for homicide. Homicides were the leading cause of death for young Colombian males as well as the number-one cause of mortality and YPLL (67.4% of the total). In 1938 the homicide rate was 15 per 100,000 inhabitants; in the 1950s, despite the violence that marked this period, the rate was 55 per 100,000; in 1991 it reached 88 per 100,000; in 1994, 78 per 100,000; and in 1995, 72 per 100,000.

The phenomenon of violence in Colombia has been analyzed extensively taking into account various interpretations of its causes, principals, and scenarios. Notable among the hypotheses are the following:

• There is a culture of violent response to conflict. Indeed, Colombia has a long history of civil wars and guerrilla movements, which may have infused society with the tendency to resolve conflicts by force instead of by dialogue and consensus building.
• Violence is being unleashed by urban growth. It should be pointed out, however, that the homicide rate in Santa Fe de Bogotá, which has the highest population density in the country, is lower than in medium-sized cities such as Manizales, Cúcuta, and Bucaramanga, where it is around 100 per 100,000 inhabitants; some smaller cities have rates around 300 per 100,000. The highest rate (800 homicides per 100,000) is found in Apartado, a locality on the Pacific Coast where the Colombian population is predominantly of African origin.
• Violence is a response to poverty. Nevertheless, an analysis of cities by per capita income and frequency of homicides showed that there was no correlation, because the poorest cities were not the most violent ones.

• Colombians are violent by nature. This hypothesis is not supported by the wide variations between the different cities in Colombia, and genetics cannot explain the rapid rise that has occurred since 1980.

• Violence is related to illicit drug trafficking. Perhaps this hypothesis comes closest to an accurate explanation, because drug trafficking is the most important change that has taken place in Colombian society in the past 15 years. It is of interest that the areas with the highest homicide rates are Antioquia, Guaviare, Putumayo, and Valle del Cauca.

The possibility of risk factors that trigger or condition violent responses in society has been studied in some of the Colombian cities. Among the factors that have been identified are the following:

• Alcohol: In Santa Fe de Bogotá, blood alcohol levels were tested in 92.6% of homicide victims and 55.7% were found to be positive (ethanol levels above 15 mg/ml). According to studies conducted in Cali, 25% of homicide victims were intoxicated. Similar results, with a higher proportion of intoxicated victims, have been reported for Medellín as well as the rest of the country. Measures such as restricting the sale of alcohol in public places or "semi-dry" laws have had positive results in Cali and, more recently, in Santa Fe de Bogotá, where there was an 18% decrease in the proportion of persons who died violent deaths that tested positive for alcohol.

• Firearms: According to the Colombian Institute of Legal Medicine and Forensic Sciences, 80% of the homicides that occurred in Cali, Medellín, and the rest of the country in 1994 were attributable to firearms. That same year, according to data from the Prefecture of Santa Fe de Bogotá, 156,283 permits were issued to carry guns in that city. An evaluation of the gun control policy instituted in Cali in 1994 showed a significant reduction in homicides by firearms.

• Judicial system: Data from Desarrollo, Seguridad y Paz show that it was possible to identify the aggressors in only 6% of the homicides that took place in Cali in 1993, and only a few of them were punished. The National Police estimate that it was possible to apprehend the murderer in only 17.2% of homicides, which does not necessarily mean that they were convicted.

• Drug trafficking: This is an important factor that directly accounts for violence and also indirectly affects the other risk factors. Youth who are unable to attend school because the school system cannot accommodate them and who are unable to enter the tight, competitive labor market because of lack of education and work skills find an easy and attractive source of income for themselves and their families in the distribution and sale of drugs. Once they get involved in this business, violence becomes essential to survival.

An analysis of the scenarios and forms in which violence has occurred since the 1970s shows a picture of social disorder resulting from premeditated acts of revenge, the settling of accounts between drug trafficking leaders, terrorist plots, ordinary delinquency, confrontations over land rights, exploitation of emeralds, and other alarming manifestations of everyday violence.

This situation has displaced many Colombians who have been obliged to move away from their places of origin to protect their lives. Displacement, or involuntary migration because of violence, has caused grave consequences for individuals and families who are not directly involved in the conflicts but whose physical safety has been threatened. These groups are scattered throughout the country. Peasants have been uprooted because of common justice or private justice, and those living in abject poverty have been displaced because their situation becomes even more difficult in conflict-torn areas. It is estimated that guerrillas are responsible for 26% of the displacement; paramilitary forces, 32%; people's militias, 16%; regular armed forces, 16%; and others, 10%. Displacement is accomplished mainly by threats (49%), followed by killings (15%), holdups (8%), and other methods (28%). The main reason for displacement, however, is political violence occurring in the form of armed confrontation between guerrilla groups and the State.

An investigation of the period 1985–1994 by the Episcopal Conference revealed that 1 of every 60 Colombians was forced to migrate because of violence. It was found that 586,261 persons, comprising 108,301 households, were displaced. Of these households, 6.7% had lost a spouse or one of the children through violence before they migrated, and 1,570 orphans, abandoned children, or youth had to assume responsibility for the family. Of this population, 52.4% were living in tenements or in slums—in other words, they were concentrated in outlying urban areas under living conditions that did not compare with the way they had lived in their places of origin. For example, 69.3% had their own homes before they were displaced, and this percentage dropped to 28.7% after displacement. Before, 40.7% were involved in agricultural production, either earning wages or as owners of small or medium-sized plots of land, and 10.0% had small or medium-sized businesses; after displacement, 22.5% had become street vendors, 12.9% had become laborers, and only 10.7% continued to be engaged in agricultural activities. This situation means that every day the Colombian population becomes increasingly drawn into the vicious cycle of poverty and disease. Access to health services is another serious problem that follows in the wake of forced migration: only 22.1% of the displaced households receive medical care.

The National Comprehensive Care System, which attends to the population displaced by violence, reports that in 1995, 1996, and the first four months of 1997 it was able to extend care to 41,675 families. According to information from humanitarian organizations, during the period December 1995–1996, 53% of the displaced population were women and 54% were under 18 years of age. Women heads of families represented 36% of the total displaced population during this period.

The Government, aware of the magnitude of the internal displacement problem and its serious effects on human rights, created the National Comprehensive Care Program to attend to the needs of the population displaced by violence, and it supported development of a plan to address the factors that generate violence, thus facilitating the voluntary return of the displaced population to their places of origin. The Government also entered into the Rural Social Contract, which integrates public policies from various sectors with a view to improving the quality of life of the rural population, which is currently plagued by high levels of poverty and is largely excluded from the benefits of society.

Communicable Diseases

Vector-Borne Diseases. Since 1990 some 180,000 cases of malaria have been reported each year, and the numbers are rising. The cases are typically found in clearly established urban foci such as Buenaventura, in the Valle area, and Barranquilla, in the Atlántico area. Of the total, 38% have been attributed to *Plasmodium falciparum.* At the end of 1996, La Guajira, where *Plasmodium vivax* traditionally had predominated, had an increase in cases among males (20% of them Wayuú Indians), 80% of which were attributable to *P. falciparum.*

Yellow fever has also increased in recent years. Two cases were reported in 1994 (in the Meta and Vichada areas); in 1995 there were three cases (in Meta and Guaviare); and in 1996 there were eight cases, all in males (Meta, Amazonia, and Caquetá).

Dengue affects all age groups, especially those aged 15 to 44. Hemorrhagic dengue and dengue shock syndrome have been diagnosed since 1989, and the number of reported cases has steadily increased, as the following figures show: 302 in 1993, 508 in 1994, 1,028 in 1995, 1,757 in 1996, and 1,702 as of week 25 of 1997. To date, however, serotype D3 has not been isolated. The areas most affected have been Santander, Tolima, Valle, Norte de Santander, Meta, and Huila.

In 1995 the Atlantic coast had the heaviest rainfall in years, which brought with it an increase in the population of *Aedes taeniorhynchus* and *Psorophora confinnis* mosquitoes, vectors that have been implicated in the equine encephalitis outbreak in Venezuela that affected around 75,000 inhabitants in the municipalities of Riohacha, Maicao, Uribia, and Manaure in the La Guajira district; a high percentage of the Wayuú population were infected.

Although the recent increase in the incidence of these diseases can be explained in part by changes in weather that have provided favorable conditions for the vectors to reproduce, it is also related to decentralization and the decline in vector control programs within the framework of health sector reform.

Vaccine-Preventable Diseases. Among children under 5 years old there was a decline in diseases preventable by immunization in the period 1990–1994, as illustrated by the fact that there have been no cases of poliomyelitis since 1991. In 1994 the national committee for certification of the eradication of poliomyelitis reported that the circulation of wild poliovirus had been interrupted in Colombia, and epidemiological surveillance had been progressively developed to the point that an adequate average level had been reached in most of the geopolitical units in the country. Vaccination coverage in 1995 was 92%, and the number of reporting units increased from 868 in 1993 to 1,930 in 1996.

In 1991 a total of 11,127 cases of measles were reported; in 1994 the figure had fallen to 1,816, of which only 254 were confirmed in the laboratory; and in 1996 there were 1,070 cases, of which only 4 were confirmed. In 1993 Colombia made the commitment to eliminate measles, and in 1995 it introduced the use of trivalent viral vaccine. Coverage has consistently exceeded 90% during these years.

The Plan for the Elimination of Neonatal Tetanus, implemented in 1989, succeeded in reducing cases by 85% (from 171 in 1989 to 26 in 1996). The localization strategy was initiated in 1994, and 150 municipalities were identified as being either at risk or in the attack phase—most of them in rural areas where access was difficult or in urban locations with a sizable marginal population. Between 1993 and 1995, coverage in these areas ranged from 29% (in small municipalities with fewer than 1,000 births a year) to 75% (in cities with more than 3,000 births a year). The principal risk factors for the occurrence of neonatal tetanus continue to be the mother's negative vaccination history, home birthing, and poverty.

Cholera and Other Intestinal Diseases. There have been outbreaks as well as isolated cases of cholera associated with precarious living conditions in the population living on the Atlantic and Pacific Coasts and in the areas bordering on the two large rivers that traverse the country from south to north, the Magdalena and the Cauca. In 1995 a total of 1,989 cases were reported, and in 1996 there were 4,428. Most of the cases were on the Atlantic Coast, and the Wayuú people were most affected (31% of the cases).

Chronic Communicable Diseases. Tuberculosis, which has been on the increase since 1993, reached a rate of 28 per

100,000 inhabitants in 1995. Extrapulmonary forms represented 10.1% of the total, and the districts of La Guajira, Atlántico, Quindío, Arauca, Vichada, Putumayo, Amazonas, Vaupés, and Guaviare, with rates in excess of 50 per 1,000, are considered to be at very high risk. In most of these districts a large proportion of the population is indigenous.

Rabies and Other Zoonoses. Human rabies declined during 1992–1994 (with seven, five, and three cases, respectively, in those years). In 1995, however, there were eight cases. Up until that year the cases had been transmitted by dogs, but the three cases that occurred in 1996 were transmitted by hematophagous bats. Since 1994, the cases have occurred exclusively in rural areas of the country.

Acute Respiratory Infections. These infections continue to be the principal health problem in children under 5 years old. In 1994 they accounted for 23.1% of all outpatient consultations.

AIDS. The program for the prevention and control of AIDS and STDs reported 933 cases of AIDS in 1992 and 1,042 in 1996, with a cumulative total of 7,776 diagnosed cases and a cumulative mortality of 41.5% (3,226 cases). Of all the cases diagnosed, 85% were in men, and 40.5% of those were in the group aged 25 to 34. Only 2.1% of the cases affected the population under 15 years of age. Heterosexual transmission accounted for 44.0% of the cases and homosexual transmission for 27.4%. The highest percentages of diagnosed cases were in Santa Fe de Bogotá (46.4%) and the district of Antioquia (15%).

Other STDs. There was an increase in diagnosis of congenital syphilis, from 322 cases in 1990 to 406 in 1995, under the Syphilis Surveillance and Control Program launched by the Ministry of Health. However, the monitoring of STDs in prostitutes was suspended, even though it had produced a 51.6% decline in diagnoses of gonococcal infections, from 39,089 cases in 1990 to 18,915 in 1995. In contrast, diagnoses of genital herpes increased 99.3% during this same period, from 2,231 to 4,446 cases.

Emerging Diseases. The prevalence of the surface antigen for hepatitis B (HBsAg) in blood banks remained stabilized, with levels of 0.73% in 1992, 0.87% in 1993, and 0.87% in 1994. Studies conducted in the past decade showed an overall prevalence of HBsAg carriers of around 5%, with transmission occurring within the household and primarily in the indigenous population. A plan for the control of hepatitis B was implemented in 1993, which involved vaccinating both the population under 5 years of age in the endemic areas and health workers. Since 1994, hepatitis B vaccine has been included in the regular vaccination scheme for all infants under 1 year old throughout the country; hence coverage for this age group went from 36% in 1994 to 73% in 1995 and to 94% in 1996.

Noncommunicable Diseases and Other Health-Related Problems

Cardiovascular Diseases. These diseases are the leading cause of death in women, the second leading cause in men, and the primary cause of death in the group aged 45 to 64. In 1994, 44% of deaths attributed to this cause were due to ischemic heart disease, 93% of them were in persons aged 45 and older, and 56% were in men. Cerebrovascular diseases represented 28% of deaths from cardiovascular conditions, 91% of which occurred in the over-45 age group and 54% in women. Arterial hypertension is the most important risk factor for cardiovascular diseases. According to the 1987 national health study, the prevalence of arterial hypertension in Colombia as a whole was 11.6% in the population over 15 years of age. However, a study conducted in 1995 in the population of Quibdó revealed a prevalence of 35% in all persons over the age of 18 and a prevalence of 39% in the Colombian population of African ancestry—percentages significantly higher than those observed in the rest of the population (21%). The prevalence rates varied by age, from 10% in young persons to 50% in those aged 49 and over. No differences were noted according to sex. Only 16% of the persons surveyed said that they participated in some form of exercise in their free time. Somatometry showed that 50% were at least 10% overweight. A comparison between body mass index (BMI) means showed that hypertensive individuals were more obese than those who were not hypertensive ($P < 0.0001$).

Malignant Tumors. These are the second leading cause of death in the group aged 45 and over and in women. The order and types of cancer differ between the sexes. In 1994, stomach cancer was the most frequent form both in men (20.5% of all cases) and women (14.0%). The second most common site for men was the lung (13.4%), followed by the prostate (12.1%), and the lymphatic and hematic system (10.3%); for women cancer of the uterine cervix was the second most common site (11.1%), followed by the breast (9.9%) and lung (7.0%).

According to the records for 1989–1993 maintained by the National Institute of Cancerology (INC), which is the national reference center, about 70% of the diagnoses were made in the advanced stages—namely, stages III and IV. In the case of cancer of the uterine cervix, 80.9% of the cases were in stages higher than IIa, and with breast cancer 80.6% of the cases were in stages III and IV. Approximately 60% of the patients attended by the INC were from Santa Fe de Bogotá and Cundinamarca.

Among the recognized risk factors for lung cancer the most notable is the use of tobacco. The Survey of Health Knowledge, Attitudes, and Practices conducted by the Social Security Institute in 1994 showed that 33% of the adult Colombian population had smoked at some time and 21.4% were current smokers (29% of males and 14% of females). Of the current smokers, 84% smoked an average of 8.5 cigarettes a day on a daily basis. Tobacco use increases with age up to age 40, when it begins to decline. Males began to smoke at 17.3 years of age, and females at 18.2 years. Of the adolescents surveyed (12–17 years old), 19% had smoked at some time, and 13% were currently smoking an average of 3.1 cigarettes a day on a daily basis. Males began the habit at 15.1 years of age, and females at 13.8 years. The highest consumption patterns were observed on the Atlantic and Pacific Coasts and in the northern part of Antioquia.

Nutritional Diseases and Diseases of Metabolism. An indicator of improved health in the group under 5 years of age is the decline in overall malnutrition, which went from 10.1% in 1986 to 8.4% in 1995. The Pacific Coast region was most affected, with overall malnutrition at 17%. Chronic malnutrition declined from 16.6% to 15.0% during the same period; it is higher in rural areas than in cities (19% and 13%, respectively). The decline mentioned may be due to, among other factors, the campaign to encourage breast-feeding. The National Population and Health Survey found that 95% of all children under 5 years old had been breast-fed for an average of 14 months (13 months in urban areas and 10 months in rural areas) and 81.3% of infants under 1 year of age had been breast-fed from the day of birth (82% in urban areas and 80.1% in rural areas). The lowest percentage (77.2%) was in the Pacific region, and the largest percentage (83.3%) was in the Atlantic region. Despite this high coverage, however, exclusive breast-feeding through the fourth month of life is less than 10% and reaches 15% only if infants who also receive human milk and water are included.

RESPONSE OF THE HEALTH SYSTEM

National Health Plans and Policies

The 1980s saw the beginning of an active process of institutional transformation. Law 10 on the municipalization of health, drafted by the health sector, gave impetus to a series of changes aimed at strengthening the sector's territorial entities. Taking this initiative into account, the new Constitution of 1991 set out the fundamental points that gave rise to reform of the social security system. This mandate was enacted gradually under Law 60, which governs matters relating to the authority and resources of the various territorial entities, and it culminated in the enactment of Law 100 of 1993, which created the social security system in general. This mandate covers standards governing the general system of pensions, professional risks, complementary social services, and the social security system as it relates to health.

The essence of the reform of the system is provision of coverage to persons under both contributory and subsidized regimens based on a partnership scheme of income redistribution that ensures universal benefits through protection of the insured, the spouse, and minor children as well as parents and other relatives. The guiding elements of the reform are efficiency, universality, solidarity, comprehensiveness, unity, and social participation.

The reform process initially was led by the Ministry of Labor and was intended to modify the country's pension plan. During discussions it was decided to incorporate changes in the delivery of services, which had been widely debated by all segments of society. The Ministry of Health had collaborated with a group of experts and contracted for a set of specialized studies to consolidate the proposal. Given the large number of participants—including international organizations and investment banks that will be financing some of the initiatives—it is difficult to know the exact cost of developing the proposal. Committees VII of the Assembly and of the House of Representatives, supported by the Ministry of Health, were responsible for negotiating the proposal.

The important role of promotion and prevention in the new system, the significant increase in the Government's financial contributions to health, the greater spending efficiency gained from competitive arrangements, the strong participation of upper-income groups, and the solidarity inherent in the system are all factors that are expected to contribute to major progress in the quality of health care, the coverage of services, and equity.

With regard to the degree of decentralization of health services, 17 departments and 4 districts have been decentralized and are directly managing more than US$ 474 billion, which represents 70% of the national allocation, and 104 municipalities have been certified to independently manage their own fiscal budgets. The sum of US$ 2,567 million has been allocated for 26 hospitals, health centers, and jobs in the health sector to improve care for the rural population.

Health sector reform currently faces a major problem with regard to access of the population, especially the very poor and the unemployed, to health services. One of the benefit plans proposed under the reform is the compulsory health plan POS-S, which is basically designed to respond to the needs of the poorest and most vulnerable members of the population. POS-S contains initiatives to benefit the individual, the family, and the community in general. Six of these initiatives are included under the basic plan and one is a form of reinsurance against high-cost diseases. In the basic health care plan, all the actions are in the area of health promotion and disease prevention and are directed toward the community. The Government is responsible for the plan, which is territorially based, free to participants, and compulsory.

Organization of the Health Sector

Institutional Organization

To facilitate practical implementation, the general social security system for health has introduced a number of major administrative and operational changes in the sector. The new system reinforces solidarity by providing all Colombians with access to a comprehensive health protection plan, which aims to definitively achieve the goal of health for all by the year 2001. Universal and comprehensive coverage is a goal that should be met gradually by increasing benefits and expanding the base of beneficiaries. The organization of the new system is a mixed type that involves both contributory and subsidized funding. Its operation is based on four fundamental forms of support:

• The National Council on Social Security for Health, under the Ministry of Health, is a professional group that represents the main participants in the system. It is responsible for standardizing, regulating, controlling, and directing the system. The Ministry of Health relies on the sectional health services (one per department) to carry out its duties at the territorial level.

• The National Solidarity and Guaranty Fund is responsible for financing the system. It is made up of four subaccounts: compensation, solidarity, promotion, and catastrophic expenses. The law stipulates that all persons with incomes higher than the equivalent of two minimum wages are required to support the system with contributions, while the poor, the unemployed, and peasants are subsidized.

• The health promotion enterprises are the fundamental organizational nuclei of the system. They are responsible for the basic mobilization of financial resources, health promotion, and organization and delivery of medical services. These entities also have the related responsibility of managing the disabled and providing health services in the event of work-related accidents and occupational diseases as well as organizing complementary health plans, which may be public, private, partnership-based, or mixed and that compete for subscribers in the population.

• Finally, there are the institutions that provide health services—the hospitals, outpatient consultation offices, laboratories, basic health care centers, and other health service centers, plus all the professionals who, either individually or in groups, offer their services through the health promotion enterprises.

As of June 1997, 104 of the 142 secondary- and tertiary-level hospitals (87%) had been turned into social enterprises of the State, and there were 165 health partnership enterprises, 67 family compensation funds, and 30 health promotion enterprises.

Organization of Health Regulatory Activities

Law 100 reaffirms the administrative, technical, and financial autonomy of the public hospitals originally established in Law 10 of 1990 and Law 60 of 1993, and for this purpose it stipulates that public hospitals will be turned into social enterprises of the State as a special type of decentralized public entity; that staff will be governed by the provisions of Law 10, and that private law shall apply in contractual matters. In addition, Law 100 specifies, as part of the Compulsory Health Plan, that initiatives executed by the local government to promote health and prevent disease must be provided free to the entire community and should respond to the needs expressed by the people. All the system's subscribers have the right to be covered under a basic plan, which includes emergency care, hospitalization, consultations, and medication.

Regulations are currently being developed for Law 100, especially with regard to increased coverage, basic packages, promotion and prevention, and financing. The National Health Authority has been an active participant in this process. Given the complexity of the model, it has been necessary to adjust the terms both of Law 100 itself and of this law in relation to other laws of importance for the health sector, such as Law 10 and Law 60. This situation has prevented the health sector from generating initiatives leading to its incorporation in the regional integration processes.

The legal framework continues to be supervised and evaluated by the various bodies responsible for this task at the national level, such as Committees VII of the Senate and the House Representatives. These law-making bodies represent the country in the Andean Parliament and other international legislative forums.

Health Services and Resources

Organization of Services for Care of the Population

Food. A Food and Nutrition Plan has been developed, which includes the following measures for sanitary regulation: a project to update sanitary legislation, implementation of techniques to analyze risks and critical control points, a program for the epidemiological surveillance of foodborne diseases, strengthening of the laboratory network, updating of the food composition table, food safety, and programs for the prevention and control of micronutrient deficiencies, especially those of vitamin A, iron, and iodine.

Health Promotion and Community Participation. On October 1, 1996, the president of the Republic lent his support to the Healthy Municipalities for Peace strategy, calling on mayors, governors, council members, and other authorities, as well as on the community at large, the private sector, and other organizations to exert all their creative capacity to ensure that every municipality in Colombia will work for sustainable human development, conserve and protect the environment, facilitate the timely delivery of health care to the people, and guarantee the quality of care. These efforts are intended to reduce inequalities in health, and, with the participation of the community, to construct the Agenda for Local Development, Health, and Well-Being.

Environment and Sanitation. Health promotion activities come under the Basic Health Care Plan and are essentially carried out at the municipal level. Within this framework, the goal of the Plan for Environment and Sanitation for 1998 is to achieve 90% coverage with water supply systems and 77% coverage with sewerage systems, benefiting an additional 6.1 million inhabitants with safe drinking water and 6.2 million with cisterns for the disposal of wastewater.

Organization and Operation of Personal Health Care Services

According to statistical data from the Ministry of Health, the public health service network consists of 3,340 jobs in the health sector, 904 health centers, 128 health centers with beds, and 555 hospitals—397 hospitals at the primary level, 126 at the secondary level, and 32 at the tertiary level. In addition, the private sector has 340 clinics.

Under the health insurance system, the 10 public health promotion enterprises, together with the 20 authorized private and mixed enterprises, have the capacity to handle a total of 21.6 million persons. As of December 1996 a total of 13.9 million Colombians were covered, of which 66.9% (9.3 million people), according to the latest official report dated June 1996, were subscribers under the Social Security Institute, and the remaining 33.1% came under other health promotion enterprises. The subsidized program currently involves 236 entities: 18 health promotion enterprises, 49 family compensation funds, and 169 health partnerships, which as of December 1996 had 5.9 million subscribers. Of this total, 33.1% belonged to the health partnerships, 53.2% to the health promotion enterprises, and 13.7% to the family compensation funds.

Inputs for Health

Essential Drugs and Medications. One of the benefits of the reform has been seen in the area of drugs. Decree 677, promulgated in 1995, establishes a complete frame of reference for all matters related to the use and quality control of pharmaceutical products. The National Institute for the Surveillance of Drugs and Food (INVIMA) was established that same year, and a bureau of Pharmaceutical and Laboratory Services was created within the Ministry of Health with the responsibility of setting policy for the sector and promoting the development of services for pharmaceutical care and the rational use of drugs.

The list of essential drugs cited in the Compulsory Health Plan (about 300 principles and 435 presentations) has become an important element in managing the system, both from the therapeutic standpoint, by guaranteeing use of the best drug for each illness, and from the administrative perspective, by handling a moderate quantity of items throughout the entire pharmaceutical care chain. This list has resulted in some changes in the inventory of drugs used in Colombia; consolidated the production, sale, and prescription of essential drugs; and hindered the entry of other products (especially "novel" ones) on the national market that are less effective and safe as well as more expensive.

In November 1995, 2 years after the reform was initiated, essential drugs accounted for 70% of the drugs prescribed in the public hospitals, and more than 60% of all prescriptions specified the generic name. In that same year Colombia adopted the Good Manufacturing Practices (GMP) standards of the World Health Organization. The pharmaceutical laboratories, in turn, had to present INVIMA with a program of technological change that would guarantee complete retooling of their productive practices in order to bring them in compliance with GMP within a period of no more than four years. The various programs for controlling the quality of products on the market are still reporting rejection rates of nearly 4%.

Human Resources

In another positive response to the reform, a study was conducted and a national plan was prepared for the development of human resources in the sector. The study, carried out in 1994, showed the distribution of human resources by category as presented in Table 1.

However, with the passage of Law 30 and Law 115 of 1994, which authorized educational institutions to create new programs, there has been a haphazard proliferation of study programs and private vocational schools at the technical and auxiliary levels, which attempt to respond to the needs of the

TABLE 1
Human resources in the health sector, by occupational category, Colombia, 1996.

Occupational category	Number	Rate per 10,000 population
Medicine	35,640	9.4
Nursing	16,560	4.4
Dentistry	21,240	5.6
Bacteriology	10,800	2.9
Physical therapy	3,744	1.0
Nursing auxiliaries	41,760	11.0
Health promoters	8,699	2.3
Total	138,443	36.5

Source: Colombia Ministry of Health, 1996.

sector. Some of these programs, especially the informal ones in technological areas, have an unclear curriculum and were created before regulations were in place to govern the practice of the new vocations.

The Ministry of Health offers training to develop health assistance in some of the priority areas. A study conducted in 1995 by the Expanded Program of Textbooks and Instructional Materials (PALTEX) of the Pan American Health Organization revealed that in general no prior assessment of training needs is made, nor is any evaluation done of its impact. This finding led to formulation of the National Human Resources Development Plan in 1996, which was intended to control the erratic growth of training programs, the lack of clear guidelines, and a series of other problems that might be considered to fall under three major headings:

- Imbalance between the availability of human resources in different occupational categories and the demand for their services, attributable in part to the absence of a clear policy of human resources planning and in part to the shortage and questionable reliability of information.
- Inconsistency between socioeconomic and epidemiological profiles, on the one hand, and occupational profiles, on the other, and incongruity between these profiles and pedagogical objectives, materials, strategies, and methods.
- Insufficient recognition of the importance of human resources management for productivity and quality of care and of critical areas such as job-relatedness, motivation, working conditions, performance evaluation, continuing education, and constructive supervision.

The National Council on Human Resources Development, created in 1977, is composed of representatives of the Ministries of Education, Health, and Labor, and it has working bodies at two levels—the National Executive Committee and the Departmental Committees—which are responsible for proposing policies on basic formation, continuing education, and the dynamics as well as the distribution of human resources in the health sector. As of the end of 1996, this Council had regulated the basic formation of the following categories: health promoters, family and community health assistants, health assistants in dental offices, nursing assistants, assistants in dental hygiene, clinical laboratory assistants, administrative assistants, information assistants (health statisticians), environmental health promoters, pharmacy assistants, and assistants in oral health and dental mechanics.

Expenditures and Sectoral Financing

According to Law 60, enacted in 1993, the subsidized program relies on the following sources of funding: 15% of the municipalities' share of current national income, fiscal allocations to the departments, national income assigned to the departments, resources from ECOSALUD (gambling taxes), voluntary contributions from the municipalities and departments, royalties from new oil wells, contributions from the compensation funds, value-added tax destined for social programs, tax on firearms and ammunition, and copayments and prorated fees from the members and their families. If the contributions from private sector insurance schemes are added, the share that health represented in the gross domestic product (GDP), not counting private expenditures by families, increased from 2.07% in 1990 to 3.18% in 1994 and 4.71% in 1996.

Two more subaccounts have been incorporated into the social security system: the Compulsory Traffic Accident Insurance account, which receives payments from every automobile owner in the country and channels them into the emergency network to care for victims of hit-and-run accidents, and the Work-Related Accidents and Occupational Diseases account, which is fed by contributions from employers based on the degree of risk to which their workers are exposed.

During 1996 the health institutions continued to receive subsidies that were at least the same as in previous years. This per capita income, calculated on the basis of the uninsured population, represents considerably less than the value of the per capita unit of pay (PCP). Its calculation is based on a detailed analysis of family incomes over time. These funds are a potential source of fees for the health system. A study was conducted on the trend of the PCP over the past decade, and its composition was established on the basis of specific beneficiary groups and their distribution by age and geographic location. Perhaps the greatest challenge to the financial stability of the system is controlling fee evasion; the health promotion enterprises are responsible for membership and building up enrollment and not for controlling underpayment of fees by higher-income members, who often underreport their income.

Private household expenditure on health was estimated at 3% of GDP in 1993, which means that in that year Colombians spent a little more than 6% of GDP on health. Of total private household expenditure, about 40% was for medication, 14% for office visits, 20% for hospitalization, 5% for diagnostic tests, and 20% for other items. Because essential drugs are included in the Compulsory Health Plan and must be referred to by their generic names, the private market has deferred to the institutional market of the health promotion enterprises and the health service delivery institutions. This means that the negotiated unit prices have fallen significantly. The hospital cooperatives, which cover about 80% of the public hospitals, have been very effective and efficient in organizing essential supplies for the public hospital system, offering average discounts of 79% on drugs and ensuring strict quality control of the products. Total social spending by the State as a percentage of GDP increased from 8.59% in 1990 to 10.65% in 1992 and 15.67% in 1996.

External Technical and Financial Cooperation

The nonreimbursable technical cooperation and funding for all sectors received by Colombia from multilateral and bilateral sources in 1990–1995 showed an uneven pattern, going from US$ 88 million in 1990 to $180 million in 1993 and then dropping to $70 million in 1994 and $80 million in 1995. During this period, the largest share of resources (27%) went to the agricultural sector for projects to eradicate unlawful crops; followed by 18% for environmental protection; 12% for health, basic sanitation, education, culture, and recreation; 11% for science and technology; 9% for industry; 6% for justice; and 5% for modernization of the Government.

Two factors have affected the level of priority that donors assign for providing nonreimbursable financial assistance, which have translated into smaller contributions: first, the financial situation of some of the cooperating organizations, in particular the specialized agencies and other organizations of the United Nations, and second, the fact that Colombia has reached social and economic levels that allow it to be classified as a country with a medium level of development.

Of the US$ 80.9 million in nonreimbursable technical and financial assistance received by Colombia in 1995, 56.6% came from multilateral sources. The largest amounts were received from the World Food Program (44.6%), the European Union (21.2%), and the United Nations International Drug Control Program (16.3%). Bilateral sources accounted for the remaining 43% received—from Germany, 19.6%; Spain, 12.47%; Canada, 4.98%; and other countries, 6.35%.

Pursuant to the priorities contained in the National Development Plan, social programs received 47% of the total contributions granted to the country in 1995, followed in order by the agricultural sector (16%), environmental protection (15%), and institutional development programs as part of the decentralization process (9%). With regard to the regional programs, the contributions were allocated, by order of importance, to education (24.3%), ethnic groups (24.2%), activities under the Alternative Development Plan (15.9%), and children (11.90%). Colombia has both received and contributed technical collaboration in the areas of health, tourism, science and technology, agriculture, institutional development, and management of international technical cooperation.

Since the end of 1994 the Government has assigned increasing importance to international cooperation, inasmuch as it is a key resource that contributes to economic and social development as envisaged in the National Development Plan. In March 1995 a policy document was issued, which called for international cooperation in institutional management by coordinating the demand for this cooperation, and which established priorities for the technical assistance the country receives from different sources. Areas identified as being of interest were social development, the elimination of poverty, and sustainable environmental development, to be carried out in tandem with territorial development and modernization of the Government.

COSTA RICA

GENERAL SITUATION AND TRENDS

Socioeconomic, Political, and Demographic Overview

Costa Rica has an area of 51,100 km² and a population of 3.36 million inhabitants (1995). It is divided into seven administrative provinces and 81 cantons and, for planning purposes, nine regions. The country has enjoyed sustained economic growth and political stability, and has had no army for 49 years. These factors have enabled Costa Rica to make significant social progress.

The economic crisis of the 1980s made it necessary to redesign the development model, which focuses on promoting exports and tourism and modernizing state institutions in the 1990s. In 1994, the per capita gross domestic product (GDP) was US$ 2,150, rising by 4.7% in 1995. At the end of 1995, the public foreign debt was US$ 3,255 million. Servicing the debt as a percentage of GDP fell slightly with respect to the previous decade. In 1995, the foreign debt was equal to 37.5% of GDP, a much lower figure than the average from the previous decade (67%), which reduces the vulnerability of the economy to foreign indebtedness.

The country's domestic debt doubled in the period 1992–1995 to 38.5% of the GDP in 1995. The domestic debt equaled 40% of the foreign debt in 1992 and 82% in 1995. This situation has brought changes in the operation of the State and has led to cutbacks in public spending. The fiscal deficit, which was 7% of GDP in 1994, fell to 5% in 1995. Despite these policies, the State increased social investment in education, health, and social welfare by between 4.5% and 8%.

It is estimated that 14.7% of households in 1995 lived in poverty, without sufficient income to cover the cost of a basic basket of food and nonfood products. In 1989, that proportion was 21.9%. Approximately 80% of poor households are located in rural areas. The Brunca and Chorotega regions are the poorest, with 36% and 33% poverty, respectively. The State has a national plan to combat poverty and protection

mechanisms for the poor (access to goods and services, subsidies, housing, etc.), and it has identified 16 areas of extreme poverty, which are receiving priority attention.

The economically active population (EAP) in 1995 numbered 1.22 million, of whom 3.8% had no education and 13.7% had a university education. Women make up 30% of the EAP and young people between the ages of 12 and 19, 13%; in the population aged 5 to 17, 13% work, but 34% of that group does not receive any remuneration for their work. Open unemployment reached 5.2% in 1995, affecting most significantly those with the least education, young people, and the elderly. Among the poor, 10.9% to 12.5% live in extreme poverty and 36% of the openly unemployed are women. According to the results of the 1995 household survey, the poorest quintile of families (20%) receives 5.5% of the country's total income, whereas the richest quintile receives roughly 49.1%.

The Costa Rican economy has always been dependent on the use of natural resources. During the 1980s, the GDP fell roughly 1.5% annually as a result of deforestation, soil erosion, and the unsustainable development of the gulf of Nicoya. There was no clear policy for managing natural resources. Costa Rica has roughly 6% of the world's biodiversity, and 25% of its territory consists of protected areas. It currently has a conservation strategy for sustainable development to deal with serious environmental problems: water and air pollution, primarily in the San José metropolitan area; solid waste effluents; and erosion and destruction of the forest reserve (which covered 56% of the country in 1960 but only 32% in 1990). In the past decade, Costa Rica has had the highest pesticide consumption in Central America—roughly 4 kg per inhabitant per year, which is some 6 to 10 times the world average.

In 1991, the national dietary caloric availability was 2,261 kcal per person and it was higher in rural (2,355 kcal) than in urban (2,170 kcal) areas; 56% of all calories come from rice, fats, oils, and sugars. Rice and beans, which are the mainstay of the Costa Rican diet, provide 30% of the calories and 34% of the protein consumed.

At the end of 1995, 99.6% of the population had access to water suitable for human consumption, 95.7% had a sewerage system or a system for sanitary disposal of excreta, and 93% had electricity (83% of which was generated by hydroelectric plants).

Education is free and compulsory through the ninth grade, and the illiteracy rate is 7%. In 1994, illiteracy in persons over 13 was estimated at 8.8% in rural areas and 3.6% in urban areas. School enrollment rates are very high, and the dropout rate in cycles I and II was 4.2% in 1994 and 5% in 1995; the number from the latter year is the highest in recent decades. The dropout rate in middle school also increased in 1995 (16.1%) compared with 1994 (14.6%), and it was triple the primary school dropout rate. In 1994, public schools in marginal urban areas had a dropout rate eight times higher than the national average.

The housing shortage is a problem—in 1994 it was estimated at 160,000 units; 75% of urban dwellings and 60% of rural ones are considered to be in good condition; 91% of urban dwellings have basic services, compared with 81% of rural dwellings.

The last national census was conducted in 1984. According to estimates from the Department of Statistics and Censuses, the population density in 1995 was 65.8 inhabitants per km². The annual growth rate fell from 3.0% in 1992 to 2.2% in 1995. Slightly over one-third of the population (34.4%) are children under 15, and 4.7% are over 65. Women make up 49% of the population, and 56.3% of the country's inhabitants live in rural areas.

In 1996, international immigration was just under a quarter of a million people—51% from Nicaragua and 66% from other Central American countries. The number of temporary and permanent undocumented immigrants is difficult to quantify. These immigrants do not always have access to the social benefits that are available to citizens, and their standard of living is, therefore, usually lower than that of the rest of the population.

Life expectancy at birth in the period 1990–1995 was 75.2 years and it is estimated at 75.6 for the period 1995–2000 (78.1 in women, 73.3 in men). The total fertility rate was 3.3 children per woman between 1985 and 1990 and 3.1 in 1990–1995. The crude birth rate was 25.4 per 1,000 population in 1992 and 23.9 per 1,000 in 1995. Roughly 80,000 births have been registered annually in the 1990s, with a male-to-female ratio of 1.02.

Mortality Profile

The total death rate was 3.8 per 1,000 population in 1992 and 4.2 per 1,000 in 1995. Of the 13,278 deaths registered in 1994, 62.9% were persons aged 60 and over, 57.2% of whom were men. The causes of death have not changed considerably in recent years. The five leading causes are chronic diseases and unintentional injuries ("accidents"). Only 2.1% of deaths were attributed to ill-defined causes.

The leading cause of death was cardiovascular disease, with a rate of 10.5 per 10,000 population in 1990, 12.6 in 1994, and 12.4 in 1995. Ischemic heart disease was responsible for 47.2% of those deaths. The second leading cause of death was neoplasms, with a rate of 7.5 per 10,000 in 1990, 8.1 in 1994, and 8.4 in 1995. In 1994, stomach cancer ranked first among neoplasms for both sexes, with prostate cancer ranking second for men and breast and cervical cancer in second and third place for women. External causes occupied third place as a cause of mortality, with respective rates of 4.4, 4.9, and 5.0 per 10,000 population in 1990, 1994, and 1995. This group of causes is responsible for the most years of potential life lost (YPLL), with 21.8% of all YPLL in 1994. Diseases of the respiratory system ranked fourth as a cause of death in 1995, with a rate of 4.6 per 10,000. Diseases of the digestive system ranked fifth, with a rate of 2.7 per 10,000.

The infant mortality rate was 15.3 per 1,000 live births in 1990 and 13.0 per 1,000 in 1994. In seven cantons, infant mortality exceeded 20 per 1,000 and eight cantons had a rate of 15 to 20 per 1,000. In 1994, 69% of deaths in children under 1 year of age (8.9 per 1,000) occurred during the neonatal period. Disorders originating in the perinatal period are the leading cause of infant mortality, with a rate of 6.4 per 1,000, followed by congenital anomalies, at 3.6 per 1,000.

Maternal mortality was low, ranging from 15 to 39 per 100,000 live births between 1990 and 1994. Among its causes, eclampsia ranked first.

Morbidity Profile

The Costa Rican Social Security Fund (CCSS) regularly surveys the reasons for outpatient consultation. The last survey was in 1992, when there were 6.13 million consultations and an annual average of 1.94 consultations per inhabitant; 64.6% of the consultations were by women. Respiratory diseases ranked first as a reason for consultation, followed by hypertension. In the 20- to 44-year age group, the leading cause was respiratory diseases, followed by back problems in men and gynecological disorders in women. Women received twice as many checkups (without any clear disorder) as men.

According to a sample of three hospitals, one of which is a national hospital, in 1995 respiratory diseases, injuries, childbirth, and asthma were the most frequent reasons for visits to emergency services.

The CCSS recorded 297,941 hospital discharges in 1994; 68.4% of those were women. The importance of gynecological and obstetric problems as a reason for hospitalization is evident in that 84% of the discharges in the 15- to 44-year age group were women; in children under 15, 57% of discharges were boys and in older adults there were similar proportions of men and women. One-tenth of discharges were for emergencies, which heavily burdened the services and involved terminal care.

In general, the number of discharges has remained stable since 1991. In 1994, the most frequent diagnoses at discharge were gynecological and obstetric causes, perineal trauma, intestinal infections, asthma, and hernias. In children, the leading causes were acute intestinal infections, asthma, chronic tonsillitis, and acute appendicitis. In adults 45 and over, hospitalizations for diabetes mellitus, inguinal hernias, prostate hyperplasia, and ischemic heart disease predominated.

SPECIFIC HEALTH PROBLEMS

Analysis by Population Group

Health of Preschool Children (Children under 5)

In 1995, it was estimated that there were nearly 400,000 children under the age of 5, or 11.9% of the total population; 80,306 live births and 1,064 deaths in children under 1 year were registered that year, with an infant mortality rate of 13.3 per 1,000 and a neonatal mortality rate of 8.5 per 1,000 live births. Disorders originating in the perinatal period were the leading cause of death in children under 1, with a rate of 6.5 per 1,000, followed by congenital anomalies, at 3.7 per 1,000, and lung diseases, at 1.3 per 1,000. Infectious and parasitic diseases were responsible for a mere 4.4% of infant mortality, with a rate of 0.6 per 1,000.

In 1994, the CCSS registered 25,772 hospital discharges of children under 1 (8.7% of all discharges), of which boys constituted 56.2%. The leading causes of hospitalization recorded at the time of discharge were healthy newborns, jaundice, intestinal infections, and acute respiratory infections. In 1992, there were 242,641 consultations by children under 1 at the CCSS, which is 4% of all consultations for that year; 15% of the consultations were for checkups, with no pathological cause.

In 1995, the deaths registered in the group between 1 and 4 years of age corresponded to 1.3% of all deaths, with a mortality rate of 5.9 per 10,000. Congenital anomalies were the leading cause of death in this group, followed closely by infectious and parasitic diseases and diseases of the respiratory system.

The population aged 1 to 4 received 610,783 consultations, or 10% of the total. That number is almost evenly distributed between boys and girls: 7% were checkups; 16,801 hospital discharges were registered, or 5.6% of the total, and 41% of those discharged were girls. In this age group, the leading

causes of hospitalization recorded at discharge were intestinal infection, asthma, bronchopneumonia, and inguinal hernias.

National studies indicate that children under 5 in urban areas have an average of 3 bouts of acute respiratory infection per year; in rural areas the number climbs to an average of 5 to 8.

Health of Schoolchildren and Adolescents

In 1995, 11.7% of the population was between 5 and 9 years of age; 10.9% was between 10 and 14; and 9.8% was between 15 and 19. The 5-to-14 age group accounted for 1.6% of all mortality in the country and had the lowest specific rate of mortality: 3 per 10,000. The leading causes of death were external causes—injuries and poisonings—followed by neoplasms and diseases of the nervous system.

In children between 5 and 9, 493,213 consultations were registered, and the leading reason for consultation was respiratory problems. The 10-to-14 age group accounted for 292,737 consultations, or 4.8% of the total, and the leading reasons for consultation were acute upper respiratory infections, followed by mental disorders in males and dermatoses in females; roughly 6% of the consultations in this group were checkups. In the 15-to-19 age group, 320,768 consultations were registered, or 5.2% of the total; 75.4% were women. The leading reasons for consultation in adolescents were related to menstruation, acute disorders of the upper respiratory system, gastroduodenitis, and obstetric complications; 15.7% of consultations in women were checkups, without a clear pathological disorder. In men in this group, the leading cause of consultation was acute disorders of the upper respiratory system; 5.9% were checkups.

The group between 5 and 9 years was responsible for 4.4% of all hospital discharges; 59.9% were boys, for whom asthma was the leading cause of hospitalization, followed by chronic tonsillitis, which was also the leading cause in girls, followed by asthma.

In the population between 10 and 14 years of age, 9,176 discharges were recorded, or 3.1% of all discharges; 54.5% were males, in whom the leading causes of hospitalization were acute appendicitis, chronic tonsillitis, congenital anomalies, concussions, and asthma. In females, the leading cause of hospitalization was also acute appendicitis (8.7% of discharges) followed by normal deliveries (5.5%), chronic tonsillitis, premature deliveries, and asthma. Obstructed labor was the seventh leading cause of hospitalization in this group; unspecified complications of abortion was tenth.

In the population between 15 and 19 years of age, 25,184 hospital discharges were registered, or 8.8% of the total; 84.7% of these discharges were women, in whom the most frequent reasons for hospitalization were gynecological and obstetric causes—normal (33%), premature (11%), or dystocial (6%) deliveries; unspecified complications of abortion (5%); and others (4%).

The mortality data for the group aged 15 to 19 are not broken down and are therefore presented in the description of mortality in the adult population.

Health of Adults

In 1995, the population between 20 and 59 years old was estimated at 1.64 million, or 48.8% of the total population. The population 60 years and over was estimated at 233,000, or 6.9% of the total population, made up of 109,000 men and 124,000 women.

The leading causes of death in the group between 15 and 34 years old were external causes—injuries and poisonings—followed by neoplasms. In women the third leading cause of death was cardiovascular disease, and in men it was endocrine and metabolic diseases and immunological disorders.

In the 35-to-49 age group, the leading causes of death in women were neoplasms, followed by cardiovascular disease and external causes. In men, external causes ranked first and cardiovascular disease was second.

In the group aged 50 to 69 years, the leading causes of death in women were neoplasms, cardiovascular and blood diseases, and diseases of the hematopoietic organs. In men between 50 and 69, the predominant causes of death were cardiovascular disease, endocrine and metabolic diseases, immunological disorders, and external causes.

In the group aged 70 and over, mortality was 644 per 10,000 in women and 850 per 10,000 in men. The leading causes of death in both sexes were cardiovascular diseases, neoplasms, and diseases of the respiratory system.

In 1992, 3.27 million consultations of persons between the ages of 20 and 59 were registered, or 53% of the total, with an average of two consultations per inhabitant.

In the 20-to-44 age group, 73% of all consultations were by women, 15.6% of which were for checkups. The leading causes of consultation were inflammatory diseases of the uterus, vagina, and vulva, followed by acute upper respiratory infections and direct obstetric complications. In men between 20 and 44, checkups accounted for 4.7% of the total, and the leading causes of consultation were acute upper respiratory infections and upper and lower back problems.

In the group between 45 and 59 years of age, still according to the 1992 data, there were roughly 870,000 consultations, or 14.2% of the total, 69.8% of which were by women. The leading cause of consultation was hypertension, followed by diabetes in women and upper and lower back problems in men; the third leading cause was joint disorders in women and diabetes in men. Approximately 4.5% of the total were checkups

without a pathological cause; that proportion was somewhat higher (4.9%) in women.

The group 60 years and over accounted for 14.2% of all outpatient consultations at the CCSS (869,000). This group averaged 3.7 consultations per person per year, and women accounted for 61.4% of the consultations. Hypertension was the top reason for consultation, followed by diabetes mellitus and joint disorders.

According to available data on hospital discharges, 48.1% of the total in 1994 were discharges of persons between 20 and 44 years of age. Of the 143,000 discharges in this group, 83.9% were of women, in whom the 10 leading causes of hospitalization were related to reproduction. Normal deliveries were responsible for 21.5% of the discharges, obstructed labor for 8.0%, and premature deliveries for 7.3%. In men, the leading causes of hospitalization were acute appendicitis and inguinal hernias, which combined account for less than 10% of all discharges. This illustrates the wide variety of causes of hospitalization for this subgroup.

In the group between 45 and 59 years of age, there were 25,000 discharges, or 7.1 per 100 persons in this group. They accounted for 8.3% of all discharges; 59.3% of those discharged of women, in whom menstrual disorders were the leading cause of hospitalization (5.6%), followed by cholelithiasis (4.9%) and diabetes mellitus (4.5%). In men in this group, diabetes mellitus, inguinal hernias, and ischemic heart disease were the three leading causes of hospitalization, accounting for 4.7%, 4.0%, and 3.1% of all discharges, respectively.

In the group 60 and over, the CCSS registered 38,410 discharges, or 4.4 per 100 persons in this group and 12.9% of all discharges. Slightly over half (51%) were men, in whom the leading causes of hospitalization were prostate hyperplasia (7.2%), ischemic heart disease (5.7%), cataracts (4.6%), and chronic obstructive pulmonary disease (4.5%). In women, the leading causes of hospitalization were diabetes mellitus (7.8%), cataracts (5.6%), chronic obstructive pulmonary disease (4.8%), ischemic heart disease, and fractures of the neck of the femur (3.4%).

According to the 1993 reproductive health survey, 75% of sexually active women use contraception. Of these, 28% use modern methods, 21% have been sterilized, 16% use barrier methods, and 10% use traditional methods. With regard to pregnant women, 75% begin prenatal checkups during the first trimester and 97% of deliveries are in hospitals; 56% of deliveries are attended by physicians and 41% are attended by nurses.

Workers' Health

It is estimated that occupational health services coverage is low—around 25% for salaried workers and practically zero in the informal sector, which represents approximately 30% of the working population. Agricultural workers—especially those in banana, melon, and rice production—are at high risk of exposure to pesticides. This trend is on the rise, although this may be due in part to decreased underregistration, which was estimated at 43% that same year. Some studies indicate that the risk of accidents for female agricultural workers is 1.7 times higher than for male workers. In 1995, 978 cases of acute pesticide poisoning were registered.

Health of Indigenous People

The indigenous population represents 1% of the country's population and is distributed among eight groups (the Bruncas or Borucas, Cabecars, Teribes or Terrabas, Bribris, Huetars, Malekus or Guatusos, Chorotegas, and Guayamis) totaling 35,850 persons. The Talamanca, Buenos Aires, and Guatuso cantons, where these people live, have high rates of infant mortality, birth, and total mortality compared with the national average. They also have major shortages of housing and basic services, such as drinking water and electricity. In 1995, steps were taken to diminish the social marginalization of these groups, extending social security and establishing the Department of Indigenous Education and the Technical College in the primarily indigenous Amubri de Talamanca community.

Analysis by Type of Disease or Health Impairment

Communicable Diseases

Infectious and parasitic diseases were responsible for some 2.4% to 2.7% of all deaths registered between 1992 and 1995, with an annual mortality rate of 0.9 to 1.1 per 10,000 population. They do not generate a large volume of outpatient services; acute intestinal and respiratory infections are a major cause of hospitalization only in children under 5. However, in recent years, several communicable diseases have re-emerged.

Vector-Borne Diseases. Malaria has flared up since the late 1980s, registering 6,951 cases in 1992, with an annual parasite index (API) of 7.9 per 1,000 population. Since 1991, malaria has shifted from the Pacific coast to the northern region and the Atlantic coast, coinciding with the development of the banana industry, deforestation, and migratory movements of temporary workers, which are factors that hinder case follow-up and control. The risk of contracting malaria in the Huetar Atlántica region is triple that in the rest of the country. There were 4,515 cases registered in 1995 and 5,480 in 1996, with an API of 4.8 per 1,000. *Plasmodium vivax* was

the infectious agent in 99.9% of the cases up through 1995. Infections caused by *Plasmodium falciparum* are imported cases (in 1996, 65 cases were recorded). In Costa Rica, no deaths from malaria had been registered in over 20 years; however in 1996 two deaths from cases caused by *P. falciparum* were recorded.

Since 1992 the *Aedes aegypti* mosquito has been detected in localities where it had never previously been found, such as the Meseta Central, at altitudes over 700 m above sea level, including the San José metropolitan area. In 1994, rates of infestation of up to 32.2% were detected in the south central region. The most frequent reservoirs are tires and, in the summer, water storage containers.

In late 1993 there was a sudden dengue outbreak, with 4,612 cases; 13,929 cases were reported in 1994 and 5,135 in 1995, including the first case of dengue hemorrhagic fever in the Chorotega region. In 1996, 2,309 cases and the first two deaths from dengue were registered. The circulating serotype that started the epidemic was serotype 1. Two cases of serotypes 2 and 4 were detected, which subsequently were not isolated again. In 1995, serotype 3 was detected in several regions of the country; in 1996 its presence increased, coinciding with the number of case fatalities. The majority of cases were in areas with high population density, in the 20- to 40-year age group, and in women (42% of the cases were in persons working in domestic occupations, and 17% were in students).

Vaccine-Preventable Diseases. A measles epidemic that began in late 1990 in Guanacaste subsequently spread to the rest of the country and did not subside until December 1993. In that period, 9,292 cases and 56 deaths were registered. Many cases were in adolescents and young adults; however, the incidence and case-fatality rates were higher in children under 1 year of age. In 1994, 103 cases and no deaths were registered; in 1995, 250 cases were reported, 86% of which were ruled out as measles. In 1996, 148 cases were reported, 84% of which were ruled out.

In the period 1992–1996, rubella exhibited a downward trend. Laboratory confirmation has been available since 1995. That year 67 cases were confirmed—7 in the laboratory and 60 clinically. In 1996, 37 cases were confirmed—15 in the laboratory. During these years, there were no cases of congenital rubella syndrome.

Since 1973, no cases of poliomyelitis have been registered, and eradication of the circulation of wild poliovirus was confirmed in 1994. In the period 1990–1995, there were no known cases of diphtheria, and the last case of neonatal tetanus was reported in 1988. The incidence of whooping cough has been low since 1991, with a downward trend, dropping from 1.1 per 100,000 population in 1992 to 0.2 per 100,000 in 1996, with only one death, in 1995, in the entire period.

Cholera. Cholera was detected in Costa Rica in January 1992. That year 12 cases were reported. In 1996, 36 cases were recorded, 19 of which were imported. As of 1996, 123 cases had been reported, 74% of which were imported. That year multiple antimicrobial resistance of *Vibrio cholerae* in all the isolates was detected, as was the first death from cholera. The most affected area was the northern border. In 1992, the predominant biotype was El Tor, Inaba serotype; the Ogawa serotype was predominant in later years.

Chronic Communicable Diseases. Tuberculosis has shown a dramatic increase recently, with incidence rates of 11.4 per 100,000 in 1992 and 19.0 per 100,000 in 1996. Despite this overall increase, the incidence of tuberculous meningitis in children under 5 is stable and low. The Pacific Central (Puntarenas) and Huetar Atlántica (Limón) regions are the areas most affected by this disease. Twice as many cases are diagnosed in men as in women. Roughly 90% of cases are pulmonary tuberculosis. In 1994, 80 deaths from tuberculosis were registered, representing 25% of all deaths from infectious and parasitic diseases that year. In 1995, the national mortality rate from tuberculosis was 2.1 per 100,000; in Limón it reached 7.0 per 100,000. The country does not have a registry of tuberculosis patients by cohort; therefore data on the effectiveness of treatment or the efficiency of the program are not available. Furthermore, there are no data on the link between tuberculosis and HIV.

Leprosy is no longer a public health problem. In late 1996, there were 158 registered cases. However, the cases are concentrated in the central Pacific coast, Huetar Atlántica, and Huetar Norte regions, all three of which have prevalence rates of over 1.2 per 10,000; 78% of the cases are multibacillary; the ratio of men to women is 2; and cases in children under 15 are unusual. In 1996, disability, primarily of the hands, was detected in 35% of the diagnosed cases.

Rabies and Other Zoonoses. No cases of human rabies have been registered for almost 30 years. The last case of canine rabies was reported in 1987. Epidemiological surveillance activities, vaccination of dogs, and joint activities along the northern border are being carried out. There are no efficient reporting and surveillance systems for other zoonoses.

AIDS and Other STDs. The first known cases of AIDS in Costa Rica, in the first half of the 1980s, occurred in hemophiliacs. In 1985, cases began to be recorded in homosexuals, and in the 1990s heterosexual and vertical transmission have emerged, with a growing trend in recent years. Parenteral transmission was never significant (0.6% of the cases are in intravenous drug users and another 0.6% were people exposed through blood transfusions). In recent years, 100% of transfusions have been screened for HIV.

In 1990, 94 AIDS cases were diagnosed, jumping to 207 in 1995. According to preliminary data from 1996, 202 cases of AIDS were registered, with an incidence rate of 5.3 per 100,000; 90.5% of the cases were in men. For men, the group most widely affected was homosexuals (37.4%), followed by heterosexuals (20.6%) and bisexuals (19.6%). From the onset of the epidemic through 1996, 1,156 AIDS cases and 621 deaths were registered in Costa Rica. The average survival period once the infection has been diagnosed is from 18 to 24 months.

There has been a gradual reduction in the reporting of cases of other STDs, particularly gonorrhea, whose incidence plummeted from 433.8 per 100,000 population in 1982 to 123.7 in 1990 and 68.6 in 1995. The incidence of syphilis also decreased from 99.8 per 100,000 in 1983 to 54.3 in 1990 and 44.7 in 1995. The persistence of congenital syphilis is noteworthy. In recent years, some 90 to 150 cases have been registered annually.

Noncommunicable Diseases and Other Health-Related Problems

Nutritional Diseases and Diseases of Metabolism. The 1996 National Nutrition Survey showed the following distribution in boys and girls aged 1 to 6, according to the Waterlow classification: 92% normal; 2% acute malnutrition; 5.7% chronic malnutrition; and 0.3% acute and chronic malnutrition.

The body mass index was used to assess the preschool population, yielding the following results: 16.4% had a nutritional deficit and 14.9% were overweight. Excess weight occurred in 16.3% of the girls and in 13.6% of the boys. Differences in nutritional deficiencies according to sex were not observed.

The proportion of infants with low birthweight was 6.3% in 1990, 7% in 1994, and 6.1% in 1995.

Despite prevention programs, 1,292 cases of endemic goiter were reported in 1994; 91% were in women, 63% of whom were of childbearing age.

Diabetes mellitus is the ninth leading specific cause of death; in 1994, it was responsible for 258 deaths. It is the eighth leading reason for medical consultations in men and fourth in women. In hospital discharges, it appears as the fourth leading cause of hospitalization; in 1995 it was cited in 4,421 discharges, mostly women.

Cardiovascular Diseases. Cardiovascular disease is the leading cause of death in Costa Rica, with a mortality rate of 12.5 per 10,000 population in 1994. Total deaths from cardiovascular disease increased between 1992 and 1994 at an annual rate of 4.4%. In 1994, they represented 31% of all deaths in the country. Together with neoplasms, they are responsible for half of all deaths; add injuries and diseases of the respiratory system and they account for three of four deaths in Costa Rica. It is estimated that 15% of the Costa Rican population over the age of 15 is hypertensive. In the 1992 survey of causes of medical consultations, hypertension ranked second in both men and women.

Among cardiovascular diseases, the leading cause of death is ischemic heart disease, followed by cerebrovascular disease and then diseases of pulmonary circulation and other forms of heart disease.

In 1994, ischemic heart disease was the third leading cause of hospitalization in men between 45 and 59. In the population 60 and over, it ranked second in men and fourth in women.

Deaths from cardiovascular disease usually occur at relatively advanced ages; therefore they rank fourth as a cause of YPLL. Cardiovascular diseases produce half as many YPLL as unintentional injuries or accidents, which rank first as a cause of YPLL.

Malignant Tumors. Malignant neoplasms are the second leading cause of death. In the period 1992–1994, they were responsible for 8.1 deaths per 10,000 population annually and were the third leading cause of YPLL. The most frequent forms are neoplasms of the stomach, lung, prostate, breast, cervix, and uterus. In general, mortality from malignant neoplasms remained stable in the period 1985–1995, except for prostate cancer in men, which increased, and stomach cancer in women, which decreased.

In general, the incidence of cancer in the period 1985–1994 remained stable, although in women there was a downward trend in cancer of the stomach, lung, cervix, and hematopoietic and reticuloendothelial systems and an upward trend in breast cancer. In men, the incidence of lung and prostate cancer increased and that of the stomach and the hematopoietic and reticuloendothelial systems decreased.

Neoplasms were the sixth leading cause of hospitalization in the period 1988–1995. Lymphomas, leukemias, and cancers of the stomach and reproductive system are the most frequent cause associated with hospital discharges of men. In women, the most frequent types of cancer as a cause of hospitalization are those of the reproductive system, particularly cervical cancer.

External Causes. Unintentional lesions or accidents (injuries and poisonings) ranked third as a cause of death. In 1994, they produced 12.2% of deaths and 21.8% of YPLL and were the leading cause of loss of healthy life (measured by the combined morbidity and mortality indicator). The corresponding mortality rate was 48.9 per 100,000.

In 1994, mortality from traffic accidents reached a rate of 17.5 per 100,000. The average age of those deaths was 39

years; deaths from motor vehicle accidents involving pedestrians were the most common (44%), followed by collisions between vehicles. Injuries from motor vehicle accidents involving pedestrians were responsible for 47.1% of deaths from external causes. In 1995, the highest mortality (9.2 per 10,000) from these causes was registered in the province of Limón, where external causes were the second leading cause of death.

In 1994, homicide and intentionally inflicted injuries were responsible for 183 deaths, at an average age of 34, and 3% of YPLL; 54% of these deaths were caused by firearms and 38% were stabbings.

In 1994, there were 162 suicides, at an average age of 37, and 2.5% of YPLL. The most frequent instruments of suicide were poisoning (37%), hanging (30%), and guns (30%).

Domestic Violence. The health sector does not have a registry for health problems stemming from domestic violence. Partial data, obtained from government institutions that assist the victims of violence, are presented here.

In 1994, the Office of Women's Affairs, a judicial arm of the Ministry of the Interior, reported treating 2,299 women who were victims of violence. In 1995, the number of complaints rose to 5,597; by May 1996, 4,221 complaints had already been registered. This increase may be related to the establishment of a National Plan against Family Violence in 1995 and the promulgation of a law punishing assaults on women. According to this same source, in 1995 and through May 1996, 715 complaints were handled from young people between 15 and 20 who were victims of domestic violence.

In the first quarter of 1997, the National Children's Foundation (*El Patronato Nacional de la Infancia*), a government agency specializing in the protection of children, reported treating 24,044 children and adolescents. The leading reasons for treatment were family and conjugal conflicts (5,423 cases), abandonment (5,639 cases), child support (1,727 cases), administrative institutionalization (2,566 cases), and abuse (3,332 cases; 1,209 were physical abuse, 2,021 sexual abuse, and 102 psychological abuse).

The National Geriatrics Hospital is the only center that has begun recording domestic violence against the elderly. In 1995–1996, 92 cases of abandonment were handled, 87 of which involved women. In 1997, a protocol for detecting domestic violence was implemented, and an increase in the detection and treatment of cases was reported.

Within health sector reform, the treatment of domestic violence has been introduced as part of the modified care model.

Oral Health. In the last national study in 1992, there was a DMFT (decayed, missing, and filled teeth) Index of 4.9 in the 12-year-old population. The lowest and highest values were found in Limón, with a DMFT of 4.0, and in Puntarenas, with a DMFT of 6.0.

Natural Disasters and Industrial Accidents. Between 1992 and 1996, the geological instability of the country, climatic phenomena, and damage to the ecological balance caused by the urban-rural distribution and economic development have led to floods, landslides, earthquakes, volcanic eruptions, and other disasters. In that period, the 1992 earthquake in Pejibaye and the August 1993 tropical storm Bret were declared national emergencies. In 1995, there were 32 floods resulting from hurricanes or other storms. In 1996, the flooding in Limón and in the south left a death toll of nine. That same year, as a result of hurricane Cesar, there were floods in the central and southern Pacific coast that affected 451,496 people, leaving 4,560 persons in shelters and 39 dead. In October 1996, the floods caused by hurricanes Lili and Marco caused seven deaths in Guanacaste and the northern area of the country.

RESPONSE OF THE HEALTH SYSTEM

National Health Plans and Policies

The national health policy and the strategic plan of the health sector for the period 1994–1998 incorporate the social policies of the national development plan. That plan states that the State will play a central role in order to ensure favorable conditions for improving health and delivering services, based on the following criteria: solidarity of financing; equitable access; universal coverage; high levels of quality, opportunity, and flexibility; efficient use of resources; and compassionate treatment of patients.

Health sector reform includes the following areas:

1. Leadership in health. Using a multisectoral approach, the Ministry of Health has assumed a leadership role in the national health system that goes beyond the sector. It has four strategic functions: management and leadership in health; regulating the development of health; monitoring health; and scientific research and technological development.

2. Adaptation of the model of care. This means adjusting care at the primary level in order to handle local health problems appropriately and in a timely manner, promoting community participation, and trimming public spending. The model uses health teams that provide basic services, subdivided into five comprehensive care programs for children, adolescents, women, adults, and the elderly.

3. Adaptation of the system of financing. This includes (a) redesign of the financing model; (b) standardization of the contribution system; (c) efficiency in collections; (d)

development of a system to improve resource allocation and administration; (e) joint private participation options in health management, financing, and services; (f) development of a system of costs, statistics, and evaluations; and (g) sale of services. The intent of this adaptation is to meet the objectives of efficiency and sustainable financing by promoting equity in the distribution of social burdens and benefits, encouraging people to subscribe to the social security system, reducing tax evasion, and streamlining the use of resources by establishing modern and efficient controls.

Organization of the Health Sector

Institutional Organization

According to a decree promulgated in 1983, the health sector consists of the Ministry of Health, the Ministry of National Planning and Economic Policy, the Ministry of the Presidency, the Costa Rican Institute of Water and Sewerage Systems, the CCSS, and the University of Costa Rica. In 1989, the decree on the General Regulations of the National Health System was proclaimed, expanding the sector to include participation by municipalities, private services, communities, and other universities.

The agreements defining sectoral reform include the 1993 Loan Agreement and Health Sector Reform Project with the World Bank and the 1994 law on the loan contract between the Government of Costa Rica and the IDB to finance the steering role of the Ministry of Health, improve the physical infrastructure of health centers and health posts, and build the Alajuela hospital.

The Ministry of Health is playing a leadership role within the framework of sectoral reform, with strategic management, leadership, and regulatory functions; the CCSS is responsible for service delivery. Financing for maternity and health insurance is tripartite, with contributions based on wages from employers (9.25%), the State (0.25%), and workers (5.5%). In the case of voluntary beneficiaries, workers contribute 13.25% and the State contributes 0.25%. The poor are covered by the State. A small sector of the population uses private health services, whose supply has increased in recent years. There are no data on the demand for and coverage of private services. The CCSS must cover 100% of the population. Currently 90% of the population is insured; the rest is covered by the State.

The decentralization process is being implemented through a financial resource allocation model for the three levels of care, based on separation of the financing and service delivery functions, through contracts between the central level and the hospitals and health areas. Furthermore, administrative deconcentration implies the creation of health areas with decentralized functions for managing human resources, procurement, and the budget.

Private participation in the national health system is regulated by the General Health Act and the General Health Regulations, which define private services as an additional component of the system. Regulating health facilities has begun as a pilot project, with an accreditation process for public and private maternity hospitals, adhering to the minimum standards set by the Ministry of Health.

Certification and practice in the health professions are regulated by the respective professional associations, each of which is established by law, and to which the State delegates the functions of certification and monitoring of professional practice. There is currently a public debate on the constitutionality of this situation, with proposals that this function be reconsidered by the Ministry of Health as the representative of the State.

Sanitary controls for and registration of drugs, food, and hazardous toxic substances are the responsibility of the Department of Drugs and Narcotics Controls and Registries of the Ministry of Health. Health regulation and surveillance, which includes the monitoring of air and soil quality, housing, chemical safety, and hazardous waste, are the responsibility of the Environmental Sanitation Division of the Ministry of Health. These are basic aspects of a priority public health program known as the Program to Protect and Improve the Human Environment. The surveillance system is being organized, and the formulation of national standards on water quality and regulations governing effluents and the recycling of wastewater have already been completed. Food is included in this program. However, the development of a System of Sanitary Controls and Registries that would include food protection is being discussed. There are currently no health controls or registries for biomedical equipment and materials.

Health Services and Resources

Organization of Services for Care of the Population

Health Promotion. Since 1995, the Ministry of Health has had a National Program for Health Promotion and Protection in place that promotes social participation and links together its education and mass communication components. The influence of this program became evident in situations such as the cholera threat and the dengue epidemic, as well as in the implementation of participatory intersectoral projects, such as the ecological and healthy cantons program, the health worker education centers, and the program for community health educators.

Vaccination Programs. In 1995, the ongoing vaccination program had national coverage of over 84% for all vaccines, although there is great disparity among cantons. In 1993, coverage in the most backward cantons was improved as a result of the vaccination campaigns. In 1997, coverage with the three-dose oral polio vaccine was over 80% in 67 of 81 existing cantons; coverage with the diphtheria, tetanus, and whooping cough (DTP) vaccine was under 88% in 72 cantons; and coverage with the measles vaccine in 1-year-olds exceeded 88% in 72 cantons. At present, all newborns in CCSS medical units receive the BCG and hepatitis B vaccines, which represents 99% coverage at the national level.

Epidemiological Surveillance. In 1996, there was little epidemiological surveillance for a number of reportable diseases and for pesticide poisoning. Entomological surveillance is conducted to combat malaria and dengue, and monitoring of water quality is the responsibility of the special basic sanitation program.

Investigating and detecting suspected cases of disease or circumstances subject to epidemiological surveillance are carried out at the local level, and notification using a standardized form is the responsibility of the local levels of the Ministry of Health, the CCSS, hospitals, and laboratories. The information flows vertically within each institution up to the central level of the Ministry. There is little coordination at the local and regional levels of the two institutions, and there is insufficient capacity for data analysis at those levels. However, there is a growing operations research capability and response capacity to the problems identified—for example, rapid response to epidemic outbreaks. The data are consolidated periodically at the national level and are published in the *Weekly Epidemiological Bulletin*.

The capacity for diagnosing dengue, cholera, leptospirosis, meningococcal meningitis, measles, and rubella is ensured by the national reference laboratory. A research center (ICMRT) linked to the University of Louisiana, in the United States, which offers diagnostic services to the CCSS, has the capacity to diagnose hepatitis and cytomegalovirus. Diagnosis of malaria is concentrated in the laboratory at the central level, although in 1996 it began to be decentralized to some local services in priority areas. The AIDS Control Department has a diagnostic and reference laboratory for public and private laboratories that diagnose HIV and for blood banks. There is diagnostic capacity for *Escherichia coli* and rotavirus in the National Children's Hospital.

Deaths in children under 1 began to be monitored in 1996 and maternal mortality was monitored in 1997. There are standards and instruments for investigating every death in each establishment. Surveillance of pesticide poisoning was implemented experimentally in some areas in 1995, and in 1997 it began to be extended to the entire country.

Water Supply, Sewerage Systems, and Solid Waste Disposal. By law, the Costa Rican Institute of Water and Sewerage Systems (AyA) is responsible for designing and building water and sewerage systems. It also manages the systems in the major cities, which are home to half the country's population. The Basic Sanitation Unit of the Ministry of Health provides assistance to the rural population in the digging of shallow wells and building latrines. Municipalities have the primary responsibility for water and sanitation, and many of them manage their systems without the AyA. There are also several hundred administrative committees for rural water supply systems, which are formed and trained by the AyA.

The AyA administers 141 water supply systems, which cover approximately 63% of the population. In addition, there are 2,214 water supply systems operated by 150 municipalities, 1,664 community committees, and 400 private businesses. The quality of the water in these systems is unknown and is neither controlled nor monitored by the Ministry of Health.

With respect to wastewater, it is estimated that the effluents from only 3% of the population are treated before being discharged. The Tárcoles river receives raw sewerage from the metropolitan area in addition to virtually untreated wastewater, most of which is from tanneries and from the food, coffee, and textile industries.

The Ministry of Health has sought to substantially increase water and sanitation coverage in the country. In order to reduce the deficit to virtually zero, the Basic Environmental Sanitation Project was implemented in 1993 and was financed with national resources from the Joint Institute for Social Assistance and the Social Development and Family Allowances Fund, channeled through PAHO.

The municipalities are legally responsible for solving the problem of domestic solid waste. The Executive Unit for Solid Waste of the Ministry of the Environment and Energy collaborates with the municipalities in this area. Some private firms also provide urban services for refuse collection and elimination in controlled sanitary landfills. Solid waste from hospitals is the responsibility of the CCSS and, for the time being, is sent to landfills or municipal dumps.

With regard to solid waste collection, coverage reaches 62% of the population. Roughly 62 municipalities (70%) deposit their solid waste in dumps, 55 of which are in the open air throughout the country. According to the National Waste Management Plan, approximately 11,764 tons of waste are generated daily in Costa Rica, 86% of which is agroindustrial waste, 13.6% is ordinary waste, and 0.4% is hazardous waste (household, industrial, pesticide, fertilizer, and hospital waste). Hospital waste is almost always sent to municipal dumps, burned in the open air, thrown away, or sold.

Prevention and Control of Air Pollution. The Ministry of Health is responsible for monitoring and controlling air pollution in general, and the Ministry of the Environment is responsible for environmental protection. There are no air quality standards. The current standards for regulating the emission of contaminants were prepared to support an environmental management program in the metropolitan area.

The main measures adopted by the Ministry of Health to reduce the emission of air pollutants include the installation of emission control equipment in the main industries, sampling conducted by specialized laboratories, direct sampling from chimneys, and the corresponding analyses. The Environmental Control Department verifies the efficiency of contaminant removal and requests improvements and controls when necessary. Furthermore, the Ministry of Public Works and Transportation, through the Transit Police, conducts a program for controlling motor vehicle pollution, for which it has equipment for direct measurement of emissions from vehicle exhaust pipes. In 1994, regulations on vehicle emissions were promulgated.

The year 1996 marked the eighth anniversary of a 1988 executive decree and was the deadline for the Refinadora Costarricense de Petróleo (Costa Rican Petroleum Refinery) to produce only unleaded gasoline, which is currently the only type produced.

The "Ecomarchamo" program, whose purpose is to reduce vehicle emissions, is under the jurisdiction of the Ministry of the Environment and Energy, the Ministry of Public Works, and the Transit Police. The Environmental Sanitation Bureau, a unit of the Ministry of Health, operates a network to monitor air quality in the San José metropolitan area. The work of the National University in laboratory studies and testing has been very important and has been conducted with the technical and financial support of ProEco, a nongovernmental organization financed with Swiss funds.

Several years ago, a decree was issued prohibiting smoking in public places. Furthermore, the CCSS and the Ministry of Health are conducting educational programs and advertising campaigns in this regard. In order to improve air quality in closed spaces, there are regulations governing ventilation in buildings. The occupational safety and health regulations and the regulations governing enclosed spaces also include guidelines on ventilation to prevent health problems. There are also regulations on the use and control of asbestos and products that contain asbestos, which are aimed at reducing harmful pollution from construction activities.

Food Safety. There is no defined policy on food safety or plan of action to coordinate the institutional food protection programs. By law, the responsibility for the coordination, orientation, execution, supervision, and evaluation of the programs lies with the Ministry of Health. Other participants are the Ministry of Agriculture and Livestock, through the Plant Health, Meat Inspection, and Animal Quarantine Departments, and the Ministry of Economics, Industry, and Commerce, through the National Office on Standards and Units of Measure, which regulates metrology, labeling, and quality control. All these institutions have well-equipped laboratories.

The country has technical policy instruments for food regulation, and the Ministry of Health is a member of the Joint FAO/WHO *Codex Alimentarius* Commission. Costa Rica has also signed the World Trade Organization agreements on health. The University of Costa Rica and the Costa Rican Institute for Research and Teaching in Nutrition and Health have conducted several studies of fresh livestock products, particularly with regard to pesticides, hormones, and heavy metals.

Through an agreement between the National Institute of Learning and the Ministry of Health, continuing education courses with national coverage were established for food-handlers. Basic education programs also include basic aspects of food-handling. Food vending on the street is not a major health problem, although it is on the rise.

The Program for Supplementary Feeding in educational centers has broad coverage, especially in rural and marginal urban schools.

Organization and Operation of Personal Health Care Services

The CCSS consists of a central level responsible for institutional policies, a regional level made up of seven regional medical service offices, and a local level comprising health areas and sectors. At the tertiary level, the CCSS has three national general hospitals and six national specialized hospitals. At the secondary level, there are 7 regional hospitals, 13 peripheral hospitals, and 38 type 3 and 4 clinics (with three or four basic medical specialties). The primary level is made up of 103 clinics, to which the sectors with basic teams for comprehensive health services and health areas are being added, as well as health centers and health posts transferred by the Ministry of Health. Each level of care covers a given territory, and the facilities make up a clearly defined service network with levels of care based on the degree of complexity and response capacity. The system for transfer and return of patients among peripheral, regional, and national hospitals has been defined. Outpatient clinics offer a service to transport patients to national or regional hospitals when warranted by the patient's condition or the distance between establishments.

The strategy for strengthening the primary care level has the goal of forming 800 health sectors with basic comprehensive care teams. In July 1996, 306 sectors were already in operation, covering 1.13 million inhabitants. This infrastructure is

located mainly in priority areas, because of their lesser socioeconomic development. The Ministry of Health still operates some health centers and health posts, mobile medical and dental units, dental school clinics, comprehensive health care centers, school lunchrooms, and comprehensive child health and nutrition centers. The majority of these services are being integrated or will soon be integrated into the CCSS.

Preventive oral health services traditionally have been provided by the Ministry of Health to schoolchildren and pregnant women, whereas the CCSS offers more complex services to direct insurance subscribers and less complex procedures to their dependents. In recent years, dentistry programs have been established in three private universities, and private practice has proliferated in this area, offering more complex services than the public sector.

Psychiatric care in the country is provided in all the national and regional hospitals and type IV clinics, as well as in some peripheral hospitals. The main psychiatric center is the National Psychiatric Hospital, with 800 beds, 600 of which are for chronically ill patients. Another hospital geared exclusively to the chronically ill has 300 beds. Attempts currently are being made to decentralize care and favor keeping the user closer to his/her community and family. A process of openness and deinstitutionalization has also begun. Drug addiction is treated on an outpatient basis by the Institute on Alcoholism and Drug Dependence. There are three schools of psychology, two of which are private; a state school of social work; and a graduate specialization in psychiatry at the national university.

Since 1994, adolescents have actively participated in the planning and execution of activities and projects targeted to this age group.

Reproductive health services, which were traditionally the responsibility of the Ministry of Health, were transferred to the CCSS to be provided by the basic care teams. The Costa Rican Demographic Association, a nongovernmental organization with external financing, supports CCSS services with family planning offices and activities to detect cervical and breast cancer.

The CCSS has a comprehensive care program for the elderly and a geriatric hospital. For the academic training of specialists there is a graduate program in gerontology and geriatrics and a master's program in gerontology at a state university.

The Official Drug List is an integral part of the National Drug Formulary. In the CCSS, drugs are selected on the basis of demographic criteria, morbidity and mortality statistics, special program requirements, and available infrastructure and equipment. Their effectiveness and safety, as determined in clinical trials, are also taken into account as well as their price at the time the purchases are made. In 1997, the CCSS allocated 7.55% of its budget for drugs, for a total of US$

49.49 million. In addition to procurement at the central level, the medical units, which are usually hospitals, are authorized to make cash purchases. Per capita spending on drugs in the CCSS was US$ 14.46 in 1989 and US$ 16.15 in 1997. In the latter year, the country had 161 pharmacies.

Hospital medical equipment is very centralized in the three national hospitals, which have over one-third of the total; the 13 peripheral hospitals have only one-fifth. One in 10 pieces of equipment in the country is not in good condition, and over 6% of equipment is underutilized. In general, surgical and emergency units are considered to be well equipped and well structured. However, space is sometimes lacking in intensive care units. Furthermore, the procurement and use of equipment is not coordinated.

Human Resources

There are no clear policies or coordinated human resources programs for health. In 1995, for every 10,000 Costa Ricans there were 12.7 physicians, 3.8 dentists, 9.6 nurses, 3.6 pharmacists, 20 nursing auxiliaries, 0.3 sanitation engineers, 2.5 community assistants, and 0.6 nutritionists. Education for the health professions is provided in several public and private teaching, university, and para-university centers. In 1989, the university established a master's degree in public health, which has trained primarily staff members of the Ministry of Health and the CCSS.

Sector institutions have assumed the responsibility for continuing education and training, and the Center for Strategic Development and Information on Health and Social Security plays a very important role in human resources education for health services. Since 1995, it has held courses for regional and local personnel in basic concepts of epidemiology, local health management, and computer science. Since 1989, the education of health services managers and administrators has been emphasized.

The Costa Rican Institute for Research and Education in Nutrition and Health, which basically conducts clinical research, and the School of Public Health of the University of Costa Rica, where research on education is carried out, are the institutions that conduct the bulk of health research.

Expenditures and Sectoral Financing

Total public expenditure on health in 1996 was US$ 889.28 million. In that same year, public expenditure in health as a percentage of GDP was 9.8%, 0.7% of which corresponded to the Ministry of Health, 8.0% to the CCSS, 0.5% to the Costa Rican Institute of Water and Sewerage Systems, 0.4% to the National Insurance Institute, and 0.2% to the municipalities. Public expenditure in health in 1996 was distributed in the following manner: 81.9% for the CCSS, 6.4% for the Ministry of Health, 5.3% for the National Institute of Water and Sewerage Systems, 4.2% for the National Insurance Institute, and 2.1% for the municipalities.

In Costa Rica, the public sector has been the predominant sector in financing and delivering health services, which is a trend that has remained stable. Up-to-date information on private sector participation is not available. The latest available data are from a 1987 household survey, in which it was estimated that private health expenditure totaled US$ 77.2 million, equivalent to 23% of the spending of the Ministry of Health and the CCSS.

External Technical and Financial Cooperation

The CCSS has a modernization and hospital infrastructure development program financed by the World Bank. Cooperation projects are also under way with the IDB for institutional strengthening of the Ministry of Health, development of the steering role of the sector, and upgrading of the health services infrastructure for primary care. With other agencies of the United Nations, such as the UNDP, UNICEF, UNFPA, and PAHO, there are broad cooperation programs for healthy communities, service delivery, the steering role, the quality of care and disease prevention, and the control of environmental degradation.

CUBA

GENERAL SITUATION AND TRENDS

Socioeconomic, Political, and Demographic Overview

The situation in Cuba since 1989 has been characterized, above all, by a profound economic crisis, which has affected virtually all spheres of national life. The severity of the crisis is evidenced by the fact that between 1989 and 1993 the country's gross domestic product (GDP) fell 35% and exports declined by 75%. The two determining factors underlying the crisis are well known. One is the dissolution of the Soviet Union and the socialist bloc, with which Cuba had maintained 85% of its foreign trade prior to 1989, and the other is the economic embargo the Government of the United States of America imposed on Cuba more than 30 years ago, which was strengthened in 1996 with the approval of the Helms-Burton Act, aimed at blocking foreign investment in Cuba and severely curbing foreign trade.

In the face of this new situation, the Cuban Government has introduced a series of adjustments and restructuring measures aimed at halting the decline and reviving the economy. The Cuban process seeks to achieve sustainability and efficiency without undoing the social gains of the Revolution, to preserve to the greatest extent possible the levels of equity that have been attained, and to prevent loss of employment and livelihood for the population.

The measures implemented include promoting international economic collaboration and foreign investment in Cuba; creating agricultural and industrial free markets that operate on the basis of supply and demand; expanding private enterprise or self-employment; developing new land and cattle cooperatives; introducing a broad-based tax system that taxes state and private activity; progressively reducing subsidies to state-run enterprises; strengthening the system of rationed distribution of goods at subsidized prices, with an emphasis on the most vulnerable groups;

downsizing and decentralizing the central government; and reforming and modernizing financial, banking, and business systems.

In addition to the increase in production and export capacity in traditional items such as sugar, nickel, fish, cement, and tobacco, an effort has been made to develop new sectors with tremendous potential for generating foreign currency revenues, such as tourism, mining, biotechnology, and the pharmaceutical, electronic, and sugar industries.

In 1994, the downward trend of the economy reversed and modest growth in the GDP (0.7%) was reported. In 1995 the GDP increased by 2.5%, and in 1996 it grew significantly by 7.8%. That same year, per capita GDP went up 7.5%, and the minimum wage, the earnings of the population, and the distribution of income all improved. In addition to other positive indicators, it should be noted that the budget deficit fell to 2.4% of the GDP (compared with 33% in 1992 and 3.6% in 1995), total exports grew 33%, labor productivity increased 8.5%, investment went up 54%, personal consumption rose 4%, and collective and government consumption increased 4% and 2%, respectively. The value of the peso, which averaged 60 pesos per United States dollar in 1994 and 32.1 pesos in 1995, dropped to 19.2 pesos per dollar in 1996, which points to a gradual revaluation of the currency. Although the negative trend seems to have reversed and the economy appears to be growing, the country still faces difficulties as a result of unfavorable foreign borrowing terms, especially high short-term interest rates.

On the political front, noteworthy developments include efforts to extend the decentralization of the government (including decentralization of the National Health System) and the economic sectors; to promote and develop popular participation in decision-making processes at all levels through development of grassroots entities within the political structure—the popular councils and municipal governments; and to strengthen the Parliament and its commissions, including health, sports, and the environment commissions, as the legislative organ of the State.

For an 8-month period beginning in June 1997, the country was immersed in a process of general elections in which the population voted, freely and by secret ballot, for the delegates to the municipal and provincial assemblies and for representatives to the National People's Assembly.

As of 30 June 1996, the estimated population was 11,005,866, and the population density was 99.3 inhabitants per km². The birth rate has declined steadily, reaching a low of 12.7 in 1996, with a reduction of about 30% for the decade. Fertility rates have also decreased. The general fertility rate dropped from 66.1 per 1,000 women aged 15–49 years in 1985 to 46.7 in 1996. At the same time, the group aged 60 and over continued to increase in absolute terms as well as proportionally and in 1996 made up 12.7% of the population. In 1992, persons under 15 years of age made up 22.4% of the population and in 1996, 22.0%. The general mortality rate was 7.0 per 1,000 inhabitants in 1992 (the highest rate during the period 1986–1992) and it reached 7.2 in 1996. Projected life expectancy at birth for the five-year period 1995–2000 is 75.48 for both sexes, 73.56 for males, and 77.51 for females.

Whereas infectious and parasitic diseases were the main causes of death 30 years ago, today the vast majority of deaths are due to chronic and degenerative diseases and accidents. The leading causes of death for all ages are heart disease, malignant neoplasms, cerebrovascular disease, and accidents. These four causes are responsible for 65% of all deaths.

From the political-administrative standpoint, the country is divided into 14 provinces and 1 municipality with special status (Isla de la Juventud). These areas have populations ranging from 0.5 to 1 million—except the city of Havana, which has slightly more than 2 million inhabitants, and Isla de la Juventud, which has 77,429 inhabitants. The urban population has increased from 69.0% in 1981 to 74.5% in 1995, according to intercensus estimates of the National Statistics Bureau of Cuba. The population under 15 in rural areas is proportionally larger than in urban areas (24.3% and 21.5%, respectively). The reverse is true of the populations aged 15–59 years (64.2% and 65.4%, respectively) and 60 and over (11.5% and 13.2%, respectively).

Mortality Profile

Analysis of the mortality profile according to six major groups of causes and by urban and rural populations in 1996 reveals that adjusted mortality rates in urban, rural-urban, and rural areas were 649.1, 617.4, and 490.6 per 100,000 inhabitants, respectively, with a mortality ratio of 1.3 between the highest and lowest rates. In general, this pattern holds for all groups of causes, with the exception of conditions that originate in the perinatal period and violence, both of which account for more deaths in rural-urban areas. Provisional data from 1996 indicate that the mortality rates per 100,000 inhabitants associated with five major groups of causes are as follows: diseases of the circulatory system, 311.4; malignant neoplasms, 141.0; external causes, 79.3; infectious and parasitic diseases, 51.4; and all other causes, 136.4.

For a number of years, general mortality has been characterized by a marked predominance of causes associated with chronic noncommunicable diseases. Mortality from diabetes, for example, has risen steadily, increasing from 9.9 per 100,000 in 1970 to 11.1 in 1980 and 23.4 in 1996, with a larger proportion of deaths occurring among women.

SPECIFIC HEALTH PROBLEMS

Analysis by Population Group

Health of Children

Perinatal mortality has decreased significantly, from 14.2 per 1,000 live births in 1992 to 12.4 in 1996, a 13% decrease for the period. Hypoxia, asphyxia, and other respiratory disorders continue to rank among the leading causes of mortality of the neonatal component.

Low birthweight, after declining steadily until 1989, when the rate was 7.3%, began to climb again, reaching 9.0% in 1993. The national program for the prevention and control of low birthweight was subsequently revised and updated, and by 1996 the level had dropped back to 7.3%. The pattern has been similar in all the provinces of the country.

Infant mortality in 1992 represented 2.1% of total mortality in all age groups; in 1996, this proportion dropped to 1.4%. The five leading causes of death in children less than 1 year old accounted for 83% of all infant deaths in 1996. Most deaths were due to conditions originating in the perinatal period, with a rate of 3.2 per 1,000 live births, followed by congenital abnormalities, with a rate of 2.1, and sepsis, influenza and pneumonia, and accidents with rates of 0.5, 0.3, and 0.3, respectively. Mortality from the latter three causes has decreased markedly.

Infant mortality continues to fall: from a rate of 10.2 per 1,000 live births in 1992, it decreased to 7.9 in 1996. In that year, the rates ranged from 9.7 to 6.0 in the western provinces and from 9.2 to 7.6 in the eastern provinces. Of the five central-eastern provinces (Villa Clara, Cienfuegos, Sancti Spíritus, Ciego de Ávila, and Camagüey) Camagüey and Villa Clara had the lowest rates (5.4 and 5.9, respectively). The highest and lowest provincial rates reported in 1990 were 13.6 and 7.6

per 1,000 live births, and in 1996 they were 10.3 and 5.1, which confirms the downward trend of these rates across the country.

Mortality from all causes in the group aged 1–4 years remained stable at 0.6 to 0.7 per 1,000 people in this age group during the last five-year period. The five leading causes of death in this age group are, first, accidents, with a rate of 1.9 per 10,000 inhabitants in 1996; second and third are malignant neoplasms and congenital abnormalities, with rates of 0.6 and 0.8, respectively. Pneumonia, which ranked second as a cause of death among preschool children in the early 1980s, was the fourth leading cause in 1996. Meningitis ranked fifth, with a rate of 0.2 per 10,000.

The crude death rate for all causes in the group aged 5–14 years, which has the lowest mortality in the country, remained at 0.4 per 1,000 children in this age group in 1987, and it dropped to 0.3 in 1996. Accidents were the leading cause of death with rates of 14.7 per 100,000 in 1992, 17.0 in 1994, and 14.8 in 1996. In the latter year, accidents caused 14.8 deaths per 100,000 children aged 5–14 (242 deaths), which was approximately 44.8% of all deaths in this age group and more than double (60%) the number of deaths due to the next four causes: malignant tumors, 4.9 (80 deaths); congenital abnormalities, 2.8 (45 deaths); influenza and pneumonia, 1.0 (16 deaths); and heart disease, 0.9 (15 deaths). Accidents were the leading cause of death in the 5–14 age group, accounting for 38.8% of all deaths in this group, more than in 1992, when the number was 34.5%. Within this group of causes, traffic accidents accounted for 73.4 years of potential life lost (YPLL) per 100,000 people in the group aged 1–4 and 36.7 per 100,000 in the group aged 5–14 years; a greater proportion of males were affected in both age groups.

Health of Adolescents and Adults

Accidents remain the leading cause of death for individuals up to 49 years of age, with a rate of 38.9 per 100,000 in the group aged 15–49 years in 1996, slightly higher than the value of 37.9 reported in 1992, and they are one of the principal health problems of adolescents and young adults. Other important problems in these two groups are the high incidence of sexually transmitted diseases (STDs) and the increase in viral hepatitis type A, the incidence of which increased from 161.2 per 100,000 in 1992 to 217.0 in 1996.

The crude death rate for all causes in the group aged 15–49 years was 1.7 per 1,000 in 1996. Accidents were the leading cause of death in 1996, and they accounted for 20.4% of all deaths in this age group. As in 1992, malignant neoplasms ranked second, with a rate of 28.8 deaths per 100,000 inhabitants. Heart disease ranked third (20.4 per 100,000); suicides

and self-inflicted injuries (18.2) and homicide (10.2) ranked fourth and fifth.

Health of Women

The number of women employed in the public sector increased from 669,100 in 1975 to 1,429,900 in 1990, when 40% of all workers were women. Health care for women and children and the work of the Maternal and Child Health Program are considered top public health priorities.

The average number of prenatal medical visits per woman increased from 17.2 in 1992 to 23.6 in 1996. The average number of well-baby visits per child under 1 year of age increased from 13.4 in 1992 to 23.5 in 1996, which, combined with the visits due to illness, brings the average number of medical visits per infant to 35.0 in 1996.

The rate of induced abortion decreased from 70.0 per 100 deliveries in 1992 to 59.4 in 1996. The Family Planning Program is seeking to expand the variety of contraceptives available, increase their use, and enhance their quality. The prevalence of contraceptive use is estimated at 79%. Maternal deaths due to complications of pregnancy, childbirth, and the puerperium decreased from 3.3 per 10,000 live births in 1992 to 2.4 in 1996.

Mortality from all causes among women aged 50–64 was 8.4 per 1,000 women in 1996. The five leading causes of death were malignant neoplasms (236.8 per 100,000), heart disease (222.3), cerebrovascular disease (79.2), accidents (42.2), and diabetes mellitus (38.9).

Health of the Elderly

In 1996, 84.7% of all deaths occurred among persons aged 50 and over. The over-60 age group accounted for 76.3% of all deaths, and the group aged 65 and over accounted for 68.9%. There has been a rising trend in the number of accidental falls among persons of both sexes aged 60 and over, and they are more frequent among women.

Mortality from all causes in the group aged 65 and over was 54.9 per 1,000 in 1996. The five leading causes of death were heart disease, with a rate of 1,803.9 per 100,000; malignant neoplasms (968.0); cerebrovascular disease (631.3); influenza and pneumonia (378.6); and diseases of the arteries, arterioles, and capillaries (330.2).

Morbidity from communicable diseases in older adults decreased in 1996 compared with the previous year, as did morbidity from acute diarrheal diseases, which fell 6%. On the other hand, medical consultations for acute respiratory infections increased to a rate of 28,212.7 per 100,000 inhabitants. The incidence of tuberculosis in 1996 was also lower than in

1995, although, proportionally, the rate is highest in this age group.

Workers' Health

The country's socioeconomic situation influenced the activity of the workers. Initially, certain occupational risks decreased because of paralysis of the work force in some sectors, which led to a reduction in accidents, especially fatal accidents; however, other risks increased as a result of job changes, reintegration of workers into the work force, and redefinition of duties in factories and other workplaces. The reorientation of many activities toward agriculture and the increase in self-employment have created new challenges for the public health sector in terms of protecting the health of workers. There are two principal occupational disorders linked to urban and industrial environments—hearing loss from excess noise and skin diseases.

Occupational accidents have shown a downward trend. Between 1992 and 1995, the incidence declined from 8.2 to 5.3 per 1,000 workers. During 1995, there were 20,805 disabling injuries, 33,000 fewer than in 1992, and the number of fatal accidents decreased to 72. Of the deaths that occurred, 70% were males, and the largest proportion occurred in the 21–40 age group.

Health care for workers is provided through the National Health and Epidemiology Network by 2,217 general practitioners who work on-site in factories and other workplaces, which helps to strengthen primary health care for workers, with an approach that emphasizes prevention, health promotion, and risk assessment.

Analysis by Type of Disease or Health Impairment

Communicable Diseases

Cholera and Other Intestinal Diseases. The incidence of intestinal infectious diseases has increased in recent years due to the influence of environmental and health-sanitation conditions. Between 1989 and 1996, morbidity from hepatitis A increased from 24.5 to 189.0 per 100,000 inhabitants. In 1996, 90.9 medical visits per 1,000 inhabitants were reported for acute diarrheal disease. Morbidity from typhoid fever increased during the period 1989–1996, rising from 0.5 to 0.7 per 100,000 inhabitants at the national level. Mortality from acute diarrheal diseases, some of which are of infectious origin, increased from 4.2 per 100,000 in 1992 to 5.0 in 1996, accounting for 0.7% of all deaths that year.

Implementing the measures needed to control this situation has been made a priority within the health system. In re-

sponse to the ongoing threat of a cholera outbreak, vigorous efforts are under way to strengthen the surveillance system, put in place mechanisms to halt the spread of the disease should any cases occur, and prevent the creation of conditions that would be favorable for an epidemic. To date, however, no cases of cholera have been reported in the country.

Vaccine-Preventable Diseases. Five cases of tetanus were reported in 1992 and four were reported in 1996. The effectiveness of the Cuban immunization system is reflected in the elimination of three diseases (poliomyelitis, diphtheria, and measles) as well as in the suppression of two serious diseases (tuberculous meningitis and neonatal tetanus) and the disappearance of two serious complications (mumps meningitis and congenital rubella syndrome). Fifteen cases of measles were reported in 1992, but none has been reported since 1994. No cases of rubella or mumps were reported in 1996. The level of immunization coverage for all vaccine-preventable diseases is satisfactory: more than 95% at the national level. By the year 2000, the country intends to immunize the entire population under 20 years of age against hepatitis B.

Acute Respiratory Infections. Respiratory infections, especially acute, short-lived infections, are by far the leading causes of morbidity in Cuba. Although they are relatively benign and seldom fatal, the high incidence of these diseases nevertheless leads to increased absenteeism from work and school and more visits to the doctor. About 60% of these visits are for children under the age of 15, and 41.7% of these are children between 1 and 4 years of age. In 1996, the total number of medical visits for this cause totaled approximately 5 million. In the past three years, the number of affected infants and preschoolers has increased, as has the number of affected persons over the age of 60.

Tuberculosis. Tuberculosis was the leading cause of death in the country early in this century. In 1961, it was still among the 10 leading causes of death. During the 1980s, mortality and morbidity from this disease declined throughout the country, and by 1990 the incidence had fallen to 5.1 per 100,000 inhabitants. However, in recent years the number of cases has risen to 12.0, 14.2, and 13.3 per 100,000 in 1994, 1995, and 1996, respectively. The largest concentration of cases is found in the group aged 65 and over and the pulmonary form of the disease is most common, with a total rate for this age group of 38.9 per 100,000 in 1996—35.0 for the pulmonary form and 3.9 for extrapulmonary tuberculosis. In 1994 the activities of the Tuberculosis Prevention and Control Program were stepped up, and at present improvements in detection and diagnosis of the disease are being noted in the majority of the provinces, which have reported a slight decrease in incidence.

Leprosy. The prevalence of leprosy has declined steadily since 1989, and by 1993 it had fallen to a level of less than 1 per 10,000 inhabitants. During 1994, the prevalence was 0.7 and in 1995 it dropped to 0.62 per 10,000 inhabitants. In 1996, the rate was 0.57, and the ratio of new cases detected to those who have completed treatment appeared to have stabilized. However, in late 1996 four provinces, three of them in the eastern region of the country, reported rates higher than 1 per 10,000 inhabitants. The indicators for measuring the level of transmission point to a slow decline. Given current rates, the disease is no longer considered a public health problem.

Vector-Borne Diseases. No indigenous cases of malaria were reported in the period 1992–1996. With regard to dengue, no indigenous transmission occurred between October 1981 and December 1996. Since January 1997, dengue cases have been reported in the country's easternmost region, in the municipality of Santiago de Cuba. A total of 2,946 cases were confirmed by serological tests; of these 205 were hemorrhagic dengue. Among children, morbidity was very low and only one case of hemorrhagic dengue was reported. Twelve deaths occurred, all in adults. Serotype 2, genotype Jamaica, was identified as the infectious agent in the outbreak. Transmission occurred with infestation indices of less than 2%.

Rabies and Other Zoonoses. The incidence of leptospirosis, which has shown a rising trend since 1986, peaked in 1994 (25.8 per 100,000 inhabitants), an epidemic year, after which the incidence declined markedly as a result of the application of prevention and control measures throughout the country. The actions undertaken, which were aimed, above all, at protecting the groups at highest risk, included vaccination and chemoprophylaxis, environmental sanitation, and improving the quality of diagnosis as well as efforts to eliminate the rodent vectors. By 1996 the incidence had been reduced to 12.9 per 100,000 inhabitants. The prevention and control activities are ongoing.

After a 10-year period during which no human cases of rabies were reported, the disease reappeared in 1988. Between that year and 1995, six fatal cases of rabies occurred in humans. No cases were reported in 1996. Of the reported cases, five were transmitted by nonhematophagous bats and one by a feral cat. There were no significant outbreaks of canine rabies during that period. In 1996, 30,202 reports were received of humans being bitten by animals; most cases involved dog bites.

Pediculosis and Scabies. Since mid-1994 an unusual increase in medical visits for pediculosis and scabies has been observed. The situation grew worse in 1995, prompting the development of an emergency action plan, which was implemented in 1996. The basic strategy was aimed at ensuring rapid diagnosis and appropriate treatment, control of foci,

active case-finding, ongoing education and involvement of the community, and availability of medications. Various institutions and agencies took part in these activities, but the joint efforts of the Ministry of Education and the Ministry of Public Health were crucial. As a result of these efforts, despite a better system of diagnosis and active case-finding, outbreaks of pediculosis and scabies fell 23% and medical visits for these causes decreased 5%. The reduction was even greater in schools, where most cases occurred.

AIDS and Other STDs. Between 1986, when the seroepidemiological detection program was launched, and the end of 1996, 1,468 HIV-positive individuals were detected; of these, 534 developed AIDS and 381 died. More males than females are infected, and most of the infected males (65%) are homosexual/bisexual. The incidence is highest in the group aged 15–19 years, followed by the 20–24 age group. The majority of HIV-infected individuals acquired the infection in Cuba; only slightly more than 15% became infected abroad. Active case-finding reveals that most new cases are detected in contacts of HIV-positive individuals (33.7%), in persons with STDs (15%), and in prisoners (14.1%). The Cuban strategy for addressing this problem includes conducting studies of the groups at highest risk, carrying out epidemiological investigation of 100% of cases, performing analyses of hospital admission records (as well as outpatient care records since 1993), and implementing a comprehensive program of health education for the general population.

Reports of sexually transmitted diseases are on the increase especially in the case of syphilis and gonorrhea, the rates for which in 1996 were 143.7 and 368.7, respectively, per 100,000 inhabitants. Work is currently under way to upgrade the prevention and control program, improve diagnosis and case reporting, and carry out educational activities and promote safe sexual behaviors.

Infectious Neurological Syndromes. The incidence of meningococcal disease has continued to decline since the initiation of vaccination in the country in 1986. The rate in 1989 was 3.8 per 100,000 inhabitants, but by 1996 it had dropped to 0.5 per 100,000. Other bacterial meningoencephalitides are associated with endemic levels of morbidity. As for viral meningoencephalitides, an epidemic increase began in 1995 and extended into the first months of 1996. Three types of enterovirus were identified in the samples studied: Coxsackie A9, Echo 30, and Coxsackie B5.

Noncommunicable Diseases and Other Health-Related Problems

In the past 20 years, the relative importance of noncommunicable diseases and injuries due to violence has increased and these two groups of causes now account for the largest proportion of deaths in all age groups. Three causes account for the largest proportion of years of potential life lost (YPLL) in the groups between 1 and 64 years of age: accidents, malignant neoplasms, and heart disease, with rates of 10.3, 7.3, and 5.5, respectively, per 1,000 inhabitants.

Cardiovascular Diseases. Cardiovascular diseases are the leading cause of death in Cuba, with a crude death rate of 205.9 per 100,000 inhabitants in 1996. Although this number is higher than in 1989 (189.3 per 100,000 inhabitants), the trend, based on age-adjusted rates, is downward. Within this group, the primary cause is acute myocardial infarction, with a rate of 112.7 (more than 50% of all deaths from cardiovascular disease). Males are at greatest risk of dying from heart disease; in 1996 the rate among males was 222.2 per 100,000 inhabitants, compared with 189.4 for females. When mortality from the six major groups of causes is calculated, these diseases are included in the group of circulatory system diseases, which account for the highest mortality in the groups aged 65 and over and 40–64, with rates of 2,776.6 and 205.5, respectively, per 100,000.

A small degree of excess male mortality from this cause is observed, particularly in the case of acute ischemic heart disease; the risk of dying from acute myocardial infarction is greater among males than females (male/female ratio: 1.3). The largest number of deaths occurs among persons over the age of 65, who account for 85% of all deaths from this cause.

Cerebrovascular disease has been the third leading cause of death for several years. In 1996, the crude death rate from this cause was 72.7 per 100,000 inhabitants, higher than in 1989 (64.3 per 100,000). Nevertheless, standardized rates indicate a downward trend. In 1989, the number of male deaths exceeded the number of female deaths according to mortality rates for both sexes, but in 1996 the male/female ratio was 0.9. Most of these deaths (79.5%) occur in the over-65 age group.

According to data from the World Health Organization (WHO), mean blood pressure in the Cuban population, compared with other countries, is in the medium-low range. Maintenance or reduction of these levels could have a beneficial effect on the population in the medium and long terms by reducing the frequency of cardiovascular and other diseases. The prevalence of high blood pressure (30.6%) is high but similar to that of other countries; one in three Cubans aged 15 or over suffers from hypertension. A national survey of risk factors in 1995 detected 12% new hypertensives. Of all the hypertensive patients interviewed, only 45.2% were being monitored regularly.

Malignant Tumors. For the past 26 years, malignant neoplasms have been the second leading cause of death in all age groups. The crude death rate from this cause increased from 128.8 per 100,000 inhabitants in 1990 to 137.3 per 100,000 in 1996; however, the adjusted rates for the same years went down from 116.6 to 111.0 per 100,000 inhabitants. The number of deaths from malignant tumors varies according to sex; the rates per 100,000 are 156.1 for males and 118.3 for females. The highest rates occur in the groups aged 50–64 and 65 and over. Mortality rates adjusted for place of residence show higher rates in urban areas (121.5 per 100,000 inhabitants) than in rural-urban areas (117.3) or rural areas (94.5). YPLL per 1,000 people aged 1–64 years ranged from 6.7 to 7.6 between 1980 and 1996.

The incidence of all forms of cancer, including both crude and adjusted rates, decreased during the three-year period between 1992 and 1994. The adjusted rate fell from 176.8 per 100,000 inhabitants in 1992 to 159.2 in 1994. The incidence by sex declined more markedly in females (from 164.7 per 100,000 in 1992 to 142.2 in 1994) than in males (from 189.8 to 177.9 per 100,000 during the same period).

For the period 1985–1993, the five most frequent cancer sites were the lung, prostate, skin, bladder, and colon for males and the breast, skin, cervix, lung, and colon for females. Comparatively, during the three-year periods 1988–1990 and 1991–1993, there was an increase only in adjusted rates of colon cancer among men (9.3 to 9.9 per 100,000 inhabitants) and breast cancer among women (29.8 to 31.7 per 100,000 inhabitants). The rates fell for the other sites.

In 1996, as part of the Early Cervical Cancer Treatment Program, 1,023.913 women aged 20 and over were screened, yielding a screening rate of 26.0%. Of the positive cases, 88% were detected at stage 0 and 11% were detected at stage 1. The mortality rate increased from 6.2 per 100,000 in 1995 to 6.8 per 100,000 in 1996. The incidence during the period 1991–1993 was 4.9 per 100,000 inhabitants, similar to the previous three-year period. The program has not produced the expected results.

The preventive activities assessed in the national risk factor survey of 1995 (Pap smear, breast examination and self-examination, among others) reflect a moderate level of performance. Among the women over the age of 30 surveyed, 26.6% had performed a breast self-examination in the preceding 12 months, and 53.5% had performed a self-examination on at least one occasion.

Chronic Obstructive Pulmonary Disease and Bronchial Asthma. These disorders are among the leading causes of death in all age groups. They occur in both sexes similarly and are most frequent among persons over the age of 55. In 1995 the crude death rate from these causes for both sexes was 22.4 per 100,000 inhabitants, higher than in 1989 (16.7). Mortality from bronchial asthma has shown a rising trend. In 1996 the crude death rate from asthma was 5.3 per 100,000 inhabitants, higher than the rate of 4.4 registered in 1989 and similar to the rate of 5.5 recorded in 1995. More females than males die from asthma, and this excess female mortality has become more marked in the past three years. In 1996 the death rate among males was 4.4 per 100,000, and among females it was 6.1. According to specialists, this pattern is linked to women's greater exposure to harmful environmental factors (domestic fuels), which exacerbates asthma attacks, coupled with difficulties in the provision of medical care and outpatient monitoring for asthmatic patients. A plan aimed at reversing this trend is currently being implemented as part of the new program for the treatment and control of asthma.

Accidents. Accidents remain the fourth leading cause of death for all ages and the leading cause in the group aged 1–49 years as well as the primary cause of premature death as measured by YPLL (10.0 per 100,000 people aged 1–64 years). Mortality from accidents has shown a slight rising trend, based on adjusted rates. The largest proportion of accidental deaths are due to motor vehicle traffic accidents, with a rate of 19.7 per 10,000 inhabitants in 1996. Within this group, deaths of cyclists increased steadily between 1990 and 1995. There is a marked sex differentiation. Accidents are far more common among males, in particular those aged 40 and over. Among females, mortality from this cause is much lower, and the age groups most affected are those between 20 and 29 years old, with a rate of 9.1, and 70 and over, with a rate of 13.2. Falls are the most frequent cause of accidental death among females, with rates of 17.9 per 100,000 women in 1992 and 19.9 in 1996, much higher than the female rate of death from traffic accidents (8.0).

Diabetes Mellitus. Diabetes mellitus was the seventh leading cause of death for all ages in 1996, with a rate of 23.4 per 100,000 inhabitants. It causes more deaths among females than males (31.4 per 100,000 inhabitants in 1996 compared with 15.5 per 100,000 for males). There are also differences among urban and rural populations, with adjusted rates of 22.2 and 13.4, respectively, per 100,000 inhabitants. Based on the records of family physicians, it is estimated that the prevalence of the disease in 1996 was 19.3 per 1,000 inhabitants.

Suicide. Deaths from suicide and self-inflicted injuries decreased from 21.1 per 100,000 inhabitants in 1992 to 18.2 in 1996. During the period 1981–1996, suicide was greater among males in all but one age group; in the group aged 10–19, the rate was greater among females.

Epidemic Neuropathy. An outbreak of epidemic neuropathy has been ongoing since 1992. The epidemic began in the western region and spread to the rest of the country in early 1993. From 1994 to 1996 the disease showed an endemic pattern, and by the end of 1996 a cumulative total of 54,640 cases

had been reported, yielding a case rate of 496.5 per 100,000 inhabitants. Of the reported cases, 41.3% were the optic form of the disease. The epidemiological pattern by age, sex, and severity of the various clinical forms has not varied. The clinical optic form is most frequent among males in the group aged 45–64 years, and the peripheral form predominates in females aged 25–44. In a follow-up analysis of all cases reported since 1992, 47,994 patients were evaluated (88.4% of the total) and 39,754 were given a clinical discharge (82.8%); 8,729 were found to have sequelae (18.8% of all patients evaluated). The patients with sequelae to the peripheral form have been included in the Community Rehabilitation Program, and those with sequelae to the optic form (impaired vision) are receiving rehabilitation services in three specially equipped centers located in the cities of Santiago de Cuba, Pinar del Río, and Havana. Doctors continue to treat the disease with A, E, and B-complex vitamins, and a national campaign is under way to promote two vitamin supplements.

Oral Health. In 1996 there were more than 17 million visits to the dentist in Cuba, which makes the rate 1.6 visits per person. Of these visits, more than 85% were for general dentistry services provided in the framework of primary health care. During the year, 3,361,122 persons were examined; 51.7% of them were under the age of 15 years. Of all those examined, 28.4% were found to have good oral health. Of those under 15 years of age, 31.8% had good oral health. The preventive program continues to be carried out at the national level, and during the year 24,103,414 fluoride rinse treatments were administered to children aged 5–14 years and 1,324,971 topical fluoride treatments were given to children under the age of 4 years. Oral cancer was detected in 1,922 of the patients examined.

According to the findings of the National Oral Health Survey carried out in 1995, 43.6% of children aged 5 and 6 years old are free of dental caries, while the DMFT (decayed, missing, filled teeth) index for 12-year-old children is 1.86 times higher than the target proposed for the year 2000.

Natural Disasters. The most recent natural disaster was Hurricane Lili, which struck Cuba on 17 October 1996 and caused severe economic damage to housing and agriculture. Nevertheless, thanks to the population's preparedness and the preventive evacuation of some 200,000 people, no human lives were lost. To enhance the country's capacity for disaster management, a disaster medicine center was established in June 1996.

Behavioral Disorders. In 1995, the National Institute of Hygiene, Epidemiology, and Microbiology, in collaboration with the National Statistics Bureau, conducted the first national survey of risk factors and preventive activities for noncommunicable diseases. This was a representative survey of households in each province of the country and the special municipality of Isla de la Juventud. The study population consisted of urban dwellers (75% of the Cuban population) over the age of 15.

Systematic efforts to prevent and control tobacco use, which have been under way since 1985, have succeeded in halting the rising trend of tobacco use and reducing its prevalence. During the five-year period 1990–1995, tobacco use decreased. The current prevalence of tobacco use is 36%. The percentage of males aged 15 and over who smoke regularly is 48.1%, and that of females is 26.3%.

Frequency of consumption and quantity consumed were the criteria used to evaluate consumption of alcoholic beverages. The results can be considered acceptable in terms of the population as a whole, given that 55% of those surveyed reported not having consumed any alcoholic beverage in the preceding 12 months or having done so fewer than five times. Men aged 20–29 and 40–59 are the groups at highest risk.

Nutritional Diseases. The nutritional situation, evaluated on the basis of body mass index, compared favorably with that in 1982 and is related to apparent levels of consumption per capita in the period 1992–1995, according to data from the National Statistics Bureau. However, a larger proportion of people with chronic energy deficiency and underweight was noted in those aged 20–59 years and, to an even greater extent, in those over the age of 60, although the levels vary from region to region within the country. Overweight and obesity are more frequent among women and tend to increase with age.

The nutritional status of children aged under 1 and 1–4 years, based on the weight-for-height indicator, has remained stable and is similar to that found in previous years. In 1996, 1.8% of children under the age of 1 year were below the third percentile. In the group aged 1–4, the proportion was 0.8%. Since 1996 the country has established sentinel sites where height-for-age is assessed, because it is considered necessary to measure the effect of the nutritional situation on the linear growth of these age groups.

Iron deficiency anemia is the most common nutritional problem in Cuba. It affects more than 40% of women in the third trimester of pregnancy, around 50% of infants between 6 and 11 months of age, between 40% and 50% of children aged 1–3 years, and between 25% and 30% of women of childbearing age. A project to enrich flour with iron is being developed.

In 1995, the National Food and Nutrition Institute (INHA) conducted a national study of iodine intake levels. Analysis of iodine excretion in the urine of schoolchildren revealed mild to moderate deficiencies in the areas studied, especially in mountainous areas. In accordance with the criteria of the In-

ternational Council for Control of Iodine Deficiency Disorders, the United Nations Children's Fund (UNICEF), and WHO on iodine deficiency, the populations in the regions identified exhibited manifestations of deficiencies of this micronutrient. For this reason, to ensure adequate levels of iodine intake, the Ministry of Industry, in coordination with the INHA, other institutions of the Ministry of Public Health, and other State agencies, has begun to produce iodized salt.

Vitamin A intake, as measured by analysis of data on apparent consumption and nutritional surveillance, is also low. There are no national studies on serum levels of this nutrient, but work is under way to enrich foods with vitamin A as a preventive measure. Intake of vitamin B continues to fall below recommended levels.

RESPONSE OF THE HEALTH SYSTEM

National Health Plans and Policies

In 1991, the Ministry of Public Health drafted a document entitled *Objetivos, propósitos y directrices para incrementar la salud de la población cubana 1992–2000* ["Objectives, Aims, and Guidelines for Improving the Health of the Cuban Population 1992–2000"], which defines health goals and objectives to be achieved by the year 2000. In 1996 five strategies and four priority programs were identified. The strategies include reorientation of the health system toward primary care and the family doctor and nurse program, which is considered the pillar of the system; revitalization of hospital care; revitalization of high-technology programs and research institutions; development of a program on natural and traditional medicine and remedies; and care with an emphasis on system objectives, such as dentistry, optical services, and health transport. The priority programs are those on maternal and child health, chronic noncommunicable diseases, communicable diseases, and care of the elderly.

As a fundamental part of the changes of the revolutionary period, since the 1960s the Government has introduced several important reforms in the health system. Reform of the health sector in Cuba can be said to be more an ongoing process than a temporary or finite phenomenon. Nevertheless, a number of factors in the current context justify a fresh approach to health reform, including the effects of the economic crisis of recent years on the health situation and on health services, changes in the national context and the transformation that has been under way in the country since 1989, the process of State reform, and the contradictions inherent in the health system.

The Ministry of Public Health has developed a strategy for responding to existing, emerging, and reemerging problems. The strategy seeks to increase the efficiency and quality of health services; to ensure the sustainability of the system, especially in financial terms; and, although a high level of health equity has been achieved, to work to eliminate the small reducible inequalities in health care and in the use of health services in different regions and population groups. The strategy emphasizes promotion of health and prevention of disease in the framework of strengthening primary health care and family medicine, decentralization, intersectoral action, and community participation, as well as improvement of services at the secondary and tertiary levels.

The process of decentralization and the creation of a new structure of government that allows for more grassroots involvement (through the popular councils) has encouraged active participation of the social sectors in health management at the local level. In 1995, as an outcome of the integrative policy for the development of the National Health System, health councils were established at the national, provincial, municipal, and popular council levels. These health councils are made up of representatives of the various social sectors and civic organizations and are headed by a government representative at each level. They have facilitated intersectoral collaboration and have increased the capacity for social participation in the identification and solution of health problems in the community. The country, as part of the "health initiative" process aimed at mobilizing national and international resources to support reform and modernization of the sector, has developed a master investment plan that sets out the basic problems, outlines strategies and actions for addressing those problems, and recommends a series of investment projects for resolving or mitigating them.

Currently, a revamping of the National Health System is being considered with a view to making more efficient use of resources and investments. Among other changes, it has been proposed that the number of hospital beds and teaching institutions be reduced and that some products made by the pharmaceutical industry be eliminated.

Organization of the Health Sector

Institutional Organization

In Cuba the State assumes full responsibility for the health care of its citizens. Health is considered the key ingredient for quality of life and is seen as a strategic objective in the development of society.

In 1983 the Parliament adopted the Public Health Law, which lays out the general activities to be carried out by the State to protect the health of Cuban citizens. The law establishes the organization of the sector and the services to be provided by the State, with the Ministry of Public Health as the lead agency, and it specifies the functions of health authorities at the provincial level. It also regulates the delivery of health care and contains provisions relating to the social nature of the practice of medicine, application of a preventive approach in the provision of services, appropriate use of science and technology, priority attention to maternal and child health care, outpatient and inpatient hospital care, transplants of organs and tissue, control of epidemics, government health inspections, health and epidemiological prophylaxis, and health education. The Public Health Law is complemented by other legislation, including environmental laws, basic sanitation regulations, a decree-law on international health regulations, and law and regulations on occupational health and protection of workers.

Despite the development attained by the sector in recent years, the Public Health Law needs to adapt to new factors and determinants, which have modified the public health environment, both internally and externally. Among these factors is the new health strategy, which is oriented toward primary care and is embodied in the family doctor and nurse program, development of new programs for the incorporation of high technology in the sector, and the need to adjust the National Health System to the economic changes taking place in the country without compromising its basic principles.

Because this goes beyond the scope of the Public Health Law, it has been determined that a new judicial framework should be adopted to allow for greater intersectoral action and community participation. Since 1995, the Health Commission of the Cuban Parliament, in conjunction with the Ministry of Public Health, has been in the process of revising the existing legislation.

Organization of the National Health System. The National Health System is organized at three levels (national, provincial, and municipal), which mirror the country's administrative structure. The National Assembly (Parliament) and the provincial and municipal assemblies have permanent working commissions. In addition, the National Health Commission also deals with issues relating to sports and the environment and advises the leadership of the National Assembly and Council of State in these areas. Local organs of government in the provinces and municipalities have a commission that is responsible for health-related issues at that level. In the Cuban Parliament, the Commission on Health, Sports, and the Environment is the highest-level regulatory body charged with oversight of the various government institutions responsible for these areas.

The national level is represented by the Ministry of Public Health, which serves as the lead agency and fulfills methodological, regulatory, coordination, and control functions. Directly under the Ministry are university centers, highly specialized medical research and care institutions, the Union of the Medical-Pharmaceutical Industry and its laboratories, and firms that market and distribute medical equipment, as well as one firm that imports and exports drugs and high-technology medical equipment.

The provincial level is represented by the provincial public health offices, which are under the direct financial and administrative authority of the provincial administrative councils. The principal units under the responsibility of the provincial governments are the provincial and intermunicipal hospitals, blood banks, provincial health and epidemiology centers, training centers for health professionals and mid-level health technicians, and the network of commercial pharmacies and optical shops.

At the municipal level are the municipal public health offices, which come under the financial and administrative responsibility of the municipal administrative councils. The units overseen include polyclinics; rural, local, and municipal hospitals; municipal health and epidemiology units and centers; oral health clinics; social welfare institutions for the elderly and persons with mental or physical disabilities; maternity homes; and other establishments. The nuclei of municipal activity are the popular councils, a set of small communities that form an organ for coordination with certain executive authorities, thus giving concrete expression to the concepts of administrative decentralization and public participation in decision-making and in the government of the nation. The councils work in close coordination with the municipal health system.

Organization of Health Regulatory Activities

Since 1993, the country has been working to develop an integrated surveillance system. Health trend analysis units have been created from the national to the municipal level. The function of these units is to integrate all monitoring and surveillance information in the context of each program, department, service, or strategy of the health system. At the same time, they conduct rapid assessments and epidemiological investigations in relation to the principal health problems, undertake a quarterly analysis of the health situation at each level, and follow trends and make forecasts for the short and medium terms. During the past year, an evaluation component has been added.

The Regulatory Bureau for Health Protection, created in 1996, is the highest official health regulatory institution in the country. Its mission is to ensure, together with other agencies, fulfillment of the specific objectives, functions, and faculties approved in the legislation on monitoring and surveillance of all products that may affect human health; regulate and monitor the approval, execution, and evaluation of biomedical research projects or any other type of research involving human

subjects; and evaluate, register, regulate, and control domestic and imported drugs, medical equipment, disposable materials, and other health care products.

The National Drugs Program was established in 1991 with a view to ensuring more rational use of drugs and improving the quality of medical care. This program was considered necessary because of drug shortages, which resulted from economic constraints and a consequent reduction in imports, and the lack of control over the prescribing, dispensing, and circulating of pharmaceutical products, as well as the persistent practices of self-medication and polypharmacy (administration of excessive medication). In 1994, the program was reformulated and measures were implemented to require a medical prescription for most drugs (exceptions include common antipyretics and analgesics and oral contraceptives); to regulate prescriptions written by doctors according to their medical specialties; to assign patients to drug distribution units in their area of residence; to strengthen the work of the pharmacotherapeutic committees; and to maintain the regulations on distribution of consumer products intended for long-term or lifelong use.

A special effort has been made to revise the essential drugs list, as a result of which it has been possible to reduce the number of active principles to 343 distributed among 29 drug classes with 439 dosage forms. In addition, there are traditional and natural medicinal products. The official drug control center is responsible for ensuring that products meet international quality standards. It is recognized internationally as the agency authorized to evaluate and register drugs, receive information, conduct inspections, analyze and authorize products for marketing, grant and revoke production licenses, and suspend the circulation and sale of drugs when necessary.

Health Services and Resources

Organization of Services for Care of the Population

Health Promotion. The health promotion strategy in Cuba stresses planning and execution of local projects, community organization, participation of all productive and nonproductive sectors, and the political will to support the development and implementation of health promotion activities.

The maximum expression of this strategy is the healthy communities movement, which seeks to pool local resources to promote health, with a solid basis of political support and the participation of various social sectors and the community within a specific territory, which permits coordination of political, technical, and community objectives.

The Cienfuegos Comprehensive Health Promotion Project was implemented in 1989 with the participation of the government of the city of Cienfuegos. The project was recognized by PAHO as an innovative experience in the Region. The national [health promotion] network, composed of 28 municipalities, was created in December 1994, and within two years it had expanded to include 51 municipalities. The Ministry of Public Health and the Cuban Parliament have made development of the network a priority objective. The project also has the support of PAHO.

Another important aspect of health promotion is mass communication. Special air time is allotted for this purpose on radio and television and on national networks as well as local stations. Alliances have been forged with professionals in these media and there are now specialized health journalists in both. All health programs incorporate a health education component, and to ensure their effectiveness health professionals are systematically trained in educational methodologies, especially those who work in the area of primary health care. The production of educational materials has increased, although difficulties persist because of the country's economic situation.

Water Supply. Cuba's hydraulic potential, although it is not uniform in density throughout the country, is sufficient to ensure the provision of water for household, agricultural, and industrial activities; 1,200 m³ of water per person per year is available for all uses. Of the total volume of water supplied to the population, 72% is of underground origin, and 28% is from surface sources; 68.3% of the total population (7.5 million) receives water from aqueducts, 89.3% in urban areas and 10.7% in rural areas. The rest of the population is served by other means (tank trucks and others), especially in rural areas. Nevertheless, the quantity and quality of the water supply have deteriorated substantially. With regard to quantity, water service is available for an average of 13 hours a day, with sizable differences among provinces, which has a negative effect on sanitation and control of vectors. Water quality is affected by the lack of treatment, which, in turn, is due to shortages of chlorine in its various forms and aluminum sulfate; in addition, chlorination equipment is frequently out of order. To correct this situation, various measures have been taken since 1994, including chlorination in about 50% of existing facilities and putting family doctors in charge of dispensing chlorine powder to families in the highest-risk areas. By directive of the central Government, in 1997 water supply systems will be upgraded in 371 rural communities with a total of 119,838 inhabitants, of which 300 are served by water tank trucks, 63 require treatment to make the water potable, and the remaining 8 need expansion of services.

Sewerage Systems. Coverage of liquid waste disposal is 91% for the country as a whole, and 34.2% of the total population has sewerage services. All dwellings constructed in areas without sewerage—most of which are concentrated in

rural areas—have individual collection and treatment systems, mainly latrines and septic tanks. Problems with sanitary disposal of excreta and liquid waste persist, collection systems are overburdened and in poor condition technically, and back-ups and breakage of sewer lines continue to occur frequently, with the consequent overflowing. All these problems increase the risk of contamination of drinking water supply systems. The provincial water supply and sewerage authorities have adopted measures for the organization and optimization of resources, but the results obtained have been insufficient to solve the problem.

Solid Waste Disposal. The situation with respect to solid waste is similar to that of liquid waste. Collection and final disposal of solid waste has been affected by transport and fuel supply problems that began in 1992 and continue to the present. This situation has given rise to the appearance of microdumps, especially in cities. Other solutions have been sought, including the use of animal-powered garbage wagons, cleanup of refuse dumps, and sanitary controls, but none of these measures has been sufficient.

To improve the health-sanitation situation, in 1994 a comprehensive national sanitation plan was implemented with civil defense participation. Supervision and control teams were created with a view to ensuring a water supply of adequate quality and quantity, proper treatment and final disposal of solid and liquid waste, and correct application of vector control and sanitation measures.

Prevention and Control of Air Pollution. Air pollution is not a major problem in Cuba, although some areas, especially Havana and other cities, are affected by air pollution from industrial activity: cement factories, thermoelectric power plants, and chemical plants, and, to a lesser extent, use of fuels for domestic purposes. In recent years, there has been an increase in the use of crude oil and petroleum products with a high sulfur content, which has increased the potential for pollution, with the associated health risks and ecological and economic damages. The national air pollution monitoring system, part of the surveillance system, has been seriously impaired by lack of resources; of 18 monitoring stations, only 6 are operating, and there are irregularities in the information they generate. The national air pollution monitoring program is aimed primarily at identifying and controlling the problems of each source of pollution, by updating inventories and inspection and identification of the areas at highest risk for air pollution and by improving the capacity of the system at the primary care level for the detection, assessment, and control of environmental risk factors.

Food Safety. Cuba has been working to reduce the number and frequency of illnesses due to consumption of foods contaminated with germs that are harmful to health. Biological, chemical, and toxicological studies, as well as strengthening the technical components and the efficacy of official health inspections, were some of the objectives. In addition, the hazard analysis critical control point (HACCP) methodology—which combines the scientific approaches employed in addressing the health and epidemiological problems surrounding food safety—was also adopted.

The food surveillance laboratory network comprises 14 health and epidemiology centers at the provincial level and 33 at the municipal level. The data processed by these centers are produced through sampling conducted in 136 health centers and 470 health areas within the system. The sampling plan was developed bearing in mind the risks posed by various foods and the existing resources in each province, and corrective health measures were introduced in areas where contaminated foods were found.

Food Aid Programs. In 1993, food intake in Cuba dropped 30% compared with 1989. The availability of foods fell below the level needed to meet the nutritional requirements of the basic market basket. In 1994 household food consumption increased by about 6%, mainly as a result of increased availability of agricultural and livestock products, foods supplied by independent producers, sales made with foreign currency in specified shops, and production of foods in work and educational centers for on-site consumption. All these measures, combined with growth in the production of various agricultural products, led to an improvement in the food situation compared with that in 1993, although some levels of availability remain unsatisfactory.

There are of three general types of national food safety programs: (1) programs aimed essentially at monitoring and assessing the food and nutritional status of the population and adopting preventive or curative health measures according to the situations at hand; (2) programs that seek to increase the production of foods, both quantitatively and qualitatively; and (3) social policy programs targeted to the entire population, addressing product availability, and especially the food and nutrition needs of vulnerable groups.

Organization and Operation of Personal Health Care Services

The National Health System comprises a network of institutions that are easily accessible and provide coverage to 100% of the population. In 1996 the system included 66,263 hospital beds (6.0 per 1,000 inhabitants) and 14,265 beds in social welfare institutions (1.3 beds per 1,000 inhabitants). Medical care is provided through a network made up of 281 hospitals, 11 research institutes, 442 polyclinics, and a contingent of family doctors practicing in workplaces and schools

in the community. In addition, there are 164 health posts, 209 maternity homes, 26 blood banks, and 4 health spas. Oral health care is provided in 168 dental clinics. Social welfare services include 190 homes for the elderly and 27 homes for disabled persons of different ages and with various types of impairment. The family doctor and nurse program serves 97% of the Cuban population.

Hospital admissions have shown a downward trend in recent years. In 1996, admissions totaled 1,419,895 (12.9 per 100,000 inhabitants). In the same year, there were 77,499,250 medical visits (7.0 per person) of which 57,563,213 were outpatient visits (5.23 per person) and 19,936,037 were emergency room visits (1.8 per person). The ratio of outpatient to emergency visits was 2.9.

Family doctors, who number 28,350 and provide 97% of the national coverage, provided 74% of the outpatient consultations. Traditional and natural medicine services were expanded, as were outpatient surgical services, and in 1996 home health care services also increased, which reflects the growing trend toward an outpatient health care model.

More than 100 operating rooms that had been closed because of physical resource problems were refurbished and put back into service, and the country slowly began to recover its surgical capacity. The number of surgical operations, which had decreased from 777,737 in 1990 to 598,329 in 1995, rose to 811,895 in 1996.

The integrated emergency system was enhanced in all provinces of the country. Within primary health care services, 33 emergency care subsystems are currently functioning and 18 more are being implemented. The objective is to reduce the case fatality rate in these services and bring down hospital mortality in minimum care services so that the services that provide care for gravely ill patients can provide adequate coverage. In addition, the medical emergency system was implemented in all the provinces and in the special municipality of Isla de la Juventud. Evaluations have shown the effectiveness of this system, which has reduced morbidity among hospital staff by an average of 40%.

The number of dental visits per person in 1996 (1.6) was higher than that reported in earlier years of the 1990s, which points to a recovery of this indicator in terms of use of oral health services by the population.

The National Disability Prevention, Treatment, and Rehabilitation Program seeks to reduce the frequency of disabilities or impairments through the creation of a grassroots rehabilitation structure. Within this structure, the family doctor and nurse are key figures, as the professionals who detect risks or incapacitating illnesses. They are supported by a multidisciplinary team that includes physiatrists, psychologists, social workers, and physical therapy and physical fitness technicians.

Mental health services are oriented not only toward the biomedical aspects of mental health, but also toward promotion of health, prevention of mental illness, and social rehabilitation. Pediatric hospitals provide child psychiatry services. Outpatient care for adults is available at all the polyclinics in the country. Cuba has 981 practicing psychiatrists, 173 of whom specialize in child psychiatry, as well as some 800 psychologists. One of the country's immediate objectives in the area of mental health is to increase the capacity to provide mental health services at the primary care level and to reduce hospitalization of psychiatric patients, facilitating the social reintegration of long-term patients.

The population of Cuba is one of the four oldest in Latin America and the Caribbean (12.7% of the population is 60 years old or more), and projections for the years 2000 and 2025 are that this proportion will increase to 14% and 21%, respectively. Therefore, it will be necessary to adapt and increase the operating capacity of the system to care for older adults in order to maintain the vitality of this important age group as long as possible and avoid hospitalization and diseases. To this end, in 1996 the program on health care of the elderly was restructured. The program has three subprograms: a community subprogram, social institutions (homes for the elderly), and the hospital subprogram. These programs seek to enhance the level of health, thereby reducing morbidity and mortality, complications, and sequelae.

Human Resources

In 1996, the country had 60,129 physicians—that is, 54.6 per 10,000 inhabitants; 9,600 dentists (8.7 per 10,000 inhabitants); and 76,013 nursing personnel (69.1 per 10,000 inhabitants), 12,716 (16.7%) of whom were university-trained. Since 1990, the number of mid-level personnel entering the health professions has decreased, although they will continue to be graduated in order to meet the requirements of development plans, in particular the growing demand for primary care personnel. The adverse economic conditions of the period 1992–1994 were reflected in the availability of human resources, and in late 1993 a reduction in the availability of mid-level technicians was observed, particularly in the area of nursing. Since 1995, economic recovery has led to greater stability of personnel. With regard to the training of upper-level specialists in the field of public health, the policy designed during the 1990s continued to be applied. That policy seeks to reduce the numbers of students entering schools of medicine and dentistry and to stabilize admissions to nursing degree programs. The total number of mid-level technicians in 1996 was 192,781. The number of students entering mid-level technical training programs has gradually decreased in recent years as the number of these technicians has risen to meet the demand in the country's network of health institutions.

Inputs for Health

Cuba was plunged into a profound economic crisis just as it was implementing a major investment program for the development of its medical and pharmaceutical industry. Nevertheless, after 1993, the worst year of the crisis, a period of recovery began, especially in the production of drugs for domestic use. Total production of drugs remained at similar levels throughout the period, except in 1993, when it dropped considerably. Domestic consumption increased 13.2%. The production of biologicals and reagents increased substantially during the period. Drug marketing was oriented toward meeting the needs of the population and supporting the priority programs of the Ministry of Public Health.

Expenditures and Sectoral Financing

Cuba's health system is financed out of the state budget, the purpose of which is to ensure the achievement of development objectives, while encouraging greater efficiency in the provision of the necessary resources. The population receives free preventive, curative, and rehabilitation services, which range from primary care, routine medical attention, and dentistry to hospital care requiring the use of highly sophisticated medical technologies. In addition, all necessary diagnostic testing and drugs are provided free of charge to pregnant women and to persons receiving outpatient care in the context of certain programs.

Out-of-pocket expenditures for families include drugs prescribed for outpatient treatment, hearing aids, dental and orthopedic apparatuses, wheelchairs, crutches and similar articles, and eyeglasses. The prices for all these items are low and are subsidized by the State. Low-income segments of the population receive monetary and material assistance, including prostheses and drugs.

Despite the economic difficulties of recent years, spending on public health has increased steadily, which reflects the political will to maintain the successes achieved in this area. In 1994, health spending, which includes current health expenditures by all agencies in the country, totaled 1,061.1 million pesos, 17% higher than in 1989. This absolute increase was accompanied by a relative increase in public health spending as a proportion of GDP, total spending, and public spending. In 1994, health spending represented 7.8% of the GDP, 7.5% of total spending, and 14.6% of public spending.

In the period 1992–1996, there was a significant decrease in investment, which in 1994 represented only 3.1% of total spending. The health system did not suffer serious damage as a result of this situation, however, because considerable investment had been made in the sector during the 1980s.

With regard to the structure of current spending, about 60% is devoted to payment of wages, and this figure has tended to grow in absolute terms as a result of the incorporation of new professional and technical personnel into the sector.

In the early 1990s, 141.1 million pesos were being spent on drugs. By 1994, this number had declined to 123.8 million. However, the 1994 value does not take into account 60 million pesos spent on vitamin supplements supplied free of charge to the population to control the neuropathy epidemic that affected the country in the period 1992–1996. In 1995, spending on drugs began to increase again (135.3 million pesos), but the amount spent remained insufficient to meet the needs of the system.

Between 1990 and 1994 spending on hospital care decreased while primary health care expenditures increased. In 1994, primary health care accounted for 36% of current expenditures and hospital spending accounted for 45%, in comparison with 32% and 52.7%, respectively, in 1990.

The decisive factor for ensuring the sustainability of the National Health System is foreign currency financing for the sector. Since 1993, all imports of supplies by the Ministry of Public Health must be financed out of the foreign currency budget that the State allocates for this purpose.

In 1989 foreign currency spending by the health sector totaled US$ 227.3 million. By 1994 this figure had dropped to only US$ 90.1 million. In 1996, although it increased to US$ 126.5 million, this amount was insufficient to cover necessities. This severe reduction in foreign currency financing seriously affected supply. For example, production of drugs by the domestic pharmaceutical industry dropped by more than one-third between 1990 and 1993. The reduced availability of foreign currency financing has also had an impact on the ability of the health sector to procure disposable medical supplies used in health care units and for diagnostic procedures, as well as in optical and dental services.

Cuba has received little foreign aid to maintain the vitality of its health system because its access to traditional sources of financing is seriously hindered by the United States of America's blockade. The country has received humanitarian aid totaling around US $20 million annually. In recent years, various means have been identified and developed for acquiring foreign currency directly by and for the health sector.

External Technical and Financial Cooperation

With regard to multilateral cooperation, Cuba has entered into agreements with United Nations agencies specializing in health: PAHO/WHO, UNICEF, the United Nations Food and Agriculture Organization (FAO), the United Nation's Population Fund (UNFPA), and the United Nations Development Fund (UNDP). Since 1989, this collaboration has played a very important role in that Cuba, in addition to obtaining the benefits of being a member country, has strengthened its relations with institutions of excellence and has been able to disseminate some of its own advances and technologies. In addition, Cuban experts have been able to participate in the work of these agencies. Multilateral cooperation has been oriented toward the development of human resources, family planning, development of the pharmaceutical industry, research on various health problems, procurement of vaccines, and educational activities.

Cuba has depended on the collaboration of Canada, Chile, Spain, France, Italy, Mexico, and Sweden for conducting research and human resources training projects and for providing input.

DOMINICA

GENERAL SITUATION AND TRENDS

Socioeconomic, Political, and Demographic Overview

The Commonwealth of Dominica became independent from Great Britain in 1978. It is the largest of the Windward Islands, and it lies between the French dependent territories of Martinique and Guadeloupe. Dominica extends for 790 km²; its landmass is of volcanic origin and its topography is the most mountainous in the Commonwealth Caribbean. The island has lush forests and an abundance of rivers.

Dominica is divided into 10 regions, or parishes. The most populous is the Parish of St. George, where the capital city, Roseau, is located. According to the 1991 Population and Housing Census Report, the population of St. George was 20,365, or 28.6% of the country's total population.

Dominica is the only Eastern Caribbean territory with an indigenous Carib population, which is estimated to be around 2,000 persons. The Carib people are mainly concentrated in a reservation of some 3,000 acres that stretches for 13 km along the eastern coast and up into the ridges behind.

Dominica has a long democratic tradition of changing governments through elections; elections held in June 1995 marked Dominica's first change in government in 15 years. The Prime Minister is the head of the Government and the President is the Head of State. The Parliament is the government body for debate and enactment of legislation.

In its inaugural budget presentation in 1995, the new political directorate emphasized its commitment to stimulate the country's faltering economy and stated its vision for sustained and balanced growth in the agriculture, industry, tourism, and service sectors. Through a series of national consultations, the Government has enlisted the opinion of all involved stakeholders in the development of a socioeconomic development reform strategy.

Parliament has recently passed a resolution to reform the health care delivery system. Specifically, reforms would introduce a national health insurance scheme and increase user fees as a way to improve local health care services and make the health care system more efficient, without discriminating against anyone who is unable to pay for services.

Dominica's economy has been traditionally described as small, open, and especially vulnerable to external shocks. Between 1992 and 1995, the gross domestic product grew in real terms at an average annual rate of just 2.1%. In comparison, during the 1986–1990 period, GDP increased at an average annual rate of 5.6%. This flattening of the economy was due in large measure to the poor performance of the banana industry, which dominates agricultural output: banana exports fell by 30.9% between 1994 and 1995.

The communication sector is the fastest growing sector of the economy, having registered real growth of 12.0% and contributed 8.8% to the GDP in 1995. Real expansion in the communication sector is followed closely by gains in the banking and insurance sector and in the construction sector, in that order. In terms of overall contribution to the GDP, however, the dominant sectors have been agriculture (despite registering negative growth for each of the last three years), government services, wholesale and retail trade, and banking and insurance, in that sequence.

The real per capita GDP of Dominica rose from US$ 2,000 in 1992 to US$ 2,047 in 1995—a 2.4% increase over the period. This represents an economic deterioration when compared to the 1988–1991 period, which showed an 8.1% increase.

The 1995 poverty assessment survey for Dominica showed that 27% of households live in poverty and are unable to adequately meet their basic needs, including their nutritional needs. The assessment concluded that despite considerable improvements in specific living conditions such as access to water, sanitation, electricity, health, education and the availability of television, "there was a great deal of poverty and an intensifying of poverty and vulnerability."

The unemployment rate in Dominica has been estimated officially at 9.9%, using the 1991 Housing and Population

Census as the basis for analysis. This represents a significant improvement over the figure of 18.6% reported in 1981.

There is no compulsory education policy. However, both males and females have historically maintained a relatively high level of school enrollment. For example, in 1993 (the last year for which complete data are available), 91.6% of the age group 5–19 years old were registered in the school system, a percentage that has been more or less consistent for the past decade. The population's level of education attained breaks down as follows: 67.1% completed primary school education, 15% completed secondary and post-secondary education, and 1.7% reached university or completed an advanced-level education and training.

The 1991 census report also found that, although the population aged 15–19 years old totaled 7,756, only 2,798 (36.0%) of them were enrolled in the school system, a fact that is largely the result of the limited number of available slots at the secondary level. Thus, almost two-thirds of the population terminate their formal education at the primary school level, at about the age of 15 years. The report indicated that 10.5% of the adult population had no formal education and could, therefore, be regarded as functionally illiterate. This illiteracy is evenly distributed among the sexes.

The total number of households was 17,310 in 1980 and 19,374 in 1991, an increase of 16.5% in the period between the last two census years. Most of these households were owner-occupied (72.0%), with 19.2% private-rented. In 1991, 5.1% of households had one room, 31.4% had two rooms, 22.4% had three rooms, 23.4% had four rooms, and the rest had five or more rooms.

The 1991 National Population and Housing Census counted 12,231 households, of which (63.1%) were headed by males and 7,143 (36.9%) were headed by females. There are no data on the number of single-parent families, but it can be safely assumed that the vast majority of households headed by women are single-parent homes.

Dominica is an extremely versatile producer of agricultural goods, which are used for local consumption and export. In terms of volume, the main agricultural crops produced since 1992 have been bananas, citrus, coconuts, and root crops, in that order. Combined, they account for 20.3% of GDP. Even so, Dominica is not self-sufficient in food production, especially in food high in protein. This is demonstrated by the fact that the importation of meat and meat products, milk and cheese, and fish and fish products amounts to more than US$ 7.4 million (2% of GDP) annually. This is an area that is targeted for attention under the national agricultural diversification thrust.

The 1991 National Population and Housing Census showed a revised final count of 71,373 persons, a decline of 2,420 (3.3%) since the 1980 census. This drop has been largely due to emigration, which has been a characteristic demographic feature of Dominica since 1960. The cities of Roseau and Portsmouth had populations of 15,853 and 4,644, respectively, with the remainder spread out among rural villages.

The Central Statistical Office has projected the population at the end of 1995 at 74,707, with males (52.3%) being slightly more numerous than females (47.7%). The population is relatively young, with 40% under the age of 15 years. The mid-year population was estimated by the Central Statistical Office at 71,892 in 1992 and at 74,729 in 1995.

During the 1983–1989 period, emigration caused a negative population growth. The flight had its greatest impact in 1989 when net migration returned a deficit of 2,355. Since 1992, emigration has slowed, with a positive net migration of 479 seen in 1994—the only such occurrence in more than 20 years. A deficit of 960 was recorded again in 1995. The most popular destinations are now the United States Virgin Islands, the British Virgin Islands, and the French Territories of Guadeloupe and Martinique.

In 1991, the total fertility rate was reported at 3.0 children per woman, decreasing from 4.2 in 1981. Projections put the corresponding figure for 1995 at 2.9. The group aged 25–29 years old is the most highly reproductive, with an age-specific fertility rate of 141.4 per 1,000 women, followed by the age group 20–24 years old (129.7) and the age group under 20 years old (114.6). The mean age at childbearing is 26.8 years. The crude birth rate declined from 25.5 per 1,000 population in 1992 (1,835 live births) to 20.1 in 1995 (1,501 live births), with a rate of 22.8 for the four-year period. There is no underregistration of births.

The crude death rate for the 1992–1995 period was 7.6 per 1,000 population, with annual rates of 7.9 in 1992 (566 deaths), 7.7 in 1993 (562 deaths), 7.2 in 1994 (529 deaths), and 7.8 in 1995 (584 deaths). There is no underregistration of deaths.

During 1992–1995, infant mortality rates per 1,000 live births were 14.2 in 1992 and 1993 (26 infant deaths in 1992 and 25 in 1993), 22.5 in 1994 (36 infant deaths), and 16.0 in 1995 (24 deaths), with a rate of 16.5 for the entire period. The high value of 22.5 recorded in 1994 was due to a decrease in the number of live births (1,599 that year, compared to 1,757 in 1993) concomitant with an increase in the number of infant deaths.

Life expectancy at birth, for both sexes combined, has been projected at 67.8 years for the period 1990–1995 (64.1 for males, 71.4 for females), an increase of 1.1 years over the 1985–1990 estimate of 66.7 years (63.5 for males and 69.8 for females). During the 1995–2000 period, life expectancy is expected to reach 68.8 years (64.8 in males, 72.8 in females). These estimates and projections were prepared by the United Nations Economic Commission for Latin America and the Caribbean, Demography Unit, Trinidad and Tobago.

Mortality Profile

During the 1991–1994 period there were 2,175 deaths, of which 12.3% were assigned to ill-defined causes. Of the remaining 1,907 deaths from defined causes, 717 (37.6%) were attributed to diseases of the circulatory system. Within this cause group, hypertensive diseases (ICD-9, 401–405) and heart diseases (415–429) were foremost, with 296 and 269 deaths, respectively. A total of 381 (20.0%) deaths from defined causes were ascribed to neoplasms; 130 deaths (6.8%), to external causes; and 123 deaths (6.4%), to communicable diseases.

An analysis of the distribution by sex of deaths from the predominant cause group of diseases of the circulatory system indicates that women (437 deaths) were considerably more affected than men (280 deaths). However, there was a fairly even distribution between the sexes for neoplasms, with 183 deaths in women and 198 in men. External causes affected men much more than women, with 112 and 18 deaths, respectively.

SPECIFIC HEALTH PROBLEMS

Analysis by Population Group

Health of Children

The 1995–1999 National Health Sector Plan identifies children 0–5 years old as one of the priority groups. In fact, this cohort has been targeted for special attention in every major health policy document since 1980. Not surprisingly, considerable improvements have been recorded in child health care over time.

Prenatal care programs follow prescribed standards. In addition, there are adequate facilities and trained personnel to carry out an intranatal care program; child health clinics are available for the ongoing care of young children and the monitoring of high-risk infants; and health promotion programs are offered to parents and guardians.

Thanks to an aggressive expanded program of immunization that is delivered through public and private health facilities, coverage among infants has reached 100%. Apart from measles, vaccine-preventable diseases have disappeared from the morbidity statistics in Dominica. The number of measles cases reported has been very small, 1 to 2 cases per year between 1992 and 1995.

Undernutrition among young children (0–59 months), as determined through weight-for-age criteria proposed by the Caribbean Food and Nutrition (CFNI) Growth Chart, has been extremely low since 1991, hovering at an annual average of 1.4%. Indeed, in 1995 there were no cases of severe under-

nutrition reported. On the other hand, obesity has climbed as high as 8.7%, and may point to a reason for concern in the future.

Most newborns in Dominica weigh at least 2,500 g at birth; still, an annual average of about 7% of newborns exhibit a weight under 2,500 g at birth. The number and percentage of newborns with low birthweight in each of the years between 1992 and 1995 was 138 (7.5%), 97 (5.5%), 108 (6.7%), and 108 (7.1%), respectively.

The leading reported causes of mortality among children under 5 years old were prematurity, congenital anomalies, and respiratory distress syndrome. An average annual number of 32 deaths occurred in this age group between 1992 and 1995, with an average annual age-specific death rate of 2.8.

Health of Adolescents

The adolescent age group generally is very healthy in Dominica, save for the incidences of teenage pregnancy and sexually transmitted diseases, including AIDS. Contrary to popular belief, teenage pregnancy is neither a new nor a worsening phenomenon. Indeed, the number of births to teenage women declined from 20% of all births in 1992 to 14.2% in 1995—the lowest on record.

A total of 399 cases of sexually transmitted diseases including syphilis, gonorrhea, and HIV/AIDS, was reported in 1994; because data are not available by age group, no informed statement can be made on the incidence and prevalence of sexually transmitted diseases among this age group.

Health of Women

Women of childbearing age (15–44 years old) have been identified as one of the vulnerable groups in the 1995–1999 National Health Sector Plan. As a result, specialized programs relating to prenatal and postnatal care and family planning services have become institutionalized.

Pregnant women have universal access to care in Dominica, which is available through a generous distribution of clinics and health centers. Only 540 of the women seen for prenatal care at health centers in 1995, however, sought care by the 16th week of pregnancy (33.3% of a total of 1,501 births), which is below the recommended levels in the maternal and child health protocol. In 1994 there were 518 women seen by the 16th week (32.3% of 1,599 births), in 1993 there were 531 (36.4% of 1,757 births), and in 1992 there were 640 (34.8% of 1,835 births). This statistic must be interpreted with caution, since it is reported that a significant though unknown number of pregnant women in Dominica make their first prenatal visit to private physicians, rather than to the public health sector. About 70% of all deliveries occur at Princess Margaret Hospital, with the remainder taking place at the home or in a health center.

Records show that the number of women of childbearing age who are currently using family planning methods increased from 5,578 (38% of women 15–44 years of age) in 1992 to 5,739 (44%) in 1995. Of current users, 62% in 1992 and 66% in 1995 attended government health centers; these are the consolidated figures from government health centers and the nongovernmental Dominica Planned Parenthood Association. The most popular methods in 1995 were oral contraceptives (58%) and injectables (34%).

A total of three deaths related to complications of pregnancy, childbirth, and the puerperium (ICD-9, 630–676) were recorded during the 1992–1995 period. Although this number is minimal, the target of zero maternal deaths was only reached in 1993.

Health of the Elderly

The elderly (population older than 60 years old) accounted for 9.8% of Dominica's population at the end of 1995; 73.2% of all deaths occurred among this age group. Morbidity and mortality patterns in Dominica are influenced strongly by common conditions that commonly affect the elderly, particularly hypertensive diseases, heart diseases, malignant neoplasms, cerebrovascular accidents, and endocrine and metabolic diseases.

There are no specialized health care programs for the elderly, but they are exempt from payment for using the health services at all levels. The elderly also benefit from routine hypertensive and diabetic clinics that are conducted islandwide.

Analysis by Type of Disease or Health Impairment

Communicable Diseases

Vector-Borne Diseases. The only vector-borne disease of significance in Dominica is dengue fever. After a relatively uneventful period in 1994, when only three cases were confirmed, an epidemic occurred in 1995, with 148 laboratory-confirmed cases reported. Dengue serotypes 1 and 2 have been identified as causative agents. The combined total of laboratory confirmed and clinically diagnosed cases in 1995 was 297; four of these were confirmed as dengue hemorrhagic fever. The continuing endemicity of dengue fever is due to the high prevalence of the *Aedes aegypti* mosquito. In 1995, the household index of the vector was reported as 15.42%, and the Breteau Index was estimated at 30%.

Intestinal Infectious Diseases. In 1994, gastroenteritis (395 cases in children under 5 years old), typhoid fever (8 cases), dysentery (7 cases), and tuberculosis (11 cases) were the most common infectious diseases. Significantly, three of the leading conditions are related to fecal contamination and personal hygiene practices.

Chronic Communicable Diseases. Tuberculosis remains a public health concern, and a set of protocols have been established for finding cases, tracing contacts, and providing treatment. No association has been drawn between the incidence of the disease and the presence of AIDS.

AIDS and Other Sexually Transmitted Diseases. There is considerable underreporting of sexually transmitted diseases. For example, in 1994 there were 307 laboratory-confirmed cases of syphilis, while only 36 cases of gonococcal infections were reported. Local expert opinion is that reporting on sexually transmitted diseases is not very reliable.

A total of 53 new cases of AIDS were reported between 1992 and 1995. Most of the cases (54%) occurred in the age group 20–29 years old, with a male/female ratio of 3:1. A continuing program of HIV testing, surveillance, and education and counseling is in place.

Noncommunicable Diseases and Other Health-Related Problems

Malignant Tumors. Neoplasms caused 20.0% of deaths from defined causes in Dominica in the 1991–1994 period. The main sites (as demonstrated by pathology confirmations, rather than by registered causes of death) are breast (112 of a total of 439 laboratory confirmations), cervix (78 confirmations), stomach (65 confirmations), and skin (49 confirmations). The peak incidence for malignant neoplasms is reported in the age group 55–64 years old.

Screening for cervical cancer is offered in Dominica through the facilities of the pathology laboratory at the Princess Margaret Hospital. The services are available to all women at risk upon referral, although the public health sector targets especially active family planning clients. A total of 15,136 Pap tests were examined between 1992 and 1995 and, apart from 1992 when a somewhat inflated figure of 4,642 smears were done as a result of a special campaign, a consistent pattern of 3,497 examinations were completed each year, on average.

Diabetes and Hypertension. The best statistics on clinic visits indicate that diabetes and hypertension are the most common reasons for health care demand. There are an estimated 4% diabetics and 18% hypertensives in the general population, and they account for increasing numbers of visits to Ministry of Health clinics and health centers. In 1994, there were 10,123 visits by diabetics (a 20.3% increase from 1993) and 24,705 visits by hypertensives (a 28.5% increase from 1993).

Mental Disorders. The 1995 Mental Health Report estimates the age-adjusted prevalence of schizophrenia in Dominica as 0.9%, with 68 new such patients being registered in that year. The major causes of mental illness are related to schizophrenia and depression. A total of 2,166 mental health outpatient visits were recorded in 1995, compared with 2,148 in the previous year.

In 1995, 8.7% of the total 652 admissions to Princess Margaret Hospital Psychiatric Unit presented with a diagnosis of alcoholism, 7.6% with cannabis psychosis, and 2% with cocaine abuse. The 1995 Mental Health Report concluded that 90% of all patients seen at the prison psychiatric clinic had a history of drug abuse, but much more work must be done to determine the size and scope of the problem of substance abuse in Dominica.

A Draft Mental Health Policy has been formulated and is awaiting ratification. This document addresses services and legal and advisory frameworks.

RESPONSE OF THE HEALTH SYSTEM

National Health Plans and Policies

In the 1995–1999 National Health Sector Plan, the Government of Dominica reaffirms its commitment to the belief that "all citizens have the right to attain the highest possible level of health in order to be able to work and live in accordance with acceptable standards of human dignity at an affordable cost." The plan continues to emphasize the shared responsibility between the Government and the community in achieving lasting improvements in the quality of life.

The gains in health status achieved from sustained public health interventions are well recognized and documented. The current strategy further emphasizes preventive health care and pursues the following priorities: applying the principles of health promotion to program planning, implementation, and evaluation; reforming the health sector to meet the special challenges involved in institutional strengthening, the mobilization and efficient use of resources, and human resource development; improving the health infrastructure through an ongoing process of retrofitting and maintenance; and strengthening the community's participation and intersectoral linkages. The thrust toward health sector reform is directed toward cost recovery, cost containment, reconfiguration of the management system, and more accountability. The

priority groups have been defined as children aged 0–5 years old, pregnant and lactating mothers, women of childbearing age, adolescents, the elderly, and the underserved population in urban and rural areas, such as indigenous populations.

Chronic diseases have been targeted for special attention, given their prominent place among the morbidity and mortality statistics. Health promotion is considered to be pivotal in the delivery of these programs.

Organization of the Health Sector

In 1979, Hurricane David brought massive devastation to Dominica's health infrastructure, precisely at a time when the health services reorganization was being planned in light of the Declaration of Alma Ata. A model primary health care system was fashioned out of this adversity.

The main thrust of the reorganization divided the island into seven health districts, each with its own management team responsible for organizing the delivery of health services at that level. A Central Technical Committee provides policy, advisory, and technical support services to these District Health Teams.

Under this arrangement, primary health care has its own budget, which has been disaggregated by district and is based on programming needs and priorities. Some authority and responsibility have devolved to the District Health Teams as a way to enhance program delivery. As a result, various program areas now operate better with one another and activities are more goal oriented. This process also encourages greater community input. The reorganization of primary health care services has proceeded well, and the system has once again been endorsed by the 1995–1999 National Health Sector Plan.

The broad objectives for the development of health and health-related services are set out in the above-mentioned plan, and involve strengthening local health systems to meet the specific needs of communities, including prioritizing programs and allocating resources more efficiently; exploring new avenues for generating resources to sustain the sector; managing information within the sector effectively; improving the quality of secondary care by instituting structural changes, infrastructural improvements, human resources training, and better care; and streamlining the functional relationships between main administration and peripheral services regarding personnel and financial and supplies management. It is anticipated that these objectives will be accomplished through the careful harnessing of all available national, regional, and international levels. Further, close links will be maintained with regional governments and with organizations such as PAHO and CARICOM, in order to access required technical and other forms of assistance.

Health Services and Resources

Organization of Services for Care of the Population

Health Promotion and Community Participation. Dominica's Ministry of Health has a Health Education Unit responsible for developing and managing public information and education efforts on health issues. The Unit trains various other staff in the principles and practice of health education, plans and implements health education programs and activities with community groups, produces and presents mass media programs on relevant health and health-related topics, and produces graphic materials.

Because the Government of Dominica acknowledges that health promotion is one of the most effective weapons to combat health problems and promote healthy lifestyles, it has endorsed the Caribbean Charter on Health Promotion that was launched in 1994. As a result, one of the program priorities identified in the 1995–1999 National Health Sector Plan is the application of the principles of health promotion to program planning, implementation, and evaluation. Insufficient intersectoral cooperation and inconsistent community participation have hindered the application; the media's awareness and interest on the subject, however, will help offset this obstacle.

A national directive holds that communities and individuals should be involved in the development process. Thus, whether at the national development planning level or at the health sector reform level, deliberate efforts have been made to involve communities in the decision-making process. The community's involvement in the drafting of a National Socioeconomic Development Strategy, the public debate that was encouraged on the new initiatives for health sector financing, and community members' active role in the work of District Health Teams have all been hailed as success stories in community participation. Many persons in Dominica, however, view community action merely in terms of coalescing around a given issue, rather than as an ongoing pursuit.

The 1995–1999 National Health Sector Plan, by commiting itself to "fostering a copartnership with the community," keeps faith with the practice of community participation in health. At the same time, it acknowledges that "new strategies must be sought to achieve meaningful social mobilization."

Environmental Protection. The Government of Dominica is commited to "preserve the environment in its most pristine form," and it pursues several strategies to that end. For example, the Government controls land use practices, which includes the protection of forest reserves from exploitation. Environmental impact assessments and hydrogeological studies are required in all physical development projects, and these projects must be formally approved by the National Physical Planning Board. Waterways are protected from chemical pollution, particularly regarding chemical contamination from agriculture. Sand mining is closely controlled through a zoning process, and it is restricted in beaches.

Typhoid fever is perhaps the most worrisome environmental health problem in Dominica. During the 1991–1995 period there were 44 confirmed cases of typhoid fever, for an annual average of 9 cases. The main source of contamination has been traced to food handling practices linked to inadequate sewage disposal methods. Most reported cases came from Marigot, Portsmouth, and Grand Bay, where sewage disposal has been a ongoing problem.

Drinking Water Supply, Sewerage, and Waste Disposal. According to the 1991 Population and Housing Census Report 77.5% of households had direct access to piped water supply from the national system, which is operated and maintained by the Dominica Water and Sewerage Authority. The water supply is routinely treated to maintain bacteriological quality. Significantly, neither springs nor rivers were mentioned as sources of domestic water supply; also noteworthy is the fact that private water supplies maintained by 12% of households may or may not be treated.

There are many serious concerns over the state of sewage disposal in Dominica. First, fully one-quarter of the total number of households (25.5%) have no approved form of sewage disposal. And although this figure represents an improvement over that in 1981, when the corresponding figure was 40%, it remains unacceptable. The situation is even more grave in some west coast villages, where as much as 60% of households have no sewage disposal facilities. The high water table creates practical difficulties in drilling holes to erect toilet facilities, while the population density of these areas compounds the problem.

The predominant means of sewage disposal is the water closet (36.8%), followed by the pit latrine (35.4%). Given the status of sewage disposal in the country, it is hardly surprising that gastroenteritis was the leading notifiable infectious disease (181.2/100,000 population) in 1994.

The proper management of solid and liquid waste is a priority. About 55% of the population are served with an organized communal solid waste collection and disposal service. The serviced area runs from Portsmouth in the North to Scottshead in the South, including the capital city of Roseau. This service is expected to be extended nationwide by 1998 under a new solid waste management initiative. A new landfill site at Fond Cole has been earmarked for development with a projected lifespan of 15 years.

Food Safety. The Government's policy regarding food safety involves ensuring that all foods intended for human consumption are sound, wholesome, and fit for use. Therefore, the food protection and safety program aims at achieving the highest standards in the selection, preparation, storage, and display of any food offered for human consumption.

In 1995, there were 2,340 food handling establishments in Dominica, including grocery shops, restaurants, bakeries, hotels, and food manufacturing plants. The greatest concentration of food handling establishments is in the Roseau Health District (47.1%), followed by the Portsmouth Health District (20.1%) and the Marigot Health District (13.1%). The Ministry of Health's Environmental Health Division estimates that 82% of all food handlers in the country were medically examined and registered.

A major function of the food safety program is the inspection of locally produced meats intended for sale, especially beef and pork. In 1995, a total of 1,329 animals slaughtered for meat were inspected by the Environmental Health Division. It is estimated that this number represents between 55% and 60% of all animals slaughtered for this purpose.

In practice, only about 25%–30% of all imported foods are routinely inspected. Reportedly, this deficiency is almost entirely due to human resource limitations; there is no officer with exclusive responsibility for port health services. Most of the laws governing food safety are outmoded and in need of revision. A process of review has been in process for many years but remains incomplete.

Workers' Health. The occupational health and safety programs encompass the assessment and approval of new industrial establishments, routine inspection of plant operations and maintenance, and the monitoring of outdoor occupations such as construction work. These programs are jointly implemented by the Environmental Health Division of the Ministry of Health, Education, and Sports and the Ministry of Labour and Immigration. The 1992 Employment Safety Act stipulates that all injuries and accidents at the workplace should be reported to the Labour Division. The number of such cases reported between 1991 and 1995 ranged between 2 and 8 incidents per year. It has been suggested that there is considerable underreporting.

Disaster Preparedness. Dominica has suffered the brunt of at least three destructive hurricanes in recent history, which have wrought enormous damage to the country's economic, physical, and social infrastructures. This risk has made the country critically aware of the importance of emergency preparedness.

A National Disaster Preparedness Committee has coordinated the development of a National Disaster Plan and holds responsibility for its periodic update. The health sector, for its part, has produced a Health Disaster Plan that details actions to be taken at every level in the event of any emergency situation. While it is fair to conclude, therefore, that emergency preparedness planning is well entrenched, it is also true that

very little has happened in terms of simulation exercises to practice and sharpen responses. This is one of the objectives that the health sector has committed itself to pursue on an annual basis. New emphasis also is being placed on mass casualty management at the pre-hospital and casualty stages.

Organization and Operation of Personal Health Care Services

Health services in Dominica are basically organized in two levels—primary health care services and secondary care services. The country's well-organized health care delivery system adequately responds to the population's needs. Coverage at the community level is provided through a network of 7 health centers and 44 clinics strategically located throughout the island. The services are provided with no direct cost to the consumer.

The country's seven health districts are used as the structure for organizing the delivery of primary health care services. Each health district is provided with a network of Type I clinics that serve, on average, a population of 600 persons within a five-mile radius. Primary care nurses deliver health district services, and they undergo a two-year training program to prepare them to work at this level of care.

Types II and III health centers offer comprehensive services; the district's administrative headquarters are located at Type III health centers. Staffing at this level includes the district health officer, district nurse midwife, and other support staff. A polyclinic at Princess Margaret Hospital provides general medical care, accident and emergency services, and specialist outpatient referral services to the entire population.

Secondary health care services are provided through Princess Margaret Hospital, which currently has a capacity of 195 beds. As a rule, medical services at the Hospital are accessed through inpatient, outpatient, and casualty facilities.

The activity level at Princess Margaret Hospital remained relatively constant during 1992–1995: there was an annual average of 7,867 admissions and an annual average of 7,901 discharges. In 1995, there were 7,858 discharges, with an average length of stay of 7.8 days. Apart from obstetric conditions, the major causes of hospital admissions were heart conditions, hypertensive disease, diabetes, and upper respiratory tract infections. The hospital provides both acute and chronic disease care.

Inputs for Health

Essential Drugs and Medical Supplies. Dominica is a full participant in the Eastern Caribbean Drug Service, a regional pooled procurement service for pharmaceutical and medical supplies. Participation has resulted in an average of 25% savings on items purchased, as well as in improvements in the quality, reliability, and availability of essential drugs and supplies. About 10% of the health budget is allocated to the purchase of drugs and medical supplies. The range of drugs available within the government service is determined by a National Formulary Committee, which reviews the National Formulary biennially in order to rationalize and update the list of drugs, including essential drugs, that should be available within the system.

Legislation relating to prescription drugs, drug registration, and license to dispense drugs is outdated and in urgent need of review. The country has no drug inspector responsible for enforcing the legislative provisions.

Human Resources

Human resources available for health care delivery in Dominica have remained constant since the turn of the decade, with no significant changes in either the categories or the numbers of health personnel available, although deployment of staff to strengthen primary health care services has been favored somewhat. The new categories of Primary Care Nurse and Community Health Aide, as well as the institutionalization of a legislative and administrative framework within which Family Nurse Practitioners can function, reflect this orientation.

In 1995, the ratio of personnel (public sector posts) per 100,000 population were as follows: 46.8 for medical doctors, 8.0 for dentists, 28.1 for pharmacists, 311.9 for nurses, 108.4 for nurse assistants, 26.8 for laboratory technologists, 22.8 for environmental health officers, and 5.4 for radiographers.

Training of Human Resources. Two institutions in Dominica offer training for health care professionals—the government-run School of Nursing and the private, offshore Ross University Medical School. The program in the School of Nursing is tailored to the specific needs of Dominica's national health service, whereas the curriculum at Ross University leans toward external market demands.

Recently, the expansion in human resources for health has been limited by the controls placed on public sector spending precipitated by the economic downturn and the structural adjustment program. Even with the availability of adequate financing, however, targeted human resource expansion and development may prove difficult, since the optimum needs of the health sector in terms of number, mix, and deployment are yet to be defined. This will be an important challenge in the future.

Expenditures and Sectoral Financing

The actual government expenditure in the health sector has averaged 13.2% of total recurrent budget for the 1992–1995 pe-

riod. This ranks health as the third largest consumer of government resources, behind administration (21.3%) and education (16.4%). In 1995, 39% of the total recurrent expenditure on social and community services was allocated to health. These figures relate to public sector expenditures only, since private sector expenditure is not captured. In terms of the GDP per capita expenditures on health, an increase was recorded from EC$ 245.37 in 1991 to EC$ 312.73 in 1995. The total government recurrent health expenditure in health for 1995 was US$ 8,870,000, which represents approximately 13.5% of the total government recurrent expenditure.

Expenditure in the health sector is still skewed in the direction of secondary care, with hospital and laboratory services consuming about 50% of the financial resources for health. The allocation that falls under primary health care has shown only a marginal increase, from 22.3% in 1992 to 22.9% in 1995. It must also be noted, however, that environmental health services account for 7.7% of the health expenditure, thereby increasing overall expenditure on primary health care services. Almost three-quarters (72.9%) of the total expenditure on health is directed towards personal emoluments, with the remainder applied toward all other operating costs.

A schedule of user fees for bed charges, use of operating theater facilities, and diagnostic services exists for persons seeking secondary care at Princess Margaret Hospital. As a way to attain equity in health, all persons under 17 years old, prenatal women, the indigent, and persons suffering from communicable diseases are exempt from user charges. Of the total public health budget, only 5.5% is recovered from direct user charges; the remainder is financed through the consolidated fund.

External Technical and Financial Cooperation

There are few prospects for bilateral international partnership for health, with the possible exception of cooperation with the Government of France, which has remained strong. Most international partnerships that have emerged over the past decade have been multilateral and have involved other Caribbean countries.

The Government's response to this situation has been to infuse health and environment considerations into all of its economic and social development initiatives and to strengthen regional ties. For example, the World Bank funded a regional Organization of Eastern Caribbean States Solid Waste Management Project that will benefit Dominica and that has been promoted as improving tourism, health, and the environment. Dominica also continues to participate in the Caribbean Cooperation in Health (CCH), which offers a platform for a regional approach to health services delivery, including shared services. In this regard, CARICOM and PAHO have been invaluable collaborators.

DOMINICAN REPUBLIC

GENERAL SITUATION AND TRENDS

Socioeconomic, Political, and Demographic Overview

The Dominican Republic occupies the eastern two-thirds of the Caribbean island of Hispaniola, which is located west of Puerto Rico. Its only border is with Haiti. The Dominican Republic has an area of 48,400 km², and its population was estimated at 7.8 million in 1995. For political and administrative purposes, the country is divided into three regions and seven subregions, which together contain the 29 provinces and the National District.

The Dominican economy has undergone profound changes in the last two decades. Until the mid-1970s, traditional export products, mainly from agriculture, represented 60% of the total value of the country's exports. Over the last two decades the service sector has led the economy, particularly economic and financial services related to tourism and industrial free-trade zones, which by 1995 accounted for more than 70% of exports. The shift came with major dislocations and economic and social imbalances. The macroeconomic adjustments of the 1980s served to substantially reduce social spending and redirect expenditures toward investment, especially in infrastructure. Annual per capita expenditures on education during 1987–1990, adjusted for inflation, were 40% of what they had been in 1980, and the expenditures on health were 7.5% lower. Together, the health and education sectors received less than 5% of public spending between 1986 and 1990.

The exchange rate of the Dominican peso against the United States dollar went from RD$ 1 per US$ 1 in 1980 to about RD$ 12 in 1990. The price of the basket of basic family goods increased by more than 400%, and the consumer price index rose 467%. The minimum wage went up only 29%, which, adjusted for inflation, was actually a reduction of 42%. The unemployment rate reached 27%, and per capita caloric intake fell 7%. As a result, there were numerous public protests, as well as increased emigration by the economically active population.

The end of 1990 brought another economic adjustment program. In 1992 the gross domestic product (GDP) began to recover, and by 1996 it was maintaining an average annual growth rate of more than 5%. In 1996 the GDP rose 5.4%, with an increase of 6.9% estimated for 1997. Per capita income reached US$ 1,824 in 1996. Stable prices, rising wages in the private sector, and a public sector salary increase in May 1995 restored the real minimum wage and the wage in dollars to levels that in January 1996 were 14% higher than in 1980, and there were further increases in 1997. Since 1992, annual inflation has remained fairly low. It was 3.7% in 1995, 0.9% in 1996, and an estimated 4.4% in 1997. The free market exchange rate remained fairly stable at around RD$ 14 to US$ 1 during 1996 and 1997. External and internal debt servicing rose substantially, reaching more than RD$ 2,400 million in 1995.

This stability and macroeconomic growth have improved the purchasing power of the working population, and absolute poverty appears to have diminished. On the other hand, reduced public spending for education and health has affected family budgets, unemployment rates (which stood at 15% in 1996–1997), and the percentage of population linked to the informal economy and nonwage-earning activities, and has thus led to a considerable increase in relative poverty and the number of people who are in need. At the same time, the economy has become extremely vulnerable to and dependent on external factors outside its control. The public domestic debt, estimated at about US$ 400 million in mid-1997, has been burgeoning, and this has tended to inhibit private domestic investment.

The fiscal system is considered to be very fragile because of its dependency on the international price of oil and the collection of customs fees, which have been declining as a result of international agreements. Oligopolistic distortions in the financial system lead to high interest rates for external capital. Foreign exchange earnings come mainly from tourism and from exports from the free-trade zones. Those earnings are vulnerable to international processes outside the country's control, such as interest rate changes in international financial markets, political decisions on preferential treatment in the United States market, and choices made by international travel agencies. Domestic industrial production relies heavily on government protectionist policies and is unprepared to compete internationally. Another factor that contributes to the country's vulnerability is its meager investment in human development. An enormous backlog in social spending has accumulated. There are major deficiencies in education and health, deteriorating basic public transportation and electricity services, and a highly inequitable distribution of income that poses an ongoing risk for social and political instability and holds down productivity.

The country also is experiencing several structural limitations at the political level—inadequate institutional development, an unreliable and inefficient judicial system, a centralized administration, a bloated bureaucracy sustained by a culture of patronage, complex procedural requirements, and public institutions that are technologically out of date. The widespread consensus on the need for structural reforms brought a new generation and a new political outlook to the Presidency in August 1996. The new administration was inaugurated amidst a climate of high hope for economic and political changes.

Population

Between 1990 and 1995, annual population growth was 3.0%, with the 0–14-year-old age group making up 35% of the population and the 65-and-older age group only 4%. Urban population was estimated at 50% in 1980 and 65% in 1995.

During the same period, life expectancy at birth rose from about 44 to 65 years. The total fertility rate declined from 7.4 to 3.1 children per woman of childbearing age, and the birth rate dropped from about 50 to 27 per 1,000 population.

Since the 1970s, emigration has been an important survival strategy for the Dominican people. It is estimated that at least 700,000 Dominicans have left the country over the last 30 years. The most reliable information available indicates that there were 300,000 immigrants living in the country in 1994. A 1991 study found that there had been a great deal of internal migration, with 34% of the population changing residence at least once in their lifetime and 9% having done so in the last five years.

The first attempt to classify the Dominican population in the different regions from the standpoint of health and living conditions was made in 1992–1993, based on information from the 1991 Demographic and Health Survey (ENDESA 91). The provinces were grouped into seven health strata according to the proportion of families with unmet basic needs. Countrywide, family needs were "mostly unmet" in 33.7% of the households surveyed; in 38.4% of the households they were "met to some extent"; and in the remaining 28% the needs

were "mostly satisfied." In the provinces of stratum VII, the basic needs were mostly unmet for 70% to 89% of the families. The analysis found that 14.8% of the urban population and 66.3% of the rural population lived in provinces where needs were considered to be "mostly unmet." These same provinces were home to 33.7% of the country's population and accounted for 19% of the national income at the time of the study.

Most of the extremely poor communities were located in the southeastern and northeastern areas of the country, along the border with Haiti.

The Secretariat for Public Health and Social Welfare, working together with the Autonomous University of Santo Domingo, conducted a study of primary economic activity and accumulation of goods and services during 1990–1994. This research showed that in the poorest provinces there was a predominance of subsistence farming; negative population growth; low levels of vaccination coverage, drinking water availability, and hospital utilization; and many deaths without medical attention or diagnosis of the cause of death.

Mortality Profile

The estimated general mortality rate has gradually declined, falling to 5.5 per 1,000 population for the 1990–1995 period. It is expected to be 5.2 per 1,000 population for 1995–2000. Decreases have occurred in both sexes and in all age groups. This trend is related to longer life expectancy at birth, which rose from 53.6 years in 1960–1965 to 69.6 in 1990–1995 and is projected to be 70.9 for 1995–2000.

The crude mortality rate registered in 1994 was 2.7 per 1,000 population (3.1 in males and 2.3 in females). During 1990–1994, cardiovascular diseases were the most frequently reported cause of death, with registered rates remaining fairly stable at about 80 per 100,000, although this disease group as a proportion of total registered mortality increased slightly, from 29.2% to 33.9%. Communicable diseases, which were the second leading cause of death in 1990, at 46.6 per 100,000, fell to fourth place in 1994, at 27.1 per 100,000. As a percentage, they went from 16.8% to 11.5% of total deaths. Such external causes as accidental injuries and violence rose from third to second place, even though the rate dropped from 33.9 to 30.2 per 100,000; as a percentage, they increased slightly, from 12.2% to 12.9%. Malignant neoplasms, which ranked fourth in 1990, with a rate of 27.7 per 100,000, moved up to third place, with a rate of 28.0 per 100,000, while proportionally they went from 10.0% to 11.9%. Perinatal causes remained in fifth place, with rates of 14.8 in 1990 and 12.6 per 100,000 in 1994, and a 5.4% proportion in both years. In 1994, diseases of the circulatory system were the leading cause of death among females, accounting for 38.2% of registered deaths, followed by malignant neoplasms, 13.6%; communicable diseases, 11.9%; and external causes, 5.8%. Among males, cardiovascular diseases represented 30.7% of all deaths; external causes, 18.0%; communicable diseases, 11.3%; and malignant neoplasms, 10.8%.

These data indicate a downward trend in deaths due to communicable diseases. Deaths from external causes are on the rise, and the percentages for malignant neoplasms and perinatal diseases remain more or less stable. Nevertheless, caution should be exercised in considering these and all the other diagnosis-based mortality figures cited here. It is estimated that underregistration of deaths was nearly 50% in 1994 and the proportion of registered deaths attributed to ill-defined symptoms and conditions was about 15% between 1990 and 1994.

To estimate the potential impact of public health efforts, indicators for the Dominican Republic were compared with the highest values in countries having a similar level of economic resources. Cuba, Ecuador, Guatemala, Nicaragua, Panama, Paraguay, and Peru were selected for this comparison because in each case their per capita GDP adjusted for purchasing power was similar to that of the Dominican Republic. The values for the Dominican Republic were also compared against the highest values attained by countries in the Region. For life expectancy at birth, the reducible gap between the values for the Dominican Republic and the highest values for the other countries of Latin America was narrowed from 33% in the 1960–1965 period to 15% for 1990–1995. The gap between the Dominican Republic and the highest values for countries with a similar level of economic resources decreased from 22% in 1960–1965 to 12% in 1990–1995. For mortality, in 1985–1990 the gap between the Dominican Republic and the highest values in the countries selected for comparison was around 42%, and it was 50% relative to the highest values in the Americas. This means that some 19,000 deaths could have been prevented in 1994. The gap is widest for children under the age of 5 and becomes progressively narrower until it is quite small in the older age groups. Thus, the greatest potential for reducing mortality and increasing life expectancy is among children under 5 years of age.

SPECIFIC HEALTH PROBLEMS

Analysis by Population Group

Health of Infants (under 1 Year Old)

The registered infant mortality rate was 19.1 per 1,000 live births in 1990 and 11.5 per 1,000 in 1994. In 1994, infants under 1 year old accounted for 10.9% of all registered deaths. According to two estimates—one by the Latin American Demographic Center (CELADE) and PAHO, and another based on the ENDESA 96 health survey—underregistration may be some 72% to 75%. That would make the actual infant mortality rate between 42 and 47 per 1,000.

The rate of decline in infant mortality appears to have slowed in the last decade. There are also significant differences between regions. Registered infant mortality per 1,000 live births was 26.4 in urban areas and 29.1 in rural areas during 1991–1996. Estimated rates ranged from 45 per 1,000 in the National District up to about 70 per 1,000 in the more impoverished areas. By educational level of the mother, the rate ranged from 85 per 1,000 for mothers without any formal education to 20 per 1,000 for women with some level of higher education.

In infants under 1 year of age, 30% of the deaths were from communicable diseases, 44.8% from conditions originating in the perinatal period, 3.2% from diseases of the circulatory system, and 2.9% from external causes.

In 1990–1995 the proportion of low-birthweight babies delivered in 25 of the country's major hospitals was 9.2%, a decrease from earlier levels.

Health of Preschool Children (Aged 1 to 4)

According to CELADE estimates, in 1990–1995 the mortality rate among children aged 1 to 4 fell to 4 per 1,000, with a slightly higher rate in males than in females (4.0 and 3.6 per 1,000, respectively), whereas ENDESA 96 estimated an overall rate of 11 per 1,000. In 1990 this age group accounted for 5% of all registered deaths, but by 1994 it was only 3.4% of the total.

As for the leading causes of death in 1994, communicable diseases represented 37.7% of the total; external causes, 17.6%; diseases of the circulatory system, 5.0%; and malignant neoplasms, 2.5%.

By more specific diagnoses, intestinal infectious diseases represented 15.9% of deaths; nutritional deficiencies, 15.3%; acute respiratory infections, 12.5%; unspecified injuries, 9.4%; and congenital abnormalities, 5.5%. These rankings were similar in both sexes, except for external causes, for which males had a slightly higher proportion.

Health of School-Age Children (Aged 5 to 14)

School-age children had an estimated mortality rate of 0.7% per 1,000 in 1990–1995. In 1990 this age group accounted for 2.4% of all registered deaths, and by 1994 that had dropped to 2.0%. External causes were responsible for 41.4% of all deaths (29.3% in girls and 50.7% in boys); "other causes," 25.5% (32.9% in girls and 19.8% in boys); communicable diseases, 15.1% (17.4% in girls and 10.6% in boys); diseases of the circulatory system, 10.7% (12.0% in girls and

9.6% in boys); and malignant neoplasms, 7.3% (8.4% in girls and 6.4% in boys).

By more detailed diagnoses, unspecified injuries headed the list and were followed, in turn, by nutritional deficiencies, intestinal infections, and diseases of pulmonary circulation and other heart diseases.

Health of the Population Aged 15 to 44

The estimated mortality rate for persons aged 15 to 44 fell to 1.8% per 1,000 population in 1990–1995 (2.05 per 1,000 in males and 1.5% in females). In 1990 this segment of the population accounted for 19% of all deaths.

Of the deaths, 26.9% were due to "other causes," 16.8% to cardiovascular diseases, 9.3% to external causes, 11.1% to communicable diseases, and 8.1% to malignant neoplasms. Among females, "other causes" accounted for 33.9% of the deaths; cardiovascular diseases, 22.6%; malignant neoplasms, 14.7%; communicable diseases, 14.5%; and external causes, 14.0%. Among males, almost half, or 48.8%, of the deaths were attributed to external causes, 23.3% to "other causes," 13.8% to cardiovascular diseases, 9.3% to communicable diseases, and 4.7% to malignant neoplasms.

By more specific diagnostic groups, among women tuberculosis was the leading cause of death in 1990, but by 1994 this disease had dropped to second place. In first place for women in 1994 were diseases of pulmonary circulation; ranking third were injuries from traffic accidents, followed by cerebrovascular and ischemic heart disease. Complications during pregnancy, labor, and the puerperium, which in 1990 accounted for 6.9% of deaths, by 1994 were down to 5%. In men, mortality due to traffic accidents was in first place, followed by homicides, other injuries, and diseases of pulmonary circulation and other heart diseases.

The registered maternal mortality rate was 45 per 100,000 live births in 1990 and 30.7 per 100,000 in 1994. The corresponding estimated rate for 1990 was 110 per 100,000, which would imply underregistration on the order of 59%. Indeed, more recent estimates based on the ENDESA 96 survey indicate the real maternal mortality rate might have been as high as 200 per 100,000 live births over the 1983–1994 period.

More than 97% of pregnant women have two or more prenatal medical consultations, and 95% have their babies delivered in institutions.

Teenage pregnancy is a serious problem. In 1996, about 23% of the women between 15 and 19 years of age had had at least one pregnancy, and this proportion appears to be increasing. Adolescent pregnancies are more common in rural areas, in lower-income districts where sanitation is poor, and among women who have had little schooling. Around 45% of the women of childbearing age, and 64% of those who declare they have a partner, practice some form of birth control, which for 64% of these women is sterilization. Only 20% use contraceptive pills, and 9% use other modern methods. The percentage of women who use sterilization as a form of contraception is declining, but efforts still need to be made to further decrease the use of this practice, which is quite widespread in the country's family planning and obstetric services.

Domestic violence against women is a major problem. Police authorities report a growing number of charges filed, particularly cases of sexual violence, including rape, with most victims being children and adolescents.

Health of the Population Aged 45 to 64

Estimated mortality rates for persons aged 45 to 64 fell to 8.3 per 1,000 population during 1990–1995 (9.6 and 7.0 per 1,000 in males and females, respectively). In 1994 this group accounted for 20.4% of all registered deaths.

Data for 1994 show that cardiovascular diseases were the leading cause of death and represented 39.7% of all deaths in this age group. In second place were "other causes," which accounted for 25.4% of the deaths, followed by malignant neoplasms, 18.8%; external causes, 9.6%; and communicable diseases, 5.7%. Among women, 41.3% of all deaths were attributed to cardiovascular diseases, 25.9% to malignant neoplasms; 23.8% to other diagnosed causes, 5.1% to communicable diseases, and 3.8% to external causes. Among men, cardiovascular diseases caused 38.6% of all deaths, other diagnosed diseases, 26.4%; malignant neoplasms, 14.4%; external causes, 13.5%; and communicable diseases, 7.3%.

By more specific diagnoses, the leading causes of death in women were cerebrovascular diseases, followed by ischemic cardiopathy, chronic liver diseases, genital neoplasms, and diabetes mellitus. The most frequent causes of death in men were ischemic cardiopathy, cerebrovascular diseases, and chronic liver diseases, in that order.

Health of the Elderly (65 and Over)

The estimated mortality rate for persons 65 and older for 1990–1995 was 52.8 per 1,000 population (48.4 per 1,000 for women and 57.4 per 1,000 for men). Deaths of persons aged 65 and over represented 40.5% of all registered deaths.

In 1994 the leading diagnosed cause of death in this age group was cardiovascular diseases, which accounted for 52.4%. Ranking next were "other causes," 23.0%; malignant neoplasms, 15.0%; communicable diseases, 6.5%; and external causes, 3.2%. The rates were similar for both sexes. According to more specific diagnoses, the leading causes were, in order, diseases of pulmonary circulation and other heart diseases, ischemic cardiopathy, hypertension, cerebrovascular diseases, and diabetes mellitus.

Analysis by Type of Disease or Health Impairment

Communicable Diseases

Communicable diseases, along with nutritional deficiencies, are the country's leading health priorities. In 1994 communicable diseases accounted for 16.8% of all diagnosed deaths. Notable among the communicable diseases are diarrheal diseases, which in 1994 represented 4% of all diagnosed deaths and 30.4% of the deaths from communicable diseases. More than half (51.3%) of the deaths from acute diarrhea occurred in infants under 1 year of age, and 16% were in children aged 1 to 4 years. Diarrheal diseases were the second leading cause of diagnosed mortality in infants under 1 year of age (15%) and ranked in first place among children aged 1 to 4 (16%), followed by nutritional deficiencies. According to data from the ENDESA 96 survey, only 39.1% of all diarrheal episodes were treated with some form of oral rehydration, although in recent years this proportion has gone up slightly. As far as cholera is concerned, even with close surveillance of diarrheal cases and the thorough investigation of suspicious cases of diarrhea, not a single case of the disease was diagnosed during the current pandemic.

In 1994 acute respiratory infections accounted for 3.6% of all diagnosed deaths and 30.9% of the deaths from communicable diseases. Acute respiratory infections were the sixth-ranking diagnosed cause of mortality in infants under 1 year of age and the third-ranking cause in children aged 1 to 4. Episodes of diarrhea and respiratory infection were the most frequent reasons for medical consultation, emergency treatment, and hospitalization in 1995.

Tuberculosis accounted for 2% of all diagnosed deaths and 15% of the deaths from communicable diseases. Meningitis was responsible for 0.6% of all diagnosed deaths and 5.2% of the deaths from communicable diseases.

Remarkably few vaccine-preventable diseases were diagnosed as causes of death. Since 1992 there has been a steep decline in mortality due to these diseases. No cases of wild poliovirus have been reported. Although the incidence of measles was 102.4 per 100,000 population in 1992, there were no confirmed cases in 1995 or 1996. No autochthonous cases of neonatal tetanus were diagnosed in 1996, and the international requirements for declaring it eliminated have been partially met. The incidence of diphtheria has been lower than 1.0 per 100,000 population in the last four years. No cases of whooping cough were registered in 1995 or 1996. Tubercular meningitis continues to decline, with an incidence of less than 1.0 per 100,000 population in 1996.

Every year some 300 cases of bacterial meningitis are reported, 60% to 70% of them in infants under 1 year of age. The most common agents are *Haemophilus influenzae* B (about 50%), *Streptococcus pneumoniae* (around 15%), and, less often, *Mycobacterium tuberculosis* and *Neisseria meningitidis* serogroups C and B.

Sexually transmitted diseases are a serious health problem. More than 10,000 new cases are reported each year. Nevertheless, in recent years there has been a marked decline in the reported frequency of cases, probably linked to measures to prevent HIV transmission. In 1995 the rates were as follows: gonorrhea, 34.5 cases per 100,000 population; syphilis, 24.4; chancroid, 3.4; and lymphogranuloma, 0.8. One-third of the women of childbearing age interviewed in the ENDESA 96 survey reported they had had a sexually transmitted disease in the last 12 months, although 82% of them indicated that it had been a vaginal infection.

Since 1983, when the first case of AIDS was reported in the Dominican Republic, the incidence of this disease has risen annually, reaching a rate of approximately 5 per 100,000 population by 1995. More than 70% of the cumulative total of cases were among heterosexuals. The male/female ratio was 2:1, and continuing to equalize. Homosexuals and bisexuals accounted for 10% of the cases and drug users for 3%. Of the cumulative total, 11.3% of the cases among women and 3.4% of those among men were associated with blood transfusion. Recently it has been estimated that more than 80% of all transfused blood is being screened for HIV and hepatitis B.

In recent years there has been an increase in the prevalence of HIV infection among pregnant women in patients seen at venereal disease clinics and, to a lesser extent, in sex workers. Some estimates indicate that by the year 2000 there will be about 50,000 HIV carriers in the country.

The epidemiology of malaria has changed considerably in recent decades. The incidence of the disease is closely related to fluctuations in the construction industry. The number of cases linked to agriculture has gradually decreased. Other factors that may affect the situation have to do with the control program itself, such as its operating capacity and the resources allocated to it. In 1991 there were 377 cases of malaria without a single death, but by 1995 the number of cases had increased to 1,808, and in 1996 there were slightly more than 1,400 cases. All were attributable to *Plasmodium falciparum*, and the majority of them were treated successfully with chloroquine. The areas most affected have been border communities and regions where large construction projects have altered the local ecology and attracted workers from neighboring countries.

Rabies is endemic, due to foci in the wild (mongooses), numerous street dogs, and extensive impoverished urban areas. Up until the 1970s the epidemiological pattern was cyclic, with major outbreaks every four or five years. Since then, the annual frequency has been related more to control measures, vaccination coverage of dogs, epidemiological surveillance, and perifocal control efforts. In recent years the number of cases in dogs has remained at around 5 per 100,000 (canine population) and the number of human cases at about 2 per year, with both of these indicators trending upward.

Hepatitis B is considered to be moderately endemic in the Dominican Republic. In 1996 about 4% of the samples taken from blood donors were positive.

Periodic coproparisitology studies in schoolchildren indicate a growing incidence of giardiasis; a positive rate of 13% was reported for the capital region in 1994. In the eastern part of the country there are known foci of bilharziasis.

The prevalence of leprosy has been decreasing steadily, and in 1996 it was below the internationally established threshold level for it to be considered a public health problem. Except in a few areas, this disease can be considered under control.

There are no foci of yellow fever, but dengue is endemic because of the high proportion of urban households infested with *Aedes aegypti*. In 1993 there were 60 new confirmed cases, 226 in 1994, and 249 in 1995, followed by a drop to about 50 in 1996. It is not known which of the virus serotypes are in circulation. The number of cases of dengue hemorrhagic fever also increased in 1994 and 1995, to 46 and 38 cases, respectively. The number of deaths declined from five in 1994 to only one in 1996.

Given its geographic location, climate, heavy tourist travel and migratory movements, and widespread poverty, the country is extremely vulnerable to the introduction and circulation of infectious agents and to outbreaks of epidemics.

Noncommunicable Diseases and Other Health-Related Problems

Nutritional deficiencies are the number-one concern among noncommunicable diseases and illnesses. In 1994 nutritional deficiencies were responsible for about 10% of the deaths in infants under 1 year of age, 15% in children aged 1 to 4, 6% in those aged 5 to 14, 5% in the population aged 15 to 44, 1% in the group aged 45 to 64, and 2% in persons over age 64. In 1996 the rate of overall malnutrition in children under 5 years of age was estimated at 6% and the rate of chronic malnutrition at 11%. In the country's poorest regions the rate of chronic malnutrition in children under 5 years old ranges from 17% to 20%, and in the capital region it is 6%.

In 1994 the prevalence of anemia and low levels of serum retinol in the age group under 15 years old was found to be 31% and 19%, respectively.

Cardiovascular diseases are the leading causes of death in the general population. In 1994 they were responsible for 79.4

deaths per 100,000 population and 33.8% of all diagnosed deaths, while hypertension and heart failure were the two primary causes for hospitalization.

In 1994 malignant neoplasms accounted for 11.9% of all diagnosed deaths, with a rate of 28.1% per 100,000 population. In women, neoplasms are most often located in the genitourinary organs, the respiratory system, and the breast. Screening for cervical cancer reaches fewer than 10% of the women of childbearing age.

External Causes

In 1994 such external causes as accidental injuries and violence accounted for 12.9% of all diagnosed deaths, for a rate of 30.2 per 100,000. According to police records, external causes made up 15.6% of hospital emergency cases in 1992. Health sources indicated that in 1995 external causes were the principal reason for emergency care in adults and the fourth-ranking cause for hospitalizations nationwide.

RESPONSE OF THE HEALTH SYSTEM

National Health Plans and Policies

The policy that has guided the Secretariat for Public Health and Social Welfare since 1992 is the primary health care strategy. This policy recognizes that health is a fundamental right exercised through free and equal access to the actions that seek to satisfy it. The policy also mandates that the State give priority to the most disadvantaged and vulnerable groups. Central to the policy are democratization, universal health services, equity, humanistic modernity, effectiveness, and efficiency. The main strategies are dispersion and decentralization, societal participation, intra- and intersectoral coordination, and the development and management of knowledge.

However, before these broad policies can be put into practice, many problems need to be solved and many changes must be made in the organization, operation, and allocation of resources in health sector institutions. In mid-1997 the Secretariat set as its highest priority a reversal of a longstanding shortfall in social spending, and declared that the reduction in infant and maternal mortality was its primary objective. In order to attain this goal, the Secretariat has proposed a nationwide mobilization with the participation of all sectors of society, and for a comprehensive plan to strengthen preventive and curative care for children and pregnant women. This goal will be achieved primarily by strengthening health services at the provincial level. At the same time, priority will be given to national programs for immunization, malaria, dengue and other vector-borne diseases, tuberculosis, and rabies. New specialized programs will also be developed for health and tourism, care of the disabled, and environmental health.

Health Sector Reform

There is an awareness in Dominican society that the State is in need of major reform. So far, responses have included creating the Presidential Commission for State Reform and Modernization in 1996, and in 1997 appointing a new Supreme Court that is empowered to modernize and overhaul the judiciary. Reforms have begun in other areas, including in the financial and tariff sectors, the health sector, and the education sector with a Ten-Year Plan for Educational Reform. The new Presidential commission has laid down general guidelines for these processes as part of the overall effort to achieve humane and sustainable development within the context of the new international realities. Health and education are essential aspects of this social reform.

In 1995 a new interinstitutional National Health Commission was created by Presidential decree and given the express mandate to draft a set of proposals within a year for reform of the sector and to promote the overall modernization of the health sector. An Office of Technical Coordination was created to conduct the background studies for these reforms. The office received broad technical and financial support from the Inter-American Development Bank and the World Bank until 1997, when the office went out of existence.

In 1995 the Chamber of Deputies' Commission on Health drafted a General Law on Health, which took into account extensive input from public sector technical teams and civil society. Although the bill was approved by the Chamber of Deputies, it met with opposition in the Senate and was not passed. In a parallel move, a committee appointed by the President in 1996 drafted a proposed reform of the social security system. This proposal, presented as being endorsed by employers, workers, and the government, went to the Congress for consideration and approval, but later met with opposition from some business sectors.

In 1997 a new Presidential decree was issued that created an Executive Commission on Health Reform directly under the Presidency, abolishing all preexisting committees, commissions, and offices, and giving this new body the express mandate to take steps to reform the health sector.

The drinking water, sanitation, and solid waste sectors have recently embarked on a reform and modernization process. It draws its guidelines from the National Drinking Water Plan for Scattered Rural and Marginal Urban Areas and the National Social Development Plan. Both plans give priority to improving living conditions for the most disadvantaged populations.

A National Food and Nutrition Plan that was approved in 1995 is currently being put into place but with much diffi-

culty. In 1997 its implementation was delegated to the Secretariat of Agriculture. One component of this plan is quality control and epidemiological surveillance of foodborne diseases, which is the responsibility of the Secretariat for Public Health and Social Welfare.

Several important trends have been taking shape in the reform process, notable among them the decentralization of the Secretariat, the strengthening of provincial levels, and coordination between government health agencies at the local level. Also, emphasis is being placed on giving greater administrative autonomy to hospital units, tranforming the central-government role largely to that of standards-setting and fiscal control, and modernizing processes at all levels, including technological updating of information systems. However, there is somewhat less consensus regarding which interventions should be guaranteed for the entire population.

Organization of the Health Sector

Institutional Organization

According to the Public Health Code, the Secretariat for Public Health and Social Welfare is the agency in charge of health services and is responsible for applying the Code. The Secretariat provides health care, health promotion, and preventive health services and is structured on three levels: central, regional, and provincial. The role of the central level is essentially standards-setting. Eight regional offices direct the services and oversee the health areas, or units, at the provincial level. The health areas have rural clinics that each cover from 2,000 to 10,000 inhabitants and are staffed with medical interns or assistants, nurse's aides, a supervisor of health promoters, and the health promoters themselves. Most of the provincial capitals have either a second- or third-level hospital with outpatient, inpatient, and around-the-clock emergency services. Some of the provinces also have health subcenters with inpatient beds, emergency services, and general adult medical care, as well as pediatric and pregnancy care.

The Secretariat's programs are structured at the central and regional levels. The most fully developed are those for the control of malaria, dengue, and other vector-borne diseases and for the prevention and control of rabies and zoonoses; the national tuberculosis program; immunization; family planning and reproductive health; and basic sanitation. There are epidemiological services at the national level and also units at the regional and local level.

According to estimated data from the User Satisfaction Survey (ESU 96), more than 85% of the population that uses child vaccination services, 60% of the women who seek prenatal care, and around 60% of those who participate in well-child programs do so through the services of either the Secretariat or the Dominican Social Security Institute (IDSS).

IDSS is an autonomous institution that covers risks from disease, disability, old age, death, and on-the-job accidents incurred by employed workers. In 1994, 6.5% of the general population and 15.4% of the economically active population were affiliated with IDSS, and its expenditures represented 0.7% of the GDP. Since 1990 there has been pressure to completely overhaul social security policy, but to date no reform of IDSS has been accomplished.

The Hotel Social Fund is an autonomous nonprofit public organization dedicated to the social welfare of workers in the hotel and restaurant sector. Its governing body is composed of workers, employers, and government representatives, and its financing is also tripartite. The funds are used for pensions and social services, including medical care. The population it covers is very small.

Affiliation with the Aid and Housing Institute is compulsory for civil servants, including military personnel below a certain salary level. Again, financing is tripartite, and its mandate includes pensions, housing construction, and such social services as primary medical care. The Institute's coverage is very low. The Armed Forces Health Services cover police and military personnel and their families and reach approximately 2% of the population. They have a highly sophisticated central hospital that also provides emergency care for civilians (volume unknown). The activities of these institutions are subject to little if any coordination, which leads to duplication of effort, reduced efficiency, and poor quality in the response this sector gives to the health problems of the population.

Private medical contracts are a form of health insurance developed by private medical centers to expand their client base and guarantee a steady flow of income. Through this system the clinics in the major cities have been able to attract large numbers of workers whose income levels would not otherwise allow them direct access to the services. The range of services varies depending on the specific plan but usually includes medical care and outpatient maternity care, and hospitalization in some cases. Prescription drugs are only covered during hospitalization. Laboratory services include only basic tests. In the case of more complicated diagnoses the contracts cover between 50% and 75% of the cost. The plans usually do not include regular checkups, preventive medicine, or care for mental disorders or chronic diseases. According to the ESU 96 survey, approximately 3.2% of the population has these medical contracts.

Almost all the life insurance companies offer their clients supplementary health insurance. These programs are geared to high-level officials and other upper-income persons. The premiums are higher than for the medical contracts mentioned above, but the plans are more flexible, with more freedom to choose one's physician or hospital. It is estimated

that this type of insurance covers approximately 2.5% of the population.

Of the self-administered health insurance programs, the most well-known is the Teachers' Medical Insurance, a cooperative subsidized by the national government. Since 1995 it has contracted private medical services for public teachers. The cooperative entity that administers it is nonprofit and has an interest in keeping costs down. Generally the services offered by these insurance programs are similar to those provided by the private medical contracts, although there may also be some preventive medical services as well as greater hospital and diagnostic coverage.

Some nonprofit private services are provided by clinics and hospitals managed by nongovernmental organizations. For example, some institutions or foundations offer low-cost services for such specialized problems as diabetes, cardiovascular diseases, skin diseases, cancer, or rehabilitation. A number of these institutions receive sizable government subsidies through the Secretariat for Public Health, and they also may be paid directly by users. Programs of this kind have greatly increased in number, and they are located mostly in the two largest cities, Santo Domingo and Santiago. When the institutions receive financial assistance from the Secretariat, they are required to submit a report on expenditures, but there is no surveillance of their activities or results.

Private for-profit services have been growing rapidly in recent decades. They are provided in facilities ranging from highly sophisticated private hospitals to small centers operating under uncertain conditions, usually located in outlying urban or semirural areas. There is no legal control over the creation or set-up of these services, and as a result it is difficult to know how many there are. According to the ENDESA 96 health survey, almost half the respondents who had requested outpatient care during the previous month, as well as half of those who had needed to be hospitalized during the preceding six months, had used services of this kind.

The public sector is thought to provide a high proportion of the preventive and health promotion services. According to the ESU 96 user survey, only 6.4% of the people who sought vaccination services obtained them in private for-profit centers.

More than three-fourths of the persons interviewed in the ESU 96 user survey believed that health is one of the top three priority areas in which the Dominican Government should be involved; 38.1% felt it should be the number-one priority. Of the respondents, 53% said that health services generally worked poorly and should be completely overhauled. A majority had a negative opinion of the Secretariat's hospitals and a very favorable opinion of private clinics. The aspect that contributed most to their unfavorable opinion of the public services was the waiting time, not only in outpatient clinics but also in hospitals and surgical services. The inability to choose one's doctor and the fact that the patient is treated by a series of different physicians during subsequent visits were also considered negative aspects of the public services.

Organization of Health Regulatory Activities

Public health regulation is very weak. The existing health care standards are 10 or 20 years old, and health professionals are certified by union-like professional associations.

In 1996 the Secretariat for Public Health and Social Welfare, working with the Private Clinics Association, began to develop an accreditation system for hospitals and private clinics, but the initiative has run into serious difficulties. It has only been possible to reach agreement on a few of the definitions, and nothing concrete has emerged from the process. There is also an effort under way to regulate and accredit public and private laboratories.

The Secretariat's Drug and Pharmacy Division is responsible for evaluating and registering drugs, as well as for inspecting drug manufacturing laboratories and pharmacies. There are pharmacological standards and procedures in effect to regulate drug registration, and an automated information system has been set up. Nevertheless, the regulatory inspection of pharmaceutical businesses is a weak link in the program. The Dr. Defilló National Public Health Laboratory is responsible for the analytical control of drug quality, but its operations are hampered by the poor state of its infrastructure and equipment. There is no department in the Secretariat responsible for the scientific or technical aspect of drugs. In the area of food regulation, efforts to apply the FAO/WHO code have been relatively ineffective.

Health Services and Resources

Organization of Services for Care of the Population

Drinking Water and Sewerage Systems. The country's rapid population growth, massive migration to urban areas, and increasing numbers of people living in poverty have resulted in serious deficiencies in the coverage and quality of water and sanitation services. It was estimated that in 1993 the drinking water supply reached 65% of the population—80% of those in urban areas and 46% of the persons in rural areas. Of the country's 8,463 rural communities, only about 2,100, or 25%, had drinking water services, while sanitary sewerage disposal services covered only 16% of the entire population and 28.0% of the urban population.

Drinking water and sewerage services represent a large share of the Government's social expenditures. The system is highly dependent on subsidies to finance its current costs and investment needs, and it operates at a significant deficit be-

cause of shortcomings in marketing, extensive water loss in aqueducts, and fee schedules that do not reflect costs. Institutional weaknesses, staff turnover, and deficiencies in operating and maintaining systems all hamper the sector's ability to meet the basic sanitation needs of the population.

Disease Control and Prevention Programs. The Expanded Program on Immunization (EPI) coordinates activities with both public and private institutions. Vaccines are procured through the EPI Revolving Fund, with the exception of hepatitis B vaccine, which is purchased directly from the suppliers. Every shipment that arrives is subject to quality control, and samples are taken in the warehouses to monitor the status of the vaccines.

During the 1992–1996 period the government developed combined vaccination strategies based on guidelines aimed at meeting the regional targets to eradicate and control vaccine-preventable diseases. Vaccination programs have been established for all the EPI vaccines, to immunize all newborns in hospitals and health centers against tuberculosis, hepatitis B, and poliomyelitis. In addition, national vaccination days have been held to reach new population groups, such as those under 15 years of age, and protect them against measles.

Vaccination coverage has exceeded 80% since 1993. Between 10% and 20% of the vaccines are administered by private providers. There is no government reporting system.

Epidemiological Surveillance Systems and Public Health Laboratories. The epidemiological surveillance system operates at the national level through the General Directorate of Epidemiology and surveillance units in the specialized programs. In addition, in each of the eight health regions there is a regional epidemiological unit, and in each of the 38 health areas there is at least one professional responsible for epidemiological duties. Also, each of the main hospitals has an epidemiology unit that is responsible for surveillance. The system has evolved and improved considerably since 1996, and it is expected to be strengthened even more after the National Epidemiology Institute starts up its activities, probably in 1998.

The compulsory reporting system relies on weekly passive and compulsory reporting of suspected cases of any of the diseases on the list drawn up for this purpose. For some diseases, such as bacterial meningitis, a special surveillance subsystem has been developed.

The epidemiological surveillance system is composed of subsystems that cover the following areas: (a) diseases for which reporting is compulsory; (b) acute febrile conditions; (c) infant births and deaths and deaths of women of reproductive age; (d) harbors and airports, and (e) specialized programs.

The subsystem for the surveillance of acute febrile conditions consists of 40 sentinel posts located in secondary and tertiary health care facilities whose task is to detect any suspected cases of malaria, dengue, measles, and other acute febrile diseases that could lead to epidemics.

The subsystem for the surveillance of live births and maternal and infant deaths is based on regulations issued in 1997 that require immediate reporting of these events. It covers all the public and private health establishments in the country. Its mandate is to monitor high-risk newborns during the first year of life and to investigate the extent to which infant and maternal deaths could be avoided.

The subsystem for the surveillance of harbors and airports is responsible for the early detection of suspected cases of diseases with high epidemiological risk, and the application of international sanitary regulations.

The surveillance subsystem for malaria and dengue relies on passive reporting through the health establishments and sentinel posts in the surveillance subsystem for febrile conditions, and it also actively seeks out febrile patients in areas where cases have been detected. The epidemiological surveillance subsystem connected with the immunization program is responsible for compliance with the standards established in the poliomyelitis eradication plan and has gradually incorporated the surveillance of other vaccine-preventable diseases. It also oversees immunization coverage at the municipal level. In addition, there are surveillance subsystems for rabies and tuberculosis.

Most of the surveillance support is provided by the Dr. Defilló National Laboratory, although the Central Veterinary Laboratory, the National Anti-Rabies Center, the National Malaria Eradication Service, and the main hospitals also contribute to this effort.

Solid Waste Collection and Urban Cleanup Services. These services are the responsibility of local communities. In almost all the cities, coverage is minimal, collection is sporadic, and solid waste is disposed of in open-air pits. The administrative units in these services are weak and suffer from shortages of equipment, funding, and specialized personnel. Trash collection in the National District was privatized in 1992, and since then services have improved in the residential areas. There are no special procedures or standards that apply to hospital solid wastes.

Control of Environmental Risks. The lower-income areas surrounding the main cities lack water supply, sewerage, or trash collection services. Many of the dwellings there are overcrowded, constructed of cast-off materials, and located near pollution sources.

Sewage runoff and liquid and gas pollutants from industry and agriculture come under the responsibility of several different institutions, including the Secretariat for Public Health and Social Welfare, the National Water Supply and Sewerage

Institute (INAPA), the municipal councils, the Secretariat of State of Agriculture, the National Bureau of Forestry, and other entities, none of which has specific policies or programs. There is also no specific legislation or adequate coordination, and resources to oversee these activities are very limited.

There is considerable pollution of groundwater and of beaches near the coastal cities. The generation of electricity in government, industrial, commercial, and home-based installations, powered by all kinds of fuels, pollutes the air and causes disturbing levels of noise in the cities.

Workers' Health. The Secretariat for Public Health, the IDSS, the Secretariats for Labor, Education, Agriculture, and Public Works, and the municipal governments share responsibility in this area. According to the limited information available, the high number of disabilities, workplace injuries, and occupational diseases is cause for concern. Programs geared toward preventing these problems have not been extensively developed; the reality is that workers are unprotected and ill-prepared to deal with these risks.

Disaster Preparedness. The Dominican Republic is located in an area exposed to cyclones, earthquakes, and floods—phenomena that have taken a significant toll in terms of economic damage and loss of life. A coordination office has been created in the Secretariat for Public Health to oversee implementation of the national plan for disaster preparedness.

Health Promotion. The Secretariat for Public Health has encouraged the establishment of local development programs, the most advanced of which is in the province of Salcedo. There, excellent results have been achieved in the improvement of environmental sanitation and the reduction of deaths from such causes as gastroenteritis, from which there have been no registered deaths since 1994.

The Department of Healthy Communities was established within the Secretariat in 1997 to coordinate local development initiatives, strengthen provincial development councils, and create healthy communities.

Food and Nutrition. The National Food and Nutrition Plan is currently being redrafted, with the goal of building food security and encouraging the formulation of projects to mobilize resources to carry out the Plan.

Oral Health. During 1995, 445 dentists and 197 dental assistants working for the Secretariat for Public Health performed a total of 324,977 clinical dental interventions in 174,699 consultations. Prevention measures, basically consisting of fluoride rinses, currently reach only 10% of the schoolchildren between 6 and 14 years of age.

Organization and Operation of Personal Health Care Services

According to data from the Secretariat for Public Health, in 1996 there were a total of 1,334 health facilities in the country, of which 730 (55%) came directly under the Secretariat, 184 (14%) under IDSS, 417 (31%) under the private sector, and 3 (0.2%) under the armed forces. There were 15,236 hospital beds, of which 7,234 (47%) belonged to the Secretariat, 1,706 (11%) to IDSS, 5,796 (38%) to the private sector, and 500 (3%) to the armed forces. These numbers represent a bed/population ratio of 1:500. However, there is a discrepancy among different sources on the number of beds available.

In 1996 the total number of outpatient consultations provided by facilities under the Secretariat came to 5.8 million, or 0.8 consultations per inhabitant, of which 2.2 million were emergency consultations, or 0.3 per inhabitant. There were 372,000 hospital discharges, or 50 per 1,000 population. No comparable current data are available for IDSS or other public institutions.

The ENDESA 96 survey showed that 97% of all pregnant women had had some form of prenatal care by physicians, and the average was 7.6 prenatal visits. Of these women, 88% had four or more visits, and 94% began their visits during the first six months of pregnancy. A large proportion of the deliveries were institutional. During 1991–1996, 95% of all deliveries took place in medical facilities, with differences by region and social level. For example, 99% of the women with university education delivered in medical centers, compared with 82% of those who were illiterate.

Inputs for Health

In 1996 the value of the private sector drug market was US$ 186.4 million, while in the public sector purchases by the Government's Essential Drugs Program were estimated at US$ 15 million. Adding to these amounts the expenditures by IDSS and the armed forces, the annual average per capita expenditure on drugs is estimated at US$ 30.

The Essential Drugs Program is responsible for buying and distributing drugs for public sector institutions based on the product list prepared by the Secretariat for Public Health.

The country has 84 drug laboratories that produce drugs and related products financed with domestic capital and one laboratory financed with multinational funds.

There is no reliable record in the Dominican Republic of equipment available in the public and private health facilities. However, the country has made sizable investments not only to equip the large network of existing services but also to periodically update the equipment on hand. There are recognized problems in the area of maintenance, and the average life of the equipment is far shorter than it should be. These

problems have been getting worse in recent years as international contacts have increased and the country has received or is in the process of receiving large donations and purchasing equipment under favorable terms. This new equipment has come from different sources, different companies, and with different technical specifications, but without any commitment from the suppliers for training or maintenance.

At the beginning of 1997 the "Health Plaza," a Government-owned complex located in Santo Domingo, began operating. It contains hospitals for maternal and child care, geriatrics, and traumatology, plus an advanced diagnostic center. A sizable investment has been made in this complex, which has 430 new beds and highly advanced technology. However, at the moment there is no clear decision as to how these installations will be linked with the rest of the health system, and the matter is now being vigorously debated.

Human Resources

In 1994 the Secretariat for Public Health and Social Welfare had working for it 5,626 physicians, 376 dentists, 1,008 bioanalysts, 8,600 nurses and nurse's aides, 6,127 health promoters and supervisors, and 372 pharmacists. No current information is available on the number of professionals in the country by profession and category.

It is estimated in 1995 that the total number of job positions with the health sector's two main employers, the Secretariat and the IDSS, came to about 62,100. That included all professional, technical, and administrative categories.

Only partial, out-of-date information is available on the labor supply for the sector. In 1996 15 of the country's 27 universities and 7 institutions of higher learning offered degree programs in the health sciences.

Enrollment for the degree program in nursing has been gradually declining, from 1,339 in 1984 to 641 in 1990, and currently the University of Santo Domingo offers this program tuition-free as an incentive to attract students. There has been an increase in postgraduate programs. Five universities offer master's degrees related to health, and four of them offer a total of 28 medical residency programs. There is also a rise in the number of specialists in relation to the number of general physicians. In addition, intermediate technical training programs (in radiology, rehabilitation, laboratory science, etc.) have grown significantly. In all these training programs there are serious problems relating to access and accreditation.

Research and Technology

Even though the National Science and Technology Council was created in 1983, as yet there is no explicit policy regarding research and scientific and technical information. This situation has hampered the development of research on health human resources. In actual practice, research projects have been undertaken more in response to funding opportunities and personal or institutional priorities than to explicit priorities related to national needs.

Since 1994 the Secretariat for Public Health and Social Welfare has provided direct or indirect support for research relating to infectious diseases, parasitology, cancer of the cervix, diabetes mellitus, and cardiovascular diseases. Also, with financial support from IDB and the World Bank, a study of the health situation was conducted on the disease burden and the public health benefits from activities that are part of health system reform and reorganization.

The lack of a clear policy on research, of an agency responsible for taking the lead, and of funding for research planning makes it very difficult to allocate funds to research projects or create greater awareness of the importance of research and the need to improve its quality.

There is no policy regulating the utilization of new technologies. Some of the local development programs have evaluated appropriate technologies, but there is no control and no evaluation of whether their use has had an impact.

In recent years there have been important cooperative efforts in the area of health information. The country now has libraries and documentation centers specialized in health, with trained personnel and regularly updated sources of bibliographic information. A network of hospital libraries has been created, as well as a system to exchange specialized information. At the local level, basic book collections and small specialized libraries have been created with support from PAHO and the European Union.

Expenditures and Sectoral Financing

There are no recent reliable estimates of private expenditures on health. According to the ENDESA 96 survey, 37% of the households had required some form of medical care in the preceding 30 days. The average expenditure per household in terms of outpatient consultations during this period came to the equivalent of US$ 8.80, and to US$ 154.70 in the case of hospitalization. Those who used public services had much lower expenditures (US$ 29.50) than those who used private services (US$ 252.00). It is interesting to note that, according to the survey, those with family incomes in the lowest 20% spent more on private care than did those in the top 20% income bracket. This was true both in terms of outpatient care (US$ 30.60 versus US$ 29.70) and hospitalizations (US$ 320.10 versus US$ 242.90).

Total public expenditures on health in 1995 were estimated at US$ 214.39 million, or US$ 29 per capita. Although the figure increased in absolute terms, the per capita inflation-adjusted expenditure on health was lower in 1991 than in 1980. Between 1992 and 1995 there was a slight recovery. As a percentage of GDP, expenditures on public health have remained level, fluctuating between 1.1% and 1.8%. However, as a proportion of total public expenditures, health rose from 7% in 1985 to 9.5% in 1990, and then fell to 7.8% in 1991–1992, where it remained through 1995. The share of the total expenditures on health made by Secretariat for Public Health and Social Welfare went from 86% in 1979–1982 to 64% in 1987–1990 and 56% in 1991. During these same years the Presidency of the Republic increased its share of health spending from 2% to 28% and then to 38%. In the Secretariat the ratio of expenditures on tertiary versus primary health care increased from 8.7 in 1988 to 11.0 in 1992. In 1991, total direct expenditures for consultations, hospital beds, and other hospitalization costs were 60% to 70% less than in 1980.

External Technical and Financial Cooperation

External financing of public expenditures on health declined from an average of 6.8% during 1983–1986 to 1.9% in 1987–1991. Although there is no reliable current information available, the share has probably increased since then, given the leveling-off in overall public spending and the growth in projects funded by various bilateral cooperation agencies.

The Expanded Program on Immunization has received support from UNICEF, the U.S. Agency for International Development (USAID), IDB, Rotary International, and PAHO/WHO. Those organizations have been working together on an EPI coordinating committee for several years.

Family planning and reproductive health programs have received financial assistance from the United Nations Population Fund and USAID. The latter has provided significant funding for AIDS prevention activities, mainly to private nonprofit institutions. Up until 1996 the national public sector program received technical and financial cooperation through PAHO/WHO. Since 1997, when the UNAIDS program started up, external funding for the Dominican program has been considerably reduced.

A number of national and local programs and projects have received support from the European Union; the German aid agency, GTZ; the Spanish International Cooperation Agency; the Japan International Cooperation Agency (JICA); and Italy.

There are numerous international nongovernmental organizations that carry out health activities in the country, most of them in support of local organizations that work in lower-income urban and rural areas.

ECUADOR

GENERAL SITUATION AND TRENDS

Socioeconomic, Political, and Demographic Overview

Despite a severe economic and political crisis, during the 1990s Ecuador succeeded in strengthening its democratic constitutional regime and assuming its identity as a multicultural, multiethnic, and multilingual society. The administration that took office in August 1992 undertook to restore the macroeconomic equilibrium and modernize the State. For this purpose it created the National Modernization Council under the Office of the President, which negotiated the first privatizations of public agencies and presented proposals for decentralization, reducing the size of the State apparatus, and reforming social security.

During 1992–1995 inflation fell from 54.6% to 22.9%, monetary reserves increased from US$ 1,300 million to $1,600 million, and the fiscal deficit declined from 7% to 3% of gross domestic product (GDP). Seasonal migrations from the countryside to the towns and from the towns to the large cities swelled the ranks of the informal work sector, which represented 60% of the urban economically active population (EAP) in 1994. Net unemployment went from 3.6% in 1990 to 6.9% in 1995. Between 1991 and 1994 underemployment remained at approximately 48.0%. In July 1996 a worker's total income, as established by the National Wage Council, amounted to US$ 154, including a minimum living wage of $27 and additional compensation mandated by law (in 1990 the corresponding amounts were $130 and $65, but purchasing power was greater).

The lack of political support in Congress, coupled with increasing resistance on the part of the public, put a halt to the plan for privatization. In November 1995 a plebiscite rejected the constitutional reforms proposed by the President, following which the administration attempted to ameliorate some of the effects. The Ministries of Health, Education, Housing, and Labor went through a financial crisis when social spending was cut from 7.8% of GDP in 1992 to 5.18%.

A new administration took office in August 1996, and there were high hopes that it would promote social programs with broad popular outreach and immediate effect. However, the leadership style and the announcement of an economic plan based on convertibility of the currency, along with aggressive privatization, fiscal austerity, and severe adjustment measures, sparked the mobilization of civilian society against them. The President was replaced by an interim government elected by Congress to serve until August 1998, which was legitimized by plebiscite in 1997. The aims of this government were to combat corruption, strengthen national unity, reduce unemployment (estimated at 10% in 1997), stabilize the economy, lay the foundation for economic and social development, and prepare for political transition to an elected government for the 1998–2002 term.

In 1997, Ecuador's population was estimated at 11,936,858, of which 55.4% lived in urban areas. The population growth rate was 2.1% in the last intercensal period (1982–1990), and the annual rate for 1995–2000 is estimated at 1.9%. In 1995 the population under 15 years of age represented 36.4% of the total, as opposed to 38.9% in 1990. In the year 2000 this age group will represent 33.8% of the total population. In 1995, 49.8% of the population lived in coastal regions, 44.8% in the mountains, 4.6% in the Amazon region, 0.1% on the islands, and 0.7% in areas without geopolitical boundaries.

The national birth rate, corrected for delayed birth registrations (50% of the total) was 23.7 per 1,000 inhabitants in 1995, representing a decline of 7.8% with respect to 1990 (24.7 per 1,000). According to the Demographic and Maternal and Child Health Survey (ENDEMAIN-94), total fertility decreased from 4.0 children per woman in 1985–1990 to 3.6 in 1989–1994 (4.6 in rural areas and 2.9 in urban areas). The decline is explained in large part by the increased years of schooling for women, their growing participation in the work force, migration from the countryside to the cities, and family planning programs. The indigenous population, on the other hand, continues to have high fertility rates, as observed in mountain provinces such as Bolívar, where the rate is 5.12 children per woman, and on the Pacific coast in districts such as Esmeraldas, with a rate of 4.66 children per woman.

Eight percent of the men and 12% of the women are illiterate; 30% of indigenous-language speakers are illiterate, compared with 10% of Spanish-speaking individuals. Only 53% of the indigenous population attends primary school, 15% is in secondary school, and fewer than 1% is enrolled in institutions of higher learning.

It is estimated that 63% of the total population was affected by some degree of poverty in 1995, compared with 54% in 1990; 40.3% of the total population has at least one unmet basic need, ranging from 60.8% in rural areas to 27.0% in urban areas. Forty percent of the total population is poor and 15% is indigent. The provinces that are poorest and have the highest percentage of households with unmet basic needs also have the lowest indexes of urbanization and, paradoxically, the lowest registered death rates. This can be explained by underregistration, which has not yet been quantified at the provincial level.

Based on data from the 1990 Population Census, it is estimated the indigenous population at that time stood at 910,146 (9.4% of the total) and was concentrated in the rural areas of the Ecuadorian Amazon region and the mountains. The exact locations of the various ethnic groups have not yet been mapped. Statistical data from 1994 indicate that the most numerous group is the Quichua, who live mainly in the mountains (66,964) and the Amazon area (72,528). Other ethnic groups in the Amazon area are the Shuaras (36,634), the Aschuaras (4,000), the Huaoranis (1,200), the Cofanes (627), and the Siona-Secoya (600). Along the coast there are 5,000 Chachis, 1,000 Tsachelas, and 27,648 Quichuas. No figures are available for the Ecuadorian population of African origin, which is concentrated along the coast and in two mountain provinces.

In the rural mountain and Amazon areas, it is estimated that 76% of the children live in poverty, a figure that reaches 80% for indigenous children and adolescents. In coastal areas, among the rural Ecuadorian population of African origin, 70% of those under 18 years of age are living in poverty. In these areas, as well as along the borders with Colombia and Peru, the situation is aggravated by migration of adult men to the cities or to other countries in search of work. Pichincha and Chimborazo have most of the emigrants from the other provinces (29.5% apiece). It is estimated that a million Ecuadorians are living abroad, mainly in the United States of America.

Life expectancy at birth in 1990–1995 was 68.8 years for the general population (66.4 years for men and 71.4 years for women); for 1995–2000 the estimate is 69.9 years (67.3 for men and 72.5 for women). The increase reflects the work that has been done in health education and health promotion, which has benefited children in particular.

Mortality

The figures on general mortality differ depending on how this indicator is measured. The accepted rate for 1995 is 5.17 per 1,000 inhabitants, which allows for underregistration of 16.4%. The estimate of underregistration, based on tables from the Latin American Demography Center (CELADE), is too high (30.3% for males and 33.4% for females) because when the tables were prepared they did not take into account the probable effect of actions undertaken on behalf of children. The percentage of deaths with medical cause-of-death certification was 84.5%, an increase of 3.3 percentage points relative to 1992. Deaths due to signs, symptoms, and ill-defined conditions accounted for 13.4% of the deaths in 1995, compared with 14.3% in 1990.

The highest mortality rates for both sexes and for all age groups were due to diseases of the circulatory system, followed by external causes in men and communicable diseases in women. The latter cause group was the one that declined the most between 1990 and 1995 in both sexes and in all age groups (from 97.0 to 79.2 per 100,000 inhabitants in men and from 84.8 to 68.4 per 100,000 in women). In that same period, the most notable drop in deaths from communicable diseases was in infants under 1 year old, with gains on the order of 400 lives per 100,000. Mortality rates from malignant tumors remained stable in men (59 per 100,000) and increased in women, from 67.3 to 71.2 per 100,000, and were highest in the population over 60 years of age. Mortality from diseases of the circulatory system declined somewhat more in women than in men, particularly among older adults. Death rates from conditions originating in the perinatal period dropped more for females than for males (110 and 72 fewer deaths per 100,000 live births, respectively). During the same time period, mortality from external causes increased slightly for males (from 99.5 to 103.8) and decreased slightly for females (from 29.1 to 26.1), underlining that there are gender-specific differences.

Between 1990 and 1995 the leading causes of death in the general population remained the same, but their rank changed: cerebrovascular diseases dropped from first to second place as the rate fell from 25.6 to 23.1 per 100,000 inhabitants; pneumonia, on the other hand, rose from third place to first, with a rate of 27.2 per 100,000; intestinal infectious diseases moved from second to ninth place and the rate dropped to half; traffic accidents remained in fourth place, with a decline in the rate from 19.4 to 15.8 per 100,000; and malignant tumors of the stomach remained in seventh place, showing a slight increase from 11.7 to 12.7 per 100,000. Deaths due to homicide and injuries purposely inflicted by other persons went from ninth to sixth place, with a 50% increase, and were responsible for 55,443 years of potential life lost (YPLL), 50,200 of them in men. A total of 1,191,882 YPLL are estimated to have been caused by deaths occurring before the age of 70—713,785 of these in men.

SPECIFIC HEALTH PROBLEMS

Analysis by Population Group

Health of Children

ENDEMAIN-94 estimated infant mortality for the country as a whole at 44 per 1,000 live births, with large differences among the provinces: in Chimborazo, where the population is predominantly rural and indigenous, the estimated rate was 100 per 1,000 live births, whereas in Pichincha and Guayas, where the two largest cities (Quito and Guayaquil) are located, the estimated rates were 32 and 33 per 1,000, respectively. As in 1990, the leading cause of death in the infant population was hypoxia, asphyxia, and other respiratory disorders; diarrheal diseases moved from second to fourth place and the rate dropped to less than one-third—an improvement attributable to the use of oral rehydration; pneumonia remained in third place.

Acute respiratory infections were responsible for 37% of the deaths in infants from 1 week to 11 months of age and for 32% of deaths in children from 1 to 4 years old; they accounted for 28% and 24% of hospital discharges, respectively. Congenital anomalies went from eighth to sixth place, although in 1995 the mortality rate from this cause had dropped to half.

Of the 8,234 registered deaths in children under 5 years of age in 1995, 2,622 were in infants less than 1 month old; 1,916 of these were newborns under 1 week old. A total of 2,926 fetal deaths were reported. If it is assumed that the rate of underreporting of infant deaths remained stable, then there was an appreciable decline in infant mortality as well as in the group under 5 years old between 1990 and 1995. Mortality rates per 1,000 registered live births, adjusted for late registration of newborns, were 30.3 for children under 5 years of age, 20.4 for infants, 7.0 for early neonatal, 2.6 for late-born neonates, 10.7 in the postneonatal period, 17.9 for those in perinatal stage I, and 20.5 for those in perinatal stage II.

In children under 5 years of age, acute respiratory infections and acute diarrheal diseases were the principal causes of morbidity. Of the children surveyed, 19% had had diarrhea during the two weeks prior to ENDEMAIN-94, and 59% had suffered from an acute respiratory infection. In 1994 and 1995, among children less than 5 years old these infections, together with diarrheal and vaccine-preventable diseases, malnutrition and anemias, meningitis, malaria, and septicemia, accounted for between 60% and 70% of all hospitalizations and between 70% and 80% of outpatient consultations in the Ministry of Public Health.

In the group 5 to 9 years of age the sharpest decline in deaths was under the heading of infectious diseases, especially diarrheal diseases and respiratory infections. In 1995, accidents were the leading cause of death for both sexes. Violent causes, including accidents, were responsible for 285 deaths and affected males disproportionately (male/female ratio, 1.7:1). Nevertheless, certain types of non-fatal aggression, such as sexual abuse, affected mostly girls 5 years of age and older.

The group aged 5 to 9 tends to fall between programs for children, which are typically geared to those under 5 years of age, and programs for adolescents. As a result, little information is available on causes of illness and reasons for outpatient consultations for this age group. Data on hospital discharges, the only available information, show a preponderance of injuries resulting from violence and accidents; there is also an increase in chronic diseases compared to 1990.

Health of Adolescents

In 1990 the age group 10-to-19 years old represented 23.4% of the population. Early entry into the work force, migration, and lack of cultural acceptance, among other factors, provoked conflicts for adolescents, which were expressed in problems relating to their reproductive and mental health and their possibilities for growth and development. Of all the deaths in 1995, 4.2% were among adolescents. In both the 10-to-14 age group and those aged 15 to 19 the leading cause of death for both sexes was accidents and violence, with 971 reported deaths, which represents a rate of 37.6 per 100,000 population. Males were predominant (716 males and 255 females; 2.8:1 ratio).

In adolescent females, the main external causes of death in 1995 were: suicide, 76 deaths (66 in the group aged 15 to 19) and traffic accidents, 48 deaths (30 in the 15-to-19 age group). There were 23 maternal deaths, representing a maternal mortality rate for this group of 76.8 per 100,000 live births—lower than the rate for 1990. For adolescent males, the leading causes of death were accidents, especially traffic accidents, with 191 deaths (126 in those over 15 years of age), homicides, 143 deaths (134 in the over-15 group); and suicide, 50 deaths (44 in those over 15).

According to a 1995 survey, prevalence of the use of illicit drugs was 3.2% in the group aged 12 to 19, and prevalence of the use of alcohol and tobacco was considerably higher. Partial surveys conducted in the 1990s, which corroborated the national data gathered at the end of the 1980s, showed that tobacco use in adolescents was 14.9%, with no difference by sex. In 1995 it was estimated that, at the national level, 48.5% of all adolescents 11 to 13 years of age had consumed some type of alcoholic beverage; the figure increased to 73.9% in the population aged 14 to 16 and to 87.1% among 17-year-olds, with no significant differences according to sex. Ten percent of all adolescents had been intoxicated before they were 10 years old.

Health of Adults

The leading causes of death in adults from 20 to 59 years of age are cardiovascular and cerebrovascular diseases, malignant tumors, and accidents and violence. In 1995 the leading cause for men aged 20 to 44 was accidents and violence, with 3,046 deaths, or 52.3% of the total (5,828) from all causes in this age group. Deaths from violence have homicides (936) and traffic accidents (653) as the most important causes. Other causes, in descending order, were cardiovascular and cerebrovascular diseases (535 deaths, or 9.2% of the total), malignant tumors (257, or 4.4%), and tuberculosis (252, or 4.3%). For women in the 20-to-44 age range the leading cause also was accidents and violence, with 486 deaths, or 18.1% of the total, followed by malignant neoplasms (425, or 15.8%), cardiovascular and cerebrovascular diseases (398, or 14.8%), tuberculosis (154, or 5.7%), and maternal causes (145, or 5.4%).

In 1995 a total of 170 maternal deaths were registered. The national rate adjusted for late registrations was 62.7 per 100,000 registered live births, a number that reflects significant underregistration. The average for the 1991–1995 period was 110.1 per 100,000 live births, with significant regional differences: in three provinces the rate exceeded 200 per 100,000, whereas in two provinces it was around 75 per 100,000. ENDEMAIN-94 estimated maternal mortality at 159 per 100,000 live births for the 1988–1994 period, and PAHO/WHO set the number at 120 per 100,000 in 1995. National organizations committed to reducing maternal mortality have adopted what they consider to be the realistic figure of 150 per 100,000. Maternal mortality, in addition to being related to poverty, is associated with shortcomings in the health services. In 1995 the proportion of professionally attended deliveries nationwide was 66.5%, but with substantial differences between the cities (84.3%) and the rural areas (41.9%). The differences are even more marked if Guayaquil (94.2%) or Quito (89.5%) is compared with the rural mountain areas (38.8%). Gynecological and obstetric morbidity has been reported to the National Epidemiological Surveillance System since 1994. While overall deliveries remained at a steady level (106,726 attended in 1996), cesarean sections, at 36,285, increased 33%, and abortions, at 12,310, were up 14%.

The leading cause of death in men from 45 to 59 years of age was accidents and violence (849 deaths, or 23.2% of the total), followed by cardiovascular and cerebrovascular diseases (663 deaths, or 18.1%), malignant neoplasms (392, or

10.7%), diabetes mellitus (169, or 4.6%), and tuberculosis (115, or 3.1%). In women of this age group the leading causes, in order, were malignant neoplasms (638 deaths, or 26.2% of the total), cardiovascular and cerebrovascular diseases (551, or 22.7%), diabetes mellitus (158, or 6.5%), and accidents and violence (147, or 6.0%). The most frequent site of malignant neoplasms was the uterine cervix, which accounted for 176 deaths in 1995. Detection programs have been targeted toward this high-risk age group.

Health of the Elderly

In 1995 the two leading causes of death in the group aged 60 and over were cardiovascular and cerebrovascular diseases and malignant neoplasms. In men of this age group the former category accounted for 3,455 deaths, or 27.1% of the total, and malignant neoplasms accounted for 1,848 deaths, or 14.5%; other major causes were accidents and violence (848 deaths, or 6.7%), pneumonia (750, or 5.9%), and diabetes (503, or 3.9%). In women aged 60 and over the proportions were similar: cardiovascular and cerebrovascular diseases headed the list (3,322 deaths, or 27.4% of the total), followed by malignant tumors (2,010, or 16.6%), pneumonia (803, or 6.6%), and diabetes (788, or 6.5%).

In general there are not enough policies, programs, services, or human resources in the field of gerontology. The Ministry of Public Health's services for the 60-and-over population, in addition to being limited, are nonspecific and lack the components of promotion, education, self-care, and rehabilitation. The Ecuadorian Social Security Institute (IESS) has established a program that focuses on mutual support groups and mental health.

Family Health

With a total fertility rate of 3.5 for 1990–1995 and a national average of five members per nuclear family unit, Ecuador's families, especially in the cities, have undergone a major transformation in recent decades, characterized by shrinking size, less community participation, not as much bonding with the extended family, and rising rates of separation and divorce, which have created a high proportion of single-parent families.

The average annual marriage rate for 1990–1995 was 6.3 per 1,000 inhabitants, and the divorce rate was 6.1 per 10,000 inhabitants. In other words, for every 10 new marriages there was one divorce. This figure does not reflect the true situation, however, because consensual unions, which tend to be more stable, are very common, especially in the rural coastal areas; there are also multiple marriages and tacit separations that, even though no divorce is involved, leave many women as heads of families who live in inadequate economic and social conditions.

Efforts to respond to family problems, although they have been considerable, have often focused on specific aspects such as protecting abused children and women or responding to urgent health needs of poor individuals and families. The work of the National Child and Family Institute is one of the most notable examples. Some private institutions, including nongovernmental organizations, are working in this field, especially in the areas of mental health, legal aid, health care, and social work in homes with high levels of family violence. In 1993 the child abuse prevention network (REDPANM) and the committees of women to deal with family violence carried out important work. Since 1993 there has been a law on violence against women and families. Some religious orders, such as the Salesian priests, have long-term programs for aiding and rescuing street children.

Workers' Health

In 1992, of the total EAP, only 1,101,131 (30%) were covered by occupational hazard insurance through their affiliation with the IESS. No attempt is being made to investigate or report the leading causes of disease and death in this group. Data available for 1990 show that over the previous 10 years the annual incidence of accident-related deaths among workers belonging to the IESS declined from 226 to 162, whereas in the unaffiliated population the number increased from 226 to 430. The leading work-related diseases were occupational deafness, pesticide and other chemical poisoning, diseases of the bronchi and lungs, dermatoses, cancer, disturbances of the locomotor system, infections and contagious diseases, and eye diseases. Since 1994, work-related accidents have been reported to the National Epidemiological Surveillance System. Between 1994 and 1996, approximately 5,000 cases were reported each year.

According to a study conducted by the International Labor Organization (ILO) and UNICEF, in 1990 some 800,000 children and youth between the ages of 8 and 18, or 30% of the total minor population of 2.5 million, were working, and this proportion increased to 38.7% in 1996. More minors (310,000) were working in rural areas than in cities, and under worse conditions. Only 23% of the minors who worked attended school. Ecuador participates in the international effort for flexible employment conditions, which calls for open contract arrangements, a reduction of benefits, the end of collective contract bargaining in the public sector, the rotation of workers, and the option of paying for overtime on an hourly basis. As a result, greater risks to the health of the working population can be foreseen.

Health of the Disabled

In Ecuador, 13.2% of the population suffers from some form of disability. Given the link between disability and poor living conditions, low income, and difficult access to health services, the incidence of disabilities is greater in marginal urban areas and in rural areas. There is no systematized national register of disabilities, but prevalence surveys provide at least a basic understanding of the situation. It is estimated that 48.9% of all Ecuadorians have some form of impairment and 2.4% are handicapped. The proportion of disabilities is slightly higher in men than in women (13.5% versus 12.9%), and it is greater in cities than in rural areas (13.5% versus 12.4%). Handicaps are clearly more prevalent in urban areas (2.8% versus 1.6%), because of the severe injuries caused by accidents and violence.

In children under 5 years old the predominant impairments have to do with psychological development (35.9%), followed by those that are language-related and psychosocial (20.3%) and those that are musculoskeletal (16.2%).

Health of Indigenous People and Other Minorities

Chief among the leading causes of death and disease in the indigenous population are those related to poverty: acute respiratory infections, acute diarrheal diseases, and malnutrition. Hypoxia and complications of delivery and the puerperium are the leading causes of infant and maternal death, respectively. The rate of infant mortality is higher in the indigenous populations than in the rest of the population; whereas the national rate in 1994 was 22 per 1,000 registered live births, in the Colimbuela and Cumbas communities it was 83.3 and 66.7, respectively. Infant mortality is related to malnutrition, diseases caused by lack of food safety, inadequate maternal and child care, unsanitary surroundings, and insufficient coverage by the health services. In 1995, for every 1,000 births there were 70 deaths before the age of 1 year, and for every 100,000 births, 198 mothers died. In the mountain regions where the population is largely indigenous, 85% of all deliveries were not attended medically. Chronic malnutrition in children under 5 years of age reached 69% in some of these areas, compared with the national figure of 49.4%.

Among black children in Esmeraldas, malnutrition is estimated at between 60% and 70%. The health situation of populations living near the borders with Colombia and Peru is critical, especially among those living in the eastern region. Chronic childhood malnutrition is 65%, and infant mortality rates exceed 50 per 1,000 reported live births. The most common diseases are parasitoses, intestinal infections, diarrhea, and anemia.

The predominantly rural location of indigenous groups is directly related to their difficult access to resources and services. The already low health service coverage in rural areas reaches its most critical levels in the Amazon region, where health professionals visit indigenous communities along the river banks once every three months at best. Some indigenous communities, such as the Awa Coiquier, the Chachi, and the Ttsachila, have no access to basic health services. The knowledge and practices of indigenous medical care cover their needs to some extent, and one of the goals of their struggle for self-determination is for their informal health agents (midwives, herbalists, shamans, *yachags,* etc.) and the people themselves to gain recognition as human resources capable of monitoring and caring for their health while integrating aspects of Western medical knowledge that will enable them to improve the health and living conditions of their communities.

Analysis by Type of Disease or Health Impairment

Communicable Diseases

Vector-Borne Diseases. In 1996, 12,011 cases of malaria were reported, or one-fourth as many as in 1993. The highest rate was in Esmeraldas (1,175.0 per 100,000 inhabitants). In the Amazon region, the province of Sucumbíos had a rate of 936.9 per 100,000. Since 1993, when *Plasmodium falciparum* infections were responsible for 46% of the cases in the country, the percentage of infections due to this parasite has been on the decline. In 1996 it represented 16% of the cases in the coastal area. The principal vector is *Anopheles albimanus.* In the Amazon region, *Anopheles triamilatus, Anopheles punctimacula,* and *Anopheles trinkae* may be involved in the transmission of malaria.

The coastal provinces were also the areas most affected by dengue, with 12,796 cases in 1996, a marked increase since 1992. The highest incidence was in Cañar, with 1,078.0 cases per 100,000 inhabitants, followed by Manabí, with 365.0 per 100,000. In the subtropical mountain areas, only two provinces, Cotopaxi and Loja, reported cases between 1995 and 1996, as opposed to eight provinces in 1990. No cases of dengue were reported in the Amazon region in 1995 and 1996.

In the 1992–1996 period, Chagas' disease was diagnosed in 12 provinces located in the mountains, along the coast, and in the Amazon region. The incidence in Pastaza increased from 2 per 100,000 inhabitants to 3.6 between 1992 and 1995, and in Sucumbíos it went from 4.5 in 1994 to 12.7 in 1995. In the blood banks, 95% of the donations are screened. The principal vectors are *Triatoma dimidiata* and *Rhodnius ecuadoriensis.* The reports received—only 13 cases in 1996—do not re-

flect the true situation, because it is estimated that some 500,000 persons are infected, mainly in Guayas, El Oro, and Manabí.

Cutaneous leishmaniasis is the most prevalent form of the disease. Its incidence increased slightly, to 1,655 cases in 1996, with reports received from 18 of the 21 provinces. In the Amazon region, which had the highest incidence, the rate fell from 143.6 per 100,000 inhabitants in 1992 to 62.8 per 100,000 in 1996, whereas in the mountains it increased from 8.72 to 10.35 per 100,000, and along the coast, from 6.9 to 11.43 per 100,000. The provinces most affected in 1996 were Zamora-Chinchipe, Morona-Santiago, and Bolívar, with rates of 211.2, 109.0, and 86.7 per 100,000 inhabitants, respectively.

Of the 12 provinces that reported 27 cases of onchocerciasis in 1992, only 6 filed reports in 1996, for a total of 10 cases. The main foci were located in Esmeraldas; however, no new cases were reported there in 1995 or 1996. The goal of the program, which is based on the mass distribution of ivermectin, is to eliminate onchocerciasis by the year 2000.

Cases of jungle yellow fever have been reported in the Amazon region in the 1990s. In 1994 and 1995 no cases whatsoever were reported in the country, but in 1996 there were eight in Morona-Santiago. In Sucumbíos, where there was transmission of the jungle form of the disease in 1992, a focus of *Aedes aegypti* was detected in 1996. Of 24 cases of the hemorrhagic syndrome investigated in Morona-Santiago, 2 were seropositive for the oropuche virus; none of the patients had had a recent infection or prior exposure to the dengue or yellow fever virus.

Vaccine-Preventable Diseases. No cases of poliomyelitis have been reported since 1990. Between 1992 and 1996 the number of confirmed cases of measles dropped from 4,356 to 40, and cases of neonatal tetanus went from 71 to 37. In 1996, vaccination coverage of infants under 1 year of age was higher than in any of the preceding five years (BCG, 100%; OPV3, 89%; DTP, 88%; and measles, 79%). During the same period, cumulative coverage with two doses of tetanus toxoid was 54% in women of reproductive age in 49 areas at risk for neonatal tetanus, compared with 20% in 1992. In 1995–1996 some cases of neonatal tetanus were detected in marginal urban areas of Guayaquil among mothers originally from indigenous areas of the province of Chimborazo who had migrated to the city only a few days before delivery.

There were epidemic outbreaks of diphtheria in 1994 (565 cases) and 1995 (145 cases) in the adult population in the provinces of El Oro and Pichincha. In 1996, however, only 22 cases were reported, which indicates that the incidence of this disease is on the decline. In 1966 a total of 136 cases of whooping cough were reported, compared with 320 in 1992.

The earliest year for which information has been available on hepatitis B is 1994, when 443 cases were reported. In 1995 a total of 564 cases were reported, and in 1996 the figure was 569.

Reported cases of rubella have increased considerably since 1994, when the national system for the surveillance of rash and fever diseases began to operate. Cases went from 760 in 1992 to 4,797 in 1995. In 1996 the figure was 1,436, but this apparent drop was actually due to the fact that the disease was categorized under "other rash and fever diseases" in the reporting system of the Measles Elimination Plan. Since the end of 1996 the laboratories at the National Institute of Hygiene in Guayaquil and the National Institute of Health in Bogotá have been processing serum samples with suspected measles in the search for cases of rubella.

Cholera and Other Intestinal Diseases. Cholera has declined sharply since 1991, when the first case was detected and the number reached 46,320. In 1994 the disease was detected in 17 of the country's 21 provinces. In 1996 a total of 1,060 cases were reported in 12 provinces, with 59% of the cases occurring in Imbabura. During 1992–1996 the case fatality rate from cholera remained lower than 1%.

The incidence of diarrheal diseases has remained stable. There were 193,352 cases in 1996. These diseases are one of the leading causes of morbidity, especially in children under 5 years of age. In 1995, of the 1,390 deaths from enteritis and other diarrheal diseases, 33.1% occurred in infants under 1 year old.

A total of 14,887 cases of salmonella were reported in 1996, for a rate of 127.3 per 100,000 inhabitants—almost 50% more than in 1992. The disease was reported in all the provinces except the Galápagos Islands. During 1992–1996 the highest incidence in the coastal provinces ranged from 160 to 325 per 100,000 inhabitants; in the mountain provinces the rate for Bolívar was the highest, at 1,025.9 per 10,000 in 1995.

Food poisoning of all types fell from 8,742 cases in 1995 to 6,992 in 1996. In the latter year, intestinal infectious diseases were the leading reason for the hospitalization of men (16,467 cases) and the third most common reason among women (15,076).

Acute Respiratory Infections. There were 598,558 cases of respiratory infections in 1996, capping a trend that has been rising steeply since 1992, when 138,684 cases were reported. The largest increase occurred between 1993 and 1994, when surveillance began to focus on children under 5 years of age. In Quito, in a 1995 sampling of 195 children who consulted health services with a cough or other respiratory difficulties, 15.9% had pneumonia, 2.6% had serious pneumonia, and the rest had acute respiratory infections without pneumonia. In 45% of those cases antibiotics were administered unnecessarily. Pneumonia was diagnosed in 6,373 hospital-

izations of men and 5,194 of women, for rates of 11.1 and 9.1 per 10,000 inhabitants, respectively.

Rabies and Other Zoonoses. Between 1992 and 1996, the human rabies endemic reached epidemic proportions in 1992–1993 and 1995–1996. Of the 65 cases reported in 1996, 20 were in the province of Pichincha and 13 were in Guayas. The remaining 32 cases were scattered among 11 provinces. Dogs are the principal source of human rabies infection.

Human cysticercosis increased from 111 cases in 1992 to 336 in 1996. Brucellosis went from five to nine cases. The incidence of foot-and-mouth disease remained stable, with an annual average of 100 bovine herds affected by vesicular diseases clinically compatible with foot-and-mouth disease. In 1996 the rate of affected bovines was 0.39 per 1,000; morbidity was 2.95 per 10,000; internal morbidity was 21.8%; and case fatality was 5.3%. A control project is being undertaken jointly by the public and private sectors (Ministry of Agriculture and Federation of Livestock Raisers) with a view to eradicating the disease.

AIDS and Other STDs. In 1996 there were 186 new reported cases of AIDS/HIV infection, and the cumulative total since 1984, when the first case was reported, was 1,279 infected persons; 608 were classified as cases of AIDS, of whom 432 had died. Between 1992 and 1996 the annual incidence of AIDS/HIV infection increased from 0.6 to 1.6 per 100,000 inhabitants. Between 1984 and 1996 three provinces reported 92% of the cases in the country: Guayas, with 69%; Pichincha, with 12%; and Manabí, with 11%. Heterosexual transmission accounted for 37.7% of the infections; homosexual transmission for 29.2%; and bisexual transmission for 19.4%. Most of the 1,279 people infected were between 19 and 39 years of age, and more than 80% of them were men. In 1996, 21 persons were accidentally infected by HIV at a dialysis unit in Guayaquil—the one that serves the most people in the country. The provinces of Imbabura, Sucumbíos, Pastaza, and Morona-Santiago are the only ones that have not reported any cases of HIV infection, nor have any cases of AIDS been found in these provinces or in Bolívar, Cotopaxi, Zamora, and the Galápagos Islands.

Gonorrhea has been on the rise in recent years, with 7,703 cases reported in 1996. That year a total of 1,541 cases of syphilis and 87 cases of congenital syphilis were reported.

Chronic Communicable Diseases. Pulmonary tuberculosis showed a generally rising trend, with 7,938 new cases (67.91 per 100,000 inhabitants) in 1996. Cases were reported in all provinces, including the Galápagos Islands. The highest rates during 1992–1996 were in provinces in the Amazon region, such as Pastaza and Napo, with 302.4 and 291.3 per 100,000 inhabitants, respectively, in 1996. In the mountains the highest rates were in the provinces of Bolívar (314.24 in 1995), Cotopaxi (280.49 in 1996), and Cañar (138.89 in 1996); Guayas and Esmeraldas had the highest rates on the coast (101.75 and 119.14, respectively, in 1994).

During 1992–1996 the national incidence of tuberculous meningitis remained steady at less than 1 case per 100,000 inhabitants. Six provinces reported cases every year. The highest rate (3.3) was in 1992 in Azuay, a mountain province that had the highest annual rates in the five-year period except for 1996. In 1996 the Amazon region had the highest rate, with 16.2 per 100,000 inhabitants in Pastaza. Also in that region, the province of Zamora reported cases in 1996 for the first time in the decade, with an incidence of 2.19 per 100,000 inhabitants.

There were 151 cases of leprosy reported in 1996. The average rate for the five-year period was 1.16 per 100,000 inhabitants. The only provinces with cases of leprosy in 1996 were Guayas (with the largest number), El Oro, Los Ríos, and Manabí on the coast, and Pichincha in the mountains. Of the new cases, 71% were multibacillary (46.5% of them clinically lepromatous).

Noncommunicable Diseases and Other Health-Related Problems

Cardiovascular Diseases. An important risk factor for cardiovascular and cerebrovascular diseases, which together accounted for 9,262 deaths in 1995 (80.8 per 100,000 inhabitants), is arterial hypertension, which is also associated with other chronic degenerative problems. In 1966 there were 25,850 cases of hypertension reported in outpatient consultations, which reflects a declining trend since 1992. Surveys conducted in various groups over 15 years of age in the past 20 years (none of them representative of the country as a whole) revealed estimated prevalences ranging from 4% in the rural mountain population to 13% in urban areas. Hypertensive disease was responsible for 2,216 deaths in 1995 (19.3 per 100,000).

In 1996 there were 2,035 reported cases of rheumatic fever—2.4 times as many as in 1992. Surveys of the prevalence of streptococcal throat infections in schoolchildren showed rates ranging from 7% to 19%. In 1995 rheumatic fever caused 66 deaths, 37 of these in females and 29 in males.

Ischemic heart disease, which was responsible for 1,330 deaths in 1995 (11.6 per 100,000 inhabitants) and occurred more frequently in men than in women (1.4:1), together with cerebrovascular disease, with 2,645 deaths in 1995 (23.1 per 100,000), has not received any direct response from the public health institutions beyond the care provided in the clinical and surgical services.

Malignant Tumors. Taken as a group, malignant tumors are an important cause of death. In 1995 the most frequent site was the stomach, which accounted for 804 deaths in men (14.0 per 100,000 inhabitants) and 644 in women (11.2 per 100,000). In males, tumors of the prostate were responsible for 333 deaths and lung cancer was responsible for 250. Prostate hyperplasias (4,436 cases) ranked ninth as a reason for hospitalization of men. In women, tumors of the uterine cervix (plus unspecified tumors of the uterus) caused 676 deaths, and breast cancer was responsible for 243.

Nutritional Diseases and Diseases of Metabolism. The only data available on protein-energy malnutrition in children under 5 years of age come from direct measurements taken through the Ministry of Public Health's Food and Nutrition Surveillance System (SISVAN), and they are representative only of the families that use the Ministry's services. They reveal the following rates: in infants under 1 year of age, 10.7% had low weight-for-age—i.e., between –2 and –3 standard deviations (SD)—and 2.5% were below –3 SD; of the children 1 to 4 years old, 21.1% were between –2 and –3 SD and 4.94% were below –3 SD. The mean incidence of low weight-for-age in infants under 1 year of age was 13.26% for the country as a whole and reached a high of 25.60% in the province of Carchi. Eight of the 18 provinces covered by SISVAN were above the median. In very poor provinces such as Chimborazo, the prevalence of low weight-for-age in children 1 to 4 years of age was 40%, compared with a national average of 26%. Six of the 18 provinces covered were above the national average. The system does not break down the information on children with retarded growth between –1 and –2 SD. ENDEMAIN-94 estimated the national incidence of low birthweight at 13.9% with the rate in rural mountain areas at 23.0%; SISVAN has set the figure at 8.9% among children born in the health units.

A 1988 diagnosis of the nutritional and health status of the Ecuadorian population showed that 69% of the children under 1 year of age, 20% to 46% of those under the age of 3, and 10% to 22% of those aged 3 to 5 had iron-deficiency anemia. In 1996 a study based on a representative sampling of schools in poverty-stricken areas indicated that 37% of the schoolchildren had anemia and the prevalence was higher in first graders (45%) than in sixth graders (22%). Iron deficiency is a serious public health problem in the entire country, and it primarily affects infants and toddlers, schoolchildren, and pregnant women.

In 1993 serum retinol deficiency (lower than 20 µg/dl) was reported in 17.7% of the children between 12 and 59 months of age in populations living in poverty, with prevalences ranging from 9.6% to 25.6%. Several studies have confirmed that vitamin A deficiency is a moderately serious problem and is mainly found in certain extremely poor areas.

The system for the surveillance of iodine deficiency reports that in 1995, 94% of the salt samples collected had iodine levels greater than 20 ppm. In that same year the consumption of iodized salt in the rural population reached a level of 97%, and in 16 of 17 sentinel health posts the median concentration of ioduria was somewhat higher than 10 μg/dl. These figures indicate a mild risk for iodine deficiency disorders in the general population.

According to ENDEMAIN-94, between 1990 and 1994, 95% of all live-born infants were initially breast-fed; 36% of those breast-fed babies began to nurse during the first hour of life and 43.5% began to nurse during the first day. The median duration of exclusive breast-feeding was 2 months in the country as a whole, varying from 3.8 months in the rural mountains to 1 month on the coast.

Obesity (body mass index over 25), dyslipidemia, arterial hypertension, and non-insulin-dependent diabetes mellitus, among other chronic diseases associated with diet and inadequate lifestyle, are on the increase and affect the population at all socioeconomic levels. Coexisting alongside nutritional imbalances and deficiencies, they make for an overlapping epidemiological picture. This situation is also observed in schoolchildren: a 1995 study showed that 19% of the schoolchildren in Quito were obese, and 22% had mixed dyslipidemias. Diabetes began to be reported in outpatient consultations in 1994; 7,044 cases (62.8 per 100,000 inhabitants) were reported that year, and in 1996 there were 7,526 cases (64.3 per 100,000).

Accidents and Violence. Accidents and various forms of violence were responsible for 7,465 deaths in 1995 (65.1 per 100,000 inhabitants), predominating in men at a ratio of 4:1. These deaths represent an estimated 192,148 and 44,805 years of potential life lost (YPLL) in men and women, respectively. Traffic accidents and homicides are mainly responsible for these deaths, especially in the male population. Ground transportation accidents increased from 8,906 in 1994 to 10,743 in 1996. Surveys conducted in various cities in the 1990s, coupled with national police records, show that most victims of transportation accidents are pedestrians and mass transportation riders. These sources also describe the important effects of negligence and alcohol abuse as causes. Accidents in the home, which are also on the rise, totaled 12,239. Outpatient treatments for violence and abuse reported in 1994, 1995, and 1996 were 3,708, 4,025, and 3,265, respectively. Fractures were the second leading reason for hospitalization of males, with 14,136 cases, and the fifth reason for women, with 6,295 cases.

Behavioral Disorders. These disorders are a growing reason for consultations, especially depression, which in 1996 headed the list with 4,521 consultations (38.7 per 100,000 inhabitants), followed by epilepsy and alcoholism. Consulta-

tions for drug dependency are rare. Mental illness was the reason for 5,291 hospitalizations of men in 1995 (9.2 per 10,000 inhabitants). Alcoholism has a prevalence of 7.7% in the population over 15 years of age. Tobacco use is associated with 6.0% of general mortality. At the beginning of the 1990s the estimated prevalence of habitual smokers among adults was 21.6%, with a male/female ratio of 2.4:1; the prevalence among adolescents was 14.9%, without any significant difference between the sexes. It was established in 1995 that in the population aged 12 to 49 the lifetime prevalence of tobacco use was 51.6%, and for the consumption of alcohol in that age group the lifetime prevalence was 76.4%. With respect to the preceding month, however, the prevalence of tobacco use was 28.3% and the consumption of alcohol was 51.2%. In the month preceding the survey, 19.7% of the persons interviewed had consumed alcohol to excess—i.e., they had gotten drunk on more than one occasion. Since 1989 the Interinstitutional Committee Against Tobacco Use has been carrying out coordinated actions, especially educational initiatives, aimed at children and adolescents. Tobacco advertising and the establishment of smoke-free areas are controlled by law, but compliance is undermined by the ineffectiveness of the boards of health.

Prevalence of the use of illegal drugs was 3.2% in youths between the ages of 12 and 19, 6.0% in the population aged 20 to 29, 7.7% among those in the 30-to-39 age group, and 3.3% among persons aged 40 to 49. There is a striking difference between the sexes in the rates of illegal drug use: 10.3% among men versus 0.9% among women, or a ratio of 11.4:1.

Oral Health. According to an epidemiological study conducted in Quito in 1993, the average index of decayed, missing, and filled teeth (DMFT) was highest in the group aged 45 and over (26.5), followed by the groups aged 35 to 44 (20.3), 25 to 34 (14.8), 15 to 24 (8.6), and 6 to 14 (2.1). The presence of missing teeth is highest in the groups over the age of 25. In 1996 an epidemiological study of oral health in public schoolchildren aged 6, 7, 8, 12, and 15 in urban and rural areas showed that at the age of 6 years 87% of the children had caries and at age 12 the rate was 85%. The DMFT index in the group of 6-year-olds was 0.22, and in the 12-year-olds it was 2.95. A reduction observed compared with the indexes for 1988 (DMFT 0.70 and 5.00, respectively).

Natural Disasters. Because of its geographic location on the Pacific ring of fire, Ecuador is exposed to various natural disasters, such as floods, earthquakes, volcanic eruptions, and droughts. The drought that has affected the provinces of Loja and El Oro in the southeast since 1995 has become a national emergency. In this area, otherwise ideal for agriculture, the scarcity of rain and the lowering of the river levels has seriously hurt the local economy and forced many residents to emigrate. At the same time, the agricultural areas on the coast are flooded every year, and the 1997 floods affected all the coastal provinces. High surf caused major damage in the province of Esmeraldas in the north of this region. By the end of March 1997 the heaviest rainfall in 10 years was recorded, which in the province of Guayas flooded 80% of the territory, caused two deaths, was responsible for countless missing persons, and left some 12,000 people affected by the damage.

RESPONSE OF THE HEALTH SYSTEM

National Health Plans and Policies

In 1992 measures were proposed for modernizing community management and financing in order to improve health coverage and the quality of care. The private sector was encouraged to participate in the administration of public health services, and incentives were offered in the form of mechanisms for recovering costs through special endowments in the hospitals and primary health care services, such as selective charges for services with the concurrence of community health committees. These changes have had only limited implementation.

Decentralization of services by means of health areas, which constitute the basic unit of organization, and local management of health services under the Ministry of Public Health, has been encouraged. The 180 areas in the country include health centers and subcenters and district hospitals, which are the first level of referral in the development of local health systems.

In June 1993 the project Strengthening and Extension of Basic Health Services in Ecuador (FASBASE) was launched in 41 priority areas. This project is based on the primary health care policy that has been promoted by the Ministry of Public Health since 1988. Beginning in 1995 it has included a component for improving emergency services in urban areas. As of mid-1997 work began on developing a new project, Modernization and Development of Integrated Health Services Networks (MODERSA).

Health Sector Reform

The social security reform proposed by the National Modernization Council during 1992–1996 included the reform of medical services. By eliminating the compulsory inscription of formal workers in the public insurance system (IESS), it was possible to set up competition between public and private providers. The National Health Council, presided over by the Ministry of Health, introduced an alternative national proposal involving the participation of all institutions in the public and private sectors and of civilian society at the central, provincial, and local levels. Basically, it calls for the organization of a national health system in which the Ministry of Health is both leader and regulator, assumes responsibility for public health actions, and implements a health insurance scheme to expand medical care coverage based on the principles of equity and partnership and on decentralized management.

The ongoing reform debate has given rise to numerous initiatives and proposals—for social security, a Social Front, a physicians' union, organizations of women and indigenous people, nongovernmental organizations, etc. Some basic points of consensus have been found for developing a government policy on the subject and for its progressive implementation.

The health reform process did not progress as had been hoped for during the administration that came into office in 1996, since the work of the National Health Council was suspended. In May 1997 a vote was put to the people, and the results committed the Government to convening a constitutional assembly by the end of that year that would give viability to the reform of the State, including the health sector.

Organization of the Health Sector

Institutional Organization

The health sector is composed of various public and private institutions, both nonprofit and for-profit, which are very loosely coordinated by the National Health Council and operate on the basis of agreements and standards regarding the application of technical mechanisms such as the standardized clinical history form and guidelines for maternal and child care developed by the Ministry of Public Health.

The public subsector consists of the Ministry of Public Health, the IESS, the Public Health Service of the Armed Forces and Police, the National Child and Family Institute, and the Ministry of Social Welfare. Private autonomous institutions with a social mandate may also be included—most notably, the Guayaquil Welfare Board, the Guayaquil Child Protection Society, and the Society to Combat Cancer. Altogether, the public subsector attends to the needs of approximately 59% of the population, especially in terms of hospital care. It is estimated that the Ministry of Public Health covers 31% of the population; social security, 18%; the Guayaquil Welfare Board, the Society to Combat Cancer, and other nonprofit private institutions, 10%; the Armed Forces and Police, 1%; and various private for-profit enterprises, 10%; the remaining 30% do not receive any formal medical care.

The Ministry of Public Health is the official State agency responsible for developing policies and public health standards. It is also the largest provider of comprehensive health benefits and has the broadest network of services. Social security is handled by the IESS, which provides services through individual membership programs for workers in the formal sector, representing 28% of the country's economically active population. Family membership for workers in rural areas comes under Farmers Social Security, which provides social benefits (burial, disability, old age) and primary medical care. The Armed Forces and Police have outpatient services and hospitalization for their members and families and operate as does social security. The Guayaquil Welfare Board and Child Protection Society serve the medium- and low-income population in the coastal region. The Society to Combat Cancer provides specialized diagnostic services and treatment in the country's large cities. The Red Cross responds to emergencies and regulates the blood banks. The Undersecretariat of Environmental Sanitation in the Ministry of Urban Development and Housing and the *municipios* that regulate and carry out sanitation activities are also considered part of the public health sector.

Private for-profit organizations have hospital establishments of varying levels of complexity, physicians' offices, and auxiliary diagnostic and treatment services for the population that is able to pay for them. They include both insurers and private prepaid medical enterprises. A considerable portion of the population—mainly those with limited resources and especially people living in rural areas—use traditional medicine.

Since 1996 the Special Health Committee of the National Congress has been analyzing various health-related bills on issues such as provision of vaccines, and it has been studying proposals on the regulation of private health care and prepaid medical plans, as well as on decentralization and popular participation, which call for participation by the *municipios*, provincial councils, and community health action organizations.

The principal agencies in the sector—namely, the Ministry of Public Health and the IESS—use different decentralization models. The Ministry's model is based on health areas that constitute small service networks with set geographic and population catchments and on a scheme of technical decentralization and deconcentration of certain administrative activities and budgetary planning and execution. The budgetary law in effect since 1994 authorizes the establishment of budgetary entities at the health area level, as long the health area has staff technically competent to do the work required. The health areas carry out their intervention plans to the extent of their decision-making authority based on the concept of primary health care and with a strong component of community participation. Even though the health areas are limited to units under the Ministry of Public Health, the concept is in keeping with the proposal for the organization and development of local health systems. The IESS, for its part, is decentralizing its administrative aspects at the level of large re-

gions. This subsector has a complex structure because its primary objective is to manage various types of insurances and benefits—of which health is only one.

Organization of Health Regulatory Activities

Health Services Delivery. Although the Constitution of the Republic gives the Ministry of Health responsibility for regulation, direction, and control of the entire health sector, in reality each of the institutions in the sector provides its services in accordance with its own policies, objectives, and resources. There are some broad problems that affect all of them, such as insufficient intra- and interinstitutional and intersectoral coordination, inadequate utilization of resources, under-par delivery of services at the different levels of care, and lack of a management information system. The FASBASE project is standardizing the benefits provided at the primary level so that all units can be linked within a comprehensive health services network (MODERSA).

Certification and Practice of the Health Professions. Under the Health Code currently in effect, the Ministry of Public Health's Public Health Control Bureau is the agency responsible for regulating provision of health services in general. It also maintains a registry of occupational titles and controls the practice of university-trained professionals in the health sciences. An amendment to the Health Code currently under study includes a proposal for the codification of all legal aspects related to medical practice.

Control of Medical Technology, Drugs, and Other Supplies. Three somewhat overlapping mechanisms are used to handle the public drug supply: procurement through the National Drug and Medical Supply Center (2% to 6% of the total value); direct imports (10% to 20%), mainly by the IESS, the Society to Combat Cancer, and the Guayaquil Welfare Board; and local purchases (74% to 88%). Lack of definition of the scope and responsibilities of the various entities involved in setting, reviewing, and controlling prices has hampered regulation of the drug market and the health services. No mechanisms are in place to protect the consumer.

The quality control of drugs has improved noticeably in both the private and the public sectors thanks to the application of Good Manufacturing Practices and also to export and production opportunities being offered to third parties under license. Between 1993 and 1997 72% of the plants operating in the country were inspected, and 90% of the staff involved in compliance with this standard have been trained—a prerequisite since 1994 for operation, sanitary registration, and export procedures in keeping with the World Health Organization model.

Ninety-five percent of all health equipment and supplies are imported. There is no system for the registration of these products. In general, the equipment, especially when it involves highly sophisticated technology, is underutilized in both the public and the private sectors.

Environmental Regulation. The Presidential Advisory Commission on the Environment, created in 1993, has promoted the development of basic environmental principles, general environmental policies, and the Ecuadorian Environmental Plan, which identifies the major environmental problems, the most endangered geographic areas, the productive activities that have the greatest impact on the environment, and the factors that restrict environmental management. There are environmental units in several of the Ministries and agencies. In each case their work is geared toward decisions and institutional actions based on a harmonious balance of economic, social, and environmental interests, and they are concerned with standardizing, monitoring, and controlling the use and management of natural resources and the quality of the environment. The National Law on the Environment will constitute the general framework for environmental management.

The Environmental Unit of the National Development Council (CONADE), with support from the Inter-American Development Bank (IDB), executes projects and drafts policies that incorporate environmental strategy in the national development plans. There are two sectoral environmental policies: one on drinking water and basic sanitation, and the other on environmental education for sustainable development. Provisions have been developed that strengthen environmental requirements in connection with the use of hydrocarbons, and these are expressly included in new contracts. The major cities (Quito, Guayaquil, and Cuenca) have introduced vigorous urban environmental policies calling for strengthening their environmental units and laboratories, implementing programs to prevent air pollution (Quito), and issuing and enforcing municipal ordinances to reduce industrial pollution from both fixed and mobile sources. Studies have been carried out on the management of chemical substances, and there is a national plan to promote their rational use. The Consultative Committee on Chemical Substances and the National Toxicology Commission have promoted the development of a draft law on chemicals. The private sector, through the Association of Importers and Formulators of Agricultural Chemicals, participates in the National Program on the Rational Use of Agricultural Chemicals. The Industrial Association, for its part, supports activities that promote the appropriate management of industrial chemicals.

Food Safety. The Ministry of Industry, Commerce, Integration, and Fishing, working through the Ecuadorian Institute of Standards, is the agency responsible for sanitary standardization and quality control of food. The Institute is the focal point for the Codex Alimentarius Commission and carries out its duties in coordination with the Ministries of Health and Agriculture as well as with the other official and private entities involved in the entire food production chain.

Health Services and Resources

Organization of Services for Care of the Population

Of the 205 existing *municipios* in 1997, 7 were taking part in the Healthy *Municipios* Movement: Tena, Riobamba, Portoviejo, Ibarra, Cuenca, Loja, and Quito. The movement's line of action centers around development activities, one of the fundamental axes of which is health. Some of these municipalities, although they are not formally enlisted in the movement, are carrying out activities that deserve special mention. For example, tourism is of interest to the *municipios* of Ibarra and Vilcabamba; the concept of sustainable development guides actions taken by the *municipios* of Tena and Cuenca; and Quito gives consideration to spatial and organizational development in its work in the areas of health and environment, education, communication, transportation, public safety, and social mobilization and participation. Some of the academic centers—such as the Chimborazo Polytechnic School and the University of Loja—have proposed to offer training and workshops that examine health promotion and its relationship to the work of local governments. The Provincial Nucleus for Health Sector Reform in Cuenca is considering a participatory proposal that envisages turning Azuay into a "healthy province."

Disease Prevention and Control Programs. The Ministry of Public Health executes national programs for prevention, control, or eradication of the main public health problems. The initiatives address problems such as tuberculosis, public health dermatology (including leprosy and leishmaniasis), tropical diseases (malaria, Chagas' disease, dengue, and onchocerciasis), rabies, AIDS and other STDs, chronic noncommunicable diseases (especially cancer), and cholera; the National Vaccination Program is also included among the initiatives. The strategy of Comprehensive Care for Diseases Prevalent in Childhood (AIEPI), initiated in 1996, is mainly designed to improve the treatment of children with acute respiratory infections and diarrhea and to reduce mortality in high-risk areas. The control of streptococcal infections and prevention of rheumatic fever, included in the programs on epidemiology and control of respiratory diseases in children, were removed from the list covered by AIEPI because of the low incidence of streptococcal angina in children under 5 years of age.

For the control of diseases not covered by the National Vaccination Program there is a proposal to introduce new vaccines, following a risk assessment and determination of the urgency for intervention in different areas of the country and for different age groups. These are the vaccines against hepatitis B and *Haemophilus influenzae* type B and the trivalent viral vaccine against measles, rubella, and parotitis. The project calls for epidemiological surveillance of the corresponding diseases.

Epidemiological Surveillance and Public Health Laboratory System. Between 1992 and 1995 there was an obvious lack of systematized epidemiological information at the various levels of care under the Ministry of Public Health. Almost all the programs had their own surveillance and information systems, none of which were coordinated with one another. In 1996 the National Epidemiology Bureau, working together with provincial epidemiologists and knowledgeable officials, succeeded in implementing a standard form for compulsory weekly reporting of communicable diseases (EPI-1) as well as a form for the monthly reporting of confirmed cases of those diseases (EPI-2). In 1997 surveillance was standardized, reports were being duly submitted, and other health institutions (IESS, the Police health services) were incorporated in the surveillance system with a view to improving the existing system and promoting epidemiological research.

Hospital reporting is partial and haphazard. The standards for statistics and clinical records are currently being reviewed along with the information system on the resources and services of the Ministry of Health, which, in addition to training health unit staff in these areas and in the management of ICD-10, will increase available knowledge about the general public health situation.

The Surveillance and Epidemiological Control System does not utilize the information from the reference laboratories at the national level. The information stored in the laboratory systems of the National Institute of Hygiene, the Red Cross, and the hospitals is not processed or utilized to its full potential. Analysis of this information at both the national and the provincial level is planned once the National Epidemiological Surveillance System is fully integrated.

Environmental Quality Control. Water resources are increasingly being contaminated by coliforms and sediment produced by the uncontrolled dumping of various effluents into waterways that flow through cities or areas devoted to oil exploration, mining, agroindustry, or agricultural exports. There has been a large increase in air pollution, especially in the major cities such as Quito and Guayaquil; this is due to emissions from automotive vehicles and industries. In Quito,

the level of total suspended particulate matter has exceeded the standard of 60 $\mu g/m^3$ since 1979, and the levels have been rising progressively, up to 300 $\mu g/m^3$ in 1994, or five times the maximum acceptable limit. Dust sediment has exceeded the limit of 1 ($\mu g/cm^2$) per 30 days. Sulfur dioxide has not yet exceeded the accepted limit, but levels are rising. Levels of lead in the air in Guayaquil (in 1990) and Quito (in 1991) were close to the maximum allowable limit of 0.5 $\mu g/m^3$. Blood lead levels in a sampling of pregnant women, newborns, schoolchildren, and street vendors in Quito were above the maximum permissible limit of 10 $\mu g/dl$.

Because of the rapid growth of the urban population, housing and basic services have not been able to keep up with demand, especially in the large cities (Quito and Guayaquil) and the medium-sized ones (Machala, Esmeraldas, Portoviejo, Ambato, and Loja). The housing deficit is estimated at 500,000 dwellings in the urban sector and 700,000 in rural areas.

A 1993 study of drinking water and basic sanitation led to a new policy for modernizing the sector and to the National Rural Basic Sanitation Plan (SANEBAR), which is expected to provide universal coverage in rural areas by the year 2005.

In an effort to reduce air pollution from automobile emissions, the ECUAIRE network has provided monitoring data for Quito, Guayaquil, Cuenca, and Ambato since 1976. In 1996, with support from the U.S. Environmental Protection Agency and the World Health Organization, the network was evaluated and a program was designed for improving it. In Quito an automated monitoring network was put into operation (US$ 2,000,000), and it now controls automobile pollution. The National Program for Eliminating Lead in Gasoline, in effect since 1996, covers various environmental sectors. Between 1993 and 1996 the Environmental Advisory Commission developed strategic projects and basic programs for overcoming environmental problems and combating their causes. Citizen organizations monitor and report activities that are damaging to the environment. In addition, the mass media have stepped up their environmental campaign. With the support of the Environmental Advisory Commission, the Ministry of the Environment is implementing an ongoing environmental management process that will contribute to sustainable development. With resources from the World Bank, the Environmental Management Technical Assistance Project is supporting initiatives by the Government, the municipalities, and nongovernmental organizations through the Environmental Technical Assistance and Rehabilitation in Ecuador project, the Amazon Region Environmental Management Plan, Municipal Environmental Management, and Environmental Management in the Guayaquil Gulf Area.

Drinking Water Supply and Sewerage Services. In 1996 water supply services reached 69.7% of the population, and sewerage services reached only 41.7%. The urban populations had better coverage levels (81.5% and 61.4%, respectively) than people living in rural areas (50.9% and 10.4%). Between 1992 and 1996 programs were implemented to build latrines for 1,841,000 inhabitants, which benefited 9.1% of the urban and 26.3% of the rural population.

Management of Municipal Solid Waste, Including Hospital Waste. In the country as a whole the collection of solid waste corresponds to an average of 51.6% (69.6% in the cities and 7.5% in rural areas) of all the waste actually produced. Much of this waste is deposited in dumps, ravines, and estuaries. In 1995 Guayaquil, the city with the largest population, improved and expanded its waste collection system. The new system for the collection, transport, and final disposal of solid waste in sanitary landfills is supplemented by a different system of management of hospital waste. Quito has implemented a transfer station, improved its dumping sites, and promoted the development of microbusinesses in the community for the collection and transport of waste, thus extending coverage to 85% of the population. Medium-sized cities such as Cuenca, Riobamba, Loja, and Ambato have master plans for solid waste management including hospital waste. Since 1994, when the Interinstitutional Committee on the Management of Hospital Waste was established, at least 2,000 workers responsible for health and cleanup have been briefed and trained. At least 20 public and private hospitals are executing programs for the handling of solid waste, and operating procedures for health establishments throughout the country were issued in January 1997.

Food Safety. The Ministry of Health, through the Bureau of Pharmacy and Sanitation Control, Food Control Division, implements policies on food quality control. At the operational level, the provincial health directorates and the health areas inspect food that has been industrially processed, while the municipalities, through the municipal hygiene directorates, monitor the food sold by street vendors. Microbiological analysis of food is performed in the laboratories of the Ministry of Health's Izquieta Pérez Institute of Hygiene and Tropical Medicine. In 1996 the National Epidemiology Bureau inaugurated the System for the Epidemiological Surveillance of Foodborne Diseases as part of the hemisphere-wide surveillance system for foodborne diseases, carried out and coordinated by PAHO's Pan American Institute for Food Protection and Zoonoses (INPPAZ). The Ecuadorian Consumer's Tribunal (a member of the International Organization of Consumers Unions), plays an important part in the promotion of food quality control and consumer protection; it publishes a bimonthly magazine.

Health Promotion, Food Aid, and Disaster Preparedness. The program under way in Cañar, which promotes dairy farming development as part of the integrated rural development effort that targets small dairy farmers, now covers 4,000 families. Primary health care and improved basic sanitation in the provinces of Esmeraldas, Manabí, Chimborazo, Azuay, and Cotopaxi—designed to aid pregnant women, nursing infants, and children—reach 76,920 persons. Some 500,000 schoolchildren are currently benefiting from the national program to improve instruction in priority areas. Comprehensive support directed toward women in the marginal urban areas of Quito covers 31,800 families.

In the area of disaster preparedness, moderate progress has been made under a program the Ministry of Public Health has been running for several years. Its activities have consisted mainly of regular drills in hospitals to test contingency plans, coordination among health sector agencies, and introduction of disaster mitigation in public health activities. At the end of 1996, the civil defense promoted new initiatives to improve coordination among the various agencies. Several universities have included the subject of disasters in their curricula. The Ecuadorian Red Cross and other nongovernmental relief organizations have programs on disaster preparedness.

A declining trend in international food aid was seen in 1990–1995: the World Food Program reduced its contribution from US$ 1,671,176 in 1992 to $91,596 in 1994, in part because of the country's reduced management capacity. The principal donors have been Canada, the United States of America, and the European Union. In recent years the World Food Program has been the only source of food donated for direct distribution; its cooperation represents 36% of total food aid.

The 1980s saw a mushrooming of nongovernmental health organizations. Their activities focus on community development, women's development, health care, research, and training. In general they perform their work independently and have not yet coordinated it with the Ministry of Health.

The for-profit private sector provides care to the population by charging various fees in different types of establishments, from outpatient services to highly complex, technologically sophisticated hospital and diagnostic and treatment services.

Organization and Operation of Personal Health Care Services

Health Services. In 1995 there were 3,462 health establishments, 2,988 (86.3%) without beds and 474 with beds. Of the former, 51.4% came under the Ministry of Public Health, 32.6% under the IESS and Farmers Social Security; and the remaining 16% under other institutions in the health sector. Of the establishments with beds, 26% belonged to the Ministry of Public Health, 62.7% were in the private sector, and the rest corresponded to other institutions. The total number of health establishments in operation includes general, specialized, and canton hospitals plus private clinics. Those without beds include health centers and subcenters, health posts, and doctors' clinics. Most of the establishments with beds are located in the cities, whereas 57.1% of those without beds are in the cities and 42.9% are in rural areas.

In terms of hospital beds, as of 1995 the normal number was 18,873. There were 17,804 available beds, distributed as follows: Ministry of Public Health, 7,812 (43.9%); Guayaquil Welfare Board and Child Protection Society, 2,580 (14.5%); IESS, 1,839 (10.3%); Ministry of Defense, 916 (5.1%); Society to Combat Cancer, municipalities, and Police health services, 624 (3.5%); and the private sector, 4,033 (22.6%).

In 1995 the output of hospital-based health services, measured as discharges, was 50.8 per 1,000 inhabitants; bed availability was 1.6 per 1,000 inhabitants, as it had been since 1988; the occupancy rate was 53.1%; and the average length of stay was 5.9 days. The rate of hospital deaths per 1,000 discharges was 18.1, compared with 0.9 deaths per 1,000 in the total population. There were 9,719,664 consultations for morbidity and 3,040,414 for preventive health, a 3.2:1 ratio. The number of emergencies attended was 1,205,207.

The National Medical Emergency Network, which aims to reduce morbidity and mortality due to medical emergencies, has been in operation since 1995. Attention has been given to strengthening public health care services, communications, and transport in Quito, Guayaquil, and Cuenca. A plan is being considered to include services for cerebrovascular emergencies, which by default have devolved on private sector facilities that do not have the capacity to meet the needs of most of the population, especially in terms of quality of care.

Specialized Services. A total of 2,319,824 interventions were reported in dental services, of which 1,231,608 were first-time visits and 1,088,216 were follow-up consultations. This represents 10.7% coverage of the total population and 1.9 consultations per patient. No information is available on the number of patients requiring rehabilitation care. Some efforts have been made at the national level to address the problems of the disabled; however, this segment of the population has limited access to the services and facilities.

Inputs for Health

Drugs. Of 32 drug-producing factories in Quito and Guayaquil, 28% belong to transnational enterprises that manufacture 60% of the products consumed locally and the rest make adaptations of products for local consumption (65%) and for third parties (35%). Between 25% and 30% of Ecuador's drug production is exported to Latin American countries. In the 1990s the drug market saw an average annual growth of 4.5% in terms of quantity and 22% in terms of value. Imports, which are favored by the pricing policy, take care of 30% to 40% of the market's needs and increase each year at a rate of 10%. The value of the drug market averages US$ 220 million a year, or some 70 million units sold, of which 61% are brand-name products and 36% are new items. Almost all the products are imported. Generic drugs are used only 3% of the time, despite the fact that there are facilities for registering them. Procurement by the subsector consisting of the IESS, the Armed Forces Public Health Service, the Police health services, and the Ministry of Public Health accounts for 10% to 15% of the market; private institutions (Society to Combat Cancer, Guayaquil Welfare Board, clinics, and hospitals) represent 35% to 40%; and some 3,900 private pharmacies, most of which have no professional direction, make up the rest of the market.

The market for medical supplies is valued at US$ 30 million, and encompasses an indeterminate number of providers. For many this is a part-time activity, concentrating on sales of reagents for clinical analysis, radiodiagnostic elements, and biomedical materials. Registration procedures for these supplies are not sufficiently stringent and often they are marketed informally. Specialized hospitals purchase them directly, and frequently patients have to bear the resulting costs.

The Government reduced its investment in drugs between 1985 and 1993 from 3.5% to 3.1% of total expenditure by the Ministry of Public Health. Only 21.5% of the population has access to drugs. In urban areas, monthly household expenditures on health increased from 42% of household income in 1991 to 54% in 1995, and half of this amount is for drugs.

A process of quality assurance in regard to infrastructure and methodology has helped to offset a notable reduction in trained staff due to government downsizing. The cutbacks brought on the introduction of prior evaluation and postregistration control, and these standards, on which consensus was reached, have played a decisive role in improving quality assurance in the area of drugs.

Immunobiological Products. Local production of BCG, DTP (diphtheria, tetanus, whooping cough), DT, and tetanus toxoid vaccines by the National Institute of Hygiene and Tropical Medicine takes care of 30% to 40% of the annual demand, and the rest of the biologicals have to be imported to meet the needs of the Immunization Program. The measles and poliomyelitis vaccines, which are not produced in the country, are imported through the PAHO/WHO Revolving Fund, as are diphtheria and tetanus antitoxins. Ecuador has suffered from periodic vaccine shortages due to delays in payment to the Fund; these shortages affected the normal development of vaccination activities in the operating units and ended up alienating users. In 1997 a law was passed that will solve this problem.

In 1995 the National Institute of Hygiene took over the Regional Program on Good Manufacturing Practices and the

Vaccine Quality Control Program. However, the infrastructure needs substantial improvement in areas of production and quality control. This situation is expected to improve with financial support from the Government of Japan.

Reagents. Given the level of technological development, it is not possible to produce laboratory supplies to meet the national demand. Marketing is based on the specific needs of the laboratories, which means that the supply is necessarily limited. At the same time, the few companies that market these supplies do not offer the needed technical advisory services, which means that they are simply vendors of products.

Human Resources

Availability by Type of Resource. In 1995 the number of employees in health institutions by occupational category per 10,000 inhabitants was as follows: physicians, 13.3; nurses, 4.6; dentists, 1.6; midwives, 0.7; nursing aides, 11.8. In considering these rates, the unequal distribution of human resources should be kept in mind—larger concentrations are found in the mountain region. The 15,212 physicians working in health establishments were distributed as follows: 16 per 1,000 inhabitants in the mountains, 11.5 on the coast, and 8.1 in the Amazon region. This pattern is similar in the various specialties. This phenomenon is related to the distribution and location of the universities that provide human resources for the health sector. Also, the concentration of resources is related to the economic development of the provinces: 63.2 % of all health personnel are found in the country's most developed provinces—namely, Guayas, Pichincha, and Azuay, with 28.6%, 27.7%, and 6.9%, respectively—65.8% of the physicians, 50.4% of the dentists, 68.5% of the nurses, and 54.9% of the midwives are in these provinces. It also is true that there is a high concentration of human resources (90% of all health personnel) in urban areas. In 1995 there were 1,788 dentists, 5,212 nurses, and 13,511 nursing aides.

Health Personnel Training. Recently the development of health professionals has focused on primary care and family medicine. Between 1994 and 1996 two new private universities joined the educational process by offering curricula leading to a degree in medicine. Emphasis has been placed on graduate-level professional education in the areas of public health, epidemiology, and health management. Most experience in the training of researchers has been in graduate-level university programs, especially in the health sciences, where health administrators have also been trained. The clinical specialties have a research component in their curricula; 50% of the graduate-level programs in the universities have well-structured scientific activities.

Continuing Education for Health Workers. Most of the in-service educational programs are sponsored by the professional unions, which plan various events in the different specialties. Most of them have the support of private companies and the endorsement of the universities. However, there are no records of the number or type of events offered or the number of persons trained. In the official sector, programs are carried out by the institutions based on the development interests of the services. The Ministry of Public Health trains personnel only in the application of technical standards and as part of the regular activities of the FASBASE project. Since 1997, personnel from other areas have been included in the programmed events. An unfavorable factor in the Ministry of Public Health has been the limited support that training has received in general, to the point that the National Training Institute (INAC) disappeared from the organizational structure in 1994. However, an effort has been made in the Ministry—with support from cooperating agencies (PAHO, United Nations Population Fund, U.S. Agency for International Development, CARE, the Embassy of the Kingdom of the Netherlands, nongovernmental organizations, and universities)—to develop a program to improve the quality of health care services that involves formulation and development of teaching materials and tools for management training based on adult education methods. The National University of Loja is working on an innovative continuing education plan that will integrate mainly the educational and health care sectors under the Ministry of Health.

Labor Market for Health Professionals. There is a gap between the supply and the demand for human resources. In the 1980s, of 1,000 aspiring physicians, only 245 graduated, of which 122 were able to secure a residency in a health institution and only 75 finally obtained a position in the sector's labor market. Of 1,000 aspiring dentists enrolled in the first year of dental school, 326 graduated and only 50 were able to find a job. In nursing, of 1,000 students enrolled in the first year, 150 graduated and 141 found jobs. Salaries do not keep up with inflation, which leads to a rapid decline in purchasing power and ultimately to labor disputes based on demands by the various professional groups and other workers in the public health institutions. The dispute beginning in mid-April 1997 lasted for more than 11 weeks.

Research and Technology

The development of science and technology has been weak, as evidenced by the limited number of publications and the few patents granted. The government budget for research is scarcely 0.1% of the gross national product (GNP) and there is no structured national science and technology system. Many of the research projects are based on the investigators' personal interests, and most of the studies are carried out in the public sector, mainly in the universities. Activities tend to involve technological adaptation more than the generation of new knowledge. Projects in the areas of biotechnology, health, and nutrition are the most common.

With IDB support, a mixed organization has been established for the development of policies on science and technology. This foundation has a board of directors that consists of representatives of the vice-presidency of the Republic, universities, the Ministry of Education and Culture and the Ministry of Industry, the chambers of commerce, and the scientific community. One of the problems that has been identified in this area is the shortage of human resources committed to research.

Scientific Documentation. Access to scientific documentation has been facilitated by the creation of computer information networks. However, as a result of the economic crisis, the publication of scientific or any other type of literature has declined considerably. The few scientific journals that continue to be published, such as those of the universities, are issued late.

Expenditures and Sectoral Financing

Each of the sector's institutions has its own source of funding, depending on the population it serves. The Ministry of Public Health is financed with government funds derived from general taxes, income from oil exports, special taxes and contributions, and international cooperation. Medical care under the IESS is financed mainly by contributions from employees and employers totaling 3.4% of the payroll. In recent years, given the low funding levels of health benefits, internal transfers have been made from the pension fund. In 1994 the estimated deficit due to sickness and maternity came to US$ 100 million, which was offset with pension funds. Farmers Social Security is financed with a three-way contribution representing 1% of the payroll, as follows: 0.35% of the value of the payroll of insured urban workers, 0.35% contributed by the employers, and a 0.30% contribution by the government, to which is added a symbolic monthly contribution by heads of households representing 1% of the minimum living wage. In other words, this system is subsidized by the IESS General Program and the State. The Guayaquil Welfare Board receives a contribution from the Government's general fund, which may not exceed 5% of its budget; basically, it is financed by proceeds from the National Lottery, income from investments, and partial recovery of the cost of health and other services. The Society to Combat Cancer has fiscal allotments and receives income from direct

taxes on transactions in the financial system. Private services are financed by direct payments from families, which constitute the major source of health care financing in the country, given the difficulties involved in the funding of public services.

Information on health care spending is not very recent, reliable, or complete, especially as far as the private sector is concerned. The data available indicate that public spending on health as a percentage of total government expenditure fell from 5.5% in 1992 to 4.6% in 1996. In addition to the meager amount, the distribution of these moneys is clearly inequitable and their utilization is inefficient and centralized.

Private spending increased, on the other hand, while government spending was declining, thanks to the fiscal crisis and adjustment programs that greatly reduced allocations to the social sector (from 7.8 % of GDP in 1992 to 5.2% in 1996). In the Ministry of Public Health, spending as a percentage of GDP fell from 1.0% in 1985 to 0.75% in 1995. Within the public sector, there is an immense difference between the per capita expenditure for each general IESS beneficiary (US$ 117 in 1994) and that of the Ministry of Public Health ($15), as well as that of a beneficiary under the Farmers Social Security ($17). In general, the IESS expenditures on medical benefits have remained steady, with a slightly rising trend, despite the serious financial crisis it has been going through for the past several years and the increase in demand, especially from its beneficiaries in the rural farming sector. Pursuant to legislation that has been in effect since 1981, steps have begun to be taken to implement a plan for the partial recovery of costs in public hospitals by charging a fee for office visits, diagnostic examinations, and other benefits that previously were offered free.

According to recent household surveys conducted by the National Institute of Statistics and Census (INEC), as of 1995, 54% of private or direct spending went for drugs, compared with 42% in 1991. The next highest category was spending on office visits—22% in 1995 compared with 26% in 1991. Spending on hospitalization in 1995 represented 9%, much lower than it was in 1991 (25%), which may reflect a drop in demand because of the rising costs (both direct and indirect) and the growing trend in self-medication. In addition, 9% went for equipment, including prostheses and other related items, compared with 5% in 1991; the purchase of private insurance represented 6% in 1995 versus 2% in 1991.

According to a survey of living conditions conducted by the Ecuadorian Professional Training Service (SECAP), in the poorest households the average expenditure on health in 1994 represented 17% of total family consumption, whereas in the urban sector it was 12%, and for middle- and upper-income groups the proportion was no higher than 5%. The survey also showed that 3.8% of the families spent more than 30% of their total monetary income on direct payments for health services. These figures reveal a profoundly inequitable distribution of spending and financing in the health sector.

External Technical and Financial Cooperation

During 1992–1997 several technical and financial cooperation agencies provided key support for the health sector in Ecuador, including the following: PAHO/WHO, the International Bank for Reconstruction and Development (IBRD), the IDB, USAID, Belgian Cooperation, the Netherlands Cooperation Agency, and similar institutions in other European countries.

The World Bank granted loans for development and implementation of the FASBASE project to extend coverage and improve basic services for the most vulnerable urban and rural groups. Of the total amount of US$ 102 million (including 30% in funds from the national Government), the sum of $25 million had been executed as of July 1997. The MODERSA project, for the organization of service networks including hospitals, received $30 million from the World Bank. The Environmental Management Technical Assistance project, in turn, has $15 million from the World Bank ($5 million from the national Government).

IDB has contributed nearly US$ 2 million toward a proposal to restructure the IESS medical care system and modernize the management of its hospital system. The Bank also contributed $1 million to the National Modernization Council for a project to update the drinking water and sanitation sector. The formulation of policies for science and technology

has been funded in the amount of $30 million, of which $23 million comes from an IDB loan and $7 million from the national Government.

The National Rural Basic Sanitation Plan (SANEBAR) has received support from the Government of Spain in the amount of US$ 30,000, and the program for cholera prevention, public health education, and latrine-building received $400,000 from the Government of Sweden. The program for the control of cholera and diarrheal diseases, in turn, benefited by a contribution from the European Union to strengthen laboratories that do clinical analysis and epidemiological surveillance.

USAID has provided approximately US$ 2 million for projects to improve management capacity in the Ministry of Public Health, information systems, the cost and quality of services, and maternal and child care programs.

Belgian Cooperation contributed US$ 1 million to support consolidation of the endemic goiter control program with the design and implementation of alternative primary health care models.

The second phase (1997–2000) of the project to assist in formulation of the national drug policy (Ecuador/PAHO/WHO/Netherlands) has benefited from a donation of US$ 900,000 for the development of drug treatment programs in the southern part of the country. The Netherlands provided $1.6 million toward the subregional project for the control of violence against women, which was in its second year in 1997.

The "Healthy Spaces" project, initiated in 1997 in four depressed cantons in the province of Loja, has received nearly US$ 4 million from the Netherlands Cooperation Agency.

EL SALVADOR

GENERAL SITUATION AND TRENDS

Socioeconomic, Political, and Demographic Overview

In mid-1995 the Salvadorian economy began to decelerate. In 1992 and 1993 the gross domestic product (GDP) had attained a real growth (adjusted for inflation) of more than 7%, but in 1994–1995 it grew only 6%, and by 1996 the rate had fallen to 3%. This reduction in the growth rate was associated with a reduction in internal demand and a slow-down in exports of goods and services as well as a major shift in the business outlook. The result was a sizable cutback in gross domestic investments by the private sector, which went from 16.6% of GDP in 1995 to 11.9% in 1996.

During 1990–1995 the driving force behind economic growth was the internal demand generated by the steady increase in consumption. This was financed with the influx of foreign currency following the Peace Accords, the growing stream of money sent home by Salvadorians residing in the United States and Canada—about US$ 1 billion a year—and the expansion of credit in the private sector.

As a result of the stabilization policy, inflation dropped to 7.4%, the lowest it had been since 1975. The policy of free convertible currency remained in place in 1996, and the nominal exchange rate was 8.75 Salvadorian colones per US$ 1.00. Net international monetary reserves increased to US$ 1,100 million, the equivalent of 81% of the monetary base or five months' worth of imports. This was possible because of a reduced deficit in the balance of trade and in the current account of the balance of payments. Domestic savings and investments have returned to levels of 16% and 18% of GDP, respectively, similar to the levels of the 1970s.

The deceleration clearly affected the economy of the working population. According to a report of the Central American Monetary Council, the rate of open unemployment in 1996 was 10%, whereas two years earlier it had been as low as 7.7%. Nominal minimum wages did not change in 1996, but when the figures are adjusted for inflation, they declined by 6.7%.

In the political arena, the most noteworthy developments in recent years have been the advances toward reforming and modernizing the State, the progress in political and electoral participation, and the end of the period for compliance with the Peace Accords.

Currently, the national debate between the Government and the sociopolitical sectors centers around the second phase of the structural reform, or modernization of the State. This has required changes that have entailed greater participation on the part of private enterprise, without which it would have been difficult to implement this reform consistently and continuously. Strategies have been discussed for improving social conditions and the national competitive position; maintaining macroeconomic stability; developing modern institutions; increasing the competitive position of the private sector; reforming health, education, and other public services; and finding new ways to participate in the international economy. One of the principles that guides the modernization process is the idea that the government should not be a producer of goods and services. In this vein, the Government has pressed for privatization of many agencies.

At the same time, the period for implementation of the Peace Accords has come to an end, and most of the commitments—the programs for transfer of land, the incorporation of former combatants into productive life, political reform and reform of the judicial sector, changes in the police and armed forces, and political and electoral reforms—have been fulfilled.

If the indicators from the Multipurpose Household Survey conducted in 1991–1992 are compared with those from 1995, it can be seen that the percent of the population who had not finished a single year of schooling went from 26% in 1991 to 21.5% in 1995, and those with more than six years increased from 23% to 28.5%. Net primary school enrollment increased from 79% in 1989 to 94% in 1996, while the primary school dropout rate fell from 15% to 6% in the same period, the rate of grade repetition went from 8% in 1990 to 6% in 1996, and illiteracy declined from 42% in 1989 to 23% in 1996.

There is a serious problem of overcrowding in makeshift shacks and rural shanties. The most common types of housing are the single-family dwelling (while communal living arrangements decrease), rural shanties, and makeshift urban shacks.

There are major gaps and marked inequalities in basic sanitation between urban and rural areas. Coverage is very low, and the services provided are usually deficient. The data available (1995) indicate that 53% of the population has access to the public water supply. Coverage of the urban population is 86% (80% with household connections and 6% through access to a public tanks) and of the rural population, 17% (16% with household connections and 1% through access to a public tank). Excreta disposal is available to 69% of the population: 57% of the urban population is connected to a sewerage system and 25% has access to latrines, while in rural areas 56% of the population depends on latrines.

In 1994, expenditures on education represented one-tenth of total public spending, and the trend has been rising since 1990. On the other hand, expenditures on housing were only 0.5% in 1995, whereas in 1985 the figure was almost 6%.

Real social expenditure, at constant prices, was 17% less in 1994 (₡1.2 billion) than it was in 1985 (₡ 1 billion). The same was true of real spending on education. Only in the area of health did real spending grow—from about ₡ 280 million in 1985 to almost ₡ 400 million.

Poverty indicators have significantly improved, from levels of about 60% in 1990 to 47.5% in 1995.

As part of its strategy to combat poverty, the Government has promoted a policy of local development aimed at stimulating the economy for small producers by encouraging them to work together in alliances at the local level so that they can compete with local businesses.

The war, which lasted from the 1970s until 1992, when the Peace Accords were signed, caused an abrupt change in Salvadorian population dynamics. During those years, higher mortality in men, combined with migration to other countries and the separation of couples, all contributed to lower fertility.

In 1997 the population was estimated at 5.91 million inhabitants, of whom 49.0% were males and 51.0% were females. The annual population growth rate was 2.1%.

Of the country's 14 departments, the most heavily populated is San Salvador, where 30.7% of the population resides. The concentration of urban population is steadily increasing. In 1996, 56.7% of the population was living in urban areas and 43.3% in rural areas. In 1995 the urban population growth rate (2.6%) was double the rate in rural areas (1.3%). The Salvadorian population is predominantly young, and for every 100 persons of working age there are 72 who depend on them. In 1996 children under 5 years of age represented 13%

of the population; those aged 5 to 14 years, 24%; those aged 15 to 19, 12%; those 20 to 24, 11%; those 25 to 59, 34%; and seniors aged 60 and over, only 6%.

Emigration began to accelerate in the 1970s and continued to increase until it peaked at around 69,000 a year between 1980 and 1985, after which it tapered off and settled down to some 11,000 emigrants a year between 1990 and 1995. It is estimated that during that period the rural population experienced a net annual rate of emigration—either to other countries or to urban areas in El Salvador—of 13 per 1,000 population.

Total fertility in 1990–1995 was 3.1 children per woman in the urban population, and in rural areas, 4.2. For 1995–2000 an average total fertility of 3.2 children per woman is projected.

The crude birth rate in 1990 was 30.1 per 1,000 population, and in 1996 it was 28.3 per 1,000.

Mortality

During 1990–1995 it is estimated that there were approximately 36,000 deaths per year, for a crude annual mortality rate of 7.0 per 1,000 population.

In 1994 a total of 30,541 deaths were registered, with underregistration estimated at around 21%. Diseases of the circulatory system were the leading cause of death, representing 33% of the total. These were followed by external causes, 19% (83% of them in males, with accidents and homicides heading the list); neoplasms, 14.2%; communicable diseases, 10% (with intestinal infectious diseases predominating); and conditions originating in the perinatal period, 4.3%. Except for neoplasms, mortality from all these causes was higher among males.

Of all the deaths occurring in 1994, those in infants under 1 year of age represented 9%; in children aged 1 to 4 years, 2%; 5 to 9 years, 1%; 10 to 19 years, 4.6%; adults 20 to 59 years, 36.2%; and those 60 and over, 47.2%.

Estimated life expectancy during the period 1985–1990 was 63.4 years for both sexes, 59 years for men and 68 years for women; in 1990–1995 it increased to 67.1 years, or 63 years for men and 71 for women.

SPECIFIC HEALTH PROBLEMS

Analysis by Population Group

Health of Children

Infant mortality ranges from 32 to 55 per 1,000 live births. In a study of hospitals managed by the Ministry of Public Health and Social Welfare, the mortality rate in 1994 was 22.8 per 1,000 live births. It is generally accepted that the most realistic estimates are those based on the National Family Health Survey (FESAL-93), which set infant mortality at 41 per 1,000.

In 1994 there were 2,653 deaths in children under 1 year of age, approximately 12% fewer than in 1992.

FESAL-93 found higher infant mortality in rural areas, attributable to the high rates of postneonatal mortality (22 per 1,000 versus 13 per 1,000 in urban areas).

In 1994 the cause of 49% of deaths in children under 1 year of age was conditions originating in the perinatal period—29% of them due to retarded fetal growth, malnutrition, and immaturity; 19% to hypoxia, asphyxia, and other respiratory conditions; and 1% to diseases of the mother that affect the fetus and the newborn. In 29% of the deaths in children under 1 year old the cause was communicable diseases; intestinal infectious diseases predominated (57%), followed by pneumonias (29%).

In the group aged 1 to 4 years there were 600 deaths in 1994, and the leading cause was communicable diseases, representing 47% of the total. Of these cases, 60% had intestinal infections. External causes were responsible for 16.3% of the mortality in this group.

With regard to outpatient office visits in 1996, according to morbidity reported by the Ministry of Public Health, acute respiratory infections were the leading cause in infants under 1 year of age, representing 22% of all visits. Second came intestinal parasitic diseases, at 6% of the visits; third were ill-defined intestinal infections, at 4.0%.

In the group aged 1 to 4 years the leading cause of morbidity in office visits during 1996 was acute respiratory infections, representing 41% of all first consultations. Intestinal parasitic diseases accounted for 10%, and ill-defined intestinal infections, 7%.

In this same 1-to-4 age group, the leading reasons for hospitalization in the units under the Ministry during 1996 were pneumonia and bronchopneumonia, which were cited in 19% of all discharges; ill-defined intestinal infections, 13%; asthma and unspecified bronchospasm, 10%; and acute respiratory infections, 4%.

In 1994 there were 302 deaths in children aged 5 to 9 years, 41% of them due to external causes and 20% due to communicable diseases. Among external causes, accidents stood in first place and accounted for 49%, with a much higher frequency among males. Homicides, also mostly in males, represented 7% of deaths from external causes. Among the diseases responsible for most mortality in this age group were intestinal infections, pneumonias, nutritional disorders, and anemia. This distribution pattern of mortality has not changed in recent years.

In the population aged 5 to 14 years, acute respiratory infections were the reason for 30% of all first consultations, followed by intestinal parasitic diseases at 15% and urinary infections at 3%.

Health of Adolescents

In 1994 approximately half of all mortality (46%) in adolescents 10 to 14 years of age was due to external causes. Accidental injuries, homicides, and suicides have been the leading causes of death, with proportions of 55%, 22%, and 20%, respectively, and, except for suicide, occurring predominantly among males.

Diseases of the circulatory system were responsible for 18% of the deaths in the 10-to-14 age group.

In the group aged 15 to 19, external causes ranked first, at 67% of the total; within this category, homicides and unintentional injuries headed the list. In terms of distribution according to sex, there was a marked predominance of homicides in males, whereas suicide predominated in females.

The second-leading cause of mortality in adolescents aged 15 to 19 was cardiovascular diseases; in third place was "all other diseases," among which complications of pregnancy and delivery was the main cause of death.

Of all sexually active women aged 15 to 24, only 4.4% had used contraceptives in their first encounter. Adolescent pregnancy poses problems not only because of the resulting illegitimate births, but also because of the age of the couple; about 30% of these adolescent women are involved with men at least 6 years their senior.

Of the almost 1,300 crimes that take place every month, 69% are committed by adolescents and young people under 25 years old, and many of them are repeat offenders.

According to the 1992 census, 52% of the adolescent population is enrolled in primary school, 7% in high school, and fewer than 1% in institutions of higher learning; 41% either have no schooling or started their schooling late.

The 1988 Assessment of the Food and Nutrition Situation revealed that only 8.5% of families had an adequate intake of iron, and adolescents were among those most affected by iron deficiency. The 1990 National Survey of Endemic Goiter in Schoolchildren revealed iodine-deficiency goiter in 25% of the schoolchildren between 7 and 14 years of age. The prevalence was considerably higher in rural areas (31%) and among girls (28%) as opposed to boys (21%).

Drug use among adolescent students is on the increase. In a study conducted by a national foundation in 1992, alcohol and tobacco were the principal drugs consumed by this age group in the capital, followed at some distance by stimulants and tranquilizers, marijuana, and cocaine. The latter were much more common in upper-class adolescents, whereas in the more disadvantaged groups inhalants are more common.

Health of Adults

In the population aged 20 to 59, a total of 11,056 deaths were registered in 1994. External causes were responsible for

35% of the deaths, and within this category homicides accounted for 50% of the deaths, suicides for 27%, and unintentional injuries for 21%. Whereas suicides predominated in women, homicides and unintentional injuries were more frequent in men.

Diseases of the circulatory system and the category "all other diseases" tied for second place, each with 22%. Under "all other diseases," the leading cause was mental disorders, with alcoholism heading the list.

Malignant neoplasms were responsible for 14.7% of all deaths. The most frequent sites are the digestive organs and peritoneum at 24% of the total, and genitourinary organs at 19%, with a higher rate among females.

In the population 15 to 44 years of age, acute respiratory infections took first place in 1996 as a reason for office visits, representing 11% of all first consultations. Urinary tract infection came second, at 6%.

The leading reasons for hospitalization in 1996 among the population aged 15 to 44 who received care in units run by the Ministry of Public Health were complications of delivery and the puerperium, which were cited in 18.3% of all hospital discharges.

El Salvador's estimated maternal mortality rate in 1993 was 119 per 100,000 live births.

In establishments run by the Ministry of Public Health and Social Welfare, prenatal monitoring of pregnant women increased from 44.6% in 1992 to 55.5% in 1996. In the Salvadorian Social Security Institute (ISSS) coverage of the eligible population (14% of the total population) increased to 98% in 1995, and the average number of office visits per pregnant woman was 5.1.

The percentage of pregnant women enrolled in the Ministry's prenatal monitoring program before the 12th week of pregnancy was 37.3% in 1995 and 38.3% in 1996.

It is estimated that in the private-care population (10% of the total population) prenatal care coverage is over 95%.

In the population covered by the Ministry, the proportion of hospital deliveries increased from 37.1% in 1992 to 42.1% in 1996, and with the ISSS it rose from 10.9% in 1992 to 14.0% in 1996. In that same year it is estimated that the private sector attended 10.0% of all deliveries. If these three sectors are added together, hospital deliveries that year were on the order of 66.3% of the total.

The incidence of cesarean section deliveries under the Ministry increased from 20.0% of all deliveries in 1992 to 22.9% in 1996.

Deliveries at home attended by trained traditional midwives increased from 20% in 1992 to 23% in 1996.

In 1992, in the services under the Ministry, 69% of deliveries were attended by medical personnel, 16% by nurses, and 16% by nursing auxiliaries; in 1995 the proportions were 93%, 3%, and 4%, respectively. In the ISSS and the private sec-

tor, 100% of the deliveries were attended by medical personnel that year. Deliveries attended by trained personnel increased from 68% in 1992 to 79% in 1996.

Health of the Elderly

In 1992 El Salvador had some 379,000 people aged 60 and over, 53.7% of them women and 46.3% men. Of this population, 55% lived in urban areas and 45% in rural areas; 53.4% were illiterate, 23.5% were in the economically active population, 20.8% were retired, 29.9% had no income, and 25.8% did not receive money from family members who were living abroad.

In 1994 there were 14,443 deaths in this age group, and nearly half of them were due to cardiovascular diseases. The second leading cause of mortality was neoplasms, at 20%. In third place, the category "all other diseases" accounted for 18% of the deaths; of these, 10% were due to diabetes, and 69% of the deaths from this disease were in women.

The six reasons most frequently cited in 1996 for the hospitalization of patients in this age group in units under the Ministry were, in descending order, chronic obstructive pulmonary disease, chronic renal insufficiency, pneumonia and bronchopneumonia, diabetes mellitus, abdominal hernias, cerebrovascular diseases, and cataracts.

Analysis by Type of Disease or Health Impairment

Communicable Diseases

Vector-Borne Diseases. In 1995 there were 9,529 cases of dengue fever and 129 cases of dengue hemorrhagic fever—it was considered an epidemic year. Serotypes 3 and 4 were isolated, and July and August were the months when the incidence was highest. In 1996 a total of 795 cases of dengue fever and 1 case of dengue hemorrhagic fever were reported. Incidence was highest in the eastern area of the country. During 1991–1995 all four dengue serotypes were in circulation, and in 1995 serotypes 3 and 4 were in circulation simultaneously.

The Salvadorian population living in malarious areas was nearly 5.5 million in 1996. A total of 2,798 cases were registered in 1994, 3,358 in 1995, and 5,884 in 1996, and the annual parasite index increased from 0.52 in 1994 to 1.0 in 1996. All cases were due to *Plasmodium vivax*.

Of 55,069 blood samples submitted for quality control during 1996, 2.2% were seropositive for Chagas' disease. The most recent entomological survey, conducted in 1997, showed only the presence of *Triatoma dimidiata*, with a household infestation rate ranging from 2% to 47%. In 1995 a study carried out in the departments of Santa Ana, Ahuachapán, and

Sonsonate indicated the presence of *T. dimidiata* in 86% of the dwellings examined, and 63% of the vectors were infested with *Trypanosoma cruzi*. In 1996 a study of 200 pregnant women in the department of Chalatenango showed a seroprevalence of 5%.

Leishmaniasis due to *Leishmania chagasi* is a major public health problem in the department of San Vicente. In 1996 a total of 129 cases were detected—94% in rural areas, 65% in females, and 47% in the group aged 5 to 14 years.

Vaccine-Preventable Diseases. Vaccination coverage with both BCG and three doses of DTP in infants under 1 year old was 100% in 1995 and again in 1996. In 1995, coverage with three doses of oral polio vaccine was 94%, and in 1996 it was 100%. In September 1994 El Salvador was declared free of wild poliovirus. Measles vaccination coverage was 93% in 1995 and 97% in 1996. Two doses of tetanus toxoid were given to 82% of women of reproductive age.

There were 12 cases of whooping cough in 1994, 4 in 1995, and 3 in 1996. No deaths from this disease were registered during the three-year period, nor were there any cases of diphtheria, and there was only one case of measles, which was reported in 1996. The incidence of neonatal tetanus has decreased considerably: in 1994 there were nine cases and four deaths; in 1995, three cases and no deaths; and in 1996, five cases and one death.

As of 1997, national vaccination campaigns were being carried out at a rate of three per year.

Cholera and Other Intestinal Infectious Diseases. In 1991, the year when cholera was first introduced in the country, a total of 945 cases were reported and the case-fatality rate was 3.5%. During the next four years the number of reported cases was 8,106, 5,525, 15,280, and 6,447, respectively, with case fatality rates of 0.6%, 0.2%, 0.3%, and 0.1%. In 1996 only 182 cases were registered, and the case fatality rate was 1.1%.

In 1996 parasitic intestinal diseases were the second leading cause of morbidity, with 233,406 registered cases and an incidence rate of 4,745 per 100,000 population.

Reported cases of diarrheal disease in 1996 came to 146,188, with an incidence of 2,972 per 100,000. That year diarrheal diseases were the third leading cause of morbidity.

Acute Respiratory Infections. In 1994, pneumonia was the cause of 31% of all deaths from communicable diseases, and the populations most affected were infants under 1 year of age and the elderly. In 1995 pneumonia was the second of the 10 leading cases of hospital mortality, with 371 deaths per 14,684 hospitalizations, or a case-fatality ratio of 2.5%.

In 1995, acute respiratory infections were the leading cause of morbidity, accounting for 721,538 office visits; pneumonia

ranked in fifth place, with 99,472 cases. Again in 1996 acute respiratory infections and pneumonia had the same respective rankings as causes of morbidity, accounting for 795,758 and 98,428 office visits, respectively.

Rabies. A total of 15 cases of human rabies were reported in 1993, 13 in 1994, 7 in 1995, and 12 in 1996.

AIDS and Other STDs. A cumulative total of 1,789 AIDS cases were reported between 1984 and December 1996. From 1991 onward there was a steady increase in the annual incidence, which went from 2.5 per 100,000 population in 1992 to 7.6 per 100,000 in 1996. In 1996 there were 417 reported cases of AIDS and 264 persons were diagnosed as HIV-positive.

In 1996 there were three cases of AIDS in men for every two cases in women.

The predominant route of HIV transmission is sexual contact, which accounted for 88.5% of the cases during the period from 1991 to 1996 (75.8% of the cases due to heterosexual exposure and 7.2% and 5.5% due to homosexual and bisexual exposure, respectively). Other routes include vertical transmission from mother to child, 4.1% of cases; intravenous drug use, 1.2%; and blood transfusions, 0.6%.

In the period 1991–1996 there were 80 registered cases of AIDS in children under 12 years old; 50% of those were in infants less than 1 year old. From 1984 until 1996 a total of 1,514 HIV-positive cases were diagnosed in blood banks and public and private laboratories. Of this total, 89% were from urban areas.

The annual incidence of acquired syphilis remained stable between 1992 and 1996 because prevention has not been assigned high priority. In 1992 the incidence of syphilis was 33.6 per 100,000 population, and in 1995 it was 25.6 per 100,000.

The incidence of chancroid in 1992 was 48.6 per 100,000 population, and in 1995 it was 14.7 per 100,000. Lymphogranuloma venereum had incidence rates of 7.4 per 100,000 population in 1993 and 4.2 per 100,000 in 1995. Even though the incidence and prevalence of gonorrhea remains high, the reports reflect a slight decline between 1993 (81.8 per 100,000) and 1995 (79.5 per 100,000). The incidence of genital herpes has remained stable in recent years: in 1993 there were 21 reported cases per 100,000 population and in 1995, 23 per 100,000. The incidence of urogenital trichomoniasis was estimated at 260 per 100,000 population in 1993, 362 per 100,000 in 1994, and 296 per 100,000 in 1995.

Chronic Communicable Diseases. In 1996 the incidence of positive sputum for tuberculosis was 67.3 per 100,000 population. The rate of patients treated was 64.3 per 100,000 population; patients cured, 51.9 per 100,000; patients abandoning treatment, 8.5 per 100,000; and treatment failures, 0.4 per

100,000. The disease exhibited a declining trend in 1995 and 1996, and it was especially marked in the latter year.

Leprosy is in the elimination phase. There are a total of 20 chronic cases and 9 new cases on the register. All the patients are adults. Five of the old cases and two of the new ones have been diagnosed as multibacillary.

Noncommunicable Diseases and Other Health-Related Problems

Nutritional Diseases and Diseases of Metabolism. FESAL-93 measured the weight and height of children under 5 years old throughout the country. The proportion with low height-for-age was 22.8%, or a decline relative to the 31.7% estimated in 1988, and the proportion with low weight-for-age fell from 16.1% to 11.2%. Chronic malnutrition in rural areas, at 28.1%, was greater than in the urban population, for whom it was 13.6%. The percentage of retarded growth in children under 5 years old was five times greater in children of mothers without any formal education (33.6%) than in those whose mothers had 10 or more years of schooling (7.1%). Chronic malnutrition was much more prevalent in the socioeconomically disadvantaged population (31.4%) than in those at the middle level (18.7%), and in this latter population it was greater than at the upper level (9.4%). There were no notable differences between girls and boys.

With regard to acute malnutrition, indicated by low weight-for-height, FESAL-93 revealed that for 1.3% of the children under 5 years old the weight-for-height was lower than the median height by 2 standard deviations.

In 1993 the overall prevalence of malnutrition—i.e., low weight-for-age—was 11.2% at the national level, but the proportion in rural areas (14.0%) was twice as high as in the urban population (7.2%). The percentage of low weight-for-age in children of mothers with little education was five times higher than for mothers with 10 or more years of schooling. The overall prevalence of global malnutrition was 4.8% in children under 1 year old but increased to 14.4% in those aged 12 to 35 months and then declined to 10.6% in children aged 35 to 59 months.

A study conducted in February and March 1994 in 78 high-risk *municipios* to establish a baseline for the National Nutrition Program showed higher prevalences of malnutrition than those reported by FESAL-93. The rate observed for overall malnutrition was 14.9%; for the chronic form, 25.5%; and for the acute form, 3.8%. According to a food intake analysis, in these 78 *municipios* 58% of the pregnant women were not meeting their caloric needs and 40.5% were not getting enough protein.

Iodine, vitamin A, and iron deficiencies are important public health problems for the country. The 1990 National Survey of Endemic Goiter in Schoolchildren reported that endemic goiter was found in 24.8% of schoolchildren aged 7 to 14 years (28.4% in girls and 20.8% in boys) and is a serious problem. The prevalence in rural schoolchildren (30.6%) is greater than in their urban counterparts (20.7%). In 1996, 90% of the salt produced in the country contained a biologically significant amount of iodine (>20 mg/kg).

The 1988 Assessment of the Food and Nutrition Situation found that vitamin A intake was insufficient for a very large proportion of the population. More than 70% of children in rural areas consumed less than half the recommended dose. In a 1994 study to establish a baseline for the National Nutrition Program, it was estimated that the intake of vitamin A was insufficient to meet the physiological needs of 95% of pregnant women, 96% of nursing mothers, and 99% of children aged 6 to 36 months.

Also in the 1988 assessment of the food and nutrition situation, only 8.5% of the families had an adequate intake of iron. The investigation showed that in the metropolitan area the greatest source of iron intake for the population was products of animal origin, whereas in rural areas the iron came mainly from beans, and the average intake of this nutrient was much less. In 23% of the children under 5 years of age their levels of hemoglobin were indicative of anemia (<11 g/dl). The group most affected was adolescents aged 12 to 17, 51% of whom had anemia. According to the 1994 survey for the National Nutrition Program, in the 78 *municipios* studied the diet of 93% of pregnant women, 68% of nursing mothers, and 85% of children aged 6 to 36 months lacked sufficient iron to meet their needs.

According to FESAL-93, fewer than 25% of the 3-month-old babies had been breast-fed exclusively; most of them were receiving supplements to their mother's milk. The most common supplement for babies under 3 months of age was water; consumption of gruel or solid food was minimal. The average duration of exclusive breast-feeding was estimated at less than 1 month, that of complete nursing at 2.8 months, and that of any type of nursing at 15.5 months.

The proportion of breast-fed babies declined from 93.1% in 1988 to 91.2% in 1993, attributable mainly to changes in the population of the metropolitan area. During the same period there were minimal increases in the average duration of breast-feeding. The proportion of breast-fed babies was lower in the metropolitan area (86.4%) than in rural areas (94.0%). The incidence and duration of breast-feeding were lower in families at higher educational and socioeconomic levels. Women working outside the home did not have as high a rate of breast-feeding as housewives. For babies born in hospitals the percentage of breast-feeding was lower than it was for those delivered by midwives. The lowest figures for breast-feeding were found with babies born in private or Social Security hospitals.

Cardiovascular Diseases and Neoplasms. In 1994 cardiovascular diseases were the number-one cause of death, accounting for 33% of the total, and they were predominant in men, who accounted for 51.8% of all deaths from this cause.

Neoplasms were the fourth cause of death in 1994, representing 14.2% of all deaths, 60.4% of them in females and 39.6% in males. The most frequent sites of malignant neoplasms as a cause of death were the digestive organs, at 30.2%. It is estimated that in 1996 in the country as a whole there were a total of 5,436 first consultations because of malignant neoplasms. The leading site was the uterine cervix, at 43% of the total, followed by the stomach, at 14%.

External Causes of Morbidity and Mortality and Behavioral Problems. Unintentional injuries, or "accidents," and violent deaths together represented the third leading cause of death in 1994 (19% of all deaths), with a predominance in males, at 84% of all deaths. Almost 90% of the deaths from external causes were in the age groups ranging from 15 through 59 years of age.

In 1995 a total of 4,210 sexual crimes and 9,912 cases of domestic violence were registered. The Institute of Forensic Medicine reported 667 cases of domestic violence, in which 84% of the victims were women; they were almost always assaulted by a companion, husband, or father.

In 1994 the Ministry of Public Health reported 1,961 cases of pesticide poisoning; in 1995, 1,439 cases; and in 1996, 1,469 cases. The poison investigation form was introduced in 1996, and 506 cases of poisoning (59% in males), 40 of them (8%) resulting in death, were investigated. In 50% of the cases, attempted suicide was the reason for the poisoning; in 19% the poisoning was the result of occupational exposure; and in 1% of the cases, homicide. Organophosphates were the cause of 27% of the reported poisonings; fumigants (phosphoamines), 23%; herbicides (bipyridyls), 16%; and carbamates, 14%.

It is considered that the most frequent mental health problems are depression and anxiety syndromes, and alcoholism.

Disabilities. In 1992 there were 81,721 disabled persons, 53.3% of them males. Slightly more than half of them (50.9%) resided in urban areas. The impairments reported were blindness (22.2%), deafness (17.6%), mutism (4.3%), mental retardation (16.2%), loss of an upper extremity (15.5%), loss of a lower extremity (13.9%), or more than one impairment (10.3%).

In 1993, a census of persons disabled as a result of armed conflict, promoted by the United Nations Development Program and the European Union, counted a total of 12,114 who were physically disabled from the armed conflict, of whom 83% were men (11% were women and sex was not recorded for the remainder).

Natural Disasters and Industrial Accidents. El Salvador's geographical location and its geology give rise to frequent geological and meteorological phenomena that often cause heavy loss of life and property. Flooding is common in the lower part of the Lempa and Grande de San Miguel basins, especially from July to September.

There is a preference for groundwater because approximately 90% of the surface water is highly contaminated by organic waste, agrochemical products, industrial runoff, and extensive erosion caused by unchecked deforestation. Because of the seasonal variation in rainfall, 97% of the annual precipitation takes place during the rainy season from May to October, when 84% of all the country's water resources are produced. As a result, water is scarce during the dry season.

In 1997 the SILCA industry had a chemical spill when liquid gas was being transferred from a container truck to individual drums. Because proper safety precautions had not been followed, some 500 people were poisoned; 20 of the cases were serious.

In the metropolitan area of San Salvador, which has 13 *municipios* and a population of 1.5 million, trash collection coverage is very low, reaching only about 60% of the households. Some 600 tons of trash pile up uncollected every day, which has led to the creation of illegal dumps in vacant lots, public thoroughfares, and ravines. In the rest of the country's *municipios* the situation is even worse.

Measurements taken in the metropolitan area of San Salvador point to a clearly rising trend in atmospheric concentration of suspended particulate matter from the burning of fuel by vehicles and factories, agricultural slash-and-burn practices, and trash incineration.

The use of leaded gasoline was prohibited starting in June 1996, and emissions of CO, CO_2, and hydrocarbons began to be regulated in diesel engines as of January 1998.

A major cause of indoor air pollution is the use of firewood as fuel; because of the size and layout of rural dwellings, families cannot avoid inhaling the smoke.

It is believed that accidents in the workplace are greatly underreported, because ISSS counts only those cases for which official reports are filed by employers. In 1992 a total of 14,056 work-related accidents were reported, and in 1996, 18,225. From 1992 to 1996, most accidents occurred in the manufacturing and construction industries and in areas related to commerce.

Between 1992 and 1995 a total of 540 deaths from work-related accidents were reported. The most frequent occupational illnesses were lung diseases, contact dermatitis (from touching cement), and lead poisoning.

RESPONSE OF THE HEALTH SYSTEM

National Health Plans and Policies

The Comprehensive Development Plan for the five-year period 1994–1999 calls for thorough reorganization and modernization of the public sector in the context of the Government's Public Modernization Program. In the health sector, the general policy set by Ministry authorities is "to improve the level of health of the Salvadorian population through modernization of the sector and the development of interinstitutional programs that focus on comprehensive health care for individuals and the reduction of risks and damage to the environment." In this context, the following principal strategic components have been identified.

Reorganization and restructuring of health sector institutions based on transforming the bureaucratic organization into an organization that generates innovation and added value.

Decentralization of health program and administrative systems by transferring the functions of planning, administration, procurement, and resource allocation for health services delivery from the central level to other public or private entities, while endeavoring to ensure that the organizational structures are prepared for their new responsibilities.

New approaches to health services delivery to improve their currently limited population coverage. The plan is to provide services by using new approaches that will guarantee free access by the entire population to a basic package of prevention-oriented health services. The Ministry of Public Health and Social Welfare will also guarantee access to a package of essential clinical services, including second-level care such as delivery care, general surgery, outpatient treatment, and hospitalization in the four basic specialties; emergency treatment for trauma and poisoning; and treatment of tuberculosis and acute infections referred from the primary level of care. The indigent population will be subsidized by the State and the rest of the population will have access to these services based on a formula that combines direct installment payments and a compulsory minimum health insurance program.

Revision of the Legal Framework. The aim of revising and updating the legal framework in the health sector is to ensure that El Salvador has the legal instruments that will enable it to strengthen the State and the institutions that comprise it in terms of their normative and regulatory function as it applies to the sectoral level (public and private entities).

Social Participation. The decisive role of civil society in the management of its own affairs is recognized. This includes giving it the protagonist role that it should have in the administration of social welfare programs. Social participation, in its multiple manifestations, should be encouraged and facilitated as one of the most important strategies for the production of health. A pilot plan is currently under way to delegate technical and administrative responsibility to primary-level health establishments by assigning these establishments to nongovernmental organizations. For example, in the case of the health unit in the *municipio* of San Julián, Sonsonate Department, the provision of services is the responsibility of the Salvadorian Health Foundation.

Organization of the Health Sector

Institutional Organization

The public subsector is composed of social security, the services of the Ministry of Public Health and Social Welfare, and other health sector services. The Ministry has a national network of 427 services, broken down as follows: 16 hospitals, 14 health centers, 313 health units, 32 health posts, 11 community posts, 8 dispensaries, and 33 rural nutrition centers. As far as hospital beds are concerned, the Ministry has 2,964 and ISSS has 1,583.

Eighty percent of the total national population is assigned to the Ministry, although actual coverage is lower than that.

The following entities also belong to the public subsector: the National Telecommunications Association (ANTEL), the Electric Lighting Company (CEL), Teachers' Welfare, and the Military Health Service. These institutions, which cover workers (or their respective members) and their families, together provide health services to 2.3% of the population. Both the public health services of CEL and of Teachers' Welfare function as a mixed group with public financing and services provided by private entities.

Social security, represented by ISSS, provides coverage to workers in private enterprises and government employees, along with their respective beneficiaries, and takes care of 17% of the population. ISSS has 10 hospitals, 35 medical units, and 24 community clinics.

The private system has second- and third-level hospitals and clinics, which are concentrated in the country's three main departments.

Nongovernmental organizations in the health sector usually provide basic health services. Several of them use health counselors for extramural activities.

ISSS offers mainly curative care, which is provided by university-educated professionals (physicians, dentists, etc.) based on the needs of its subscribers. The unit costs are higher in ISSS than in the Ministry—as much as four times higher in some cases.

ISSS medical services are provided free to its subscribers and there is no restriction on use of the services, nor are there any mechanisms for preventing abuse. Since 1996 there has been an effort to establish community clinics, which are intended to fulfill a function similar to that of the Ministry's first level of care, with an emphasis on prevention.

Recently, steps have been taken to form committees of patients with chronic noncommunicable diseases that are of epidemiological interest—for example, diabetes and arterial hypertension. ISSS also has established specific programs relating to diseases of institutional interest, such as its diabetes and tuberculosis programs.

According to data from the Ministry of Public Health and Social Welfare, between 1994–1995 and 1995–1996 the total number of medical consultations in the country went from 2.4 to 3.2 million, and dental consultations went from 265,000 to 369,000. There were 275,700 hospital discharges in 1994–1995 and 280,400 in 1995–1996. In the same years, surgical interventions numbered 123,700 and 113,800, respectively, and there were 65,000 and 69,000 attended deliveries.

Organization of Health Regulatory Activities

Authorization to practice a given health profession is granted by an oversight board composed of professionals from that discipline. There are boards for medicine, dentistry, chemistry/pharmacy, psychology, veterinary medicine, clinical laboratory science, and nursing.

The Superior Public Health Council is responsible for regulating the use of drugs. The mechanisms for regulating and controlling the importation of drugs are based on the Health Code and the Pharmaceutical Specialties Regulations.

Private pharmacies and health establishments purchase drugs directly. Drug quality control is handled at the national level by the Ministry of Public Health. A recent change in legislation on the use of drugs specifies that tranquilizers and other psychotropic agents may be sold only upon presentation of a prescription signed by a physician specifically authorized to prescribe those drugs.

The Ministry coordinates the surveillance of processed foods with support from the Consumer Protection Bureau within the Ministry of Economy and from the universities, where additives and chemical and biological contaminants are studied as part of thesis research.

Responsibility for regulating and controlling food quality is being assumed by the food production sector itself, using its own laboratories and with the support of other entities such as the Salvadorian Foundation for Economic and Social Development (FUSADES) and the universities. The Ministry oversees compliance with technical standards.

The Epidemiological Surveillance System has been established and mechanized in the 18 departmental health districts. Reports from penal institutions, nongovernmental organizations, the ISSS, and private hospitals have been incorporated into the network. Also, statisticians from the districts and departments have been trained in the use of computer programs for epidemiological surveillance.

Health Services and Resources

Organization of Services for Care of the Population

The Ministry of Public Health and Social Welfare has implemented comprehensive health care programs in rural areas. One of the priorities of the Healthy Schools Program is basic sanitation, including installation of sanitary structures such as latrines, manual pumps, and drinking water treatment systems. The Community Health Program has given water supply and sanitation coverage to communities whose schools benefited from the Healthy Schools Program.

In 1996, the Ministry and the Government of Switzerland signed a cooperation agreement to carry out a project to monitor and study water quality, and in 1997 the Ministry entered into a technical cooperation agreement with the Executive Secretariat for the Environment under which the Ministry's Department of Environmental Sanitation assumes responsibility for the Environmental Unit and participates in the Environmental Impact Assessment System and the National Environmental Information System.

In addition, the Critical Areas Program is being carried out under an agreement between the Government of El Salvador and the Inter-American Development Bank. This program focuses on solid waste, air pollution, and water pollution. Recently, general provisions have been formulated with regard to automobiles that have problems with catalytic converters, and drivers are fined if their vehicles are found to have any problems that increase pollution.

The program dealing with occupational and environmental aspects of pesticide exposure in Central America got under way in 1997, in coordination with PAHO and with support from the Danish Cooperation for International Development (DANIDA). This program focuses on strengthening the health sector in order to better respond to problems caused by pesticides and includes occupational, epidemiological, toxicological, educational, environmental, and research aspects.

Organization and Operation of Personal Health Care Services

Various activities have been undertaken to improve the population's nutritional status. There is an intersectoral food security plan coordinated by the Ministry of Agriculture that sets policies on prices, production, and credit. The Nutritional Surveillance and Growth Monitoring Program comes under the Ministry of Public Health and is executed at the community level by health promoters, who assess children's nutritional status and take the necessary steps to help improve nutritional status or recover its optimal level. There also are programs in place to train volunteer nutrition counselors, fortify food with essential micronutrients, and distribute food supplements to vulnerable families.

In 1996 the Ministry of Public Health launched the National Nutrition Education Program with a view to improving families' food and nutrition practices. The program has three components: nutrition for pregnant women, breast-feeding and diet for nursing mothers, and nutrition for infants. In 1995, the Healthy Schools Program was established, which has helped to identify and treat cases of malnutrition.

Various actions have been taken to prevent iodine deficiency disorders. Supplementation with iodized oil and Lugol's solution is provided for 8% of the school population covered by the Healthy Schools Program (some 240,000 schoolchildren). Preventive care began to be given in 1997 to the population in areas where there was a high prevalence of iodine deficiency. In 1993, the law on salt iodization was reviewed, updated, and ratified; a cooperation agreement was signed by the Government, the salt industry, and external cooperation agencies (World Bank, PAHO/INCAP, and UNICEF), and iodized salt was gradually put on the market.

With regard to iron deficiency disorders, steps have been taken to intervene with ferrous sulfate supplementation for pregnant women, children under 5 years of age, and schoolchildren. Since 1996 all wheat flour produced in the country has been fortified with iron, folic acid, and B-complex vitamins.

To combat vitamin A deficiency in the Salvadorian population, the Ministry distributes vitamin A supplements to children 1 to 6 years old and to nursing mothers. Sugar also is fortified with vitamin A. In 1994, a law was passed on the fortification of sugar with vitamin A, and in 1995 the corresponding regulations and technical standards were developed. According to the Ministry, in 1995–1996, 85% of a series of sugar samples had retinol levels higher than 6 mg/kg and 61% exceeded 10 mg/kg. This means that the program's quality and coverage have improved considerably, although the optimum goal has not yet been reached. In a household survey conducted in 1995, retinol was found in 80% of the sugar samples taken. The target is for at least 90% of the samples to have retinol levels of 5 mg/kg.

Human Resources

For every 10,000 inhabitants, El Salvador has 9.1 physicians, 5.4 midwives, 3.8 nurses, and 2.1 dentists.

The public system has 3,473 physicians, 334 dentists, 5,274 nurses, 2,367 administrative staff, 3,404 service and maintenance staff, 1,499 health promoters, and 536 environmental health inspectors. ISSS has 1,621 physicians, 176 dentists, 1,973 nurses, 244 laboratory technicians, 87 X-ray technicians, and 40 health promoters.

Sixty percent of all physicians, nurses, and dentists are concentrated in the capital, and 70% of all specialized physicians are working in establishments at the second level of care such as hospitals and health centers in the public system, the ISSS, and the private sector. The rest of them work in establishments at the first level of care under hourly contracts.

To reduce the human resources problem in the national health system, training has been given to workers in technical, financial, administrative, strategic planning, and information areas, and efforts have been made to integrate training entities with the Ministry's activities so that occupational profiles can be updated as needed in order to provide better primary health care. The Interinstitutional Human Resources Development Group is composed of representatives from the universities and a delegate from the Ministry.

The impact of the budgetary adjustment in terms of the health labor market for the Ministry's workers has been quite acceptable compared with other institutions.

The Ministry has made some recent changes in the management of human resources. There has been greater participation in the areas of human resources, and activities have been decentralized in each hospital and department. Decentralization has enabled human resource program heads to participate in decision-making, in development of plans of work, and in administration of resources under their jurisdiction.

Expenditures and Sectoral Financing

The 1997 operating budget for the Ministry of Public Health and Social Welfare was US$ 151.30 million, distributed as follows: expenditure on preventive health services (including drugs and medical and surgical supplies), 33%; expenditure on outpatient and hospital services (including drugs and medical and surgical supplies), 59%; secretariat, 6%; and investments, 2%.

The ISSS operating budget for 1997 was US$ 49.74 million, of which 21% corresponded to pharmaceutical expenditures; spending on medical, surgical, and laboratory supplies, 2%; and payroll and miscellaneous (77%).

External Technical and Financial Cooperation

In 1996 the Ministry's Department of External Cooperation received international or foreign aid amounting to over

US$ 44.5 million; 86% of this aid was received through the execution of 57 projects. Funds were contributed by Germany, Canada, Denmark, the Netherlands, Luxembourg, Norway, Sweden, Switzerland, INCAP, the OAS, United Nations World Food Program (WFA), UNICEF, EU, the World Bank, Social Investment Funds, USAID funds to promote social development projects at the national level, the Spanish International Cooperation Agency, GTZ, and the United Nations Population Fund. The largest contribution was from the Government of Sweden, in the amount of US$ 1,083,000, followed by the Netherlands, which provided US$ 347,000. The largest contributions from international agencies and banks were from the Social Investment Funds, in the amount of US$ 20,226,000, and the World Bank, which came to US$ 11 million.

FRENCH GUIANA, GUADELOUPE, AND MARTINIQUE

GENERAL SITUATION AND TRENDS

Socioeconomic, Political, and Demographic Overview

The French Departments of French Guiana, Guadeloupe, and Martinique, have been integral parts of France since 1946. Although located in the Region of the Americas, they enjoy special protection measures and receive European structural funds designed to assist developing European regions.

The population of the Departments remained stable between the 1960s and 1980s. There were pronounced migrations to France in this period owing to the shortage of labor, which offset a vigorous but waning birth rate. Since the mid-1980s and the beginning of the employment crisis in France, repatriation movements have started with the return of adults or young retirees.

The 1990 census showed an average annual population growth of 1.1% in Martinique, 2.1% in Guadeloupe, and 5.8% in French Guiana for the 1982–1990 period. This growth continues, and in 1996 the population density was 248/km^2 in Guadeloupe, 353/km^2 in Martinique, and 2/km^2 in French Guiana. Population estimates in 1996 were 422,090 inhabitants in Guadeloupe, 383,340 in Martinique, and 151,780 in French Guiana. The population of French Guiana is the youngest, with 36% under 15 years of age, compared with Guadeloupe and Martinique where this age group represents 26.5% and 24% of the population, respectively. In 1994, life expectancy in French Guiana was 78.2 years for women and 71.2 years for men; in Guadeloupe it was 80.2 years for women and 72.7 for men; and in Martinique it was 82.4 years for women and 79.5 for men.

A portion of this population growth is due to immigration from neighboring developing countries. In French Guiana, one-third of the population is foreign; in Saint-Martin (Guadeloupe), the special free-port status and growth in tourism have virtually quadrupled the population in eight years, with a foreign population of about 50%.

Since 1986 fiscal incentives have boosted the building, public works, and hotel sectors. Unemployment rates in Guadeloupe were 27% in 1986, 26.1% in 1993, 26.1% in 1995, and 29.3% in 1996; in Martinique the unemployment rates for these four years were 31%, 25%, 26.1% and 27.2%; in French Guiana the rates were 22%, 24.1%, 23% and 22.4% for the same period.

Registered unemployed and underemployed persons account for half of the active population of the Antilles (Guadeloupe and Martinique), and 44% in French Guiana. On the basis of the 1990 census, a survey conducted by the National Institute of Statistics and Economic Studies (INSEE) defined the high-risk population as households occupying makeshift accommodation without water in or near their dwellings and those with an unemployed head of family. An estimated 22% were considered to be high risk in Guadeloupe, 18% in Martinique, and 30% in French Guiana. Table 1 presents socioeconomic indicators for the three Departments.

Morbidity and Mortality Profile

Among the specific health problems affecting the three French Departments are a high prevalence of sexually transmitted viral infections and an endemic level of dengue with epidemic outbreaks. Among noncommunicable diseases, there is a high prevalence of sickle cell anemia and a high frequency of diabetes and hypertension and their complications (particularly chronic kidney failure). With the exception of cervical and prostate cancers there is a low incidence of malignant tumors. Traffic accidents contribute enormously to years of potential life lost (YPLL).

In 1995, there were 5,383 deaths in French Guiana, Guadeloupe, and Martinique. The most recent information on causes of death is from 1993, since analysis is conducted by the National Institute of Health and Medical Research in Paris. This analysis is independent of the INSEE collection of data from the registry of births, marriages, and deaths.

TABLE 1
Socioeconomic indicators for French Guiana, Guadeloupe, and Martinique, 1982 and 1990.

	French Guiana		Guadeloupe		Martinique	
	1982	1990	1982	1990	1982	1990
Households with running drinking water	69.1%	84.4%	70.1%	89.8%	78.8%	94.3%
Households with electricity	80.4%	87.8%	77.2%	89.4%	72.3%	90.3%
Households with sewage disposal[1]	34.3%	44.3%	24.5%	36.3%	22.5%	38.0%
Proportion of overpopulated dwellings[2]	24.6%	24.0%	26.7%	17.1%	26.2%	14.8%
Average number of persons/household	3.3	3.4	3.7	3.4	3.8	3.3
Urban population	...	64.3%	...	91.4%	...	84.6%
Literacy rate	72%	...	82%	...	85%	...

[1]These figure do not include dwellings equipped with individual septic tanks.
[2]Dwellings having fewer rooms than the number of occupants.
Source: National Institute of Statistics and Economic Studies (INSEE), 1982 and 1990 reports.

Infectious and parasitic diseases are, in the YPLL classification, the second most common cause of death in French Guiana among both sexes. In the Antilles, they are the fourth cause and account for only 6% to 7% of YPLL. In Guadeloupe, AIDS accounts for 6.5% of deaths in infants under 28 days old. Guadeloupe is the Department most seriously affected by problems during the perinatal period. In all Departments, the most frequent causes of death in the perinatal period are anoxia and other respiratory diseases.

Injury and poisoning (particularly road traffic accidents) are the primary cause of death among men, contributing to over one-third of YPLL among the male population in the three Departments. Among women, these causes occupy first place in French Guiana and are the third most common cause of death in Guadeloupe and Martinique.

While cardiovascular disorders are the largest contributor to mortality in the Departments, their importance should be viewed in light of the late age at which death occurs. These disorders occupy second place in YPLL in the Antilles, and third place in French Guiana.

In the Antilles, malignant tumors are the principal cause of death among women in terms of YPLL and the fourth most common cause in French Guiana. Cancers are the fifth leading cause of death among men in French Guiana (accounting for 4% of YPLL), and occupy second place in Martinique (18%) and third place in Guadeloupe (13%).

RESPONSE OF THE HEALTH SYSTEM

National Health Plans and Policies

The Secretariat of State for Health forms part of the French Ministry of Labor and Social Affairs. A number of other Ministries are also involved in health activities, including the

Ministries of Home Affairs (drug abuse programs), Environment, Agriculture (food safety), Youth and Sport (health activities), and National Education (school health).

A 1992 law provides that all persons residing in France and in French Departments have the right to financial assistance for medical treatment costs in case of need. Access to medical attention for the poor is organized by the Department in which they live. The Department pays either the entire cost or the "ticket moderateur," which is a portion ranging from 0% to 65% depending on the nature of the illness, the care provided, or the type of medication. The costs of care to the homeless are paid by the State.

Health insurance is provided by the social security system, a State-sponsored mechanism financed with compulsory contributions from salaries. The patient pays the entire cost of treatment directly to the treatment provider and is reimbursed by the health insurance. The amount reimbursed is calculated on the basis of rates negotiated between care providers and social security. A growing proportion of the population voluntarily takes out additional insurance to finance non-reimbursable portions. To prevent the patient from having to pay in advance, direct payment by insurers is widely used in the Departments, especially in hospitals and pharmacies. In such cases, the care provider is paid directly by health insurance and the patient pays only the "ticket moderateur."

Organization of the Health Sector

Institutional Organization

The State has responsibility for general public health, including community-wide disease prevention, sanitation surveillance, border health control, and the control of major diseases and drug and alcohol addiction. The State oversees training of health personnel, helps define their conditions of work, monitors observance of quality-control regulations and health safety in treatment centers, and regulates pharmaceutical products. Moreover, it supervises the adequacy of treatment and preventive arrangements and regulates the volume of treatment provided. The central Government oversees the functioning of public hospitals, appoints their directors, establishes their budgets, and organizes their staff recruitment. Finally, the State supervises social welfare, its financing, the rules for population coverage, and financial responsibility for treatment.

A prefect directs the State's decentralized services that come under the authority of each of the Ministers concerned, particularly in matters of health. At the local level, a prefect has jurisdiction over the Departmental Bureau of Health and Social Affairs in each Department, and an Interregional Bureau of Social Security, which is common to the three Departments and headquartered in Martinique.

Under the 1983 decentralization law, certain State medical and social responsibilities were transferred to the Presidents of the General Councils in each Department. These include: maternal and child welfare, immunization, tuberculosis control, sexually transmitted diseases (excluding AIDS), cancer, leprosy, child social welfare, and part of the assistance to the elderly and to disabled adults. The mayors may have certain responsibilities for sanitation and immunization, and chair the boards of directors of public health establishments.

Residents of the French Departments enjoy unrestricted access to a wide range of primary and secondary medical services. In 1991, the University Hospitals and Regional Cancer Control Centers in France provided 61,000 hospital days to 4,500 patients from the French Departments, which represent an estimated 11% of hospital activity in Guadeloupe, 3% in Martinique, and 15% in French Guiana. More than 25% of those days were for treatment of cancer patients, followed by patients suffering from cardiovascular disorders and genitourinary diseases. The social security system reimburses hospital expenses, but pays airfares for only a small proportion of patients requiring medical treatment not available in the Departments.

Public and private hospitals provide full hospitalization, ambulatory treatment, and outpatient consultations. Inpatient care is divided into short-term treatment (acute conditions), follow-up (convalescence, readaptation, and functional rehabilitation), and long-term care (designed essentially for the elderly). Private practitioners provide most ambulatory or home care, although patients may also avail themselves of outpatient services at hospitals or treatment centers.

The public and private sectors differ in some regards. Teaching and research are part of the specific missions of the public hospitals. They are obliged to accept all patients and employ only salaried staff. Physicians in private hospitals charge fees.

Since 1985, public establishments have been financed primarily through a grant made by the State on an annual basis and paid by the health insurance scheme. Private establishments are funded through lump-sum payments and daily rates fixed by the regional health insurance offices. Their funding is thus proportionate to their activity, which is not the case for public hospitals.

Organization of Health Regulatory Activities

Environmental Protection. Environmental control is the responsibility of the State services at the departmental level. Drinking and bathing water quality (sea water and water in swimming pools) and wastewater treatment are subject to regular inspections.

Food Security. Food-poisoning surveys are conducted jointly by the Departmental Bureau of Health and Social Affairs and the veterinary department (Ministry of Agriculture.) The Departmental Bureau of Competition, Consumption, and Fraud Eradication (Ministry of Finance) effects quality control of food products and food conservation.

Health Technology. Equipment is monitored on a national scale. Only equipment approved at the national level may be installed in health establishments, based on a health map that defines ratios of bed capacity and major equipment to the number of inhabitants.

Health Services and Resources

Organization of Health Services for Care of the Population

Health Promotion. The French Center for Health Education devises campaigns on a number of health and hygiene topics, which are taken up by the Departments. In addition, the National Medical Insurance Scheme institutes prevention and screening campaigns (e.g., cancer of the uterus and breast). The Departmental Bureau of Health and Social Affairs may launch campaigns using locally produced materials that are better suited to the inhabitants of the Departments.

Programs for Disease Prevention and Control. Residents of the French Departments have access to regular examinations during their school years and in the workplace. Maternal and child welfare services are available to pregnant women and young children. It is obligatory for the Depart-

271

mental Bureau of Health and Social Affairs to report certain infectious or communicable diseases.

Organization and Operation of Personal Health Care Services

Service Networks. "Town-hospital" networks, which make it possible to improve coordination between hospital doctors and private practitioners, have been established for poisonings and hepatitis C. In addition to these networks centers for HIV information and care have been set up in each region.

Ancillary Diagnostic Services and Blood Banks. Blood transfusion units operate nationally under the French Blood Agency. Regionally, a physician monitors proper blood-transfusion practices.

The Antilles and French Guiana have 50 medical biology laboratories in the private sector and 18 in the public sector. There are 22 private and 8 public laboratories in Guadeloupe, 3 private and 2 public in French Guiana, and 25 private and 8 public in Martinique. The prefect can authorize the operation of private laboratories taking local conditions, personnel qualifications, and available equipment into account. The public laboratories pertain to the hospitals.

Specialized Services. Psychiatry in France is organized in geographically defined sectors. Each adult psychiatry sector covers a population of approximately 70,000; there is one child psychiatry unit to three adult units.

There are two administrative units for the disabled: the Departmental Special Education Commission reviews all applications for placement of the disabled under 20 years of age, as well as requests from their families for financial assistance. For those over 20 years of age, it is the task of the Technical Guidance and Vocational Reclassification Commission in each French Department to classify disabled workers and provide vocational orientation, as well as to assess the allocation of financial assistance and direct them to a specialized institution.

Since 1984, the French prison population has received medical coverage equivalent to that of the general population.

Inputs for Health

Drugs and Immunobiologicals. There are 308 pharmacies in the Antilles and French Guiana (140 in Guadeloupe, 139 in Martinique, and 29 in French Guiana) and 7 wholesale distributors (2 in Guadeloupe, 2 in Martinique, and 3 in French Guiana). All pharmaceutical products, including vaccines, are imported from France. Usually, drugs are avail-

able by doctors' prescription and the patient is reimbursed by a health insurance agency. A system of direct payment by insurers relieves the patient from having to advance the cost. The authorities set the price of reimbursable drugs. Generic drugs have yet to find a significant niche in the French drug market. The price for drugs in the Departments is adjusted to offset transportation costs. In the last 20 years there has been a sharp increase (approximately eightfold) in expenditures for medications by households in the French Departments.

Quality control for pharmaceuticals is based on the use of health surveillance systems, warning systems, application of manuals of good practice, continuing education of pharmacists (soon to be compulsory), and pharmacy inspections in each region. Drug advertising is controlled for the public and for physicians. Information campaigns on drugs and their correct use are periodically organized by the authorities.

Medical Equipment. Major medical equipment requires authorization of the minister or the prefect of the region. Certain equipment is shared by all three Departments. For example, an MRI scanner is located in Martinique and a lithotriptor in Guadeloupe.

Human Resources

Training. Doctors are trained in the medical schools attached to the university hospitals. A tertiary cycle of medical studies exists with a training capacity of 5 specialists and approximately 100 general practitioners per year in the Departments. This takes place through an agreement between the University of Bordeaux II and the Antilles-French Guiana Training and Research Unit, which is attached to the University of Antilles-French Guiana.

The Fort-de-France and Pointe-à-Pitre teaching hospitals serve as supervised practical training facilities for medical students. A school in Martinique, attached to the Fort-de-France university hospital, trains 14 midwives a year; a school for operating room nurses at the Lamentin Hospital in Martinique trains 10 nurses a year; and there are two schools for ambulance staff, one in Martinique and the other in Guadeloupe. There is also a school of nursing in each of the Departments, training a total of 61 nurses per year. Other health professionals are trained in France.

Continuing medical education is provided for salaried doctors in the health establishments where they are employed, and has been compulsory for private doctors since 1996. This training is managed by Regional Councils for Continuing Education and the National Council for Continuing Education.

Health Personnel. As of January 1997, the ratio of private doctors in the Departments was 66 general practitioners and 40 specialists per 100,000 population. Private doctors are paid for each consultation, while other health professionals may be salaried or may practice privately and be paid for each consultation.

Health Research and Technology

The National Institute of Health and Medical Research has a unit in Guadeloupe devoted to hemoglobinopathy. The Institute has Research Guidance Committees in each Department.

External Technical and Financial Cooperation

To ensure access to care for the destitute, Physicians of the World, a nongovernmental organization, provides free medical consultations. Likewise, the AIDES Association, in partnership with State authorities, is involved in the fight against AIDS.

Specific projects are assisted through the Inter-ministerial Fund for the Caribbean. The Fund, which receives approximately 10 million francs (US$ 1.8 million) annually, is administered by an inter-ministerial delegation responsible to the prefect of Guadeloupe, and is designed to support bilateral cooperation projects involving at least one Department and a neighboring foreign country. One-sixth of the Fund is devoted to health. Health facilities, particularly the Fort-de-France and Pointe-à-Pitre teaching hospitals, negotiate cooperative activities with neighboring countries in the areas of training, telemedicine, and on-site visits by health practitioners to administer treatment.

FRENCH GUIANA

French Guiana occupies 90,000 km² on the northeast coast of South America, bordered by Suriname on the west and Brazil on the east and south. Dense equatorial forest covers 90% of the territory. The main modes of access to the interior are waterways, and most communities are accessible only by motorboat. A few isolated communities have authorized landing strips.

In 1994, the fertility rate was 110.5 births per 1,000 women of childbearing age. Between 1982 and 1992 it increased by 4% among mothers 10–14 years old, and by 14% among mothers 15–19 years old. The birth rate was 29.2 resident births per 1,000 in 1995, the mortality rate was 3.9 deaths per 1,000 inhabitants, and the infant mortality rate (average for 1991–1993) was 15.3 per 1,000 live births.

SPECIFIC HEALTH PROBLEMS

Analysis by Population Group

Health of Children and Teenagers

The perinatal mortality rate in French Guiana has remained at around 30 per 1,000 live births for the past 10 years. In 1995, neonatal infections, congenital malformations, and toxemia of pregnancy were the main causes of death during the perinatal period. The infant mortality rate was reduced three-fold in 20 years, falling from 50 per 1,000 in the 1970s, to an average of 15 per 1,000 in recent years. The three main causes of hospitalization in the 1992–1993 period were premature births and low birthweight (48%), infectious diseases (17%), and acute respiratory infections (6%).

The Departmental Maternal and Infant Protection Unit has a system for permanent recording of information for the perinatal period in all public and private maternity clinics, and in the departmental health centers. It consists of records of pregnancy results and fact sheets on the causes of perinatal deaths, as recommended by WHO.

The ratio of stillbirths to newborns weighing 500 g and 1,000 g was 22.6 per 1,000 and 16.7 per 1,000, respectively, in 1995. Early neonatal mortality was 9.8 per 1,000 for births at 500 g and 8.6 per 1,000 for those at 1,000 g. The premature birth rate has been stable at 12% since 1993. The proportion of newborns with a birthweight of less than 2,500 g is 11%.

In 1995, 67.3% of women sought fewer than the seven consultations provided by law during pregnancy, 53.3% sought fewer than six consultations, and 19.7% sought three consultations or fewer. The situation among minors is alarming: 79% sought fewer than seven prenatal consultations.

Between 1981 and 1983 deaths among 1–4-year-olds were due mainly to external causes and trauma (67 per 100,000) and diseases of the central nervous system (40 per 100,000). In the 1988–1990 period the leading causes were infectious diseases (37 per 100,000), external causes and trauma (30 per 100,000), and respiratory diseases (18 per 100,000). The main causes of hospitalization in this age group are infectious diseases (18%), cranial trauma (13%), and chronic illnesses of the upper respiratory tract (11%).

Among children in the 5–14-year age group, the three main causes of death in the 1988–1990 period were: external causes and trauma (12 per 10,000), infectious diseases (6 per 100,000), and circulatory diseases (4 per 100,000). The main reasons for hospitalization for children between the ages of 5 and 9 were broken limbs (14%), cranial trauma (12%), and appendicitis (12%). Among 10–14-year-olds appendicitis was the main cause (18%), followed by broken limbs (14%), and normal delivery (12%).

Early pregnancies, drug abuse, and AIDS and other STDs appeared to be the main health problems among adolescents. In the past decade, approximately 8% of mothers have been under age 18. In 1992, one-third of this group showed signs of pathology during pregnancy. Of the AIDS-affected population, 11.3% are under 20 years old.

Health of Adults

Between 1988 and 1990 the main causes of death among women in the 15–34-year age group were suicide (20%), road traffic accidents (10%), and AIDS (10%); for women ages 35–64 the main causes were malignant tumors (30%) and cerebrovascular diseases (16%). Among men ages 15–34 the main causes were traffic accidents (20%), AIDS (10%), suicide (8%), and homicide (6.3%); for men 35–64 years old malignant tumors predominated (11%), followed by AIDS (10%), cerebrovascular diseases (9%), and road traffic accidents (9%).

Health of the Elderly

Between 1988 and 1990, the most frequent causes of death among those over age 65 were cerebrovascular diseases (10% in men, 23% in women), respiratory diseases (7%), infectious diseases (7%), and malignant tumors of the digestive system (7%). The most common chronic illnesses in this age group are severe hypertension (19% in men and 36% in women), diabetes (15% in both sexes), and tumors (15% in men and 9% in women).

Analysis by Type of Disease or Health Impairment

Communicable Diseases

Vector-Borne Diseases. The incidence of malaria in French Guiana is high: 5,892 biologically confirmed cases were registered in 1995. The three types most frequently encountered were *Plasmodium falciparum, P. vivax,* and *P. malariae.* The two areas of malaria transmission in French Guiana are the two large border rivers (Maroni and Oyapock) where transmission is permanent, and the coastal zone, with sporadic and limited transmission. Since the malaria-infected areas are very distinct, it is difficult to define the global evolutionary trend.

Beginning in 1994, there was an outbreak of the disease in the Upper Maroni (Maripasoula) region. Migratory movements, mainly from Brazil and Suriname, connected with gold mining along the rivers have contributed to this rise in malaria transmission.

In 1992, a study revealed a 68% *in vivo* failure rate of chloroquine malaria treatment (62% *in vitro*), with 24% resistance to quinine. These findings were confirmed by *in vitro* chemosensitivity conducted at the Pasteur Institute (1993–1996), which also indicated resistance to halofantrine.

The dengue vector in French Guiana is *Aedes aegypti* and the 1, 2, and 4 virus types circulate in an endemic-epidemic mode. An epidemic wave caused by the dengue-2 serotype was observed from July 1991 to October 1992. During that period 40 cases of dengue hemorrhagic fever were registered, including six deaths. In December 1995, this serotype reappeared mainly in Cayenne. There has been a new outbreak of the disease since the last quarter of 1996 with distribution of dengue-1 in Kourou and dengue-2 in Cayenne.

Cholera and Other Intestinal Diseases. Together with malaria, diarrhea is the principal reason for consultation and observation in the departmental health centers. Typhoid breaks out in small epidemics, mainly in the communities in the Maroni region.

The first case of cholera was reported in French Guiana in 1991. Between December 1991 and November 1994, 22 cases of cholera were reported, 55% of which originated in rural areas. No case of cholera has been reported in French Guiana since November 1994.

AIDS. Since the beginning of the epidemic, 588 cases of AIDS have been reported in French Guiana. Women account for 38.4% of all cases; 30–39-year-olds are the most affected age group (38.8%), followed by the 40–49-year age group (17.7%), and the 20–29-year age group (15.6%). Transmission in 79.2% of cases is heterosexual. While mother-to-fetus transmission is a striking aspect, representing 58 cases (9.9% of all cases), transmission in a drug-abuse context is very low (2%). Of the cases reported, 57.8% died as of 31 December 1996.

"Tritherapy" or multi-drug treatment of AIDS began in August 1996, and patients have access to viral-load measurement. In 1997 French Guiana embarked on a "strategic programming" process to address this high-priority disease.

Tuberculosis and Leprosy. In 1995, 69 cases of tuberculosis were registered. The predominance of the disease among males in 1994 (male-to-female ratio of 2.2:1) appears to have tapered off (male-to-female ratio of 1.16:1 in 1995). Two-thirds of tuberculosis cases are found among immigrants from Brazil, Haiti, and Suriname. The tuberculosis/HIV co-infection rate was 19% in 1995. Poverty and marginality, which have been exacerbated since 1993 in French Guiana, are factors that probably encourage transmission of tuberculosis.

In French Guiana, 15 to 20 new cases of leprosy are detected each year. The paucibacillary forms predominate (nearly 80%). Since 1986, the incidence of leprosy has dropped by half and ranges from 0.08 to 0.15 per 1,000. Prevalence has shown a steady decrease, from 3.2 per 1,000 in 1985 to 1.1 per 1,000 in 1995.

Noncommunicable Diseases and Other Health-Related Problems

Nutritional Diseases. Protein-energy malnutrition mainly affects the black population of the Maroni region, particularly in babies being weaned. There are 15 to 20 hospitalizations per year for severe infant malnutrition (kwashiorkor, marasmus, and mixed forms) at the Saint Laurent Hospital in Maroni. Infant protein-energy malnutrition in the black population is linked to a number of factors, mainly reduced interest in breast-feeding and belief systems regarding infant feeding.

Malignant Tumors. Cancers are the leading cause of death in the 35–64-year age group. In men, the cancers mainly affect the digestive system, the prostate, and the respiratory system. In women, the most frequent are tumors of the digestive system (37%) and cancer of the uterus (20%).

Behavioral Disorders. French Guiana has conducted few studies on its inhabitants suffering from mental disorders. Hospital data, however, indicate a general increase in activity in recent years, especially in child and juvenile psychiatry. The data reveal a high percentage of forcibly hospitalized patients (30.6% in 1993, while the national average was 21%); a lack of suitable structures for stabilized illnesses or handicaps, resulting in hospitalizations not justified in terms of psychiatry; and the onerous burden of health coverage for drug addicts. In 1993, drug addicts accounted for 22.6% of hospitalizations and 73% of forcible hospitalizations. Fifty percent of hospitalized drug addicts have an associated severe psychiatric disorder.

According to a recent study on drug addicts treated at the care establishments, 7% used crack cocaine, 59% are between the ages of 20 and 34, and 66% are out of work (compared with 14% of addicts with stable jobs).

There is a dearth of information on alcohol-related morbidity, but 3% of all deaths appeared to be alcohol-related.

RESPONSE OF THE HEALTH SYSTEM

Health Services and Resources

Organization of Services for Care of the Population

Water Supply, Sewerage Systems, and Solid Waste Disposal. The drinking water made available to 85% of the pop-

ulation, which is concentrated on the coast, is generally of high quality. The communities in the interior have water of mediocre, if not extremely poor quality; their treatment centers are either inadequate or have facility maintenance problems. The most serious problems affecting water quality are bacteriological parameters, the presence of aluminum, by-products of chlorination, and the occasional presence of mercury.

Sewage facilities for domestic wastewater are not very effective in French Guiana. It is estimated that only 30% of the wastewater produced is treated. French Guiana has no organized treatment or recycling facility for domestic wastes. Landfills are the only means of waste disposal, and there are only two controlled landfills, both located in the urban area of Cayenne. In addition there are some 20 crude communal landfills and more than 100 random dumping grounds. Most of the landfills are installed without prior impact studies, often on unsuitable sites.

Control of Vector-Borne Diseases. Malaria control is the province of the Departmental Disinfection Bureau and comprises vector control by spraying homes (walls), impregnating mosquito nets with long-lasting insecticides, attacking the parasite pool with active detection techniques, and treatment of parasite vectors. The surveillance system is based on compulsory notification of cases of local and imported malaria and on active and passive detection. The Disinfection Bureau and Pasteur Institute of French Guiana also conduct entomological surveillance. The Pasteur Institute is responsible for entomological studies on malaria vectors and their sensitivity to antibiotic products.

Since the Second Consensus Conference on Malaria (Cayenne, October 1995), recommendations for treating malaria in French Guiana exclude chloroquine as a first medication and concentrate on the use of quinine in association with doxycycline, halofantrine, or mefloquine.

The Pasteur Institute is the National Reference Center for surveillance of dengue and yellow fever and is responsible for identifying viral strains. The current surveillance system is based on the positive seroreactions requested by doctors. The Disinfection Bureau's vector control relies on different activities such as: control of larval deposits by periodic visits to homes; visits and treatment of close contacts of positive seroreaction cases; and larva control and imagocide among the close contacts of seropositive patients. Imagocide activities are stepped up when there is a resurgence of dengue cases. Health education campaigns are organized through the media, the national education department, and associations to encourage public participation in the elimination of larval deposits.

Immunization. Given its geographical situation and the risks of infection with yellow fever virus, immunization in

French Guiana is compulsory from the age of 12 months, with a booster shot every 10 years. All of the Department's health centers have been equipped to perform this immunization since 1995. Compulsory vaccination is performed free of charge in the health and prevention centers. Besides the compulsory vaccinations (BCG, DTP, polio, and yellow fever), the General Council covers measles, mumps, and rubella immunization, and provides immunization against hepatitis B for groups with high risk of infection.

Mental Health Programs. The regional psychiatry plan, decreed in 1996, defines goals for the next five years. Priorities were the creation of new sector divisions (three for adult psychiatry, and one for child-youth psychiatry); extension of access to care, particularly for the inhabitants of isolated communities; and measures to cover psychiatric emergencies and dangerous patients.

Organization and Operation of Personal Health Care Services

The coastal area of French Guiana has three urban centers—Cayenne, Kourou, and Saint Laurent du Maroni—home to nearly 80% of the population. The coast enjoys developed health facilities (three hospitals and three private clinics), a network of private doctors, and prevention facilities administered by the General Council. The population of the interior is distributed mainly along the two border rivers and in the outback. In the remote rural areas where there are no private doctors or hospitals, there is a network of public health clinics administered by the General Council. Access to treatment, including medicines, is entirely free in these facilities.

There are two public hospitals, one is in Cayenne (with 526 beds, 80 of which are devoted to psychiatric patients), the other is in Saint Laurent du Maroni (104 beds). There is a nonprofit private clinic in Kourou (65 beds), and three nonprofit clinics in Cayenne (with 81, 45, and 36 beds). There are no cardiac surgery, neurosurgery, or serious burn facilities in French Guiana, making medical evacuation to the Antilles or France a necessity. There are 9 medical health centers and, in the remote areas, 17 satellite health centers staffed by health workers. The health centers provide nursing care and medical consultations and maintain beds for patients needing observation. The territory has been divided into 12 health zones, which more or less follow the administrative borders. Doctors usually travel in canoes along difficult routes (up to six hours in a canoe within a single health zone). Health teams may transfer a patient to the coastal hospitals. Canoe, airplane, helicopter, or ambulance are the modes of evacuation, depending on the center's location and the degree of urgency. Evacuations are done for consulta-

tions or specialist examinations, planned hospitalization, and medical emergencies.

Since 1993, the social security service has shared in the operation costs of the departmental health centers, prorated on the estimated percentage of insured persons residing in a community.

GUADELOUPE

Guadeloupe is an archipelago of eight inhabited islands; the two largest, separated by a sound, are Basse-Terre and Grande-Terre. The other islands include Les Saintes and Marie Galante to the south, Désirade to the east, and the French section of Saint Martin and Saint Barthélemy some 230 km to the north.

SPECIFIC HEALTH PROBLEMS

Analysis by Population Group

Health of Children

Child health in Guadeloupe has improved considerably in the 1992–1996 period. This improvement is most marked in regard to infant mortality. Perinatal mortality has dropped to an average rate of 10.1 per 1,000 live births over the 1994–1996 period, but the stillbirth rate remains high (7.4 per 1,000). The number of infant deaths between 7 and 28 days has stayed the same (1.9 per 1,000) in this period. Infant mortality has dropped from 10.4 per 1,000 in 1992 to 7.9 per 1,000 in 1995. The main causes of infant mortality are conditions arising in the perinatal period (50%), congenital anomalies (16%), and infectious and parasitic diseases (12.5%).

Child mortality in the 1–4-year age group during the 1987–1992 period was due to accidental causes in 42% of cases. This percentage is essentially the same for both sexes. Other causes of death were infections (12.6%) and malformations (12.3%).

At 3 years of age, 77% of children were enrolled in kindergarten and underwent health examinations. During the 1994–1995 school year, 1.4% of the children examined had language problems requiring specialized treatment. Out of every 1,000 children, 8 suffer from confirmed hearing impairment and 18 from confirmed sight impairment (7 had confirmed strabismus).

Half of deaths in the 5–14-year age group are caused by accidents: 47% among girls, and 52% among boys. Tumors are the next most common cause of mortality in this age group (11.5%), followed by diseases of the nervous system (9.3%).

Health of Teenagers and Young Adults

Teenagers and young adults (ages 15 to 24) represent 16% of the population in Guadeloupe. This group has a 48% unemployment rate. In the 15–19-year age group, 86% are registered in schools. A study of deaths for the 1987–1990 period shows that 2.7% occur in this age group. With an annual average of 62 deaths, the mortality rate for this group is 0.7 per 1,000 (1.2 per 1,000 among men and 0.3 per 1,000 among women).

Traffic accidents cause 1 in 3 deaths in this age group. They are followed in descending order by: ill-defined and other accidents and their late effects (28%), tumors (7.3%), and diseases of the circulatory system and disorders of the nervous system and the respiratory tract. Teenagers are most affected by accidents involving two-wheeled vehicles with, respectively, 37% of deaths and 47% of serious injuries on average per year. The 15–24-year age group also accounts for a high proportion of automobile accident victims (21% of deaths and 26% of seriously injured).

A study conducted in 1993–1994 at the University Hospital in Pointe-à-Pitre revealed 71 admissions for attempted suicide among teenagers aged 15–19 years. The risk factors identified included a previous history of psychological problems (42%), frequent failure at school (50%), a high incidence of broken families (76% were children of divorced couples), and a history of attempted suicide by close relatives (7.5%). Past incest or rape were other risk factors frequently reported. Repeated suicide attempts are widespread (30% of cases), with recurrences within an average of 4.5 months.

Illnesses fully covered by the health insurance scheme during the 1989–1991 period accounted for 4% of all hospital admissions in this age group. The main cause of admissions was mental disorders (46% of cases), followed by congenital and valvular heart disease (7.6%), hemoglobinopathy (7.5%), and diabetes and progressive scoliosis (6.2%).

In 1992, 5.4% of pregnancies occurred in girls under 18 years of age. However, between 1982 and 1992 the fertility rate dropped from 45 to 29 per 1,000 in the 15–19-year age group and from 149 to 98 per 1,000 for the 19–24-year age group.

Health of Adults

The principal medical causes of deaths among adults between ages 15 and 60 for the 1987–1990 period were cardiovascular disorders (33%), tumors (19%), trauma (12%), ill-defined causes (7%), diseases of the digestive system (6%), and diseases of the respiratory system (5%). The order of causes differs for the 15–34-year-old age group: accidental causes, road traffic and other accidents are the first two causes of death, followed by suicides and HIV infection.

Eight hundred deaths occurred before the age of 65 in the 1987–1990 period. The main causes of these premature deaths are accidents, diseases of the circulatory system, and tumors. About one-half of these deaths were avoidable: 228 by a change in high-risk behavior, and 196 with better screening and/or proper attention by the health system.

The hospital morbidity survey conducted in 1992–1993 in the short-term facilities shows hypertension, diabetes, and alcoholism to be the diseases most frequently associated with hospitalization.

Health of the Elderly

At the time of the 1990 census, inhabitants age 60 and older represented 11.7% of the total population; in 1995, this sector of the population was 12.3%. Virtually everyone age 60 and over lives at home, due to the protection provided by the traditional lifestyle and the existence of a state home care policy. Cardiovascular disorders are the main cause of mortality (43%), followed by tumors (20%) and ill-defined morbid conditions (9%). Diabetes and hypertension account for 56% of coverage for chronic illnesses, followed by cancer, cerebrovascular accidents, and progressive chronic arteriopathy.

Reproductive Health

The fertility rate in Guadeloupe fell by 27% between 1984 and 1994. Rates for women in the 15–19- and 20–24-year age groups dropped by one-third, and in the 25–29-year age group by one-quarter. The fertility rate has remained constant among women 30 and older.

Data from family planning and education centers show that 75% of the clients used oral contraceptives, 8% an intrauterine device (IUD), and 17% other methods. The perinatal mortality survey conducted in 1984–1985 suggests an abortion rate of 26% among the female population of childbearing age. In 1994, the abortion rate was 30 per 100 conceptions. The maternal mortality rate was 51.4 per 100,000 live births for the 1987–1990 period.

Family Health

The most salient characteristic of the Guadeloupan family is the role played by single-parent families (one-third of all families); in 86% of cases a woman is the head of household. One-third of children under age 17 are brought up in single-parent families. Special measures seek to encourage child care while parents are at work (help in opening day-care centers

277

and financial assistance for parents using registered care providers); to provide needy families with financial assistance for their children's basic needs; and to enable children to attend school at an early age.

Health of the Disabled

In 1992, a random sample from the Departmental Commission for Special Education records shows that moderate and slight mental retardation were the most common disabilities (a rate of 5.1 and 4.8 per 1,000, respectively), followed by peripheral motor disabilities (1.3 per 1,000), extensive motor disabilities (1.2 per 1,000), and multiple disabilities (1.2 per 1,000).

Analysis by Type of Disease or Health Impairment

Communicable Diseases

Vector-Borne Diseases. There are 4–5 imported cases of malaria in Guadeloupe every year. There were serious outbreaks of dengue fever in the second half of 1992 and 1994. Dengue-2 virus was isolated in 1994. Seven cases of dengue hemorrhagic fever were recorded in 1995, three of them fatal. Seropositivity is more than 30% during epidemic outbreaks.

The only form of schistosomiasis encountered is *Shistosoma mansoni* (intestinal bilharziasis). The main transmission sites were eradicated through a biological campaign against the mollusk vector *(Planorbis).*

Vaccine-Preventable Diseases. No cases of poliomyelitis or diphtheria were recorded in recent years. The measles surveillance network set up in 1992 did not report any cases confirmed by serology between 1992 and October 1996, when an epidemic broke out. By the end of March 1997, 85 cases had been confirmed by serology, 79% in schoolchildren between 10 and 19 years of age. There were no cases in children under 1 year old. Of the confirmed cases, 17% had been vaccinated.

No cases of neonatal tetanus have been discovered in the 1992–1996 period. Two deaths from tetanus occurred in 1994: one was an 80-year old woman and the other an unvaccinated female foreigner.

Influenza syndromes as a whole were monitored by the network of sentinel doctors, and influenza surveillance with a nasopharynx search for the virus was instituted in March 1996. This confirmed the existence of an epidemic early in October 1996, and the presence of the H3N2 strain of the type-a virus was established.

Blood donation samples taken in 1989 showed a 2.9% prevalence of hepatitis B. These encouraging results were ob-

tained through rigorous donor selection procedures established to increase the security of blood transfusion products. Positive hepatitis C tests from blood donation samples fell from 21.8% in 1990 to 0.9% in 1993 and to 0.07% in 1996.

Cholera and Other Intestinal Diseases. There were no cases of cholera in Guadeloupe, and diarrheal diseases are no longer a public health problem, owing to the high quality of the water system and to food-product controls.

Acute Respiratory Infections. The rate for acute respiratory infections is 0.5 per 1,000 among children under age 5. A 1993 study conducted on schoolchildren aged 6–12 years showed a 13.6% prevalence of asthma in the Basse-Terre region.

Rabies and Other Zoonoses. No case of rabies has ever been discovered in Guadeloupe. Leptospirosis is endemic in Guadeloupe, with 5–6 cases occurring per year. Nineteen cases, including two deaths, were reported in 1996.

AIDS and Other STDs. As of 31 December 1996, a total of 731 cases of AIDS had been reported in Guadeloupe. The proportion of affected women is high. Transmission is heterosexual in 63% of cases, and the mother-to-fetus infection rate is 3%. The 20–39-year age group accounts for 53% of the cases, and 59% of total cases have died. In 1994, an HIV seroprevalence rate of 2% was found among 1,469 persons tested at screening centers.

A survey conducted in 1996 at the family planning centers and the anti-venereal facility showed a 14.3% prevalence rate for *Chlamydia trachomatis* in the under-25 age group.

Tuberculosis and Leprosy. In 1990 and 1991 a tuberculosis outbreak resulted in 18.3 and 16.2 cases per 100,000 population, respectively. This was followed by a decline in the global incidence of tuberculosis, stabilizing at an average rate of 10.8 per 100,000 inhabitants between 1994 and 1996. This reduction in incidence is visible mainly among women. No cases were detected among children under age 15. The BCG immunization rate is 90% among 1-year-olds. The two groups most affected are those over age 65 and 24–44-year-olds (28 and 16 per 100,000, respectively). One-quarter of new cases of tuberculosis occur among the foreign population. Half the cases are contagious and show the presence of Koch's bacillus on direct examination. The tuberculosis/HIV co-infection rate is 27%. The study of antibiotic resistance conducted by the Mycobacteria Center of the Pasteur Institute revealed one case of multidrug resistance.

The leprosy incidence rate (7 new cases in 1995 and 10 in 1996) remains low. In the last two years, 14 of the 17 cases occurred among males. All new cases have been found among persons over the age of 15. The bacillogenic forms predominate (9 in 17 cases). In 1995, there were some 700 cases in the active files, 20% of whom were in treatment and 80% under post-treatment surveillance.

Noncommunicable Diseases and Other Health-Related Problems

Diabetes. Given the estimated 6.6% prevalence of diabetes and the many complications associated with this disease, in 1996 a five-year action plan was developed to address this health problem in Guadeloupe.

Cardiovascular Diseases. An average of 740 deaths resulted from cardiovascular diseases each year during the 1987–1992 period, making it the leading cause of death (33% of all deaths). Cardiovascular disorders cause one death in five in those under age 65. Cerebrovascular disorders cause an average of 320 deaths per year, accounting for 43% of deaths from cardiovascular diseases.

Hypertension is the condition most often requiring hospitalization. Cerebrovascular accidents account for 9% of admissions for circulatory diseases. In 40% of these cases, hospitalization exceeds 10 days. Cardiovascular disorders constitute 41% of all illnesses for which the patient receives full coverage by the health insurance system.

Malignant Tumors. Cancer is the second most common cause of mortality. Prostate cancer in men, cancer of the cervix in women, and stomach cancer in both sexes are quite frequent. Hospital admissions for cancer account for 5% of all hospitalizations.

Accidents and Violence. Road traffic accidents pose a priority public health problem in Guadeloupe. Annually, an average of 98 people die and 568 sustain serious injuries (requiring more than six days in hospital). Sixty-three percent of deaths from road traffic accidents are in the 15–44-year age group. Pedestrians and drivers of two-wheeled vehicles account for 22% and 33% of traffic deaths, respectively. The 15–44-year age group accounts for 69% of those seriously injured.

In 1993, there were 1,565 victims of accidents at work; 10% were serious or fatal.

The main victims of domestic accidents are children under age 5. The principal causes are poisoning by household products, falls, and burns. In 1996, there were 423 reports of child abuse. In 87% of the cases reported to the judicial authorities, removal of the victim was immediate because of extreme violence and/or sexual abuse.

Alcohol, Tobacco, and Drug Use. An annual average of 150 deaths were attributed to alcohol-related problems between 1987 and 1990. The male-to-female ratio of alcoholism is 8:2. Chronic alcoholism is the fourth most frequent cause of premature death (under age of 65), and the third most common pathology associated with hospitalization. Of alcohol-related pathologies, alcoholic psychosis accounts for about 45 deaths a year. The annual average deaths from cancer of the upper digestive tract and cirrhosis of the liver are 55 and 50, respectively.

An average of 150 tobacco-related deaths were recorded during the 1987–1990 period. Of the victims, 60% were men and 40% women, although breakdown varies according to the pathology group. Cancer of the trachea, bronchus, and lungs is increasing, especially in women.

There has been a transition from dependence on marijuana to dependence on crack cocaine in Guadeloupe. There has been an increase in the number of drug addicts treated by the health and social services and in the number questioned about drug use and trafficking. The population using drugs is young (62% were under age 30 and 47% under age 25 in 1994), mainly male (92%), and often falls into the inactive population group (two-thirds of cases). In 1994, the two most commonly used substances were marijuana (64%) and crack cocaine (26%).

Natural Disasters. Guadeloupe is situated in a high-risk zone for natural disasters such as hurricanes, volcanic eruptions, and earthquakes. Hurricanes pose a yearly threat. In 1989, Hurricane Hugo caused considerable damage, as did Hurricanes Luis and Marilyn in 1995.

RESPONSE OF THE HEALTH SYSTEM

Health Services and Resources

Organization and Operation of Personal Health Care Services

The Guadeloupe health system is organized around 25 health establishments; 10 are in the public sector (one regional university hospital center, five hospitals, one psychiatric hospital, two local hospitals, and one long-term care hospital) and 15 are private, for-profit clinics on Basse-Terre and Grande-Terre. As of January 1996, the capacity for short-term medical, surgical, and gynecological/obstetric care was 1,146 beds in public and 900 beds in private facilities. There were 417 beds in public hospitals and 21 in private clinics for psychiatric admissions, with 214 public and 209 private beds available for follow-up and rehabilitation.

Certain specialized care is provided on the two main islands, including: emergency admission and treatment, resuscitation, neonatal care and resuscitation, treatment of chronic kidney failure (322 patients were on dialysis and 7 kidney transplants were performed in 1996), and gynecological/obstetric medical treatment.

MARTINIQUE

Martinique is the northernmost of the Windward Islands; Dominica is its closest neighbor on the north, and Saint Lucia is its neighbor to the south. The island covers an area of 1,130 km² and is mountainous, with Mont Pelée, a dormant volcano rising to 1,400 m, its most prominent physical feature. The administrative and commercial capital is Fort-de-France.

SPECIFIC HEALTH PROBLEMS

Analysis by Population Group

Health of Children

The infant mortality rate in Martinique was halved in 10 years to 5.8 deaths per 1,000 live births in 1995. Perinatal mortality stood at 11.4 per 1,000 total births in 1996. The premature birth rate was 8% in 1996. The proportion of newborns under 2,500 g was 9.4% and those under 1,500 g was 1.3%. In 1995, 699 infants (12% of all births) were hospitalized in the neonatal wards, of whom 2.6% died during the neonatal period. The main causes of death were extreme prematurity and infections.

An average of 60 deaths per year occurred among children between the ages of 1 and 4 (2.8% of all deaths) in the 1987–1990 period. The deaths were attributed to external trauma, ill-defined illnesses, diseases of the nervous system, diseases of the respiratory system, and tumors.

A 1997 survey on immunization coverage in 1-year-olds showed 83% coverage with BCG, 97% with three DTP and polio doses, and 78% with hepatitis B vaccine, which was introduced into the immunization program in 1994.

School attendance is obligatory beginning at 6 years of age. However, one-fourth of 2-year-olds attend school, and nearly all children attend from age 3 onward.

On average, there were 35 recorded deaths each year for the 1987–1990 period among 5–14-year-olds (1.6% of all deaths). More than half were due to external trauma, and tumors. Hospital admissions for this age group were for three main causes: respiratory diseases (24%), diseases of the digestive system (18%), and trauma and poisoning (9%). There was an increase of allergic diseases, including asthma. Some 400 to 500 cases of chickenpox are reported each year, principally among primary school-age children.

Health of Adolescents and Adults

There is almost 100% school enrollment among 15–19-year-olds, and 42% for the 20–24-year age group. Unemployment was highest among 20–24-year-olds, with 52% in 1996.

In the 1987–1990 period an average of 45 deaths occurred each year among 15–24-year-olds, with a male-to-female ratio of 3:1. Road accidents and other violent forms of death predominate among men (69% of deaths in this age group); tumors account for 8% of deaths. Among women in this age group, the external causes of trauma, primarily suicides, predominate (46% of deaths).

Deaths before age 65 account for 29% of all deaths, with a higher prevalence among men (35%) than women (21%). External causes of trauma (accidents, suicide, and violence), tumors, diseases of the circulatory system, and alcohol-related disease account for 75% of these deaths. The preponderance of tumors and disorders of the circulatory system is higher among women than men, while the converse is true for trauma and alcoholism. Nearly half of these deaths appear to be avoidable. In men, they could be avoided by altering high-risk behaviors, while more effective coverage by the health care system would lower the rate for women.

The 1992–1993 hospital morbidity survey showed that for women between the ages of 15 and 64 more than one-third of the hospital stays were related to maternity. This was followed by genitourinary diseases (11%) and digestive ailments (9%). Among men of the same ages, 21% of hospital admissions followed trauma or poisoning, whereas 14% were due to diseases of the circulatory system. Diseases for which social security covers hospitalization for patients between age 15 and 34 include mental disorders (37%), diabetes (9%), sickle cell anemia (8%), and cardiac failure (8%). Diabetes, severe hypertension, and mental disorders are the main conditions requiring hospitalization in the 35–64-year age group.

Health of the Elderly

In 1996, 15% of Martinique's population was 60 or over. The main causes of death for those age 60 and older are cerebrovascular diseases, prostate cancer, and cardiac failure in men, and cerebrovascular diseases, cardiac failure, and diabetes in women. Cancer, hypertension, and diabetes are the most commonly observed pathologies. Hospital admissions increase sharply with age, and adults over age 65 represent 23% of all short-term hospital stays.

The elderly population is still well integrated into the family in Martinique. In the 75–85-year age group, 37% still live at home. The population aged 75 and over live in urban and peripheral urban areas, 28% of them in the capital.

Efforts to reduce unhealthy housing have provided this population group with improved basic sanitation conditions. Only 16% of those age 60 and over have no indoor toilets, and 6% have no source of potable water. Two-thirds own their own homes and 2% live in institutions or as boarders with families.

Reproductive Health

The number of women of childbearing age was estimated at 104,200 in 1996 (52% of the female population). The fertility rate was 1.8 children per woman in 1994, compared with 2.1 in 1990. The birth rate in 1995 was 14.4 per 1,000. Deliveries by girls under age 15 are unusual (1 delivery in 1,000). Deliveries by girls under age 18 account for some 2% of births.

Contraception is accessible to all women either through the private medical system, the Maternal and Child Welfare Service, or family-planning centers. During 1996, the Martiniquan Association for Family Information and Guidance, a private family-planning center, was consulted by 11,312 women, 95% of whom were seeking contraceptives. The pill is prescribed for 78% of women; IUDs are used by 18% of women.

Seven prenatal visits for pregnant women are fully covered by the health care system. The proportion of women rarely or poorly monitored (under four visits) ranges between 7% and 8.5%. In 1996, virtually all births took place in either a hospital or clinic, and 0.3% at home. The public hospitals attend to 68% of deliveries, while 32% take place in private clinics. The cesarean-section rate is 14% in the public sector and 16% in the private. The proportion of multiple pregnancies is stable, at 1.3% in 1996. The maternal mortality rate was 54 deaths per 100,000 births for the 1987–1993 period.

Abortions, which have been legal up to the 10th week of pregnancy since 1982, approximate 2,000 a year. In 1994, 23 abortions per 100 conceptions were recorded. A study of the 1992 statistical records shows that most abortions occur among women between 20 and 30 years of age, with minors representing 5%. These women are most often single (72%) and 62% are students or gainfully employed. Two-thirds had had previous pregnancies and one-fifth had undergone a prior abortion. Abortion is not officially practiced in the private sector, but it does occur owing to the long waiting lists in the public sector. An estimated 20% of abortion requests are not granted.

Health of the Family

The 1990 population census showed that household size in Martinique had decreased sharply, with 14% of households with 6 people or more compared with 30% in the 1974 cen-

sus. In addition, various generations cohabit less often than in the past. In 1990, nearly 4 out of 5 households had a very simple structure: people living alone (21%), adults alone with children (16%), and couples with children (32%) or without children (10%). Also, 39% of children were in single-parent homes. This situation is linked to tradition (women bring up their children alone) and to a more recent development (the breakup of couples). Moreover, 77% of children under age 7 come from homes where both parents (or the single parent) practice a profession.

Health of the Disabled

The disability prevalence rate among children age 10–19 years is 12.6 per 1,000. The most frequently observed impairments are intellectual (36%) and other psychological deficiencies (21%). There are approximately 100 children acutely affected and suffering from multiple handicaps. Over half of these children have been placed in specialized institutions or receive institutional monitoring. The number of disabled adults (over age 20) is estimated at 15,000. Over 5,000 receive a disabled adult allowance. Fewer than 3% live in specialized institutions.

A 1994 survey revealed that visual impairment affected an estimated 5% of the disabled population between 20 and 60 years old.

Analysis by Type of Disease or Health Impairment

Communicable Diseases

Vector-Borne Diseases. In Martinique malaria is entirely imported and its annual incidence is low. No cases of yellow fever have been recorded. In 1995 and 1996 yellow fever immunizations were given to 3,164 and 3,951 persons, respectively, by the Departmental Hygiene Laboratory.

Dengue epidemics occur annually. The annual incidence of dengue-2 and -4 was approximately 2 cases per 10,000 inhabitants in 1993, increasing to 14 per 10,000 in 1995 owing to pronounced hurricane activity. There were 9 cases per 10,000 inhabitants in 1996. These cases were all confirmed by serology. The upsurge of cases takes place in August–September, peaking in December–January. In 1995, three cases of dengue hemorrhagic fever were recorded, with one death. In 1996, 14 cases were reported, but there were no deaths.

Vaccine-Preventable Diseases. No cases of poliomyelitis, diphtheria, or whooping cough have been reported to the health authorities for more than 10 years. Recorded cases of measles mainly affected children with an average age of 9. In

1995, 8 laboratory-confirmed cases were reported, and 13 in 1996. The immunization coverage survey conducted by the departmental authorities in January 1997 showed it to be 90% for the Department as a whole. There have been no cases of neonatal tetanus since the end of the 1970s. However, cases of tetanus do occur among the elderly (11 per year), owing to their loss of vaccine immunity. Since 1990, the measles, mumps, and rubella triple vaccine was applied in systematic immunization campaigns. Influenza syndromes have been reported to the Departmental Bureau of Health and Social Affairs by the sentinel doctor network since 1995. In 1996, 10,064 cases were reported.

In February 1992 a decree mandated testing for HBsAg during the sixth month of pregnancy. A seroprevalence survey conducted in Martinique on a sample of 492 women who gave birth in 1993 revealed a prevalence of 0.6% for HBsAg. A second survey conducted by the Maternal and Child Welfare from August 1992 to June 1993 on 1,000 pregnant women showed a prevalence of 1.13%. Hepatitis C affects an estimated 3,000 persons in Martinique. As of March 1996, 44 patients had been admitted to the chronic hepatitis C unit.

Cholera and Other Intestinal Diseases. There have been no reported cases of cholera in Martinique.

Salmonella is the most common etiological agent of food poisoning (68.1% of sources for which a causal agent was identified). The number of cases of *Salmonella typhi* is steadily decreasing, confirming the disappearance of major epidemics of typhoid and paratyphoid fevers long considered to be the most important communicable disease in Martinique. An average of 14 cases are reported per month, most (30 cases) occur in the month of August.

Between August 1995 and July 1996, 14 cases of ciguatera were admitted to hospital and an additional 32 cases were reported but not admitted. The annual incidence rate is 1.2 cases per 10,000 inhabitants. With high incidence throughout the year, viral gastroenteritis epidemics are the prime cause of diarrhea in Martinique. There has been a 90% reduction in cases of hookworm and 80% in cases of threadworm in the last six years owing to a higher level of hygiene, preventive activities, and Departmental Bureau of Health and Social Affairs screening. High-risk population groups (military recruits and farm workers) are systematically screened, but because of their risk status, screening results cannot be applied to the population at large. Polyparasitism (hookworm and threadworm or *Schistosoma mansoni*) were detected in 5% of the cases.

Tuberculosis and Leprosy. The incidence of tuberculosis fell from 66 cases in 1982 to 33 in 1995. A retrospective study of all 178 tuberculosis cases from 1990 to 1995 shows a drop in the average age of patients, from 57.5 years of age in 1991 to 48.4 year of age in 1995, probably due to HIV co-infection.

The most frequent form of the disease is pulmonary (82%). Out of 169 cases documented, 6% have suffered a relapse. Most cases (92%) are found in Martiniquans. While the number of tuberculosis sufferers infected with HIV has been falling since 1993, HIV-positive individuals are at 900 times greater risk for contracting tuberculosis. The extra-pulmonary forms of the disease are encountered particularly in HIV co-infection.

Out of 195 cases of leprosy followed by health institutions, in the active population, 92% were seen during 1996. Of the 458 patients under observation without treatment, 79.2% were examined in 1996.

AIDS. The AIDS epidemic in Martinique poses a priority public health problem. As of 1 January 1997, 402 cases of AIDS had been reported; 26% in women and 74% in men. Since the onset of the epidemic, 262 people have died of AIDS. HIV seropositivity is not subject to any notification, and only known AIDS cases are reported.

There were 44 new AIDS cases reported in 1992, 43 in 1993, 49 in 1994, 38 in 1995 and 35 in 1996. The epidemic has stabilized and is probably on the decline. Heterosexual infection is 82% among women and 60% among men, or 64% for both sexes combined. This predominance is not due to under-representation of other transmission groups, but is caused by the increase in heterosexual transmission. A survey conducted in 1994 on sexual behavior in the Antilles and French Guiana revealed the significance of constant multiple partners in the French Departments. No socioprofessional class or age group has escaped the AIDS epidemic in Martinique.

Because of exceedingly strict regulation regarding blood-transfusion, the virus is no longer transmitted by that route. Improved coverage of seropositive pregnant women has reduced transmission of the virus from mother to child to approximately 10%; there are currently 14 infected children.

Martinique has a departmental AIDS control scheme. Funds allocated for AIDS control amount to 6 million francs for prevention, and 20 million francs for treatment. The treatment provided in Martinique is progressive. Tritherapy began in June 1996, and some 250 patients receive bi- or tritherapy. There are approximately 400 persons monitored for seropositivity at all stages, and the viral load of patients is now routinely measured.

Noncommunicable Diseases and Other Health-Related Problems

Nutritional Diseases and Diseases of Metabolism. No diseases linked to nutritional deficiencies have been recorded for over 10 years. However, a higher socioeconomic level has brought about changes in eating behaviors, with the ensuing excess-linked diseases (obesity, diabetes, and high choles-terol). An average of 85 deaths from diabetes are recorded each year (4% of all deaths). Diabetes accounts for 22% of hospital-izations that are fully covered by the social security system.

Cardiovascular Diseases. Cardiovascular disorders are the leading cause of mortality in Martinique. An average of 740 deaths, 30% of all deaths, were recorded each year in the 1990–1992 period. The impact of cardiovascular disorders on premature deaths (i.e., deaths between the ages of 1 and 64) is the same for both sexes, representing 21% of premature deaths.

The Social Security Code provides for coverage of 30 "long-term" diseases, or those requiring protracted or expensive treatment. Cardiovascular disorders, primarily acute hyper-tension and cerebrovascular accidents, account for 40% of long-term admissions each year. Cardiovascular disorders also account for 8% of all short-term admissions, placing them in fourth place among reasons for hospitalization. Hypertension is estimated to occur in 20% of the general population.

Malignant Tumors. Every year some 500 deaths from ma-lignant tumors are recorded; tumors are responsible for one-quarter of deaths among men and one-fifth of deaths among women. Standardized cancer mortality rates dropped by 10% in the 1980s. All cancer cases have been recorded in Mar-tinique since 1981. Cancer incidence in Martinique is lower than that found in other regions and countries of the world.

The prostate cancer rate among men is high and on the in-crease. Ear, nose, and throat cancers are particularly wide-spread, while the incidence of broncho-pulmonary cancers is low. Among women, the incidence of cancer of the cervix is very high and breast cancer somewhat low. The incidence of cancer of the esophagus and stomach is high for both sexes, while there are few colon and rectal cancer cases. The cancer registry shows that between 1981 and 1990 there were 153 cases of oral cancer among men and 30 among women.

Accidents and Violence. There was an annual average of 51 road accident deaths between 1991 and 1994. Mortality rates have leveled off since 1992 but the number of serious in-juries is increasing. Of all road accident deaths in 1994, 34% were drivers of two-wheeled vehicles, 48% were driving cars, and 19% were pedestrians. Serious road accident victims in-volving two-wheeled vehicles are more common among teenagers and young adults. The under 15-year age group comprises the most victims among pedestrians.

In 1993 there were 2,722 work accidents. Eight deaths oc-curred (six involving travel), and 112 accidents had late effects.

An average of 40 suicides per year were recorded in the 1987–1990 period (1.9% of deaths). The suicide rates are higher among men over 65. The suicide mortality rate in-creased among men, but dropped slightly among women

since the 1982–1984 period. There was an annual average of seven homicides in the 1987–1990 period.

Substance Abuse. During 1990–1992, an average of 131 alcohol-related deaths were recorded each year, accounting for 6% of all deaths. Alcohol-related deaths account for 9.2% of all male deaths compared with 2.2% of all female deaths. The 45–64-year age group is the most affected.

During the 1990–1993 period, an annual average of 147 deaths attributable to tobacco were recorded (7% of all deaths).

Marijuana has long been the most widely consumed illicit drug in Martinique. Crack cocaine entered the scene in the early 1980s and is currently widely used, alone or in conjunc-tion with marijuana. In November 1995, the health and social services treated 198 drug addicts. Illegal drug activity dou-bled between 1992 and 1995.

Behavioral Disorders. Mental disorders are a major public health problem. Psychiatric treatment of adults in Mar-tinique is concentrated in a single hospital. A study of diag-noses of hospitalized patients reveals a considerable propor-tion of schizophrenia and other psychoses. There are 470 beds for psychiatric hospitalization.

The child and juvenile psychiatry units provide a network of community services in Martinique. A day clinic with 15 places for autistic and similarly affected children under 11 years of age has been in operation since 1993.

Oral Health. A survey of children aged 6–10 years shows that 30% suffer from tooth decay. This is most often encoun-tered in families living in a vulnerable social situation. There is no fluorine in the water in Martinique and supplementa-tion by fluoridated salt or fluorine pills is necessary.

Sickle Cell Anemia. Sickle cell anemia is the most com-mon genetic disease in the Antilles. The detection coverage rate in Martinique is 99%. Two studies have shown that 10% of the population bore some sickle cell trait, 0.17% of the sub-jects being SS and 0.24% SC. One union in 65 poses a risk, and 15 to 20 children will be born annually with a phenotype that triggers a major sickle cell syndrome. In addition, 600 children (i.e., nearly 10%) will be born with the sickle cell trait.

RESPONSE OF THE HEALTH SYSTEM

Health Services and Resources

Organization of Services for Care of the Population

Health and the Environment. Water for consumption is subject to intensive controls and is of high quality. Some 23 parameters are regularly checked and warning procedures are in place in the event that contaminants exceed certain levels. The pesticides used in agriculture must conform to national standards. Pesticides have not been found in the drinking water supply. Industrial medicine covers poisoning prevention; in the last 10 years cases of poisoning have fallen by 90%, standing at present at five cases per year.

Organization of public services regarding health and environmental issues involves six State units, as well as local communities. Special groups are encouraged to study specific environmental problems.

Atmospheric pollution in Martinique is limited to that caused by automobile emissions in urban centers and along major highways. Burning of sugar cane fields or rum production produce very low levels of pollution, and there is virtually no industrial air pollution. New cars are required to be equipped with catalytic exhaust systems. An increasing number of automobiles use unleaded gas (approximately 30%).

Organization and Operation of Personal Health Care Services

The regional health organization plan in Martinique includes an "emergency" and "resuscitation" section. It comprises three public hospitals (including one teaching hospital), and three private clinics. The public sector offers 1,831 beds for short-term hospitalization, 114 beds for follow-up and functional rehabilitation, and 101 beds for medium-term care. The private sector provides 100 beds for short-term care, 39 for follow-up and functional rehabilitation, and 61 for medium-term care. Specialties are provided in all categories and offer a full range of treatment.

Ambulatory care provided includes home dialysis, alcohol and cancer control centers, and a multiple-addiction center.

Emergency medical care is given special attention in the regional health organization plan. The current organization is based on a single emergency telephone number, through which calls can be made free of charge.

GRENADA

GENERAL SITUATION AND TRENDS

Socioeconomic, Political, and Demographic Overview

Grenada lies at the southern end of the Windward Islands and comprises three sister islands: Grenada, Carriacou, and Petit Martinique. Grenada is situated between 12° North and 60° West and is about 100 miles north of Venezuela and 90 miles southwest of Barbados. The country's total land area extends for 133 mi².

The capital, St. George's, is located in the parish of St. George, and has an approximate population of 31,994 (33% of the total population). In 1991, the parish of St. Andrew had a population of 24,135 persons (25% of the population), followed by St. David, with 11,011 (12%); St. Patrick, with 10,118 (11%); St. John, with 8,752 (9%); and St. Mark, with 3,861 (4%). According to the 1991 population census, 6% of the population, or 5,000 persons lived in Carriacou and 726 persons lived in Petit Martinique.

The gross domestic product (GDP) at factor cost in constant 1990 prices was US$ 195.1 million in 1995 (about US$ 1,980 per capita), which represents a 5.3% increase from the 1992 figure, when it was US$ 185.3 million (US$ 1,920 per capita). Annual inflation between 1992 and 1995 averaged 2.6%. The tourism sector grew annually at a rate of 10% over the period.

Tourism was the most vibrant sector between 1992 and 1995—its percentage contribution to the GDP increased by 23.3%, moving from 7.3% to 9.0%. Stay-over visitors jumped from 87,554 to 108,007 during this period, an increase of 23.4%. In 1995, there were 446 cruise ships that came to the island, up 3.5% from the 1992 figure; they brought 249,879 visitors, representing a 27.6% increase over the number in 1992.

Agricultural production of traditional crops such as cocoa, nutmeg, and bananas had mixed success between 1992 and 1995. Cocoa production increased by 17%, nutmeg's de-

creased by 24%, and bananas's decreased by 32%. The combined production of these crops fell by 26.1% between 1996 and 1995, primarily due to a 57% drop in banana production. Other agricultural crops had fairly stable production during the period.

Telecommunications were significantly enhanced between 1992 and 1995, with the most modern services and communication technologies available by the end of that period. The single electricity generating plant was privatized in 1994, and there are plans for expanding its capacity.

The rate of inflation has remained relatively unchanged, increasing slightly from 2.1% in 1995 to 3.1% in 1996. Based on the findings from the 1996 Labour Force Survey, 6,835 persons between the ages of 15 and 60 years old were unemployed, for an unemployment rate of 13.6%. The survey also revealed that women accounted for 68% (4,844) and persons 15–29 years old accounted for 56% (3,826) of the total unemployed population.

The Government changed in 1995, when the New National Party replaced the National Democratic Congress. The new administration is committed to establishing a statutory body to manage the entire public health care system. As the first step in this process, a board of directors will be created to manage the General Hospital.

Total public sector recurrent expenditure in 1996 was US$ 68.1 million, slightly higher than the US$ 68 million spent in 1995, and 7.5% higher than the US$ 63.3 million spent in 1992. Health expenditures were US$ 8.2 million in 1992, US$ 8.0 million in 1993, US$ 8.2 million in 1994, US$ 8.7 million in 1995, by 10.7% (US$ 9.6 million) in 1996. This shows that health expenditures increased approximately 17% from 1992 to 1996, which more than doubled the 7.5% national increase on all expenditures over the same period. In 1996, per capita recurrent health expenditure was US$ 97.10.

Grenada implemented a structural adjustment program between 1992 and 1994. Reforms focused on reducing public sector expenditure; stimulating private sector growth; providing incentives for projects related to tourism, manufacturing, and informatics; and facilitating the privatization of Government assets. During that period, the value of Government services as a percentage of GDP declined from 19% to 16.6%, decreasing further to 15.9% in 1995.

The adult literacy rate was estimated at 85% in 1996. During the 1994–1995 academic year, 3,448 children between the ages of 1 and 5 years old were registered in 73 public preschools. In that same year, there were 2,595 new admissions into the primary school system, resulting in 23,017 students enrolled in the 58 public primary schools; there were 869 teachers, with a student-to-teacher ratio of 26:1 in the public primary schools. There also are 16 private primary schools in the country. During the same academic year, 1,448 students were registered at the 19 secondary schools for the first time, resulting in a total enrollment of 7,260, with 41% males and 59% females. There were 381 secondary-school teachers, with a teacher-to-student ratio of 1:19. Between 1992 and 1995, there were 1,039 dropouts from the primary school system (59% males and 41% females) and, during that same period, there were 403 dropouts from the secondary school system (44% males and 56% females).

Population

Grenada's estimated population in mid-1995 was 98,500, 50.8% female and 49.2% male. The population structure was very young, with 47,313 persons (or 48.3% of the total population) below the age of 20 years. With life expectancy currently estimated at 68 years for men and 72 years for women, the population group aged 60 years old and older is expected to increase over the next decade.

Total live births have declined over the last decade, dropping from 3,107 in 1985 to 2,372 in 1992, and 2,286 in 1995. The crude birth rate decreased by 27%, declining from 34.0 per 1,000 population in 1985, to 24.6 per 1,000 population in 1992, and to 5.3% to 23.3 per 1,000 population in 1995, for a 5.3% decline. The crude death rate has been fairly stable; it was 8.2 per 1,000 population in 1995. The rate of natural increase in the population ranged between 20 and 26 for most of the 1980s, and was estimated between 15 and 17 per 1,000 population during the 1992–1995 period. The total fertility rate over the period averaged 3.2 children per woman of childbearing age.

In 1995, 28% of mothers delivered their first baby, 19% delivered their second child, and 16% delivered their third, a pattern similar to that observed in 1994. In the latter year, 26.1% of births were to women aged 20–24 years old, and teenage mothers accounted for 16.9% of all births, a change from 1992 percentages of 28.6% and 18.3%, respectively.

Mortality Profile

The quality of mortality data has improved in recent years, and there are ongoing efforts to build on those gains. For example, as a way to improve the completion of death certificates, seminars will be conducted with physicians to bring the reporting system in line with the requirements of the *International Classification of Diseases.*

In 1992 and 1995, leading causes of death included diseases of pulmonary circulation and other forms of heart disease, with 131 deaths and 119 deaths, respectively, and with corresponding rates per 100,000 population of 136.2 and 120.8. Other leading causes of death during these same years were cerebrovascular disease, with 94 and 114 deaths, respectively, and mortality rates of 97.7 and 115.7 per 100,000; malignant neoplasms with 72 and 95 deaths and mortality rates of 74.8 and 96.4; ischemic heart disease, with 30 and 51 deaths and mortality rates of 31.2 and 51.8; diseases of the urinary system, with 22 and 33 deaths and mortality rates of 22.9 and 33.5; endocrine and metabolic diseases, with 25 and 32 deaths and mortality rates of 26.0 and 32.5; certain conditions originating in the perinatal period, with 21 and 38 deaths and mortality rates of 21.8 and 38.6.

Morbidity

During 1992–1995, there were 31,440 admissions to the General Hospital, with an average length of stay of 6.1 days and a bed occupancy rate of 60%. Admissions and discharges from the General Hospital are categorized by service and diagnosis, but only data on service are regularly compiled into a report.

The older population is primarily affected by diabetes, hypertension, and coronary or cardiovascular diseases and their complications. For persons screened in the district health services over 1992–1995, between 8.5% and 14.1% were diagnosed with diabetes mellitus and between 10.5% and 11.7%, with hypertension.

Data on morbidity—which is limited to information about persons seeking treatment in the public primary health care system and reflects only notifiable diseases—show that the main causes of infant morbidity continue to be respiratory tract infections, gastroenteritis, and diarrhea. Data for 1996 show that the main causes of morbidity in children 0–4 years old also are respiratory tract infections (4,772), gastroenteritis (957), and diarrhea (550). Between 1992 and 1996, reported data show an alarming increase in gastroenteritis in children, increasing by 60% in children under 5 years old and by 73.5% in those older than 5. Better monitoring has contributed to the increase in reported cases in 1996, however.

SPECIFIC HEALTH PROBLEMS

Analysis by Population Group

Health of Children

Between 1992 and 1995, there were 119 deaths in children under 1 year of age, with 48% of these deaths occurring within the first day of life. The leading causes of death were congenital anomalies of the heart and circulatory system, hypoxia, birth asphyxia, other respiratory conditions, slow fetal growth, and fetal malnutrition and immaturity. In the same period, 27 children aged 1–4 years old died, with the leading causes of death in this cohort being diseases of the nervous system, the respiratory system, and the digestive system. In the age group 5–9 years old, 16 children died during the period.

The proportion of low-birthweight babies ranged between 9.7% and 10.6% of total births in 1992–1995. The infant mortality rate in 1992 was 10.5 per 1,000 live births, increasing to 14.4 per 1,000 and 14.6 per 1,000 in 1993 and 1994, respectively, and decreasing to 12.7 per 1,000 live births in 1995. The neonatal mortality rate was 9.9, 9.8, and 7.4 per 1,000 live births for the years 1993, 1994, and 1995, respectively.

According to data on the estimated population of children under 5 years old and the number of first visits to well-baby clinics, more than 80% of this age group is seen by trained personnel in the public sector. On their first visit in a given year, children are weighed and measured—during the 1992–1995 period, between 1% and 2% of children who came for their first visit were found to be either underweight or overweight. No information is available for children who visit private doctors exclusively. In 1995, the Ministry of Health instituted a campaign to encourage more breast-feeding. A total of 1,154 infants were seen at age 3 months, and of these, 397, or 34.4%, had been solely breast-fed for the first three months of life.

Health of Adolescents

In 1995, the country had an estimated 21,000 persons between the ages of 10 and 19 years old, and most were attending primary or secondary school. Data for 1996 show that 2,503 teenagers were employed.

Fertility rates among teenage women have continued to decline, dropping from 92.9 per 1,000 to 82.4 between 1992 and 1995. Teenage pregnancies decreased by 9.7%, from 433 to 391 births, representing 18.3% and 17.1% of total births in those years. In 1994 and 1995, 75% of teenage mothers delivered their first babies and 5% recorded their third or subsequent deliveries. The number of births registered by mothers under age 15 years increased from 8 in 1994 to 17 in 1995.

There were 45 incarcerations of teenagers in 1995, 60% of which were for theft. There were 10 deaths within this age group, representing about 1% of total deaths.

Health of Women

It is estimated that approximately 78% of pregnant women attended prenatal clinics held in community health facilities and were seen primarily by a nurse. Only 5% to 7% of these women, however, registered their first visit before the 12th week of pregnancy, while 80% of those who attended did so by the 16th week of pregnancy or later. Some pregnant women visited a private physician prior to seeking attention at public prenatal facilities.

In 1995, 948 post-natal women requested family planning services in the district health services. Of these, 65% requested advice pertaining to family-planning options; 25% requested condoms; 7%, sterilization; and the rest sought advice mainly regarding intrauterine devices or injection. The Grenada Planned Parenthood Association also provides family planning services; in 1996, the Association provided services to 1,266 women, compared to 1,729 in 1995.

Health of the Elderly

Mid-year data indicate that persons 60 years old and older represent 10.8% of the total population (10,648 persons)—59% were women and 41% were men. Data also showed that 31% of households were headed by persons 60 years old and older, 53% of them by women and 47% by males. Among the elderly, 30% live alone, a percentage that is equally distributed between the genders. In 1996, 8.9% of the labor force (38,078 persons) were 60 years old and older, of which 59% were men and 41%, women. There are 13 homes that care for the elderly (1 public and 12 private), and a nongovernmental organization also works specifically with this age group.

Health of the Disabled

The National Council for the Disabled is the main body responsible for activities pertaining to this population group; it is charged with providing support for physically and mentally disabled persons and their parents. During 1997, the Council investigated the number of persons with disabilities in the country.

Analysis by Type of Disease or Health Impairment

Communicable Diseases

Vector-Borne Diseases. As a way to keep the spread of dengue fever in check, the mosquito control program continues to try to reduce the *Aedes aegypti* population. The main methods used are chemical control throughout the country, focusing on high-risk areas, and health education programs that encourage the public to maintain a clean and healthy environment. Source reduction and biological control with a heavy emphasis on community participation are being increasingly used.

After having had no cases of dengue fever in 1992 and an average of fewer than 10 in the following three years, there were 21 cases in 1996.

Rabies. The environmental health department continued to work toward reducing the incidence of rabies through the annual vaccination of domestic animals throughout the island, in an effort to break the link between the transmission of the rabies virus from the mongoose to man.

Vaccine-Preventable Diseases. In 1996, immunization coverage of children under 1 year old was lower than the expected standard for the country, showing an overall decline compared to previous years—80% were immunized against diphtheria, tetanus, whooping cough, and poliomyelitis and 85% were immunized against measles. A senior community health nurse has been charged with coordinating the program, and better monitoring is being put in place. All health centers have been visited in order to review how the target population is identified within each district, and staff were given guidance on possible improvements.

Legislation enacted in 1980, and currently being reviewed and updated, mandates that all children under 13 years old must be immunized against diphtheria, whooping cough, tetanus, measles, and poliomyelitis. There have been no reported cases of neonatal tetanus in the last two decades; immunization coverage of women attending the public prenatal services in 1995 exceeded 80%. The Ministry also provides immunization against mumps and rubella as part of the program, and the reintroduction of immunization against tuberculosis is being considered.

AIDS and Other Sexually Transmitted Diseases. The AIDS epidemic continues to progress slowly in Grenada. The cumulative total of reported HIV-infected persons stood at 141 at the end of 1996, with a male-to-female ratio of 2:1. Of these, 7 were pediatric cases, 3 of which died. All the pediatric cases have been linked to vertical transmission during pregnancy. In 1996, 19 new HIV-infected cases have been reported;

3 pediatric cases were reported that year. This is the first year in which more than one case has been reported. In 1996, 17 cases of AIDS were reported, resulting in a cumulative total of 96 cases—70 men and 26 women—of which 71 died.

The number of cases of syphilis reported to the Ministry of Health dropped from 127 in 1992 to 54 in 1996, a reduction of more than 57%. In 1996 there were 112 gonorrhea cases, more than double that of the previous year. These figures may understate the true numbers, since most persons tend to seek a private physician to treat these diseases. It is imperative for private doctors to provide this information so that the Ministry of Health can better assess the situation.

Noncommunicable Diseases and Other Health-Related Problems

Environmental Health, Water Supply, Sewerage Systems, and Solid Waste Disposal. The Ministry of Health's Environmental Health Department is responsible for controlling water pollution; improving wastewater treatment; ensuring that the population has access to an adequate supply of safe drinking water; improving systems for the disposal of excreta and other substances harmful to human, animal, and plant life; and improving the country's food hygiene. The department is staffed by 14 environmental health officers.

Grenada has no national policies or organized programs to combat coastal pollution, but is cognizant of the various international agreements protecting the Caribbean Sea from pollution. Legislation pertaining to environmental health is being revised, and the anti-litter act is currently being processed.

The 1991 Census of Population and Housing indicates that 50.2% of Grenadians had their water supply piped into their dwellings, another 13.4% had water piped into their yards, 7.5% had private catchments, and 21.1% used public standpipes. The National Water and Sewerage Authority estimates that in January 1994, the percentage of households with pipe connections was about 59%, which means that about 85% of the population has access to potable water—96.4% in St. George's and 76.1% in the rest of the country.

The Ministry of Health is responsible for monitoring water quality, but its resources are insufficient to do so. The National Water and Sewerage Authority currently handles the monitoring, and submits periodic reports to the Ministry through the Chief Medical Officer. The Ministry is working to acquire its own quality monitoring capabilities through the Caribbean Environmental Health Institute (CEHI) and in conjunction with resource personnel provided by the Produce Chemist Laboratory.

According to the 1991 census, 59% of households used pit latrines, 33% used septic tanks, 3% were linked to a sewerage system, and 3.9% (more than 850 households) had no toilet facilities. The St. George's Sewerage system was upgraded in 1992, and in 1993, the Grand Anse Sewerage project was put in place.

The introduction of the 1995 Solid Waste Act established the Solid Waste Management Authority, a statutory body intended to accomplish a more efficient system of removal and disposal of garbage. These functions previously carried out by the MOH are now privatized and contractors have the responsibility to keep the country clean. The MOH will continue its regulatory role in its monitoring of solid waste management in the country.

Food Safety. The Ministry of Health continues to upgrade the food handling and processing situation with the objective of reducing foodborne diseases. Several workshops have been held and will continue to be held for itinerant vendors to provide information and support for better food-handling practices.

Nutritional Diseases. The Grenada Food and Nutrition Council is a statutory body managed by an intersectoral Board of Directors and ultimately responsible to the Minister of Agriculture. The Council works closely with the Ministry of Health to implement joint programs and conduct district- and hospital-level research.

There is no active monitoring of the prevalence of iodine or vitamin A deficiencies in Grenada.

In 1996, the Council launched a project to monitor iron deficiency anemia in the population. The project will develop a protocol for the treatment of anemia and investigate the causes of the high prevalence of anemia in different population segments. Preliminary results show that between April and September 1996, 30% of pregnant women attending prenatal clinics for the first time during their pregnancies had hemoglobin levels under 10 g/dl, and that 34% of those attended clinics in the rural parish of St. Andrew. Of the total 626 children under age 1 year who were screened, 55% showed hemoglobin concentrations under 11g/dl, indicating that iron deficiency anemia in children of this age group was a problem throughout the island. Of the 2,667 children aged between 4 and 5 years old who were checked, 39% had hemoglobin concentrations under 11g/dl.

Staff in the maternal and child health program check the hemoglobin levels in infants to estimate the incidence of anemia in that population. In 1995 and 1996, the program was improved so that every health center could conduct the screening. Of the 2,680 infants who made their first visit to the maternal and child health service in 1996, 629, or 23.5%, had hemoglobin levels under 11g/dl.

This iron deficiency screening will be expanded to cover other age groups, and the data will be used with other Min-

istry data to monitor the prevalence of iron deficiency anemia.

It was difficult to get an accurate picture of the country's nutritional situation, because the information on local food production and consumption was limited.

Behavioral Disorders. Since its establishment in 1986, the National Drug Avoidance Committee has worked to "shape policies and oversee the implementation of action programs aimed at reducing the demand for drugs and alcohol." A national master plan for the 1997–2001 period has been completed. The plan assesses the country's drug problem, proposes a strategy for dealing with it, and outlines activities to be implemented, resource requirements, and persons responsible for various parts of the plan.

The committee has compiled drug-abuse data in collaboration with the police, the prisons, and the Ministry of Health, which has supplied information about Carlton House, a substance abuse rehabilitation center, and Rathdune, the acute psychiatric unit in the General Hospital.

RESPONSE OF THE HEALTH SYSTEM

National Health Plans and Policies

Grenada's health policy aims at ensuring that every Grenadian has access to quality health services. The Government has embraced primary health care as the main strategy for improving the population's health status and attaining "health for all by the year 2000"; it also has adopted the goals and targets established through the Caribbean Cooperation in Health initiative as the priorities for its health services.

The country has undergone an epidemiological transition that has moved chronic diseases ahead of communicable diseases as causes of morbidity and mortality. This change is placing greater demand on the health sector's limited resources. It should be said, however, that despite the demand, everyone in Grenada has access to public health services, regardless of their ability to pay.

The Government is decentralizing the health services and placing them under the management of a board of directors established by law. As part of an effort to introduce a national health insurance program, the financing of the health services also is being reviewed. The insurance program would create an equitable way of injecting new resources into the health sector, contribute to improve the quality of care, and help to reduce the dependence on the central government for health sector financing. The proposal for implementing the health insurance program is being reviewed to ensure that it responds to Grenada's needs and that both health care providers and the public understand it fully.

In conjunction with the Ministry of Finance's Central Statistical Office, the Ministry of Health will undertake a community health needs assessment in 1997, which will become the basis for developing a national health plan for 1998–2002. The plan, which will be formulated through an intersectoral approach involving broad public consultation, will chart the health sector's direction. Projects designed to strengthen health programs and ensure the orderly development of the health sector will be identified. The Ministry's organizational structure will be one of the first issues to be addressed in preparing the plan, since it will affect the overall management system. In addition, strategies will seek to establish an environment in which health workers can be as productive as possible to facilitate infrastructure development and to improve the quality of care provided to the population. More complete information will be gathered on the population of each health district, in order to have a clearer view of the population's health profile. Finally, indigents who cannot pay for health services will be identified, and special provisions will be put in place so that they, too, have access to health care.

Because every health worker is considered to be a health educator, further staff training is planned, as is the organization of activities to reach the community effectively. The school health program will be particularly emphasized, because it is one of the best ways to effectively reach the country's youth to help improve their lifestyles.

Organization of the Health Sector

Institutional Organization

Grenada is divided into seven health districts. Six of the districts have a health center, which is the major primary care facility, and an additional 30 medical stations distributed throughout the country are usually the first point of contact within the health system. All facilities are within easy access to the entire population, and most are in satisfactory physical condition.

The community health services function as the Ministry's front line for health service delivery. Each health district is assigned a District Medical Officer; several categories of nurses, including family nurse practitioners, public health nurses, district nurses, and community health aides; dentists and dental auxiliaries; pharmacists; and environmental health officers.

Secondary care is provided through a network of hospitals. The acute care facilities in the public sector include a 240-bed at St. George's General Hospital and two rural hospitals, Princess Alice, with 60 beds and the Princess Royal, with 40. The General Hospital is in disrepair, and the Government plans to refurbish it; the design is under way, and financing for the project is being secured.

A 20-bed acute psychiatric unit is located on the grounds of the General Hospital, and it serves as the entry point for those seeking psychiatric care and support. There also is an 80-bed psychiatric hospital (Mt. Gay), which handles chronic patients, and a geriatric facility with 120 beds; occupancy rates usually exceed 100% at both. Carlton House provides support and assistance to substance abuse patients.

As part of its rationalization study of health facilities, the Ministry will analyze utilization levels to determine whether it would be better to have fewer, better equipped, and better staffed facilities. The study also will recommend a maintenance schedule for all facilities based on their current state and realistic projections of financial resources.

The health sector's basic organization has remained unchanged in recent years. Most program heads are based at Ministry of Health headquarters, as are those for administrative, planning, health promotion, and budget and expenditure.

In 1992, the budgets for Carriacou and Petit Martinique health services were consolidated under one program, which has led to better monitoring of resources and a more integrated management and delivery of health care services in the two sister islands. An administrator for the consolidated program was appointed in 1996.

Between 1992 and 1996, there were four ministers of health, five chief medical officers, five permanent secretaries, and three medical officers of health. This turnover in the Ministry has broken continuity, which, in turn, has hindered overall health sector management. In order to achieve its goals, the Ministry of Health has relied heavily on department heads for preparing and implementing program plans and budgets.

Organization of Health Regulatory Activities

A Medical Board chaired by the Chief Medical Officer is responsible for granting medical licenses to practice medicine in Grenada. Nurses must register with the Nursing Council. Once granted, medical licenses need not be renewed annually, and the doctor need not pursue continued education or prove to be physically fit to practice. A pharmacy council monitors the importation and distribution of pharmaceuticals to the public and private sectors and registers pharmacists and pharmacies on an annual basis.

Health Services and Resources

Organization of Services for Care of the Population

Health Promotion and Community Participation. The Ministry of Health relies on health promotion as one of its main approaches for improving the overall health of the public. The Health Education Department, a well-established unit within the Ministry, has been working toward improving the health sector's links with other sectors. Several workshops have been held for health workers, teachers, religious and community leaders, and NGO members to ensure that every health worker knows that he or she is a health educator and shows a commitment to an intersectoral, community-based approach to health promotion.

The Health Education Department has involved the community in the planning of health activities, including participating in the health needs assessment, the organization of community health fairs, and the participation discussions about issues such as AIDS and chronic diseases. As a way to help institutionalize health and family life education in schools, a health education curriculum is being developed with the Ministry of Education.

To date, the community has only been minimally involved in the planning and implementation of national health activities, and its involvement varies considerably from district to district. In its planned revitalization of the primary health care program, however, the Ministry will involve the community in the development and implementation of health programs.

Several NGOs are involved in health promotion programs in the community. For example, the Grenada Planned Parenthood Association conducts a youth outreach program through which counselors visit schools and community groups to speak on family life and sex education issues. Three times a year, they also conduct a 15-week program for adolescents and school dropouts that teaches them coping skills and helps them with academic work.

Moreover, health promotion continues to be the primary mechanism used to foster lifestyle changes to avoid health problems, especially those targeting better diet and more exercise. Public and private groups will be integrally involved in planning programs targeting lifestyle changes.

Diabetes and hypertension, both of which are prevalent in the country, are conditions that have been linked to a person's lifestyle. The Ministry of Health's Education Department has emphasized programs that provide information pertaining to these chronic diseases, particularly those that can lead to positive lifestyle changes. The Department also relies on radio programs, community forums, health fairs, and programs in schools as part of its work.

A family life education curriculum has been developed for secondary schools, but not all schools have put it in place. Teaching the curriculum is left up to the discretion of the principal or teacher; many parents strongly object to their children being taught "sex education."

The Ministry also works closely with NGOs in programs aimed at influencing the public's behavior. For example, the Grenada Planned Parenthood Association, which primarily focuses on providing family planning services, also operates a youth center staffed by a nurse, who conducts clinics, and a youth officer, who conducts outreach programs in schools and communities and has a weekly radio magazine program. They also provide training in a range of skills to slow learners and school dropouts.

Information Systems. Information systems providing public health data are not functioning properly. As a result, from 1992 to 1994, efforts were made in collaboration with PAHO to strengthen the areas of communicable diseases, nutritional surveillance, and environmental health. Because information from the private sector is limited, health situation analysis in some important areas may be distorted.

Organization and Operation of Personal Health Care Services

Consultants conduct specialist clinics in pediatrics; ears, nose, and throat; and mental health at the district level. The District Medical Officer refers persons seeking care in other specialties to the General Hospital, but there are long delays before receiving services. Referrals for admission to the General Hospital also are made through the Accident and Emergency Department. No established follow-up system is in place to inform the district medical team when a discharged patient returns to the community, and this is an area that also will be given high priority in the future.

Inputs for Health

Grenada procures most of its pharmaceuticals and medical supplies through the subregional program managed by the Eastern Caribbean Drug Service. The procurement cycle ensures that regional standards are reviewed annually and revised periodically, and that essential drugs are available on a timely basis. Persons under a doctor's care can obtain medication from a public pharmacy at a much lower cost, and patients who are unable to pay can be exempted from the fee at a doctor's request.

Pharmacists dispense medication at doctor's clinics, but referrals to the main dispensary in the capital or to the private sector are sometimes necessary.

Human Resources

In 1996, there were 50 physicians employed in the public health sector, and most of them also worked in private practice; 10 were District Medical Officers who conduct clinics at the community level. There are 36 doctors who work primarily in a hospital setting, 16 of whom are consultants and the rest, junior doctors. Fifteen doctors work exclusively in the private sector, most of them as general practitioners. There are 6 physicians per 10,000 population.

Several categories of nurses work in the public health system—173 nurse/midwives work in the three hospitals; 50 work at the district level, including public health nurses, family nurse practitioners and district nurses; and 9 work in the mental and geriatric facilities. There are 24 nurses per 10,000 population.

Legislation giving family nurse practitioners the authority to prescribe medication in accordance with their training has not yet been enacted, which is a source of frustration for these health workers. The Ministry of Health is reviewing draft legislation.

The public sector employs 26 pharmacists, most of whom are based in the community, the procurement division, and at the hospitals. There are 18 private pharmacies staffed with 21 pharmacists. Grenada has 4.8 pharmacists per 10,000 population. Shifting the pharmacy school from the Ministry of Health to the Ministry of Education is being explored, but up to 1997 the Ministry of Health retained some administrative responsibilities. The school trains pharmacists for the public and private sectors through a three-year program; 13 pharmacists graduated from the program between 1992 and 1995.

Seven dentists are employed in the public sector, but they all have private practices as well; another seven work exclusively in private practice. The country has 1.4 dentists per 10,000 population. Five dental auxiliaries work with the dentist in the public sector, mainly with the school population.

In 1996, the Ministry of Health implemented a performance appraisal system. It also has developed a training program that will target staff at all levels of the system who work in priority areas. Training areas will include management, public and interpersonal relationships, and the promotion of a better understanding of the public service.

St. George's University School of Medicine provides annual scholarships to Grenadian nationals, but caters primarily to non-nationals. In 1997, Grenada was among four countries whose medical schools met eligibility criteria to participate in the United States of America's Federal Family Education Loan Program. In 1996, the school added a Faculty of Arts and Sciences, which offers undergraduate training in several disciplines, including pharmacy and nursing and physician's assistants.

Research and Technology

The Windward Island Research and Educational Founda-

tion was created in 1994 and registered in Grenada as a non-profit organization in November 1996. The Foundation's programs are designed to conduct collaborative research projects with scientists from local and international institutes on the epidemiology and control of communicable diseases, particularly zoonotic infections, noncommunicable diseases, and on health systems and conservation ecology.

Expenditures and Sectoral Financing

The health sector has consistently received more than 12% of the annual Government recurrent budget, and public health recurrent expenditure is estimated to have represented about 4.5% of GDP over the 1992–1996 period. The main hospital accounted for 40% of all health expenditures, and district health services—including community health services, environmental health, and dental department programs—accounted for approximately 26%. Wages and salaries in the sector accounted for approximately 70% of health expenditures on human resources.

The Ministry of Health prepares annual budgets for recurrent expenditures and capital expenditure that are coordinated by the Finance Officer and the Planning Officer, respectively. Each program head must fully justify budgetary requests and outline expected results, and staff at all levels participate in the budgetary process. Because the Government uses a line-item system for estimating its budget, it is difficult to monitor and price the various activities undertaken. The Ministry intends to continue having all departmental heads very involved in the planning and budgeting process, and focused on using the budget estimates as a management tool. Financial allocations by the Ministry of Finance usually are below the Ministry of Health's original request, a constraint that usually translates in budgetary reductions in such areas as maintenance and procurement.

The health sector in Grenada is underfinanced—the population's demand for resources is growing faster than the resources available for the sector. This is evident by the need for funds to rebuild the General Hospital; the insufficient funds for maintenance of other health facilities; and the inability to adequately pay health workers, especially physicians. The Government is presently reviewing the health sector's financing. In order to advance reforms, a financial model will have to be developed, showing current financing sources and the effect of the new funds generated by the proposed health insurance program. This process will entail in-depth discussions with the Ministry of Finance to determine necessary changes in the allocation of resources to the health sector. It should be noted that a major constraint in carrying out a financial reform of the health sector is the limited understanding of the level of health expenditure in the private sector, which has grown in terms of numbers of physicians, pharmacies, and small hospitals.

External Technical and Financial Cooperation

Most international assistance provided to Grenada, excluding capital projects, is included as a component of the Ministry of Health's budget. During 1994–1996, however, some international assistance to the Ministry was not included in the total expenditure component. For example, Grenada participated in a USAID-funded health care policy, planning, and management project, which facilitated dialogue among officials of the Ministries of Health and of Finance and the social institutions in the member states of the Organization of Eastern Caribbean States. In addition, medical personnel from various organizations and groups from the United States and Canada have worked with local personnel to provide attention, and personnel teams from the United States military have assisted with refurbishing medical facilities and providing medical and dental care.

GUATEMALA

GENERAL SITUATION AND TRENDS

Socioeconomic, Political, and Demographic Overview

The Republic of Guatemala has a land area covering 108,889 km², bordered on the north and northeast by Mexico, on the east by Honduras and El Salvador, on the northeast by Belize, and on the south by the Pacific Ocean. It is divided politically and administratively into 22 departments, which include 330 *municipios*. The departments are grouped into eight regions. In 1995 the population was estimated at 9.98 million, with an annual growth rate of 2.8%. Sixty-five percent of the population lives in rural areas, where 80% of the people live in settlements of fewer than 500 inhabitants.

During the present decade Guatemala has been slowly resuming its economic growth rate. Between 1990 and 1996 the gross domestic product (GDP), adjusted for inflation, increased at rates of 3% to 5%, and the GDP per capita grew only 0.1% to 1.9%. In 1994 the per capita gross national product (GNP) was US$ 1,190.

Total unemployment has remained steady at around 37%. Open unemployment, which was 6.5% in 1990, dropped to 2.5% in 1993 and then rose again to 5% in 1996. Inflation fell considerably during 1990–1996, as evidenced by the fact that the annual variation in the consumer price index went from nearly 60% to between 8% and 14%.

The fiscal policy succeeded in keeping the public sector deficit under control: in 1990 it was 4% of GDP, whereas by 1996 it was only 1.2%. This reduction was due more to austerity in spending than to an increase in revenue from taxes, despite the reforms that have been made in this area, including an increase in the value-added tax from 7% to 10%. However, these favorable macroeconomic indicators are not matched by a decline in poverty, which afflicts three of every four Guatemalans.

According to data from 1989, the proportion of the population living in conditions of poverty was 75% for the country as a whole, with 58% living in extreme poverty. Both poverty and extreme poverty are higher in rural areas and among the indigenous population, 93% of whom were living in poverty and 91% in extreme poverty in 1989. By contrast, among the nonindigenous population the proportions were only 66% and 45%, respectively.

In 1994 the literacy rate was 71% in men and 57% in women, with an overall national rate of 64%. The total rate of enrollment in primary school was 79% in 1991, 83% in 1992, and 85% in 1995.

The northern, northeastern, and southeastern regions are relatively less developed than the rest of the country. Almost half the population lives in these regions, and the population is largely indigenous. Twenty-two percent of the people live in the national capital.

The birth rate was 37.3 per 1,000 population in 1995, and total fertility was 5.1 children per woman (6.2 in rural areas and 3.8 in the urban population). The fertility rate in the indigenous population remained steady between 1986 and 1995, whereas in the nonindigenous group it dropped from 5.0 children per woman in 1987 to 4.3 in 1995. In 1994 under-registration of births was estimated at 3%.

In 1992 life expectancy at birth was 62.4 years for men and 67.3 years for women; by 1995 it was 64.7 for men, 69.8 for women, and 67.1 for the population as a whole. In 1995 females represented 49.5% of the population and women of reproductive age, 22%. The Guatemalan population is very young: 45% are under 15 years of age and only 3% are older than 60.

Indigenous peoples, classified linguistically into more than 21 different groups, represent 43% of the country's population. Speakers of Quiché represent 29% of the total indigenous population; Kakchiquel, 25%; Kekchí, 14%; Mam, 4%; Pocomchi, Pocomam, and Tzutuhil, 24%; and other languages, 4%. About 32% of the indigenous population speaks only a Mayan language.

Since 1987, when the process of voluntary individual repatriation began, there has been a steadily increasing return of

Guatemalans who had been living for years in neighboring countries, especially Mexico. It is estimated that some 20,000 people returned between 1993 and 1995 and since 1996, after the Peace Accords were signed, people have been returning in much larger numbers. For the most part, those who have come back have made their homes in remote jungle areas, where they are living in precarious conditions without basic services.

Mortality Profile

In 1995 the crude death rate was 7.4 per 1,000 population. During the period 1985–1995 infant mortality was 51.0 per 1,000 live births (neonatal mortality, 26.0 per 1,000; post-neonatal mortality, 25.0 per 1,000).

In 1994 a total of 65,535 deaths were reported, for a crude death rate of 6.8 per 1,000 population. Of all deaths, 27.3% were in infants under 1 year old; 3.9% in children 1 to 4 years of age; 2.7% in the population aged 5 to 14; 21.8% among those aged 15 to 59; and 36% in the 60 and over bracket.

Of all the deaths reported in 1994, 58% were males and 42% were females; 24% occurred in hospitals, 66% at home, 8% in public places, and 2% in nursing homes. The leading causes of death were pneumonia and influenza (16.5%), conditions arising in the perinatal period (13.8%), intestinal infectious diseases (8.9%), and nutritional deficiencies (5.7%). Infectious diseases, deficiency diseases, and conditions related to pregnancy and delivery accounted for about 45% of the deaths.

In 1994, 57% of the deaths were reported or registered by physicians, 28% by other health personnel, and 10% by persons outside the health sector; in 4.5% of cases it was unknown who certified the death. Underreporting of death was estimated at 2.8% in 1993.

SPECIFIC HEALTH PROBLEMS

Analysis by Population Group

Health of Children

In 1994 the perinatal mortality rate was 14.2 per 1,000 live births, and that same year a total of 17,907 deaths were reported in infants under 1 year of age (27.3% of all deaths). Infant mortality was 48.3 per 1,000 live births, and the leading causes were conditions in the perinatal period (50.5%), pneumonia (17.0%), intestinal infections (8.8%), and malnutrition (2.3%). The percentage of low-weight newborns (less than 2,500 g) was 7.8% in 1993. In 1995, 50.5% of infants breastfed exclusively until 4 months of age and 32% did so until the age of 6 months.

Mortality in children 1 to 4 years of age was 2.3 per 1,000 in 1995. The leading causes of mortality in this group, according to 1994 data, were pneumonia (26.0%), intestinal infections (24.3%), and nutritional deficiencies (10.0%).

Health of Adolescents

In an estimated population of 2.4 million adolescents aged 10 to 19, a total of 2,148 deaths were reported in 1994, corresponding to a mortality rate of 88 per 100,000. The leading cause in this group was external causes, with a rate of 20.4 per 100,000. Within this category, firearms were the leading cause (8.9 per 100,000). Bronchopneumonia (7.0 per 100,000) and intestinal infections (4.6 per 100,000) came next. In this age group mortality was much higher among males (60.5% of all deaths as opposed to 39.5% for females, corresponding to rates of 104.6 and 70.8 per 100,000, respectively). The leading cause of death in male adolescents was injuries from firearms and other types of injuries; in female adolescents the most frequent causes were bronchopneumonia and intestinal infections.

According to a study conducted by the Childhope organization in 1990, Guatemala has two types of street children: those who work in the street, and those who live in the street. For the former group the street is their place of work but they maintain a more or less permanent relationship with their home. Those who live in the street, on the other hand, have broken ties with their families and the street is their source of sustenance, their social environment, and the center of their lives. Both groups share the same strategy for obtaining income: they find activities—not necessarily "labor"—which for the first group become a form of work but for the second are a means of survival. These youths carry out their activities in places frequented by potential clients (markets, main roads and intersections, parks, shopping centers, and places known for night life, usually prostitution), where they compete with adults and other youths for their essential space. The Childhope study conducted a census between May and September 1990 that identified about 500 street children, 63% of them boys and 37% girls, between the ages of 4 and 17. The larger proportion of boys may be explained in part by the fact that many of the girls were being exploited sexually and were in closed places rather than on the street.

Health of Adults

In the group aged 20 to 24 years the mortality rate was 177 per 100,000 in 1994. The leading cause of death was external causes, including injury inflicted by firearms, followed by other injuries and unintentional deaths, and attacks with sharp instruments, with rates of 30.7, 23.3, and 8.4 per

100,000, respectively. Bronchopneumonia came next, with a rate of 7.4 per 100,000. Of the total deaths in this age group, 72% were in males, for whom the most frequent cause was injury inflicted by firearms or other means. In women the leading causes of death were bronchopneumonia and intestinal infections.

According to a 1994 estimate of years of potential life lost (YPLL) in adolescents and young adults (10 to 24 years old), if deaths due to violent causes were eliminated, YPLL would be reduced by 21% in the group aged 10 to 14, by 50% in the group aged 15 to 19, and by 49% in the group aged 20 to 24.

During 1990–1995 maternal mortality was estimated at 190 per 100,000 live births, based on data from the second national maternal and child health survey (1995), which used the sisterhood method of collecting information. The latest year for which routine information is available is 1994, when maternal mortality was reported at 96 per 100,000. Underreporting is estimated at approximately 60%. The five leading causes of maternal mortality were complications of delivery (30%), retention of the placenta (14%), puerperal sepsis (11%), eclampsia (11%), and abortion (7%).

The percentage of pregnant women who received prenatal care given by trained personnel rose from 34% in 1992 to 54% in 1995, when 45% of all prenatal monitoring was done by physicians, 8% by nurses, and 26% by midwives. Among indigenous women and in rural areas, prenatal care was more frequently given by midwives and nurses. Physician care was most frequent among nonindigenous and urban women.

In the country as a whole, 37.8% of all deliveries were attended by trained personnel (physicians, 34.1%; nurses, 3.7%). As with prenatal care, physician-attended deliveries were much more frequent in urban areas (60% of all deliveries) than in rural areas (18%). By contrast, midwives attended 53% of the rural deliveries and only 31% of urban deliveries.

The proportion of women who received at least one dose of tetanus toxoid during pregnancy was 55% in the country as a whole (49% among indigenous women and 60% among nonindigenous women).

In 1995 it was estimated that in the total population of women of reproductive age 5% used traditional contraceptive methods and 26% used modern methods such as female sterilization (14.5%), contraceptive pills (3.5%), intrauterine devices (2.4%), hormone injections (2.3%), condoms (2.2%), or male sterilization (1.5%). It is estimated that currently, of all women living in sexual unions, 69% do not use any contraceptive method. In the indigenous group only 9.6% of the women use any family planning method; in the nonindigenous group the proportion is 43.3%.

Nearly a million people travel every year from the highlands to the large plantations on the southern coast in search of work. This mass annual mobilization poses a major obstacle to organizing preventive or curative health care.

In a 1996 sample survey of this migrant population, 80% were under 40 years old, 98% were males, and 75% were indigenous. The great majority (85%) stayed from November to the following April on plantations that gave them jobs cutting cane or harvesting coffee or cotton. Only 30% said that they earned enough money to support their household. Health problems, cited in 80% of the people surveyed, were acute respiratory infections, malaria, fever, diarrheal diseases, headache, dengue, and cramps.

According to the 1994 census, 0.7% of the Guatemalan population had some form of disability—physical in 60% of the cases, sensory in 36%, and mental in 3.1%. By sex, 58% of the disabled were males and 42% were females.

Analysis by Type of Disease or Health Impairment

Communicable Diseases

Vector-Borne Diseases. The malarious area covers 80% of the national territory (20 of the 22 departments). In 1994 there were 21,996 reported cases of malaria and 90 deaths, and in 1995 there were 23,608 reported cases and 108 deaths. In 1996 there were 21,556 cases of clinical malaria, of which 7,795 were confirmed. The annual parasite index in the endemic area was 2.4 per 1,000. Of the confirmed cases in 1996, 86% corresponded to *Plasmodium vivax* and 0.7% corresponded to *P. falciparum.*

In 1994 there were 2,384 reported cases of classical dengue and in 1995 there were 3,886. In 1995 there was one reported case of hemorrhagic dengue in Escuintla. By 1996 the numbers had risen to 3,704 cases of classical dengue and 19 cases of the hemorrhagic type, with no deaths. That year the Guatemalan Social Security Institute (IGSS) reported 500 cases of classical dengue.

Vaccine-Preventable Diseases. In 1994 there were 68 reported cases of measles and 34 deaths from this cause, 28 of which were in children under 5 years old. In 1995 there were 64 reported cases, and by 1996 there was only 1 confirmed case. In 1994 there were 74 reported cases of whooping cough, with 73 deaths; there were 62 cases in 1995 and 66 in 1996. There were no reported cases of diphtheria in 1994 and there were 2 cases in 1995. With regard to neonatal tetanus, 18 cases were reported in 1994, with 7 deaths; there were 8 cases in 1995 and 12 in 1996. No cases of wild poliovirus have been reported since 1990. The Expanded Program on Immunization was established in the country in 1982. By 1996, vaccination coverage of infants under 1 year old was 73% for the three doses of oral polio vaccine, 73% for the three doses of DTP, 70% for measles vaccine, and 77% for BCG; coverage was 8% for tetanus toxoid in women of reproductive age.

Cholera and Other Intestinal Infectious Diseases. In 1994 a total of 84,932 cases of acute diarrheal disease were reported, with 5,842 deaths from this cause; in 1995 there were 83,643 cases and 6,784 deaths. There has been a decline since 1992, when 99,737 cases were reported, which can be attributed to preventive measures and investments in resources to increase coverage and to water quality surveillance, which started in 1991 in response to the cholera epidemic.

Intestinal parasitic diseases are one of the leading causes of morbidity nationwide. In 1994 there were 154,911 reported cases, for a rate of 15.1 per 1,000 population, and 442 deaths attributed to this cause. No data are available that distinguish among the different causes of parasitic disease.

In 1994 there were 16,779 reported cases of cholera, but this number dropped to 8,280 in 1995 and to 1,572 (106 confirmed) in 1996. The respective case fatality rates were 0.9%, 1.2%, and 0.9%. The department that had the highest morbidity in 1995 was El Progreso, with 276 cases per 100,000 population.

Chronic Communicable Diseases. In 1994 there were 3,365 reported cases of tuberculosis, for an incidence of 33 per 100,000. By 1995 the incidence had fallen to 17.3 per 100,000. There were 523 deaths that year. During the 1991–1997 period there were 77 reported cases of leprosy, all of them in adults—66 multibacillary and 11 paucibacillary.

Acute Respiratory Infections. Acute respiratory infections continue to be one of the leading causes of morbidity and mortality in the country. In 1994 there were 138,550 reported cases, and in 1995, 178,355 (which represents an incidence of 18 per 1,000). In 1994, 10,846 reported deaths were attributed to pneumonia and influenza, which were the leading causes of total mortality and the second-ranking cause of hospital mortality that year. Pneumonia was the second leading cause of mortality in children under 1 year old (17% of deaths) and the leading cause in the group aged 1 to 4 years (26%). It was also the leading cause of death in women aged 15 to 49 (12% of all deaths in that age group).

Rabies and Other Zoonoses. In 1994 there were 13 reported cases of human rabies, and in 1995 there were only 9. In 1996 some 8,000 people were bitten by animals suspected of having rabies, 8 persons died, and 178 cases were reported of rabies in animals. The zoonosis section conducted nationwide rabies vaccination campaigns. No information is available on brucellosis, leptospirosis, teniasis-cysticercosis, and equine encephalitis, although all these diseases are known to exist in Guatemala.

AIDS and Other STDs. As of 30 September 1996 the Ministry of Public Health and Social Assistance had reported a cumulative total of 1,371 cases of AIDS in Guatemala since 1984. Of this total, there were three times more cases in men than in women, which have also been on the increase. Sexual transmission was responsible for 93% of the cases, 67% of which were due to heterosexual transmission. Given the serious reporting difficulties, it would be risky to estimate the incidence of AIDS and the mortality from this disease in Guatemala. The data available indicate that the annual incidence is on the order of 5 cases per 100,000 population. The treatment of AIDS patients is very limited, and only people with high incomes can afford the antiviral and other drugs for opportunistic infections, of which tuberculosis is the most common (30% of opportunistic infections diagnosed).

Diagnosed cases of syphilis in 1994 came to a total of 308. No information is available on other STDs.

Foodborne Diseases. In 1994 there were a total of 257,680 reported cases of foodborne disease, with a morbidity rate of 2,580 per 100,000 population and a mortality rate of 25 per 100,000. In most cases the etiologic agents and foods involved were unknown.

Noncommunicable Diseases and Other Health-Related Problems

Nutritional Diseases and Diseases of Metabolism. In 1994 mortality from malnutrition was 45 per 100,000 population nationwide. In the Sentinel School Program, initiated in 1994, low height for age in children under 6 years of age was found in 64% of the girls and 75% of the boys; low weight for height was found in 11% of the girls and 17% of the boys; and low weight for age was found in 45% of the girls and 54% of the boys. According to the same study, in 1994, 84% of the girls and 83% of the boys under 9 years old were suffering from malnutrition.

In the 1995 National Survey of Micronutrients the excretion of urinary iodine in schoolchildren, both girls and boys, was used to measure possible dietary deficiency of this micronutrient. The results showed that the situation is good, with an average iodine excretion of 211 µg/ml in rural areas and 248 µg/ml in the urban population (normal excretion was considered to be 100 µg/ml).

In 1995 the prevalence of anemia was 35.4% in women of reproductive age, 39.1% in pregnant women, and 26.0% in children from 1 to 5 years old. The prevalence of vitamin A deficiency in children aged 1 to 5 was estimated at 15% nationwide.

Malignant Tumors. In 1994 there were 2,329 reported deaths from malignant tumors (3.6% of all deaths). The most frequent sites of origin were the stomach (36%), liver or bile duct (36%), and bronchus or lung (10.5%). In women aged 15 to 49, the most frequent sites were the uterine cervix (40%), stomach (27.5%), liver (14.0%), breast (10.9%), and bronchus (3.7%). In men the five leading sites were the stomach (41.3%), liver (31.5%), bronchus and lung (10.5%), pancreas (6.9%), and prostate (3.5%). In 1994 mortality from cancer of the uterine cervix in women over 15 years of age was 4.4 per 100,000.

Accidents and Violence. In 1994 there were 1,720 reported deaths caused by trauma, poisoning, and other injuries and external causes; 85% of these deaths were in men and 15% were in women. The mortality rate from injuries caused by motor vehicles was 0.92 per 100,000 population.

In 1996 the IGSS reported that it had attended a total of 37,676 accidents—85% of them non-work-related and 15% work-related accidents. The most common sites of these accidents were places of business (67%), public thoroughfares (23%), and the home (9%).

Estimated mortality from homicide in the population over 15 years of age was 47 per 100,000 population in 1994.

Oral Health. In 1991 the Department of Oral Health in the Ministry of Public Health and Social Assistance studied a sampling of 11,000 schoolchildren and youths aged 2 to 18 from 157 randomly selected educational centers. The average index of decayed, missing, or filled teeth (DMFT) was 7, and 80% of the students said that they had a toothbrush or something similar.

Behavioral Disorders. There are no nationwide data for psychiatric morbidity. It is estimated that one-fourth of the population may have some kind of emotional disorder, and this proportion may be as high as 35% in areas of armed conflict.

RESPONSE OF THE HEALTH SYSTEM

National Health Plans and Policies

In 1994 a formal negotiation process got under way following the agreement to reinitiate the peace talks. The Peace Accord was signed on 29 December 1996 by representatives of the Government and the guerrilla forces. This new state of peace led to a thorough institutional modernization of the State with a view to substantially improving efficiency and management capacity, addressing the delicate question of public finances, and effectively implementing social programs that would support the processes of peace and economic development.

Health policies come under the program for economic modernization of the Government, which includes reforms aimed at increasing State income, controlling the national debt, and raising expenditure in the social sectors. An important complement to these policies has been the reforms in the allocation of funds to the *municipios.* Of the amounts that the Government gives to the municipalities—namely, 8% of the national budget—at least 90% is supposed to go for programs in education, preventive health, infrastructure, and public services to improve the quality of life.

The 1996–2000 Social Development Plan reviews and examines the goals and objectives set forth in previous development plans and incorporates the commitments assumed at the recent Central American presidential summits, especially with regard to sustainable development and social integration.

The Government has formulated a set of health policies for 1996–2000, which incorporate, orient, and support various aspects of the reform and the peace accords. These policies address seven areas: (a) reorganization, integration, and modernization of the health sector; (b) increased coverage and improved quality of basic health services, with emphasis on the prevention and control of priority problems; (c) improved management of hospitals; (d) promotion of health and a healthy environment; (e) increased coverage and improved quality of drinking water and extended coverage of basic environmental sanitation in rural areas; (f) social participation and oversight as part of public management of the services; and (g) coordination of international technical cooperation to support the activities determined to have priority in the health policies and in the sectoral reform process.

The overall framework of State reform includes reform of the health sector, with the political aim of bringing about a comprehensive transformation in the social production model for health. Above all, it undertakes to achieve an organized social response so that the sector's interventions will have an effect on the fundamental causes of disease and not merely their effects on health.

The health sector reform that got under way in 1994 has the following specific objectives: (a) to increase the coverage of basic health services, focusing on the poorest segment of the population; (b) to increase public spending and expand the sources of financing for the sector to ensure its sustainability; (c) to rechannel the allocation of resources; (d) to increase the efficiency of the public sector's performance of its duties and the production of its services; and (e) to generate an organized social response founded on a broad base of participation.

Along with this process a financial reform is also taking place that envisages economic modernization of the State, maintenance of a stable macroeconomic situation, and creation of the fiscal capacity necessary to increase social spending.

Organization of the Health Sector

The health sector is made up of both public and private institutions, nongovernmental organizations, and a large sector of traditional medicine surviving from the Mayan culture, which is found mainly in rural areas among the indigenous population.

At the national level, institutional coverage of the population is as follows: Ministry of Public Health and Social Assistance, 25%; IGSS, 17%; Military Health Service, 2.5%; nongovernmental organizations, 4%; and the private sector, 10%. Less than 60% of the population has the benefit of some form of health service coverage, and this coverage has not increased substantially since 1990, when it was 54%. This was one of the reasons why the Government decided to change the traditional care model by reforming the sector. A Comprehensive Health Care System (SIAS) was designed, which is now being implemented and intends to provide basic health care to the entire population that currently is without access to health services. Existing resources will be used for this purpose within a context of community organization and participation that will generate and bring about changes in the health situation.

The SIAS concept is based on the delivery of specific, simplified, and ongoing health services provided by volunteers with the support and supervision of institutional personnel. These community participants are expected to work closely with a health team that provides them with technical, logistic, and decision-making support and whose members, unlike traditional health personnel, work in close contact with the community.

With regard to health care for individuals, specifics have been formulated for minimum health services and national coverage according to the communities' epidemiological profile. The following activities are included: (1) care of pregnant women through prenatal monitoring, administration of tetanus toxoid, provision of ferrous sulfate, and care during delivery and the puerperium; (2) child health care, vaccination, control of acute respiratory infections and diarrheal diseases, and nutritional evaluation and care of children under 2 years of age; (3) emergency and acute disease care (diarrhea, cholera, respiratory infections, malaria, dengue, tuberculosis, rabies, STDs, and others, depending on the local epidemiological profile).

The expanded health services are directed toward the 58% of the population already covered by health services and are provided by institutional personnel who, in addition to the minimum services listed above, offer care for women of reproductive age, early detection of cancer, and family planning; care for infants and preschoolers under the age of 5; emergency care and treatment of illnesses; and environmental protection, sanitation standards, and project development and management.

A national educational reform is currently under way, known as the National Self-Management Program for Educational Development (PRONADE), which began in 1996 with a pilot teacher training program in 39 teaching centers throughout the country. PRONADE's aim is to prepare enough bilingual teachers (in Spanish and an indigenous language) so that by the year 2000 all children in Guatemala will have had a basic primary education.

Development of Health-Related Legislation

The purpose of the new Health Code is to ensure viability and implementation of the changes that have been ushered in with health sector reform. It incorporates innovative aspects, including the definition and concept itself of "health sector," and it creates the National Health Council, an entity that advises the Government and the Ministry of Public Health and Social Assistance on regulating the development and infrastructure of health services with regard to formation and utilization of human resources and the health care service network. The Code specifically includes and gives priority to health promotion and protection.

In November 1996 a law was enacted to prevent, punish, and eradicate domestic violence. Its text defines domestic violence, the scope of application of the law, the presentation of claims, the institutions responsible for receiving them, safety measures, duties of the State, etc.

The law to protect the elderly, also enacted in 1996, is intended to safeguard the rights of the elderly and promote their quality of life.

Health Services and Resources

Organization of Services for Care of the Population

Water Supply, Sewerage Systems, and Solid Waste Disposal. In 1994 water supply systems reached 92% of the urban population and 54% in rural areas. Sanitation coverage (sewerage systems) in urban areas was 72% (65% with drainage or a septic system and 33% with latrines), whereas in rural areas it was only 52%. This means that 3.7 million people had no supply of drinking water and 4.2 million did not have adequate sanitation services.

There are 16 wastewater treatment plants in the metropolitan area, but only 4 of them are in operation. Of the 329 municipalities in the rest of the country, 286 have a sewerage system, but only 15 have a wastewater treatment plant. The rest of them dispose of wastewater without treating it.

Nowhere in Guatemala is there a system for the final disposal of solid waste. In the urban areas it is estimated that 47%

of the population has the benefit of solid waste collection. The rest of the people burn, bury, or toss out their trash. In rural areas only 4% of the population has the benefit of trash collection services. The waste that is collected, in both urban and rural areas, is deposited in dumps with no further treatment.

The sector is currently going through a reorganization process that will include the promulgation of a law on water (now a bill in Congress) that will make it possible to regulate and conserve drinking water sources.

There is a Water Quality Surveillance, Control, and Monitoring Program that operates at the departmental level and is promoting the development of quality standards for drinking water as well as technical standards for regulating the disposal of wastewater. To increase environmental management capacity, authorities from 80 of the 330 *municipios* in the country were given training in the formulation of plans for collection, transport, and disposal of solid waste.

Environmental Protection. Air pollution in Guatemala is mainly from motor vehicles, which increase in number each year. A 1995–1996 study conducted in Guatemala City by the San Carlos University and the Central American Ecological Program showed that atmospheric concentrations of particulate matter, nitrogen dioxide, and ozone all exceeded WHO standards.

A standard for leaded gasoline was issued in 1991 by the Ministry of Energy and Mines, which regulates gasoline imports to ensure that lead concentrations do not exceed 130 mg/l.

Guatemala is an agricultural country, with 32% of its territory devoted to farming. Almost 2 million people live in direct contact with pesticides. In 1994 a total of 5.7 million kg (0.5 kg per capita) of pesticides were imported. The Ministry of Public Health and Social Assistance periodically checks for traces of pesticides in food for human consumption. Of 72 samples analyzed in 1995, only 2 had levels exceeding the limits set by FAO/WHO.

The use of pesticides results in a sizable number of accidental work-related poisoning cases each year. Although the exact number of acute cases of pesticide poisoning is unknown, according to IGSS reports there were 282 cases in 1993, 237 in 1994, and 80 in 1996. Nearly 90% of the cases were in men, and three-fourths of them were day laborers. The pesticides most often involved in acute cases of poisoning are the organophosphates.

Several public and private institutions conduct training and education programs aimed at the prevention of poisoning. In 1994 a total of 1,400 persons were trained in programs offered by the Ministry of Public Health and Social Assistance, the Ministry of Agriculture, Livestock, and Food, and the Agrochemical Union.

Food Poisoning. Food poisoning continues to be a frequent cause of morbidity and mortality. Adulteration is one of the main problems, especially in dairy products. In 1993, 53% of the dairy product samples collected met established standards. In 1993 in microbiological tests of food sold by street vendors, the quality was satisfactory in 60% of the samples taken in the capital and in 52% of those taken in the interior.

The System for the Epidemiological Surveillance of Foodborne Diseases is currently being revamped, because there is considerable underregistration due to insufficient reporting. Moreover, diseases such as cholera and others that can be transmitted by food are not reported as foodborne diseases.

Public Health Information and Statistics. The System for Epidemiological Surveillance of Maternal Deaths began to be implemented in the metropolitan region of Guatemala City in 1991, and in 1995 it was also introduced in the departments of Huehuetenango and Baja Verapaz. The data are gathered by health workers who have been briefly trained for the purpose, and the resulting information has provided useful support for the decision-making process.

In 1996 the Ministry of Public Health and Social Assistance decided to implement the Health Information Management System (SIGSA), which is based on the policy of expanded coverage and incorporates information as part of the Comprehensive Health Care System. An integrated information system, SIGSA includes modules on health statistics, finance, planning, supplies, human resources, and hospital management. Its aim is to give added analytical capacity to personnel at various levels so that their decisions will be based on timely and pertinent information.

The Ministry has also begun to implement the Geographical Information System and the *International Classification of Diseases,* Tenth Revision.

Organization and Operation of Personal Health Care Services

In 1993 the Ministry of Public Health and Social Assistance had 19,385 employees and a network of some 3,861 health establishments, including 35 hospitals, 32 type A health centers, 188 type B health centers, 785 health posts under the Ministry of Health, 24 health posts under the Military Health Service, and 2,642 establishments, including State pharmacies, municipal drug dispensaries, etc. The private sector has some 2,000 establishments, but they cover only 10% of the population.

According to 1995 data, there are 12,725 hospital beds in the country as a whole, or 1.1 per 1,000 population.

The IGSS has 24 hospitals, 4 of them specialized. IGSS coverage is limited at the national level, because it has health posts and first aid stations in only 9 departments and offices for consultation in 10. Its hospitals are mainly located in Guatemala City, but it has also opened hospitals in Escuintla and Suchitepéquez in recent years.

The health posts of the Ministry and the IGSS are covered by auxiliary personnel. The Ministry's health centers have permanent medical staff but are open for only eight hours per day. The health posts and centers have very limited decision-making capacity and there is no effective system in place for referrals and counterreferrals.

The hospitals of the Ministry and the IGSS have specialists on contract who work four hours per day. The national specialized reference hospitals are located in Guatemala City.

Health of Former Combatants. Some 3,400 former guerrilla combatants (URNG) have been resettled in seven encampments in the interior in the departments of Quiché, Alta Verapaz, Escuintla, and Quetzaltenango. They are mostly adults under 30 years of age; 15% to 20% are women, and there are also some children. A bimonthly program was started on 3 March 1997 that will carry on the process of social reintegration through training and vocational programs. There are also programs for comprehensive medical care and oral health. The health teams comprise a URNG physician, who heads up the team; a physician from Médicos del Mundo, a nongovernmental organization, four dentistry students, a health promoter from the Universidad Misionero de los Pobres, a health promoter from the URNG, and a dental health promoter, also from the URNG.

Mental Health. Mental health has not been given high priority in Guatemala, but for the past two years a group of governmental and nongovernmental agencies has called attention to the problem and to promotion of development of a national mental health program.

The Ministry has a 350-bed national psychiatric reference hospital that offers outpatient consultation as well as daytime hospitalization. The IGSS has a 25-bed psychiatric unit to which cases from its affiliates are referred, and it also offers outpatient consultation. The Ministry has outpatient psychiatric clinics in three of its national-level hospitals located in Guatemala City. There are 10 Ministry psychologists and 10 IGSS psychologists in the metropolitan area who provide services in health centers and peripheral polyclinics. The IGSS has a community psychology program in the department of Escuintla.

For human resource development there is a postgraduate program in psychiatry for Ministry and IGSS personnel that turns out about five psychiatrists a year. In 1995, 20 Ministry and IGSS professional nurses were trained in psychiatry and mental health.

The Ministry's Mental Health Department is essentially a technical and normative office that plans and coordinates mental health programs at the national level, including one that covers former combatants and provides mental health care in the units near the resettlement camps.

Inputs for Health

Essential Drugs and Medications. Drugs are marketed through a network of 52 public pharmacies, 80 municipal drug dispensaries, and 1,920 privately owned pharmacies. There are 900 pharmacists and 1,100 pharmacy technicians. A total of 8,172 pharmaceutical products are registered, of which only 12% are in circulation. There are 81 national and 9 foreign laboratories that manufacture drugs. There is one official laboratory for drug quality control and there are four private ones.

In 1995 a total of US$ 159 million was spent on drugs, of which $13 million (8%) corresponded to the Ministry of Public Health and Social Assistance, $19 million (12%) to the IGSS, and $127 million (80%) to the private sector.

The most widely used therapeutic groups of drugs are anti-infectives, anti-inflammatories, and drugs for gastritis and peptic ulcers. Since 1996 there has been a multisectoral committee on drug policies that includes participants from the Ministry of Public Health and Social Assistance, the IGSS, the Ministry of Economy, the association of drug manufacturers and importers, and PAHO.

The Ministry of Public Health and Social Assistance has a Division of Food and Drug Registration and Control, which registers drugs; grants licenses to pharmaceutical establishments; performs physical and chemical analyses; monitors the production, marketing, and dispensing of narcotics; and authorizes advertising related to drugs.

According to a study conducted in 1993 in a sampling of Ministry health posts throughout the country, 70% of the posts had stocks of the 27 drugs that the Ministry has designated "essential."

Human Resources

In 1993 there were some 51,000 persons working in the health sector, of whom 26% were community volunteers, 17% were in the private sector, and 57% were in the public sector. The Ministry of Public Health and Social Assistance had 19,385 employees, distributed as follows: 12.4% professionals, 8.8% technicians, 26.5% auxiliaries, and 52.3% administrative and general service staff. The IGSS had approximately 8,000 regular employees and 1,300 supernumeraries. Of this total, 50.5% had administrative and miscellaneous duties.

According to 1993 data, for every 10,000 Guatemalans there are 9 physicians, 3 professional nurses, 11 nursing aides, 20 midwives, and 1.3 dentists.

Approximately 80% of physicians, 56% of professional nurses, and 50% of nursing aides are located in the metropolitan region, where there are 28 physicians and 4.9 professional nurses per 10,000 population. The rural areas, where 65% of the population lives and where the high-risk groups are concentrated, are largely covered by nursing aides, rural health technicians, midwives, and volunteer community health promoters.

Nearly 80% of IGSS health personnel are found in the metropolitan region. The concentration of human resources in the metropolitan area and the shortage in the hospitals of physicians with the basic specialties seriously undermines decision-making capacity at the rural outpatient and hospital levels. The current distribution of human resources is a reflection of a centralized health care model that is heavily inclined toward curative medical care.

With regard to administrative training, institutional staff are trained for specific operational processes, but they are not trained in managerial aspects of the health system.

In the field of public health, all the country's departments have epidemiologists with varying levels of training. There is a shortage of sanitary engineers and specialists in health economics, even at the central level of the Ministry. Education for the health professions is given at the University of San Carlos (USAC), Francisco Marroquín University, and the University of Valle. The latter two institutions are private, while the USAC belongs to the State. In 1995 a master's degree program in public health was introduced at USAC that will train staff from various government institutions in management, environmental studies, research, and epidemiology.

Expenditures and Sectoral Financing

Public spending on health in 1995 was equivalent to 1.2% of the GDP. The percentage of the Government's general budget devoted to health in 1991–1994 came to 18.1%. In 1996 public spending on health amounted to 13% of total public spending, whereas in 1992 it had been 6.6%.

The budgetary allocation for the Ministry of Public Health and Social Assistance in 1996 equaled US$ 195.98 million, and in 1997 the figure was US$ 203.57 million. The IGSS allocation in 1994 amounted to US$ 199.27 million, and in 1995 it was US$ 227.23 million (exchange rate for 1996 and 1997: 6 quetzals = US$ 1).

In 1996, unlike other years, public spending on health was redirected and a large proportion (43.8%) was allocated for primary health care, or local health services, while 24.6% was designated for the hospital network.

The Ministry's Sectoral Planning Unit currently has a set of peace-related proposals, of which the following are of interest:

• Comprehensive Health Care System for Critical Departments and *Municipios* in the Peace Zone, for which the Ministry has a budgetary allocation equivalent to US$ 13.81 million and a supplementary foreign investment of US$ 26.3 million.

• Drinking Water and Sanitation for Rural Areas of Priority *Municipios* in the Peace Zone, which envisages a government investment of US$ 12.65 million, a community contribution of US$ 5.06 million, and a foreign investment of US$ 12.65 million.

• 24-hour First-Level Medical Emergency Units in the metropolitan area of Guatemala City, with a Ministry expenditure of US$ 232,000 and a foreign investment of US$ 659,000.

GUYANA

GENERAL SITUATION AND TRENDS

Socioeconomic, Political, and Demographic Overview

Guyana extends for 215,000 km² along the northeastern coast of South America. It is the only English-speaking country in South America and is a member of the Caribbean Community (CARICOM). Because of its historic, economic, and cultural ties with the English-speaking Caribbean, Guyana's economic and social conditions are more often compared with Caribbean countries than with countries in South America. In October 1992, a new Government was elected to office, marking the first change of ruling political party since the country's independence from Great Britain in 1966.

The 1980s witnessed a massive outward migration of skilled personnel to other Caribbean countries and North America because of the devastation of the Guyana economy and a dramatic decline in living conditions.

In 1996, the mid-year population was estimated at approximately 770,000 people. Males represented 49.2% and females represented 50.8% of the total population. The 0–14-year-old age group represented 36.8% of the population, the 15–64-year-old age group represented 59.3%, and those 65 and older represented 3.9%. The population growth rate was 1.1% in both 1995 and 1996, significantly down from the 1992 rate of 2.8%.

Amerindians or indigenous persons account for approximately 6.8% of the total population. Persons of East Indian descent account for 49.5% and those of African descent account for 35.6%. The remaining 15% are made up of Portuguese, Chinese, and persons of mixed descent.

In the 1992–1993 Household and Expenditure Survey, 68.9% of the total population was classified as rural. Approximately 61.3% of the total population resided in 2 of the 10 administrative regions. Georgetown, the capital, is located in Region 4 (Demerara-Mahaica), which has 41.4% of the country's population. Region 6 (East Berbice Corentyne) is the second largest region, with 19.9% of the population. Approximately 51% of the Region 4 population is urban, compared with 28% in Region 6. Region 10 (Upper Demerara-Berbice) has 5.5% of the total population, and approximately 80% is urban. The population of Region 2 (Pomeroon-Supenaam) is 5.8% urban, and is the only other region not classified as 100% rural. Most of the estimated 49,713 Amerindians lived in the rural areas of Regions 1, 2, 7, 8, and 9.

The average household size is 4.28 persons. Region 4, which has 67.4% of the total urban population, has the smallest average household size (4.02), and Region 9 (Takatu Essequibo), has the largest average of 5.96.

In 1992, the illiteracy rate was estimated at 4% (2% for males and 6% for females); 52.5% of the population had attained the primary-school level, 34.5% had attained secondary-school level, and 10% had attained a level higher than secondary education. Despite the seemingly favorable literacy rate, questions exist as to the functional literacy level of the population, particularly in relation to school dropout rates.

In 1990, 12.5% of the country's population had no access to health services, an increase from 11% during 1987–1989.

Data from the Bureau of Statistics indicate that 89.6% of the urban population and 45.2% of the rural population had drinking water supply services. The Bureau of Statistics also reports that 91.8% of the urban population and 80.4% of the rural population had sewage and excreta disposal services.

Guyana's public sector monthly minimum wage was US$ 63 in 1997, up from US$ 52 in 1996, and US$ 25 in 1992. The monthly cost of a basic diet of 2,400 calories ranges from US$ 33, or 64% of the 1996 minimum wage in Region 6, to US$ 42, 79% of the minimum wage in Region 10. As part of efforts to provide relief for the poor, the personal income tax threshold was increased from US$ 107 per month in 1996 to US$ 129 per month in 1997.

In order to assist the elderly, in 1997 Government pensions were adjusted to ensure that they fall no lower than 50% of the minimum wage in force.

The poor are seriously affected by a chronic shortage of housing and the negative effects of poor sanitation, limited access to piped water, flooding, and other such conditions in the unplanned housing areas that have sprung up around the country.

Average income and living standards have declined for nearly two decades, the burden of which was borne principally by the poor and underprivileged. Guyana's external public debt burden in the early 1990s was just over US$ 2 billion. In 1989, the Government of Guyana embarked on an economic recovery program concurrently with an International Monetary Fund/World Bank-supported structural adjustment program to transform Guyana's state-dominated economy to a more market-oriented one. Toward this end, the Government removed restrictions on imports, relaxed foreign exchange controls, and began to privatize many state corporations.

Fiscal policy has been severely constrained by the high internal and external debt burden. In 1996, the external debt stood at US$ 1.5 billion or US$ 1,947 per capita. With total domestic and scheduled external debt services estimated at 61.2% of current revenues in 1996, very little revenue is available for expenditures on the social sector. From 1995 to 1997, the Government took aggressive steps to secure debt relief of US$ 600 million through direct negotiations with its official bilateral creditors. These negotiations were held under the auspices of the Paris Club, the United Kingdom, and Trinidad and Tobago.

Guyana's abundance of natural resources and the Government's commitment to economic reform enabled the country to return to the path of economic growth in a short time after the introduction of the economic recovery program. Economic and social indicators for the 1992–1996 period suggest that living conditions are improving, despite the fact that the percentage of the population living below the poverty level is, by conservative estimates, just above 40%.

The sugar, rice, and bauxite industries account for a significant portion of the country's gross domestic product (GDP). Consequently, problems in the bauxite industry, together with problems in export markets for sugar and rice are serious causes for concern.

Guyana's per capita GDP was US$ 766 in 1996, compared with US$ 680 in 1995 and US$ 454 in 1992. The average for the period 1991–1994 was US$ 504. The growth rate of real GDP was 7.9% in 1996, up from 5.1% in 1995, and 7.7% in 1992. The average rate for the 1991–1994 period was 7.7%. Inflation, which was extremely high in the late 1980s and early 1990s because of the structural adjustment programs, has declined from a high of 101.5% in 1991. In 1995, inflation had fallen to 8.1% and in 1996 to 4.5%. The average rate for the 1991–1994 period was 27.1%.

In 1997, the Government published a draft of its National Development Strategy. A major objective of the Strategy is to provide conditions for the private sector to expand and flourish in order to create more and better paying jobs in the economy. Ensuring human development is the principal guiding orientation of the Strategy, which addresses four broad national objectives: rapid growth of incomes of the population in general; poverty alleviation/reduction (rapid growth of the incomes of the poor); satisfaction of basic social and economic needs; and sustaining a democratic and fully participatory society.

The National Development Strategy acknowledges the fact that the population in interior regions of the country has tended to be marginalized, especially the Amerindian groups. It puts forth new approaches for addressing the country's most basic social problems in areas such as health, education, housing, poverty alleviation, the role of women, and the role of Amerindians.

Mortality Profile

Life expectancy in Guyana was 64 years in 1994, compared with 64.9 in 1992. For females it was 67.7 years in 1992, compared with 62.1 years for males. The crude birth rate was 29.2 per 1,000 population in 1996 and 29.8 in 1995, up from 25.6 in 1992. The crude death rate was 7.3 per 1,000 population in 1996 and 7.1 in 1995, up from 6.6 in 1992. The fertility rate was 2.8 children per woman in 1994, the same as in 1992. The infant mortality rate as reported by the Bureau of Statistics was 27.8 per 1,000 live births in 1995 and 28.8 in 1994, significantly lower than the 1992 figure of 42.9. The Maternal Child Health Unit at the Ministry of Health reports, however, an infant mortality rate of 33.2 per 1,000 live births in 1995.

The estimates of the crude birth and death rates provided above are reported by the Bureau of Statistics and represent the official estimates used by the Government. Estimates reported by the Statistics Unit of the Ministry of Health differ from the official estimates although both sets are based on data collected from the General Registrar's Office. Ministry of Health estimates tend to be slightly higher. The differences between the two sets of figures are a source of much concern.

There were 5,098 deaths in 1995 compared with 4,372 in 1994 and 4,003 in 1992. The 60 and older age group accounted for the most deaths: 2,291 (45%) in 1995, compared with 1,882 (47%) deaths in 1992. The 20–59-year age group had the second highest number of deaths with 1,797 (35%) in 1995, compared with 1,416 (35%) deaths in 1992. In 1995, there were 737 (14.5%) deaths among children under age 5, up from 488 (12.2%) deaths in 1992, ranking this group third in number of deaths.

SPECIFIC HEALTH PROBLEMS

Analysis by Population Group

Health of Children

According to the Health Statistics Unit (Ministry of Health), there were 18,360 live births in 1995, of which 15.3% had low birthweight (<2,500 g). Of the 72,740 children under 5 years old who enrolled at clinics in 1996, 13,215 (18.2%) were assessed as moderately malnourished at least once during the year. The percentage of moderately malnourished children under 1 year of age was 21%. The percentage for children 1–2 years old, 3–4 years old, and 4–5 years old were 17%, 17%, and 12%, respectively. The number of children diagnosed as severely malnourished was 683 (less than 1%), with a rate of 2% for infants under 1, 1% for children 1–2 years old, and less than 1% for children 2–5 years old. A 1996 survey completed by the Ministry of Health assessed vitamin A, beta-carotene, iron, and iodine status in the population. The nutritional status of 288 children 0–4 years old was assessed and 34 (11.8%) of the children showed levels of undernourishment and stunting, and only 3 (1%) of the children were overnourished.

In 1996, of the 17,726 infants attending clinic at three months, 5,844 (33%) were breast-fed exclusively, 9,910 (56%) were partially breast-fed, 1,246 (7%) had stopped breast-feeding, and 611 (3.5%) were never breast-fed. The breast-feeding status of 1% of the children was unknown. Clinical data for 1995 showed that 30.5% of infants were being fully breast-fed at three months, with prevalence ranging from 18% in Region 4 (East Coast) to 79% in Region 9.

In 1995, the stillbirth rate was 22.9 per 1,000 total births. The perinatal mortality rate was 36.9 per 1,000 live births, while the neonatal mortality rate was 17.5 per 1,000 live births.

Between 1992 and 1996, vaccination rates for BCG, DTP, OPV, measles, and MMR were above 80% in most cases. In 1996, BCG coverage was 88.4%, DTP coverage was 83%, and OPV3 coverage was 83%. Measles vaccination, which was replaced by MMR in 1996, had a 1995 coverage rate of 84.1%. Special efforts were made in 1995 and 1996 to introduce MMR in line with measles reduction activities in the Caribbean. Introduced in late 1995, MMR coverage in 1996 was 96%, up from 76.7% in 1995.

For the 0–4-year-old age group, the five leading causes of illness treated at reporting clinics during 1996 were: acute respiratory infections, with 12,975 cases (43.2% of total cases); worm infestation, with 3,506 (11.7%) cases; diarrheal diseases, 2,689 (9%) cases; scabies, 1,036 (3.5%) cases; and accidents and injuries, 844 (2.8%) cases. Together, these five cause groups accounted for 70.2% of all cases treated in 1996.

In 1995, there were 736 deaths in the 0–4-year-old age group, compared with 649 deaths in 1994, and 488 deaths in 1992. The five leading causes of death for this age group in 1995 were: certain conditions originating in the perinatal period with 277 deaths (representing 37.6% of the deaths of this age group); intestinal infectious diseases, with 169 deaths (23%); other diseases of the respiratory system, 69 deaths (9.4%); congenital anomalies, with 57 deaths (7.7%); and nutritional deficiencies, with 38 deaths (5.2%). The top five causes were responsible for 610 or 82.9% of the 736 deaths in 1995, 532 (82%) deaths in 1994, and 348 (85.5%) deaths in 1992. Females accounted for 314 (42.7%) deaths in 1995, compared with 258 (48.5%) deaths in 1994, and 204 (58.6%) deaths in 1992.

The primary school-age population (5–9 years old) comprises approximately 11% of Guyana's population. In 1995, there were 41 deaths in this age group, compared with 43 deaths in 1994, and 22 deaths in 1992. The five leading causes of death in the 5–9-year-old age group in 1995 were: "other accidents," including late effects, with 7 deaths (representing 17.1% of deaths in this age group); "other violence," 6 deaths (14.6%); congenital anomalies, with 4 deaths (9.8%); diseases of the nervous system, with 3 deaths (7.3%); and accidental poisoning, with 3 deaths (7.3%). Together these five causes were responsible for 23 (56.1%) deaths in 1995. Females in this age group accounted for 18 (43.9%) deaths in 1995, compared with 18 (41.9%) deaths in 1994, and 7 (31.8%) deaths in 1992.

Health of Adolescents

Adolescents in the 10–14-year-old age group comprise 12% of the population, and those in the 15–19-year-old age group comprise 11.5%.

In 1995, there were 29 deaths among 10–14-year-olds, compared with 31 deaths in 1994, and 39 deaths in 1992. The five leading causes of death for this age group in 1995 were: "other violence," with 9 deaths (representing 31% of deaths for the group in 1995); "other accidents," including late effects, 5 deaths (17.2%); traffic accidents, 3 deaths (10.3%); infectious intestinal diseases, 2 deaths (6.9%); and diseases of pulmonary circulation, 1 death (3.5%). The five leading causes were responsible for 20 deaths (68.9%) in 1995, 14 deaths (45.3%) in 1994, and 9 deaths (23%) in 1992. Females accounted for 7 deaths (24.1%) in 1995, compared with 14 (45.2%) in 1994, and 20 (51.3%) in 1992.

In 1995, there were 97 deaths in the 15–19-year-old age group, compared with 71 deaths in 1994, and 67 deaths in 1992. The five leading causes of death in this group in 1995 were: "other violence," with 16 deaths (representing 16.5% of deaths in this age group); "other accidents," including late effects, with 14 (14.4%) deaths; suicide and self-inflicted injury, with 10 deaths (10.3%); transport accidents, with 7 deaths (7.2%); and diseases of blood and blood-forming organs, with 6 deaths (6.2%). The top five causes were responsible for 53 or 54.6% of the 97 deaths in 1995, 38 (53.6%) in 1994, and 25 (37.3%) in 1992. Females accounted for 40 deaths (41.2%) in 1995, 30 (42.3%) in 1994, and 32 (47.8%) in 1992.

The five leading causes of illness treated in the 15–19-year age group at reporting clinics during 1996 were: acute respiratory infections, with 19.8% of total cases; accidents and injuries, 12.5% of the cases; malaria, 5.5%; worm infestation, 3.3%; and diarrheal diseases, 3.0%. Together these five cause groups accounted for 44.1% of all cases treated in 1996 and 42.8% of all cases treated in 1995. "Symptoms, signs and ill-defined or unknown conditions" accounted for 16.4% of the cases in 1996 and 16.6% in 1995.

Health of Adults

In 1996, of 17,496 women receiving prenatal care for the first time during a pregnancy, 11% were under 15 years of age, 10% between 15 and 17 years old, 81% between 18 and 34 years old, and 7% were 35 years and older. Of these, 25% of the women had 0 parity, 59% had a parity of 1–4, and 16% a parity of 5 or higher. Only 32% of the women sought care during the first 20 weeks of pregnancy, 61% had been pregnant for 20 weeks or more, and for 7%, the length of gestation was unknown. Of 15,856 women who received prenatal care for the first time during a pregnancy, 14% had had an abortion, 14% had had more than one abortion, 68% never had an abortion, and 4% would not give any information. Of the 1,869 women with high-risk conditions diagnosed or identified for the first time during a pregnancy, 29.2% had high blood pressure, 18.1% tested positive for syphilis, 1.7% tested positive for sickle cell, 4.9% had malaria, 14.7% had pre-eclamptic toxemia, 5.4% had diabetes, and 26% had conditions classified as "other."

In 1995, women under 20 years of age accounted for 3,786 (20.6%) of the 18,360 live births, while women under 16 years old accounted for 102 (0.6%).

The four leading causes of maternal mortality were toxemia of pregnancy; hemorrhage of pregnancy and childbirth; complications of the puerperium; and other complications of pregnancy (excluding abortion), labor, and delivery. Together, these four causes were responsible for 28 deaths in 1995, 22 deaths in 1994, and 9 deaths in 1992.

The maternal mortality rate among admissions in 1996 at Georgetown Public Hospital was 148 per 100,000; in 1995 it was 201 per 100,000, and in 1994, 310 per 100,000. The significant reduction in maternal deaths may be attributed to more timely recognition of life-threatening illness by medical staff as a result of ongoing training. There has also been a reduction in hospital staff turnover in the past three years.

Of the 12,603 clients attending family planning services for the first time in 1996, 5,469 (43%) used oral contraceptives; 479 (4%), IUDs; 1,313 (10%), condoms; and 990 (8%), other methods. In 1996, 758 abortions were performed at Georgetown Public Hospital.

The Guyana Responsible Parenthood Association, a nongovernmental organization that provides sex and reproductive health services with support from several international donors, has clinics in Georgetown and several regions. It had 183 new clients for its Pap test service introduced in September 1996.

For the 20–64-year-old age group, the five leading causes of illness treated at outpatient departments of reporting clinics were: acute respiratory infections, hypertension, accidents and injuries, arthritis, and diabetes mellitus. Together, these five conditions accounted for 52% of all cases treated in 1996 and 45.2% of all cases treated in 1995. Symptoms, signs, and ill-defined or unknown conditions represented 15% of total cases in 1996 and 13.7% of cases in 1995.

The three leading discharge diagnoses in 1995 for the Georgetown Public Hospital were normal delivery (18% of total discharges), direct obstetric causes (7.4%), and abortions (3.9%).

In 1995, there were 1,797 deaths in the 20–59-year-old age group, compared with 1,526 deaths in 1994, and 1,416 deaths in 1992. In 1995, the five leading causes of death in the 20–59-year-old age group were: endocrine and metabolic diseases, 285 deaths (15.9%); ischemic heart disease and cerebrovascular diseases, each accounting for 173 deaths (9.6%); diseases of other parts of the digestive system, 165 deaths (9.2%); and diseases of pulmonary circulation, 111 deaths (6.2%). Together, these five causes were responsible for 50.5% of the deaths in 1995 and 49.6% of deaths from defined causes in 1995, 43% of deaths in 1994, and 36.7% of deaths in 1992. Females accounted for 35.4% of deaths in this age group in 1995 compared with 37.6% in 1994, and 35.8% in 1992.

Health of the Elderly

Persons 60 years and over, of whom 52.7% are female, represent 5.9% of the population. Of these older adults, 20,127 (20.5%) were National Insurance Scheme pensioners in 1996, compared to 17,559 (19.6%) in 1992.

For the age group 65 years old and older, the five leading causes of illness treated at reporting clinics in 1996 were: hypertension (26%); arthritis (11.6%); acute respiratory infections (9%); diabetes mellitus (9.6%); and accidents and injuries (4%). Symptoms, signs, and ill-defined or unknown conditions represented 10.8% of total cases in both 1995 and 1996.

In 1995, there were 2,291 deaths in the 60 years and over age group, 1,939 deaths in 1994, and 1,882 in 1992. The five leading causes of death for this age group were: cerebrovascular disease, with 515 deaths (22.5% of deaths in 1995); ischemic heart disease, 331 deaths (14.5%); diseases of pulmonary circulation and other forms of heart disease, 253 deaths (11%); endocrine and metabolic disease, 179 deaths (7.8%); and other diseases of the respiratory system, 172 deaths (7.5%). The top five causes were responsible for 63.3% of the deaths in 1995, 63.7% in 1994, and 60.8% in 1992. Females accounted for 48.7% of the deaths in 1995 compared with 48.1% in 1994, and 46.3% in 1992.

Family Health

According to data in the 1993 Household Income and Expenditure Survey, females headed 29.5% of households. The proportion is much higher in the depressed urban areas than in the rural areas. Afroguyanese women account for approximately 50% of all female-headed households, compared with East Indians (35.2%) and Amerindians (2.6%).

According to the 1996 Guyana Human Development Report, the increased incidence of female-headed households can be attributed to several factors, including: high rates of migration, which contribute to a breakdown in social mores and familial ties; the inability of the majority of the population to earn enough to maintain a domestic unit; higher divorce rates; and an increase in the number of women in the labor force, providing them with a greater degree of independence from male support. Approximately half (51.8%) of women heading households report their main activity as home duties. Women are strongly represented among the category of working poor, employed as household help, manual labor, and members of the nonprofessional ranks of the public services. It is therefore likely that many female-headed households find it difficult to afford the food, housing, medical supplies, and other inputs that contribute to good health.

Workers' Health

In 1995, based on information compiled by the Ministry of Health and the National Insurance Scheme, among employees (aged 16–59) registered by sex and average age, it is estimated that 44% of the insured labor force was female compared with 44.8% in 1992. Of the self-employed registrants, 47.4% were female in 1995 compared with 27.8% in 1992.

According to Ministry of Labor, Occupational Health, and Safety statistics, there were 3,848 reported industrial accidents in 1996. Of the accidents, 90% occurred in the agricultural sector; manufacturing accounted for 7%; mining, for 1.7%; and forestry, construction, communication, commerce, and electricity, for 1.3%. The 1996 figure represents a 26% reduction from the 5,174 accidents in 1995 and a decrease of more than 50% from the 1993 figure of 8,383. Despite the decrease in total accidents, the number of fatalities increased substantially; there were 11 fatalities in 1996, compared with 5 in 1995, and 8 in 1993. Only 3 of the 11 fatal accidents in 1996 were related to agriculture. Mining accounted for two accidents, commerce for two, electricity, gas, and water for one, and communications for one.

Health of Indigenous Populations

The Amerindian population is estimated to represent 6.81% of the total population and comprise most of the population in the remote interior of Regions 1, 8, 9, and a significant portion of Region 7. They have the highest incidence of poverty, with approximately 85% falling below the poverty line. The geographic isolation of many of the communities poses major problems in achieving equitable access to both health and educational services.

Malaria, tuberculosis, diarrhea, and respiratory infections are the leading forms of morbidity among the Amerindian population. By 1992, it was estimated that one-third of the Amerindian population was afflicted with malaria, with 60% of the cases attributable to *Plasmodium falciparum*. Diarrheal diseases affect the entire population, especially younger children. The prevalence of this disease stems primarily from contaminated water sources because of the lack of latrines, persistent flooding in the riverine areas, and inadequate methods of waste disposal.

In 1992, there were 556 cases of cholera, resulting in eight deaths in Guyana. These cases occurred among the Amerindians in the northwestern province that borders Venezuela. Environmental conditions and movement across borders accounted for the spread of the disease.

Analysis by Type of Disease

Communicable Diseases

Vector-Borne Diseases. In 1996, there were no cases of yellow fever, dengue, Chagas' disease, or schistosomiasis reported in Guyana, although vectors for all these diseases are present.

In 1996, malaria was the second leading cause of morbidity in the country, with 34,075 cases reported, or 44.2 cases per

1,000 population. In 1995, the number of reported cases was 59,311, or 77 cases per 1,000 population, as compared to a rate of 52.3 cases per 1,000 population in 1992. The percentage of positive slides was 13% in 1996, 20.4% in 1995, and 24.9% in 1992.

In 1996, *P. falciparum* accounted for 52.7% of cases, and 50% of cases in 1995, compared with approximately 60% of cases in 1992. The main vector is *Anopheles darlingi*. Males account for approximately 70% of the cases annually, reflecting the link between the disease and occupations in gold and diamond mining and logging.

Region 1, which was the most seriously affected during the 1988–1992 period, continued to be the most affected in 1995, accounting for 35.6% of reported cases. However, in 1996 Region 1 accounted only for 16.5% of the cases reported, surpassed by Regions 8 and 9, with 20.3% and 26.2% of the cases, respectively. There were 37 malaria deaths reported in 1995 (65% males) and 23 deaths (61% males) in 1992.

Vaccine-Preventable Diseases. Since 1991, an Expanded Program on Immunization (EPI) was established to report the prevalence of rubella and has shown yearly improvement. In 1996, 166 cases of rash and fever were reported in Guyana, of which 77% were confirmed as rubella either by laboratory or epidemiologically. In the first quarter of 1997, of the 69 cases of rash and fever reported, 51% were confirmed as rubella. A retrospective study completed for the years 1992–1996 showed 15 congenital rubella syndrome (CRS) compatible cases and 1 serologically confirmed case of CRS in 1996.

Regarding other vaccine-preventable diseases, measles has not been detected since 1992; yellow fever has not been reported since the 1970s; whooping cough was last reported in 1991; there have been no cases of neonatal tetanus reported since 1988; and no cases of poliomyelitis have been reported in recent years. Two cases of tetanus were reported as of mid-year 1997.

Cholera and Other Intestinal Diseases. In an outbreak of cholera, 556 cases were reported between November 1992 and early January 1993. No further cases of cholera have since been reported in Guyana. Vigilance has increased in the territories bordering Venezuela, where outbreaks continued to be reported in 1996 and 1997. In 1995 there were 257 deaths from intestinal infections, 8 of which were due to typhoid fever, 4 to amebiasis, and 245 classified as "other and ill-defined intestinal infections." In 1994, there were 203 deaths from intestinal infections, of which 10 were due to typhoid and 193 classified as "other and ill-defined intestinal infections."

Chronic Communicable Diseases. Tuberculosis cases have risen from 296 in 1995 to 303 in 1996 (38.27 per 100,000

to 40.19 per 100,000). Although the number of cases increased in 1996, the number of cases identified by sputum analysis has decreased because the service was unavailable in some areas. In Region 4, the major urban center in the country, where 52.98% of cases were found, only 11.8% were confirmed by sputum analysis, 73.5% were diagnosed by chest radiographs, and 3% were identified by pathological methods.

Major risk groups for tuberculosis are Amerindians, HIV-positive persons, the elderly, and young adults. In 1996, Afroguyanese accounted for 40.4% of the cases and Amerindians accounted for 24.2%.

In 1996, 32 deaths due to tuberculosis were recorded at Georgetown Public Hospital and the chest clinic, compared with 43 reported deaths in 1995, and 29 deaths reported in 1994.

In 1996, there were 21 new leprosy patients (13 males and 3 females), compared with 48 (28 males and 20 females) new patients in 1992. The incidence per 10,000 population dropped from 0.6 in 1992 to 0.3 in 1996. Two leprosy deaths were recorded in 1995 (one male and one female) and two in 1994 (one male and one female).

Acute Respiratory Infections. Acute respiratory infection was the leading cause of illness seen at outpatient departments in 1996. It was the leading cause of morbidity in the 0–19-year-old age group, the second leading cause in the 20–44-year-old age group, and the third leading cause among persons 65 years and older. Acute respiratory infections accounted for 50% of illnesses diagnosed in infants under 1 year of age and for 39% of illnesses in children 1–4 years old.

Rabies and Other Zoonoses. A rabies outbreak in cattle was identified in Region 3 in August 1996, and 45 cases (deaths) were confirmed. A vaccination campaign was conducted and 500 animals were vaccinated. There has been no rabies in dogs or humans. In 1996, 20 cases of equine encephalitis in Region 6 were diagnosed based on clinical signs and symptoms. A vaccination program was carried out in the affected area.

AIDS and Other STDs. Between 1987 and 1995 there were 1,241 reported cases of HIV and AIDS, of which 796 were AIDS cases. Females accounted for 34.4% of the cases. In 1992 there were 162 AIDS cases, of which 55 (34%) were females; in 1994 there were 105 cases (46.7% female), and in 1995 there were 192 cases (42.2% female). Of those affected, 76.8% were under 39 years old. Region 4 accounted for 71.3% of the reported cases, with an incidence rate of 29.3 per 10,000 population. Region 10, with 7.1% of the cases (a rate of 22.2 per 10,000 population), had the second largest prevalence rate. Of the cases reported since 1989, 45% were persons whose major risk factor was heterosexual contact. This population increased to 77.8% in 1992 and to 85% in 1995. In 1995 there were 132 reported AIDS deaths, of which 48 (36.4%) were female, an increase from 75 deaths (36% female) in 1994. Deaths from AIDS-related complex decreased from 31 (32.3% female) in 1994 to 23 (30.4% female) in 1995. Up to the end of 1995, the National Blood Transfusion Service had screened 20,472 units of blood for HIV and 275 units (1.34%) tested positive. The seroprevalance of HIV among blood donors increased to 1.6% in 1992 but dropped to 1.5% in 1995 with no discernible trend in the intervening years. The lowest seroprevalence between 1989 and 1995 was 0.9% (in 1989) and the highest was 1.6% (in 1992 and 1994).

A survey was conducted by the Ministry of Health in 1995 of pregnant women who attended two health centers in Georgetown for the first time. Of the 70 samples collected, five (7.1%) tested HIV-positive. In a survey conducted in 1989 of 51 commercial sex workers, 22 (43.1%) tested HIV-positive. In a second sample of 108 sex workers in 1993, 27 (25%) tested HIV-positive.

In 1995, the following sexually transmitted diseases were diagnosed: 625 cases of gonorrhea (85.4% male); 325 cases of syphilis (85.5% female); and 856 cases of nongonococcal infections. The figures underestimate the prevalence of STDs in the country since they only include persons treated at the Genitourinary Medicine Clinic at the Georgetown Public Hospital. There were eight reported deaths from venereal diseases in 1995; five were the result of syphilis.

Noncommunicable Diseases and Other Health-Related Problems

Nutritional Diseases and Diseases of Metabolism. A 1996 survey by the Ministry of Health assessed vitamin A, beta-carotene, iron, and iodine status in the population. Of the 269 pregnant women and 438 adults aged 15–30 tested for hemoglobin, 52% and 42.2%, respectively, were found to have deficient hemoglobin levels. Severe iodine deficiency in the 5–14-year-old age group was higher in females (3.9%) than males (2.5%), while 2.1% of the 285 pregnant women tested had severe iodine deficiency.

In 1995 there were 65 reported deaths from nutritional deficiencies, compared with 51 deaths in 1994. In 1995, 37 of the deaths occurred in infants under 1 year old.

Cardiovascular Diseases. In 1995, cardiovascular diseases accounted for 1,966 deaths (38.6% of all deaths), compared with 1,650 deaths (37.7%) in 1994, up from 1,613 (40.3%) in 1992. Cerebrovascular diseases were responsible for 699 deaths (13.7% of all deaths) in 1995, 593 (13.6%) deaths in 1994, and 640 (16%) deaths in 1992. Ischemic heart disease was responsible for 518 deaths in 1995, 456 deaths in 1994, and 386 in 1992. Diseases of pulmonary circulation and other forms of heart disease were responsible for 373 deaths in 1995, 345 in 1994, and 288 deaths in 1992. Hypertensive disease was responsible for 208 (4.1%) deaths in 1995, 193 (4.4%) deaths in 1994, and 252 (6.3%) deaths in 1992. Atherosclerosis was responsible for 22 deaths in 1995, 27 deaths in 1994, and 19 deaths in 1992. Rheumatic fever and rheumatic heart diseases were responsible for 9 deaths in 1995, 13 deaths in 1994, and 8 deaths in 1992. Cardiovascular diseases accounted for 992 (50.5%) male deaths and 974 (49.5%) female deaths in 1995.

Malignant Tumors. Malignant tumors were responsible for 319 deaths in 1995 (156 males and 163 females). Malignant neoplasms of digestive organs and peritoneum accounted for 110 of those deaths, and neoplasms of genitourinary organs accounted for 106. Together these two groups accounted for 67.7% of deaths due to malignant tumors in 1995, 66.1% in 1994, and 67.1% in 1992. Women accounted for 27 of the 33 deaths due to neoplasms of bone, connective tissue, skin, and breast in 1995, 21 of the 22 deaths in 1994, and 21 of 25 deaths in 1992. Statistics from the Georgetown Public Hospital indicate that in 1996 there were 65 discharges attributed to malignant tumors, of which 44 were females. Females accounted for 14 of the 16 discharges due to neoplasms of bone, connective tissue, skin, and breast, and for 20 of the 21 discharges for malignant neoplasms of genitourinary organs.

Accidents and Violence. Accidents and violence accounted for 525 (10.3%) of reported deaths in 1995, up from 474 (10.8%) deaths in 1994. Males accounted for 78.2% of those deaths in 1995. There were 96 deaths due to suicide and self-inflicted injuries, of which males accounted for 74 deaths (77.1%) in 1995 and 91 deaths (69% male) in 1994. There were 42 homicide deaths, of which 86% were male in 1995, down from 49 deaths (73% male) in 1994. In 1995, there were 54 deaths due to motor vehicle traffic accidents (83.3% male), compared with 23 deaths (78% male) in 1994. Statistics from the Police Department suggest that these figures underestimate the number of deaths due to violence and injuries.

Behavioral Disorders. Data on the prevalence of mental health problems in Guyana are not available. However, in April 1994, of the 272 patients at the Psychiatric Hospital in Fort Canje, Berbice, 150 (55.1%) were men and 122 (44.9%) were women. The majority suffered from schizophrenia, while the rest were destitute with or without pathology. In 1996, mental disorders ranked eighth among the 10 most common causes of discharges from Georgetown Public Hospital, with 400 discharges for the year.

Oral Health. The national dental program is essentially a tooth extraction service. It does not have the materials to offer more advanced care. In 1996, the service reported 86,782 extractions and 208 fillings. The number of prophylaxis decreased consistently from 1993 to 1995, but dramatically increased in 1996 when 5,102 prophylaxis were reported, compared with 867 in 1995, 3,012 in 1994, and 1,270 in 1993.

Natural Disasters and Industrial Accidents. The most recent major disasters in Guyana are associated with human error rather than with natural phenomena. This prompted the Government to re-examine the overall management of the environment and disaster management, and to establish an Environmental Protection Agency.

In August 1995, Guyana recorded its worst-ever environmental disaster when a breach occurred in the tailings pond used to store cyanide-laced water and waste at the Omai Gold mines. The Omai and Essequibo rivers were severely affected by the discharge, and many dead fish were sighted following the spill. By the time the breach was contained, 4.2 million cubic meters of tailings had escaped from the pond. Public reaction to news of the disaster was massive. According to the report of a Government-appointed inquiry commission, the contamination had both environmental and economic impacts.

In 1996, severe flooding due to extensive breaches in sea defense dams affected thousands of homes and farms in several communities in the upper Demerara and Upper Berbice regions. This resulted in damage to rice fields and other crops, along with the death of cattle. There were no human deaths or major health emergencies created by the flooding, and the impact was primarily economic. A United Nations Development Program (UNDP) report on the flooding indicated that 9 of the 10 administrative regions were affected by heavy flooding as a result of high tides and rainfall, and poor or non-existent drainage. The Government announced a state of emergency in July 1996. International agencies, nongovernmental organizations, and foreign governments contributed to relief efforts.

RESPONSE OF THE HEALTH SYSTEM

National Health Plans and Policies

The 1994 version of the National Health Plan prepared by the Ministry of Health identifies and analyzes many of the problems facing the health care system, identifies priority areas of health care, and raises concerns that must be resolved in the course of establishing a national health policy. Malaria, sexually transmitted diseases, acute respiratory infections, vaccine-preventable diseases, and perinatal problems have been identified as priorities. The next set of pressing problems includes malnutrition, accidents and injuries, diabetes, hypertension, dental caries, mental health, drug abuse, and skin conditions (primarily scabies among children). The plan defines objectives and targets for expanding primary health care, improving secondary and tertiary health care, and strengthening the management of the health sector.

The Ministry of Health, with the assistance of the Attorney General's Chambers, has embarked on a major revision of outdated health legislation.

Health Sector Reform

Proposals in the 1997 National Development Strategy addressing health sector reform emphasize health promotion. The strategies proposed to improve the physical, social, and mental health status of all Guyanese are to: promote a better home, work, and general living environment; ensure that health services are as accessible, affordable, timely, and appropriate as possible, given available resources; ensure that health standards are developed, implemented, monitored, and updated; empower individuals to take responsibility for their own health through health promotion and disease prevention; enhance health personnel effectiveness through continuing education, training, and management systems; invest and share responsibility with communities, organizations, institutions, and ministries; and collaborate with other countries.

Organization of the Health Sector

Institutional Organization

The institutions, organizations, agencies, and individuals involved in health care delivery in Guyana can be classified into seven broad categories: (1) Government Ministries—particularly the Ministry of Health and the Ministry of Public Works, Communication, and Physical Development; (2) Government agencies such as the National Nutrition Council, the Guyana Water Authority, and the Guyana Sewage and Water Commission; (3) quasi-public institutions such as the Guyana Sugar Corporation and the LINMINE and BERMINE bauxite companies, that provide health care services for employees and their dependents; (4) the National Insurance Scheme, to which all employed and self-employed persons are required to make contributions, a portion of which is used to cover some health benefits; (5) nongovernmental organizations, a variety of which are involved in health delivery; (6) a private sector that includes six private hospitals; a large number of private medical and dental practitioners, pharmacists, and traditional healers; and private insurance companies that offer health insurance; (7) international donor agencies including the Inter-American Development Bank, The World Bank, the European Union, PAHO, and the United Nations Children's Fund.

Health services in the public sector are provided at five different levels. Levels I and II include health posts and health centers, Level III includes district hospitals, Level IV comprises regional hospitals, and Level V includes the Georgetown Public Hospital and specialty hospitals.

Organization of Health Regulatory Activities

The Ministry of Health is responsible for the regulation of health policies and legislation, the establishment and enforcement of standards for the delivery of health care and the protection of public health nationally, accreditation of all health facilities, identification of human resource needs in the health sector, development and placement of health personnel, and promotion of health leadership.

A Standards Unit was created in the Ministry of Health in 1991. However, only a few standards have been established to date and the lack of resources makes monitoring and enforcement difficult. There are numerous other entities with an interest in standards development and enforcement. These include the Guyana Medical Council, the Guyana Nursing Council, the Guyana Medical Association, the Guyana Nursing Association, the Public Service Union, private hospitals, the Pharmacy and Poison Board, the Guyana Pharmacy Association, the Private Hospital Inspection Board, the Central Board of Health, and the Government Analyst Department. Adequate mechanisms to ensure effective coordination of these agencies are, however, not in place.

Health Services and Resources

Organization of Services for Care of the Population

The Minister heads the Ministry of Health. Reporting to the Minister is the Permanent Secretary, who is the Chief Executive Officer of the Ministry. The Ministry is organized into three major sections, the heads of which report to the Permanent Secretary. These include the Chief Medical Officer, the Hospital Administrator of Georgetown Public Hospital, and Administrative Services, which oversee finances and personnel.

The Chief Medical Officer is responsible for the supervision and coordination of health service delivery. Five major divisions carry out this task: the Department of Disease Prevention and Control, the Regional Health Services, Standards and Technical Services, the Planning Unit, and the Health Education and Health Science Education Directorate. Several other agencies and organizations are also involved in health education activities. These include the health education divisions within Georgetown City Council, the Guyana Sugar Corporation, the Ministry of Labor, private sector firms, and a variety of nongovernmental organizations including church and community groups.

The Ministry of Health and the municipalities have retained responsibilities for traditional environmental health concerns, while a variety of agencies are responsible for monitoring the environmental health impacts relating to business and industry.

Tuberculosis Control. The mission of the tuberculosis program is to reduce the mortality, morbidity, and transmission of the disease until it no longer poses a threat to public health in Guyana. Case-holding posed the major challenge to the program in 1996. Even though supplies of drugs were adequate, only 38.3% of infectious tuberculosis cases reported from June 1995 to June 1996 completed the six-month treatment course, 43.1% defaulted during the first four months of treatment, while 16% remained on treatment after the six-month treatment period. This trend is unsatisfactory and steps are being taken in 1997 to introduce the Directly Observed Treatment Strategy (DOTS) in selected regions of the country in collaboration with community agencies.

Vector Control. The Vector Control Service is responsible for the control of malaria, filariasis, leishmaniasis, and dengue fever, and is the Ministry of Health's main device for the diagnosis and treatment of malaria in Guyana. The unit presently collaborates with the primary health care system. Activities accomplished in 1996 include passive case detection in Georgetown and at all population centers in the interior; the enhancement of diagnostic capabilities in Region 8 with the training of community health workers in malaria microscopy; and residual house spraying with DDT in areas of high malaria transmission to supplement the other activities.

Oral Health. The mission statement of the Oral Health Program aims to provide appropriate preventive, restorative, surgical, orthodontic, periodontal, endodontic, and prosthodontic dental care to the population through the National Health Service, utilizing both professional and para-professional staff. However, dental service work was almost exclusively focused on extractions. In 1997, the Government began the design of a preventive dentistry program with the support of various donor agencies. The European Union provided funding for a new facility for expanded dental service in Georgetown.

A National Oral Health Education Program for primary schoolchildren was launched in 1995. The program aims to reduce the prevalence of oral diseases by increasing children's awareness of the importance of oral hygiene, emphasizing that they take responsibility for their own oral health.

The American Dental Association in collaboration with Health Volunteers Overseas and the Guyana Dental Association has scheduled a program that includes a national oral health survey, continuing education for dentists and dental nurses, and oral health education. With the assistance of the Ministry of Health's Planning Unit, a five-year and annual work program for dental services was developed.

Maternal and Child Health and Family Planning. The situation regarding maternal and child health and family planning in Guyana has been strengthened over the last three to four years. A manual outlining norms and standards for maternal and child health was prepared, drawing on the existing 1973 manual, the 1993 Maternal and Child Health Strategy for the Caribbean, and consultation with persons working in the field. The manual was introduced to the staff in 1996 in a series of workshops.

In 1995, a simplified and computerized maternal and child health data collection instrument was introduced, allowing data to be summarized in a timely manner and returned to the respective Regions for prompt intervention. Regional supervisors received training in the use and interpretation of these data and, in turn, trained local staff members.

In the area of family planning, there have been special efforts to increase the involvement of men. A number of seminars conducted across the country geared toward men were well received. The three nursing schools continue to train nurses in family planning. However, the impact of this training is reduced because many nursing graduates emigrate or join the private sector soon after completing their studies.

Expanded Program on Immunization. In 1996, an MMR vaccine follow-up campaign was conducted as part of the strategy to eradicate the indigenous transmission of measles. Between April and September 1996, 76,384 children aged 12 to 59 months were vaccinated with MMR.

In order to ensure adequate immunization coverage for EPI target diseases, community health workers in remote communities received additional training in administering vaccines to their community members, which they do on a monthly basis. Quarterly EPI evaluation meetings continue, where targets are assessed and achievements and constraints in the program are reviewed.

Nutritional Surveillance. Using clinic-based services, in 1996 the Nutritional Surveillance Program provided nutritional assessments, breast-feeding promotional activities by clinic staff, iron/folate supplements to pregnant women at-

tending prenatal clinics, and a supplementary feeding program targeting pregnant and lactating mothers. The National Breast-Feeding Committee coordinates the establishment of regional committees on breast-feeding promotion. The Committee also developed a national policy on breast-feeding practices, which was approved by the Cabinet in 1997. A school-feeding program provides a mid-morning snack at nursery and primary schools in the Regions. Other accomplishments included the production of a Nutrition Surveillance Bulletin.

Hospital Standards. A major achievement of the Standards Department in 1994 was the inspection of private hospitals for the first time in more than seven years. Recommendations with respect to licensing were made to the Minister of Health and a set of minimum standards for hospital operations were developed. During 1996 and continuing in 1997 steps were taken to establish a quality assurance program for the clinical laboratory and to enhance infection control monitoring. These services support the quality control unit at the Georgetown Public Hospital. Staff continuity remains as a problem, affecting the sustained improvement in setting and implementing standards.

Environmental Health. The Environmental Health Service has suffered from a consistent decline in the number of qualified environmental health officers over the past several years for reasons associated with the country's economic conditions. To address this problem, a cadre of persons was trained to a lower level of skill to assist environmental health officers in their work program. These environmental health assistants were taught basic field inspection and health education skills in a one-year training program. Two one-year programs have been conducted, with 29 graduates, 25 of whom are still employed with local government and other agencies.

Another persistent environmental health problem has been the management of solid wastes in Georgetown.

Veterinary Public Health. The Veterinary Public Health Unit is located within the Ministry of Health and its main areas of activity are food hygiene and protection, zoonoses prevention and control, and health education. Currently, food hygiene and protection covers seafood and poultry, but not red meat. In 1996, the Unit developed a Food Safety Plan of Action and prepared for the introduction of the HACCP system in the fish and seafood industry. During the early part of 1997, surveillance activities for foot-and-mouth disease, rabies, and bovine tuberculosis were carried out in various regions.

Health Promotion and Community Participation. The Ministry of Health recognizes health education and promotion as the strategic approach for the planning and delivery of health care in Guyana. To this end, the Directorate for Health Education and Promotion was proposed for inclusion in the new structure of the Ministry of Health, which is awaiting approval from the Public Service Ministry. The Ministry relies heavily on resources from international agencies (PAHO and UNICEF) for activities that include training of health workers and community groups in using health education and promotion.

With funds from the World Bank, the Ministry of Health embarked on a Primary Health Care Project in three regions that focuses on health development through community participation and action. In other regions, community organizations are being developed to assist in reducing the incidence of malaria and tuberculosis. In all of these areas, community response has been enthusiastic.

The primary health providers in the Amerindian communities are the community health workers, individuals who complete an 18-month training program conducted by the Ministry of Health. Their efforts are supported by visiting services from medex (paramedical personnel) and, occasionally, physicians. The terrain, transportation, and supplies are constraints to optimum service delivery.

Programs for the Disabled. People with disabilities indicate that there has been very little advancement made in their socioeconomic situation over the past five years. Rehabilitation professionals and planners agree that while the demand is increasing, the availability of services is decreasing, especially at the secondary and tertiary levels where there is a shortage of institutional and specialist care.

A serious access problem faces persons with disabilities in rural areas, since rehabilitation institutions are concentrated in the capital and larger towns. Several agencies provide aspects of rehabilitation for children with disabilities; services for adults are provided through the physiotherapy service of the Ministry of Health and the Guyana Society for the Blind.

At the community level, the nongovernmental, externally funded Guyana Community-Based Rehabilitation Program has reported success in widening access to basic but essential rehabilitation through service delivery to children and adults with disabilities. The program, which uses volunteers for the delivery of services, has gained the active participation of the family and wider community in the rehabilitation process, thus ensuring the utilization of all available community resources and sustainability of programs. Inherent in such a program is the need for an effective referral system between the community and other levels of rehabilitation care.

To address the inadequate supply of rehabilitation professionals, in 1997 the Ministry of Health initiated a training program for rehabilitation assistants, a new category of mid-

level, multi-disciplinary technicians. The training program will include components on speech, occupational, and physical therapy. The assistants will work under the supervision of professionals in clinics as well as in the community.

A draft National Policy on the Rights of People with Disabilities in Guyana was submitted to the Government for consideration. This document was formulated using United Nations Standard Rules of Equalization of Opportunities for Persons with Disabilities as a guide.

Organization and Operation of Personal Health Care Services

Health care services are delivered across five different levels. There are 39 health posts found in Regions 1, 2, 7, 8, 9, and 10 that provide mainly health promotion and preventive care in remote areas. There are 194 health centers throughout the country that provide mainly preventive care, as well as some promotion, curative and rehabilitative care. Eighteen district hospitals with 420 beds provide basic inpatient and outpatient care along with selective diagnostic services. There are four regional hospitals with 717 beds in Regions 2, 3, 6, and 10. They provide general inpatient and outpatient services, diagnostic services, and specialist services in obstetrics and gynecology, general medicine, general surgery, and pediatrics. The Georgetown Public Hospital has 601 beds and provides a wide range of diagnostic services and specialist inpatient and outpatient referral services. It is intended to provide high-cost specialized treatment and sophisticated diagnostic tests. There are three specialty hospitals including a psychiatric hospital in Berbice, a leprosarium at Mahaica, and a geriatric hospital in Georgetown. In addition, there are six private hospitals in Georgetown and five company hospitals located in Regions 1, 4, and 10.

Inputs for Health

In the public sector, drugs and medical supplies are purchased from a variety of sources including UNIPAC, a unit of UNICEF that provides drugs and medical supplies to governments at competitive prices. The Guyana Pharmaceutical Corporation produces some drugs and medical supplies for the local market. Private procurement and distribution of drugs and medical supplies is also extensive.

The Government Analyst Department must certify pharmaceuticals entering the country for use in both the public and private sectors. The Ministry of Health uses the Caribbean Regional Drug Testing Laboratory (established to allow Member States of CARICOM to benefit from cost-effective arrangements) to test the supplies it purchases. Distribution is done by the Ministry of Health or Regions, or it is con-

TABLE 1

Distribution of human resources by category of service, Guyana, 1997.

Health occupation	Central	Regional	Quasi-public	Municipal	Private	Total
Physician	—	43	—	—	—	43
General medical officer	50	—	6	1	26*	83
Consultant	9	—	—	—	18*	27
General dentist	9	9	—	—	14*	32
Dental surgeon	—	—	—	—	—	—
Pharmacist	8	7	3	—	111*	129
Professional nurse[1]	293	312	25	12	115*	757
Other health professionals[2]	48	8	2	—	30*	88
Midwife (12-month training program)	48	109	5	—	3	165
Medex (18-month training program)	8	31	24	—	1	64
Health technician[3]	8	3	—	—	9	20
Nursing auxiliaries[4]	80	—	18	1	64	163
Other auxiliaries[5]	112	111	—	4	8	235
Nursing assistants	245	267	20	—	10	542
Total health personnel	918	900	103	18	409	2,348
Administration and general services	32	10	2	—	9	53
General service and administrative technicians[6]	131	30	3	—	124	288
General service and administrative auxiliaries[7]	406	100	59	7	144	716
Total general service and administration	569	140	64	7	277	1,057
Total personnel	1,487	1,040	167	25	686	3,405

[1] Includes registered nurses, Registered Nurse/Registered Midwife, health visitors, public health nurses, and health service tutors.

[2] Includes physiotherapists, medical technologists, radiographers, and X-ray technicians.

[3] Includes technicians (dispensers, multipurpose, orthopedic, biomedical) and physiotherapist assistants.

[4] Includes nursing aides.

[5] Includes assistants (dental, orthopedic, laboratory, dispenser, clinic) community health workers, and environmental health assistants.

[6] Includes secretaries, receptionists, clerks, typists, office assistants, accountants, and statisticians.

[7] Includes maintenance workers, drivers, porters, attendants, guards, maids, laundresses, cooks, seamstresses, and tailors.

tracted out to the private sector. Guyana has a draft National Drug Policy, but it has not been fully implemented.

A shortage of funds and human resources interrupts the supply of essential drugs, affecting both remote health facilities and Georgetown Public Hospital. On average, approximately 70% of essential drugs are stocked in the health centers and hospitals. In 1997, a revised essential drug list was introduced. The Ministry of Health is developing an essential drug list and a formulary for the Georgetown Public Hospital and other health facilities.

The cost and importance of drugs and medical supplies makes the availability of adequate storage facilities critical. However, there are not enough facilities in Guyana, and those that do exist are below standard.

Human Resources

Table 1 summarizes the distribution by category of health sector personnel.

Research and Technology

Guyana depends almost entirely on foreign imports for health technology. The development and maintenance of systems to monitor the quality, condition, location, and utilization of biomedical and other equipment are considered to be priorities. A preventive maintenance program is being established with the assistance of external agencies.

Expenditures and Sectoral Financing

Since 1990, government allocations to health have increased. In 1996, G$ 2.88 million (US$ 20.5 million) was spent on health, compared to G$ 0.4 million (US$ 10.1 million) in 1990—more than a sixfold increase in six years. In 1996, health expenditures accounted for 6.3% of the national budget, compared with 8.3% in 1995, and 5.3% in 1992. For 1992–1995, the increase in health spending was due primarily to capital expenditures, which accounted for 42% of total expenditures in this period, compared with 17% in 1990. The increase resulted from the construction of the Ambulatory Care, Surgical, and Diagnostic Center at Georgetown Public Hospital, and the 63% decrease in capital expenditures from 1995 to 1996 was due to the completion of this project.

Government health expenditure per capita also increased during recent years. While the figure amounted to G$ 538 (US$ 13.6) in 1990, it came to G$ 3,741 (US$ 26.56) in 1996. These figures are quoted in nominal prices, so part of the increase is attributable to inflation.

The inflation factor is largely eliminated when public health expenditures are seen in relation to GDP. In 1996, government health expenditures amounted to 3.45% of GDP, a decrease from more than 4% in previous years. In 1995, the figure was as high as 5.17%. Again, the relatively high figures for the years 1992 to 1995 can be explained by the capital costs of the construction at Georgetown Public Hospital. However, compared to the 1990 figure, estimated real levels of expenditures on health have still shown significant improvement, even when excluding the construction costs.

Traditionally, government and quasi-public institutions have been the dominant providers of health care in Guyana. In recent years, however, the decline in the quantity and quality of government services has made the independent private sector's contribution more important. In 1994, the private health sector comprised some 14 physicians with full-time practices. Approximately 15 others worked with the Ministry of Health but also maintained part-time practices. In addition, there were some 20 physicians working full-time at six private hospitals, all located in Georgetown.

A new approach to health care financing, which includes the identification of user fees for certain services, is currently being designed by the Ministry of Health. Only three types of user fees are in place in the public health sector: fees for physiotherapy services, laboratory pregnancy tests, and rooms in private wards. Fees for rooms have been recently adjusted based on the amount private hospitals charge for a similar room, but fees for physiotherapy and pregnancy tests have not been adjusted in years, and do not reflect true costs.

In 1996, 30.85% of government health expenditures were used on drugs and medical supplies. In the 1997 budget, 30.96% has been earmarked for this expense. In theory, this amount could meet national needs, but due to inefficient procurement and distribution systems, drugs and medical supplies are not reaching a large portion of the population.

External Technical and Financial Cooperation

The United Nations Development Program's contributions to the health sector from 1992 to 1996 amounted to US$ 1,097,473. In 1996, the contribution was US$ 269,141, distributed through the United Nations volunteers Multi-Sectoral Project. The focus of this project with respect to the health sector is to provide technical assistance to enhance health service delivery as well as to strengthen the capacity of national counterparts working in the health sector. The project financed the contracts of 12 specialists in the areas of pediatrics, orthopedic surgery, anesthesiology, obstetrics and gynecology, general surgery, ophthalmology, speech therapy, and quality assurance. Some of the specialists are providing formal training at the School of Medicine, University of Guyana. A number of nurses have also benefited from training in midwifery and ophthalmic and pediatric nursing.

HAITI

GENERAL SITUATION AND TRENDS

Socioeconomic, Political, and Demographic Overview

The Republic of Haiti occupies the western third of the Island of Hispaniola, which it shares with the Dominican Republic. The country is divided into nine departments ("départements"), 133 municipalities ("communes"), and 561 districts ("sections communales"). The country's roads are in poor condition, and sea transport is used extensively among coastal cities.

Water supply and basic sanitation services are still very deficient. No city has a public sewerage system, and there only are isolated wastewater treatment units throughout the country. Solid waste management is a serious problem; bad excreta disposal practices are polluting almost all 18 water sources supplying Port-au-Prince. Drainage systems are inadequate and any major storm produces serious flooding. The growing number of motor vehicles and their inadequate maintenance have created a serious air pollution problem in Port-au-Prince.

Every year, approximately 20,000 tons of arable land are lost to the sea due to deforestation and erosion. This phenomenon is aggravated by charcoal production throughout the countryside and heavy agricultural pressure on steep slopes.

The major trends in the Haitian economy over the past decade indicate a steady decline in the actual gross domestic product and a net rise in unemployment. Economic sanctions that were imposed in 1991 further deteriorated the economy. The gross domestic product in 1994 had decreased back to its pre-1980 level. This was paralleled by a population growth rate of 2.1% and a steep decline in per capita income from 1990 to 1995. The 4.2% growth rate in GDP reported for 1994–1995 could not offset that indicator's 25% decrease during the embargo (1991–1994), thus maintaining Haiti's position as the poorest country in the Western Hemisphere. According to World Bank figures, per capita GDP was US$ 220 in 1994, equivalent to US$ 896 adjusted according to

purchase power parity (PPP), making it one of the lowest in the world.

The inflation rate averaged 25.4% between 1991 and 1994 and rose to 27% in 1995. The unemployment rate is estimated at 70%.

Ongoing reforms reflect the Government's commitment to establish an open market economy that calls for economic structural adjustments such as privatization of state-run services and enterprises, decentralization, streamlining of public spending and public sector employment, and an effective tax policy.

Population projections, developed by the Haitian Institute for Statistics and Information Technology in conjunction with the Latin American Demographic Center, estimated the population of Haiti at 7,180,296 inhabitants in 1995. Persons younger than 15 years of age account for 40% of the total population; children under 5 years of age account for 15%. Persons of working age, between the ages of 15 and 64 years, represented 56% of the population. Approximately 25% of the population were women of childbearing age (15–49 years of age). The population aged 65 years old and older accounted for only 4% of the total.

Projections for 1995–2000 place the crude birth rate at 34.1 per 1,000 and the crude death rate at 10.72 per 1,000. The fertility rate was estimated at 4.8 children per woman. Based on these estimates and an anticipated population growth rate of 2% per year, it was estimated that the population will reach 8 million by the year 2000. Haiti has one of the highest population densities of all Latin American countries, with 260 inhabitants per km^2 as of 1995 and 885 inhabitants per km^2 of cultivated land.

The percentage of urban population in 1994 was 33%, the lowest in the Hemisphere. However, it has increased in recent years with rapid proliferation of shantytowns in Haitian cities (Le Cap-Haïtien, Gonaïves, Les Cayes). More than one-third of the total population (34.7%) lives in the capital, Port-au-Prince. The rural exodus has overburdened the housing situation, particularly in Port-au-Prince. Haphazard housing construction resulted in the erection of many dwellings in drainage areas, river beds, and protected water resource developments.

There were major migratory movements between 1991 and 1994. Internal migration to the countryside occurred after the coup in September 1991, with approximately 200,000 persons fleeing Port-au-Prince to take refuge in rural areas. Since 1995, there has been an increase in internal migration back to Port-au-Prince, accompanied by a decline in illegal migration. The number of Haitians living abroad is estimated at more than 2,000,000, mainly in the USA, Canada, France, and the Dominican Republic.

Legal, administrative, and cultural factors affect the quality and the completeness of birth and death registration in Haiti.

There is no systematic method to collect, process, and disseminate information on mortality. Nearly one-half of all deaths occur within the first 5 years of life. According to a survey on morbidity, mortality, and use of services conducted by the Child Health Institute in 1994–1995 (EMMUS-II), 74 out of each 1,000 live births die before their first birthday, and approximately 131 never reach their fifth birthday. In 1987, an earlier study (EMMUS-I) put infant mortality at 101 deaths per 1,000 live births.

There has been a steady improvement in net enrollment ratios at the primary school level over the past decade. Enrollment climbed from 37.2% to 44.1% between 1988 and 1991, and the estimate for 1995 is 51.4%, with similar values for males (51.8%) and females (48.2%), but this has been accompanied by a shrinkage in the average size of school facilities and the growing numbers of poor-quality schools and overcrowding. School attendance by lower income children is limited by the cost of school fees and curtailed by child labor.

French and Creole are the two official languages, but Creole is the everyday language used by all segments of society.

The individual perception of illness in Haiti is grounded in a highly complex cultural heritage. There are various types of traditional healers, including spiritual healers. Improper feeding practices have important deleterious effects on health (e.g., administration of purgatives to newborns during the first days after birth and feeding newborns with porridge or solid foods). Forty-two percent of newborns are bottle-fed within the first month; it is estimated that less than 1% of children are completely breast-fed by 6 months of age.

SPECIFIC HEALTH PROBLEMS

Analysis by Population Group

Health of Children

The leading causes of child mortality in Haiti are diarrheal diseases, acute respiratory infections, and malnutrition. Major causes of hospitalization for children 0–14 years old in 1995 were prematurity (23%), pneumonia (16%), malnutrition (8%), meningitis (8%), typhoid (6%), and gastroenteritis (5%).

In 1991, the Center for Research on Human Resources conducted a survey in three cities in three different departments. The survey provided an overview of the plight of children (boys and girls under 18 years of age) in especially difficult circumstances, including several groups: children employed as domestics, abandoned children, orphans, incarcerated juvenile offenders, child prostitutes (male and female), abused children, and street children.

The term "street children" refers to children whose only home is the streets and who only find food and shelter there. In 1991, the number of street children in Haiti ranged from 1,500 to 2,000 in Port-au-Prince, more than 100 in Le Cap Haïtien, and just under 100 in Les Cayes. Most of them are boys, but the number of girls appears to be increasing, accounting for 18% of the children surveyed in Port-au-Prince. The mean age of these children is about 11 years; 55% of them are aged 12 to 18 years old, and 14% are 5 years old or less. Their health problems include headaches, fatigue, insomnia, and anxiety. They are particularly vulnerable to tuberculosis, anemia, skin diseases, and sexually transmitted diseases. Many of these children are drug users (53% of the inner-city sample).

Another group studied are boys or girls who are engaged by a family to help with the household chores in exchange for food, lodging, education, and health care; they are called "restavek." In 1991, this category included an estimated 130,000 children. Between 60% and 80% are female and 82% live in urban areas. These children are from low-income backgrounds (56%–86%, depending on the area). Most of these children are placed in households with monthly incomes of less than 1,250 gourdes (US$ 80); they are not properly cared for and are less likely to receive medical care. Major health problems for this group include sexual abuse. Four out of five children reported having been beaten.

Health of Adolescents (Age Groups 10–14 and 15–19 Years Old)

A study conducted in 1992 in Cité Soleil (the main slum of the capital) by the Research, Culture, Health and Sexuality Team revealed that many young residents were sexually active by 13 years of age. The use of contraceptives is extremely rare within this age group. According to data from EMMUS-II, only 4.4% of those who were sexually active at the time of the survey had used a modern method of contraception, and 8% of all births were to teenage mothers aged 15 to 19 years of age. A previous survey found that 4.6% of the teenage pregnancies resulted in a premature birth (compared with 2% for other age groups). The risk of developing eclampsia was twice as high among teenagers under 20 years of age.

Adolescents accounted for 15% of birth-related deaths, and nearly 4% of them had induced abortions with rates higher in the cities (6.3%–7%) than rural areas (2.5%). Between 1991 and 1992, the Child Health Institute conducted a seroprevalence study of post-partum HIV-1 infected women, which revealed that 7.4% (1 out of 13 sexually active teenagers) was seropositive for HIV in metropolitan areas, compared to 4.1% (1 out of 28) in rural or semirural areas. Other diseases also figure prominently in the health of adolescents. Typhoid accounted for some 64% of admissions to the Haitian State University Hospital (HUEH) pediatrics ward of children aged 9–14, and meningococcemia accounted for 28%.

Health of Women

Women accounted for roughly half of the total population (51%). Data from EMMUS-II underscored the extent to which males were underrepresented in urban areas, with women accounting for 55% of the population. In the field of education, girls and boys have equal opportunities to attend primary school, but women in the age group 16 to 24 years old appeared to be at a disadvantage compared with their male counterparts. At the primary school level the gross number of years of schooling for girls is 0.5–2.1 years lower than for boys. Women also enter the job market at an early age; roughly 10% of young girls aged 5–9 years and 33% of girls aged 10–14 may be considered economically active. Women accounted for 70%–75% of the work force of the country's assembly plants. Despite existing legislation, workers had little protection against work-related accidents and illnesses and no occupational health benefits. Maternity benefits were limited to a very small part of the concerned population.

Because of food insecurity and short intervals between births, chronic malnutrition, including anemia, was widespread among women of childbearing age. The main indicators include high prevalence of low birthweight (estimated at 15%), of anemia among women (ranging from 35% to 50%), of body mass index under 18.5 kg/m2 (estimated at 18%), and of high maternal mortality rate (estimated at 456 per 100,000 live births).

In 1995, a national study on violence against women was conducted by the Center for Research and Action for the Promotion of Women. From a randomized sample of 14 municipalities, out of a total of 133, 1,705 families were randomly selected and 550 men and 1,354 women participated. A total of 1,935 cases of violence were reported: violence was classified as physical (33%); sexual (37%), with rape representing 13% of the total; political (2%); social (2%); psychological (2%); and unspecified (25%). Most victims of violence are young women (81% of all documented cases of violence involved women aged 10–34).

Although women played a critical role in caring for the health of their families and children and accounted for the majority of health care personnel (25% of physicians, 85% of nurses, and 92% of auxiliary personnel), there were no preventive health programs targeted specifically toward women, such as regular examinations for the early detection of cervical and breast cancer.

According to a study conducted by the Albert Schweitzer Hospital, cancer strikes more women than men (55% of cases are women). Cervical cancer is the most common form of cancer in women. According to the study, only 6% of all ectocervical squamous cell carcinomas were in situ carcinomas, due to the lack of early detection. Women are increasingly victims of HIV infection; 53% of female partners of infected males are HIV carriers.

For the 1990–1995 period, life expectancy in Haiti was estimated at 58.3 years for women and 54.9 for men. The general fertility rate is 4.8 children per woman for women aged 15–49 years old. Most women indicated that they wanted to give birth to only three children.

Some 71% of the female respondents interviewed during EMMUS-II reported having been attended by a professional or a traditional birth attendant during childbirth. Of the women interviewed, 80% had given birth to their last child at home. Fifty percent of women living in Port-au-Prince generally give birth in a hospital, compared with only 31% of births in other urban areas and 9% of births in rural areas. The leading causes of maternal deaths are: obstructed labor (8.3%), toxemia (16.7%), and hemorrhage (8.3%). The high maternal mortality rate is mainly the result of inadequate prenatal care.

According to EMMUS-II, an estimated 68% of pregnant women had at least one prenatal examination by a health care professional and 66% received at least one dose of tetanus vaccine. There are large disparities between data for mothers with at least a primary school education (94% received prenatal care and 74% were vaccinated against tetanus) and women with no formal schooling (53% received prenatal care and 58% were vaccinated against tetanus). There also are vast disparities between urban and rural areas.

Among pregnant women, 34% had four or more prenatal examinations, 26% had 2–3 examinations, and 8% had only one examination; 32% of women gave birth without any prenatal care.

The most popular methods of contraception were the birth control pill, female sterilization, injections, and condoms (3% each). Among sexually active women, 13% used a modern method of contraception and 4% relied on traditional methods. Among sexually active men, 17% used a modern method (6% used condoms) and 16% relied on traditional methods. There are large contrasts between urban and rural areas (a ratio of 2:1). Variations are also evident for women with a primary or secondary school education compared with women with no formal schooling (a ratio of 3:1). Among sexually active women, 43% expressed a desire to use future birth control methods. Among male respondents, 40% indicated the same inclination. There are limited data available on abortion.

Health of the Disabled

Haiti had an estimated disabled population of 800,000, most of them adults. The country has 85,000 blind persons. In 1995, eye care clinics treated 25,000 patients, 600 of whom underwent surgery. Major causes of blindness among adults examined are cataracts (34%), infections (13%), and glaucoma (9%), while blindness in children primarily is due to infections (45%), cataracts (8%), and glaucoma (5%). An unprecedented 50 cases of blindness as a complication of measles were reported in 1995. During that same year, the Saint Vincent School, a specialized care facility for disabled children, treated 2,058 affected by motor and neurological disabilities. According to the data from Saint Vincent School, the most frequent disabilities are club foot; orthopedic problems, some of which are due to polio; deformities; hydrocephalia; sequelae of meningitis; sequelae of neonatal anoxia; congenital deformities; and infantile cerebral hemiplegia.

Health of Prisoners

The prison population is exposed to various risk factors associated with overcrowding. The total number of prisoners rose from 1,500 in June 1995 to more than 2,817 in December 1996. In the National Penitentiary, 200 to 300 inmates share a single room measuring 400 m²; in another facility, 13 inmates may share a space of 5 m². There are a few women and minors in the detention center, although there is a special prison for women and minors (Fort-National) in Port-au-Prince. Dilapidated facilities, a shortage of clean water, and extremely poor sanitation conditions magnify the widespread and serious health problems that affect the prison's population.

An epidemic of beriberi broke out in November 1995 at the National Penitentiary, striking 84 out of 1,000 inmates. Ten inmates died, representing a fatality rate of 12%. These inmates were fed completely on prison meals. Subsequently there were two smaller outbreaks in March and June 1996. Several actions have been taken to address this problem.

The National Prison Administration, established in 1995 and attached to the Ministry of Justice, operates 18 prison facilities. In October 1994, a project to support prison reform was undertaken by UNDP with assistance from USAID and the Government of France. UNICEF helped to improve conditions for juvenile offenders in detention facilities, mainly through advocacy; PAHO and other agencies are involved in the health and nutrition component of the project. Existing health posts have been upgraded, and new ones were established in most detention facilities between 1995 and 1996 (e.g., a 20-bed dispensary at the National Penitentiary for a target population of more than 1,000 inmates). Twenty health auxiliaries were appointed.

Analysis by Type of Disease or Health Impairment

Communicable Diseases

Vector-Borne Diseases. Malaria is considered a public health problem in Haiti, especially in rural areas. In some areas, malaria shows evidence of year-round transmission; in others, transmission is seasonal, coinciding with the rainy season. *Plasmodium falciparum* is prevalent throughout the country. The last confirmed indigenous cases of *Plasmodium vivax* infection occurred in 1983. Most cases of malaria transmission occur in coastal areas at altitudes below 300 m, particularly in the heavily populated rice-growing areas in the south and Artibonite. The disease remains confined to certain foci, with some areas showing a positivity index of 5%–10%. Estimates made in 1988, as part of an effort to map out a strategy for malaria control, amounted to 250,000 annual malaria cases, with a 1% case fatality rate. Slide positivity indexes for the 1991–1994 period are unusually high, ranging from 31.2% to 42%.

Chloroquine is still the preferred drug for malaria treatment. There have been no documented cases of resistance to its 4-aminoquinolines. Chloroquine sensitivity tests conducted in 1995 found no chloroquine-resistant strains of *P. falciparum*. Given the widespread use of chloroquine, high priority will continue to be placed on surveillance operations for the parasite's sensitivity to this drug. Its main vector, *Anopheles albimanus*, is resistant to organochloride compounds (DDT).

Dengue is considered an endemic disease. The vector of the disease, *Aedes aegypti*, is found throughout the country, and extremely high infestation rates have been reported over the years, particularly in urban areas. Data collected 10 years ago by the Department of Public Health put the seroprevalence rate at 3%. In 1994, an outbreak of dengue was reported in Port-au-Prince among U.S. soldiers attached to the multinational force. Serotype 1 isolates were found in patients suffering from febrile illnesses. Serotypes 1, 2, and 4 are currently found in Haiti, while serotype 3 has never been identified. The omnipresence of the vector poses a constant threat of outbreaks of dengue hemorrhagic fever.

Lymphatic filariasis, found in scattered urban foci, mainly in the north and Gulf of La Gonâve, is still a serious public health threat in Haiti. *Wuchereria bancrofti,* transmitted by *Culex quinquefasciatus,* is becoming meso-hyperendemic in coastal areas. Its effects were most visible in boys and men, who generally develop elephantiasis of the scrotum. Studies conducted by the United States Centers for Disease Control and Prevention indicate that more than 20% of the population of most coastal cities, including Léogâne, Petit-Goâve, Arcahaie, and Limbé, are carriers of the microfilaria. Many men over 15 years of age in the Léogâne region suffer from hydrocele; 5% of the local population suffers from elephantiasis of the foot.

Vaccine-Preventable Diseases. In August 1994, Haiti was declared free of poliomyelitis by the International Certification Commission on Polio Eradication, and since then no cases of flaccid paralysis have been confirmed as poliomyelitis. However, vaccination rates remain very low (30% in 1995).

Between 1989 and 1994, the average attack rate for measles was 24 per 100,000 persons. A countrywide measles epidemic broke out in July 1991. Since the national vaccination campaign in 1994–1995, no cases of measles have been confirmed. The routine vaccination rate in infants younger than 1 year old in 1995 was estimated at 75%.

In February 1996, one case of diphtheria was confirmed by culture. The patient was a 9-month-old infant who had been administered only one dose of the DPT vaccine. No cases of whooping cough were reported in 1995. The vaccination rate for DPT3 was 30% in 1995.

Regarding neonatal tetanus, 78 cases were reported in 1995 for the whole country. During the first six months of 1997, 31 cases of neonatal tetanus were reported by 39 sentinel sites from the nine departments.

Hepatitis B surface antigen was found in 5.5% of donors tested in 1990. In 1996 serosentinel studies conducted by the Child Health Institute and GHESKIO Centers, at facilities in nine locations (one by department), found hepatitis B surface antigen in 2%–7% of pregnant women.

Intestinal Infectious Diseases. There were no reported cases of cholera as of July 1997. The epidemiological surveillance system established for acute diarrhea identified *Vibrio furnissii* for the first time in the Caribbean and Non-01 *Vibrio cholerae* isolated from a stool specimen taken from a patient with cholera-like symptoms.

From 1987 to 1994, the National Health Surveys detected a sharp decline in the incidence of diarrhea in children under 5 years old (from 43% to 27.6% for the two-week period preceding the surveys); however, values remain very high, reaching 47.7% in the age group 6–11 months old. Diarrheal diseases are the leading cause of illness and death in children under 5 years of age, often associated with acute respiratory

infections and malnutrition. According to EMMUS-II, only 31.6% (up from 16.4% in 1987) of children suffering from diarrhea were treated with a home-based oral rehydration therapy (ORT). Only 14% of children suffering from diarrhea were treated at a health care facility or by a professional.

Typhoid is endemic in Haiti. In 1991, a major typhoid epidemic was confirmed in several low-income neighborhoods of Port-au-Prince. Several epidemic foci were reported in 1992–1993, predominantly in the south. The health center of Les Cayes, which serves 100,000 area residents, reported that 12.5% of 2,500 patients examined during January 1993 suffered from typhoid. From July to December 1995, typhoid was responsible for 6% of admissions at the Haitian State University Hospital pediatrics ward. It ranked as the fifth leading cause of hospitalization.

Chronic Communicable Diseases. Between 1981 and 1990, more than 6,000 new cases of tuberculosis were notified each year to WHO; 10,237 cases or 154.7 per 100,000 were reported in 1991, date of the last notification. The incidence of tuberculosis in Haiti is estimated at 180 per 100,000 inhabitants. The high mortality rate is the result of the country's generalized poverty, malnutrition, limited access to health care, and HIV/AIDS epidemic. In a study conducted in 1992–1993, an HIV seroprevalence of 19% was found in a group of 240 tuberculosis patients. Data from 1991 show that 50% of all patients with AIDS suffered from tuberculosis. Seroprevalence studies among children, conducted in 1996, confirmed the close correlation between tuberculosis and HIV infection. Children with tuberculosis aged 16 months to 5 years have a 5.85 greater risk of being HIV-positive than children in the same age group who do not have the disease. In 1995, multidrug-resistance further complicated efforts to manage this disease.

Between 1977 and 1996, the country's two referral facilities, Providence Hospital in Gonaïves (Artibonite) and the Fame Pereo Institute in Port-au-Prince, saw 1,998 registered patients, 80.5% them being paucibacillary cases and 19.5% multibacillary cases. A breakdown of leprosy patients by age group reveals that 21% were children under 15 years of age of whom 12.6% were multibacillary cases. Of 521 leprosy cases diagnosed between 1993 and 1996, 22 cases of disabilities grade 2 and over were notified.

Acute Respiratory Infections. Data produced by EMMUS-II for 1994 showed that 20% of children under 5 years of age suffered from acute respiratory infections (ARIs) during the two weeks preceding the survey. In 1994, ARIs accounted for 25% of deaths among children under 5 years of age, and pneumonia was the number one cause of death among ARI patients. In 1994–1995, ARIs were the leading cause of patient visits to 42 sentinel facilities in Haiti.

Rabies and Other Zoonoses. Two to four cases of human rabies were reported each year between 1990 and 1995. Only one of the cases in 1993 was confirmed by the Connecticut State Laboratory in the United States. Seven cases were reported in 1996.

In 1993, 183 clinical cases of human anthrax were reported in northern Haiti. This figure rose sharply in 1994, with 622 new cases reported after tropical storm Gordon. This rising number of reported cases may have been due to improvements in surveillance operations in response to the storm. Of the 768 cases of human anthrax reported in 1995, 70.5% were from the country's southeast.

Leptospirosis appeared to be on the rise. In 1995, 64 cases of the disease were identified and 32 cases were reported during the first four months of 1996. The male-to-female ratio is 2:1, with 35% of the cases involving males between the ages of 20 and 39. The disease proved fatal in 33% of the cases.

AIDS and Other Sexually Transmitted Diseases. A cumulative total of 4,967 AIDS cases (46% of whom were female) were reported between 1982 and 1992. Official reports and notification of AIDS cases were suspended by 1992. As of 1996, the percentage of the sexually active population infected with HIV was estimated at 3%–5% in rural areas and 7%–10% in urban areas. Preliminary projections, based on different mathematical models, conclude that the number of HIV-positive individuals will reach more than 380,760 by the year 2000 and the annual number of deaths could climb as high as 27,000, including 6,000 children. HIV transmission is predominantly heterosexual (male/female ratio 1.2:1).

STDs were not included in the list of notifiable diseases, but there is a proposal to include syphilis, gonorrhea, and AIDS in the revised Code of Public Hygiene. In 1995, a national survey conducted by the Child Health Institute reported that 8% of all male respondents suffered from an STD during the 12 months preceding the survey: among them, 4% from an urethral discharge and 2% from a genital ulcer. A prevalence study of 1,000 pregnant women in Cité Soleil showed 45% of subjects suffering from at least one STD. Of the same study population, 11% had a positive RPR (Rapid Plasma Reagin), suggesting a high prevalence of congenital syphilis.

Leading causes of genital ulcers in Haiti are, in descending order: syphilis, soft chancre, invasive genital herpes (particularly when associated with HIV infection), donovanosis, and venereal lymphogranuloma. Prevalence studies of syphilis were conducted in selected Haitian population groups. Among low-risk groups, seropositivity to the VDRL test ranged from 3%–6% in 1990 and from 6%–8% in 1991 among the urban population of Port-au-Prince. In 1992–1993, seropositivity to VDRL and FTA-ABS tests ranged from 4%–12% in seroprevalence studies of pregnant women at five sentinel locations. A serosentinel survey conducted in nine sites in 1994–1995 indicated that a pregnant woman with syphilis had between 1.4 and 5.2 times higher risk of being HIV-infected than a pregnant woman without syphilis.

According to research conducted by the Haitian Group for Study of Kaposi Sarcoma and Opportunistic Infections Centers (GHESKIO), 48% of urethral discharges in Haiti are caused by gonorrhea, and only a small percentage of these discharges are caused by trichomoniasis (6%) or chlamydia infections (5%). In the remaining cases, the etiologic agent could not be identified, mostly because 70% of the patients already had been subject to self-administered treatment. From 1989 to 1992, a GHESKIO Centers study conducted at a reference clinic for sexually transmitted diseases showed that 90% of all identified gonococcal strains were penicillinase-producing *Neisseria gonorrhoeae* (PPNG).

A study on STDs causing vaginal discharges among pregnant women in Cité Soleil ranked trichomoniasis first (35%), followed by chlamydia infections (10%) and gonorrhea (4%). Of all cases of leukorrhea, 5% are associated with pelvic inflammatory disease.

Emerging and Re-emerging Diseases. In late April 1994, a meningococcemia epidemic was reported in Ouanaminthe, in the Northeast Department. By the end of November, approximately 100 cases and nine deaths had been reported. Group C *Neisseria meningitidis* was identified. In 1995, in the Port-au-Prince area, over 75% of the cases involved children between 5 and 14 years of age. The rest of the country also reported cases, with the largest number of cases seen in rural areas in the Artibonite. In all of 1995, 158 cases were reported, of which 55 died, yielding a case-fatality rate of 35%.

There were reports of sporadic cases of yaws, and a clinical, serologic survey was conducted in September 1993 in the Department of Grande-Anse. From a total of 553 subjects tested (including 231 subjects under the age of 15), 11 cases of yaws were identified. These cases were serologically confirmed by the FTA-ABS test.

Noncommunicable Diseases and Other Health-Related Problems

Nutritional Diseases and Diseases of Metabolism. In 1994–1995, EMMUS-II revealed a significant increase in the prevalence of wasting since 1990, mainly affecting children under 3 years of age. More than one-third of all children who survived their first birthday showed signs of severe growth retardation.

By age 5 years, 41% of all children were severely stunted. High rates of malnutrition and infectious diseases suggest that many preschool children are suffering from the effects of vitamin A deficiency and/or nutritional anemia. Mangoes are an important dietary source of vitamin A, and following their abundant availability, a seasonal variation has been observed in the dietary intake and deficiency of vitamin A.

A 1991 survey conducted in the Central Plateau showed a prevalence rate of 10% for all types of goiter (Grades 1 + 2) and 2.5% for visible forms of goiter. Similarly, urinary iodine in the general population was 10.3 μg/dl. Iodine deficiency problems are typically confined to the isolated inland mountainous areas.

There were three types of diabetes registered in Haiti: type 1, or insulin-dependent diabetes (10% of total); type 2, or non-insulin-dependent diabetes; and type 3, or malnutrition-related diabetes ("tropical" diabetes). The prevalence ranges from 2%–8% for different parts of the country. Half of all amputations performed in the State University Hospital in 1987 concerned patients with diabetes.

Cardiovascular Diseases. These diseases accounted for 40% of patient admissions at the State University Hospital in 1996, mainly cerebrovascular accidents and ischemic heart disease. Two surveys suggest a 13%–15% prevalence of high blood pressure in the adult population 18 years and older.

Malignant Tumors. Three problems hindered cancer treatment. The low level of awareness, the limited access to biopsies or surgical procedures outside Port-au-Prince, and the extremely limited treatment options. Cancer treatment in Haiti is limited to surgical resection or excision. Chemotherapy is costly and unavailable. The National Cancer Institute, a nonprofit foundation established in 1988, is subsidized by the Ministry of Health. It operated Haiti's only radiation therapy service, which has been inoperable due to obsolete equipment. The Institute's main radiation therapy resource is a Janus cobalt-60 unit, which is virtually devitalized. The National Cancer Institute statistics showed that the most frequent type of cancer treated was cervical cancer, representing 60% of the total for the period 1988–1990 and 40% for the period 1991–94. Breast cancer ranked second with 15% and 30% respectively. Nasopharynx occupied the third position with 10%–15% of the cases. The total cases of cancers treated by the institution averaged 250 per year from 1988 to 1994.

Several health care facilities are partially involved in the detection, diagnosis, treatment, and care of patients suffering from cervical cancer/dysplasia. These facilities are operated by the public, the private nonprofit, and the private profit-making sectors.

Accidents and Violence. Violence is a major public health problem in Haiti. Political violence decreased dramatically since 1994. Many casualties are associated with criminal violence resulting in gun and knife injuries or fatalities. The widespread problem of domestic violence was the focus of a 1995 national survey on violence against women.

Data reported by the Haitian State University Hospital for 1995 showed that a higher incidence of traffic accidents occurred in December, as compared with the rest of that year. The total annual number of dead and injured was 2,393; males were more affected than females (1.7:1). Frequent domestic accidents resulted in serious burns mainly affecting children. In addition, Haiti is regularly the scene of fires and shipping accidents, such as the Neptune tragedy in February 1993, which caused 1,500 deaths.

Behavioral Disorders. Over the past few years, there has been an increase in reported mental disorders precipitated by the sociopolitical crisis, unemployment, violence, social unrest, and drug use (marijuana, cocaine, and crack cocaine). In the main psychiatric center, 25% of patients suffered from acute disorientation and 20% from paranoid schizophrenia. The most prevalent disorders among children and adolescents were hyperactivity and learning disorders. There were many cases of drug addiction among patients 16–25 years of age, although they often present themselves for psychiatric reasons that are secondary to drug abuse. A private hospital with 300 beds reported that more than 60% of admissions were attributed to manic-depressive psychoses, and the remaining 40% to chronic schizophrenia.

Oral Health. There were 32 dentists per 10,000 inhabitants. Surveys estimated decayed/missing/filled teeth (DMFT) for 12-year-old children around 1. The high HIV prevalence among the sexually active population of urban areas (7%–10%) and the dangerous practices of the traditional dentists who treat most of the population are factors that have an impact on oral health in the country.

Natural Disasters. Tropical storm Gordon struck Haiti in November 1994, claiming 1,122 lives. It destroyed 3,550 homes, seriously damaged several water supply systems, killed thousands of livestock, and damaged vast acres of food crops. The storm affected the health services through increased demand for and redistribution of limited resources. Widespread flooding, both in rural (the south in November 1995, and the south and northwest in February 1996), as well as urban areas (beachfront areas of Port-au-Prince) caused extensive damage. Drought regularly affects the country's northwest.

RESPONSE OF THE HEALTH SYSTEM

National Health Plans and Policies

In March 1996, the Ministry of Health introduced a health policy that recognizes a fundamental right to health and the State's obligation to guarantee access to health care for all.

This policy is based on equity, social justice, and solidarity. Health sector reform was designed as part of the State's decentralization effort to ensure equal access to a minimum package of services. However, scarce available resources and the constraints imposed by the economic structural plan make the application of the health policy a great challenge for the Government.

Health Sector Reform

The Ministry of Health defined the following priorities:

- Strengthening the Ministry of Health at central and departmental levels, including developing human resources and managerial capacity; using new health financing modalities, undertaking hospital reforms, updating health legislation, reviewing the policy on essential drugs, developing the health information system, pursuing intersectorial coordination, and implementing community health units based on decentralization and community participation.
- Developing primary health care aimed at delivering a minimum package of health services to the population, including comprehensive child care that targets acute respiratory infections; comprehensive health care for women with emphasis on pregnancies and reduction of maternal mortality; vaccination; access to essential drugs; prevention and control of communicable diseases; targeting emerging and re-emerging diseases such as tuberculosis, STDs, and AIDS; controlling meningococcal infections and vector-borne diseases; eradicating measles, neonatal tetanus, and leprosy; and improving medico-surgical emergencies and dental care.
- Strengthening health promotion activities to encourage the population to assume responsibility for its health and adopt a healthy lifestyle—programs included health information dissemination, health education, and social mobilization, particularly in the prevention of communicable diseases, violence and accidents, school health, and pathologies linked to poor nutritional habits.
- Improving environmental health, including access to potable water, food hygiene, control and disposal of excreta and atmospheric pollution as well as the prevention and mitigation of disasters.

Organization of the Health Sector

Institutional Organization

Haiti's health system includes the public sector, the semi-public sector, and the private sector.

The public sector was seriously affected by the country's political crisis, which led all foreign aid to be channeled through nongovernmental organizations (NGOs). The Ministry of Health is structured into central, departmental, and community levels. Through its central directorates and units, it sets standards. Planning, monitoring, and supervision are the responsibility of the heads of the nine sanitary departments. One-third of the country's 663 health institutions belong to the public sector.

The semi-public or mixed sector encompasses nonprofit institutions that are supported mainly by NGOs. Staff is paid in whole or in part by the public sector, but is managed by the private sector.

In 1994 there were 49 hospitals and 61 other inpatient facilities, with an estimated 90 beds per 100,000 population; occupancy rates have not been available at the central level for a long time. Of the country's total health care facilities, 32% are operated by NGOs (Table 1). The private, profit-making sector is comprised of physicians, dentists, and other private practice specialists who mostly work in Port-au-Prince and in private health care facilities.

The high cost for services at these facilities makes them unaffordable to most of the population. Public and private establishments function completely independent of one another with very little networking. Differences in access to adequate health care are further magnified by the uneven geographical distribution of centers and hospital beds.

Social security benefits are limited to formally employed people. In 1995, the Insurance Agency for Occupational Accidents, Illness, and Maternity (OFATMA), an autonomous body under the umbrella of the Ministry of Social Affairs, provided insurance coverage to 2,500 public and private firms. In 1996 it covered 60,000 workers, an increase from 40,000 covered in 1994. A few private firms provide limited coverage.

The estimated per capita expenditure in health for 1995 was G15.7 (US$ 2.0); it represented a decrease compared with that of 1990, which was G24.8 (US$ 3.4). Total per capita expenditure on health reached US$ 9, representing 3.5% of GDP in 1995. According to these estimates, in 1996 the government budget represented about 16% of the total expenditure; external donor agencies, which are mostly channeled through the Ministry of Health and NGOs, 28%; NGOs, 20%; and private expenditures, 36% in 1996.

Organization of Health Regulatory Activities

Health legislation originally enacted in 1981 remains in effect, but a new legal administrative framework is being drafted.

The Ministry of Health established criteria for the operation of medical and paramedical education facilities. Two private nursing schools and 10 training facilities for auxiliary nurses

TABLE 1
Breakdown of health care facilities, by category and sector, June 1994.

| Department | Hospitals | Category | | | | Total | Sector | | | |
		Inpatient facilities	Outpatient facilities	Clinics	Asylums		Public	Private	Mixed	Not specified
Artibonite	4	11	16	52	1	84	37	26	20	1
Centralga	2	1	10	31	0	44	20	15	7	2
Norde-Anse	2	9	5	41	3	60	28	6	26	
North	1	10	10	30	1	52	19	10	23	
Northeast	1	4	1	16	0	22	10	3	9	
Northwest	1	7	4	46	1	59	18	16	25	
West	33	9	82	109	2	235	54	127	54	
South	4	8	7	51	1	71	25	4	42	
Southeast	1	2	4	29	0	36	23	9	3	1
Total	49	61	139	405	9	663	234	216	209	4

Source: PAHO/WHO, list of facilities by geographic area.

obtained operating licenses. The Ministry's pharmacy service issues a certificate to pharmacy students after completion of a four-year training program with a one-year internship.

The pharmacy service regulates all matters related to pharmaceuticals, which mainly involves the inspection of private pharmacies. Haiti has no drug registration, control of drug imports, or inspections of drug manufacturers. Drugs that normally required prescriptions are easily accessible and commonly sold by street vendors.

Between November 1995 and June 1996, an outbreak of acute renal failure affected 100 children, and the majority died. A multiagency investigation revealed that the condition was due do the ingestion of a locally produced acetaminophen syrup contaminated with imported diethylen glycol. To address the situation, the Ministry of Health endeavored to improve quality control monitoring through regular inspection of manufacturers, importers, suppliers, and pharmacies. Because there was no national quality control laboratory, all samples had to be sent abroad for analysis.

In November 1995, the Ministry of the Environment elaborated the National Action Plan of Environment, designed to deal with various environmental threats to freshwater, seawater, air, and soil.

Health Services and Resources

Organization of Services for Care of the Population

Health Promotion and Social Communication in Health. Several large-scale, public awareness campaigns involving various sectors were launched, some of which are highlighled below. A social marketing campaign for condoms, managed by PSI with AIDSCAP funding since September 1992, resulted in the sale of 14 million condoms. The "baby friendly hospitals" initiative that UNICEF and PAHO jointly launched in 1994 to promote breast-feeding resulted in the certification of two hospitals as baby friendly in 1996. The national campaign for the eradication of measles, which was implemented in 1994–1995, achieved a 98% vaccination coverage. The national campaign for the promotion of breast-feeding that was launched in August 1995 reached the majority of the population. The observance of "Tuberculosis Day," "International Women's Day," "Safe Water, the Environment, and Health Day," "World No-Tobacco Day," "Mental Health Day," and "AIDS Day" receives media coverage.

School Health. The Ministries of Public Health and of Education, with external financial and technical assistance, are working together to develop school health policies appropriate for Haiti, including early detection of hearing and vision problems; promotion of oral health and detection of dental caries; nutritional surveillance; detection of iron deficiency and diseases caused by intestinal parasites; early detection of poor posture; health education and promotion, including sex education; and the prevention of STDs.

Workers' Health. Haiti has no national health program for workers, but workers who receive coverage from the Agency for Occupational Accidents, Illness, and Maternity were given annual examinations to detect tuberculosis and syphilis. The Agency has a 30-bed hospital in Port-au-Prince that granted appointments to an average of 30 outpatients a day.

The Center for the Promotion of Women Workers is an NGO that offers a preventive health program to women workers in general and female assembly plant workers in particular. The program encompasses educational forums, AIDS prevention, and the operation of a women's health clinic for prenatal care. Another NGO, the AIDS Control Group, conducts educational programs directly in factories.

Programs for Disease Prevention and Control. Haiti follows a strategy for the integrated management of child health, integrating health care interventions, providing quick and efficient screening for prompt referrals to better equipped facilities, and using every opportunity to have children visit health care facilities to promote preventive health measures against childhood illnesses.

In 1992, NGOs throughout the country allocated funds for the planning and implementation of vaccination programs in which regular staff members from public health facilities participated.

A vaccination campaign against measles was carried out between November 1994 and June 1995, resulting in the vaccination of 2.8 million children, which represents 98% of the target population of children between 9 months and 14 years of age. A countrywide network of four to five storage and distribution units for vaccines and supplies for immunization in each department was established. This process will be completed with the establishment of an active distribution system with motorized couriers.

In 1996, 200 clinics provided diagnosis, treatment, and follow-up of tuberculosis patients. The cure rate varied considerably from one department to another, ranging from 40% to 78%. Improvements in cure rates are most likely the result of the increasingly widespread use of the short-course therapy. Training activities conducted from 1993 to 1995 targeted 828 health care workers. In 1995, the emergence of several cases of drug-resistant tuberculosis made it necessary to use costly second-line drugs. This significantly raised the cost of treatment for a drug resistant patient from US$ 45 to US$ 3,000.

Regarding malaria, the country pursues a primary health care strategy that involves the elimination of deaths and the reduction of morbidity rates by emphasizing early detection and timely treatment. The vector control component includes provisions for community participation. The Ministry of Health undertook the task of training all health care personnel in the prevention and control of malaria. Upon completion in 1997, a total of 3,500 health workers will have been trained.

Since 1991, AIDS control efforts have been supported technically and financially by four organizations, including: PAHO, USAID, WHO (GPA) and the French Cooperation, and UNFPA. This support has bolstered activities implemented by roughly 20 NGOs in the areas of serosentinel surveillance for HIV infection, IEC campaigns, production of IEC materials, training of health workers and community leaders to care for AIDS and STD patients, clinical and psychological care of patients suffering from STDs/AIDS in a reference center in Port-au-Prince and in three hospitals based in both urban and rural areas, financial aid and nutritional assistance for AIDS patients and their families in Port-au-Prince, distribution of condoms, and supply of drugs and materials for the prevention and control of STDs.

The Ministry of Health, PAHO, the GHESKIO Centers, and AIDSCAP NGOs have been developing simplified algorithms for the treatment of STDs. On January 1, 1996, UNAIDS officially began to operate in Haiti. The national program for the control of AIDS and other STDs was launched by the Ministry on World AIDS Day, December 1, 1996.

The Ministry of Agriculture's Health Protection Unit is responsible for administering the strategy for the control of zoonoses. The Unit's Animal Health Service of has five veterinarians and 90 workers deployed throughout the country. Health officers are actively involved in efforts to control stray dogs and are working with Ministry of Agriculture personnel to conduct vaccination campaigns.

Anthrax control efforts are based on a strategy to contain outbreaks. In addition, in cooperation with an NGO, a nationwide campaign for the vaccination of 500,000 head of livestock began in 1995. By February 1996, more than 218,000 animals were successfully vaccinated against anthrax in all nine departments.

Regarding rabies control efforts, a national vaccination campaign for dogs and cats was implemented by the Ministry of Agriculture in 1995 with assistance from the United States Army, the Ministry of Health, and PAHO; the country is estimated to have approximately 100,000 dogs. More than 54,072 doses of vaccine were administered between July and August 1995, mostly in the metropolitan area.

Efforts to control micronutrient deficiencies mainly entail short-term supplementation interventions, including universal distribution of high-dose vitamin A prophylaxis of 100,000 UI to children 6–12 months of age and 200,000 UI to children 12–72 months old at vaccination sites, universal distribution of vitamin A supplements (200,000 UI) to mothers within one month after delivery by community health workers or traditional birth attendants, iron-folate supplementation for those diagnosed with anemia, and targeted iodine capsule distribution in specific areas. PAHO, working with UNICEF, is involved in long-term strategies to build the local capacity to iodize salt and to produce and promote solar dried mangoes rich in vitamin A.

Foodborne diseases remain a public health challenge, due in part to the limited personnel involved in the inspection process and deeply-rooted cultural factors. The Ministry's Directorate of Health Environment and Epidemiology is responsible for control activities related to food safety. The laboratory attached to the Faculty of Agronomy is involved in testing products destined for export.

TABLE 2
Trends in water supply and basic sanitation coverage levels, Haiti, 1990–1995.

Service and location	1990	1993	1995
Water supply in the capital	53%	34%	35%
Water supply in smaller cities (72)	58%	40%	45%
Water supply in rural areas	33%	23%	39%
Basic sanitation in urban areas	43%	41%	42%
Basic sanitation in rural areas	16%	14%	16%

Epidemiological Surveillance Systems and Public Health Laboratories. Until 1991, only four diseases—poliomyelitis, neonatal tetanus, AIDS, and cholera—had specific surveillance systems in place. Between late 1992 and 1995, several NGOs supported the establishment of a simplified epidemiological surveillance system that relies on monitoring simple operational indicators for principal diseases gathered through a network of private or semi-public sentinel facilities. This basic system was later complemented by a strengthened epidemiological surveillance system for specific diseases.

In September 1996, the Ministry of Health created a committee to design and support the implementation of a new National Health Information System. The committee's 16 members include representatives from the Ministries of Public Health, of Finance and Planning, and of External Cooperation; one NGO, and three technical cooperation agencies.

Drinking Water Services and Sewerage. The political crisis and ensuing trade embargo have greatly impaired the water supply and sanitation sector. Ongoing investment projects in this sector, totaling US$ 163 million, were interrupted. With no maintenance, the water supply infrastructure deteriorated rapidly, and service coverage levels in the capital fell by nearly 30% between December 1990 and December 1994 (Table 2). The crisis also disbanded the National Water and Sanitation coordinating committee and national water agencies. In October 1994, almost all projects that had been suspended in November 1991 were resumed, and since then, increasing amounts are being invested in the water supply and sanitation sector.

Municipal Solid Waste Management Services. Nearly 30% of the daily volume of solid wastes produced in Port-au-Prince is collected by the Ministry of Public Works and the municipality; an autonomous government agency in charge of solid waste management shut down in 1993. Service was more reliable in smaller cities, where collection was ensured by local services run by the Ministries of Public Works and of Health. Disposal of hospital waste also is poor.

Food Assistance Programs. Food aid is very important for Haiti, where growing numbers of households face escalating food security problems. Main donors were USAID, the European Union, and the World Food Program of the United Nations. Many NGOs and bilateral agencies also were involved in relief food distribution.

Organization and Operation of Personal Health Care Services

Ambulatory Services, Hospitals, and Emergency Services. Ambulatory care is delivered through outpatient facilities, clinics, and outpatient services in most hospitals; services vary greatly from one structure to another.

In 1993, a pilot project for emergency care was launched with the assistance of PAHO and physicians attached to the French Emergency Ambulance Service (SAMU). The project will lay the foundation for a countrywide emergency services network that would provide services ranging from screening and first aid (level 1) to specialized treatment (level 4). Four health centers in the metropolitan area are equipped with emergency units. In addition, the Haitian Red Cross and several new hospitals are establishing their own ambulance service and emergency telephone and radio communications. Training in emergency medical care was organized for health personnel throughout the country: 314 physicians, nurses, and health auxiliaries and 72 paramedics working in the public and private health sectors received the training. The experience is expected to serve as the basis for the formulation of a national plan for emergency care. The Ministry of Health includes emergency medicine/surgery in the minimum package of health services.

Auxiliary Services for Diagnosis and Blood Banks. The only medical testing laboratories are located in a few private or semi-public hospitals in the main cities, and they generally only conduct basic laboratory tests. A total of 122 public and private nonprofit institutions have diagnostic facilities for malaria, and 200 diagnostic centers are part of the tuberculosis control network, equipped to perform sputum examinations. There were no organized quality control services.

Since 1986, when the blood transfusion service operated by the Haitian Red Cross took over all the country's blood transfusion services in hospitals located in major cities, blood has been screened for HIV infection. At the blood transfusion center in Port-au-Prince, blood donations also are systematically tested for hepatitis B (surface antigen) and syphilis (serologic testing for acquired syphilis). Lack of resources has hindered screening of hepatitis C.

Because Haiti is considered to be highly endemic for HIV infection and syphilis and mesoendemic for malaria and hepatitis B, blood transfusions were kept to a strict minimum. A national blood transfusion policy was developed by the Haitian Red Cross since early 1996.

Specialized Services. Rehabilitation services for persons with disabilities are scarce and most disabled persons are cared for by relatives at home. A few establishments provide services in the area of prevention (2), special education (3), specialized care (8), vocational training (4), and social mainstreaming (4). The majority of disabled persons do not receive specialized re-education or social rehabilitation services.

The main institutions for the disabled include the Saint Vincent School for infants and youths up to 18 who suffer from motor or sensory disabilities. The school is equipped with a workshop for the manufacture of orthopedic devices and artificial limbs. The Special Education Center, the only institution for the mentally retarded (500 new cases per year), operates a school for 80. A vocational center and workshop provides training for 40 girls and 40 boys aged 6 to 18 years old; Montfort Institute, with branches in Cap Haïtien, Port-de-Paix, and Saint-Marc, serves 450 deaf-mute children, 300 of whom are Port-au-Prince residents; and The Haitian Society for the Blind and the National Committee for the Rehabilitation of Disabled Persons provide outreach services and work to increase public awareness of problems faced by disabled persons.

According to the new health care policy, dental health is part of the package of health services. The current status of oral and dental health care in Haiti is marked by shortages of manpower and equipment. Some NGOs attempt to bring affordable, community-based solutions to oral and dental health problems.

Most of the population believes that psychiatric disorders are caused by supernatural influences, which leads at least half of all patients to seek out the services of a "houngan," a male voodoo practitioner. Haiti has very few facilities that provide psychiatric care—a 300-bed public psychiatric hospital, a 60-bed specialized public psychiatric facility, and three private clinics, including a 300-bed facility. Since 1988, the situation has improved due to the availability of increasing numbers of specialists and introduction of new forms of treatment.

There were no nationwide programs for the treatment of diabetes and hypertension. An NGO in Port-au-Prince provided prevention activities, medical care, access to drugs at a reasonable price, and rehabilitation services. Early detection of diabetes was impeded by several factors: the shortage of diagnostic tools and equipment, which were virtually nonexistent in rural areas; insufficient health facilities; low awareness among the general population; and the lack of an early detection policy.

TABLE 3
Population distribution, deployment of health care personnel, and beds per 100,000 population, by department.

Department (% population)	Physicians	Nurses	Auxiliaries	Beds per 100,000 population
West (34%)	561 (73%)	527 (67%)	674 (37%)	56
Southeast (7%)	21 (3%)	42 (5%)	42 (2%)	42
North (11%)	31 (4%)	52 (7%)	178 (10%)	66
Northeast (4%)	15 (2%)	11 (1%)	67 (4%)	102
Artibonite (14%)	69 (9%)	33 (4%)	218 (12%)	45
Central (7%)	14 (2%)	9 (1%)	105 (6%)	62
South (9%)	30 (4%)	61 (8%)	264 (14%)	135
Grande-Anse (9%)	13 (2%)	22 (3%)	160 (9%)	89
Northwest (6%)	19 (2%)	29 (4%)	136 (7%)	38

Source: Ministry of Public Health and Population and PAHO/WHO. Health situation analysis. Haiti, June 1996.

Inputs for Health

Physical Infrastructure. The health care infrastructure and medical equipment are seriously impaired by a lack of maintenance and timely repairs. The deterioration in the condition of installations and equipment in public health care facilities was compounded by the nation's three-year-long crisis. Between October 1994 and March 1996, a total of US$ 1,310,525 was spent on rehabilitation projects in 46 health care facilities and 5 hospitals, including the Haitian State University Hospital. A total of US$ 8,278,610 was invested for the partial rehabilitation of 88 health care facilities and 5 hospitals, including the University Hospital.

Access to Health Care. A total of 663 health facilities are located throughout the country. According to EMMUS-II most women in urban areas live close to health care facilities (79%–98% in Port-au-Prince and 62%–87% in other cities). The situation in rural areas is quite different. In 1991, an estimated 40% of population had no access to primary health care services. Disparities are also evident in the deployment of health professionals throughout the country. Approximately 73% of all physicians, 67% of all nurses, 35% of all health care facilities, and 52% of all hospital beds are concentrated in the West Department and serve one-third of the total population. Table 3 shows the distribution of population, health care personnel, and beds per 100,000 population by department, revealing the disparities in access to health care in Haiti.

Socially and economically deprived people living in rural areas seldom visit a health professional. Some progress has been made in making essential drugs available and affordable in most public and private facilities and nonprofit organizations. Cost recovery mechanisms finance a social fund to provide care for destitute patients.

Because the population widely relies on traditional medicine, efforts have been made to bridge the gap between traditional and modern medicine. For example, in 1995 the Ministry of Public Health and Population issued a health policy paper stating that relations with traditional health practitioners would be encouraged and that the integration of traditional medicine into the national health care system would be worked out in conjunction with traditional health practitioners.

Essential Drugs, Immunobiologicals, and Reagents. There were 4 drug manufacturers, 50 importers and suppliers, and 200 authorized private pharmacies in the Port-au-Prince area.

In 1992, with help from national and international partners, PAHO created an essential drug program (PROMESS) to distribute essential drugs and medical equipment in Haiti as part of humanitarian assistance; the Ministry of Health has chaired the board of PROMESS since 1996. The Ministry has approved approximately 400 essential drugs. Drugs for PROMESS were financed by internal cost recovery funds and by subsidies from international donors.

In order to promote the use of essential drugs, the Ministry developed training in essential drugs management for field-level personnel. Government peripheral warehouses, supplied by PROMESS, facilitated the distribution of drugs and medical supplies to health institutions in the countryside. Medicinal herb manuals in Creole are disseminated by a few NGOs.

UNICEF imported EPI vaccines and provided them free of charge; vaccines were stored at and distributed from the PAHO warehouse. Only a few reagents, such as stains for TB control, were prepared locally.

Health Technology. Health technology was extremely limited in Haiti. Radiology and radiation therapy services were concentrated in Port-au-Prince and in a few provincial hospitals, and most of the equipment was outdated. Well-trained technicians were rare, and dosimetry services and protective measures in and around X-ray rooms were unreliable. In general, modern diagnostic imaging equipment was located in the private sector. A Port-au-Prince private facility received its first CT scanner in 1995. Kidney dialysis services in Haiti were limited to two units in a private hospital.

Communications. A radio communications network known as the "a radio health network" was established in 1993 by PAHO/WHO in conjunction with health sector NGOs. It has proven invaluable, both for routine regulatory activities (logistics, administration) and for emergencies. The radio

network has 15 affiliates. Five VHF relay stations provide coverage for approximately 70% of the country.

Human Resources

Availability by Type of Resource. The Ministry of Health is one of the country's largest employers, with a staff of approximately 8,900 (19% of the civil service.) Of these, 38% are medical and paramedical personnel, with the other 62% representing administrative and support staff. There were large disparities in the nationwide deployment of MOH personnel. Department hospitals suffered from shortages of trained managers and personnel such as obstetricians/gynecologists, anesthetists, pediatricians, surgeons, orthopedists, midwives, and nurses.

There are approximately 11,000 traditional birth attendants who attend nearly 80% of all childbirths. Despite an attempt in June 1995 to redeploy physicians from Port-au-Prince to rural areas, the needs at the departmental level remained largely unsatisfied.

Several professional associations regulate and set standards for different types of medical and paramedical personnel. The Haitian Medical Association, founded in 1948 and reorganized in 1973, drafted a code of medical ethics and formulated proposals for the 1990 health policy. The Association also sought to further involve private practitioners in public health. Various specialized associations were affiliated with the Haitian Medical Association.

Very few data are available on pharmacists exercising in Haiti. The Faculty of Pharmacy trains an average of 25 pharmacists per year, but as the pharmaceutical arena does not offer attractive positions, many move abroad, or join the private sector as medical representatives or as chemists in the pharmaceutical industry.

Education of Health Personnel. In 1997, there were seven public institutions, including one school of medicine and pharmacy; one school of odontology; four nursing schools, one each, in Port-au-Prince, Les Cayes, Cap-Haïtien, and Jérémie; and one medical technology institute. All four national training centers for health auxiliaries were closed. A nongovernmental, nonprofit training institute on community health and epidemiology operates in Port-au-Prince. Around 80 medical doctors receive diplomas each year as well as 150 nurses.

Prior to 1993, many medical and paramedical training facilities were opened by private profit-making enterprises. There are 2 medical schools, 10 nursing schools, more than 40 training facilities for nursing auxiliaries, and several medical technology institutes. The degrees conferred by these establishments are not always recognized by the Ministry of

TABLE 4
Public expenditure on health, fiscal years 1989–1990 and 1995–1996.

	Fiscal year	
	1989–1990	1995–1996
Ministry of Health expenses (million gourdes, current prices)	157	418
Ministry of Health expenses (million gourdes, 1990 constant prices)	157	115.2
Public expenses on health/Total public expenses	8.8%	10.7%
Public expenses on health/GDP	1.1%	1.0%
Public expenses per capita in gourdes (1990 constant prices)	24.8	15.7

Source: Andre F. Buttari J. Examen des Depenses Publiques d'Haiti, Note No. 8, Santé, March 1997.

Health. A four-year training project for traditional birth attendants (1996–1999), financed by UNDP, resumed in cooperation with the Ministry of Health.

Expenditures and Sectoral Financing

The budget of the State University Hospital in Port-au-Prince, although decreasing over the last three years, absorbed a significant amount of the public expenditure (17%); another 28% was spent on other public hospitals. Public expenditure on drugs accounted for 2% and 3% of the total amount spent in 1994–1995 and 1995–1996, respectively, but most private and public institutions used a cost-recovery mechanisms. Public expenditure on equipment represented 4%–5% of the budget; in addition, 7.4 million gourdes (US$ 510,345) was spent on equipment in 1994–1995 through external aid for that purpose (Table 4).

The Ministry of Health budget was 157 million gourdes in 1990 and 418 million in 1996, but due to inflation this represents a decrease of 27%. In constant 1990 values, the amounts are 157 and 115 million gourdes, respectively.

Government spending in health ranged between 7.1% and 10.7% of the national budget between 1990 and 1996, representing approximately 1% of the GDP. Per capita public spending in health decreased from 25 gourdes in 1990 to 16 gourdes in 1996, in constant 1990 values. The figure for 1996, however, indicated an upward trend after four years of decrease during the political crisis. Until the mid-1990s, around 90% of public expenses had gone into wage and salary payments, exhausting the working capital for health care facilities, whose services steadily deteriorated. Under the 1995 and 1996 budget, the share of wages and salaries was expected to be limited to 70%, but this was not fully implemented and their share remained at 80% in 1996.

Health sector resources were not the only resources that contributed to the national effort to improve the welfare of the Haitian population. Major contributions were made by other sectors and cabinet ministries in areas such as intersectoral planning, training, social participation, sports, environmental protection, refuse collection, water supply, housing and road construction, food and agriculture, minimum wage legislation, gun control legislation, and traffic regulations. Examples of direct contributions in health care operations over the past few years are highlighted below.

For example, the Ministry of Social Affairs, through its social Welfare Institute, addressed such issues as sexually transmitted diseases in prostitutes, provided prenatal care, oversaw the welfare of street children, and provided doctors for orphanages within its purview. The Ministry of Agriculture was actively involved in programs for the control of zoonoses, the water supply in rural areas, and the food/work program. The Ministry of Education planned school health programs and has been in charge of the schools of medicine, pharmacy, and odontology since 1995. The Ministry of Women's Affairs and Women's Rights issued a policy paper on women's health in 1995, evaluated women's prison conditions, and developed a standard medical record for use in the prison health services. A memorandum of understanding for the improvement of prison conditions was drafted and submitted for approval by four cabinet ministries (Social Affairs, Health, Justice, and Education). The Ministry also published a guide for the evaluation of women's shelters and took part in an effort to educate groups of women from grass-roots organizations on reproductive health and AIDS. The Ministry of the Environment campaigned to heighten public awareness on the importance of protecting nature and identified strategies for the control of deforestation. The Ministry of Public Works played a major role in water supply and sanitation programs and in efforts to upgrade the nation's roads. The Metropolitan Water Company, the National Water Supply Service, and the Metropolitan Solid Waste Collection Service are all attached to the Ministry of Public Works.

Charging and collecting fees in both the private and the public sector is sometimes used to provide care to clients without resources. However, the amounts cannot cover the entire cost of the services.

External Technical and Financial Cooperation

A large share of expenditure in health came from foreign aid, particularly for capital outlays and operating expenses. International aid represented more than 50% of total public spending, reaching 78% in 1994–1995. Before 1996–1997, the main donors were USAID, France, Canada, and Japan; the European Union has now become the major donor in the sector.

Most NGOs operate independently. The 100 affiliates of the association of private health institutions are scattered throughout Haiti's nine departments. This NGO provided technical assistance and served as the coordinator and spokesperson for affiliated NGOs. NGOs and the private sector have generally operated independently of the Ministry of Health.

HONDURAS

GENERAL SITUATION AND TRENDS

Socioeconomic, Political, and Demographic Overview

Honduras has a surface area of 112,492 km² and a population density of 46 inhabitants per km². In urban areas, the population density is 184 inhabitants per km². The terrain is predominantly mountainous, with 19 watersheds. The country's principal environmental problem is deforestation. Between 1964 and 1990, forests were reduced by some 25,899 km² (34%), with an annual deforestation rate averaging 800 km². It is estimated that between 1992 and 1993, as much as 7% of the forest cover reported in 1990 was lost, which indicates a deforestation rate of more than 1,000 km². The country is divided into 18 departments and 297 *municipios* with 3,730 towns and 27,764 small rural communities. With the adoption of the Municipal Government Law (1990), decentralization was strengthened and 5% of Government revenues were transferred to the municipal governments.

In 1990 a program for structural adjustment of the economy was established and policies and incentives were gradually put in place to promote the most efficient use of resources, coupled with social compensation programs, such as the Honduran Social Investment Fund, the Family Allocation Program, and the Social Housing Fund. These programs are designed to relieve the effects of the adjustment in the poorest segments of the population. The share of these three programs in social spending increased from 3.6% in 1990 to 13.6% in 1995.

The per capita gross domestic product (GDP) was US$ 702.7 in 1990 and US$ 722.0 in 1995, with an average annual growth rate of 0.58%. In the same period, the country's total foreign debt increased 23.5%, climbing from US$ 3,517.8 million in 1990 to US$ 4,343.5 million in 1995; public debt accounted for 90% of this amount.

Although the predominant economic activities continue to be agriculture, forestry, hunting, and fishing, Honduras experienced sustained growth in the manufacturing industry (export processing and assembly) in the 1990s; this economic activity generated some 50,000 jobs as of 1994 compared with about 6,000 in the mid-1980s.

The economically active population (EAP) makes up 35% of the total population. In 1995 the underemployment rates were 34% in rural areas and 17% in urban areas. In 1993 women made up 31% of the EAP: 40% of the urban EAP and 22% of the rural EAP. Twenty-four percent of households are headed by women and 65% of those are poor.

Young people of both sexes face discrimination when they enter the job market. In 1994, unemployment and underemployment affected 73% of young men and 69% of young women aged 15–19 years. Among those aged 20–29, in contrast, the percentages were 43% among males and 45% among females; in the group aged 30–44 years 29% of males and 40% of females were unemployed or underemployed.

Inflation rose from 21.7% in 1994 to 29.5% in 1995. The impact of this increase was felt especially in the cost of the basic market basket of food, which jumped 144% between 1990 and 1995. It is estimated that the national population consumes, on average, only 77% of the required daily caloric intake. During the 1980–1994 period, per capita availability of food fell 10% because production grew at a slower rate than the population.

A study by the Secretariat for Coordination and Budget, based on average per capita consumption or expenditure per month per household and the cost of a basic market basket of goods and services in March 1994, revealed that in 1994 the percentage of households that fell below the poverty line was 75.6% (54.5% of households were indigent). Only 24.4% of households were above the poverty line.

During the 1990–1994 period, illiteracy declined from 31.3% in 1990 to 22.8% in 1994; the highest percentage reduction occurred in rural areas (from 39.8% to 29.0%) and among women (from 31.6% to 22.6%). However, illiteracy in rural areas remained 49% higher than in urban areas. The average level of educational attainment for the total population in 1994 was 4.2 years; it is estimated that 60% of the EAP has fewer than three years of schooling.

The housing shortage in 1995 totaled 700,000 dwellings. Of urban dwellings, 64% are overcrowded, 33% do not have a regular supply of drinking water, and 41% lack sanitation systems. In rural areas, only 16% of dwellings are considered adequate; more than 81% have no access to drinking water, excreta disposal services, and electricity.

Based on the last population census, carried out in 1988, the estimated population in 1996 was 5.6 million (49.9% female), with a growth rate of 2.8%. In 1996 the population aged 0–4 years made up 15.7% of the total; the population aged 5–9 years, 14.2%; the population aged 10–14 years, 12.9%; the population aged 15–19 years, 11.5%; the population aged 20–24 years, 9.6%; the population aged 25–39 years, 18.9%, the population aged 40–59 years, 12.1%; and the population aged 60 and over, 5.1%. As this distribution indicates, children under 15 make up the largest proportion of the population (42.8%). The absolute numbers of persons under 15 and over 65 increased between 1992 and 1996.

There are eight culturally differentiated ethnic groups in Honduras: the Lencas, the Pech, the Garífunas, the Chortis, the Tawahkas, the Tolupanes or Xicaques, the Miskitos, and the English-speaking black population. A study conducted in 1993 with a view to characterizing the indigenous peoples of Honduras estimated the size of this population at 253,790 (5.97% of the total population). The areas inhabited by the indigenous population are often not covered by the health situation analyses that the Ministry of Public Health carries out, and they have little access and a limited basic infrastructure of services, subsistence economies, and ecological problems.

It is estimated that in 1995 urban dwellers made up 43% of the total population. Most of the urban population is concentrated in two cities: Tegucigalpa and San Pedro Sula (32.9% and 16.2% of the total urban population, respectively). This concentration is due mainly to migration from rural areas to the country's political and economic centers, whose annual growth rate is 4%. There is a significant geographic/sex differential in this migration: females tend to migrate primarily to the departments of Cortés and Francisco Morazán, especially the major urban centers in those departments (San Pedro Sula and Tegucigalpa), whereas males migrate mainly to agricultural areas. In 1995, the total estimated net rate of internal migration was –1.6% (–1.7% for males and –1.4% for females). Most migrants are between 15 and 44 years of age, and the largest proportion are in the 20–29 age group. Emigration also has been increasing: in 1989 the net emigration rate was –1.1% (–1.3% for males and –1.0% for females).

Life expectancy at birth, which was 64 years for the total population in the period 1985–1990, was estimated at 71 years for women and 66 years for men in 1996. The estimated

total fertility rate, according to the 1991–1992 National Epidemiology and Family Health Survey (ENESF), was 5.2 children per woman, compared with almost 7 in 1970. In the 1991–1992 period, the total fertility rate was 6.4 children per woman in rural areas and 4.3 in urban areas. The 1995–1996 ENESF survey reported a total fertility rate of 4.9 children per woman nationwide, 6.3 in rural areas, and 3.9 in urban areas. The birth rate per 1,000 population was 36.6 in 1992 and 33.4 in 1996.

It is estimated that about 80% of the population has access to public health care services: 60% is covered by the Ministry of Public Health and approximately 11% by the Honduran Social Security Institute (IHSS). The private sector covers a relatively low percentage (around 5% of the total population), which means that many Hondurans do not have access to any health services.

Mortality Profile

The limited development of the country's vital statistics system is reflected in the underreporting of deaths. In 1990, the last year for which information is available, an estimated 44.2% of deaths went unreported. According to estimates of the Secretariat for Planning, the crude death rate in 1996 was 5.8 per 1,000 population; a total of 32,666 deaths occurred, of which 18,510 were males and 14,156 were females. Of the total number of deaths, 15% (5,355) were reported in connection with hospital discharge figures.

In 1990, the five leading causes of death in the general population were ischemic and hypertensive diseases, diseases of pulmonary circulation, and other forms of heart disease (19.0%); accidents and violence (13.0%); diseases of the respiratory system (9.5%); intestinal infectious diseases (9.0%); and malignant neoplasms (8.2%). The leading causes of infant mortality in 1990 (1,624 registered deaths with 638 attributed to ill-defined conditions) were intestinal infectious diseases (28.2%); diseases of the respiratory system (21.8%); and certain disorders originating in the perinatal period (20.6%).

Because of the aforementioned problems with the registration of deaths, the country relies on other sources to calculate mortality figures. These include national surveys conducted on specific subjects and population censuses carried out in certain geographical areas, which provide mortality data based on various methodologies. The data on maternal mortality are considered reliable and are based on prospective studies carried out in 1990, which indicate a rate of 221 maternal deaths per 100,000 live births. The infant mortality rate decreased from 50 per 1,000 live births in 1990 to 42 per 1,000 in 1994.

Hospital deaths increased in absolute numbers from 4,433 in 1993 to 5,355 in 1996 and from 10% to 16% with respect to total deaths for those years, which were estimated at 33,300, and 32,666, respectively. The leading causes of hospital death between 1993 and 1996, based on ICD-9 classification, were diseases of the respiratory system (11.8%); ischemic and hypertensive diseases, diseases of pulmonary circulation, and other forms of heart disease (9.1%); and accidents and violence (8.2%). These three leading causes are the same (although not in the same order) as those reported in 1990. Other important causes of death were malignant neoplasms (5.7%), viral diseases (5.4%), and AIDS (5.4%).

SPECIFIC HEALTH PROBLEMS

Analysis by Population Group

Health of Children

During the 1980s, the percentage of children with low birthweight who were delivered in health facilities of the Ministry of Public Health and the IHSS ranged from 7.0% to 8.7%. The figure increased to 9.2% in 1992. The percentage of malnutrition in children under 5 increased from 48.6% in 1987 to 52.5% in 1991 and, according to the Ministry of Public Health, 2.1% of infant mortality in 1990 was associated with malnutrition, compared with 0.9% in 1980.

The percentage of exclusively breast-fed infants (in the 0- to 3-month age group) increased from 36.7% in 1991 to 42.4% in 1995. Of this proportion, 52.2% were children of low-income families, 51% lived in Tegucigalpa or San Pedro Sula, and 49.0% lived in rural areas. The proportion of children aged 6–9 months who were being breast-fed with supplementary feeding was 69.2%, and the proportion who continued to be breast-fed into the second year of life (20–23 months) was 45.4%. The average duration of exclusive breast-feeding is 2.1 months.

A comparison of the leading causes of death in children under 5, based on the last two epidemiological surveys, reveals that acute respiratory infections continue to be in the forefront, accounting for 22% of deaths in 1991–1992 and 23% in 1996. The next leading cause is diarrheal diseases, which increased from 19% to 21% during the same interval. The results of a survey on socioeconomic indicators in 1994 show that the geographic areas with the lowest rates of drinking water service coverage have the highest prevalence of diarrhea. Taking into account deaths due to prematurity as well as those due to complications of childbirth (sepsis, asphyxia, and birth trauma), perinatal conditions are a leading cause of death, accounting for around a third of mortality in the under-5 age group.

In 1994, an estimated 73.1% of children aged 5–9 years were enrolled in school. Available data for this population group relate to nutritional status and come from several height censuses of schoolchildren aged 6–9 carried out between 1986 and 1996. The proportion of malnourished children remained at 39%. In 1996, 33.3% of girls and 42.2% of boys suffered from chronic malnutrition, an insignificant change with respect to 1986. In 1996, malnutrition affected 26.2% of the urban population in this age group and 44.6% of the rural population. This situation has worsened since 1991, when the percentages were 24.4% and 40.8%, respectively. The prevalence of low height-for-age has clearly risen with age: in 1996, the rate was 28.8% for 6-year-olds, 40.7% for 7-year-olds, 50.9% for 8-year-olds, and 58.9% for 9-year-olds.

Health of Adolescents (10–14 and 15–19 Years Old)

Honduran law defines young people as those between the ages of 13 and 25 years. In 1994 this group made up 28% of the total population and 47% of the total EAP; 7.5% of the households in the country are headed by persons in this age group. In 1993, 46% of young people lived in urban areas and 54% lived in rural areas. According to the Ministry of Public Health, in 1995, 16.3% of AIDS cases in the country occurred in the group aged 10–24, 20% in the group aged 25–29, and 21% in the group aged 30–34.

According to the 1995–1996 ENESF, almost 45% of 18-year-old women are sexually active and one-half of them have been pregnant; 8.5% of 15-year-olds and about 40% of 18-year-olds are married; by age 20, 50% of women are mothers. Among women aged 15–19 years who live with a male partner, 27.6% use some method of contraception; the most frequently used method is oral contraception.

In the group 16–19 years old, illiteracy declined from 11.9% in 1990 to 8.2% in 1994. Among males, this proportion dropped from 14.4% to 10.1%, and among females, from 9.4% to 6.2% in the same period. In the Central District, there are 70 known *maras* (gangs or groups of juvenile delinquents) with some 1,500 members aged 10–25 years; most of them are male. These groups operate in the marginal sectors of the middle- and low-income strata.

Health of Adults (15–60 Years Old)

Mortality studies on women of childbearing age conducted in 1990 (IMMER-90) found that the maternal mortality rate was 221 per 100,000 live births in that year, with higher rates in departments with poor socioeconomic conditions and little access to basic health services (Gracias a Dios, Intibucá, La Paz, Lempira, Ocotepeque, Atlántida, Colón, and Comayagua). According to the same study, the leading cause of death was hemorrhage (32.8%), followed by infections (20.7%) and hypertensive disorders (12.3%). Abortion accounted for 8.7% of all maternal deaths; in 79% of these cases, the cause of death was infection. At the hospital level, the principal cause of maternal death was infection (30.4%), followed by hypertensive disorders. Together, these two causes accounted for 50% of all hospital maternal deaths, and hemorrhage caused 15.2%. The IMMER-90 estimated that 5 of every 100 deaths of women aged 15–49 were attributed to cervical cancer. In 1996, childbirth was associated with the largest proportion (70.4%) of hospital discharges in the group aged 15–49 years; 1.6% of the discharges were associated with alcohol dependency syndrome.

Although recent data are not available, improvements in other indicators suggest that maternal mortality may have declined since 1990. For example, between 1991–1992 and 1996, the proportions of women receiving prenatal care and institutional care for childbirth increased by 14% and 18%, respectively, and use of family-planning methods increased around 7% among women living with a male partner.

Health of the Elderly (60 Years Old and Older)

The aging of the population, which has come about as a result of increases in life expectancy, translates into a greater demand for health care for problems characteristic of the elderly. This, in turn, implies additional costs for health services at a time when the health care needs of the younger population are still not being fully met. There is no comprehensive information on the health status of the elderly population. Hospital discharge data from 1996 reveal that 17.9% of discharges in the group aged 50 and over were associated with alcohol dependency syndrome and 16.6% were associated with diarrheal diseases.

Workers' Health

According to estimates of the National Occupational Health Commission, which drafted a national plan on workers' health in 1992, the EAP represented an estimated 31.8% of the total population in that year. The Commission also found that working conditions often were poor and posed a threat to workers' health. Six major health problems were identified: accidents in the workplace, pesticide poisoning, noise pollution in the manufacturing sector, reproductive health of workers, widespread use of chemical products, and mental health problems (such as depression and alcoholism). Little information is available on these problems, except for some studies on pesticide levels in prepared foods and breast milk and on cholesterol levels in agricultural workers.

Health of the Disabled

In Honduras, 4.5% of the population has some disability requiring rehabilitation services. Although the age and sex distribution of the disabled population is unknown, there are isolated reports from specific institutions such as the IHSS, the general hospitals, the home for the disabled, and a Fundación Teletón, a local foundation. The latter has three centers (in Tegucigalpa, San Pedro Sula, and Santa Rosa de Copán), which served 26,139 patients between 1990 and 1995. It is estimated that in the *municipios* of Siguatepeque and La Esperanza, 4.5% and 4.8% of the population, respectively, have some disability, which has led to strengthening of the process of community-based rehabilitation.

Health of the Indigenous Population and Border Populations

The country's working-age, indigenous population comprises persons from 8 to 59 years old. Malnutrition is widespread, affecting 95% of the indigenous population under the age of 14. Of every 100 indigenous people born, 68 die of infectious diseases. In 1993, estimated life expectancy in this group was 36 years for males and 43 years for females; in the general population, life expectancy was estimated at 67 years (64.8 years for males and 69.6 for females).

In localities located along the Honduras-El Salvador border, where 71,043 people reside, the five leading causes of mortality in 1994 were respiratory diseases, intestinal infectious diseases, certain conditions originating in the perinatal period, accidents, and pneumonia in the departments of La Paz and Intibucá (Honduras), and diarrheal diseases, malnutrition, respiratory diseases, accidents, and heart diseases in the department of Morazán (El Salvador). Immunization coverage in 12 border *municipios* averages 60.3%.

Analysis by Type of Disease or Health Impairment

Communicable Diseases

Vector-Borne Diseases. The available data indicate that the number of cases of malaria increased from 70,838 in 1992 to 74,487 in 1996, with annual parasite indices (API) of 18.05 and 16.49, respectively. The disease mainly struck the country's northern and southern areas, which together accounted for 52% of the cases reported in 1996. However, the highest incidence rates per 1,000 population (46.4 in 1994 and 74.3 in 1995) occurred in the swampy region on the east. In 1996, 98.9% of all cases were due to *Plasmodium vivax* and 1.1% (1,003 cases) to *Plasmodium falciparum*. In 1995, three hospital deaths were registered, two of whom were females over the age of 50. In the period between 1993 and 1995, the largest proportion of malaria cases occurred in females aged 15–49 years (51% in 1993, 62% in 1994, and 53% in 1995).

In 1993, 2,687 clinical cases of dengue were reported. In 1994, the number was 4,687 (74% more than in 1993); in 1995, 28,064; and in 1996, 7,564. In 1995, most dengue cases (16 were cases of dengue hemorrhagic fever) were diagnosed in the central and northern areas of the country, which accounted for almost 50% of all cases. The most critical months were between August and November, the rainy season, when 86% of the cases for the year were reported. In 1993–1994, most cases occurred in women and more than half were in the population over 15 years of age.

Rhodnius prolixus and *Triatoma dimidiata* are the vectors of Chagas' disease in Honduras. The former is found in the mountainous rural areas that extend from the southern border with Guatemala north to the border with El Salvador and Nicaragua. The latter is widely distributed throughout the country, in both rural and urban areas. Fourteen clinical cases of Chagas' disease were reported in 1994, 94 in 1995, and 66 as of October 1996. A clinical-epidemiological study conducted in 1995 showed a 35% prevalence of heart disease in seropositive adolescents and adults in highly endemic areas, and data on patients who received pacemakers during the period 1994–1996 indicate that 25% had the disease; the average age of these patients was 32. A study conducted in 1996 in the *municipio* of San Francisco de Opalaca, located in the department of Intibucá (where Chagas' disease is highly prevalent), found that 17.7% of children under 5 were infected.

In 1992, 992 cases of cutaneous leishmaniasis were reported, and in 1994, 1,083. The number increased 13% in 1995, when 1,230 cases were reported, 70% of which occurred in the department of Olancho; in 1996, 1,234 cases were reported. Hospital records do not indicate the number of cases of atypical and visceral leishmaniasis, but in 1996 the central laboratory of the Ministry of Public Health reported 3,866 laboratory-confirmed cases, of which 1,678 were the ulcerated cutaneous form, 238 the mucocutaneous form, 169 the visceral form, and 1,781 the nonulcerated cutaneous form.

Vaccine-Preventable Diseases. No cases of poliomyelitis have been reported since 1989. There was one reported case of measles in 1995 and four in 1996; since 1991, no measles deaths have been registered. Immunization coverage among children under 1 year old was 91% in 1996. The rate among children under 5 increased with respect to earlier years, and in 1996 it was 97.3% for the oral polio vaccine, 96.5% for DTP, 98.7% for measles, and 100% for BCG.

In 1990 the country made a commitment to eliminate neonatal tetanus. By 1995, coverage with two doses of tetanus toxoid in women of childbearing age was 93%. Only three and four cases of neonatal tetanus were reported in 1995 and

1996, respectively, which represents a reduction of 50% with respect to 1994. In the 1990–1994 period, 63% of the cases were reported in urban areas.

A campaign to vaccinate all health workers against hepatitis B was launched in 1994. By 1995, 50% had been vaccinated and by 1996, 67.8%. In 1996, 200 cases of whooping cough were reported. There have been no cases of diphtheria since 1981, although surveillance was intensified in response to reports of outbreaks in the Region. Eleven cases of tuberculous meningitis were reported in 1994, 8 in 1995, and 10 in 1996.

Cholera and Other Intestinal Infectious Diseases. The prevalence of diarrheal diseases in children under 5 in Tegucigalpa and San Pedro Sula decreased from 25.5% in 1987 to 18.8% in 1991 and 14.8% in 1996. In rural areas, the prevalence has been variable (31.9% in 1987, 19.1% in 1991, and 21.1% in 1996). Cholera re-emerged in the country in October 1991, causing a hospital case fatality rate in children under 5 of 4.2% in 1992 and 2.0% in 1996. In 1995 there were 4,748 cases of cholera nationwide, with a case fatality rate of 1.6% (77 deaths); 56% of the cases were in males and 76% of those occurred in persons aged 15 and over. In 1996 there were 708 cases and 14 deaths, with a case fatality rate of 1.9%; 53.2% of the cases occurred in men and, of these, 40% were aged 15 and over.

Chronic Communicable Diseases. There were 45 cases of tuberculous meningitis in 1992, 23 in 1993, and 15 in 1994, with 6, 5, and 11 cases, respectively, in children under 5. The number of cases of tuberculosis reported from 1992 to 1996 was 4,267, with a morbidity rate of 83.3 and a mortality rate of 4.9 per 100,000 population in 1992. These rates were 70.6 and 5.0 per 100,000 population, respectively, in 1996.

In the period 1993–1995, tuberculosis was associated with an annual average of 1,289 hospital discharges, with a predominance of cases in males (60%) and in those over the age of 15 years. The central and northeastern regions of the country have the greatest number of cases. Extrapulmonary tuberculosis occured at a rate of 5.2 cases per 100,000 population in 1989 and 2.0 cases in 1996. All detected cases of pulmonary tuberculosis have been treated; only one drug-resistant case has been identified. Of the 416 patients who received the directly observed treatment, short-course, 380 were cured and 36 abandoned treatment (this information relates to 50% of the cases diagnosed by sputum smear microscopy during the first half of 1995).

The prevalence of leprosy remained constant at 0.1 (84 cases) per 10,000 population from 1992 to 1995; an average of 3 new cases per year were diagnosed between 1992 and 1995.

Acute Respiratory Infections. The 1991–1992 ENESF survey found that acute respiratory infections were more frequent in Tegucigalpa and San Pedro Sula (38.2%) than in other smaller cities or in rural areas (32%) and that children under 1 year were most often affected. Among 4-year-olds, the prevalence of acute respiratory infections is 25%, compared with 38% in children under 1. Thanks to the strengthening of activities to promote community management of pneumonia and to train volunteers, the case fatality rate from these infections has decreased.

Rabies and Other Zoonoses. In 1992, two cases of human rabies were reported from the Tegucigalpa metropolitan area; in 1993, no cases were reported; in 1994, one case was reported from the country's southern area; and in 1995, two cases were reported, both from the metropolitan area. All but one case involved persons under the age of 10. In 1996, no cases of human rabies were reported. The number of cases of canine rabies decreased from 14 in 1995 to 9 in 1996.

With respect to cysticercosis, a study carried out in 1995 in animals slaughtered in metropolitan meat-packing plants showed that 3% of the pigs analyzed were infected with cysticerci. The most affected departments are Olancho, Francisco Morazán, El Paraíso, and Choluteca.

AIDS. In 1993 a rate of 19.0 AIDS cases per 100,000 population was reported. In 1995, the rate was 17.7. The predominant route of transmission is through heterosexual contact (82.9%). The male-female ratio of 4:1 registered at the beginning of the epidemic has shifted steadily over the years and is now approaching parity. The 25–29 age group is most affected (21.8%), although the number of cases diagnosed in children under 5 has been increasing (from 1.9% in 1987 to 4.8% in 1996). Geographically, the largest proportion of AIDS cases are in the northern region of the country (47.6%), followed by the central region (20.4%). Of the cumulative total of 6,005 cases registered up to 1996, 1,041 have died. The percentage of infected women also has risen: from 30.3% of 752 cases in 1992 to 38% of 734 in 1996. In 1991, in San Pedro Sula the prevalence of HIV infection was 3.6% among pregnant women and 14% among prostitutes. The registered prevalence rate in pregnant women was 2.8% in 1992 and 2.5% in 1993. Among prostitutes, the prevalence was 16.3% in 1992 and 15% in 1993. In Tegucigalpa the prevalence of HIV infection among pregnant women remained constant at 0.3% in 1992 and 1993.

Candidiasis ranks first (37.7%) among opportunistic diseases, followed by tuberculosis, in both the pulmonary form (19.8%) and the disseminated form (3.6%). This association between tuberculosis and AIDS has shown a rising trend, with the rate increasing from 0.11 per 100,000 population in 1986 to 1.4 in 1996. No strains of tuberculosis resistant to conventional treatment have been detected.

Other STDs. The incidence of other STDs continues to be higher in the metropolitan region and in the northern part of the country. In the 1992–1995 period, the number of cases of these diseases dropped gradually from 2,004 to 1,026. In 1996, 1,112 cases were reported, with a rate of 19.8 per 100,000 population. According to hospital discharge records, syphilis is most frequent in women and in the group aged 15–49 years; the second most frequently affected age group is children under 1 year of age, in whom the disease is detected at birth. With regard to gonorrhea, the number of reported cases fell from 5,952 in 1992 to 2,146 in 1996.

Noncommunicable Diseases and Other Health-Related Problems

Nutritional Diseases and Diseases of Metabolism. Rates of chronic protein-energy malnutrition—stunted growth—in children under 5 remained relatively stable between 1987 (39.1%) and 1994 (39.7%). Although the problem has decreased since 1987 in the group aged 1–5 years (from 43.9% in 1987 to 36.7% in 1996), the prevalence remains high, suggesting that it is due to prolonged periods of inadequate feeding accompanied by continuous mild morbid processes. Malnutrition—wasting—has been reduced and is not currently a major problem. A rate of 1.9% was registered in 1987, 2.4% in 1991–1992, and 1.9% in 1993–1994. Rates of underweight (low weight-for-age) during the 1987–1994 period remained at around 20% (20.6% in 1987, 21% in 1991–1992, and 19.0% in 1993–1994). The most serious nutritional problems are found in the western rural areas of the country, where the prevalence of chronic malnutrition is 59.5% and that of overall malnutrition is 32.5%. This situation is closely related to the high poverty levels (96.1%) in that area.

Subclinical vitamin A deficiency affects 13% of the population aged 1–3 years. The problem is most severe in rural areas in the western and northern regions and in several urban areas. There are no current data on the prevalence of goiter due to iodine deficiency in schoolchildren (in 1987 the rate was 8.8%); however, iodine level studies conducted in 1995 in sentinel sites suggest that it is not a major problem. Deficiency of these micronutrients has been treated through a successful program of fortifying sugar with vitamin A and salt with iodine. Iron deficiency is prevalent and in 1996 affected 30.2% of children aged 1–3; 0.5% of these children were severely anemic. The problem occurs throughout the country. Twenty-six percent of women of childbearing age and 32% of pregnant women with deficient levels of hemoglobin were found to be anemic.

Cardiovascular Diseases. The only available information on cardiovascular disease is from hospital discharge and mortality records: discharge rates per 100,000 population were 99.0 in 1993 (2,030 patients), 116.6 in 1994 (4,768 patients), and 126.3 in 1995 (6,189 patients); hospital mortality rates per 100,000 population were 11.7, 14.8, and 13.6, respectively, for the same years. Women over the age of 50 made up the largest proportion of patients with cardiovascular disease discharged from hospitals. The largest proportion of deaths (38%) were due to cerebrovascular diseases. Although these data do not make it possible to identify a national trend, a rise in both mortality and hospital discharges associated with these causes has been observed.

Malignant Neoplasms. Of the 173,961 cytology exams carried out in 1995 in the country as a whole (34.8% coverage of women aged 30–59 years), 0.4% of the samples were found to be abnormal. The largest number of cases were detected in the northwestern area of the country; 53% occurred in women aged 30–49, and 25% were in women aged 50 and over. Since 1990 there has been a cancer registry in the San Felipe General Hospital (Tegucigalpa), which is the national cancer referral center and the only hospital with a cobalt-60 unit. In 1990 and 1995, 389 and 870 new cases of cancer were treated, respectively. In 1994, 60% of the cases were uterine cancer; 8% were breast cancer; 4% were cancer of trachea, bronchus, and lung; 4% were skin cancer; and 3.6% were stomach cancer. The Department of Statistics within the Ministry of Public Health reported that hospital mortality from malignant neoplasms was 60 per 100,000 population in 1993, 51 per 100,000 in 1994, and 43 per 100,000 in 1995. The principal cancer sites are the digestive system, the genitourinary system, the respiratory system, and bones and tissue.

Accidents and Violence. According to information provided by the Bureau of Criminal Investigation, violence at the community level has been increasing throughout the country. The Public Security Force reports that the homicide rate increased from 20.7 per 100,000 population in 1989 to 40.0 per 100,000 in 1995. Firearms were used in most homicides (69.6%). The age at which criminal activities begin has fallen (10 years).

Mortality from traffic accidents increased from 7.6 per 1,000 population in 1989 to 13.8 in 1994; the rate of domestic violence was 65.5 per 100,000 population in 1996 when records on this type of violence began to be kept. Crimes against minors (between 1 and 18 years of age) reached a rate of 66.0 per 100,000 population in 1996. In that same year, the reported incidence of rape was 3.0 per 100,000 women and 5.3 per 100,000 girls.

Behavioral Disorders. The age at which young people begin to use alcohol and tobacco has dropped. A study on children and alcohol carried out in eight marginal neighborhoods in the Tegucigalpa metropolitan area in 1992 revealed that the age at which alcohol was consumed for the first time ranges from 10 to 16 years and that this first experience usually takes place in the home or in a friend's house. In 78% of homes in which young people reside, some drug is used; tobacco and alcohol are the most frequently used substances. Forty-two percent of traffic accidents are associated with alcohol consumption by the driver, and 61% of occupational accidents (injuries and mutilations) occur among workers who consumed excess alcohol the previous day. Fifty-one percent of divorces occur in marriages in which one of the spouses, usually the man, is an alcoholic and exhibits personality disorders.

In a study conducted by the Honduran Institute for the Prevention of Alcoholism, Drug Addiction, and Drug Dependency on the use of alcohol and drugs among students in teachers' schools in Honduras in 1996, four of every five students reported that children and adolescents could easily obtain alcohol in their neighborhoods or communities, and approximately half the respondents (47%) reported the same about tobacco. With regard to illegal drugs, fewer than 17% said that marijuana could be easily obtained in their communities.

Natural Disasters. In 1993, tropical storms Bert and Gert affected 4,000 households, 30,000 people, and 2,000 km^2 of agricultural land in the northern region of Honduras. In November 1996 there were floods due to heavy rainfall in the Chamelecón, Ulúa, Luán, and Aguán river basins, which affected an estimated 80,840 people. Corn, beans, sorghum, rice, and banana crops worth approximately US$ 7.7 million were also lost, and several roads and about 10 bridges were damaged.

RESPONSE OF THE HEALTH SYSTEM

National Health Plans and Policies

The effort to modernize and decentralize the government has included the health sector. Between 1994 and 1997 the Ministry of Public Health stepped up the process of decentralizing functions to health areas and to municipal government agencies. The Ministry also enlisted other key players in the promotion of the process of increasing access to health services as a fundamental aspect of health reform. This process has become the Ministry of Public Health's main focus, as well as its primary response to reform pressures coming from outside the sector; for example, demands from the National Commission on State Reform, the Ministry of the Treasury, the Department of the Interior, and other agencies of the central administration involved in structural State reform, as well as from international lending institutions.

The aging of the population and changes in the epidemiological profile, coupled with increased violence, mental illnesses, drug addiction, and chronic diseases such as cancer and cardiovascular disorders, have added to the complexity of the country's epidemiological profile. In addition, the country has experienced rapid urbanization without the necessary service infrastructure; a more educated population demands timely and quality care, while at least 30% of the population has no access to even basic health services.

The national access initiative, which seeks to address these problems by extending service coverage and transforming the country's basic health institutions—under the leadership and regulation of the Ministry of Public Health—encompasses three basic strategies: adaptation of local health systems, with an emphasis on health areas; social control of the management of health systems; and development and improvement of human resources. The definition of an appropriate health policy and of basic strategies for applying that policy have strengthened the political management capacity of the Ministry of Public Health as well as its power to negotiate with the various relevant agents and its ability to enlist support at the national level. As many management and planning aspects have become decentralized, it has become necessary for central and intermediate regulatory entities, which are used to a centralized management of vertical programs, to amend their approaches. International cooperation agencies are also coordinating their actions, taking these national processes into account, and are decentralizing their cooperative activities to the most underserved health areas in order to achieve the greatest possible impact in terms of equity, efficiency, effectiveness, and social participation, which are the basic principles of Honduras's health policy.

The Ministry of Public Health has promoted specific policies, such as rapid extension of services through universal access to basic health packages; coordination of international cooperation; reorganization of the health system, with an emphasis on the local levels; environmental and health protection; health financing; food security; development of institutional and community human resources; and identification of solutions to critical problems, such as shortages of drugs and medical supplies. The 1994–1997 government plan provides for increasing the coverage of water and sanitation services in the areas at highest epidemiological risk, as well as protecting the environment through the application of the sustainable local human development concept.

Organization of the Health Sector

Institutional Organization

The health system in Honduras comprises public and private subsystems. In the public subsystem, services are pro-

vided mainly by the Ministry of Public Health, which covers 60% of the population and functions as both a service provider and a regulatory agency. The Honduran Social Security Institute serves between 10% and 12% of the population. Smaller proportions of the population are covered by the Armed Forces Health System; the National Social Welfare Agency; and the Department of Occupational Medicine, Hygiene, and Safety within the Ministry of Labor. The public health subsystem also oversees the National Autonomous Water Supply and Sewerage Service (SANAA). The private subsystem comprises 15 hospitals and an undetermined number of private physicians and clinics, some of which are financed and administered by religious groups. It is estimated that the private sector provides care to some 10% of the population.

The services provided by the Ministry of Public Health are organized in six levels of care, linked in a weak referral system. For administration and management of the services, the Ministry has organized nine health regions, which, in turn, are divided into 41 health areas; this division does not mirror the country's political-administrative division. In 1994 the Ministry's network of services consisted of 978 establishments, including 28 hospitals, 214 physician-staffed health centers, 727 rural health centers, and 9 maternal and child clinics. Of the 28 hospitals, 6 are considered national reference hospitals, 6 are regional hospitals, and 16 are area hospitals.

The public subsector has 4,803 hospital beds, 4,141 of which are in Ministry of Public Health establishments and 662 are in IHSS establishments (a rate of 0.8 public-sector beds per 1,000 population). In 1995 the Ministry of Public Health recorded 35.1 hospital discharges per 1,000 population, of which 40% were patients admitted for childbirth. The private subsector accounts for some 30% of all hospital discharges in the country. The average occupancy rate in hospitals of the Ministry of Public Health was 73%. In rural areas, the vast majority of deliveries are attended by traditional birth attendants; in urban areas, most deliveries are attended in hospitals.

To coordinate activities and avoid duplication of primary and tertiary care services, agreements for shared services have been established between the Medical-Surgical Hospital of the IHSS and the national hospitals of the Ministry of Public Health in the areas of psychiatry, ophthalmology, oncology, nephrology, intensive care, and cardiology.

Health Legislation

The current Health Code was approved in 1991. Through the Law on Municipal Government (Decree No.134-40, October 1990) progress has been made in decentralizing the health sector and in coordinating and executing measures and activities to ensure the health and general well-being of the population.

The General Law on the Environment, enacted in 1993 to encourage environmental protection, established the Office of the Environment, the National Environmental Advisory Board, and the Technical Advisory Committee to support the Ministry of the Environment and the Office of Environmental Law.

The Law on Modernization and Development of the Agricultural Sector, enacted in 1992, regulates the registration of agrochemical and biological products for agricultural or veterinary use as a way to prevent environmental risks. In 1993, regulations were adopted on the sanitary control of food sold in public places.

In 1993 a procedural law was adopted that provides special benefits for the elderly, retirees, and pensioners, including discounts on recreational activities, travel, hospitalization, and other services.

There is a health commission within the National Congress, which is responsible for studying and issuing opinions on proposed legislation to be submitted to the legislature for approval. In the context of Central American and Latin American integration movements, this commission also participates in the Central American Parliament (PARLACEN) and the Latin American Parliament (PARLATINO).

Organization of Health Regulatory Activities

Certification and Practice of Health Professionals. The health sector's work force, as are workers in other sectors, is regulated by the current Law on Civil Service, whose enforcement falls under an office of personnel and human resources. For physicians, the statute on employment of physicians regulates issues such as procedures for hiring and retaining medical personnel, work days, promotions, and salary increases. Professional associations, especially for medical and nursing personnel, are in the process of revising the regulations that govern the practice of those professions.

Drug Market. Between 7,000 and 9,000 drugs are marketed in Honduras. Of these, the Ministry of Public Health has granted marketing authorization for 5,071 products—4,011 brand-name and 1,060 generic products. The drugs consumed in the country are marketed through a network of distributors consisting of 115 wholesale dealers, 620 pharmacies, and 215 drug retail outlets.

The Ministry of Finance controls the price and markup of imported drugs. The price of domestic pharmaceutical products is not subject to any controls. Between 1992 and 1994, official price indexes for imported pharmaceutical products increased 26%, which was similar to the reported increase in health care costs (30%) in the same period.

Environmental Quality. The contamination of rivers has been investigated only where pollution is obvious. Bacteriological contamination has been detected in most water systems in rural areas. In urban areas, such as Tegucigalpa and Choluteca, drinking water often becomes contaminated because supply systems are obsolete. According to the records of SANAA, only 11 of the 55 major sewerage systems in the country have wastewater treatment systems. It is estimated that 82% of the population is provided with excreta disposal systems consisting of a sewerage system, septic tank, or latrine.

The country combats air pollution in several ways. The Ministry of the Environment, together with the Ministry of Finance and the Treasury, have carried out activities aimed at introducing unleaded gasoline in the country. The Center for the Study of Pollution continually monitors pollution from motor vehicle emissions and other pollutants. The Ministry of Public Health conducts studies on hospital waste.

The Ministry of the Environment was created in 1993 to oversee enforcement of the General Law on the Environment, formulate policies, and coordinate actions with other institutions, including the Ministry of Natural Resources, SANAA, and international cooperation agencies in order to protect the environment nationwide. The legal mechanisms for protecting health and the environment are, in addition to the aforementioned General Law on the Environment, the General Environmental Regulations, the Health Code, and the Law on Municipal Government. The latter assigns powers to municipal governments specific for managing natural resources and treating and controlling pollution, among other functions. Nearly no municipal government currently has sufficient technological capacity to implement environmental policy measures.

During 1996 the establishment of environmental quality indices was initiated in 45 cities, with a view to assessing and controlling various environmental risks through low-cost technology.

Food. Honduras has no programs for protecting food quality. Activities in this area involve quality-control measures provided for under the Health Code and various laws, such as those concerning fortification of foods with micronutrients (addition of vitamin A to sugar and iodine to salt) and enrichment of wheat flour.

Health Services and Resources

Organization of Services for Care of the Population

Health Promotion and Community Participation. The Ministry of Education coordinates sports activities designed to improve and promote healthy lifestyles. Violence has been acknowledged as a public health problem and various entities have been created to address it, including a national commission for the prevention of abuse, a governmental office on women's issues, and 20 interinstitutional regional councils on the treatment and prevention of domestic violence. In addition, there are offices specifically dealing with cases involving women and children, as well as the National Directorate to Combat Drug Trafficking.

The Honduran Congress has drafted a new code on child health and welfare, various laws aimed at controlling alcoholism and drug addiction, and a new criminal procedural code. In addition, it has adopted a law creating an institute for childhood and family issues and a special law on domestic violence. The National Commission for the Protection of Human Rights also has been strengthened, with special attention to provisions relating to juvenile offenders, abused children, and battered women. In June 1994 an agreement on support for child protection activities was signed.

Health communication activities are increasingly being incorporated into municipal health plans as a way to disseminate messages that address the population's health problems.

IHSS provides services to 14,680 pensioners and retirees throughout the country. The Retirees and Pensioners Unit of the IHSS offers seminars on preparing for retirement and courses in handicrafts, and it provides support for project management (cooperatives and microenterprises).

Disease Prevention and Control Programs. The Ministry of Public Health oversees various disease prevention and control programs, among them the programs for control of cancer, STDs and AIDS, rabies, vector-borne diseases, tuberculosis, and leprosy (the last program operated until 1996).

Epidemiological Surveillance Systems and Public Health Laboratories. The epidemiological surveillance system has maintained coverage levels of under 60% for weekly national reporting of diseases, although there are significant differences among the various health regions of the country. The system encompasses diseases under international surveillance (cholera, plague, smallpox, yellow fever, influenza, and malaria), as well as diseases under surveillance by the national disease alert system and the Expanded Program on Immunization: typhoid fever, dengue, meningitis, and encephalitis.

Most of the control programs have established their own information systems, but they are not linked together. As a result, efforts have been made to design an integrated information system that would generate information needed for timely decision-making. At the subregional level, Honduras participates in epidemiological monitoring of diarrheal diseases, amebiasis, tuberculosis, rabies, leishmaniasis, and AIDS. As part of a process of applying health situation analysis methodologies, training has been given in 76% of the health areas in preparation for municipal and area plans.

The laboratory network is made up of 28 hospital laboratories, 8 regional laboratories, and 1 central reference laboratory. Sixty-five percent of the human resources in this area work in the health regions, 26% in the hospitals, and 8.2% in the central reference laboratory.

Water Supply and Sewerage Systems. Regulatory and control functions are carried out by the National Drinking Water and Sewerage Commission (CONAPA), a decentralized technical agency of the Ministry of Public Health that has considerable operational and financial independence. Some services are currently being decentralized with the participation of the private sector; the decentralization process involves transfer of SANAA-operated systems to the *municipios.*

SANAA has adopted a pricing structure that establishes different categories of users, sets basic charges, and takes into account water use. In rural water supply systems, the community sets the charges for services. In general, the rates applied do not generate sufficient resources to ensure sustainability of service.

The two principal service providers in the country's two major cities (SANAA in Tegucigalpa and the Municipal Water Department in San Pedro Sula) suffer from relatively high rates of water losses, lack of up-to-date records of users, and lack of water meters. The rural systems constructed by SANAA include an important community participation component, and their management is delegated to administrative boards made up of users. Smaller urban systems and rural systems constructed by other public agencies and by nongovernmental organizations follow similar practices; responsibility for their operation is entrusted to the municipal governments, boards of trustees, or administrative boards. There continue to be significant discrepancies in service coverage depending on area of residence; coverage of drinking water and sanitation services is 94.5% in urban areas, compared with 63% for water and 57% for sanitation in rural areas.

Solid Waste Disposal Services. The most common method of treating household solid waste is open-air burning, which causes air pollution. Communities with greater managerial capacity and larger populations generally have systems for waste management, with a coverage level that ranges from 20% to 50% in medium-sized communities and from 50% to 80% in larger cities (Tegucigalpa and San Pedro Sula).

Food Aid Programs. Honduras has four food aid programs: the maternal and child supplementary feeding program (PAMI), the program of food and nutritional assistance for at-risk groups and promotion of food production for personal consumption, the school lunch program (PME), and the "food for work" program (PAT). These programs were incorporated in 1995 as strategies under the national food security plan. During the 1990–1993 period, PAMI served 220,907 people, distributing food through 1,153 food and nutrition centers. During the same period, PME served an annual average of 434,939 schoolchildren and in 1993–1994 covered nearly 50% of the public schools.

Organization and Operation of Personal Health Care Services

Outpatient, Hospital, and Emergency Services. The mobile surgery project is aimed at providing maximum access to health services and attending the most frequent minor surgical needs in the most remote and underserved areas of the country, especially among children. A mobile unit began operating in May 1996 and that year performed 468 surgeries— 46% at the primary level and 52% at the secondary level.

Auxiliary Diagnostic Services and Blood Banks. There are a total of 25 blood banks and transfusion services. Of the six national hospitals, only three have blood banks and transfusion services; regional and area hospitals have their own blood banks. In the Ministry of Public Health, a unit has been created to structure the organization and operation of the blood bank network. This unit and the network of blood banks are overseen by microbiologists. As of 1997 operation of the blood banks was not subject to established technical standards and procedures. Quality assurance consists of screening.

Specialized Services. The Ministry of Public Health provides dental services through 34 local oral health clinics in schools and 84 health centers and hospitals. There are four high-productivity centers. The services provided are basically curative and the vast majority are extractions. The ratio of 1.68 dentists per 10,000 population is insufficient to meet the oral health care needs of the Honduran population.

Two national psychiatric hospitals are located in Tegucigalpa. In San Pedro Sula, there is a psychiatric care clinic that refers patients to one of the two hospitals in Tegucigalpa. Each general hospital has two or three beds available for psychiatric patients.

There are two homes for the elderly, which are financed by voluntary contributions and offer basic inpatient services.

Inputs for Health

A 1% tax is levied on imported drugs. Raw materials imported for production of drugs are taxed at a rate of 5%, and products used in the production process (accessories, bottles, stoppers, cardboard boxes) are taxed at a rate of 1%.

The total supply of drugs in the Honduran pharmaceuticals market during the 1992–1995 period increased 26%. Imported drugs account for a high percentage of the national market (54.8% in 1990 and 60.7% in 1994) and represented 23% of Honduras' total imports in the period 1993–1995; their value rose from US$ 24 million in 1990 to US$ 40 million in 1996.

The public sector (Ministry of Public Health and IHSS) accounted for 27.2% of the total supply of drugs on the market in 1993 and 29.0% in 1994. The Ministry of Public Health accounted for 19.2% of the total in the network of services in 1993 and 24.8% in 1994, which is an indirect indicator that access to drugs is low. The IHSS accounted for 8.0% of supply in 1993 and 4.2% in 1994.

Vaccines for the Expanded Program on Immunization are acquired through PAHO. Spending on biological products totaled US$ 1,328,976.08 in 1996 and US$ 1,292,976.08 in 1997.

Human Resources

Type of Resource. In the public and private health sectors, there are an average of 6.5 physicians per 10,000 population (33% in the public sector); 2.4 professional nurses (48% in the public sector); 8.4 auxiliary nurses (87% in the public sector), and 0.2 dentists (18% in the public sector). This situation is more critical for some categories of technical and auxiliary personnel because training is available in the country in only four technical areas (radiology, laboratory, anesthesia, and medical records) and auxiliary nursing personnel are scarce or nonexistent in the areas of dental hygiene, nutrition, and equipment maintenance.

There are insufficient numbers of human resources in the public sector for the majority of the professions, which limits their ability to respond in a timely fashion to demands for services. The situation is exacerbated by the unequal geographical distribution of resources; in some communities in the country, the job market for health personnel is saturated, whereas in others—generally those that are most inaccessible—many positions are vacant.

Education of Health Workers. The education of health professionals is the responsibility of the National Autonomous University of Honduras (UNAH). In the period 1992–1996, an average of 272 physicians, 19 nurses, and 41 dentists were graduated each year. The education of auxiliary and mid-level technicians is the responsibility of educational establishments administered by the Division of Human Resources of the Ministry of Public Health. In 1990, several new categories of health workers were recognized: environmental health technician, teacher in public health, and nurse specialist in maternal and perinatal health; in addition, a special secondary school curriculum with a health orientation was instituted. The UNAH school of journalism is currently studying the feasibility of creating a program in health journalism.

Continuing Education of Health Workers and the Health Labor Market. The public sector, including IHSS, employs 69% of all health workers in the country. There are groups in the nine health regions that offer continuing education on topics such as the process of increasing access to health services, maternal and child health, sexuality, and AIDS.

Health Research and Technology. At present there are no complete records of all the studies conducted in the area of health. There is little applied research in health, owing to a shortage of human resources with training in research techniques, lack of financing, and, especially, the absence of a national policy on health research. The university is responsible for the majority of the activities that are carried out in this field, although some research is also conducted under the aegis of the Ministry of Public Health, IHSS, the Center for the Study and Control of Pollution, the Ministry of the Environment, municipal governments, and nongovernmental organizations as well as by independent investigators.

The majority of funding for research comes from the United States Agency for International Development (USAID), the Japanese International Cooperation Agency (JICA), PAHO/WHO, the World Bank, and the Governments of the United Kingdom and Sweden.

Expenditures and Sectoral Financing

Health expenditures, as a proportion of GDP, increased from 2.7% in 1990 to 3.0% in 1995, a rate that continues to be low. As a proportion of total public spending, health expenditure has shown an erratic pattern: from 8.1% in 1990 it dropped to 6% in 1993 and then rose to 9.2% in 1995, which is indicative of the vulnerability of the sector to the overall situation of fiscal constraints during that period. Similar fluctuations were observed in health spending as a percentage of total central government expenditures (10.4% in 1990, 9.0% in 1993, 13.4% in 1995) and as a proportion of real social spending (34.1% in 1990, 30.4% in 1993, and 38.4% in 1995).

Despite these variations, which unquestionably affected the services provided in the years in which the decline was

most marked, health expenditure per capita increased from US$ 18.9 in 1990 to US$ 21.5 in 1995. Current spending decreased from 70.9% in 1990 to 61.4% in 1995; the greatest decline occurred in the category of compensation (40.5% in 1990 and 31.0% in 1995), which resulted in a 9.5% decrease for the period, which had an evident impact on the supply, availability, and quality of public health care services.

Although the amount allocated in the health budget for procurement of goods and services increased 20%, inflation (29.5% in 1995), which led to devaluation of the lempira with respect to the dollar, has had a marked impact on the procurement of supplies, drugs, and medical and surgical materials, with negative consequences on the supply and quality of services.

Capital spending has increased significantly: from US$ 26.0 million in 1990 to US$ 41.2 million in 1995, which is a 58% increase for the period, with an average annual growth rate of 9.6%. In addition, capital spending as a percentage of total health expenditures rose from 29.1% in 1990 to 38.6% in 1995.

With regard to the distribution of expenditures by programs, although those of the Ministry of Public Health continue to be concentrated in the delivery of hospital services, this proportion dropped from 40.1% in 1990 to 28.5% in 1995, while the share of spending on the communicable disease control program increased from 18.9% in 1990 to 22.4% in 1995. The proportion of spending on studying and constructing health facilities rose from US$ 4.58 million in 1990 to US$ 10.9 million in 1995. This increase is reflected in the larger number of facilities and in improvements to the existing infrastructure.

External Technical and Financial Cooperation

Of the total resources available for the health sector during the period 1990–1995, 78% were public funds and 22% was foreign funding channeled through the Ministry of Finance and Public Credit. Bilateral cooperation accounts for 53.3% of international cooperation for health, and the United States is the largest donor (45.2%); however, since 1990 there has been a decline in the amount of bilateral assistance, which has been replaced by cooperation from agencies of the United Nations system and financial institutions such as the Inter-American Development Bank and the World Bank. In 1992, the three largest bilateral donors were the United States (US$ 38.4 million), Italy (US$ 37.4 million), and Japan (US$ 19.4 million).

JAMAICA

GENERAL SITUATION AND TRENDS

Socioeconomic, Political, and Demographic Overview

The island of Jamaica covers an area of 10,991 km² and lies about 885 kms south of Miami (United States of America) and 145 kms south of Cuba. It is the largest of the English-speaking Commonwealth Caribbean Islands, and the third-largest island in the region. The island is divided into 14 parishes and there are two major urban centers—Kingston on the southeast coast and Montego Bay on the northwest coast.

An independent state in the Commonwealth of Nations since 1962, Jamaica is governed by a parliamentary democracy based on the Westminster/Whitehall model. Parliament consists of a governor-general who represents the Queen, and a bicameral legislature. The Cabinet of Ministers forms the executive arm of government, which is headed by a Prime Minister.

Traditionally, Jamaica's economy has been based on agriculture, with sugar, bananas, and citrus the leading exports. During the 1960s, bauxite mining increased in importance as a source of foreign exchange, surpassing the agricultural sector. With the decline in aluminum prices worldwide beginning in the 1980s, tourism has replaced the bauxite industry as the leading hard currency earner. Gross foreign exchange earnings from the tourism sector in 1995 were an estimated US$ 965 million, a 5% increase relative to 1994.

In 1995, the balance of payments account showed a surplus of US$ 21.8 million, but the current balance of payments account shows a deficit of US$ 224 million. Fluctuations in the exchange rate have resulted in a value of US$ 1.00 to J$ 39.80 in 1995, dropping to J$ 34.70 in 1997. Consumer prices rose by 25.5% at the end of 1995. Wage increase demands were a contributing factor.

Special measures were introduced in 1995 in an attempt to control the fluctuation of the dollar and to slow inflation. These measures included an increase in treasury bill rates; further fiscal tightening to yield a public sector surplus of 3% of GDP; sale of foreign exchange by the Bank of Jamaica to the banking system; and implementation of a special deposit scheme for liquidity management purposes.

At the end of 1996, Jamaica's population was 2,527,600. The growth rate is estimated at 1.0, slightly lower than the previous year's rate of 1.2. Life expectancy at birth was 73.6 years—69.6 years for males and 72.9 years for females in 1990. Males represent 49.7 % of the population and females 50.3%. The proportion of the population under age 15 declined from 38.4% in 1982 to 34.3% in 1991.

Infant mortality rates have shown marked improvement over the last seven years, declining from 29.8 deaths per 1,000 live births in 1990 to 23.8 in 1996. The maternal mortality rate was 10.2 per 10,000 women in 1994. The crude birth rate was 22.8, while the crude death rate was 5.9 per 1,000 population. The dependency ratio in 1995 was 722 per 1,000 persons, slightly higher than in 1994 when it was 719. The 1995 contraceptive prevalence rate was 64, and the total fertility rate stood at three children per woman. The 1993 contraceptive prevalence survey of women in the 15–44-year age group demonstrated that fertility was highest among 15–29-year-olds.

The current leading causes of death are chronic noncommunicable diseases. Malignant neoplasms, heart disease, cerebrovascular disease, and diabetes were the leading causes of death in 1991. The crude death rate has shown marked reduction from 8.9 per 1,000 population in 1960 to 5.4 in 1992. The death rate per 100 hospital discharges in 1995 was 4.37.

The number of immigrant visas issued to Jamaicans destined for the United States in 1995 was 14,239, compared with 10,681 in 1994. A total of 3,577 persons emigrated to Canada in 1995, compared with 3,731 in 1994. The United Kingdom issued entry certificates to 242 Jamaicans in 1995, compared with 334 in 1994.

Data for 1996 suggest that in the last three years there has been a significant increase in the number of persons who had migrated from agrarian areas in western Jamaica to urban centers and who are now returning to their "rural roots." This "reverse migration" may be linked to the continuous rise in violence and the cost of living in urban centers.

The poverty severity index rose from 3.9 in 1989 to 4.4 in 1992, having peaked at 6.6 in 1991. In addition, 22% of those employed fell below the poverty line in 1993. Poverty can no longer be associated exclusively with unemployment. A new category—the working poor—has emerged. There was actually a downward trend in unemployment over the 1991–1994 period. Unemployment in this period remained steady at 9.4%–9.5% for males, but fell slightly from 22.8% to 21.8% for females. Despite lower unemployment levels, it was estimated that in 1993 28.2% of the population was living in poverty, up from 27.6% in 1989. From all unofficial indicators, it is likely that in 1994 the number further increased substantially.

Unemployment among 15–29-year-olds ranged from 20% to 31% nationwide. In Kingston, the rate was 25.8%, closely approximating the national average for population in this age group. With respect to education, 1996 data show a national average of 31% of 15–29-year-olds with a primary education; in Kingston the value was only 17.2% for this age group.

The 1994 Jamaica Survey of Living Conditions reported a 10.6% decrease in mean (and real) per capita consumption over the 1990–1993 period. The declines were 14.4% in the Kingston metropolitan area and 16% in other towns.

The Government of Jamaica has clearly stated its intention to eradicate poverty and has conducted poverty alleviation projects. Projects addressing health problems have been mainly in the area of nutrition and the environment. In 1995, approximately 40,000 individuals were targeted for nutrition assistance. Environmental projects in east-central and south St. Andrew aim to improve the health status of these inner city communities. Toilets have been built and repaired, and water pipes installed and rehabilitated in these communities.

The parishes with large urban centers, including Kingston/St. Andrew, St. Catherine (Portmore and Spanish Town), and St. James (Montego Bay) ranked better than the national average on all indicators. In St. Andrew, approximately 70% of households enjoy piped water supply, while 40% of households lack their own sanitary facilities. In Kingston, however, approximately half of households lack piped water and 60% lack their own sanitary facilities, an extremely high figure for the country's major urban center. According to the Planning and Evaluation Unit of the Ministry of Health, 84% of all Jamaicans have access to potable water.

SPECIFIC HEALTH PROBLEMS

Analysis by Population Group

Health of Children and Adolescents

According to the Economic and Social Survey, at the end of 1995 the prevalence of malnutrition in the 0–35-month-old population was 5.64%, with 5.22% moderately malnourished, and 0.42% severely malnourished. This is a slight improvement over 1994. The supplementary feeding program, which distributes locally manufactured, high-energy supplements to malnourished children through clinics, has improved the effectiveness of the nutrition intervention process by increasing the rate of weight gain and shortening the period for complete rehabilitation of malnourished children.

In 1991, there were 2,317 hospital discharges diagnosed with perinatal complications, representing 2.1% of all discharges and 9.5 per 10,000 population. Perinatal conditions accounted for 44% of all years of life lost due to premature mortality in the age group under 5 years old, and 36% of all disability adjusted life years in young children. Efforts of the Diarrheal Diseases Program have effectively maintained the case fatality and mortality rates from diarrhea in children at less than 1%. Congenital abnormalities rank second to perinatal conditions for infant mortality. The main factors that affect infant survival in the neonatal period (up to 28 days) are birth weight and the quality of prenatal and perinatal care.

An average of 51.7% of infants seen at postnatal clinics island-wide were reported to be fully breast-fed at the end of 1995. This is the same as in 1994, despite accelerated promotion of breast-feeding.

The main causes for hospitalization of infants under 1 year old in 1991 were conditions related to the perinatal period and gastroenteritis (e.g., diarrhea), followed by respiratory illnesses. Hospitalization due to respiratory illnesses ranked first for children 1–4 years old, followed by injuries and poisonings, and gastroenteritis. In 1991, among children under 1 year old, perinatal conditions accounted for 33% of discharges from public hospitals; pneumonia, bronchitis, emphysema, and asthma accounted for 10%; other diseases of the respiratory system, 8%; injuries and poisoning, 4%; gastroenteritis, 13%; and all other conditions, 32%.

Over the past five years, immunization coverage of children under 1 year old has increased steadily. Universal coverage has been achieved for BCG and over 90% has been achieved for polio (OPV), diphtheria, pertussis, and tetanus (DPT).

All parishes have achieved over 80% immunization coverage, except in the case of measles. In 1995, special surveillance activities for measles were conducted and a measles vaccination campaign aimed at children between 1 and 10 years old was undertaken. Certain logistical problems, including an inadequate number of health care personnel, supplies, equipment, and transportation have affected the immunization programs.

Poisoning, accidents, and violence are the leading cause of morbidity and mortality among children 5–14 years old, as reflected in discharge reports from public hospitals. The Peace and Love Program commenced in 1994 in primary schools to train teachers and students in conflict resolution skills and to promote nonviolence in schools and the wider community.

Also prevalent among the 5–14-year-old age group are diseases of the respiratory system including influenza, pneumonia, bronchitis, emphysema, and asthma; intestinal infections; and diseases preventable by immunization. Other areas of concern are anemia and malnutrition. According to the Survey of Living Conditions, in 1994, 16% of the 10–14-year-old age group of adolescents surveyed were anemic, with hemoglobin levels below the accepted standard of 12 g/dl for males and 15 g/dl for females.

Injuries and poisoning were responsible for 34.6% discharges from public hospitals in the 5–14-year-old age group; pneumonia, bronchitis, emphysema, and asthma accounted for 8.5%; appendicitis and hernia accounted for 3.8%; genitourinary disorders were responsible for 4.8%; complications of pregnancy, 4.1%; and all other conditions, 42.4%.

A survey on smoking published by the Medical Association of Jamaica in 1994 showed that 20% of male smokers surveyed in 1993 first started smoking under the age of 15 years.

Teenage births as a percentage of total births have decreased from 31% in 1977 to 23.7% in 1992. In 1993, 2.5% of women between 10 and 14 years old had their first birth. Results of the Jamaica Contraceptive Prevalence Survey show that the age-specific fertility rate in 1993 for 15–19-year-olds was 108 per 1,000 women. In the 20–24-year age group, this rate was 160 per 1,000 women in 1993, a decline of 1.8 compared with 1987.

Within the adolescent population of 268,530, there were 25 cases of syphilis, 195 cases of gonorrhea, and 229 nongonococcal infections. In the 10–19-year age group, 10 males and 14 females were infected with AIDS.

Health of Women

Abortion is one of the most important causes of maternal mortality in Jamaica caused by infections and complications from procedures performed under unsanitary conditions by untrained personnel. More adequate conditions with less risk of complications are the norm for upper-class women who choose to terminate their pregnancies.

There was a slight reduction in the average number of visits to health centers for prenatal care in 1994 compared with 1993. In 1994, there were 3.9 visits per pregnancy, and in 1993, 4.0 visits. First visits as a percentage of estimated births were 73.6% in 1994 compared with 72.4% in 1993. The percentage of women receiving care before the 16th week of pregnancy is approximately 68.2%. During the postnatal period, 74.4% of mothers and 75.6% of babies received care at health centers. Of the mothers visiting health centers in this period, 51.2% fully breast-fed, and 61.2% accepted family planning.

Over 80% of deliveries take place at Victoria Jubilee Hospital, the main public maternity hospital serving the Kingston/St. Andrew metropolitan area. Service is inadequate due to a shortage of personnel and beds. For example, two night nurses are often responsible for nine labor and delivery stations. The "baby friendly hospital" project carried out renovation at the hospital in 1994 and 1995 under the Debt Relief for Children Initiative, a collaboration between the Government of the Kingdom of the Netherlands and UNICEF.

Studies show that in 1994–1995, most rural parishes recorded increases in the percentage of postnatal family planning acceptors, while larger urban areas such as Kingston/St. Andrew and St. James showed no significant increase. Questions arise as to whether urban parishes are more resistant to family planning, or the women prefer to seek contraceptives at private centers.

Total new family planning acceptors as a percentage of women 15–49 years old increased slightly in 1994 to 7.5%, from 6.5% in 1993. In 1995, 40,000 clients were recruited into the Government's Family Planning Program. This was 21% below the 51,000 target. The pill remained the dominant choice with an acceptance rate of 47.8%; 28.8% chose the condom; 21.7% of clients opted for the Depo Provera Injection. Family planning visits increased marginally from 51,866 visits in 1994 to 55,918 in 1995. Tubal ligations were introduced in all hospitals by 1994 and were performed at two family planning clinics and one type-5 health center. A total of 3,830 women were ligated in 1994, compared with 3,475 in 1993. Vasectomy is not a widely used form of family planning, and no Jamaican men were reported to have been sterilized in 1993.

The five leading diagnoses for females discharged from hospital were complications of pregnancy 29,147 (33%); normal delivery 28,336 (32%); injuries and poisoning 3,958 (4.5%); genito-urinary disorders 3,716 (4.2%); and cardiovascular diseases 3,457 (3.9%). Normal delivery represented the shortest length of hospital stay (a mean of 2 days). Complications of pregnancy was the condition representing the most days of care (96,185 days).

Health of the Elderly

In 1995, there were 110,430 males and 130,020 females in Jamaica in the 60 years and older group, representing 9.42% of the population. This age group is affected mainly by chronic noncommunicable diseases. Cardiovascular diseases followed by diabetes and neoplasms were the diseases for which persons over 65 years old were most often hospitalized in 1991. Genitourinary disorders, injuries, and poisonings were also of significance. The 1994 Jamaica Survey of Living Conditions indicates that persons over 60 years old exhibited the highest prevalence of protracted illness. Additionally, 81.5% of the ill or injured sought medical care from private institutions. Females were more likely than males to seek medical care.

A study done of the elderly in August Town, Kingston, determined that their major health problems were hypertensive diseases, diabetes, arthritis, and heart disease. A larger number of obese people complained of arthritis than those who were normal or overweight. A history of heart disease was also more prevalent in obese persons.

The Golden Age Home in Kingston accepted 489 residents in 1995, 250 of whom were males. The Home provides meals and accommodation; medical, dental and nursing care; and occupational and recreational activities. Similar facilities provide long-term geriatric care in rural parishes.

The National Council for the Aged operates island-wide. In 1995, its main activities included: advocacy and policy formulation; initiation and monitoring of over 100 Golden Age Clubs that carry out income-generating protects for the elderly; caring and community projects; oversight of senior citizen day-activity centers and feeding programs; training and education; and referral and other services. Other social services include concessionary rates for the elderly on public transportation.

Since 1977, the Government has made drugs for chronic diseases available at lower cost for the elderly. Many pharmacies also discount drug prices for senior citizens.

Family Health

According to the 1993 Jamaica Survey of Living Conditions, over 45.5% of Jamaican households are single-parent families headed by women. Many of these families are included in the 21.2% of households that are below the poverty line. The Government has instituted food aid and other projects to assist these families.

The food aid program is designed to supplement the food intake of persons at risk of becoming malnourished and others who have little or no visible income. Beneficiaries are school-aged children, lactating mothers, and children 0–6 years of age whose nutritional levels need to be improved. In 1995, 3,000 malnourished children between 4 and 59 months old benefited from locally manufactured, high-energy supplements distributed through nutrition clinics. A feeding program in schools assisted 315,518 students in 1995. Students were provided with at least one meal per day in early childhood, primary, and secondary public institutions to encourage regular school attendance. In 1995, there were 270,000 persons on the Food Stamp list. This figure represented 78.1% of the overall target of 350,000, a reduction from 86.6% of the 320,000 targeted in 1994.

Children in need of care and protection are the responsibility of the Children's Services Division of the Ministry of Health.

The Adoption Board granted eight adoption orders in 1995. Other services to assist families include the Family Court System, which provides judicial and social services, and the Women's Center, which provides continuing education for mothers 16 years and under.

Workers' Health

The importance of workers' health is gaining momentum in Jamaica as a priority for the Government. An example of concerns in this area is the failure to wear protective gear in some emergency establishments, which poses health risks. In 1994, of 100 employees in such organizations visited by public health inspectors, only 16% used protective equipment. In the garment industry, out of a working population of 506 females and 61 males, only 3.5% were seen by public health inspectors to be wearing protective equipment.

A preliminary report from a 1994 study conducted by the Statistical Institute of Jamaica in collaboration with UNICEF revealed that 4.6% of children between 6 and 16 years old were employed, mostly in the informal sector, despite legislation prohibiting employment of children under the age of 12. There is a great deal of overlap in the phenomena of out-of-school youths, working children, and street children. Many from these groups sleep on the street and are exposed to the elements, physical violence, and sexual abuse. Maintaining hygiene is a problem for these children; they are generally malnourished and tend to share health related problems. They are often exploited by peers and adults because they lack the physical strength to resist.

Efforts to address the problem include work done by the Save the Children Fund (United Kingdom), which has assisted in integrating 500 street and working children into the formal school system in Spanish Town and Montego Bay. Other projects provide cooked meals and remedial education.

Informal commercial workers (called "higglers") sell goods that are generally purchased overseas. There is concern that these workers are at risk of STDs and AIDS due to the nature of their work, which involves international travel and absence from home. HIV prevalence among commercial sex workers in Kingston in 1995 stood at 11%. According to the Epidemiology Unit of the Ministry of Health, the HIV prevalence rate in migrant farm workers has remained stable at 0.1%.

Health of the Disabled

The Jamaica Council for the Disabled is responsible for administering the Government's rehabilitation program for persons with disabilities. Its responsibilities include national registration of the disabled; securing benefits and concessions for the disabled; assessment, guidance, and placement of persons in need of skills training and employment; providing accommodation and support for clients receiving vocational training; providing support for self-help projects; and catering to disabled 0–6-year-old children.

The Abilities Foundation provides training and education for disabled young adults aged 18–25. Other programs for the disabled include the National Vocational Rehabilitation Service and Early Stimulation Project, which focuses on children 0–6 years old. In 1995, 296 disabled children attended a special program addressing their needs.

Analysis by Type of Disease or Health Impairment

Communicable Diseases

Vector-Borne Diseases. A dengue fever outbreak in 1995 resulted in 1,884 suspected cases. This included 108 cases of dengue hemorrhagic fever, 3 cases of dengue shock syndrome, and 4 deaths. There were 5 reported cases of malaria in 1995 and 14 reported cases in 1996, all imported.

Vaccine-Preventable Diseases. Immunization coverage levels are about 90% for DPT, polio, and tuberculosis. Measles immunization coverage is about 77% for children under 23 months. With the exception of measles, the incidence of these diseases is very low. Between March and May 1995, there was an outbreak of rubella in the parishes of St. Elizabeth, Portland, and Kingston/St. Andrew. These parishes accounted for 65% of rubella cases reported in 1995. Five other parishes had confirmed isolated cases of rubella during the second and third quarters of the year. Of the rubella cases reported, 62% were in females.

Cholera and Other Intestinal Diseases. There have been no cholera outbreaks in Jamaica, but given the presence of the disease in South and Central America, gastroenteritis is monitored as an indicator of potential problems. Gastroenteritis increased in 1995 compared with the previous two years. It appears to be largely a seasonal problem, occurring between October and March. The main etiological factor is the rotavirus.

There were 27 cases of typhoid fever in 1995, a slight increase over 1994. The reported incidence over the past 20 years suggests a gradual decline in the endemic level of the disease, with periodic outbreaks.

Foodborne illnesses are grossly underreported and pose a problem with regard to investigations and confirmation of epidemiological information. The resulting lack of information in this area has hindered the creation of long-term control measures to address problems of specific food vehicles

and to improve food-handling techniques. Training is being conducted in the proper handling and preparation of food.

Chronic Communicable Diseases. While chronic communicable diseases in general are on the increase in the Americas, rates for many diseases have remained relatively low and stable in Jamaica. The island has a surveillance system network consisting of 44 sentinel sites and 22 hospital active sites. These sites include type-3 health centers as well as public and private hospitals island-wide. Efforts are being made to strengthen the surveillance system by including private practitioners, particularly pediatricians.

Reported cases of tuberculosis have been steady over the first half of the decade. There were 109 confirmed cases in 1994; 97% were new cases and 3% were relapsed cases. Confirmed cases of tuberculosis peaked at 121 in 1996, the highest since 1991. Of this number, five were reactivated cases, indicating that 96% of the cases were due to active transmission. Twelve (10%) were co-infected with HIV and accounted for 50% of the 14 deaths. The parishes of residence of those infected include Kingston/St. Andrew, St. Catherine, and St. Ann.

Hansen's disease (leprosy) has seen a decrease and strategies are being put in place to achieve the goal of eradication. Tuberculosis has remained almost constant at a relatively low level for the population. However, there is concern about the coinfection of HIV and tuberculosis and plans are afoot to address this in view of the worldwide trend.

Acute Respiratory Infections. Respiratory infections were second among the 10 leading causes of visits to health centers (89,733) in 1996. Pneumonia, bronchitis, emphysema, and asthma were the fourth major cause of hospitalization in 1994, with the exclusion of obstetric conditions. Asthma is becoming the major cause of illness prompting visits to emergency departments of public hospitals (28,178 cases in 1996). The most commonly affected are children in the under-5 age group. Increased environmental pollution could be a major contributor to this situation. The usual trend of increased influenza activity during the last quarter of the year was supported by anecdotal reports.

Rabies and Other Zoonoses. Epidemiological data showed that leptospirosis is a serious health problem, both in the human and animal population. A research protocol was developed in 1994 for an epidemiological retrospective assessment of the leptospirosis situation. The study is still pending. Jamaica maintains its rabies-free status.

During the 1991–1995 period, technical cooperation concentrated in supporting epidemiological surveys to assess the condition of cattle herds. Jamaica could be considered free of both bovine brucellosis and tuberculosis, and a proposal for official certification of this status was prepared at the end of

1995. Certification would have a positive impact on public health and contribute to Jamaica's economy by benefiting the beef trade.

AIDS and Other Sexually Transmitted Diseases. In 1995, there were 505 cases of AIDS reported to the Ministry of Health Epidemiology Unit in 320 males and 185 females, a 41% increase over 1994. Between 1982 (when the first AIDS case was reported) and December 1995, there have been 1,533 reported AIDS cases, representing a doubling of cases every two years. Of the total, 62.3% are males and 37.7% females. The adult male-female ratio is 1.7:1 and indicates a predominately heterosexual transmission. More women of childbearing age are affected. There is a doubling of cases every two years. Transmission categories are ranked heterosexual, homosexual/bisexual, and mother to child. There is an increase in the number of HIV positives in the prenatal clinic population, and criteria for testing prenatal clinic clients will be developed. There have been 907 AIDS-related deaths, a mortality rate of 59.2%. The total number of pediatric cases is 108. There were 73 pediatric deaths, a pediatric AIDS mortality rate of 67.6%. The adult mortality rate is 58.5%.

All parishes were affected by the epidemic: St. James had the highest case rate (155/100,000 population) and Clarendon the lowest (12/100,000).

HIV prevalence among United States visa applicants, blood donors, migrant farmers, and insurance company clients has remained between the ranges 0.5/1000 and 4/1000. However, an increase in the rate among food handlers has been observed. While HIV prevalence in female commercial sex workers in Kingston has remained the same during the past five years (11%–12%), screening has shown a seroprevalence of 22% among this group in St. James. The intervention among sex workers in Kingston had positive impacts, and a similar intervention program has begun in St. James. That 31% of the 64 HIV-positive sex workers in St. James are cocaine addicts poses a serious problem, since this population has been found most resistant to condom use.

The incidence of STDs remains high and continues to be a major concern. In the public health services, cases of chlamydia, syphilis, gonorrhea, and nongonococcal urethritis remain high, as do cases of congenital syphilis and ophthalmia neonatorum. There are also increasingly high levels of gonococcal resistance to penicillin and tetracycline, signifying the need for the use of more expensive drug therapy.

Studies in Jamaica support international research on the contribution of STDs to increased spread of HIV. It has been shown that genital ulcer disease and the inflammatory STDs (gonorrhea and chlamydia) facilitate transmission of HIV infection. Of concern, therefore, are the large numbers of genital ulcers and inflammatory STDs being seen at the Comprehensive Clinic in Kingston. After conducting a study at this clinic,

STD syndromic reporting was introduced in 1995 with respect to urethral and vaginal discharges. A treatment algorithm was developed to treat these discharges.

Noncommunicable Diseases and Other Health-Related Problems

Nutritional Diseases. The results of relatively recent surveys among children under 5 years of age provide some notion as to changes in prevalence of malnutrition over time. The data indicate that the proportion of children under 5 who are mildly, severely, or moderately low weight-for-age declined over the period 1970 to 1985. Mildly malnourished children moved from 39.0% to 31.9%, while moderately and severely malnourished declined from 10.8% to 8%. These surveys found that the weaning period of 6 to 11 months was the peak period for wasting, lowest in the age group 48 to 59 months. Stunting increased with age, implying that suboptimal intakes continued after weaning. In comparison, the 1989–1993 Jamaica Survey of Living Conditions data suggest a prevalence rate of 6.5 to 9.9% for moderately and severely malnourished children. In 1993, 9.9% of all children aged 0–59 months had low weight-for-age, 6.3% were stunted, and 3.5% were wasted. Recorded low weight-for-age wasting and stunting increased in 1993. All survey data sets highlighted the fact that rural areas show a higher prevalence of malnutrition than urban areas.

Since 1980, the Ministry of Health has had data supplied from the Monthly Clinic Summary Report Systems. Data for 1984–1987 indicate an average of 4.1% of clinic clients aged 0–35 months were classified as moderately to severely malnourished. In 1988, the Ministry of Health adopted the WHO classification, and data for 1989–1994 indicate that the percentage of children assessed as being moderately and severely malnourished averaged approximately 8.4% over the period. The clinic population is a self-selected one and does not necessarily indicate the actual prevalence of malnutrition island-wide.

Malnutrition in Jamaica occurs most frequently in households of the unemployed, among subsistence farmers in rural areas, in the lowest income urban areas, in large families with no paternal support, and among very young mothers.

Iron deficiency anemia is prevalent among pregnant and lactating women and young children. Ministry of Health clinic data for 1984–1991 indicate that, on average, some 28.9% of pregnant women tested were diagnosed as anemic. The 1985 National Health Survey estimated that 25% of children under age 5 years were anemic, with the peak incidence being in the age group 6–11 months old.

While malnutrition in Jamaica has been relatively low and is no longer a major cause of death, there are localized areas with more severe levels of malnutrition. Increased surveillance at the community level and regular monitoring of the population in these areas are needed to analyze the contributory factors and design appropriate targeted interventions.

Chronic Noncommunicable Diseases. The leading causes of mortality and morbidity in Jamaica are chronic noncommunicable diseases. Their ranking varies depending on the indicator used. In general, the ranking is as follows: cardiovascular disease, neuro-psychiatric conditions, cancers, diabetes, and nutritional disorders.

Chronic noncommunicable diseases represent a substantial portion of the illness burden. Hypertension and diabetes (123,090 and 50,783 visits, respectively) made up two of the five major causes of ambulatory visits in health centers in 1996. In 1994, cardiovascular disease, diabetes mellitus, and neoplasms were among the five first-listed causes of hospitalization. In 1990, cardiovascular disease accounted for 30% of all noncommunicable diseases.

Cancers accounted for 15% of noncommunicable diseases and 9% of total disease burden in 1990. Cancers of the breast and cervix are the most common neoplasms in women, with rates in 1991 of 22.6 and 19.2 per 1,000 population, respectively. Prostate cancer is the number one form of cancer found in men. The rate in 1991 was 28.2 and reflects a growing trend.

The crude death rate has shown marked reduction from 8.9 per 1,000 population in 1960 to 5.4 in 1992. It remained the same in 1994. The leading causes of death are now due to chronic noncommunicable diseases, a change from the 1950s when the leading causes were primarily infectious diseases. The leading causes of death in the general population for 1990 were heart diseases (114.0/100,000 population), malignant neoplasms (82.2), cerebrovascular diseases (80.1), diabetes (51.0), and diseases of the respiratory system (30.1).

Morbidity information is based on hospital utilization by diagnosis in government institutions. For 1991, the six top conditions for hospitalization were complications of pregnancy, normal delivery, genitourinary disorders, injuries and poisonings, cardiovascular diseases, and neoplasms, with diabetes mellitus ranking 10th. In 1993, the top six conditions were complications of pregnancy, normal delivery, injuries and poisoning, cardiovascular diseases, genitourinary disorders, and pneumonia, bronchitis, emphysema, and asthma.

Injuries and poisoning were the leading diagnoses (representing 14.9% of all diagnoses), according to the number of days of care provided. An estimated 124,648 days of care were provided with an average length of stay of 9.3 days. More than 70% of the cases hospitalized were male. An examination of the geographical distribution shows that the incidence of these cases is predominantly an urban phenomenon linked to poverty and other socioeconomic variables. These factors raise serious concerns regarding the use

of health care resources for conditions that are clearly preventable.

Cardiovascular diseases and diabetes mellitus predominate at both the hospitals and health centers; 8% of all discharges from hospitals and 14.3% of all clinic visits are due to cardiovascular diseases. Diabetes mellitus has the longest average length of hospital stay (15.0 days) and accounts for 5.9% of all clinic visits. An island-wide survey done in 1993 showed that the prevalence for diabetes is 17.9% and for hypertension is 21.1% (systolic reading only).

The area of chronic noncommunicable diseases is receiving greater attention, but needs to be organized as a program so that the problem can be better defined, prevention and control strategies can be established, and resources can be effectively allocated.

Accidents and Violence. Accidents and trauma are among the five leading causes of hospitalization, estimated to represent about 20% of hospital admissions and 33% of expenditures. In 1994, violence and accidents accounted for 12% of hospital discharges. Of trauma cases treated in hospitals, 48% are attributable to motor vehicle accidents; burns represent about 28%; and acts of violence, 20%. During 1996, there were 3,286 stab wounds and 1,156 gunshot wounds; the number of cases of burns by fire, chemical, or other causes totaled 1,333; there were 749 cases of poisoning. Road traffic accidents gave rise to 8,655 cases that were treated in hospital.

Violence constitutes a growing public health problem as demonstrated by the alarming increase in the rate of mortality, morbidity, and disability in the society. The overwhelming loss of potential years of life and its psychological effects on the population also are problems. The Ministry of Health has examined the cases of trauma due to accidents and violence in Jamaica in order to facilitate programs for the prevention of accidents, the prevention and control of violence, and the promotion of peaceful coexistence in which health related activities are emphasized.

Parishes with the highest level of population density had the largest number of traumas associated with violence. In 1994, Kingston/St. Andrew had 718 stab wounds and 404 gunshot wounds, while St. Catherine had 490 and 126 cases, respectively.

In 1994, the varying types of trauma that required emergency care in public sector casualty departments affected all age groups. The 16–44-year age groups (5,012) and the 5–15-year-olds (1,051) comprised the highest number of victims. The number of children under 5 years old that were victims of trauma (847) is of concern, especially trauma due to burns (499), motor vehicle accidents, and poisoning. There is a need for education about safety in the home and road safety programs that make the use of seat belts and crash helmets mandatory.

While there has been a decrease in motor vehicle accidents, they still are an area of major concern. It is estimated that for every motor fatality there are an average of nine injuries, three of them requiring major medical treatment. A Government-sponsored road safety report in 1993 ranked Jamaica as having the third and fourth highest rates for motor vehicle fatalities per number of cars and population size, respectively. Traffic accidents also are highly localized, occurring mostly in the Kingston/St. Andrew and St. Catherine areas. Most deaths involve pedestrians, the elderly, and children. Unsafe driving habits and unfit vehicles are the major causes of vehicular accidents.

Behavioral Disorders. Mental health visits account for 2% of total public health center visits, up from 1.4% in 1989. Of the 7,067 patients seen by the Community Mental Health Services, the most common diagnoses were schizophrenia (49.6%), depression (19.6%), substance abuse (9.6%), neurosis (7.0%), and organic psychosis (4.7%).

The Ministry of Health has recognized the need for community mental health services and for more information on the nature and extent of the problem. Mental health services are not integrated into general services, which contributes to an ineffective use of resources and poor patient management. Services are limited in range and are short of trained personnel to support patient rehabilitation. Finally, mental illnesses require health promotion approaches that can destigmatize and increase public awareness about the disease. A Mental Health Act designed to direct greater resources to this area is planned for 1997.

Oral Health. A successful program in salt fluoridation has been in operation since September 1987. This is evident by the decrease from 6.7% in 1984 to 1.08% in 1995 in decayed, missing, and filled teeth (DMFT) in children 12 years of age. A 1995 study showed that 63% of the sample needed no dental care, and the degree of fluorosis was negligible (0.4%). The overall dental status of the Jamaican population has improved considerably, based on the decline in extractions performed.

The Ministry of Health's Dental Health Program targets children under age 16 for comprehensive care. In 1996, there were 189,290 dental visits and 71,888 preventive procedures performed. In addition, emergency and palliative care was provided for adults. The private sector helped considerably to meet the increasing demand for prophylactic, orthodontic, restorative, and other specialty services. The ratio of dentists to population (public and private) was approximately 1:12,000 in 1996.

Natural Disasters. The last natural disasters of major significance were Hurricane Gilbert in 1988 and a 1993 earthquake that registered about 8 on the Richter Scale.

Flooding is a recurrent problem during the rainy season, causing problems with transportation, housing, and water supplies.

The Ministry of Health and the Office of Disaster Preparedness share disaster and emergency response and mitigation activities with support from the Jamaica Defense Force. The Ministry of Health is responsible for emergency medical services and the Office of Disaster Preparedness is responsible for other aspects of emergency preparedness and disaster response. Nongovernmental and voluntary organizations involved in disaster response include the Jamaica Red Cross and the Adventist Disaster Relief Agency. The Government of Jamaica has a well-organized disaster response program and the capacity to assist other countries in the northern Caribbean when they are affected by disasters.

RESPONSE OF THE HEALTH SYSTEM

National Health Plans and Policies

Jamaica has developed a large and complex public network of primary care centers and hospitals around the country, offering an extensive array of services, frequently for free or below cost. Over time, experience has shown that reliance on Government resources is insufficient to properly maintain the infrastructure and to provide adequate personnel and other essential support services. The rising costs of health care resources, which are largely imported, and devaluation of the Jamaican currency during the early 1990s have widened the gap between available and required resources.

In response to this situation, the Government is engaged in health sector reform with the assistance of several technical cooperation agencies. Major elements of the reform are: decentralization, integration of services, promotion of quality assurance standards, rational resource allocation, human resource development, greater cost sharing, increased efficiency, fostering public-private partnerships, and equity.

It is recognized that health services delivery and management must be transformed to better match the changing epidemiological conditions and the demands of health care consumers and providers, as well as to make efficient and effective use of available resources. The Ministry of Health's central office will function in more of a regulatory capacity for the entire health system rather than in its traditional role as the centralized manager of the public system. Service delivery and management responsibilities will be delegated on three levels: 4 regions, 14 parishes, and 130 health districts.

In 1997, the Government proposed a National Health Insurance plan to offer coverage for a defined set or package of hospital, laboratory, diagnostic, and pharmacy services.

Organization of the Health Sector

Institutional Organization

Over the past decade, there has been significant growth in the private health care sector. It is estimated that 75% of ambulatory care of a curative nature is delivered in the private sector, while most hospital and preventive services are provided largely in the public sector. In 1995, there were nine small private hospitals in Jamaica, which accounted for about 300 beds, and 75 private clinics. Private hospitals report approximately 50% occupancy. There are six private health insurance companies in Jamaica, covering an estimated 10%–15% of the population. Most reimbursements are for drugs (41%) and doctor's fees (24%). The pharmaceutical sector consumes 10% of total national health expenditures, 80% of which is in the private sector.

Primary care remains a top priority with the Government. In 1996, the Ministry of Health operated 364 primary health care centers, which operate at five levels of service. The higher the level of service, the wider the catchment area of the clinic. Use of primary health care centers for curative care, which represents 46% of the workload, is decreasing despite an expansion in the number of facilities and range of service benefits. Maternal and child health services, family planning, and dental services comprise the remaining 54% of services.

In 1995, curative visits to primary health care centers totaled 780,520, down from 1,005,126 in 1992. It is assumed that more services are provided in the private sector. The other services provided by primary care centers, such as preventive care and health promotion, remain important in improving the health conditions of the entire population, but most notably among children, the elderly, indigent, and individuals suffering from chronic and communicable diseases.

The public secondary and tertiary care system comprises a total of 23 acute care hospitals: six tertiary specialty hospitals, five secondary care hospitals, nine small community hospitals, and three hospitals specializing in chronic care. The University of the West Indies Hospital, with 430 beds, is a regional teaching facility. Public hospital utilization has steadily decreased over the past five years. Bed availability has fluctuated due to the Government's extensive hospital restoration program that has focused on six major hospitals. Total hospital discharges (111,002), average occupancy rate (66.6%), deliveries (36,059), outpatient visits (333,409), and casualty visits (389,855) for 1995 reflect lower use despite service expansion. The number of x-rays taken increased slightly and physical therapy treatment almost doubled, reaching 173,733.

It is estimated that public hospitals are responsible for 95% of inpatient days and 65% of costs. While the leading reasons for admission relate to normal and complicated maternity cases, trauma cases and chronic diseases account for the largest expenditures.

Organization of Health Regulatory Activities

The Ministry of Health, in its thrust to protect the environment and promote health for sustainable development, divides responsibility for the management of its environment health strategies among the Public Health Inspectorate, the Veterinary Public Health Unit, the Environmental Control and Pharmaceutical divisions, and the Pesticide Council. Their roles include the regular monitoring of the quality of food, drugs, air, and drinking water; the disposal of excreta; the management of wastewater, solid and hazardous wastes; port health; the control of vectors and pesticides; and monitoring of workers and occupational and institutional health.

The Food Safety Program targets both raw and cooked foods. Food processing, milk processors and ice cream manufacturers, hotels, restaurants, and itinerant vendors are monitored to ensure food safety. Meat also is inspected to ensure its safety for human consumption. The Food Division of the Government Chemist Department assists with the monitoring of food, especially milk samples. Of special relevance is the mushrooming of street food vendors. The Food Handler's Clinic educates clients on personal hygiene and good food handling practices.

The Pharmaceutical Services Division of the Ministry of Health, created by the Food and Drug Act of 1964, controls the authorization, importation, distribution and use of pharmaceuticals. The division ensures that all substances used as food, drugs, and cosmetics are safe and of high quality. A task force was set up to examine the classification and regulation requirements of herbal preparations, vitamins, and homeopathic medicine. The Pharmaceutical Services Division is also charged with the distribution of drugs, vaccines, and other medical supplies within the Government health system. Supply and personnel shortages are chronic, especially in primary care centers.

It is estimated that private funds currently finance 82% of pharmaceutical costs, but it is not clear what level of service this represents. The Ministry of Health has gradually relinquished the pharmaceutical industry to a quasi-public agency (Health Corporation Limited) and the private sector. There are about 275 registered pharmacies and 520 pharmacists in the country.

The National Public Health Laboratory is the Ministry of Health's central laboratory facility. It investigates and monitors food and water and serves as a referral laboratory for hospitals and clinics, as a reference laboratory for quality control purposes, and as a clinical laboratory for Kingston Public Hospital and Victoria Jubilee Hospital.

Health Services and Resources

Organization of Services for Care of the Population

Veterinary public health is the joint responsibility of the Ministries of Health, Agriculture, and a number of other agencies cooperating to prevent zoonoses and reduce the risk of foodborne diseases. The training of food inspectors, public education, and community participation are the main strategies for improving hygienic food handling and rodent control programs.

The Health Promotion Charter for the Caribbean has been the framework for health education and promotion strategies for countries in the subregion, including Jamaica, since its inception in 1993. The Charter emphasizes multisectoral multidisciplinary considerations in the formulation of health public policy. The Bureau of Health Education is the unit responsible for planning, implementing, evaluating, and coordinating health education and promotion programs in the country. Under health sector reform, the Bureau will form part of the Division of Disease Prevention and Health Promotion.

Environmental Services

The Government recognizes the critical relationships between health and the environment and sustainable economic development. It has identified three national priorities in this area: community water and sanitation, solid waste management and disposal, and occupational health. Several joint technical cooperation programs are working to strengthen human resources, infrastructure, and the institutions responsible for maintaining environmental services.

The Ministry of Health shares the responsibility for environmental health services with a number of other public, quasi-public, and private agencies such as the National Water Commission. Public health inspectors assigned to parish health departments are responsible for the enforcement of public health laws.

Over 80% of the population is connected to piped water supply systems, 12% receives treated water of questionable quality, and the remaining 7% of the population does not receive water from a public water supply network. The principal sources of drinking water are rivers, wells, and bore holes, resources that are in danger of being seriously degraded if inadequate waste disposal methods and pollution persist.

The continued use of open trench irrigation systems, poorly maintained water transmission and distribution systems, siltation, industrialization, and use of chemicals in agriculture pose threats to the natural water resources.

Management of Solid and Hazardous Waste. A major area of concern is the treatment and disposal of liquid and solid waste. In 1995, there were 26 officially recognized dump sites, all of which are located in environmentally precarious areas with regard to land, water, and air pollution. The Government is considering a national rationalization program for solid waste management, including the development of landfills. Six sites were identified as potential landfills. Of these, Riverton City is currently being converted.

Twenty percent of the population has access to sewerage systems, which exist only in the major urban areas and tourist centers of Kingston, Montego Bay, Ocho Rios, and Negril. The disposal facility for 50% of the population is the pit latrine, while 28% have access to individual septic tanks and absorption systems. There are 109 water treatment plants; 40% are in the Kingston/St. Catherine area.

Solid and hazardous waste, including industrial byproducts, and air pollution are on the rise due to increased industrial activity, urbanization, and the number of motor vehicles. In response to public complaints about air pollution, spot checks of air quality were conducted at Waterloo Road in St. Andrew, Riverton City Dump in Kingston, and Windsor Road in St. Catherine. Four mini-volume air samplers were acquired with the assistance of Government of the Kingdom of the Netherlands.

For the long term, a study on Jamaica's medical waste management recommended that dedicated incinerators be constructed in Kingston and Montego Bay; that an appropriate separation, storage, and collection system be provided throughout the medical community; and that incineration capabilities be upgraded in existing facilities.

The disposal of sewage from ships that dock in Jamaica's harbors is a matter of concern, since the country is at risk for the spread of the feco-oral diseases and cholera.

Water Quality. The major suppliers of drinking water include the National Water Commission and the Parish Councils. In 1996, there were approximately 891 formal sources of water supply providing approximately 140 million gallons per day. Of this number, 567 supplied treated water. According to the Water and Sanitation Monitoring System, 84% of all Jamaicans have access to potable water. While 96% of the urban population can access drinking water, this is true for only 69% of the rural population. Twelve percent of those without access use rainwater catchment systems and protected springs; 4% have no regular supply.

The Ministry's goal to test 15,000 samples of drinking water was surpassed. Of 16,626 water samples, rates for chlorine residue were satisfactory in 13,234 (79.6%). Of 7,012 samples taken, 1,635 (24.5%) had coliform/bacterial contamination, an increase of 2.1% over 1995. These samples were found mainly in Parish Council Supplies and household tanks. The parishes of Portland, St. Mary, Trelawny, and Hanover need to improve water treatment practices.

There is a need for intersectoral collaboration with suppliers of drinking water to provide piped water to the 16% of the population who do not have access, and to improve their chlorination practices. Similarly, citizens constructing pit latrines or sewage systems in areas with limestone soil or high water tables should seek the guidance of the Public Health Department to prevent contamination of the groundwater.

Vector Control. The vector control program is an integral part of the Ministry's efforts to prevent outbreaks of vector-borne diseases. Surveillance of *Aedes aegypti, Anopheles albimanus,* and other mosquitoes continues through inspection of breeding sites at households, in drains, and at the international airports. While the Ministry of Health conducts public education programs, treats breeding sites with larvicide, and sprays or fogs communities infested with mosquitoes, community participation is vital to ensure that drains are kept clean and that domestic water storage containers do not foster mosquito breeding. In 1996, the house indices of the *Aedes aegypti* (vector of dengue and yellow fever) ranged from 2% to 52%.

Approximately 90% of aircraft landing at the Norman Manley and Sangster International Airports spray residually or in flight.

The Pesticide Control Authority monitors and controls the use of chemical pesticides on the island through registration of pesticides; licensing of importers, manufacturers, sellers and pest control operators; authorization of sellers; and registration of premises. The Ministry of Health approved regulations to the Pesticide Act in January 1996; to date, there are 330 different pesticide products registered for use in Jamaica.

Beach and River Pollution. The Beaches and Rivers Monitoring Project was implemented in 1996. Water samples taken at Bluefields, the only bathing beach visited, revealed an unsatisfactory fecal coliform level; local experts will continue monitoring. Hunts Bay, Kingston Harbor, and three fishing beaches are monitored as control sites in assessing trace elements in fish and shrimp. While cadmium values were very low in all areas, lead was high at Hunts Bay, and the zinc level was high in all areas sampled. In three rivers monitored—Rio Cobre, Black River, and Roaring River—the chemical oxygen demand values were above expected. There was no evidence of fish life in these rivers.

Organization and Operation of Personal Health Care Services

The National Public Health Laboratory is the island's major public sector laboratory and blood banking facility. It offers services in hematology, chemistry, serology, bacteriology, histology, cytology, HIV testing, and other areas. In 1996, 738,450 laboratory examinations were performed; 17,759 units of blood were issued (down from 21,110 in 1995 due to

a decline in the donor population); 23,834 were tested for HIV; and 995 genotyping (paternity) tests were conducted.

The Ministry of Health is responsible for x-ray examination, contrast with and without ultrasonography, and other diagnostic imaging services in hospitals island-wide. X-ray services were provided for 166,268 clients; 35,875 as inpatients and 130,393 as outpatients.

The Emergency Medical Service is managed jointly by the Ministries of Health and Local Government and the Jamaica Fire Brigade and receives funding from the Inter-American Development Bank. Accidents and emergency departments in several hospitals had been upgraded, as were facilities at fire stations. Thirty-five doctors and nurses were trained in Advanced Cardiac and Trauma Life Support for adults and children. Staff of the Department of Social and Preventive Medicine trained 62 firemen to be emergency medical technicians. Ambulances are equipped for basic life support, and the Ministry of Health supplied necessary communication equipment.

The major noninvasive treatment modalities used in public sector hospitals include pharmaceuticals and physical therapy. Physiotherapy services are offered at regional general hospitals (Type A) and at general hospitals (Type B), except at Mandeville, which has a shortage of personnel. The only parish hospital (Type C) that offers this service is Falmouth. Bustamante Hospital for Children and National Chest Hospital (specialist hospitals) also offer these services. A total of 180,034 physiotherapy treatments were given to 48,844 clients, approximately 4 treatments per client.

Therapeutic radiological services are offered at the Kingston Public and Cornwall Regional Hospitals. Of the 2,633 clients who received superficial x-ray treatment, 362 were new. Beta therapy treatments were given to 109 patients (40 new clients included) at the Kingston Public Hospital, the only public sector facility that offers the service.

Physical and substance abuse therapy are offered at Sir John Golding Rehabilitation Centre for physical disabilities, Ken Royes Centre for mental ill health, Detoxification Units at Cornwall Regional and University Hospitals, Patricia House, and William Chamberlain Memorial Men's Hostel and Rehabilitation Centre for substance abuse. The Drug Abuse Secretariat established mechanisms to enhance the income-generating capabilities of recovering addicts.

Richmond Fellowship, Jamaica/Patricia House is a 24-bed residential facility for Jamaican nationals or non-nationals who have lived in the country for more than five years. The service model embraces the "therapeutic community" approach to substance abuse that focuses on individual and group counseling. During 1996, 67 clients were admitted, and 33 graduated. Funding is from the Ministry of Health, and entry is voluntary.

The William Chamberlain Memorial Men's Hostel and Rehabilitation Centre is funded and operated by the Salvation Army. This facility can accommodate 25 persons. The rehabilitation program lasts four to six months and is open only to male substance abusers. Entry is voluntary and all clients have a psychiatric evaluation at the Detoxification Unit, University Hospital, before admission.

Inputs for Health

The Pharmaceutical Division uses a Vital, Essential, and Necessary list of drugs to guide the procurement of pharmaceuticals. The third edition of the National Drug Formulary was issued in 1997. This document embraces the concept of rational drug use and will serve as a guide to doctors, nurses, pharmacists, and students of these disciplines. It is also expected to assist with the maintenance of rational prescribing practices.

Health Corporation Limited, a quasi-private company established in 1994 to ensure the efficient, cost-effective procurement and distribution of pharmaceuticals and medical supplies, has met approximately 70% of the essential needs of the public sector.

Although budgetary allocation for essential drugs has moved from US$ 3 million in 1991–1992 to US$ 8.6 million in 1996–1997, affordability remains a constant concern of the Government. To this end, there is a policy in place that fosters the use of generic drugs. Additionally, the Jamaica Drugs for the Elderly Program was launched in 1996 to alleviate hardships experienced by elderly clients in obtaining drugs for diseases such as arthritis, asthma, diabetes, glaucoma, and hypertension. Response to this program has been overwhelming, with 71,105 persons registered throughout the island. There is also private sector participation in the program of over 100 pharmacies, indicating good private/public partnership.

To increase accessibility to pharmaceuticals, the Ministry of Health collaborated with the Consumer Affairs Commission in a survey of prices on 33 prescription drugs to treat asthma, diabetes mellitus, and hypertension as well as over-the-counter drugs such as antacids, anthelminths (deworming medications), and cough and cold remedies.

Human Resources

The number of health personnel in the public sector increased from 4,220 in 1991 to 4,968 in 1995, approximately 18%. There were 417 physicians and 1,836 registered nurses in 1995. Several categories of health personnel are in short supply, and, in general, personnel are poorly distributed, with the less affluent and rural areas having less access to care.

The Government is the primary sponsor and trainer of health workers. Much training is provided overseas and funded through international cooperation. In general, there is a scarcity of training facilities and resources for health care personnel. This disparity varies with profession, but there is particular need to strengthen and create greater capacity for programs for health administrators, other management specialists, information technology professionals, and physical therapists. The growing private sector creates increasing competition for those scarce government-trained human resources. Private providers dominate in ambulatory care and pharmacy services.

In addition to strengthening existing human resources and training facilities, new categories of health workers need to be developed to coincide with different approaches to managing resources and delivering care.

Finally, there are weak economic incentives for people to pursue or remain in the selected health professions, at least in the public sector. Inadequate financial remuneration, benefits, and poor incentives contribute to a poor distribution of personnel relative to human resource needs. For example, nurses are known to avoid permanent hospital assignments, choosing instead to work in primary care or take short-term contract work in hospitals. This is a critical problem for certain professions such as laboratory and pharmacy technicians. Chronic staff shortages, low productivity, and frequent strikes are common. These problems should not be overlooked, since the health sector represents a large and growing segment of the economy, and should serve as a source of a variety of jobs in the future.

Expenditures and Sectoral Financing

The Jamaican health sector is estimated to have had about US$ 348 million in total expenditures in 1995. Depending on the source, total health expenditures consume between 5% and 8.9% of the GDP. Public expenditures are estimated to represent 35% of total health expenditures, indicating a gradual shift toward the private sector over the past decade. This is most applicable to ambulatory care, of which the private sector provides 75%. Fifty-two percent of drug expenditures are in the private sector.

Public expenditures on health represent about 6% of the Government budget. The Government provides 95% of the hospital care and funds 65% of this care. Significant but undetermined portions of public hospital funds or resources go to physicians operating in both sectors, leading to a subsidy for private physicians and patients capable of paying to use public resources.

Taxation revenue provides nearly 90% of the Ministry of Health's budget. Other sources include bilateral/multilateral funding and cost recovery programs such as user fees. The former primarily fund capital development projects, while the latter are utilized for recurrent expenditures by the collecting institutions.

In recent years, the Ministry of Health has been chronically underfunded, a problem compounded by generally unfavorable fluctuations in the Jamaican dollar. Substantial funding of services and other activities comes from extrabudgetary sources, such as bilateral and multilateral loans and grants.

With the growth of the private sector, the public now finances about 35% of the national health system. In the 1996–1997 fiscal year, actual public expenditures are estimated to have totaled US$ 157 million.

While compensation and secondary care continue to absorb the largest part of the Ministry of Health budget, trends are improving for line item categories and programs. Such expenditures decreased to 58% and 51% respectively. Primary care is allocated about 18% of the recurrent budget. Financing the maintenance of plant and equipment, currently allocated less than 1% of the health budget, continues to be a problem.

In recent years, the Ministry of Health has placed a greater emphasis on cost recovery for hospital services. The Health Sector Initiatives Program, part of the health reform movement, has implemented new management systems that have led to significant increases in money recovered from hospital patients. Unfortunately, charges bear no relationship to actual costs, and fee increases cannot keep pace with costs. On average, hospitals collect fees equal to about 5%–10% of their expenses. It is recognized that other financing sources must be developed, such as insurance programs and public-private partnerships. Revenue from all sources average 2% of total Ministry of Health expenses.

Approximately 7% of the Ministry's total budget for 1996/1997 came from bilateral/multilateral programs, consis-

tent with the 1995/1996 budget (7.4%). User fees, on the other hand, accounted for 3.2% of the recurrent budget for 1996/1997, an increase of 0.3% over the previous year. User fees were collected from three main areas—secondary and tertiary care, primary care, and health services support—totaling US$ 5,328,911 in 1996/1997. Because secondary and tertiary care have better mechanisms for collecting fees, over 95% of the user fees collected in 1996/1997 were from hospitals. While user fees are not a significant portion of the Ministry of Health budget, they do offer the collecting institutions access to ready cash to purchase supplies when necessary.

There are a significant number of volunteer organizations, local and overseas, that contribute to the delivery of health services. Visiting medical teams, arrangements with medical institutions overseas, government loans, and fund-raising campaigns are options commonly used to obtain care for Jamaican citizens and deserve further analysis. More information is needed to achieve efficient management of these valuable resources.

External Technical and Financial Cooperation

There are many varied external technical and financial cooperation activities in health and related sectors. Jamaica and the donor agencies take a multisectoral approach to improving living conditions, another factor essential to sustainable socioeconomic development. Examples include areas such as AIDS prevention, health sector reform, water safety and waste disposal, violence reduction, and poverty eradication. Bilateral/multilateral programs fund about 7% of the Ministry of Health budget.

MEXICO

GENERAL SITUATION AND TRENDS

Socioeconomic, Political, and Demographic Overview

The United Mexican States' territory extends for 1,967,183 km². The country is made up of 31 states and the Federal District, which is the seat of Government. The Government has three branches: the executive, headed by the President of the Republic; the legislature, made up of the Chamber of Deputies and the Senate; and the judiciary, headed by the Supreme Court of Justice.

In December 1994, the national currency was severely devalued, going from 3.1 to 7.5 pesos to US$ 1 and unleashing the worst economic recession in several decades. From December 1994 to December 1995, inflation soared from 7% to 52%. In 1995, the gross domestic product (GDP) was US$ 246.4 billion and the per capita GDP was US$ 3,320. In the 1995–1996 biennium, real wages fell by 22%, and employment in the formal sector shrank. Short-term interest rates shot up, aggravating the financial difficulties of families and companies already in debt. There were, however, substantial increases in the minimum wage, whose real value stayed about the same in 1995 and 1996.

In 1996, the principal macroeconomic variables yielded positive balances and the GDP, boosted by the rise in exports, grew by 5.1%; inflation was 27.7%, almost half what it was in the crisis of 1995; the exchange rate for the peso fluctuated slightly around 7.58 to US$ 1; short-term interest rates dropped to their lowest levels since December 1994; with the creation of 583,000 jobs, employment in the formal sector grew by 2.1%, representing a 71% recovery over the previous year, while the open unemployment rate fell to 10.5% (in 1995 it was 11.2%). In 1997, signs of economic recovery became widespread; the economy grew by 7% in the first half of the year, inflation continued to fall, the national current account neared balance, and the peso underwent slight fluctuations.

The North American Free Trade Agreement between Canada, the United States of America, and Mexico, which went into effect in 1994, opened new markets for exports and attracted foreign investment, particularly along the country's northern border, which became an area of economic expansion. The treaty has implications for the health sector through the relaxation of tariffs on trade in medical and food products, changes in sanitary and phytosanitary standards, regulations to protect the environment, and the increase in the mobility of people, goods, and services.

It was estimated that in 1995 the percentage of people living in poverty—i.e., without income or with income equal to or less than twice the minimum wage—was 60.4%. The states of Oaxaca, Chiapas, Yucatán, Hidalgo, and Puebla had the largest proportion of poor people (between 70% and 76%) and, coincidentally, a high proportion of the indigenous population.

Between 1990 and 1995, the number of private dwellings grew from 16 million to 19.3 million, piped water coverage increased from 79.4% to 85.7%, and drainage coverage rose from 63.6% to 74.9%. In 1995, 15.4% of dwellings had a dirt floor.

Of the 105,749 towns in the country, 52.7% were classified as extremely poor and 20.9% as very poor; 14.7% had modest income levels, while in 6.6% and 5.1% poverty levels were low and very low, respectively; 16.9% of the population lived in towns with poverty levels that were very high and high, 9.0% in towns with modest income levels, 8.3% in towns with low poverty levels, and 65.8% in towns with very low poverty levels. There is a high concentration of very poor localities in the states of Chiapas (73.6% of the localities and 36.8% of the population), Guerrero (80.4% and 33.1%), and Oaxaca (71.1% and 34.4%), all three of which have large indigenous population groups. Poverty is a predominantly rural phenomenon—7 of 10 towns with 100 to 999 inhabitants are classified as having very high and high poverty levels (9,115,601 persons). Poverty also seems to have ethnic roots—of the 13,466 towns where 40% or more of the population speaks an indigenous language, 12,870 fall under the category of very high or high levels of poverty (95.6%).

In 1995, the literacy rate for the population was 89.3% (87.6% in 1990)—91.4% for men and 87.2% for women. With regard to schooling, 71.3% of men had some degree of secondary education versus 65.2% of women. There are also marked differences between urban and rural areas.

It was estimated that in 1997 the population was 94.7 million, with 2.3 million births and approximately 425,000 deaths, which, when added to the negative migratory balance of 300,000 people, yields a net growth of slightly over 1.5 million people and an annual growth rate of 1.62%. Between 1992 and 1995, the population increased by 13% despite the drop in the natural growth rate (1.87% in 1993 and 1.72% in 1995), and the number of children per woman continued to fall (3.08 in 1992 versus 2.73 in 1996). The crude birth rate dropped from 26.78 per 1,000 population in 1992 to 24.46 per 1,000 in 1996.

Between 1990 and 1995, the percentage of the population living in localities with populations under 2,500 (rural environment) fell from 28.7% to 26.5%, and the percentage inhabiting cities of over 500,000 inhabitants rose from 22.0% to 25.0%. In 1995, 6 of 10 Mexicans lived in a city, 3 of 10 in a rural area, and 1 of 10 in a locality that was in transition from a rural to an urban environment. The urban population—i.e., the population living in towns with over 15,000 inhabitants—totaled 58.4 million (64%), and the nonurban population totaled 32.8 million (36%). The states with the largest urban population were the Federal District (100%) and Nuevo León (90.6%), and those with the largest nonurban population were Oaxaca (77.1%) and Chiapas (72.8%). The Mexico City metropolitan area is home to 16.8 million people, or 18.5% of the nation's population.

Domestic migration for 1993 was estimated at 27.5 million people (32.2% of the population), 60% of whom crossed state boundaries; the remaining 40% moved between municipalities within the same state. Some 792,000 people migrated temporarily to the United States of America in search of work in 1993; in 1995 the figure was 543,000. These workers were predominantly men (94.5% in 1993 and 1995) of economically active age (88.3% in 1993 and 89.6% in 1995 were between 12 and 44 years of age) from urban areas (57.6% in 1993 and 54.7% in 1995). Estimates put the net balance of permanent migration to the United States at 1.5 million people between 1990 and 1995 (2.5 million from 1980 to 1989); the Mexican population living in that country is estimated at between 7.0 and 7.3 million people.

The population under 15 years old fell from 38.3% in 1990 to 34.7% in 1997, and the population over 65 grew from 4.2% to 4.4%. In 1997, the average annual growth rates in the age groups 5 and under and 6 to 14 were –0.5% and 0.1%, respectively; however, that year the population from 15 to 64

years of age grew by 2.4%, and the group aged 65 and over grew by 3.9%, confirming the trend of an aging population that has been observed since the 1980s. The dependency rate dropped from 104.0 in 1970 to 68.1 in 1994, and it is estimated that in the year 2000 there will be 60.1 dependents for every 100 persons between 15 and 64 years of age. The population aged 15 to 24 reached its highest levels in history in 1997, both in absolute (19.9 million in 1997) and relative (21.2%) terms, and its distribution has changed significantly in recent decades. This population went from being a primarily rural group (60%) in 1960 to a predominantly urban one in 1997 (74%). Although the number of young people in rural areas rose from 3.9 million to 5.3 million in those 35 years, with an annual growth rate under 1%, the increase in the urban youth population was six times faster (4.9% annually), resulting in an increase from 2.6 to 14.6 million. In 1995, 46% of young people were economically active; the participation of men was double (60.8%) that of women (30.9%).

The total fertility rate, which has been declining markedly since the 1980s, fell from 3.08 children per woman in 1992 to 2.73 in 1996 (a 13.6% drop), and the states that historically had the highest fertility levels showed the greatest decline—Guerrero went from a total fertility rate of 5.6 children in 1980–1984 to 3.5 in 1991–1995, Michoacán went from 5.4 to 3.4, and Oaxaca went from 5.6 to 3.8. The 1994 National Demographic Survey found that women without schooling had an average of 4.1 children, whereas women who had passed at least one grade at the secondary level had 2.4 children. It further found that women who were not directly engaged in economic activities had more than twice as many children as those who did (3.2 and 1.4 children, respectively).

Life expectancy at birth changed little between 1992 and 1996, increasing from 72.1 to 73.3 years (73.2 to 76.4 years for women and 68.9 to 70.1 years for men); the two extremes in 1991–1995 were 65.7 years for men and 72.5 for women in Oaxaca and 70.4 for men and 76.4 for women in Nuevo León, which represents an excess mortality of 33% in Oaxaca compared with Nuevo León.

Mortality and Morbidity

The total mortality rate continues to decline, dropping from 4.8 deaths per 1,000 population in 1992 to 4.7 in 1995. The most pronounced drops were observed in infant mortality (18.7 in 1992 and 17.5 in 1995), in the 1- to 4-year group (1.3 in 1992 and 1.2 in 1995), and in persons over 65 (5.3 in 1992 and 5.2 in 1995). The Federal District had the highest total mortality rate in 1995 (5.8 per 1,000 population), followed by Puebla (5.6) and Oaxaca (5.4). The number of deaths in 1995 was greater in males than in females in infants under 1 (27,237 and 20,718, respectively); in children aged 1 to 4 (5,734 and 4,943); in children aged 5 to 14 (4,795 and 3,241); in the 15- to 64-year age group, where deaths in men were almost double those in women (105,913 and 57,247); and in persons 65 and over (97,211 and 100,785, respectively). In 1995, the national excess male mortality rate was 129.2; this indicator topped 100 in every state.

The infant mortality rate in 1995 was 17.5 per 1,000 live births, which represents a 26.8% drop over the 1990 rate. Between 1994 and 1995 the registered infant mortality rate rose (17.0 and 17.5, respectively). Health authorities think that this was due to corrections made in the number of newborns, because recorded deaths diminished in that period, and they consider the adjusted infant mortality rate to be more reliable, which shows a decline between 1994 (26.5) and 1995 (25.9). In 1995, early neonatal mortality (under 7 days) was 7.7 per 1,000 live births and late neonatal mortality (7 to 28 days) was 2.3 per 1,000, while postneonatal mortality was 7.5 and perinatal mortality was 14.5.

In 1995, maternal mortality was 5.3 per 10,000 registered live births, which is higher than in 1994, when it was 4.8, and at levels similar to those in 1990, when it was 5.4 per 10,000. The increase in maternal mortality in 1995 was attributed to better registration of deaths with the new death certificate, which investigates the preexistence of pregnancy in the deaths of all women of childbearing age. The highest maternal mortality rates in 1995 were in Puebla (11.2 per 10,000 live births), Tlaxcala (9.7), and Oaxaca (9.0).

In general, the most frequent causes of death continue to be cardiovascular disease (a rate of 64.1 deaths per 100,000 population in 1992 and 69.4 per 100,000 in 1995), followed by malignant neoplasms (50.4 and 52.6), accidents (44.1 and 38.8), and diabetes mellitus (32.6 and 36.4). Cerebrovascular disease (ICD-9, 430–438) was the sixth leading cause of death in 1992 (at a rate of 24.7) and it moved to fifth place in 1993 (a rate of 25.5 in 1995); disorders originating in the perinatal period (ICD-9, 760–779), which occupied fifth place in 1992, dropped to seventh in 1995 (a rate of 22.4), and cirrhosis and other chronic diseases of the liver ranked sixth in 1995 (a rate of 23.2).

Deaths from heart disease (ICD-9, 410–414) are more frequent in men than in women, but the difference between the sexes shrank between 1992 (a rate of 72.4 per 100,000 in men and 69.7 in women) and 1995 (76.3 and 75.4, respectively). The predominance of deaths in women from malignant neoplasms, due to the high number of deaths from cervical tumors, is being reduced, and in 1995 the rate was 54.6 in women and 50.6 in men compared with 53.1 and 46.2, respectively, in 1992. Mortality from accidents is higher in men than in women (60.3 and 17.6, respectively, in 1995), whereas mortality from diabetes mellitus is higher in women than in men (40.4 and 32.3, respectively); the same pattern holds for

cerebrovascular disease (27.1 and 23.9). The average age of death from the 10 leading causes of death did not change substantially between 1992 and 1995: for example, for heart disease it was 78.7 years in 1992 and 78.8 in 1995; for malignant neoplasms it was 61.6 and 61.9; 35.6 and 36.6 for accidents; and 66.3 and 66.2 for diabetes mellitus.

Among the diseases subject to epidemiological surveillance, respiratory infections ranked first with regard to outpatient visits in 1996, with 22.5 million new cases (a rate of 24,154.6 cases per 100,000 population), followed by intestinal infectious diarrhea, with 4.05 million cases (a rate of 4,355.2), and intestinal amebiasis, with 1.3 million cases (a rate of 1,488.6). In 1995, the information system on hospital discharges in the public sector recorded 3,619,341 discharges (3,184,007 in 1991); 65.6% of these patients were social security recipients and 34.4% were the open or uninsured population served in units of the Secretariat of Health. Of hospital discharges, 56.6% corresponded to the 15 to 44 age group, 13.8% to the 45 to 64 age group, 11% to persons over 65, 7.6% to children under 1, 5.9% to the 5 to 14 age group, and 5.1% to children aged 1 to 4. Women accounted for the largest number of discharges (68.9% of the total), and the average stay in 1995 was 4.0 days per discharge. The most frequent reasons for hospitalization in 1995 were direct obstetric conditions (17% of the total), normal deliveries (13.6%), injuries and poisonings (7.3%), diseases of the urinary tract (4.7%), diseases of the circulatory system (4.6%), fractures (3.2%), abortions (3.1%), and malignant neoplasms (2.7%), the most frequent of which are cervical neoplasms (12.1% of all malignant tumors), leukemia (11.2%), and breast cancer (9.4%).

In 1995, 88,764 deaths were reported in hospitals in the public sector; 60.2% corresponded to social security recipients and 39.8% to the uninsured population (53.8% in men and 46.2% in women). The most frequent causes of death were diseases of the circulatory system (18.4% of all deaths), certain disorders originating in the perinatal period (12.9%), malignant neoplasms (9.6%), diabetes mellitus (9.3%), cerebrovascular disease (6.1%), cirrhosis and other chronic diseases of the liver (5.3%), and infectious and parasitic diseases (4.8%).

SPECIFIC HEALTH PROBLEMS

Analysis by Population Group

Health of Children

Child health has continued to improve, as evidenced by the eradication of polio in 1991; the drastic reduction in morbidity and mortality from measles, whooping cough, diphtheria, and neonatal tetanus; and the continuing drop in mortality in infants and children under 5, as well as in deaths from diarrheal and respiratory diseases. These achievements are attributable to a combination of demographic and socioeconomic factors in addition to specific health sector interventions— high coverage of a complete vaccination program, the increased use of oral rehydration salts, and provision of a basic package of services to the population without regular access to health services.

However, child health varies throughout the country. In 1995, the central area had the highest infant mortality rate, with 22.3 deaths per 1,000 live births and the northern and southern areas had rates of 12.2 and 12.8, respectively. The states of Puebla (33.2), Tlaxcala (28.7), and Mexico (26.8) had the highest rates, compared with Durango (3.9), Sinaloa (5.9), and Guerrero (8.5), which had the lowest. In children under 5, again there are differences between the regions— the highest rate is observed in central Mexico, with 21.5 per 1,000 live births, followed by the south (17.3) and the north (14.6).

The order of the leading causes of death in children under 1 did not change between 1992 and 1995. Therefore, the most frequent causes continued to be conditions in the perinatal period, with a rate of 777.8 deaths per 100,000 live births in 1992 and 745.4 in 1995; congenital anomalies, whose rate increased from 248.8 per 100,000 in 1992 to 268.4 in 1995; pneumonia and influenza, with 184.2 in 1992 and 127.3 in 1995; nutritional deficiencies, with 61.3 in 1992 and 53.2 in 1995; and accidents, with 44.3 in 1992 and 46.0 in 1995.

According to public hospital records, in 1995 the most frequent reasons associated with discharge in children under 1 were conditions originating in the perinatal period, with 157,454 cases and 57.3% of all discharges (102,379 cases and 48.5% in 1992); diseases of the respiratory system, with 29,054 cases and 10.6% in 1995 (30,299 cases and 14.3% in 1992); infectious and parasitic diseases, with 22,766 cases and 8.3% in 1995 (27,133 cases and 12.8% in 1992); and congenital anomalies, with 20,166 cases and 7.3% in 1995 (16,459 cases and 7.8% in 1992).

Accidents remain the leading cause of death in children between 1 and 4, with rates of 25.1 per 100,000 population in 1992, 24.3 in 1994, and 22.8 in 1995, followed by pneumonia and influenza (14.7 in 1992, 16.5 in 1994, and 16.4 in 1995), intestinal infectious diseases (24.2 in 1992 and 15.4 in 1995), congenital anomalies (8.4 in 1992 and 10.4 in 1995), and nutritional deficiencies (7.9 in 1992 and 8 in 1995). With regard to morbidity, for 1995 the hospital discharge records for children in that same age group show that 32.8% of the total were for respiratory diseases (31.3% in 1992), 16.6% were for infectious and parasitic diseases (15.3% in 1992), and 10.7% were for injuries and poisonings (11.4% in 1992).

Health of Schoolchildren

The leading cause of death for this group in 1995 was accidents, with a rate of 11.8 per 100,000 population (16.2 in men and 7.3 in women), the most frequent being motor vehicle accidents (a rate of 4.9, 6.7 in men and 3.1 in women). Malignant neoplasms were in second place, with 4.3 per 100,000 (4.6 in men and 3.6 in women), the most frequent form of which was leukemia, with 2.3 (2.5 in men and 3.6 in women). The third leading cause of death in women was congenital anomalies (2.0), and in men it was homicides and injuries inflicted by another person (2.5). In fourth place were pneumonias and influenza for women (1.7) and birth defects for men (2.0). In a comparison of the leading causes of death in 1995 and 1992, the most notable aspect is the 20% reduction in the death rate from accidents (a rate of 14.8 in 1992).

In children aged 5 to 14, the morbidity data show that in 1995 injuries and poisonings were responsible for 20.5% of hospitalizations in that age group, followed by diseases of the respiratory system, with 17.1%; diseases of the digestive system, with 13.1%; and diseases of the genitourinary system, associated with 7.4% of all discharges. The order of the reasons associated with discharges did not change between 1992 and 1995, and the frequency is quite similar during those years.

In 1995, 14,324 minors were living on the street and were cared for by the National System for the Integral Development of the Family through a strategy of shared responsibility among children, the family, and the community, which includes an economic incentive—supplying of essential provisions—and medical checkups at least three times a year. Some 60 nongovernmental organizations work with these children; the exact number of minors seen is unknown.

Health of Adolescents

The majority of deaths in young people between 15 and 24 are from injuries—61.6% in 1995 (63.3% in 1991); 32.1% are due to noncommunicable diseases (29.3% in 1991) and 6.2% are due to communicable diseases (7.4% in 1991).

Analysis of the reproductive behavior of young people shows that the average age for first marriage (19 years) and the average age for the birth of a first child (21 years) have not changed in the past five years. In 1996, 16% of births were to teenage mothers. The prevalence of contraceptive use among sexually active adolescents, which increased significantly between 1986 and 1992, has remained at roughly 36% since then, far from the 60% laid out as a goal for the year 2000. A family-planning survey conducted in nine states found that 92% of the young people interviewed were in favor of using contraception; that number increased to 94% among those with secondary schooling or higher and was 87% among those who had a primary education or less. The relative frequency depended on the place of residence and ranged from 87% in rural areas to 93.7% in urban areas.

A problem of growing importance in this group is alcohol and drug use. Surveys conducted in the Federal District show that the number of young people between 12 and 18 who have consumed alcohol at some time has risen (55.8% in 1986, 65.5% in 1991, and 73.8% in 1994). The epidemiological surveillance system for addictions of the Secretariat of Health reported that the typical drug user is a male aged 15 to 19, particularly an unattached man with little education. It further shows that marijuana and inhalants are the drugs most frequently used by adolescents and that use of these substances has risen to 4% in recent years.

Health of Adults

Between 1991 and 1995 mortality in persons between 15 and 64 years of age fell from 301.2 per 100,000 population to 296.9 per 100,000. The leading cause of death was accidents, whose rate dropped from 50.7 per 100,000 population in 1991 to 42.7 per 100,000 in 1995 (the most frequent were motor vehicle accidents, which were responsible for 40% of all accidents and 43.5% of accidental deaths). Accidents are followed by malignant neoplasms, with 37.3 and 39.3 per 100,000 respectively. The third leading cause is heart disease, with 29.5 and 31.4 per 100,000 respectively, and fourth is cirrhosis and other diseases of the liver, with 26.5 and 27.2 per 100,000 respectively. Deaths from homicide and injuries inflicted by other people fell from fifth place in 1991 (25.9) to sixth in 1995 (25.3), and deaths from AIDS, which occupied twelfth place in 1991, with a rate of 3.8 per 100,000, climbed to ninth place in 1995, with a rate of 7.0 per 100,000.

According to hospital discharge records, the most frequent cause of hospitalization among persons between 15 and 44 years of age in 1995 was complications of pregnancy, childbirth, and the puerperium, which was associated with 60% of all discharges in 1995 (65.4% in 1992), followed by problems of the digestive system (7.3% in 1995 and 5.7% in 1992), diseases of the genitourinary system with 6.5% (5.3% in 1992), and injuries and poisonings with 6.2% (5.1% in 1992). For the group aged 45 to 64, the most frequent causes of hospitalization in 1995 were diseases of the genitourinary system, with 18.3% (17.1% in 1992); diseases of the digestive system, with 17.5% (17.4% in 1992); diseases of the circulatory system, with 11.7% (10.8% in 1992); and neoplasms, with 10.7% (10.8% in 1992).

The greatest amount of information on women's health is related to the reproductive issues. In 1995, there were 1,454

maternal deaths (1,477 in 1990); 87.1% were due to direct obstetric causes (92.1% in 1990), subdivided into 28% from toxemia of pregnancy, 23.6% from hemorrhage during pregnancy and childbirth, 11.6% from complications in the puerperium, 1% from obstructed labor, 1% from infections of the genitourinary system, and 21.6% from other direct causes. Coverage by the national family-planning program increased between 1987 and 1996 from 52.7% to 66.5% of women of childbearing age; the greatest increases were in women who had not completed primary school, with coverage rising from 23.7% in 1987 to 48.4% in 1995. The distribution of contraception users according to method was bilateral tubal ligation (41.3%), intrauterine device (21.9%), traditional methods (13.4%), oral contraceptives (12.7%), injections (4.6%), barriers (5.1%), and vasectomy (0.9%). The Secretariat of Health reports differences among states in terms of the use of contraceptives by women—in Baja California Sur, Nuevo León, the Federal District, Baja California, Coahuila, and the State of Mexico prevalence was over 75%; in Guerrero, Chiapas, and Oaxaca it did not exceed 56%.

Prenatal care coverage by health workers increased, and the average number of prenatal consultations by pregnant women rose from 2.2 in 1990 to 2.8 in 1996. A survey conducted in 1995 found that medical personnel followed 86.1% of pregnancies between 1993 and 1995, representing an increase of more than 50% over the past 20 years; the percentage of births attended in public hospitals rose from 54.3% to 65.8% between 1990 and 1995.

Cervical and breast cancer are public health problems that demand urgent and more effective action. Mortality from cervical cancer fell from 10.2 per 100,000 women in 1990 to 9.5 per 100,000 in 1995, and mortality from breast cancer rose from 5.3 to 6.6. A sampling of women between the ages of 15 and 49 in Mexico City found that 65.0% of the women interviewed had had a Pap test, compared with 30.2% in a rural area in the State of Oaxaca that was also studied; the principal factors identified as predictors for having that test were associated with socioeconomic and reproductive risk elements.

Health of the Elderly

The country's demographic transition in recent decades has increased the population over 65 in absolute and relative terms, posing new challenges to the health system because of this group's health needs. The proportion of hospitalized persons over 65 has steadily increased—in 1991 they accounted for 7.2%, in 1993 for 8.2%, and in 1995 for 11.0% of all hospital discharges in the public system. The most frequent causes of hospitalization in 1995 were diseases of the circulatory system (17.8% of all discharges for this age group), diseases of the genitourinary system (16.0%), diseases of the digestive system (13.8%), and diseases of the respiratory system (9.5%).

In 1995, the leading causes of death in persons over 65 were heart disease (at a rate of 1,188 per 100,000 persons) and malignant neoplasms (655.3 per 100,000), the most frequent of which were those of the trachea, bronchi, and lungs (101.0 per 100,000); stomach (75.4); and prostate (71.0). These are followed by diabetes mellitus (501.9), cerebrovascular disease (449.4), pneumonia and influenza (224.6), nutritional deficiencies (163.9), and chronic bronchitis, asthma, and emphysema (163.8).

Health of Indigenous People

In 1995, the indigenous population—defined as all persons speaking an indigenous language and members of households in which the head of household or his/her spouse speaks an indigenous language—was calculated at 9.17 million persons, with an average growth rate of 1.23% compared with 1990, which is almost half that of the rest of the population (2.13%). In 1995, life expectancy at birth for the indigenous population was estimated at 69.5 years (67.6 for men and 71.5 for women), which is more than three years shorter than that of the rest of the population. This difference is equivalent to a 30% higher mortality level and is more marked in women (36%) than in men (25%). The infant mortality rate was almost double that of the rest of the population (54 compared with 29 deaths per 1,000 live births). The average number of children born to indigenous women was 4.1, compared with 2.9 for nonindigenous women.

In 1995, the per capita years of potential life lost (YPLL) from the three leading groups of causes of death showed premature mortality of 19.0 years for indigenous men compared with 15.3 for nonindigenous men and 15.4 for indigenous women compared with 11.2 for nonindigenous women. The gap in the YPLL between the indigenous and nonindigenous population from communicable and perinatal diseases was 2.5 years for men and 2.6 for women; for noncommunicable diseases it was 0.8 year for men and 1.6 for women; finally, for accidents and injuries it was 0.4 for men, with no difference for women. Among indigenous peoples there are still differences that have not been adequately explained: there is a lower level of infant mortality among children whose mothers speak Chontal (33 per 1,000 live births), Mayan (36), Chinanteco (40), and Zapoteco (40) than in those who speak Chatino (77), Popoluca (79), Tarahumara (79), Tepehunán (80), Tzotzil (81), and Tojolabal (87). Differences are also observed in the number of children the women have; the two extremes are 3.7 children for the Chontals and 4.5 for the Tojolabals.

Analysis by Type of Disease or Health Impairment

Communicable Diseases

Vector-Borne Diseases. Malaria continues to be endemic, although the number of cases dropped by more than half between 1992 and 1996 (18.6 and 6.8 cases per 100,000 population, respectively). The last epidemic outbreak was in the 1980s; the largest number of cases (134,000) was recorded in 1995. In 1996, 6,293 cases were reported; the states with the highest incidence were Sinaloa, with a rate of 109.3 per 100,000 in 1992 and 63.5 in 1996, and Chiapas, with 107.7 per 100,000 in 1992 and 42.7 in 1996. There were 69 cases of infection from *Plasmodium falciparum* in 1995 and 60 in 1996, all of which were in the states of Chiapas and Tabasco.

There was an epidemic outbreak of dengue in 1980, with nearly 51,000 cases; in subsequent years the number of cases fell somewhat irregularly, with 14,396 cases of dengue fever and 355 cases of dengue hemorrhagic fever in 1995 and 20,056 and 884, respectively, in 1996. Over 60% of the cases in 1996 were in the 15- to 44-year age group, and 78% of the affected persons resided in six states—Veracruz (26.6% of the cases), Tamaulipas (23.3%), Colima (10.3%), Sonora and Tabasco (6.7% each), and Nuevo León (5.1%). In 1994, dengue serotype 3 was isolated; there are currently four serotypes in circulation. In that same year, *Aedes albopictus* was found in the northern states bordering Texas. The incidence rate for dengue hemorrhagic fever rose from 0.03 per 100,000 population in 1994 (30 cases) to 0.39 in 1995 and to 0.95 in 1996, the year when the largest number of cases were reported in Veracruz (358), Tamaulipas (198), and Nuevo León (85).

Onchocerciasis remained stable from 1992 to 1996, with 24,870 cases in 1992, 26,029 in 1995, and 25,889 in 1996; health authorities believe that the use of ivermectin since 1989 has helped to contain the spread of the disease. The endemic area encompasses 16,900 km^2 in the states of Oaxaca and Chiapas in the southeastern part of the country, and the at-risk population is calculated at 280,000 persons distributed in 947 localities.

Cases of leishmaniasis rose from 502 in 1992 to 1,579 in 1995 and then fell to 1,025 in 1996. There is an undetermined level of underreporting of cases.

Trypanosomiasis is increasing in frequency and virulence. The National Institute of Cardiology estimates that cardiopathies related to Chagas' disease have increased and that 15 million people are at risk of infection. It puts the annual potential number of these cardiopathies at 500. Deaths from this cause rose from 11 in 1992 to 18 in 1995, and the serological prevalence in blood banks was 0.8% in 1995. Routine screening of Chagas' disease and onchocerciasis in donated blood is conducted only in endemic localities in the country.

Scorpion bites are a problem in 16 states, and in 1992 48,465 cases were recorded, rising to 83,672 in 1995 and 108,359 in 1996. It is estimated that over 300 people die annually from this cause.

Vaccine-Preventable Diseases. Complete vaccination coverage increased from 75.3% in 1993 to 88.2% in 1996 in children under 1 and from 90.1% to 95.8% in children between 1 and 4. Poliomyelitis was eradicated in 1991, and there are no signs of wild poliovirus circulating in the country. Cases of measles fell significantly, plummeting from 27,790 in 1990 to 12 in 1995, and deaths from this cause fell from 5,899 in 1990 to 2 in 1995. Tetanus also declined, with an incidence of 0.23 cases per 100,000 population in 1992 and 0.14 per 100,000 in 1995. Neonatal tetanus showed a downward trend, with 137 cases in 1992 (a rate of 0.16 cases per 100,000 population) and 67 in 1995 (0.07 per 100,000). Isolated cases of whooping cough were reported, with a rate of 0.16 cases per 100,000 population in 1992 and 0.21 per 100,000 in 1996. In recent years no cases of diphtheria have been reported.

Cholera and Other Intestinal Infectious Diseases. The diarrheal disease rate (including cholera) has increased in recent years from 3,653.1 cases per 100,000 population in 1993 to 5,842.5 per 100,000 in 1995. Hospitalizations for this cause fell from 202.8 discharges per 100,000 population in 1992 to 102.2 per 100,000 in 1995.

Mortality from intestinal infectious diseases decreased from 22.0 per 100,000 population in 1991 to 10.5 per 100,000 in 1995. The same downward trend was seen in children under 5, from 91.8 to 77.8. The states with the highest rates in 1995 were Tlaxcala (177.0), Puebla (164.3), Mexico (135.4), and Querétaro (113.0), with children under 1 the most vulnerable group, and accounting for 70.5% and 80.2% of the deaths in children under 5 in 1990 and 1995, respectively. Men had a higher mortality rate than women. The drop in mortality in children under 5 is attributed to the increase in oral rehydration therapy at home, which was used in over 80% of cases in 1995.

The trend for cholera varied, with a mortality rate of 6.19 per 100,000 population in 1993, 4.3 in 1994, 17.94 in 1995, and 1.16 in 1996. The case-fatality rate went from 1.2% in 1992 to 0.9% in 1995 and 0.5% in 1996. Only four states did not report cases of cholera in 1996 (Baja California, Baja California Sur, Zacatecas, and Sinaloa) and the most affected states were Yucatán (2,690 cases), Veracruz (1,803), Campeche (1,719), and Tabasco (1,361).

Acute Respiratory Infections. The incidence rate for acute respiratory infections in the general population doubled between 1991 and 1995, soaring from 13,731.0 to 29,009.6 cases per 100,000 population (26,574,579 in 1995);

in 1995, the highest rates were in the Federal District, with 81,101.8 (6,540,846 patients), Campeche, with 55,245.4 (347,815 patients), and Baja California Sur, with 43,874.5 (168,678 patients).

Mortality from respiratory infections, including pneumonia and influenza, showed a downward trend, with a rate of 26.0 per 100,000 population in 1991 and 23.7 per 100,000 in 1995; that year, the greatest percentage of deaths occurred in persons over 65 (42.1%) and in children under 1 (32%). Of all deaths in children under 5 years, 39.8% were due to this cause. Between 1990 and 1995 mortality from these causes in children under 5 dropped by 32.8% and the states with the highest mortality were Tlaxcala (177.0), Puebla (164.3), Mexico (135.4), and Querétaro (113.0). A high proportion of the deaths occurred at home (30%); therefore, a training strategy for mothers has been implemented so that they can learn to identify warning signs and seek medical assistance at the health centers.

In 1995 nearly 3.5 million mothers had been trained, and over 5 million were trained in 1996.

Rabies and Other Zoonoses. The main zoonosis in Mexico is rabies, a disease that has been in decline since the end of the 1980s. Deaths for each year between 1992 and 1996 were 35, 29, 25, 31, and 22; a decline in cases of canine rabies also was reported (59.2%), falling from 2,106 in 1992 to 859 in 1996. In that period, over 10 million dogs were vaccinated per year and, although they remain the principal source of rabies infection in humans, transmission of the disease by bats and other wild species is also important.

In 1992, 5,958 cases of brucellosis were reported and in 1996 the number was 3,362. It is understood that there has been underreporting of the figures in the past three years, and it is calculated that the annual rate for the past five years is five or six cases per 100,000 population. It was determined that two-thirds of the patients (66.4%) had been infected by consuming unpasteurized milk, fresh cheese, and other dairy products, and that goats were the main source of contamination in humans. Mortality from brucellosis fell from 0.04 per 100,000 population in 1992 to 0.01 in 1996.

Concerning the taeniasis-cysticercosis complex, the adult form (taeniasis) dropped in recent years from just over 14,000 cases in 1992 (a rate of 17.2 per 100,000 population) to 3,362 in 1996 (3.8) and, although it is distributed throughout the country, slightly over one-third (37%) of all cases in 1996 were concentrated in five states in south-central Mexico (Hidalgo, Chiapas, Michoacán, Jalisco, and Tabasco). In recent years cysticercosis has been recorded with very similar morbidity and mortality frequencies in humans, with 586 cases in 1990 (261 deaths) and 601 in 1996 (293 deaths). Studies found that the national seroprevalence is 1% and that porcine cysticercosis is predominant over bovine cysticercosis.

Leptospirosis is a disease with low prevalence. Serological testing of 5,122 patients with a presumptive diagnosis of this disease between 1992 and 1996 was positive for 32%, and the most frequent serovars were *canicola, pomona,* and *icterohaemorrhagiae.*

Venezuelan equine encephalitis was verified by isolating the virus in equine outbreaks in 1993 (Chiapas) and 1996 (Oaxaca and Tamaulipas), without similar verification in human cases.

AIDS and Other STDs. Statistics on STDs in Mexico are recorded at the primary care level, and it is known that there is underreporting. The reporting of AIDS is more rigorous. The STDs that occurred with the greatest frequency in 1996 were urogenital candidiasis, with a rate of 136.4 cases per 100,000 population, and urogenital trichomoniasis, with 108.8 per 100,000. The incidence of syphilis dropped from 2.20 in 1993 to 1.51 in 1996 (1,414 cases); the same trend was observed for gonococcal infection, whose rate fell from 23.39 in 1993 to 13.57 in 1996 (12,697 cases).

There are few data on the prevalence of STDs. A 1995 study of prostitutes in Mexico City found a frequency of syphilis (RPR/FTA-Abs) of 6.4%, genital herpes (HV-2 antibodies) of 65.1%, HIV (Western blot test) of 0.6%, hepatitis B (HBc antibodies) of 3%, gonorrhea (culture) of 3.7%, and chlamydia infections (culture) of 11.1%.

As of 1 January 1997, there were 29,962 AIDS cases, of whom 16,636 had died (55.5%), 11,208 were still alive (37.4%), and the situation of 2,118 (7.1%) was unknown. A total of 25,771 cases were in men and 4,191 were in women; 83.2% of the patients were between 20 and 49 years of age (30.0% from 20 to 29; 36.0% from 30 to 39; and 17.2% from 40 to 49). Children under 14 accounted for 2.7% of the total. The mode of transmission was reported in 71.7% of the cases: 86.5% were infected through sexual activity and 13.5% through blood transfusions. Of the reported cases, 55.3% (16,431) were concentrated in the three most populous states: the Federal District, the State of Mexico, and Jalisco.

The general incidence rate for AIDS fluctuated between 3.7 per 100,000 population in 1991 (3,155 new cases), 5.7 in 1993 (5,058 new cases), and 4.8 in 1995 (4,310 new cases). The ratio of men to women in those years was 5:1, 6:1, and 7:1, respectively, and 98% of the cases in men (25,771) were in adults in the following categories: homosexuals, 27.3% (7,007 cases); bisexuals, 18.9% (4,883); heterosexuals, 17.6% (4,542); transfusion recipients, 3.7% (959); hemophiliacs, 1.0% (254); intravenous drug users, 0.7% (177); paid donors, 1.2% (315); homosexuals/intravenous drug users, 0.8% (202); occupational exposure, 0.0% (4); undocumented, 28.0% (7,227). There was also perinatal exposure of 0.8% (201). On review of the cases at the end of 1991, 1995, and 1996, a trend toward an increase in cases of sexual transmission is observed, representing 87%,

94%, and 95.7% of the total, respectively. At the start of the epidemic, the cases in women were associated with transfusions of contaminated blood and their frequency subsequently declined—the cases from this cause dropped from 59.4% at the end of 1991 to 26.1% in 1995 to 21.2% in 1996, whereas the frequency of sexual transmission climbed from 40.6% in 1991 to 76.8% in 1996.

The total cases in children under 14 numbered 795 at the end of 1996 (62.8% in boys and 37.2% in girls); infection occurred through transfusion of contaminated blood in 37.6% of the cases, through sexual transmission in 3.3%, and perinatally in 59.1%. In 1991, 85 pediatric AIDS cases were reported and there were 89 in 1996. Perinatal transmission decreased from 51 to 27 cases in those years.

Chronic Communicable Diseases. Tuberculosis occupies 15th place among the general causes of death. The mortality from this cause declined from 7.6 to 5.1 per 100,000 population between 1990 and 1995. In 1995, it caused 4,648 deaths, with tuberculosis of the lung responsible for 87%, meningeal tuberculosis for 4%, and other forms for the remaining 9%.

Morbidity from tuberculosis rose slightly from 17.3 per 100,000 population in 1990 to 17.5 in 1996, with an annual average of roughly 16,000 cases. Pulmonary tuberculosis was predominant, accounting for 87% of the cases; the meningeal forms accounted for only 1% of the cases. In 1996, 85% of new cases occurred in persons over 15 years of age; 531 patients exhibited resistance to drugs (45% of them exhibited multidrug resistance); 76% (3,372 cases) were cured; and 509 (11%) abandoned treatment.

Leprosy evidenced a clear downward trend, and the prevalence rates in 1990, 1992, and 1996 were 2.1, 2.0, and 0.4 cases per 10,000 population, respectively.

Noncommunicable Diseases and Other Health-Related Problems

Nutritional Diseases and Diseases of Metabolism. The 1988 National Nutrition Survey (ENN), which is the most recent, indicated that 41.9% of children under 5 were suffering from some type of malnutrition, as measured by the weight-for-age indicator, and that, according to the Waterlow weight-for-height and height-for-age criteria, 29.2% of the children were suffering from some type of malnutrition. The 1993 National Survey of Chronic Diseases (ENEC) survey found that 21.5% of the population between 20 and 69 years of age had a body mass index over 30 and that the greatest prevalence of obesity (over 25% of the population) was found in the northern states (Baja California, Baja California Sur, Coahuila, Chihuahua, Durango, Nuevo León, Sonora, Sinaloa, Tamaulipas, and Zacatecas).

There is no information available on the frequency of anemia in children under 5 and women; however, it has been recorded as one of the 20 leading causes of death in children under 5. Between 1992 and 1995 mortality from this cause increased in children under 1, from 6.3 deaths per 100,000 live births to 7.9, and in children between the ages of 1 and 4 from 1.7 to 2.2 per 100,000. In 1995, the states with the highest mortality from nutritional deficiencies in children under 1 were Puebla (142.3 deaths per 100,000 population) and Tlaxcala (128.8).

In 1995, of 764,618 live births weighed and registered, 91.9% of the newborns weighed 2,500 g or more. However, this information is incomplete, because not all institutions provide these data.

Two surveys identified iodine deficiencies. The first, conducted in 1991 in the State of Hidalgo, found a 6% prevalence of goiter among the 3,000 schoolchildren studied. The second study, conducted in 1994 in several parts of the country, found a 3% prevalence of goiter. Currently, salt sold for human consumption is iodized; an inspection of samples on the market in 1996 determined that 92% of the salt was effectively iodized.

The 1988 ENN reported that in the Federal District and the metropolitan area, 37% of children under 5 had a vitamin A intake below the recommended allowances; in marginalized areas of the country this percentage was as high as 53%.

Cardiovascular Disease and Other Chronic Diseases. The 1993 ENEC survey, which is the most recent, found a 23.6% prevalence of hypertension, a 7.2% prevalence of diabetes mellitus, and an 8.8% prevalence of hypercholesterolemia (levels equal to or greater than 240 (μg/dl) in the population older than 20. The prevalence of these three conditions increased with age, and in the 65- to 69-year-old age group the illnesses of this type with the highest prevalence were hypertension and diabetes mellitus (58.5% and 26.1%, respectively); the 60- to 64-year age group accounted for 17.4% of the cases of hypercholesterolemia. The distribution by gender was similar for diabetes mellitus (7.2% each) and was slightly higher in men for hypertension (28.5%) and hypercholesterolemia (10%).

The incidence of hypertension is increasing in the public health services. In 1996, 403,582 cases were reported, at a rate of 433.1 per 100,000 population (268,365 cases and a rate of 297.6 per 100,000 in 1994). The trend is the same for diabetes mellitus (249,774 cases and a rate of 268.1 in 1996 and 184,130 cases and a rate of 204.2 in 1994).

Mortality from chronic diseases is clearly on the rise. In 1992, cardiovascular disease accounted for 55,606 deaths (a rate of 64.1 per 100,000 population) and in 1995, 63,609 deaths (69.4). Diabetes mellitus was responsible for 28,304 deaths (32.6) in 1992 and 33,316 in 1995 (36.4). Deaths from

cirrhosis of the liver increased from 19,105 in 1992 (22.0) to 21,245 in 1995 (23.2).

Malignant Neoplasms. Malignant neoplasms are the second leading cause of mortality. Mortality from this cause increased by 4% between 1992 and 1995 (52.6 deaths per 100,000 population). In 1995, the most common sites were trachea, bronchi, and lungs (a rate of 6.5 per 100,000 population); stomach (5.1); and cervix (4.8). In children under 1, neoplasms ranked 17th as a cause of death (a rate of 2.9 per 100,000 live births); in the 1 to 4 age group they ranked sixth (5.3), and in schoolchildren (4.3) persons of productive ages (39.3), and older age group (655.3) they ranked second. Compared with 1992, it can be seen that mortality increased in preschool children (a rate of 4.9 in 1992) and in persons of productive age (38.0 in 1992). It remained practically the same in children under 1 and schoolchildren and declined in the older age group (671 in 1992).

Although there is no registry that documents new cases of neoplasms, in 1993 a Histopathological Registry of Malignant Neoplasms was established, to perform that function and whose basic data are anatomopathological. In 1993, this registry recorded 40,924 new cases of malignant neoplasms, 66% of which were in women—primarily of the cervix (23.5%) and breast (12.6%)—and just over 50% were in persons aged 50 and over. In 1994, 62,725 new cases of malignant neoplasms were reported, 64.7% of which were in women and 18% were in persons 60 and over. Cervical (23.2%), breast (10.2%), and prostate (4.9%) neoplasms had the highest prevalence.

Accidents and Violence. Mortality from accidents and various types of violence fell from 44.1 deaths per 100,000 population in 1992 to 38.8 per 100,000 in 1995. In children between 0 and 14, it dropped 13.3% in 1995 compared with 1990; however, in 1990 accidents occupied fifth place as a cause of death, and in 1995 moved to third. In 1995, mortality from these causes in children under 1 was 0.5 per 1,000 live births and ranked sixth as a cause of death, while in the group aged 1 to 14 it was 15.0 per 100,000, or a 6.5% reduction over the 1990 rate. Accidents were the leading cause of death for persons of that age.

The most frequent accidents in infants, preschool children, and schoolchildren were traffic accidents, followed by suffocation and drowning and accidental falls, except in children under 1, for whom the second most frequent cause was accidental poisoning. Concerning the origin of injuries due to accidents, the first place in children from 0 to 14 years are accidents in the home, which exhibited an upward trend between 1991 and 1995, followed by accidents and injuries on public roads and accidents at school. In the population 65 and over, mortality from injuries and accidents also fell from 172.6 deaths per 100,000 population in 1992 to 153.2 in 1995.

The National System for the Comprehensive Development of the Family found that in 1995 slightly more than 15,000 cases of child abuse were reported. The most frequent form was physical abuse, followed by emotional abuse; sexual abuse was in third place. Another problem documented in recent years is violence against women, which is the subject of governmental and nongovernmental research by a number of organizations. A study conducted in the Federal District on reported cases of sexual violence in the first half of 1996 found that 54% were rapes, 8.0% attempted rape, 33% sexual abuse, and 5.0% statutory rape. In addition, various studies in specific localities documented high frequencies of domestic abuse and domestic violence against women, as well as rape and violence (verbal and physical) toward pregnant women by their partners.

Behavioral Disorders (Smoking, Alcohol, and Drugs). The 1993 National Survey of Addictions (ENA) revealed that 25.1% of the respondents between the ages of 12 and 65 identified themselves as smokers, 20.3% as former smokers, and 54.6% as nonsmokers. The prevalence of smoking by gender was 38% in men and 14% in women; among former smokers, the proportion of men was also higher (25% versus 17%); and in the group of nonsmokers the proportions were 37% and 70%, respectively. Most smokers fall in the age group 16–20 years old (50%), and the highest prevalence of tobacco consumption (30%) was observed in the Mexico City metropolitan area.

The ENEC survey found that 33.4% of the population between 20 and 69 years of age were active smokers, 52.6% were nonsmokers, and 14% were former smokers. The Federal District had the greatest concentration of smokers (43.9% of all respondents). This survey also found that 66% of the urban population between 12 and 65 years old consumed alcohol (77.2% of men and 57.5% of women), among them, 41.6% drank occasionally but in large quantities (five or more glasses per time); 25% of the respondents abstained from drinking; 8% were considered former drinkers. The regions with the most frequent alcohol consumption were in the western part of the country and the Federal District, with 78.3% and 73.4%, respectively.

Concerning drug use, 3.9% of the population between the ages of 12 and 65 responded that they had used illegal drugs at some time in their life (ENA 1993). Among the nonprescription drugs most frequently used in the 30 days before the survey are marijuana (0.2%) and cocaine (0.1%); 3.3% of the interviewees had used marijuana at some time in their life, 0.5% had used cocaine, and another 0.5% had used some inhalant; 60% of the users between 19 and 34, for the most part men, reported having used an illegal drug at some time in their life. Study findings published in 1997 by the Secretariat of Health indicate that drug use is increasing in the country

and that the highest growth compared with 1986 is in cocaine use, although marijuana continues to be the most widely used drug. Drug use is no longer exclusively associated with high-income sectors. The Juvenile Integration Centers, which are nonprofit, nongovernmental, civil organizations, report that they treated more than 37,000 minors and conducted more than five million preventive counseling sessions between 1991 and 1995.

Oral Health. There are no recent data on oral diseases. Estimates for 1990 set the decayed, missing, and filled teeth (DMFT) index for children 12 years of age at 5.3, which means that the country has a serious problem of dental caries.

Environmental Problems and Their Effect on Health. For 1995, it was calculated that 62.8 million people (96%) in urban centers had drinking water coverage, and 2.6 million lacked this service. In rural localities 13.7 million people (52.5%) had that service, and 12.5 million people had no coverage. Sewerage coverage in urban areas reached 55.9 million people (85.5%), but 9.5 million did not have service; in rural areas the coverage was around 5.5 million people (20.9%), and 20.7 million people lacked service. It is estimated that 83,585 tons of waste are generated daily; 70% are collected and only 17% are disposed of in sanitary landfills. There is insufficient recycling of waste.

Another environmental health problem is exposure of the population in the Federal District to lead contamination. Lead concentration in blood dropped from 17 µg/dl in 1992 to 9 µg/dl in 1996, due mainly to the introduction of unleaded gasoline and the control of lead content in paints. The use of glazed earthenware pots is the main source of contamination.

In Mexico City, the levels of ozone and suspended particulate matter are serious problems. In 1995, for 324 days the ozone level exceeded 100 IMECAS (a scale developed to classify and communicate to the public air pollution levels in the valley of Mexico, in which 100 points is the limit for satisfactory air quality); the same year, ozone levels exceeded 250 IMECAS on 6 days. The total suspended particles exceeded the standard by 46.9% in 1992 and 15.6% in 1995; for breathable particulate fractions the standard was exceeded 8.3% of the time in 1992 and 12.6% in 1995. Nitrogen dioxide levels were studied in Mexico City, with an average of 0.037 ppm; Guadalajara had 0.032 ppm; Monterrey had 0.019 ppm; and Cuernavaca had 0.023 ppm. An increase in the incidence of asthma in the infant population and decreasing spirometric values in healthy children in Mexico City are attributed to this contaminant.

Foodborne Diseases. The most frequent foodborne diseases are paratyphoid and other salmonelloses, with 95,383 cases in 1992 (a rate of 109.9 per 100,000 population) and 151,895 in 1996 (163.0 per 100,000); bacterial food poisoning, with 49,598 cases in 1992 (57.2) and 48,267 in 1996 (51.8); shigellosis, with 12,242 cases in 1992 (14.1) and 32,256 in 1996 (34.6); and typhoid fever, with 10,440 cases in 1992 (12.0) and 9,149 in 1996 (9.8). Other, less frequently reported diseases of this origin are taeniasis (9,495 cases in 1992 and 4,649 in 1996), brucellosis (4,012 in 1992 and 5,324 in 1996), and cysticercosis (691 in 1992 and 1,157 in 1996).

Between 1992 and 1996 the national epidemiological surveillance system reported 244 outbreaks of foodborne diseases, with a total of 12,596 cases and 98 deaths. In 99 outbreaks (40.6%), the cause was identified; 75.7% were caused by bacterial agents (*Salmonella enteritidis, Escherichia coli, Staphylococcus aureus*); 8.1% by toxins (primarily *Clostridium botulinum*), 4.1% by viruses and chemicals, and 4.0% by parasites. In the remaining cases the causative agent was not identified.

RESPONSE OF THE HEALTH SYSTEM

National Health Plans and Policies

The Government's policy in the social sector, as set forth in the 1995–2000 National Development Plan, is to combat inequities among individuals, between genders and in the productive sectors and geographical regions, as a way to translate economic progress into social improvements for the population. The main health policies are geared toward reorganization of the system in order to expand coverage and provide efficient and good services to the population and to treat the disorders stemming from current epidemiological and demographic problems. To address the first of these objectives, the Health Sector Reform Program was launched in 1995; for the second objective, in 1997 the Secretariat of Health defined the priority areas in disease prevention and control, based on the development of programs, strategic lines of action, and support mechanisms, whose operation is the responsibility of the state health services.

Health Sector Reform

The 1995–2000 Health Sector Reform Program allows social security recipients to choose the physician who will treat them at the health services; establishes family insurance coverage in the Mexican Social Security Institute (IMSS), whereby persons able to pay may voluntarily enroll; transfers health services to the states to care for the uninsured population; fosters greater local participation in health through the healthy *municipios* program; expands coverage through a basic package of services for persons without access to the health services; and reorganizes the system, with the Secretariat of Health exercising leadership and regulatory roles, health care for the uninsured population being integrated and coordinated, and IMSS separating the functions of financing and service delivery to introduce competition among service providers and to simplify the health insurance system.

Decentralization of health services was carried out within the framework of what is known as the New Federalism, and in August 1996 a national agreement was signed that transfers 121,000 jobs, 7,370 pieces of real estate, and 8,495 million pesos (over US$ 1.1 billion) from the central level to the states. The Federal Government retains the authority to set health standards; regulate services and sanitary control of goods, establishments, and decentralized services; and control professional certification and accreditation of health units, generation of national statistics, and international representation of the sector. The state and municipal agencies share responsibilities for the organization, operation, and monitoring of public and private health services; sanitary control of services to the population; and fulfillment of health promotion and orientation tasks.

In 1996, the Secretariat of Health implemented a program to expand coverage, based on the provision of a basic package of health services that included 12 interventions for the population with limited or no access to medical services in rural areas; this program covered 6 million people in 18 states in 1997. In addition, in July 1997, IMSS introduced family health insurance, which people may voluntarily obtain by paying a fee of MN$ 180, which is complemented with a Government contribution (the average exchange rate in November 1997 was US$ 1 = MN$ 8.28). This insurance offers practically the same benefits as the regular system.

The Secretariat of Health has actively supported the healthy *municipios* movement with a view to expanding it and ensuring that the health initiatives carried out by the town halls or mayors' offices receive the necessary technical support. By the end of 1997, 860 *municipios*—35% of the country's *municipios*—were participating in this program; 535 of them were part of the national health network for *municipios*.

Organization of the Health Sector

Institutional Organization

Organization of the health system is still closely linked with employment sector; therefore, employees in the private sector and self-employed persons are covered by IMSS, which is financed with tripartite or bipartite contributions from employees, employers, and the Federal Government. Public sector workers are covered by the Social Security and Services Institute for Government Employees (ISSSTE) and other institutions, such as the military, petroleum, and the national university, which are financed with contributions from employees and the Government; a still undetermined segment of the population receives private care, and the remainder (over 40 million people) are treated in establishments of the Secretariat of Health and under a system known as IMSS-Solidarity, operated by that institution in specific regions. In 1995, 51% of the population had health insurance (social security in most cases). Roughly 10 million inhabitants did not have regular access to health services in 1995.

Organization of Health Regulatory Activities

The sector's legal framework basically rests on two broad laws that the Government updates periodically—the General Health Act and the Social Security Act. In 1997, several modifications to the Social Security Act went into effect. These changes were designed to revitalize the structure and practice of the pension and health care systems, by, among other provisions, reducing employer contributions and increasing Government contributions, offering family health insurance for those who wish to purchase it, and allowing for the transfer of employee contributions from their workplace to other providers when the employees so wish it, but with IMSS retaining the collection function. In that year, 52 reforms to the General Health Act also were introduced. They aim at making health deregulation more effective, introducing a new drug classification system and promoting the use of generic drugs in the private market, further specifying the Secretariat of Health's authority regarding the use of human tissue, improving the surveillance of biotechnology products, and granting authority to the Secretariat of Health to regulate labeling of alcoholic beverages and cigarettes.

Health regulation activities in the past four years have been geared toward prevention and control of disease, especially at the primary care level (diabetes mellitus, uterine and breast cancer, tuberculosis, HIV/AIDS, rabies); delivery of standardized services to special population groups (women during pregnancy, childbirth, and the puerperium; children and adolescents, to monitor their growth and development; family planning services; and psychiatric care); decentralization (delegation of authority to the states in public health, administration of blood banks, and issuing of authorizations and health permits); and the new structures and organs of the Secretariat of Health (the makeup of boards of trustees in hospitals, health institutes and jurisdictions as well as the National Health Council and National Medical Arbitration Commission).

Deregulation of the sector was implemented in 1996. That same year, the National Medical Arbitration Commission

(CONAMED) was created by presidential decree as a technically autonomous mediation agency to handle complaints about irregularities in the delivery of care or the failure to provide necessary care.

Health Services and Resources

The public sector is composed of the Secretariat of Health and social security, which have separate care institutions of all levels of complexity coordinated in networks regulated by their own controls, and procedures. The Secretariat of Health manages and coordinates the health sector; exchanges information and conducts meetings and other activities at the federal and state levels, as agreed upon among the institutions; organizes and provides medical services in keeping with the Health Care Model for the Uninsured Population in effect since 1995; and determines the activities to be conducted in health promotion, disease prevention, diagnosis, treatment, and rehabilitation. Coordination of these activities is the responsibility of the health jurisdictions, which are technical-administrative units responsible for planning, managing, and controlling health services for the population at the local level.

The basic package of health services that is provided to expand coverage consists of 75 health activities grouped into 12 basic interventions—basic sanitation at the household level; effective home-based standard case management for diarrhea; antiparasite treatments for families; identification of the warning signs of acute respiratory infections and referral to health facilities; prevention and control of tuberculosis of the lung; prevention and control of hypertension and diabetes mellitus; immunization; monitoring of children's nutrition and growth; distribution of contraceptives; care during pregnancy, childbirth, and the puerperium; first aid; and formation of health committees.

The number of outpatient clinics for the uninsured population increased from 10,443 in 1993 to 14,978 in 1997, and the hospital network grew from 329 to 372 institutions in that same period. The Secretariat of Health has 11 national institutes of health in the capital that operate in a decentralized manner and provide care at the tertiary level to patients referred from throughout the country. The social security institutes treat their members through their own service networks; outpatient clinics increased from 3,029 in 1993 to 3,208 in 1997, and the number of hospitals increased from 422 to 438. Traditional healing, whose extent has not yet been measured, is extremely widespread, particularly in areas with a high concentration of indigenous peoples and homeopathic medicine.

The volume of public services has steadily increased. Total medical consultations rose from 160 to 190 million between

1993 and 1996; hospitalizations increased from 3.6 to 3.8 million; and auxiliary diagnostic services rose from 123 to 137 million. An increase in care for both the uninsured population and Social Security members has been observed.

Because social security and the Secretariat of Health provide services consistent with their own models and schemes of care, in practice there is coverage overlap in some regions, and there are no shared criteria for technical and administrative procedures. The situation is different in the field of information, where common criteria are applied and data from different institutions are consolidated into national health statistics. In 1995, the National Epidemiological Surveillance Committee was formed, which operates a single information system in this area.

In recent years, private medicine evolved outside the scope of official policies. For 1995, it was calculated that the private supply of goods and services was responsible for half of all health expenditure, 30% of the bed count, 34% of employed physicians, and 32% of medical consultations. Private health insurance coverage is limited, and a traditional model involving direct collection of fees for services persists, with charges being as high as the market will bear. For the coming years, the private sector is expected to become more dynamic because of a return to fees that will be implemented by IMSS and because of the increase in the number of private insurance companies.

Organization of Services for Care of the Population

Health Promotion. This is a strategic approach within the priorities for disease prevention and control defined by the Secretariat of Health. The work strategies are health education, social participation, and educational communication. They are carried out along six tracks—family health, comprehensive health of schoolchildren, comprehensive health of adolescents, healthy *municipios,* health care exercises, and development of educational content. For all the above, recommended approaches and activities will have to be implemented by the health services at the operational levels, working in concert with institutions and groups concerned about health promotion. A key component is the healthy *municipios* strategy, which has fostered the political leadership of heads of *municipios* and the organized participation of society in defining priorities and executing local programs that deal with health promotion. Another project under way since 1996 is the "heart to heart project," which integrates initiatives of the private business sector, the Pan American Health Organization, and the Secretariat of Health under the aegis of the national health authority. This program is conducting a major mass communication campaign to reduce tobacco use and sedentary lifestyles and to promote healthy eating habits. The country recently adopted

the healthy schools strategy, which works to transform environments, conditions, and lifestyles in the schools.

Disease Prevention and Control Programs. Public health institutions, under the guidance of the Secretariat of Health, conducted systematic disease prevention and control programs for the principal diseases, with intervention models that combine systematic activities by the health services and limited campaigns with specific objectives to control risk factors or eliminate the causative agents of particular diseases. In 1997, the Secretariat of Health established a new priority disease prevention and control model, in which standardization, follow-up, and evaluation at the federal level are strengthened, combined with autonomous execution of the programs by state health services within the framework of institutional decentralization. In this way, 10 substantive programs with a direct impact on the health status of specific population groups were defined: reproductive health, child health care, health care for adults and the elderly, vector-borne diseases, zoonoses, mycobacteriosis, cholera, epidemiological emergencies and disasters, HIV/AIDS and other STDs, and addictions. For each of these programs, general objectives, components and strategies, impact goals, and coordination to be carried out were established; two strategic lines were also defined (health promotion and research on health services) as tools for strengthening the programs and the three support mechanisms (epidemiological surveillance, statistical information, and comprehensive supervision) that contribute information on the programs' development.

Epidemiological Surveillance Systems. In 1996, the country's epidemiological surveillance system was upgraded and integrated into different public sector institutions. The unified information system for epidemiological surveillance (SUIVE) was implemented, which generates information from the different health services at the technical-administrative levels, backed by a software package (SUAVE) for receiving, collecting, and analyzing the information obtained. SUAVE reports on new cases of disease, the 20 leading causes of disease, the unit control reports, and the weekly control reports, providing catalogs, graphs, and maps, all classified by age group and institution.

There is a morbidity registry, whose information comes from the Unified Epidemiological Surveillance System and reports on hospital discharges from health facilities. The information on mortality is based on death certificates, which are the compulsory legal mechanism for death certification. At the beginning of 1998, all health institutions in the country began to use the ICD-10 for their statistical records.

Quality of the Environment, Drinking Water and Sanitation Services, and Chemical Safety. The National Water

Commission, in close collaboration with the Secretariat of Health, is carrying out a national clean water program to ascertain the quality of the water being used for human consumption. The program monitors contaminants and levels of residual chlorine, and seeks solutions to pollution. In the Mexico City metropolitan area, a multimillion-dollar investment program is under way to improve sewerage services and wastewater treatment plants. In 1997, the sectoral analysis of solid waste was concluded in the metropolitan area, yielding extensive information on the need for projects and investment.

A multisectoral program to improve air quality is being carried out in the Mexico City metropolitan area. Its general purpose is to protect health by gradually and permanently reducing the levels of air pollution. Among other measures, the program includes ongoing monitoring of pollutants; compulsory semiannual inspection of motor vehicle emissions; control of emissions from industries, gas stations, and other establishments; factory closings; and restricting the use of automobiles in environmental emergencies. The environmental situation was studied in other large cities, such as Guadalajara and Monterrey, and similar programs to improve air quality are being devised.

All procedures for obtaining authorization to use chemical substances are carried out in the General Environmental Health Directorate of the Secretariat of Health; there is an Intersecretarial Commission to Control the Processing and Use of Pesticides, Fertilizers, and Toxic Substances (CICLOPLAFEST), which coordinates regulatory and control activities, including aspects of marketing, environment, and health.

Food Protection and Control and Food Assistance Programs. On the basis of broad studies that had been done, in 1996 the Secretariat of Health began modernizing health promotion and food control, seeking greater efficiency in fully and comprehensively guaranteeing food safety from production, through distribution, and to consumption.

There is a program for monitoring salt iodization in the market. In 1996, it reported that 92% of salt samples were properly iodized. The fluoridation of salt for domestic consumption dates back to 1994, and its distribution is limited to the regions where the water lacks fluoride. Semiannual doses of vitamin A are administered to children between 6 months and 4 years of age in 1,318 high-risk *municipios.*

There are food assistance programs for poor families. One of the most prominent, because of its scope, is the PROGRESA program, which in 1997 was under way in 524 *municipios* in 22 states, covering 400,000 families. The program provided nutritional supplements to pregnant and breast-feeding women, monetary support to mothers to improve nutrition and well-being at home, training in hygiene and caring for family health, and a basic package of health services. The National Institute

for Indigenous Culture, with the backing of the Government Secretariats, conducts programs with health, food, education, and basic sanitation activities for 59 ethnic groups located in 1,000 *municipios* and 9,500 towns and villages.

Inputs for Health

The Secretariat of Health is responsible for overseeing the quality, safety, and efficacy of the drugs that are produced and sold in the country and for regulating the marketing of those drugs. It exercises health surveillance and control basically by issuing licenses and through health registries and verification, analytical control, and evaluation of drugs. There was a major boom in the national pharmaceutical industry, composed of over 140 companies, including the national chamber, which provides over 95% of the drugs needed in the country and also exports its products.

The 1996 modifications to the regulations simplified registration procedures, and a technical cooperation agreement on certifying drug registration was drawn up between the Pan American Health Organization and the Secretariat of Health; furthermore, the obligation to identify drugs by their generic name was incorporated into the General Health Act. A basic set of 50 essential generic drugs that must be available in all medical units at the primary care level was established, along with eight vaccines and two more inputs. Additional initiatives involve the definition of a standard set of allopathic, herbal, and homeopathic drugs and the preparation of a catalog with the recommended drugs for the secondary and tertiary care levels. In 1994, the sixth edition of *The Pharmacopeia of the United Mexican States* was published (the previous edition was from 1988) and in 1995 and 1997 supplements were published that update the specifications for the manufacture of drugs marketed domestically.

Human Resources

In 1993 there were 421,581 public health workers in the health sector and in 1997 there were 463,611. There was a 14.5% increase in care for the uninsured population (174,942 workers) and 7.4% in social security institutions (288,669 workers). The number of physicians increased similarly (102,125 in 1993 and 116,047 in 1997), as did the number of nursing personnel (146,802 and 161,303), and paramedics (175,895 and 190,877). In 1996, the Secretariat of Health reported that 110,804 people worked in private medicine, of whom 51.4% were professionals and 24% were nursing personnel, and that of the 178,520 physicians in the sector, 2.8% were general practitioners, 47.9% specialists, 5% dentists; the rest were residents, interns, and others.

In 1996, 7,556 graduates (11% more than in the previous year) from the 57 medical schools fulfilled their social service requirement in the National Health System. Graduates of the Military Medical School, the Naval School, and the Air Force School, who do their social service within their own institutions, were exempted. There are 70 approved medical specialties, with an enrollment of 4,400 students for 1996–1997. The estimated programming for 1997–1998 is 5,345 graduate students in the health system.

Expenditures and Sectoral Financing

Data from the national accounting system on total health expenditure show that this figure increased through 1994, which is the last year for which figures are available, and that the estimates for 1995 and 1996, based on the total budget allocated for health, held that trend. For 1994, the total expenditure of the National Health System was estimated at between US$ 19.7 and US$ 27.3 million dollars, which are the upper and lower estimates, based on an annual average exchange rate of 3.4 pesos to $US 1. Health expenditure as a percentage of GDP for 1992, 1993, and 1994 reached 5.1%, 5.6%, and 6.1%, respectively, calculated by taking an average of the high and low figures on national health expenditure. The analysis of expenditure according to this source shows that households contribute the most, with 49% of total spending in the period 1992–1996, compared with employers, who contribute 29% and, finally, the Federal Government, which contributes 22%.

Of the total budget allocated to health, 68% was directed toward curative care (including hospitalization); 15% to administration, policy, and planning; 7% to preventive care; 6% to infrastructure; and 4% to other categories. Between 1992 and 1994 salaries consumed almost half the budget of the institutions with the greatest volume of services—48% in IMSS and 50% in the Secretariat of Health; however, in ISSSTE the figure was only 21%, and operating expenditures were the highest (51% of total expenditure). In IMSS, operating expenditures accounted for 35% of the total—the second highest—and in the Secretariat of Health they accounted for 3% of total spending for the same period.

Private expenditure is aimed predominantly at curative care, and its distribution shows that fees account for 35% of the total, drug purchases for 27%, and hospitalizations for 20%. Private out-of-pocket spending exhibited a regressive trend in all objects of expenditure—each year it represented a larger proportion than revenue. Per capita health expenditure for 1995, estimated from the budget executed by public institutions and the total population, was MN$ 499. The absolute values for private expenditure in urban areas are 10 times higher for the households with the highest income than for those with the lowest income (US$ 750 versus US$ 75 per quarter); in rural areas this difference may be 20 times ($1,294 versus $65). In urban and rural areas, the national accounts system for health reports that the totals spent for the various spending categories are similar.

Analysis of the resources utilized between 1992 and 1994 by the national accounting system through the so-called concentrated funds and funds utilized by the various institutions reveals that the sums used by social security institutions, private concerns, and establishments that serve the uninsured population increased. Social security handled the greatest proportion of resources (43%), followed by private concerns (42%). The institutions that treat the uninsured population (which are largely Government entities) used 13% of the total resources. Private health insurance represented a growing fund but was far surpassed by the others (barely 2% of the total). The participation of State governments rose to 3.7% between 1992 and 1994; however, it is acknowledged that this is probably an underestimate. Higher growth after 1996 is calculated, in view of the prevailing policy of decentralization.

The health budget continued to grow, while that of the Secretariat of Health rose from MN$ 8.893 billion in 1996 to MN$ 14.064 billion in 1997, an increase of 58% (the average exchange rate in 1996 was US$ 1 = MN$ 7.60). It should also be noted that the national budget allocated for social security, based on sectoral reform and changes to the 1997 General Social Security Act, which increased state contributions more than eightfold, grew from MN$ 2.641 billion to MN$ 21.379 billion between 1996 and 1997 and increased the State contribution to the institution's total revenue from 4.5% to 28.5%. In the field of disease and maternity, state transfers rose from 5% to 37%, substituting worker-employer contributions. The data on health resources and expenditure from the Secretariat of Defense and the Secretariat of the Navy are confidential and therefore are not available.

External Technical and Financial Cooperation

The Secretariat of Health is working to diversify international cooperation in health. To that end, in 1996 cooperation agreements were signed with the Governments of Cuba and Guatemala, and negotiations began with Belgium, Germany, Japan, the Kingdom of the Netherlands, and the Pacific Rim countries. The cooperation with Central America includes sending Mexican experts, providing fellowships in institutions in the country, and conducting health programs in border areas.

The volume of foreign financial aid in health declined notably in 1995 (US$ 4 million) with respect to 1990 (US$ 493 million), 1991 (US$ 190 million), and 1992 (US$ 7.8 million) because of the absence of large projects with international lending banks. In 1996, a five-year loan in the amount of US$ 310 million was obtained from the World Bank, of which US$ 60 million was provided that year.

Mexico's financial contributions to international organizations and bilateral health programs together dropped from US$ 25 million in 1992 to US$ 8 million per year between 1992 and 1995 and to US$ 6.5 million in 1996. This decline was especially visible in bilateral cooperation programs, which fell from US$ 17 million in 1992 to less than US$ 1 million in 1996.

MONTSERRAT

Montserrat stretches for 102 km² of mountainous terrain, and is part of the Eastern Caribbean volcanic island chain that extends from Saint Kitts in the north to Grenada in the south. It is a British dependency with its own system of government: the executive branch comprises a Chief Minister and three other ministers, all elected by the people, as well as a Governor who represents the British Government.

The prolonged eruption of the Soufriere Hills Volcano, which started in July 1995 and continues to date, was the pivotal event for Montserrat during the 1994–1997 period. The eruption has severely affected every aspect of Montserrat's economy, politics, development, and overall living conditions.

An in-depth discussion of these issues is outside the scope of this report, but a brief review of the volcanic emergency provides a useful context in which to view the territory's health conditions. It also should be noted that the upheaval and uncertainty have wreaked havoc with health service maintenance, recordkeeping, and the overall collection of information. Furthermore, the drastic population shifts compromised the quality and quantity of information that could be collected.

THE VOLCANIC EMERGENCY

The current eruption is Soufriere Hills volcano's first in more than 300 years. A series of earthquakes in 1992 may have marked the beginning of the current volcanic activity. In July 1995, the volcano first began venting ash, steam, and gases, and has continued to do so with increasing intensity. A major eruption in June 1997 resulted in 20 deaths, the destruction of many villages, and the closure of the island's only airport. Travel into and out of Montserrat was only possible from nearby Antigua via ferry or helicopter.

Over the two-and-a-half year period of volcanic activity, the dangerous area (the "exclusion zone") progressively expanded, and by the end of 1997, the southern two-thirds of the island had become unsafe. This included Plymouth, the capital and the territory's industrial, commercial, and government center, as well as the location for essential services. Plymouth's destruction and abandonment and the near total destruction of the capital's infrastructure triggered a steep economic decline. Glendon Hospital also was destroyed and is now relocated in a former school at St. John's in the territory's north.

Most of the population lived in Plymouth and its environs, and many families lost their homes. The number of persons evacuated out of the exclusion zone progressively increased over the years of the emergency, despite the fact that the territory's overall population decreased steadily as many persons fled the island. Initially, displaced persons were housed in temporary shelters in the north, but these soon became overcrowded. As new housing becomes available, however, the pressure on these shelters should significantly ease.

Most agriculture was conducted in the south, and had to be abandoned. The Government has leased or rented land in the safe zone for livestock and crop production, but farming has only been able to continue on a much reduced scale.

The tourist industry has been particularly hard hit. Earnings from this sector fell from US$ 14.5 million for the first six months of 1995, to US$ 5.9 million in the first six months of 1996. Figures for 1997 are not yet available, but these are expected to show an additional sharp decline.

The GDP was EC$ 147.32 million in 1994, EC$ 139.18 million in 1995, EC$ 116.32 million in 1996, and EC$ 115.31 million in 1997, representing negative real growth rates of 0.04% in 1994, 7.64% in 1995, 17.69% in 1996, and 1.73% in 1997.

The inablility to predict the course of the volcanic activity will seriously affect Montserrat's near and mid-term future. Good information collection, recording, and analysis are critical for effective planning and an efficient use of resources. Clear and dedicated leadership is particularly important in the present circumstances, where activities must fit available resources and where the capability to effectively respond to the emergency must be maintained.

GENERAL SITUATION AND TRENDS

Accurate population figures were extremely difficult to track in the emergency, as many residents left to spend varying periods abroad. The best population estimates show a drop from 10,402 in 1994 to 5,600 in 1997. By January 1998, the population had sunk to 3,483. There were 150 live births in 1994, 126 in 1995, and 128 in 1996. Age and sex breakdowns are not available for the period under review.

The crude death rates for the period were 9.3 in 1994, 12.1 in 1995, and 12.6 in 1996. Infant mortality rates for these same years were 13.0, 24.0, and 7.8. Data for 1997 are not available. Given the difficulties in obtaining accurate population and age breakdown figures, rates should be interpreted with caution.

In 1994, the leading causes of death for the age group 30 years old and older were heart diseases, malignant neoplasms, cerebrovascular disease, diabetes mellitus, diseases of the respiratory system, and diseases of the digestive system. In 1996, diabetes mellitus ranked first as a cause of death, followed by heart diseases, malignant neoplasms, hypertensive disease, cerebrovascular disease, and malnutrition. Malnutrition ranked as the sixth leading cause of death in 1996, and these deaths all occurred in the elderly (age group 70–99 years old). Although mortality data for 1997 are not available, deaths in that year were mostly due to severe burns caused by the eruption. These deaths were three times as high as the leading cause of death for the years reported, and are likely to remain the leading cause of death for 1997.

There were 1,302 admissions to Glendon Hospital in 1994 and 1,106 in 1995. In 1996, there were 1,166 admissions to St. John's Hospital. Diabetes, hypertension, heart disease, pregnancy, and gastroenteritis were the main causes for hospital admissions over the 1994–1996 period.

SPECIFIC HEALTH PROBLEMS

Analysis by Population Group

Among adults, diabetes and hypertension were the two most common reasons for clinic attendance over the period under review, followed by heart disease, asthma, and upper respiratory tract infections complete.

The elderly receive special attention. At the end of 1997, 126 elderly persons were housed in four homes/shelters for seniors operated by the Government and the Montserrat Red Cross, and the Red Cross is constructing another 50-bed home. There are another 180 elderly persons living in homes or community shelters who receive home help and other assistance.

Special attention has been given to the refugee shelters and their populations. Severe overcrowding early during the emergency could easily have led to health problems, but environmental health measures were put in place to manage solid waste disposal, improve toilet facilities, provide adequate potable water, and ensure food safety. District nurses added the shelters to their portfolio for home visits. A communicable disease surveillance system was put in place to monitor outbreaks. The shelter population peaked at about 1,400 in April 1996, but by the end of 1997, the number of persons in shelters had fallen to approximately 500.

Analysis by Type of Disease or Health Impairment

The number of cases of *gastroenteritis* among children under 5 years old varied from 57 in 1994, to 35 in 1995, and 42 in 1996. From 1994 to 1996 there was an average of about 100 gastroenteritis cases per year in the population 5 years of age and older (96, 93, and 112 cases, respectively).

Reported cases of *influenza* rose from 66 in 1994 to 90 in 1996.

An outbreak of *dengue fever* began in October 1994 with 327 reported cases; there were 750 cases reported in 1995 and 2 in 1996.

Montserrat has established a multisectoral *AIDS/STD* council. The territory continues to observe all regional guidelines, and blood for transfusions is screened. In the review period there were two confirmed cases of AIDS in Montserrat and no deaths.

The number of cases of *ciguatera* poisoning rose from 22 cases in 1994 to 28 in 1995, dropping to 14 in 1996.

In 1997, there were 110 patients on the psychiatric register, with the most significant mental disorders being *chronic schizophrenia, manic depression, substance abuse psychoses, and depression.*

RESPONSE OF THE HEALTH SYSTEM

Organization of the Health Sector

Primary care services have continued to be provided throughout the emergency, despite such difficulties as the need to close clinics within the exclusion zone and the loss of health personnel. Primary care clinics decreased from 12 in 1994 and 1995, to 5 in 1996, and 3 in 1997.

Plymouth's 65-bed Glendon Hospital, newly rebuilt in 1989 after Hurricane Hugo, was destroyed, and hospital services were relocated to St. John's in the north. A school building has been fitted to serve as a center for providing limited *secondary care,* mainly medical and uncomplicated elective surgery. The facility at St. John's has a bed capacity of 30, but up to 10 beds may be occupied by discharged patients awaiting to return to the community. Patients are referred to Antigua and Saint Kitts for care unavailable in Montserrat.

Hospital laboratory services are limited to simple hematology and biochemistry investigations and blood banking; no microbiological investigations are performed. The X-ray department is able to perform basic emergency investigations with a portable X-ray unit.

Health Services and Resources

Prenatal care is provided at the three district primary care clinics and by two doctors in private practice. Delivery care is provided at St. John's Hospital for low-risk pregnancies; all high-risk pregnancies are sent to Antigua or Saint Kitts. Postnatal care is provided at the three district clinics at six weeks after delivery and then at the mother's place of residence.

Family planning services are offered at the three district primary care clinics and by the two private practitioners.

The *immunization program* has continued to operate well throughout the volcanic emergency. Coverages for DPT, MMR, and polio are estimated to near 100%. Immunizations are administered at the primary care clinics and as part of the preschool physical examination program for 4–5-year-old children upon entering primary school. Of the diseases covered by the Expanded Program on Immunization (EPI) there were two suspected cases of measles reported, one in 1994 and one in 1995. There was one case of diphtheria reported in 1995. There were no reported cases of mumps, rubella, pertussis, tetanus, or polio over the period.

A retired psychiatrist and a psychiatric nurse manage the *mental health services.* The program is mainly community-based, with one clinic being held specifically for follow-up of psychiatric patients. The number of clients served rose from 100 in 1994, to 220 in 1995, and 240 in 1996, before dropping to 110 in 1997.

Organization of Services for Care of the Population

Vector Control, Water Supply, Sewerage Systems, Solid-Waste Disposal, and Pollution Monitoring. The Pest Control Unit directed most of its efforts toward the control of the *Aedes aegypti* mosquito. Integrated vector control methods were used to control all mosquitoes, flies, roaches, rats, and mice. An outbreak of dengue fever in October 1994 mobilized most of the population in an islandwide mass cleanup program for

source reduction, which helped to control the outbreak within four months.

The volcanic emergency required a massive relocation of the population to the north of the island, which set back the vector control program and led to a proliferation of many insects, pests, and rodents, especially in and around the crowded shelters.

A survey of Montserrat's water supply system in 1997 confirmed that the water supply had not been contaminated by volcanic products, but continued monitoring would be necessary. Most of the water sources were located in the south of the island, where most of the population lived before the volcanic eruption began, and water sources and storage areas in the exclusion zone were abandoned. It is estimated that adequate amounts of water can be obtained to meet future demand, with some changes in the pumping, piping, and storage characteristics of the water supply system.

A program to facilitate the construction and use of precast latrine units was implemented in 1995. A public education program on the proper maintenance of septic tank systems was also carried out in 1995.

Refuse collection was privatized in March 1995, which markedly improved solid waste management. Prior to the crisis, the Government had procured a 55-acre plot that was to be developed as a sanitary landfill site, but the site had to be abandoned because it was located in the exclusion zone. An alternative site has not been found, and a temporary site is under use. This remains as a significant problem.

Air quality is monitored by measuring the concentration of respirable dust, and is reported to the public by the Montserrat Volcano Observatory. The air quality in the safe zone in the north of the island has been consistently within acceptable limits.

Human Resources

Montserrat has experienced a flight of health staff since the volcanic crisis began. The number of registered nurses dropped from 40 in 1994 to 13 in 1998. Staffing shortfalls mostly have been offset by human resources from other Caribbean countries and the United Kingdom.

Expenditures and Sectoral Financing

Expenditure at present is heavily dependent on the United Kingdom aid budget for Montserrat. Health expenditure as a percentage of Montserrat's total budget was 16.5% in 1994, 17.5% in 1995, 13.4% in 1996, and 13.5% in 1997; health expenditure as a percentage of the total recurrent budget was 16.5%, 17.5%, 16.9%, and 16.7%, respectively.

NETHERLANDS ANTILLES

GENERAL SITUATION AND TRENDS

Socioeconomic, Political, and Demographic Overview

The Netherlands Antilles is composed of five islands: Curaçao, Bonaire, Saba, Saint Eustatius, and Saint Martin. The first two are located near the northwestern coast of Venezuela and the others are about 900 km to the northeast. The total area of the Netherlands Antilles is 800 km². The official language is Dutch, but Papiamento is the language commonly spoken on Curaçao and Bonaire, and English is spoken on Saint Martin, Saba, and Saint Eustatius. Curaçao, with an area of 444 km², is the largest of the Dutch islands in the Caribbean, and its capital, Willemstad, is the seat of the central government.

The Netherlands Antilles is an autonomous territory within the Kingdom of the Netherlands. The islands are responsible for their own political affairs and administration, except for defense, foreign affairs, the legal system, and financial and administrative oversight. A parliamentary democracy exists and elections are held every four years. The cabinet of ministers is chosen by the Parliament. There are two levels of government: the central government, with a parliament on Curaçao composed of representatives of all the islands, and the local government of each island, consisting of an island council and a legislative assembly. The Governor of the Netherlands Antilles is the representative of the Kingdom of the Netherlands; the representative of the central government on each island is the Lieutenant Governor, who has executive powers.

The service sector—especially tourism—is the mainstay of the economy. Other important sectors are manufacturing and construction. In 1993, per capita income was US$ 7,800 and the gross domestic product (GDP) was US$ 2,114.8 million. The inflation rates for the years 1992–1996 were 1.4%, 2.1%, 1.8%, 2.8%, and 3.6%, respectively.

As for educational levels, 31% of the population of Curaçao aged 24 years and over has completed primary education; 39% has completed basic secondary studies; 18% has finished advanced secondary studies (high school); and 10% has attended a polytechnic institute or university. According to the population census of 1992, only 2% of the population of Curaçao aged 24 years and over had not completed the primary level of education. Higher percentages of females completed primary school, but more males attained higher levels of education. On average, levels of education are higher among males than females, and they are higher among young people than older adults and the elderly. The difference in educational level between males and females is greatest in the oldest segments of the population.

The official unemployment rates in Curaçao for 1994, 1995, and 1996 was 12.8%, 13.1%, and 13.9%, respectively—lower than the rate reported in the 1992 census (16.9%). In 1995, unemployment was 17% among women and 9.8% among men. As for the other islands, in 1994 the unemployment rate was 5.5% on Bonaire, 4.2% on Saba, 5.8% on Saint Eustatius, and 11.3% on Saint Martin.

In 1994 and 1995 the population growth rates for the Netherlands Antilles as a whole were 2.6% and 2.5%, respectively, and for Curaçao the rates were 1.2% and 1.8%. Net migration has been positive since 1994. In 1995, the estimated population of the Netherlands Antilles was 207,333 inhabitants, with a density of 259 inhabitants per km²; 34% of the population was less than 20 years of age, 59% was between 20 and 64, and 7% was 65 and over. In that same year, Curaçao had 151,540 inhabitants (73% of the total population of the Netherlands Antilles, with a similar age distribution). Females constituted 52.9% of the population. In 1994, Bonaire had 12,533 inhabitants; Saba, 1,197; Saint Eustatius, 1,882; and Saint Martin, 37,256. Annual population growth ranged from 1.2% on Bonaire to 4% on Saint Martin. Life expectancy at birth is 77.5 years for females and 71.8 years for males.

Mortality Profile

The crude death rate increased from 5.3 per 1,000 inhabitants in 1986 to 7.1 in 1993, and standardized mortality rates ranged from 4.7 per 1,000 inhabitants in 1986 to 5.4 per 1,000 in 1993. The standardized mortality rate for males is 1.5 times higher than the rate for females. Age-specific mortality for both males and females remained stable from 1986 to 1993. A significant increase has been noted in male mortality in the 1–4 and 25–44 age groups.

In 1993, diseases of the circulatory system and malignant neoplasms accounted for 36.3% and 22.1%, respectively, of deaths from defined causes. Mortality from infectious and parasitic diseases and external causes has shown a rising trend, and deaths attributed to perinatal and ill-defined causes have tended to decrease. The rest of the causes have remained stable. Only 3.6% of deaths are attributed to ill-defined causes. In 1993, the leading causes of death were cerebrovascular diseases (13.6%), followed by diseases of pulmonary circulation and other forms of heart disease (10.0%), ischemic heart disease (9.1%), and diabetes mellitus (5.1%). Ischemic heart disease was the leading cause of death among males; cerebrovascular diseases accounted for the largest share of female deaths. Malignant neoplasms cause more deaths among males. AIDS is the eighth leading cause of death (2.9%) among males.

Age-specific mortality has two distinct patterns: for the population aged 45 years and over, the leading causes of death are chronic noncommunicable diseases, including cardiovascular diseases, cerebrovascular diseases, and diabetes mellitus; for the group aged 1–44 years, AIDS and external causes are the most common. In general, there has been an increase in deaths from external causes, which numbered 49 in 1986 and 75 in 1993 and which occurred more frequently in males than in females.

SPECIFIC HEALTH PROBLEMS

On Curaçao, the methods used for routine compilation of data by health service providers are not reliable because they do not provide a complete picture of the health status of the population. For this reason, between November 1993 and August 1994 the Curaçao Health Survey was carried out in a random sample of the noninstitutionalized adult population of Curaçao to obtain the necessary information.

The results of the study, based on the responses of the 2,248 individuals interviewed, provide information in three main areas: health status, lifestyles, and use of health services. About 10% of the adult population suffers from diabetes mellitus, and approximately half of them are unaware they have the disease; 20%–30% of the population suffers from hypertension; and 7% has glaucoma. Psychological problems are prevalent among adults and young people: 12% of the respondents in the 18–24 age group reported suffering from stress, nervousness, or depression. The elderly, women, and people in the lower socioeconomic groups are in a disadvantaged position with respect to their health. Seventeen percent of the respondents said they smoked. As for physical exercise and eating habits, 75% of all the adults do not engage in any regular physical exercise, and there are some obvious nutritional deficiencies: 37% do not eat vegetables daily and about half do not eat fruit every day. Excess weight is also a significant health problem, especially among women in lower socioeconomic groups.

Only 40% of those surveyed visit a dentist every year. The elderly on Curaçao do not make greater use of the general medical services than younger individuals, nor do individuals in the lower socioeconomic groups.

Analysis by Population Group

Health of Children

Infant mortality decreased for both sexes from 17.8 per 1,000 live births in 1986 to 11 per 1,000 live births in 1993. Neonatal mortality fell from 9.9 per 1,000 live births in 1990 to 8.7 in 1993, and perinatal mortality declined from 23.6 to 17.9 per 1,000 live births in the same period. During the 1991–1993 period, conditions originating in the perinatal period (64.5%) and congenital abnormalities (23.0%) were the leading causes of death in the first year of life. Infectious diseases were responsible for 6.6% of infant mortality. Among children aged 1–4, the mortality rate increased; there were no differences by sex, and the most common causes of death were congenital abnormalities, which accounted for 20.8% (five deaths), followed by traffic accidents (16.7%) (four deaths), and intestinal infectious diseases (8.3%) (two deaths). The mortality rate in the group aged 5–14 years remained stable during the period 1986–1993, and no sex differences were noted. Nine of the deaths (50%) reported between 1991 and 1993 were due to traffic accidents.

Health of Adolescents

In the group aged 15–24 years, mortality is twice as high among males and showed a slight upward trend in 1992–1993. External causes accounted for 42.8% (21 deaths); of these deaths, 20.4% were due to traffic accidents, 16.3% to homicide, and 6.1% to drowning.

Health of Women

During the period 1990–1991, the fertility rate remained stable at 2.4 per 1,000 women of childbearing age (15–49 years of age) as did the specific fertility rate for the group aged 15–19 years (0.05 in 1981 and 0.05 in 1991).

Prenatal care is provided by general practitioners, midwives, and obstetricians/gynecologists. Only midwives use the perinatal information system, which includes information on prenatal care, childbirth, and the puerperium. In 1994 the system contained records on 1,144 women (37% of all births). From these records it can be concluded that only 25% of prenatal visits were made before the 20th week of pregnancy and that 52% of the women began prenatal care in the third trimester. As for care during childbirth, most births (99%) take place in clinics or in hospitals. Low-risk births generally occur at maternity clinics, and high-risk cases are referred to the General Hospital. As for maternal mortality, although only 13 maternal deaths occurred between 1986 and 1993, with an average of 3,000 live births per year, this number yields a maternal mortality rate of 54 per 100,000 live births. Among the causes associated with this rate are the high prevalence of sickle cell anemia and preeclampsia.

Health of the Elderly

The population aged 65 and over doubled between 1960 and 1992, and in 1995, according to data from the Central Statistics Office, persons in this age group made up 8% of the total population. The main causes of death in this group are cerebrovascular disease, followed by heart disease (ischemic heart disease) and diabetes mellitus.

Family Health

In the last population and housing census, which was carried out in 1992, 41,272 homes were surveyed. The average number of occupants per household was 3.5, which represents a decrease with respect to the previous census, in which the average was 4.3. Women head 36% of all households; 71.3% of households consist of nuclear families, 19.1% consist of nonnuclear families, and 9.6% consist of two or more nuclear families.

Health of the Disabled

According to the 1992 census, 3.9% of the total population reported some type of disability. Of that percentage, 28.4%

had a physical disability and 22.7% had a visual disability. Of the latter group, 3.8% (212 people) were blind and 82% of blind people were 60 years of age or older.

Analysis by Type of Disease

Communicable Diseases

Dengue has been endemic on Curaçao since 1973. A surveillance system exists and activities are carried out to control vectors of the disease. An outbreak occurred in early 1993 and serotypes 2 and 4 were isolated. During that outbreak, 18% of all the cases were dengue hemorrhagic fever and one death was reported. Another outbreak occurred in 1995, and yet another was detected later the same year. This second outbreak ended in February 1996. Serotype 4 was isolated in only one case during the second outbreak. Of the cases reported in the last two outbreaks, 6.5% and 4.2%, respectively, were hemorrhagic dengue.

In 1995, 555 cases of dengue were reported, which is double the number reported in 1993. Knowledge and attitude surveys conducted in 1995 and 1996 indicated that even when the population has sufficient information about controlling the dengue vector, the knowledge is generally not put into practice. Doctors as well as the general population believe that the number of cases reported by the surveillance system underestimates the total number of dengue cases that occurred in these two years, either because physicians did not request laboratory confirmation of the diagnosis or because people are familiar with the disease and do not consult doctors.

No cases of poliomyelitis or acute flaccid paralysis have been reported. Between November 1996 and April 1997, seven cases of Guillain-Barré syndrome were reported, but all were negative for poliovirus. No cases of diphtheria, whooping cough, tetanus, mumps, or *Haemophilus influenzae* B have been reported.

In January 1997, after an outbreak of measles on Guadeloupe, surveillance was stepped up on Curaçao. As of May 1997, 14 suspected cases had been reported, and measles was ruled out in 10 of those cases.

No cases of cholera have been reported—there is no system for reporting clinical cases of infectious intestinal diseases. Laboratory reports from 1993 through 1995, which include results of studies of food-handlers, indicate that shigella, *Campylobacter*, and salmonella are the most commonly occurring microorganisms. The incidence of intestinal infections for the three years analyzed remained stable (3 per 1,000 inhabitants). The most susceptible age group was children under 1 year of age.

There is no record of outbreaks of meningitis, reporting of which is not mandatory. In 1993, 1994, and 1995, respectively, four, five, and six cases of tuberculosis were reported; three of these cases were resistant to isoniazid. Investigation of contacts is carried out for all diagnosed cases. In 1993, acute respiratory infections were the fifth leading cause of death for all age groups; there is no surveillance system for such infections. There were no reported cases of rabies or other zoonoses.

For the period 1985–1996, the cumulative total of cases of individuals infected with HIV in the Netherlands Antilles was 815, of which 466 (57.2%) were male and 349 (42.8%) were female. The majority of individuals infected with HIV are between 25 and 44 years of age (68.3%), and 97.5% of infected persons live in Curaçao and Saint Martin. Among infected newborns, the virus was transmitted by the mother, and in the group aged 25–44 years transmission was through sexual relations. All pregnant women are tested for HIV. The highest incidence occurs in the age groups that are sexually and reproductively active. The male/female ratio is 1.3:1, which suggests that transmission of the virus is predominantly heterosexual. The risk of acquiring the infection from a blood transfusion is minimal because laboratories screen all donated blood for HIV. The exact number of AIDS cases in the Netherlands Antilles is unknown; efforts are under way to establish a central registry in the Department of Public Health and Environmental Hygiene. As of October 1996, 58 people were using one or more drugs to treat HIV infection; the drugs were supplied by the pharmacy of Saint Elizabeth's Hospital in Curaçao; no data are available for the rest of the islands. In Curaçao, AIDS is a leading cause of death in the age group 25–44 years; in 1991–1993 the disease accounted for 14% of deaths in that age group.

Noncommunicable Diseases and Other Health-Related Problems

Nutritional Diseases and Diseases of Metabolism. In a sample of 981 children less than 1 year old who were selected from children seen for well-child visits in public health services in 1992, 5.4% weighed less than 2,500 g at birth. According to data from the Public Health Service of Curaçao, in 1993 about 9% of all live-born children weighed less than 2,500 g. In the same year, 3% of children under the age of 1 who were seen for well-child visits were malnourished. In the group aged 1–4 years, the highest percentage of malnutrition (low weight for age) was found among children 2 and 3 years old (5%). A study conducted by the Public Health Service (which comprised one-third of the schools on Curaçao) of two cohorts of children born in 1987 and 1984 found that 4% and

1%, respectively, were malnourished (low weight for age). More than 40% of the children with low weight for age were of normal height, which indicates only acute malnutrition; 20% of the malnourished children exhibited both acute and chronic malnutrition.

In 1993 a quantitative study in Curaçao looked at food intake in a sample of male and female children aged 10–14 years. The intake of macronutrients met Dutch nutrient recommendations for this age group; however, the average intake of micronutrients was lower than recommended. In 1996, the Department of Public Health carried out a qualitative study of eating habits among adolescents aged 16 and 17 years in a sample of 180 secondary school students on Curaçao. The findings indicate that, in general, adolescents eat fewer vegetables, fruits, and milk products than recommended; they frequently consume sweets, carbonated beverages, sugar, and fried foods; and they very often eat foods prepared outside the home.

With respect to breast-feeding, the results of the Curaçao Health Survey conducted in 1993–1994 among 236 women who had at least one child aged 0–4 years indicate that at 6 weeks of age, 73% of the children were being breast-fed; at 3 months, 42% were; and at 16 months, 16.7%.

According to the results of the Curaçao Health Survey, the prevalence of Type II diabetes mellitus is 10% in the population over 18 years of age. The prevalence increases with age, and in the group aged 45 years and over, it is 30%–35%; the number is even higher in the group aged 65 and older. Diabetes mellitus is more frequent among women than men, but the difference is not significant. The principal risk factor is obesity. More than 50% of women are obese; in the group aged 45–64 the prevalence of obesity reaches 60%. Diabetes is significantly more prevalent among those who are obese than among those of normal weight. Diabetes was the fourth leading cause of death in 1993, accounting for 5.1% of mortality. Among women, it is the third leading cause of death (17.4%) and among men it is eighth (2.9%).

Cardiovascular Diseases. The results of the Curaçao Health Survey revealed that hypertension is the most frequently reported disease (11.4% of men and 16.7% of women), and it is estimated that the actual prevalence is double the amount reported. In 1995 there were 524 hospital admissions for cardiovascular disease on Curaçao, which represents 349 admissions per 100,000 inhabitants, with an average hospital stay of 11.8 days. No heart surgery or catheterization is performed in the Netherlands Antilles; these procedures therefore were the main reason for sending patients to other countries in 1994. Ischemic heart disease ranks third among the 10 leading causes of death, accounts for 9.1% of all deaths, and constitutes the leading cause of death among men.

Malignant Tumors. Between 1982 and 1987, the incidence of malignant neoplasms in the Netherlands Antilles increased from 156 to more than 200 per 100,000 inhabitants. From 1987 to 1991, the incidence ranged from 200 to 220 per 100,000 inhabitants. This increase is attributed to the aging of the population, to improvements in diagnosis, and, possibly, to a real increase. Among males, the most frequent tumor sites are the prostate, lung, and stomach, with incidences of 40.8, 22.2, and 18.5 per 100,000 population, respectively; among females, the most frequent sites are the breast (44.8 per 100,000 inhabitants), cervix and uterus (21.5 per 1,000 inhabitants), and colon (11.4 per 1,000 inhabitants). In both sexes, 9.5% of malignant tumors are diagnosed in situ and 90.5% are diagnosed after they have progressed to an invasive stage.

Accidents and Violence. Mortality from external causes has shown a rising trend. In the group aged 1–44 years, AIDS and external causes are the most frequent causes of death, especially for males, among whom external causes account for four times more years of potential life lost. A study of mortality from external causes carried out in Curaçao showed that from 1986 to 1993 traffic accidents (motor vehicle collisions) were the leading cause of death, accounting for 20–25 deaths per year. Accidental falls ranked second (approximately 10 per year), and drownings were third. Eight suicide deaths occur per year on average and there are an equal number of homicides, although in 1993 the number of homicides doubled.

Behavioral Disorders. According to the 1992 census, 21.8% of the population aged 18 and over smoke. According to the Curaçao Health Survey (1993–1994), the prevalence of smoking among adults over the age of 18 is 17.1% (28.3% in males and 8.8% in females). The highest prevalence was found in the group aged 45–64, followed by the group aged 25–44. A 1996 study of a sample of households found that 20% of males and 9% of females smoked. The Curaçao Health Survey revealed that 20.5% of the population surveyed drinks alcohol regularly (37.9% of males and 7.5% of females) and 49.2% drinks occasionally (43.1% of males and 53.8% of females).

With regard to drug use, a 1996 study of a sample of households indicated that more males than females use illegal drugs (2% and 0.1%, respectively). The highest percentage of drug use was found in the group aged 35–49 (2%), followed by the group aged 20–34 years (1.4%). Drug use is more common among people with low and medium levels of education (1.8% and 1.4%, respectively) than among those with more education (0.3%). The highest rates of drug use were found among unemployed people seeking work (2.6%). Of the population that was not economically active, 1.3% indicated they used drugs. Among those who worked, 1% were drug users. The most frequently used drugs are marijuana and cocaine.

According to data from the Curaçao Health Survey, 20.5% of those surveyed suffer from some psychiatric disorder, and significantly more women than men have psychological problems (23% and 17.1%, respectively). There are no significant differences among different age groups, and there is a clear correlation to socioeconomic status; psychiatric disorders occur less frequently in groups with higher levels of income and education.

Oral Health. Access to oral health care on Curaçao is variable; among those insured by the Government, access is quite limited, whereas for persons with other types of insurance there is ample coverage, both quantitatively and qualitatively. Use of dental services is low, especially among the youngest members of the population, and there are obstacles to preventive care because many groups lack appropriate coverage. The oral health services available to the disabled are insufficient. According to the Curaçao Health Survey, 30.5% of the respondents have all their teeth, and 11% have no teeth; of the latter group, one-fifth (or 2.2% of the total sample) do not have false teeth.

Natural Disasters and Industrial Accidents. The Netherlands Antilles has suffered damage from hurricanes and storms, which have caused both loss of human life and material losses. Industrial accidents have been associated with oil refineries and hydrocarbon shipping centers. Explosions, fires, and oil spills have been reported. The Disaster Prevention System coordinates the activities of governmental and nongovernmental organizations in cases of emergencies and disasters.

RESPONSE OF THE HEALTH SYSTEM

National Health Plans and Policies

In 1994, the island government of Curaçao initiated a process of cost containment aimed at curbing rising health care costs. This process, known as the "New Policy," gave rise to a project to develop a new health insurance system. In response to the enormous financial problems facing the Saint Elizabeth Hospital, a meeting was organized with participants from all areas of the health sector. Subsequently, the Steering Committee for Health Sector Reform was formally established by decree of the island government in October 1994. This Committee is composed of members of the Public Health Services of Curaçao, the Department of Finance of the Executive Council of Curaçao, the Welfare Services, and the Department of Public Health and Environmental Sanitation. Additional participants include a communications official, the manager of the new health insurance project, and the manager of the subsidized institutions project. The five issues discussed at the meeting were health inspection, audits and studies of efficiency and effectiveness, regulation of the licensing of health professionals, investments in health care and the central advisory board, and budget funding.

In November 1995, the Steering Committee submitted final recommendations on the five issues discussed at the health summit to the Executive Council of Curaçao. The policy recommendations were accepted by the Executive Council, which will submit them to the Minister of Health. However, implementation of the recommendations will require the combined efforts of the central and island governments.

The goal established by the Steering Committee with regard to health care is to ensure the provision of humane, effective, and efficient health care based on criteria of equality and on the real needs of the various population groups. The following measures have been proposed as means to develop a policy on quality of care and cost containment, to increase the financial control of the health sector, and to create a clear structure with division of responsibilities. In addition, it is proposed that a Steering Committee be established at the level of the central government and that Steering Committees also be created at the level of the island governments by decree of the Executive Council of each island.

Agreements exist with the Ministry of Health and the Universities of Maastricht and Groninga in the Netherlands to carry out health studies and assess the impact of the economic measures that have been taken and the new forms of health care financing. There is keen interest in monitoring the quality of medical care.

Taking into account the results of the Curaçao Health Survey, the Government's National Health Plan assigns priority to prevention and control of chronic noncommunicable diseases as well as encouraging changes in lifestyles and habits that increase the risk of cardiovascular diseases, hypertension, and diabetes mellitus. The Ministry of Health has created three multidisciplinary working groups to develop intervention programs. It has been decided to conduct surveys similar to the Curaçao Health Survey on the rest of the islands in the Netherlands Antilles in order to better assess the health situation of each island and design appropriate intervention programs.

Organization of the Health Sector

Institutional Organization

Curaçao has two general hospitals and one surgical hospital, with a total of 618 beds: Saint Elizabeth's Hospital (540 beds), the Adventist Hospital (42 beds), and the Dr. Taams

Surgical Hospital (36 beds). There is also a maternity clinic with 23 beds, and the Institute Mon Verriet has a rehabilitation service with 12 beds. Curaçao has a total of 4.4 beds per 1,000 inhabitants. Saint Elizabeth's Hospital, which provides hemodialysis, intensive care, and neonatal services, receives patients from the other islands in the Netherlands Antilles as well as Aruba.

The entire population has access to health services. At the primary care level, there are 90 general practitioners. The new general health insurance system and the new financing models are intended to improve the quality of care and enhance equity. Curaçao has 97 medical specialists, including 12 internists, 4 cardiologists, 4 neurologists, 1 gastroenterologist, 11 surgeons, 2 urologists, 5 orthopedists, 1 neurosurgeon, 2 plastic surgeons, 10 gynecologists, 3 neurologists, 3 dermatologists, 6 anesthetists, and 2 pathologists. Health professionals are trained in the Netherlands and, occasionally, in other countries.

There are five insurance modalities: the PPK ("pro-paupere kaart"), which is totally funded by the Government and is intended for the indigent and those who are not otherwise insured because of advanced age or the existence of a chronic condition; the public insurance program, which covers 100% of health care costs for blue-collar workers and 90% for personnel in higher categories of public-sector employment; the insurance fund for retired public-sector employees; private insurance plans provided by large private companies for their own personnel; and the social security fund, which covers employees of small private companies and other forms of private insurance. Given the significant differences in coverage under the various modalities of insurance, one of the objective of the insurance system restructuring process is to reduce differences in access and quality of medical care.

Health Services and Resources

Organization of Services for Care of the Population

Various health education, promotion, and protection initiatives have been implemented in the Netherlands Antilles, especially by nongovernmental organizations. The health care system remains oriented predominantly toward curative care, however. In the "Financial Review of Health Care Costs in the Netherlands Antilles, 1993" it was estimated that on Curaçao 0.8% of total health care spending was devoted to preventive care, compared with 55% for curative care. Many of the health problems that have been identified are linked to lifestyle, socioeconomic and cultural factors, and attitudes toward health and illness. Health promotion activities in the Netherlands Antilles are centered around prevention of chronic noncommunicable diseases related to lifestyle and unhealthy habits (poor diet, lack of exercise, consumption of alcohol, and smoking); prevention of drug use and rehabilitation of users; and promotion of responsible sexual behavior (AIDS prevention) and reproductive rights. The adoption of the Caribbean Charter for the Promotion of National Health in the Netherlands Antilles was a great achievement.

Since February 1995, the Department of Public Health and Environmental Sanitation has had an Environmental Section. Sustainable development constitutes the point of departure for the Government of the Netherlands Antilles in the formulation of its plans and policies for the future, which means that protection of the environment and of natural resources must be included in socioeconomic policy plans. Five main priority areas have been selected for work in the next five years: waste and wastewater; the petroleum industry and the environment; tourism, environment, and nature; environmental management; and strengthening environmental awareness. To guide efforts in these areas, a set of national regulations and basic principles for environmental management and protection of nature were developed and presented for consideration by the Parliament. Under these legal provisions, all the islands will be obligated to formulate legislation on the environment and nature. Model draft legislation for the islands is under study.

Curaçao, Bonaire, and Saint Martin have good drinking water and sewerage systems. Desalinization plants produce water of excellent quality, although the process is quite costly. Only Curaçao and Saint Martin have wastewater treatment plants; on the other islands, the use of septic tanks is common.

Most of the islands have refuse collection services operated by private companies under the supervision of local authorities. There are problems related to the safety of the final disposal sites and projects for the construction of sanitary landfills have been developed but have not been implemented because of insufficient funding. Hospitals have services for the collection and incineration of hazardous material.

Expenditures and Sectoral Financing

Based on the most recent data available and financial records for 1992, health sector expenditures in the Netherlands Antilles currently range from US$ 150 million to US$ 167 million. For the island of Curaçao, expenditures range from US$ 128 million to US$ 138 million per year.

An important objective is to improve and standardize health financing information systems. The Netherlands Antilles has acquired the Medical Costs Information System ("ZIS systeem") from the Netherlands and adapted it for functional use on Curaçao. The total cost of the computer programs was financed by the Cabinet for the Netherlands Antilles and Aruba (KABNA) under the condition that the system be used by the BZV Foundation. The Foundation, established in February 1993 by the Government of the Netherlands Antilles and the Executive Council of Curaçao, is responsible for processing all medical care bills for public employees and their families, patients with PPK cards, and government retirees. In addition to processing payments, the Foundation centralizes medical-financial operations in order to keep track of total expenditures and exact numbers of insured individuals.

The introduction of the General Insurance Plan for Special Medical Expenses is the first step toward a general insurance system in the Netherlands Antilles. The next step will be the introduction of a general health insurance program. The Government of the Netherlands Antilles intends to submit legislation for the establishment of national health insurance by the end of 1997.

The current policy is also aimed at introducing the Medicine Provision System ("GVS systeem"). If the Government of the Netherlands Antilles and the Executive Councils of Bonaire, Saint Martin, Saint Eustatius, and Saba decide to use the "ZIS systeem," financing of a large portion of health care will become considerably easier.

NICARAGUA

GENERAL SITUATION AND TRENDS

Socioeconomic, Political, and Demographic Overview

Nicaragua is located in the middle of the Central American isthmus and has a surface area of 130,682 km². The country is divided topographically into three regions: Pacific, Atlantic, and central. The population is unevenly distributed. The majority is concentrated in the Pacific region, which occupies 15.3% of the national territory but has 61.5% of the total population (with poverty levels ranging from 5% to 24%) and 76.4% of the urban population. The central region, with 33.9% of the total area, has 32.6% of the population (with poverty levels ranging from 15% to 35%), with most inhabitants living in rural areas. The Atlantic region, which occupies 50.9% of the national territory, has only 5.9% of the total population (with poverty levels ranging from 35% to 45%).

The Government that was elected in 1990 inherited a country recovering from war, with a divided and polarized society. It had to address three major problems that demanded rapid solutions: putting a definitive end to the war, curbing hyperinflation, and laying the foundation for sustainable economic growth, which entailed resolving property ownership disputes and promoting private sector investment.

In addition to pursuing stabilization of the exchange rate and a restrictive monetary and credit policy, the core of the Government's economic adjustment program sought to reduce overall spending in the public sector to a level that could be financed out of regular revenues, foreign donations, bilateral loans, and credits from multilateral institutions. The adjustment plan also called for privatization of State-run enterprises, reduction in the number of public officials, and liberalization of international trade.

As of 1996, the Nicaraguan economy was continuing to grow at a sustained rate, as it had since 1994. This growth is a reflection of government efforts to consolidate stabilization programs with economic growth. In this context, the gross domestic product (GDP) rose for the third consecutive year, increasing 5.5% in 1996, the highest growth rate in 17 years. At the same time, the GDP per capita grew 2.3%.

Several factors contributed to growth of the GDP during 1996; the principal ones are macroeconomic stability, opening the economy to foreign investment, and the dynamics of the investment process in the private sector. The sectors that experienced the greatest growth were agriculture, fishing, manufacturing, construction, commerce, and services.

In 1996, the economically active population increased by 3.1%, similar to the previous year's growth. The employed population increased by 5.8%, and open unemployment decreased 8.8%, a trend that was consonant with the growth in the GDP. This was possible thanks to the program of public investment, the boom in industrial free trade, temporary employment programs implemented by the Fund for Emergency Social Investment, and creation of jobs in the agricultural sector.

During the first half of 1996, the average monthly inflation rate was 0.92%, higher than during the same period the previous year (0.77%). The rise in inflation began to slow in July, and by the third quarter it had dropped to an average of 0.13%; nevertheless, in the month of October the inflation rate was 2.6%, basically because of increases in the prices of beans, rice, and butane gas. In late 1996, the cost of the basic urban market basket of 53 products in the city of Managua was C$ 1,225.60—13.6% higher than in 1995.

In 1996 the wage policy in the public sector continued to be determined by the process of structural adjustment and reduction of spending that has been under way since 1991; salaries in the public sector have remained frozen. In the private sector, on the other hand, employers continued to apply a policy of market determination of wages, except for the legal minimum wage. The average nominal wage increased 9.1% at the national level with respect to the previous year, although for central government employees the increase was only 2.8%. Wages in the Nicaraguan Social Security Institute

(INSS) increased 7.6%, mainly because of adjustments in the private sector. The sectors in which wages increased the most were transportation, agriculture, and mining (23.4%, 14.7%, and 12.5%, respectively).

The volume of exports increased from an annual average of US$ 282 million in 1985–1989 to over US$ 500 million in 1995. That same year, the value of imports amounted to US$ 18 million. The per capita debt (US$ 2,600) exceeds annual per capita income (US$ 407).

The most important changes stemming from the economic policy applied during the period 1990–1996 include reduction of the foreign debt from US$ 10,220 million to US$ 5,517 million; elimination of hyperinflation, which ranged from 3.5% in 1992 to 11.1% in 1995; renewal of economic growth, which was 3.3% in 1994 and 4.2% in 1995; a fixed exchange rate with a 1% monthly margin of fluctuation; reduction of current spending in the nonfinancial public sector, from 42.5% of GDP in 1990 to 21% of GDP in 1994; growth of public investment as a percentage of GDP, from 2.5% in 1990 to 14.2% in 1994; privatization of foreign trade; reduction in the number of public employees by up to 60% in 1994; simplification of the tax system and reduction of tax rates in order to stimulate domestic and foreign public investment; completion of the privatization of State-run enterprises in 1995; opening of private banks in 1991; and establishment of a stock exchange.

The country's social policies have been guided by its economic adjustment policies and therefore have prioritized mechanisms to optimize social spending. Emergency social funds have been established to compensate for the reduction in earnings of the poorest groups, self-help activities have been promoted, and community efforts have become an important strategy for combating poverty. The Government has designed several programs to alleviate poverty, among them the Social Investment Fund, the National Reconciliation and Rehabilitation Program, the Action Fund for Oppressed Sectors, the Community Employment Fund, and the Cooperative Production Program.

Nicaragua is subdivided into 16 departments, 2 autonomous regions, and 145 rural or semiurban *municipios.* Starting in 1990, in the context of State reforms, a process of decentralization was launched with a view to strengthening the *municipios* as the principal managers of local socioeconomic development and providers of basic services. According to the 1995 census, the population totaled 4,139,486 and women made up 52% of the total. As for age structure, 45.4% of the population belonged to the group aged 0–14 years, 51.8% to the group aged 15–64, and 2.8% to the group 65 and over. The results of a quality-of-life survey carried out by the National Statistics and Census Institute (INEC) in 1993 indicated that 75% of Nicaraguan households had one or more unmet basic needs and 44% lived in conditions of extreme

poverty. In rural areas, the proportion of households in extreme poverty was 60%.

In 1996 the economically active population numbered 1,534,100 (34% of the total population), of which 58% were male and 42% were female. The unemployed population totaled 245,600 inhabitants (16.1%), of which 45% were male and 55% were female.

Life expectancy at birth increased from 48.5 years in the period 1960–1965 to 66.2 years in 1990–1995. In rural areas, life expectancy is almost 10 years lower, although females have a higher life expectancy than males. The estimated birth rate for the period 1990–1995 was 40.5 per 1,000, and the fertility rate was 5.0 children per woman.

Until the 1940s, the population grew at a moderate rate, but then the country entered a phase of demographic transition, characterized by a steady decline in total mortality, which fell from 22.7 per 1,000 in 1950–1955 to 6.8 per 1,000 in 1990–1995, and a considerable decrease in fertility, which dropped from 7.3 children per woman in 1950–1955 to 5.0 in 1990–1995. As a consequence of these changes, the natural population growth rate accelerated and remained at an annual average rate of around 3% until the end of the 1980s. Hence, the size of the national population tripled between 1950 and 1990, rising from 1.1 million people in 1950 to 3.6 million in 1990 and to 4.1 million in 1995.

Between 1940 and 1995, as a result of a steady migration from the country to the cities, the percentage of the population living in urban areas gradually increased from 30% to 57%. Nicaragua has thus become a predominantly urban country, although a large proportion of the population in the capital city is of rural origin.

Internal migration takes place, for the most part, from rural to urban areas. The department of Managua receives almost 40% of internal migrants, but it attracts fewer migrants than it did 20 years ago. In rural areas, internal migration flows toward new agricultural areas. According to INEC, 80% of these migrants lack any type of public health care services. It is estimated that in the period 1985–1995 more than 350,000 people migrated from one area of the country to another.

Most migrants to urban areas are women (60% of all migrants and 67% in the 15–29 age range, according to the 1995 census). In 1995, 59% of all migrant women worked in the commerce and service sectors, and 27% were unemployed. As a consequence of diminishing economic activity in the country starting in 1990, especially agricultural exports, the volume of migration to Costa Rica began to exceed that of internal seasonal migration. It is estimated that there are currently some 350,000 illegal Nicaraguan immigrants in Costa Rica and that 20,000–30,000 people emigrate there annually. The departments of Chontales, Boaco, Matagalpa, Estelí, León, and Granada generate more than 65% of all migration, internal as well as international.

Mortality Profile

Of all the variables of population growth, the reduction in mortality is the demographic component that has had the greatest impact on the size and age structure of the population. Underregistration of mortality in 1995 was estimated at 56%. Based on the Sociodemographic Survey of 1985 (ESDENIC-85), the total mortality rate was estimated at 10.1 per 1,000 population. The leading causes of death in the period 1990–1995 were diseases of the circulatory system, intestinal infectious diseases, and certain conditions originating in the perinatal period. The number of deaths reported by the National Vital Statistics System (SINEVI) has shown a decrease since 1985, which may indicate an increase in underreporting. However, in the groups aged under 1 year, 1–4 years, and over 45 years, the rates have remained more or less stable. For the period 1990–1995, the annual crude death rate is estimated at 6.8 per 1,000 population, with an average of 28,000 deaths annually. The percentage of deaths certified by a doctor is 50%, and the percentage of deaths attributed to "signs, symptoms, and ill-defined conditions" is 5%.

In 1984, the official statistics on maternal mortality indicated a rate of 47 per 100,000 live births, a figure that reflects significant underregistration. In 1988, based on indirect evaluations, the real rate was estimated at 87 per 100,000 live births, and in 1990 it was estimated at around 100 per 100,000. The statistical yearbooks and time series of the Ministry of Health reveal only hospital death rates, which ranged from 95 maternal deaths per 100,000 live births in 1983 to 73 in 1987, with a high of 106 in 1985. Since 1988, the reported rates have included deaths occurring in health care institutions as well as at home.

In 1991, under the Master Health Plan, it was estimated that maternal mortality was around 150 per 100,000 live births. This figure was derived on the basis of data from SINEVI, after correcting for underregistration and adjusting for the total mortality rates estimated by INEC. An analysis done in 1995 of the period 1991–1995 indicates that maternal mortality increased from 93 to 155 per 100,000 live births. This increase reflects the effort to improve data collection at the local level, but it also shows that much remains to be done in this area. The causes of maternal death are associated with conditions that generally develop in the last half of pregnancy, including hemorrhage, hypertension, and sepsis, although abortion is also an important cause. High maternal mortality rates are linked to the prevalence of several reproductive risk factors in the female population, notably the large number of children per woman and high specific fertility rates in women under 19 and over 35 years of age. Adolescent pregnancy accounts for almost 28% of all pregnancies.

SPECIFIC HEALTH PROBLEMS

Analysis by Population Group

Health of Children

The ESDENIC-85 survey estimated the infant mortality rate at 71.8 per 1,000 live births; for 1996, the rate was estimated at 58 per 1,000 live births. Infant mortality rates in the departments of Matagalpa, Jinotega, León, and Chinandega are higher than the national average; the departments of Madriz, New Segovia, Estelí, Masaya, Rivas, Chontales, and Boaco have moderately high rates, around the national average; and the department of Managua has rates below the national average.

Deaths of children under 1 year of age constituted 28.7% and 30.8% of all deaths in 1988 and 1990, respectively, and 24.1% in 1991. The trend has been downward, and for 1996 it is estimated that the proportion decreased to about 21%. The leading causes of death among children under the age of 1 year are intestinal infectious diseases, certain conditions originating in the perinatal period, acute respiratory infections, congenital anomalies, and malnutrition.

In 1995, children under 5 accounted for 5% of all deaths. In 1995, the population aged 5–14 made up about 30% of the total population and accounted for 3.5% of all registered deaths. Several communicable diseases—which are associated with poverty and unmet basic needs—continue to account for a significant proportion of mortality (31.3%), and the proportion of deaths due to accidents and violence (30.2%) and to degenerative diseases (10%) is increasing.

Health of Adolescents

The adolescent population includes the group aged 10–19 years, which makes up 25.6% of the total population. It is estimated that 38.8% of adolescents aged 15–19 are employed and that the specific fertility rate for adolescents is the highest in Central America. Normal childbirth was associated with most of the discharges among female adolescents; among males the main causes are appendicitis and fractures resulting from accidents. The main causes of death for both sexes are accidents, drowning, suicide, and self-inflicted injuries.

Workers' Health

The number of workers registered by the Department of Occupational Risks within the INSS decreased from 214,675 in 1992 to 203,489 in 1995; 3,430 and 3,275 work-related accidents were reported in those two years, respectively. The number of deaths recorded in the Registry of Work-Related Accidents maintained by the Ministry of Labor decreased from 27 in 1992 to 11 in 1996.

Responsibility for health care for workers has been transferred from the Ministry of Labor to the Ministry of Health, which has a special occupational health program within the Department of Public Health, but the program lacks an operational plan. As of the 1995 census, all persons over the age of 10 years are considered members of the economically active population (EAP). This decision reflects the economic reality of the country—which is predominantly agricultural—and the fact that many children work. Some 24,000 children aged 10–14 work in the informal sector and 6,000 work in the formal sector.

Eighty percent of chemical products used in the country are pesticides. In 1996 the rate of acute pesticide poisoning was 58 per 100,000 population, although it is estimated that up to 9.6% of cases are unreported.

Analysis by Type of Disease or Health Impairment

Communicable Diseases

Vector-Borne Diseases. Malaria cases, which had decreased from 35,785 in 1990 to 27,653 in 1991 and to 26,866 in 1992, increased to 47,798 in 1993 and to 70,235 cases in 1995, a national record. The number of cases of malaria due to *Plasmodium falciparum* also increased that year (2,926 cases and 16 deaths). The parasite distribution in 1995 was 4.41% *P. falciparum* and 95.6% *Plasmodium vivax*. One of every four cases of malaria in the country occurs in the city of Managua. Transmission is favored by factors such as rural-to-urban migration; the emergence of squatter settlements in unsanitary areas; an increase in rainfall during recent years, with the consequent formation of immense swamps in Managua's coastal areas; high turnover of the personnel who work in vector control activities; shortage of resources, including transportation and supplies; and a lack of intra- and interinstitutional coordination.

Dengue has been endemic in Nicaragua since 1985, and outbreaks of the illness have occurred in various areas of the country. As of 15 October 1994, vector control measures have been centralized and activities aimed at eliminating breeding sites in the city of Managua have been stepped up, with a view to reducing transmission of the disease. Serotype 4 was introduced into the country in 1992–1993, and serotype 3 followed in 1994, causing an epidemic with 20,469 reported cases, 1,511 hospitalizations, and 6 deaths; the departments of León and Managua were most heavily affected. In 1995, a total of 19,260 cases of dengue were reported, but the number

dropped to 2,792 in 1996 (a reduction of 82%). Only 10% to 15% of the dengue cases reported are laboratory confirmed. One of the components of epidemic surveillance that is most in need of improvement is laboratory confirmation through a system of sampling.

On 19 October 1995 the epidemiological surveillance system of León reported the death of six people who resided in the *municipio* of Achuapa, all from an acute febrile illness that quickly evolved into a severe respiratory disorder. On 6 November, the Minister of Health, with support from the United States Centers for Disease Control and Prevention, identified the causal agent and reported that the disease was leptospirosis. During the months of October and November, in the *municipios* of Achuapa and El Sauce, 17,847 patients were examined and 1,904 suspected cases of leptospirosis were detected. Between October and November the total number of probable deaths due to leptospirosis reached 48 in the country as a whole. The ages of the victims ranged from 4 to 60 years; the average age was 18. The male/female ratio of cases was 1.4:1. A large-scale study of the animal population is currently under way; preliminary results of pathological-anatomical studies indicate that 90% of the rats captured in Achuapa had leptospires in their renal tissue. In addition, serologic tests in dogs have shown high titers of antibodies to the *canicola* serovar.

Between 1994 and 1996, a total of 2,723 cases of leishmaniasis were reported: 2,605 cases of cutaneous leishmaniasis, 76 of the mucocutaneous form, and 42 of visceral leishmaniasis. Between 1988 and 1996, the parasitology laboratory of the National Diagnosis and Reference Center diagnosed 44 cases of visceral leishmaniasis in the country. The magnitude of underreporting of information was demonstrated by a study conducted by the nongovernmental organization Médicos del Mundo [Doctors of the World] of Spain, which carried out active case finding over three months in coordination with the integrated local health system (SILAIS) of Río San Juan and found 1,140 cases of cutaneous and mucocutaneous leishmaniasis in only three *municipios*. That figure was higher than the 946 cases registered by the national reporting system in 1996 for the entire year. In addition, several cases of atypical cutaneous leishmaniasis, a clinical variant of cutaneous leishmaniasis, were detected for the first time in the country in 1996.

Between 1992 and 1996 the National Blood Center of the Nicaraguan Red Cross detected 358 donors who were seropositive for *Trypanosoma cruzi;* 249 of them could not be confirmed externally because of a lack of resources.

Rabies and Other Zoonoses. An average of two cases of urban human rabies occurred per year during the 1970s, three cases per year in the 1980s, and one case per year in 1990–1996 period. The incidence of canine rabies was 150 cases per year in the 1970s, 83 cases per year in the 1980s, and 39 cases per year in the period 1990–1996. The departments of Managua, León, Masaya, Granada, and Chinandega have the highest incidence of the disease.

Vaccine-Preventable Diseases. The incidence of vaccine-preventable diseases (poliomyelitis, measles, whooping cough, diphtheria, and tetanus) has shown a downward trend in recent years as a result of the increase in vaccination coverage, which in 1996 was 94% for polio vaccine, 83% for DTP, 83% for measles vaccine, and 100% for BCG among children under 1. The last case of poliomyelitis was reported in 1982, and eradication of the disease was certified in 1994.

The last measles epidemic occurred in 1990, when 18,225 cases (37% in persons over the age of 10) and 772 deaths were reported. That year, measles accounted for 6% of all deaths from all causes at the national level. In recent years, the incidence has diminished, thanks to the implementation of elimination strategies, and it has been more than three years since a case was confirmed in the laboratory. In 1994, 587 suspected cases were reported; in 1995, 195; and in 1996, 302. However, measles was ruled out in all these cases.

The last case of diphtheria was reported in 1987. Whooping cough remains endemic, but the number of reported cases decreased from 242 in 1990 to 14 in 1996.

The number of reported cases of neonatal tetanus fell from 90 in 1980 to 17 in 1990 and to 1 in 1996. Since 1990, efforts have been under way to increase the coverage of vaccination with two doses of tetanus toxoid among women of childbearing age throughout the country and especially in known high-risk areas.

Cholera and Other Intestinal Diseases. According to SINEVI, 2,166 deaths from diarrhea were registered in 1990, 75.6% among children under 1 year old. In 1991, the cholera control campaign yielded a reduction of 45% in deaths in the various age groups compared with 1990; among children under 1, the reduction was 48%. In 1993 and 1994, the surveillance system registered 255,000 and 264,366 cases of diarrhea, respectively. Up to 1990, the number of deaths exceeded 2,000 annually; in the period 1991–1996, the number of deaths decreased to an average of 1,000 annually. In the period 1993–1995, an average of 7,677 cases of cholera and 172 deaths were reported annually. In 1996, 2,979 cases and 82 deaths were reported (a reduction of 61% with respect to the average number of cases during the period 1993–1995 and a reduction of 52% in relation to the average number of deaths during the same period).

Chronic Communicable Diseases. In the 1990–1995 period, an average of 2,836 cases of tuberculosis and 230 deaths were registered each year. The cure rate increased to 81%, and the treatment abandonment rate dropped to 7%. In 1995, the number of deaths decreased to 185, compared to the average for the period 1990–1995, with a mortality rate of 4.5 per 100,000 and an incidence of 69 per 100.000. To date, no representative studies on the prevalence of HIV infection and AIDS among tuberculosis patients have been conducted.

As of 1995, the reported prevalence of leprosy was 0.997 case per 10,000 population. There were 413 cases of the disease, distributed in 11 SILAIS, of which 45% were in Managua, 27% were in Chinandega, and 10% were in León.

Acute Respiratory Infections. During the period 1993–1995, an average of 1 million cases of acute respiratory infections were reported annually; the average number of deaths during that period was 1,200.

AIDS and Other STDs. Between 1987 and the first half of 1995, a total of 96 cases of HIV infection and 114 cases of AIDS were detected. Of the AIDS patients, 71 died during that period; 91% of those affected were under 44 years of age. Of the total number of cases, 86% were in males and 14% were in females, with a male/female ratio of 6:1. Sexual transmission accounted for 94% of the cases; 54% were in heterosexuals, 25% in homosexuals, and 15% in bisexuals. With regard to geographic distribution of cases, 54% occurred in the department of Managua; 6% each in the departments of Chinandega, León, and Rivas; 5.2% in New Segovia; and fewer than 3% in the rest of the country.

In 1995, 9 cases of congenital syphilis and 490 cases of acquired syphilis were reported, making the incidence 0.2 per 100,000 live births and 11.8 per 100,000 population, respectively.

Noncommunicable Diseases and Other Health-Related Problems

Between 1992 and 1995, mortality from cardiovascular diseases increased from 64.0 to 71.0 per 100,000 population; mortality from malignant neoplasms, from 26.6 to 28.5; mortality from hypertensive disease, from 3.1 to 10.8; and mortality from diabetes mellitus, from 8.9 to 9.6 per 100,000 population.

Nutritional Diseases and Diseases of Metabolism. According to the National Survey on Micronutrient Deficiencies carried out in Nicaragua in 1993, the caloric intake of Nicaraguan children was only 88.9% of the recommended daily allowance. The survey found that almost one of every three children suffers from vitamin A deficiency and iron-deficiency anemia; two of every three preschool children suffer from, or are at risk for, vitamin A deficiency; and one of every three adult women suffers from anemia, caused mainly by iron deficiency. The deficiencies in intake of calories, iron, and vitamin A can be attributed to insufficient availability and access, both geographic and economic, as well as to cultural attitudes that may limit the consumption of available vegetables. High rates of morbidity, especially from infectious diseases (diarrheal diseases and acute respiratory infections), also contribute to the prevalence of micronutrient deficiencies in children.

RESPONSE OF THE HEALTH SYSTEM

National Health Plans and Policies

The mission of the Ministry of Health is to ensure that the population has access to health services that respond to their real and perceived needs and that the health system emphasizes health promotion and prevention of disease through an integrated and humane approach. The major challenges that the Ministry of Health must address in order to fulfill its mission and advance the process of institutional reform are to incorporate new modalities of organization and administration, adopt new financing alternatives, modernize hospitals, promote the protection of investments in infrastructure and equipment, establish and provide a basic package of essential services, prioritize high-risk areas and groups, promote health and prevent diseases, achieve efficiency in the use of resources, and improve management control systems. Work is under way to develop a new health care model that will approach health problems through a preventive, integrated, interprogrammatic, and participatory strategy that addresses risk factors. The country's health profile indicates that priority should continue to be assigned to women and children and that greater attention should be given to adolescents and the elderly. The emphasis in health care for women is on the reproductive stage of life, and the services offered focus on family planning; care during pregnancy, childbirth, and the puerperium; and timely detection of cervical cancer and breast cancer. Health care for children includes monitoring of growth and development, diet and nutritional status, and difficult circumstances that affect child health. For adolescents, prevention of drug addiction and of early and unwanted pregnancy is stressed. Health care for the elderly emphasizes self-care, prevention, and timely treatment of complications as well as solidarity and the responsibility of society for the elderly.

The Constitution of the Republic, the law creating the Unified National Health System, and the provisions contained in various international agreements and instruments form the basic legal and conceptual framework for health care in Nicaragua. However, many laws and legal provisions have become obsolete as a result of the developments that have taken place in the health sector, heightened concern for the environment, the need for regulation of foods and drugs, and increased attention to patients' rights.

Organization of the Health Sector

The Ministry of Health is the main provider of health services. It is estimated that the social security system covers 5% of the population and the private sector covers 4%. The Ministry of Health has 873 primary health care units, with potential coverage of approximately 3 million people. Despite the progress made in enhancing the organization of the public health services system, problems persist, notably the shortage of medical and nonmedical supplies, infrastructure and equipment deficiencies, unplanned growth of the units, lack of technical-administrative guidelines, unmet demand for some services, saturation of hospital capacity, and low productivity and inadequate distribution of human resources.

During the 1980s, the infrastructure of the Nicaraguan Social Security Institute and its health resources were transferred to the State and came under the control and administration of the Ministry of Health.

Since 1992, health insurance plans funded by workers, employers, and the State have purchased health services for the insured and their dependents from organized service providers. This model has permitted greater participation by the private sector in the health services market. The INSS continues to play its traditional role as collector of insurance fees, but it has transferred responsibility for health care activities to the 32 health insurance companies. The INSS serves as facilitator and supervisor of health activities in order to assure adherence to minimum quality standards in the delivery of services. The establishment of this health insurance model has made it possible to extend coverage at the national level to 110,269 active plan participants nationwide. The INSS provides 71.3% of the total insurance coverage, reaching 290,000 persons nationwide.

Although the exact magnitude of the private subsystem is unknown, it is estimated that it covers approximately 4% of the total population. The private health care infrastructure consists of 7 hospitals with 200 beds, 200 outpatient clinics, and an unknown number of laboratories and pharmacies.

In the context of State reform, the principal institutions that make up the health sector (the Ministry of Health, the INSS, the nonprofit and for-profit private sector, the Military Health Service, and the various training institutions) are reexamining their strategies with a view to finding better responses to the health problems of the population. The Ministry of Health has introduced needed changes and has decentralized functions to its intermediate structures—the integrated local health care systems (SILAIS)—although further change is required in order to achieve equity, efficiency, and effectiveness. The social security system has been reoriented toward financing and regulating the medical insurance companies, from which it purchases a basic package of services for its affiliates. The Ministry of Health, through its health care units, provides free care for conditions not covered by the basic package. At present, no services are being provided under the health insurance model to pensioners or retirees, who continue to be covered by the Ministry of Health.

Private medicine has suffered from the country's economic crisis, competition from nonprofit centers, and the development of private services in public hospitals. This situation is exacerbated by the lack of alternative forms of organization for private health care, such as cooperatives, private medical insurance, or prepaid plans. Recently, the number of nongovernmental organizations that provide health services has grown, mainly in the fields of women's reproductive health and health education. These nongovernmental organizations coordinate their activities with the local health systems, although no official coordination mechanism exists. Both the Ministry of Health and the INSS finance services for those they insure, and both institutions regulate the operation of health establishments.

Hospitals currently face two main types of problems: shortages in the supply of basic products (drugs, materials that must be periodically replaced, and linens and clothing), a problem associated with deterioration of the physical infrastructure, and lack of motivation on the part of doctors because of extremely low salaries.

Health Services and Resources

Organization of Services for Care of the Population

Water Supply and Sewerage Systems. The water available for human consumption is sufficient to meet the population's needs. In 1996, 82.4% of the urban population and 30.1% of the rural population had drinking water service. In rural areas, the coverage level has not increased since 1992 because the services and the population have grown at about the same rate. Although much of the urban population continues to be served through household connections, 23.4% receive water from public hydrants. The number of urban and municipal water supply systems has remained at 148. In 1990, 70% of these systems obtained water from underground sources; the remaining 30% used surface sources.

The Nicaraguan Institute of Water Supply and Sewerage Systems (INAA) administers 19 sewerage systems, of which only 7 have their own treatment facilities (stabilization ponds). Lack of treatment and improper final disposal of wastewater pose a serious risk to the environment and to human health. In the city of Managua, for example, domestic and industrial wastewater is discharged on the banks of Xolotlán Lake without any treatment.

During the 1981–1992 period, the percentage of the population with sewerage services in urban areas decreased from 32% to 29.9%. However, in 1996 the proportion rose again to 32.6%.

The estimated number of housing units in the country, as of 1992, was 621,926, of which 46.6% received drinking water from water supply systems administered by INAA, 21.5% from excavated wells, 12.7% from rivers and ponds, 15.5% from public hydrants, and 3.9% from cistern trucks. As for disposal of excreta and wastewater, 21.9% of the housing units were connected to sewerage systems, 8.1% had cesspools or septic tanks, 55.7% had latrines, and 14.2% had no system.

Solid Waste Disposal. Urban sanitation services for collection and final disposal of solid waste are supplied in 69 of the 143 municipal city seats, which, in terms of urban population coverage, represents approximately 35%. With a daily per capita production of solid waste equivalent to 0.5 kg, it is estimated that the urban population produces 1,272.5 metric tons of waste per day; if only about 35% of that amount is collected and eliminated, then there are 827 metric tons of waste in urban areas that are not being properly removed. The waste collected is not being properly disposed of because appropriate environmental impact assessment criteria and techniques are not being applied for selection of sites for municipal waste dumps. In addition, waste disposal is largely unregulated, and only 13% of waste dumps have been certified as sanitary sites. Solid waste is disposed of in open-air dumps, with no planning or control, and no treatment, recovery, or recycling methods are applied.

Environmental Protection. There has been a progressive deterioration of natural resources in rural areas, mainly because of aggressive development of new agricultural lands, use of forest lands for agricultural purposes, felling trees for fuel, lack of legislation on use of land and natural resources, and inappropriate farming techniques. It is estimated that deforestation affects some 100,000 hectares of forest per year.

Organization and Operation of Personal Health Care Services

With the exception of some remote areas, the coverage of health services is adequate. The health center is the most frequent source of outpatient care. Health posts, which were designed to be the first point of contact at the primary care level, are used very little, probably because of a lack of personnel and insufficient drugs.

For operation of the SILAIS, the country has 873 service provider units at the primary care level, including 708 health posts, 165 health centers, and 589 beds. At the secondary care level, there are 24 hospitals with 3,930 beds for acute cases and 4 hospitals with 407 beds for chronic cases, for a total of 4,337 hospital beds (1 bed per 968 population).

During the five-year period between 1991 and 1995, the number of patient visits to primary and secondary health care facilities rose from 4.9 million (1.2 visits per person) in 1991 to 6.5 million (1.5 visits per person) in 1995, an increase of 30%. During the first three years of that period, the primary care level accounted for 70% of the total care provided, and in 1995 it accounted for 75%, which appears to indicate greater use of this level; the remaining 25% of care was provided at the secondary level and includes emergency care.

Maternal and child health care showed an increase in absolute figures, consistent with the growth in the target population. Although the number of first prenatal visits decreased 4% overall, the number of first prenatal visits in the first trimester of pregnancy increased 3%, and total prenatal visits showed an upward trend, with relative growth of 29%.

The percentage of hospital deliveries was 45.0% in 1995, lower than the figure of 46% registered in 1991. The highest percentage during the period was achieved in 1993, when 49% of births took place in health care institutions.

In 1995, visits to monitor growth and development increased 20% for children under the age of 1 year and 48% for children aged 1–5 years, as compared to 1991.

Inpatient services (as measured by hospital discharges) increased from 228,000 in 1991 to around 278,000 in 1995. In 1995, acute-care hospitals accounted for 87% of total discharges. The use of bed resources in these hospitals has improved markedly, as evidenced by the fact that the occupancy rate increased from 63.7% in 1991 to 74.2% in 1995, with no increase in the number of beds in these centers since 1992. Hospital discharges per 100 population rose from 5.6 in 1991 to 6.2 in 1995; childbirth was associated with approximately 30% of all discharges.

An increase in major surgeries took place as a result of improvements in operating rooms in 16 hospitals in the country. A noteworthy development was the introduction of outpatient surgery services in hospitals. Previously, the vast majority of surgical procedures were carried out in operating rooms, but beginning in 1991–1992 some procedures began to be performed in delivery and emergency rooms. The most common procedures are laparoscopies for sterilization and ophthalmologic surgeries, but cesarean sections, appendectomies, and herniorrhaphies are also performed.

The number of laboratory tests increased from 3.4 million in 1991 to 5.0 million in 1995, including tests performed at both the primary and secondary levels of care, although the

secondary level accounts for a greater proportion (59% of the total number).

Geographic access to health services is acceptable in urban areas. In Managua, only 13% of the population lives more than 30 minutes' walking distance from a health unit. The figure is 8% in other urban areas of the country. In rural areas, the situation is radically different: the percentage of the population that lives more than two hours' walking distance from a health unit is 33% in the case of hospitals, 22% for health centers, 10% for health posts, and 26% for private physicians.

A growing market of private services exists, but the Ministry of Health continues to be the main provider of services for the Nicaraguan population as a whole. A study of health care financing options identified a sizable private sector that provides care that is more costly but of better quality. Although the social security system offers medical services to approximately 5% of the population, its resources are insufficient and the basic basket of services that it provides is limited. Social security affiliates who have more serious health problems must seek care in health facilities of the Ministry of Health, but there are no agreements for the transfer of funds, so delivery of these services constitutes a de facto subsidy of the social security system.

A study demonstrated that many users pay directly for a significant proportion of the total cost of health services, even in the public sector. Widespread payment for private services, direct payment to public health care providers, and frequent purchases of drugs and supplies by users of public services result in significant out-of-pocket expenditures, which are an important source of health care financing without which the public sector would face tremendous fiscal pressure and users would receive even fewer services. The weight of these economic contributions, however, is not distributed evenly or equitably. In poor rural areas of Nicaragua, families tend to suffer more illness but seek less medical attention than those in urban areas who have higher incomes. In the rural population, the increase in payment for services in public facilities has led to a significant reduction in the use of these services, which has been only slightly offset by patients seeking care from other sources. In the urban population, on the other hand, especially in Managua, similar relative increases have led to changes in the mix of the public services used as well as greater substitution of care from other sources and only a small reduction in overall use of services.

Inputs for Health

The country's policies on pharmaceutical products promote the best possible use of low-cost generic drugs. The essential drugs list contains 234 products; 137 essential drugs are specified for health centers and 19 for health posts. Often, however, these essential drugs are not available in health centers, which leads to inefficiency in the delivery of care and tends to discredit the health services. Medical prescriptions are required for the dispensing of drugs.

In principle, drugs for the care of mothers and children and drugs used in the treatment of diseases targeted by public health programs, such as tuberculosis, malaria, dengue, and sexually transmitted diseases, can be obtained free of charge in health centers. Nevertheless, these drugs are not always available.

Recent studies indicate that the availability of drugs ranges from 60% to 70% of need. The average amount spent on drugs per episode of illness is C$ 30.00 for children aged 0–5 years and C$ 65.00 for those over the age of 6 years. Self-medication and irrational use of drugs are common. Government spending on drugs totaled US$ 32.2 million in 1989 and US$ 14.2 million in 1993.

Human Resources

The sector has 16,642 health professionals and technicians: 4,551 physicians, 4,817 nursing auxiliaries (with one year of training), 2,577 nurses, 2,499 technicians, 1,099 dentists, and 1,099 pharmacists. In 1990 there were 1 professional nurse and 2.57 nursing auxiliaries per doctor; in 1995, the ratios were 0.38 and 1.66 per doctor, respectively. The ratio of other health technicians per doctor decreased from 4.08 in 1990 to 0.69 in 1995. While the number of doctors has risen steadily, the numbers of nurses, nursing auxiliaries, and technicians are declining. The Ministry of Health no longer assumes responsibility for training health personnel, and severe budgetary constraints have limited the capacity of universities and technical schools to offer such training.

Although, in general, medical and paramedical personnel are well trained, 32% of Ministry of Health personnel have only a primary-school education or basic reading and writing skills. Low wages and inappropriate policies on promotion and retention of personnel, together with physical and financial limitations, result in high personnel turnover.

Expenditures and Sectoral Financing

Resources for health come from six main sources: grants to the Government (which finance 30.1% of total health spending), expenditures of private companies (21.2%), taxes (16.1%), loans to the Government (15.8%), expenditures by households (11.9%), and grants to nongovernmental organizations (4.9%). The uninsured population accounts for 66.1% of total health spending; the insured population, for 27%; and the population with purchasing power in the private sector, for 6.9%. By institution, Ministry of Health facilities account for 61.3% of the total; the medical insurance companies, for 27%; private hospitals, for 6.9%; and nongovernmental organizations that provide health services, for 4.8%. In 1995, health spending represented 6.6% of GDP and 16.2% of total public spending. Current spending consumes 97% of the resources, and investment accounts for only 3%.

PANAMA

GENERAL SITUATION AND TRENDS

Socioeconomic, Political, and Demographic Overview

Panama has an area of 75,517 km² and is divided into 9 provinces, 67 districts or municipalities, 3 indigenous regions, and 512 mayoral jurisdictions. The Panama Canal, an 80-km-long interocean waterway, connects the Atlantic with the Pacific across one of the narrowest places on the continental isthmus.

According to the last National Population and Housing Census, in 1990 the country's population was a little more than 2.3 million. The annual growth rate during the 1980s was estimated at 2.6%. The population density is 34.9 inhabitants per km². The estimated population in 1995 was 2.63 million, 49.5% of whom were women and 50.5% men. One-third of the population is younger than 15 years of age, 2.3% are children under 1 year of age, and 9.3% are 1 to 4 years of age. A population of 2.8 to 2.9 million is projected for the year 2000, assuming an annual population growth rate of 2.1% during the 1990s. More than half the population (53%) resides in urban areas.

The estimated birth rate for 1995 was 23.1 births per 1,000 inhabitants (29.1 in rural areas and 20 in urban areas). The total fertility rate is 2.76 children per woman.

The majority of the population is made up of nonindigenous groups (91%), which include Hispanics (the majority), descendants of African slaves, and descendants of African slaves from the West Indies. The rest of the population is indigenous (9%), divided among five groups: Kuna, Emberá and Wounaan, Ngobe-Buglé (previously known as Guaymíes), Bokotas, and Teribes.

In 1995 Panama's economically active population totaled about 1 million people, 61% of whom were in Panamá City. Women represent 37% of the economically active population. The employment rate for women increased from 37.7% in the late 1980s to 41.3% in 1994. Of the total number of employees, 75% were concentrated in the Panamá City metropolitan area. The average wage for women is 87% of that for men.

The overall open unemployment rate declined from 14.7% in 1992 to 13.7% in 1995, when 10.5% of the men and 20.1% of the women were unemployed. Unemployment is higher in urban areas (15.8%) than in the countryside (10.6%).

In 1995 the gross national product (GNP) was estimated at US$ 7,144 million, or US$ 2,746 per capita. GNP grew at an annual rate of 7% during the 1990–1994 period. However, the annual rate of increase in employment was only 4.5%; as a result, unemployment fell only 2.4% each year.

At the end of 1995, the public debt was approximately US$ 5,708 million, equivalent to 81% of the GNP and distributed in the following manner: 63%, the private banking sector; 13%, multilateral debt; 10%, bilateral debt; and 14%, foreign bond holders and assorted lenders.

Of the US$ 3,789 million in public expenditures in 1995, almost half (US$ 1,566 million) was allocated to social services. Spending on health and education was equivalent to 12.8% of the GNP or 24.4% of public spending in 1995, approximately US$ 317 per capita.

The distribution of income is very uneven. The bottom 10% of the population receives only 0.5% of the total income of the country, while the top 10% receives 42.2%. In urban areas, the bottom 40% of lower-income households receive 6% of the total income. In rural areas the poor distribution of land and the lack of access to basic services exacerbate the situation.

In 1995 it was estimated that 40% of the population lived in poverty, which represents an improvement over 1991, when the figure was calculated at 49%. It is estimated that in 1995 18.1% of the general population and 15.9% in the metropolitan region lived in extreme poverty. In districts such as La Mesa, Sambú, Las Palmas, Las Minas, Santa Fe, and Tolé, it was estimated that more than 90% of the population was living in poverty. Of the households headed by women, 71% live in poverty in rural areas and 48% in urban areas.

The total illiteracy rate was 10.7% in 1990. The rate was 15.0% in rural areas, 3.3% in urban areas, and 44.3% among the indigenous population. School enrollment for 1995 was 362,877 students, representing a net coverage of 91% of the school-age population.

Life expectancy at birth rose from 70.1 years in 1980 to 72.7 in 1990 and 73.4 in 1995. For urban areas it was 75.1 years and in rural areas, 71.5; for women it was 75.4 years and for men, 71.0 years.

The death rate in 1995 was 4.2 deaths per 1,000 population, with an estimated rate of 5.2 after adjusting for underreporting. Of the 11,168 deaths recorded in 1995, 89.4% had medical certification. The leading causes of death were accidental injuries and violence (15%), malignant tumors (14%), cerebrovascular disease (11%), myocardial infarction (7%), and other ischemic heart disease (5%). These five causes accounted for 52% of all deaths.

Deaths from cardiovascular disease increased by 2% annually during the 1990–1994 period. These diseases are now one of the three leading causes of death. Diabetes mellitus increased by 8% annually during that same period and, if the trend continues, it will become one of the leading causes of death in the adult population.

Among the leading causes of morbidity in 1995, influenza and acute respiratory infections were in first place, with nearly half of the total, with diarrhea and intestinal parasitic diseases following far behind.

SPECIFIC HEALTH PROBLEMS

Analysis by Population Group

Health of Children

According to data from the Office of the Comptroller of the Republic, the infant mortality rate per 1,000 live births was 17.2 in 1992 and 18.0 in 1994. Infant mortality in 1994, adjusted for underreporting, was estimated at 18.9 per 1,000. The regional rates of infant mortality vary greatly, ranging from 9.9 per 1,000 live births in Herrera Province to 34.6 per 1,000 in Colón Province. In a 1994 study by the Ministry of Planning and Economic Policy, the infant mortality rate among the indigenous population was 84.1 per 1,000.

Among the 1,134 deaths registered with medical certification in children under 1 year of age in 1993, the leading cause of death was disorders originating during the perinatal period (9.1 per 1,000), followed by congenital abnormalities

(4.1), pneumonia (1.3), intestinal infections (0.8), and protein-calorie malnutrition (0.6).

Neonatal mortality declined from 12.0 per 1,000 live births in 1990 to 11.2 per 1,000 in 1994. The difference in rates between urban areas (12.8 per 1,000) and rural areas (9.6 per 1,000) is undoubtedly due to underreporting. Postneonatal mortality held stable between 1990 and 1994, when a rate of 6.8 per 1,000 live births was recorded (8.4 per 1,000 in rural areas and 5.2 in urban areas).

In 1992 the death rate for children under 5 years of age was 4.9 per 1,000. The leading causes were accidental injuries, other forms of violence, intestinal disorders, and pneumonia. The Prevalence of Malnutrition Survey that health institutions conducted in 1994 showed that 5.2% of the population under 5 years of age was suffering from moderate chronic malnutrition (below normal height-for-age) and 3.4% from serious chronic malnutrition.

Coverage of growth and development monitoring for children under 1 year of age was 94%, with an average of 2.8 physician office visits. For children from 1 to 4 years of age the coverage was 40.6%, with two consultations on average.

The 5–9-year-old age group constituted 11.3% of the estimated population in 1995. According to the fourth height census, done in 1994, 17.7% of this population exhibits moderate growth retardation and 6.2% serious growth retardation. Mortality in this age group was 0.4 per 1,000 in 1994. No significant differences were observed between boys and girls.

Health of Adolescents

Persons from 10 to 19 years of age accounted for 20.3% of the country's population in 1995. In 1994 the fertility rate for adolescent women aged 10 to 14 was 3.6 per 100,000, and 87.0 per 100,000 in the group aged 15 to 19. Of the total births, 0.7% corresponded to mothers aged 10 to 14 and 18.3% to those 15 to 19 years old.

It is estimated that in 1994 0.8% of the total abortions occurred in the 10–14 age group and 17.1% in the 15–19 group. These percentages declined in 1995 to 0.6% and 15.9%, respectively.

In the 10–14 age group, mortality was 37.6 per 100,000 in 1994, with no significant differences by sex. In the 15–19 age group, however, mortality was 88.1 per 100,000, with vast difference between the sexes: 108 in males and 53 in women.

A 1996 study among high school students 12 to 18 years old in Colón Province showed that 48% of this population consumed alcohol. In Panamá Province that percentage was 45%.

Health of Adults and the Elderly

The 15–60 age group represents 59.1% of the country's population. In this group the mortality rate was 2.3 per 1,000 in 1995. In the subgroup from 20 to 44 years of age, the leading causes of death in 1993–1995 were accidental injuries, suicides, homicides and other forms of violence (15%), malignant neoplasms (14%), cerebrovascular disease (11%), acute myocardial infarction (8%), and other ischemic heart disease (5%). In the group aged 45 to 59, the leading cause of death was cardiovascular disease, followed by cancer, accidental injuries and other forms of violence, and ischemic heart disease.

In 1995 the national maternal mortality rate was 5 per 10,000 live births. It was highest in the region of San Blas, of 44 per 10,000.

In 1993, 41% of women of childbearing age utilized some method of contraception (49% oral contraceptives and 37% intrauterine devices).

Persons 60 years old and over constituted 7.5% of the total estimated population in 1995. In this group the leading causes of death in 1995 were hypertension (33%), influenza (12%), the common cold (7%), gastritis (5%), and urinary tract infections (5%).

Workers' Health

The occupational health program of the Social Security Fund has reported a drop in workplace accidents among active contributors to the Fund. In 1993 a rate of 3.4 accidents per 100 active contributing workers was recorded; in 1996 the rate dropped to 2.8. Mining and quarrying produced the highest rates of work-related accidents in recent years, with a rate of 15.4 occupational accidents per 100 active contributing workers in 1996.

Between 1993 and 1996, occupational illness rates declined from 2.4 per 1,000 contributing workers to 1.2 per 1,000. Construction produced the highest rate of occupational illness in 1996, with a rate of 5.0 per 1,000 active contributors. In total, men have 20 times as many work-related accidents as do women. With regard to occupational illnesses, there are 6 male cases for every female case.

Health of the Disabled

According to the 1990 Population Census, some 30,000 Panamanians are disabled. To deal with disabilities, the country has established the Center for the Rehabilitation of Handicapped Persons and the Panamanian Institute for Special Training.

Health of Indigenous People

There are no specific disaggregated health indicators for the indigenous population, but the provinces with a predominantly indigenous population exhibit the worst conditions. In Bocas del Toro Province mortality from diarrhea was 34.4 per 100,000 in the last four years, some five times the national rate of 6.4. In the San Blas region the country's highest incidence of cholera was recorded in 1993. It was 14 per 10,000 population, some 80 times the nationwide level. The incidence of pneumonia in 1994 was 12 per 1,000, 6 times the nationwide rate.

Vector-borne diseases also have the highest rates in the regions populated primarily by indigenous groups. In 1996 the national rate for leishmaniasis was 0.96 per 1,000 inhabitants; in Bocas del Toro the rate was 7.75 per 1,000.

In the National Vitamin A Survey conducted in 1992, a 13% incidence of low retinol levels was found (<20 μg/dl) in the indigenous population aged 12 to 59 months. The incidence in the nonindigenous population was 5%.

Analysis by Type of Disease or Health Impairment

Communicable Diseases

Vector-Borne Diseases. Malaria in Panama is concentrated geographically, occurring mainly in rural areas and in the provinces located in the far eastern and western parts of the country. In the past three years more than 85% of the cases have occurred in the regions bordering Costa Rica and Colombia. In 1996, 25 *Plasmodium falciparum* cases and 451 *P. vivax* cases were detected. This 1996 *P. falciparum* incidence represents a 78% reduction from the 111 cases reported in 1992.

On 19 November 1993, Panama reported the first case of indigenous dengue since the 1940s. A total of 14 cases were reported in San Miguelito, a densely populated section of the Panamá City metropolitan area. The seroepidemiological survey conducted in and near the community five months after the first case showed a 5.7% incidence of antibodies for dengue, mainly in individuals more than 44 years old. Subsequently, 790 cases were recorded in 1994, 3,084 in 1995, and 812 in 1996. Dengue persists primarily in San Miguelito and in the Panamá City metropolitan area. In 1995 serotypes 1 and 3 circulated, and in 1996, serotype 1. In 1995 there were three cases and one death from dengue hemorrhagic fever.

Leishmaniasis, which was stable between 1993 and 1995 with a rate of 0.6 per 1,000, flared up in 1996, with 2,577 cases and a rate of 0.96 per 1,000. Those most affected were nursing infants and children under 5 years of age. No deaths from this disease were recorded between 1992 and 1996.

393

Chagas' disease began to show a clear decline in 1993. In 1996 a single case was recorded, in Herrera Province. The last deaths from this disease were recorded in 1993.

Vaccine-Preventable Diseases. The last cases of poliomyelitis were recorded in 1972 and of diphtheria, in 1981. The incidence of neonatal tetanus has shown a marked decline since 1993. In 1993, there were four cases; in 1994, two; in 1995, one; and in 1996, none.

Whooping cough is on the decline but outbreaks still occur in remote areas. In 1993, 209 cases were recorded. There were 44 cases in 1996, all from an outbreak in Bocas del Toro Province.

In 1993, 191 cases of measles were recorded. In 1994 and 1995, there were 19 cases each year and in 1996, none. In 1993, 8,344 cases of rubella were recorded and in 1996, 1,457. In 1993, 14 cases of congenital rubella syndrome were reported and in 1996, 11 cases. There were 1,204 cases of mumps in 1996. In 1995, 1,997 cases were recorded.

In children under 1 year of age, DTP vaccination coverage was 81.8% in 1993 and 91.6% in 1996. For polio vaccine, the rate of coverage was 83.0% in 1993 and 92.3% in 1996; for BCG, 91.6% in 1993 and 100.0% in 1996; and for measles, 82.7% in 1993 and 90.2% in 1996. The rate of coverage with tetanus toxoid for women of childbearing age remained low from 1992 to 1995, at around 24%. In the 1–4 age group, 58,956 children were vaccinated with the triple vaccine against measles, rubella, and mumps in 1993, representing a coverage rate of 24.3%. In 1996, this number increased to 100,474, for a coverage of 41.2%. Certain risk groups are vaccinated against hepatitis B and yellow fever.

Cholera and Other Intestinal Infectious Diseases. Cholera last occurred in the country in 1993, when 42 cases were recorded, all of them outside the Panamá City area.

The epidemiological surveillance system recorded 87,396 cases of diarrhea in 1993 and 107,661 cases in 1996. Mortality from diarrhea has remained stable, at 6 per 100,000. The most affected regions are Bocas del Toro and Veraguas, with rates of 34 and 13 per 100,000, respectively. The age groups with the highest mortality from diarrhea are those over 75 and those under 5, with rates of 57 and 29 per 100,000, respectively. There were 3,834 cases of intestinal amebiasis in 1995, with a rate of 146 per 100,000. Children under 1 year of age were the most affected, with a rate of 5.4 per 1,000.

Chronic Communicable Diseases. Pulmonary tuberculosis is clearly on the rise. In 1990 an incidence of 33 cases per 100,000 was recorded, increasing to 39 per 100,000 in 1994, and to 49.6 in 1996. The most affected group were people 65 and older, with an incidence of 102 per 100,000. Of the 1,017 cases of pulmonary tuberculosis recorded in 1995, 62.1%

were among men and 37.9% among women. The region most affected was Bocas del Toro, with an incidence of 139.9 per 100,000 population. Mortality from pulmonary tuberculosis remained relatively stable between 1992 and 1996, with 4.5 deaths per 100,000 population. Of the 137 deaths from tuberculosis recorded in 1996, 88% were due to pulmonary tuberculosis and 4% each to miliary tuberculosis and tubercular meningitis.

In 1992 a total of 133 cases of leprosy were recorded in Panama, representing 0.5 cases per 10,000. Multibacillary forms made up 61% of the cases and paucibacillary strains, 39%. In 1996, 36 cases were detected.

Acute Respiratory Infections. Among communicable diseases, acute respiratory infections are the most frequent cause of morbidity in children under the age of 5, responsible for 10% of their recorded deaths in 1994. Pneumonia was the second cause of mortality among communicable diseases, with an incidence of 200 per 100,000 in 1994 and 156 per 100,000 in 1995. Mortality was 9.8 per 100,000 in 1995. Most affected are people from 65 to 74 years of age, with an incidence of 27 per 100,000, and those aged 75 and older, with a rate of 235 per 100,000.

Rabies and Other Zoonoses. Cases of sylvatic rabies are still reported, transmitted mainly by vampire bats (especially *Desmodus rotundus*). In 1995, 71 cases were recorded in cattle and horses, 19 of them laboratory-confirmed. In 1996, 28 cases were laboratory-confirmed. In 1995, there were two cases of human rabies in gold prospectors in Darién Province, transmitted by vampire bats.

In 1995, after an eight-year absence, Eastern equine encephalitis re-emerged (serological diagnosis). In 1996, 12 cases were clinically diagnosed.

AIDS and Other STDs. The first case of AIDS was diagnosed in Panama in 1984. As of 1995, 1,044 cases had been recorded, with a case-fatality rate of 59.1%. In the 1984–1994 period, the greatest proportion of cases (74%) were found in the 20–44 age group, with a significant percentage (4%) also occurring in children under 5 years of age. Sexual transmission remains the most frequent route of infection (84%), with heterosexual exposure in 44% of the cases and homosexual/bisexual exposure in 40%. Blood-borne transmission from transfusions accounts for 1% of cases and perinatal exposure for 5%. Panamá Province is the most affected, with 77% of the cases.

Recorded cases of other sexually transmitted diseases declined between 1993 and 1996. Soft chancre went from 4.8 cases per 10,000 in 1993 to 2.9 in 1996. Symptomatic early syphilis fell from 5.8 to 2.0 per 10,000. Congenital syphilis exhibited rates of 0.5 and 0.2 per 1,000 live births in 1992 and

1996, respectively. In 1996, the rate for cases of gonorrhea was 88 per 100,000.

Noncommunicable Diseases and Other Health-Related Problems

Nutritional Diseases and Diseases of Metabolism. In 1994, a nutritional assessment was conducted that included a random sampling of 945 children under the age of 5 seen at health centers during a particular week, also chosen at random. At the end of the assessment, children who were 2 standard deviations below the average weight or height were categorized as malnourished. A 5.2% incidence of malnutrition was found for this age group according to weight-for-age, 3.4% according to weight-for-height, and 5.2% according to height-for-age.

Studies of the indigenous population indicate that approximately one-quarter of the children under 5 years of age are malnourished.

The National Survey of Multiple Indicators, conducted in 1996 with a sample of 1,569 children under 5, showed that 91.5% of the children studied had been breast-fed at some time and that 86% of infants under 6 months of age were then being breast-fed. The proportion of babies under 4 months of age fed exclusively by breast was 32% and for those under 6 months, 25%.

In 1991, a 23.2% incidence of goiter was found in 1,603 schoolchildren from the Azuero region. In the rest of the country the incidence in a sample of 1,459 schoolchildren was 12.3%.

A Maternal and Child Survey was conducted in 1992 in Bocas del Toro, Chiriquí, Veraguas, San Miguelito, the Panamá City metropolitan area, San Blas, Herrera, and Los Santos. It found anemia (hemoglobin <11 µg/dl) in 43.4% of children under 1 year of age, 38.4% of children 1 to 4 years of age, 20.2% of schoolchildren, and 38.9% of pregnant women. In another 1992 survey using the same criterion, conducted with a sample of 929 children 12 to 59 months old, 18% had anemia.

In the National Vitamin A Survey of 1992, no concentrations of plasma retinol lower than 10 µg/dl were found among children from 12 to 59 months of age, but in 6% of this group low levels were found, below 20 µg/dl. In 1992, in the hospitals of Chiriquí and Changuinola in Bocas del Toro Province, 24 children with eye damage from vitamin A deficiency were identified.

In 1993, diabetes mellitus was the eighth most common cause of death, with a rate of 13.8 per 100,000 of population.

Cardiovascular Disease. Hypertension is the third leading cause of morbidity in the 20–59 age group and leading cause in the group aged 60 and older. In general morbidity, it occupies sixth place.

Malignant Neoplasms. In 1993, 3,128 malignant neoplasms were recorded (42.9% in men and 57.1% in women), with a rate of 123 per 100,000 inhabitants. The most affected group were people over 70 years of age, who accounted for 34.5% of the total cases. In women, cervical cancer occupies first place, with a rate of 72 per 100,000 women over the age of 15; this is followed by breast cancer, with a rate of 27.2 per 100,000 women over 15. In men, the most common tumor is of the prostate, with a rate of 27.2 per 100,000 men over 15; men over 70 account for 67% of the total cases.

External Causes. Accidental injuries or accidents, along with suicides, homicides, and other forms of violence were the second leading cause of death in 1993, with a rate of 54.4 per 100,000 inhabitants. In the provinces of Colón, Bocas del Toro, Darién, and Veraguas, these external causes ranked first among the causes of death. Of the total deaths recorded in 1993 from external causes, 81.9% occurred in males.

Deaths from external causes are increasing, with a rate of 54.0 per 100,000 in 1992 and 58.3 per 100,000 in 1994. Deaths related to traffic accidents ranked first among deaths from external causes in 1993, with a rate of 16.3 per 100,000.

RESPONSE OF THE HEALTH SYSTEM

National Health Plans and Policies

Health is the heart of the Government's policies, as set forth in the document "Social Development with Economic Efficiency." The political goals of the Ministry of Health for the 1994–1999 five-year period are as follows:

• Strengthening the leadership of the Ministry
• Promoting primary care, consolidating a comprehensive and decentralized health system organized by levels of care
• Establishing environmental health programs aimed at sustainable development
• Promoting health programs for specific demographic groups
• Developing individual abilities and responsibility for a better quality of life
• Strengthening societal participation in health promotion, disease prevention, care, and management of health
• Improving the use of regular and extrabudgetary sources and seeking other sources of financing to increase funding for the health sector
• Training individuals in the areas required to strengthen national and local health plans and programs

• Promoting health research and the dissemination of information and scientific and technical knowledge to develop the health system

Decentralization with active societal participation is one of the mechanisms for achieving efficiency in public administration. This process of adjustment, however, should make it possible for the provincial, municipal and local levels of government to assume responsibility for the planning, execution, monitoring, and evaluation of the programs and projects transferred to them.

The mission of the Social Security Fund is to guarantee comprehensive health services that deal with the biopsychosocial, environmental, and labor risks and injuries incurred by beneficiaries. This mission is based on the principles of universality, solidarity, integrity, and fairness, with quality and efficiency, within the framework of a philosophy of social enterprise.

Reformulating the public management strategy, including health policies, is an integral part of the reform and modernization of the State, which seeks to improve the efficiency and quality of the services provided by the public sector. In the health sector, decentralization is a top priority, oriented basically to primary care; this involves giving priority to neglected groups, developing the first level of care, and improving the operating and managerial capacity of the health services. The reform and modernization that the Ministry of Health promotes includes expanding comprehensive health services coverage to the entire population, financing care for the most vulnerable groups, strengthening the service network of the National Health System, developing financing mechanisms for the health system, and strengthening the role of the national health authority.

The new model for the financing, management, and delivery of health services was introduced in the San Miguelito health region in 1997. This new model seeks to provide universal coverage for the health needs and health problems affecting both people and the environment, with efficiency, quality and fairness, by integrating all the resources and potential of the public sector, the private sector, and the community. The object is to separate the financing of services from the Social Security Fund and the delivery of services from the Ministry of Health. To this end, an agency will be established to manage hospital and outpatient services.

The Social Security Fund has proposed a new model for care that guarantees fulfillment of the principles of fairness, efficiency, effectiveness, solidarity, and universality. The activities to follow through on this proposal are defined according to levels of care. At the first level, the plan is to decentralize and disperse services, operate the referral system, strengthen the response capacity of the local primary care units, prevent domestic violence and substance abuse, and promote home

care. At the second level of care, one goal is to strengthen the response capacity of the polyclinics. Other objectives are to institute outpatient surgery and to establish simple rehabilitation units; short-stay units; hospitals for one-day, intermediate, and chronic care cases; and a second-level general hospital in the Panamá City metropolitan area. At the third level, the goal is to divide the management of the Hospital Medical Complex into two units, each with a different level of complexity, as well as to create a unit for transplants and another for burn patients, and to establish a hospital-home extension.

In 1997, the 21st Century Panamanian Municipalities Network was formed. Its goal was to foster mutual support and share experiences, while promoting solidarity, cooperation, and communication between the municipalities participating in a health promotion program in their jurisdictions.

Within the framework of the Central American Health Initiative and the "Fronteras Solidarias" (Shared Borders) Program, activities are under way in the municipalities of Changuinola, Barú, and Renacimiento, in the region bordering Costa Rica, to promote health and prevent diarrheal diseases, cholera, malaria, dengue, and AIDS.

Panamanian health authorities have categorized violence as a public health problem, and an institutional plan for its prevention and control has been formulated. A multisectoral national commission is in charge of coordinating activities, and the Ministry of Health has instituted mandatory recording in the health units of suspected domestic violence.

Organization of the Health Sector

The Constitution of Panama establishes that safeguarding the health of the population of the Republic is an essential function of the State and affirms that, as part of the community, an individual is entitled to the promotion, protection, preservation, restoration, and rehabilitation of health, and also has an obligation to preserve it. In order to meet these responsibilities, the State has created a number of institutions to provide health services. Principal among them are the Ministry of Health, the Social Security Fund, the Institute of National Water Supply and Sewerage Systems, and the Metropolitan Department of Hygiene.

The health services of the Social Security Fund are under the National Bureau of Services and Medical Benefits. The insured beneficiaries of the Fund receive two types of benefits: medical benefits, aimed at comprehensive protection of the work force and provided by the national health services network of the Fund, and economic benefits for workers who are permanently or temporarily off the job for any reason (old age, disability, maternity, disease, etc.). Private institutions participate in the Social Security Fund as health service providers.

Health Legislation

The provisional draft of the General Health Act is in the analysis and consultation phase at the internal and institutional level. With regard to the Health Code currently in force, the General Health Act outlines the organization of the national health system, establishes the norms governing health—not just those having to do with disease—includes elements related to the rights and responsibilities of the population with respect to health, and establishes a frame of reference for the responsibilities of the Government, society, and individuals.

In recent legislation, domestic violence and child abuse have been defined and the creation of specialized agencies to help the victims of these crimes has been ordered.

Health Services and Resources

Organization of Services for Care of the Population

Epidemiological Surveillance Systems. The epidemiological monitoring system is organized at the local, regional, and central level. Depending on their priority, there are diseases requiring immediate notification, weekly notification by telephone, and routine weekly reporting. The diseases monitored are those included in the International Health Regulations, as well as outbreaks and epidemics, especially measles, rubella, botulism, encephalitis, viral meningitis, food poisoning, and other types of poisoning. Vector-borne diseases are the responsibility of a specific surveillance subsystem. For surveillance in border areas, there is a binational committee that meets periodically and monitors basic sanitation activities, vector control, immunization, and emerging and re-emerging diseases.

Epidemiological surveillance of nosocomial infections has been conducted since 1995. Its objective is to formulate suitable strategies to control specific hospital problems, and thus facilitate changes in detrimental behavior by staff, the application of preventive measures in patient care, and the development of programs for in-service training.

Water Supply, Sewerage Systems, and Solid Waste Disposal. Management of water resources is the responsibility of the Institute for Water Resources and Electrification and the Institute of National Water Supply and Sewerage Systems, which have initiated the preparation of comprehensive integrated plans for joint surveillance. In 1996, water quality standards were drafted, and the preparation of wastewater quality standards was also begun. The Institute of National Water Supply and Sewerage Systems and the Ministry of Health are responsible for enforcing the quality control standards for drinking water.

It has not been possible to control the sanitary handling of solid waste despite there being a plan to manage, collect, transport, and dispose of it. Dealing with solid waste is the responsibility of the municipalities, with the exception of the districts of Panamá, San Miguelito, and Colón, which have an autonomous institution, the Metropolitan Department of Hygiene, that is responsible for handling solid wastes. In 1996, the municipalities of Panamá and San Miguelito produced 845 tons of waste daily. It is transported to the Cerro Patacón sanitary landfill, where it is disposed of properly.

Hospital waste is mixed with common waste, constituting a health and safety hazard for the general population. Only sharp objects are removed and then deposited in rigid containers. In 1996, a regulation was issued establishing minimum requirements for handling hazardous waste in hospitals.

Environmental Risks. The risks generated by the use of growing quantities of chemical substances are ever-increasing. In response, the Environmental Planning Unit and the Environmental Health Bureau of the Ministry of Health were established in 1995. The priority is to conduct research and training projects that will make it possible to reduce or eliminate environmental health risks. High mortality from malignant neoplasms and congenital abnormalities could be related to the carcinogenic and teratogenic nature of the chemical substances used in agroindustrial and household activities. At the moment, measures to prevent, correct, control, and monitor these risks are very limited. A project is under way to form a national network to control the manufacture, transport, and elimination of chemical products. A national response plan for chemical emergencies is also being developed.

A law has been passed establishing automobile emission limits, and there are also norms aimed at reducing exposure to tobacco smoke in public buildings, as well as in hospitals and other health institutions.

In 1992, the Regulations for Radiation Protection were established, which control the use of devices that generate ionizing radiation.

Pharmaceutical Regulation. The Ministry of Health has drawn up a National Formulary of Essential Drugs and is currently working on a proposal for production of the basic drugs. The Social Security Fund uses the Official Drug List, which is reviewed every year by representatives from all the health professions and their corresponding professional associations.

The Ministry of Health maintains a registry of the drugs and biologicals that can be marketed in the country. The use of generic drugs is promoted.

There is only one specialized laboratory that conducts ongoing monitoring of the physical, chemical, and biological quality of drugs.

Food Safety. In 1996, the law and the norms and regulations governing meat and dairy products, seafood, flours, and the registry of foodstuffs were updated. The 1994–1999 Plan of the Ministry of Health includes a policy and plan of action concerning food safety. To monitor and control food safety, the National Commission for Food Protection was established; its representatives are from the Ministry of Health and other public and private institutions, as well as consumers.

Food handlers receive training so that they can carry out their activities with minimum risk to the population. In 1996 a surveillance system for foodborne diseases was established, for which a specific handbook has been developed. This system recorded 10 outbreaks of foodborne disease in 1995.

To carry out food testing and control, there are five regional laboratories, the central laboratory, the laboratories of the School of Medicine of the University of Panama and the Ministry of Agricultural and Livestock Development, and four private laboratories.

Organization and Operation of Personal Health Care Services

At the primary care level, Panama has 155 health centers, 112 subcenters, 376 health posts, 34 polyclinics, and 6 dispensaries. At the second and third level, there are 37 hospitals, 5 of them located in Panamá City, that offer third-level services. In total, there are 720 sites providing services of varying degrees of complexity, 19.6% of which are concentrated in Panamá Province. The Social Security Fund has 10 hospitals and 27 polyclinics.

In 1995, the Ministry of Health carried out 5.6 million health service activities, 71.2% of which were medical services, 14.8% oral health services, 10.2% nursing services, and 3.8% services provided by technical personnel. Of this total, 10.7% were provided in the five national hospitals. Of the 3.98 million outpatient consultations (38% more than in 1993), 15.7% were classified as emergencies and 5.9% were performed by specialists.

The Social Security Fund provided 4.65 million consultations in 1996 (31% more than in 1992). Of the total consultations in 1996, 12.5% were for uninsured individuals. The Fund handled 15,946 births, 18.7% of them by cesarean section.

According to the records of the Social Security Fund, it covered more than 1.6 million people in 1996, or 61.4% of the Panamanian population. Of the persons insured, 40.3% are contributors and 59.7%, dependents. Since 1992, the total number of covered individuals has risen by 19.9%, while the number of contributors has increased by 12.5%. In 1996, there were approximately five active contributors (545,500) for each pensioner (116,000).

In 1995, the nation had a total of 7,138 hospital beds, 86.5% of which belonged to the public sector and 13.5% to the private. There are 2.7 beds available for each 1,000 persons, but with a very unequal distribution. There are 7.5 beds per 1,000 inhabitants in Panamá City and only 1.7 in Veraguas and 1.4 in Coclé. The national occupancy rate for hospital beds is 61.6%, with a higher percentage in public health centers (66.3%) than in private facilities (33.1%). The national average hospital stay is 5.5 days (7.7 days in public institutions and 4.0 in private facilities). The 2,090 beds of the Social Security Fund had 77,256 patient stays in 1995.

Of the total visits for prenatal check-ups in 1994, 1.6% corresponded to pregnant women 10 to 14 years of age and 19.4% to pregnant women 15 to 19. Prenatal check-up coverage in 1995 was 89.1% of pregnant women, with an average of 3.1 consultations per expectant mother. Of total deliveries, 86.5% were done in institutions; of these, 16.6% were by cesarean section.

An important institution is the laboratory at the Gorgas Memorial Center, which conducts serological and virological analysis for dengue and functions as a reference laboratory for the Central American countries in the diagnosis of measles and poliomyelitis. This institution participates in research projects related to the re-emergence of dengue, leishmaniasis, retrovirus, anti-malarial drugs, recombinant DNA vaccines, and epilepsy.

Health Inputs

There is a procedure for registering drugs prior to marketing them, and drug control committees have been formed at the institutional level to ensure the use of high-quality, safe, and effective drugs.

The majority of the drugs purchased institutionally are imported. For their procurement, there is a national formulary of essential drugs and an official list of drugs from the Social Security Fund.

The Social Security Fund spent approximately 11% of its budget for pharmaceuticals in 1993 and 1997. In 1993 this percentage represented US$ 22.5 million and in 1997, US$ 36.2 million.

Vaccines for the Expanded Program on Immunization (EPI) are provided to the country through the Revolving Fund of the EPI.

The technical department of the General Bureau of Infrastructure and Maintenance, which is responsible for maintaining biomedical equipment and controlling the introduction of new technologies, is in the process of consolidation.

Of the total budget allocated in 1995 for investments in the Ministry of Health, only 7.1% was used for equipment for health facilities. In absolute and relative terms, this represents a significant reduction over 1994, when 49.6% of the investment budget went for equipment. In 1996, the Social Security Fund spent US$ 38.2 million for equipment, 12.2% of its health budget; US$ 5.9 million, or 1.9%, went for maintenance.

Health Activities and Professional Accreditation

The Technical Health Council is made up of representatives from the health institutions and the various health-employee associations. It accredits hospitals, clinics, and laboratories and authorizes the use of restricted medications. A draft law to establish the eligibility requirements for the accreditation of health professionals and technicians and to create a National Human Resources Accreditation Board is currently in the analysis and public comment phase.

As recommended by the Commission on Medical Specialties, 95 medical specialties were officially recognized.

Human Resources

In 1995, the Ministry of Health had a staff of 21,899 employees and the Social Security Fund had 12,344. The personnel of the Ministry of Health consisted of 3,702 physicians and dentists, 2,566 nurses, 2,704 nurse's aides, 107 veterinarians and agronomists, 944 laboratory workers, 79 nutritionists, 1,012 pharmacy workers, 471 environmental health inspectors, 541 health assistants and aides, 125 administrators, and 39 legal advisers. The remaining staff are other health management professionals and technicians. Physicians, nurses, and dentists make up 28.6% of the total staff; administrative personnel, 34.3%; and the rest, 37.1%.

In 1995, the personnel of the Social Security Fund consisted of 1,936 physicians, 227 dentists, 1,410 nurses, 1,450 nurse's aides, 316 pharmacists, 202 X-ray technicians, 343 laboratory workers, 806 professionals in other health categories, and 1,794 support staff.

In 1995, there was one physician in Panama for every 841 inhabitants, one dentist for every 4,576 inhabitants, and one nurse for every 1,025. The health regions with the fewest health workers per inhabitant are San Blas, San Miguelito, and Darién.

Every year more than 250 students enter medical school at the University of Panama, and about 60 physicians graduate. In 1994, two private medical schools were established. Their enrollment has increased rapidly, with 138 first-year students in 1996.

In 1994, a total of 85 nurses, 28 pharmacists, and 28 dentists graduated from the University of Panama.

In 1997, the country had 4,434 physicians, 1,397 dentists, 3,923 registered nurses, 756 pharmacists, and 213 public health specialists.

Expenditures and Sectoral Financing

It is impossible to estimate total health expenditures. That is because there is no information on the private sector or on individuals' direct purchases of ancillary drugs, supplies, and examinations.

In 1995, public expenditures in health totaled US$ 547 million, or 6.9% of the gross national product and 14.5% of total public expenditure. In the allocation of public expenditures for health in 1995, the Social Security Fund ranked first, with 55%. The Ministry of Health was allocated 37%, and other institutions in the social field received the remaining 8%. The total budget of the Ministry of Health was US$ 150.1 million, US$ 132.6 million of which went for operating expenses and the remainder for investment. The total operating budget of the Ministry in 1995 was almost half a million dollars lower than in 1994. Per capita public spending on health in 1995 was estimated at US$ 210.

The Social Security Fund had a total budget of US$ 868.6 million in 1996, of which it allocated US$ 313.1 million to health, or 36.1% of its budget. Of the total allocated to health, 72.9% was used for operating expenses and 27.1% for investment.

Public services for promotion, prevention, cure, and rehabilitation are financed primarily by the Ministry of Health and the Social Security Fund. The principal sources of financing for the state health system are the current revenues of the Government, workers' and employers' contributions to the Social Security Fund, and special funds received through loans and donations from international public and private agencies. Payments for community health services are also a source of revenue. Uninsured persons who receive services from the Ministry of Health at first-level care facilities are charged US$ 0.50 per consultation. That is a donation by the user to the facility, not a payment based on the true cost of the services. For cost recovery for hospitalization, surgery, and auxiliary or intermediate services, the amount charged is based on a series of tables and collected according to the user's ability to pay.

In 1995, the budget of the Ministry of Health consisted of the following sources of financing: 74.4%, public funds; 12.1%, loans from the IDB and the World Bank; and 13.5%, foreign funds from the European Union and Japan, among others.

External Technical Financial and Cooperation

External financial assistance is erratic, due in general to the country's positive health indicators. Standing out among the international cooperation agencies that have provided technical support to Panama in recent years are PAHO/WHO,

UNICEF, the United Nations Development Program, the European Union, the Japan International Cooperation Agency, and the Spanish International Cooperation Agency. All these agencies provide technical cooperation and nonreimbursable financial assistance. The IDB and the World Bank grant "soft" and long-term loans. Both support the development of the new care model and the reform and modernization of the health sector.

PARAGUAY

GENERAL SITUATION AND TRENDS

Socioeconomic, Political, and Demographic Overview

Paraguay lies at the center of South America. It has two major rivers, the Paraguay and the Paraná. The Paraguay River divides the country into two distinct regions: the west, a relatively arid plains region, and the east, a more heavily populated and wealthier region.

In addition to the capital city, Asunción, the country is divided administratively into 17 departments, which in turn are subdivided into 264 districts. Paraguay has a presidential system of government, with an executive branch and a legislative branch, which consists of a bicameral legislature.

Paraguay's transition to democracy began in 1989 with the direct election of municipal governments. Since then, several events have strengthened the democratic process and helped the country withstand the military crisis in April 1996. These events include the adoption of a new Constitution, presidential elections in 1993, municipal elections in 1996, and the decision to hold presidential and departmental elections in 1998.

The country has a surface area of 406,752 km². In 1997, the population was estimated at 5.1 million inhabitants, of which 40.3% were under 15 years of age, 56.2% were between the ages of 15 and 65, and 3.5% were 65 years of age or older. A high rate of growth of the population has been one of the defining characteristics of Paraguay's social development. Between 1950 and 1992, the country's population tripled; between 1982 and 1992, the average annual growth rate was 3.2%.

A downward trend has been noted in birth rates, which fell from 37.7 per 1,000 in 1972 to 33.8 per 1,000 in 1992. Infant mortality has also declined: from a rate of 53.1 per 1,000 in the 1970s to 43.3 per 1,000 in 1995.

Life expectancy at birth for males was estimated at 60.6 years in the 1950s. By 1996, it had increased to 68.1 years.

During the same period, life expectancy at birth for females rose from 69.1 to 71.9 years.

The total fertility rate at the national level was 4.5 children per woman during the period 1990–1995, down from the figure of 4.7 children per woman reported by the 1990 Survey of Reproductive Health.

The population density is 12.5 inhabitants per km², with considerable variation among different regions in the country. The western, or Chaco, region occupies almost 61% of the total land mass, but only 2.5% of the population lives there. In the eastern region, the population is quite unevenly distributed; there are 4,200 inhabitants per km² in Asunción, while there are 350 per km² in the Central Department and only 15–45 inhabitants per km² in the departments of Guairá, Cordillera, Caaguazú, Alto Paraná, Paraguarí, and Itapúa.

According to data from the 1992 census, 50.3% of the population is urban and 49.7% is rural. Estimates for 1995, however, indicate that 53% of the population lives in urban areas.

An important factor in Paraguay's social organization is language. Spanish is used in formal education and as the official language, but Guaraní has been a central element in shaping the country's cultural identity. Moreover, teaching of Guaraní in primary and secondary schools has been mandatory since 1994. According to data from the Population and Housing Census of 1992, almost 40% of the country's population speaks only Guaraní and about 50% speaks two languages.

As a fairly new democracy, Paraguay faces many challenges, including the absence of an agrarian policy, low wages, high unemployment, scarcity of housing, elevated school dropout rates, unmet health needs for the most disadvantaged social sectors, and exacerbation of existing inequities. Wealth is still closely linked to land ownership. Agriculture and livestock-breeding continue to be the principal productive activities, although in the past few years there has been an attempt to diversify and open up markets beyond these sectors.

The Southern Common Market (MERCOSUR), which was launched in January 1995 and comprises Argentina, Brazil, Paraguay, and Uruguay, has drawn Paraguay into the global and regional integration processes under way. The creation of MERCOSUR, however, has come at a difficult juncture in Paraguay's history, opening up new opportunities, but posing some risks. The country is faced with the challenge of integrating into a highly competitive market with trading partners who are demographically larger and socially and economically stronger.

The country's economic mainstay is agriculture, particularly cotton and soybean production for export. The agricultural sector generates 26.7% of the gross domestic product (GDP), employs 35.8% of the economically active population, and produces 90% of registered exports. Of these exports, approximately half are raw materials. Nevertheless, in the 1990s the agricultural sector has scaled down, as compared with other sectors of the economy. For example, industry and construction now account for 21.6% of the GDP, and the service sector generates 51.7%. In addition, the country derives enormous financial and energy resources from the binational hydroelectric plants in Itaipú and Yacyretá.

In the early 1990s, GDP growth rates declined steadily, bottoming out at 1.8% in 1992. According to preliminary statistics, between 1993 and 1995, the annual GDP growth rate was 4.1%, 3.1%, and 4.7%, respectively, but in 1996 the figure again dropped to 1.3%. Inflation has remained at acceptable levels: 10.5% and 8.2% in 1995 and 1996, respectively, after having reached an annual level of 44% in 1990. This reduction has come at a cost, however, because anti-inflation policies are considered one of the main factors behind the slow GDP growth rate during the past several years.

In the area of foreign trade, the country has succeeded in reversing the downward trend of international reserves seen in the late 1980s. Nevertheless, the balance of trade remains negative, and the country's trade deficit has increased over the past five years as the gap between the volume of exports (US$ 1,048 million in 1996) and imports (US$ 2,658 million in 1996) has widened.

With an average annual per capita income of US$ 1,634 (preliminary statistics for 1996) and social indicators that reveal deficits in health, nutrition, education, and housing, Paraguay ranks among the countries with medium levels of human development, based on the criteria applied by the United Nations Development Program to calculate the human development index.

The problem of unemployment in Paraguay has more to do with a shortage of jobs that pay a living wage than with open unemployment. It is estimated that three-fourths of rural workers are employed in family farming operations.

Data on unemployment from different sources are not consistent. According to the Central Bank, unemployment between 1992 and 1996 was approximately 9% and reached a level of 9.8% in 1996. In contrast, statistics from the Department of Industrial Policy within the Ministry of Industry and Commerce put unemployment at 13.7% for 1995. This figure reflects both open and concealed unemployment. Open unemployment (the proportion of job seekers who cannot find work) for that year was 5.3% in urban areas and 3.4% nationwide. Hidden unemployment (the proportion of people who, although they want or need to work, are not actively seeking employment because they believe that they will be unable to find a job that will meet their needs) reached 10.3% nationwide in 1995.

Women's participation in the labor market has increased steadily, as has the number of women obtaining higher levels of education.

According to recent studies, at least 30% of the population lives below the poverty line. This figure was obtained by estimating the cost of satisfying the food needs of each person, as well as other basic needs, and comparing it with individual or family income. In this way, a distinction is made between indigence or extreme poverty, which refers to the inability to satisfy essential food needs, and "basic poverty," which is the inability to meet all basic needs (food, clothing, housing, etc.). In rural areas, the percentage of people living under conditions of basic poverty is approximately 55%, and women and children are most often affected. Since the 1980s, levels of basic poverty have remained relatively stable in urban areas, although extreme poverty has increased from 15% to 21%.

Paraguay faces a serious housing problem. According to the 1992 National Population and Housing Census, more than half of all housing units are located in urban areas, with an average of 4.6 inhabitants per dwelling. In rural areas, the figure is five inhabitants per dwelling. The cumulative housing shortage amounts to more than 350,000 dwellings, and the annual unsatisfied demand for housing is around 15,000 units. Thirty percent of the population lives in conditions of overcrowding, which is defined as an average of three or more persons per room. As for the quality of housing, more than a third of dwellings have basic deficiencies, with marked differences between urban and rural housing. In urban areas, 23% of the housing is considered to have basic deficiencies, and in rural areas the figure is 49%.

As for literacy, 9.4% of Paraguay's population is illiterate (persons who are 10 years of age or older and have not completed the second grade are considered illiterate). The percentage is higher among females, with the exception of girls in the 10–14 age group, who have higher literacy rates than boys the same age. Illiteracy has shown a downward trend, dropping from 21% to 9.4% between 1982 and 1992, although the improvement has been less marked among females and among rural inhabitants. Primary school enrollment is as high as 95%, but grade repetition rates are high (9% at the national level and 10.4% in rural areas), as are dropout rates. Only 51% of children who began the first grade in 1986 have completed the sixth grade.

Mortality Profile

Based on records of registered deaths maintained by the Ministry of Public Health and Social Welfare, as well as the crude death rate computed by the Bureau of the Census, Statistics, and Surveys (5.43 per 1,000), underreporting of mortality is estimated at 38.7%. However, this national average conceals substantial regional variations. In 1995, in 37% of reported infant deaths, the child had received no medical attention. Of the deaths certified by doctors, the percentage attributed to ill-defined signs and symptoms was 10.3% in 1995.

The following figures on mortality rates are based on currently available data. This information reflects only deaths registered by the Ministry of Public Health and Social Welfare. The aforementioned percentage of underreporting should therefore be taken into consideration when interpreting the information.

In 1995, the Ministry of Public Health registered a total of 16,069 deaths. By cause, based on the groups of causes used in the PAHO publication *Health Statistics in the Americas,* diseases of the circulatory system accounted for 34.5% of the deaths, followed by malignant neoplasms and external causes, which accounted for 12% each. Communicable diseases accounted for 11.4% of the registered deaths, and 3.9% were due to conditions originating in the perinatal period. By age group, 12.6% of the total deaths occurred among children under 5 years of age, 2.1% among children aged 5–14, 18.9% among adults aged 15–49, 15.7% among persons aged 50–64, and 50% among people 65 years and older. In 1991, children under 5 accounted for 17.2% of all deaths, and adults 65 years and older accounted for 46.6%.

The mortality profile of the 18 health regions is fairly similar to the national profile. In 13 of the 18 regions, the leading cause of death is diseases of the circulatory system. Malignant neoplasms are either the second or third leading cause of death in 16 of the 18 regions. Likewise, external causes ranks as either the second or third cause in 12 of the regions. It is noteworthy that the leading cause of death in four of the regions (Alto Paraná, Amambay, Canendiyú, and Boquerón) is external causes.

Deaths due to accidents (codes E800–E949 in the International Classification of Diseases, 9th Revision) represent a significant proportion of total mortality. This group of causes accounts for 7 per 100 registered deaths, making it one of the primary causes of death in the country.

SPECIFIC HEALTH PROBLEMS

Analysis by Population Group

Health of Children

In 1995, 1,570 deaths were registered among children under 1 year of age; 43% were due to neonatal infections, pneumonia, influenza, diarrhea, meningitis, and tetanus. The infant mortality rate in 1991 was 24 per 1,000 live births. According to data from death certificates, this number decreased to 19.7 per 1,000 in 1995. Even when underregistration is taken into account, there are significant regional variations in the 1995 data, with rates ranging from 32.4 per 1,000 in Alto Paraná to 16.2 per 1,000 in Asunción.

In 1995, half of all registered deaths in the under-1 age group occurred during the first 28 days of life. The neonatal mortality rate was 9.8 per 1,000 live births; obstetric causes accounted for 38% of these deaths, neonatal infections for 18%, and prematurity for 15%. The postnatal mortality rate was 9.9 per 1,000 live births, and pneumonia, influenza, and diarrheal diseases were the principle causes of death. The mortality rate in the 1–4-year age group was 5.7 per 1,000 registered live births in 1995. The principal causes of death were pneumonia, diarrhea, and accidents.

The only data available on morbidity rates are figures registered by health care facilities of the Ministry of Public Health, which suffer from deficiencies in coverage and quality. For the under-5 age group, 1995 data indicate that the leading cause of medical visits was acute respiratory infections, which generated 146,971 visits. Other important causes included acute diarrheal diseases (30,729), parasitic diseases, (27,421), and anemia (16,652).

In 1995, 147 deaths were registered in the age group 5–9 years old, of which 55% were males. The first, second, and third causes of death were external causes (ICD-9, E800-E999), which accounted for 30% of the total; respiratory diseases (ICD-9, 460–519), which accounted for 13%; and malignant neoplasms, which accounted for 10%.

Among external causes, traffic accidents accounted for one of every three deaths and firearms accounted for 14%.

With regard to morbidity rates, in 1995 the principal reasons for medical visits among children aged 5–9 in establishments of the Ministry of Public Health were acute respiratory infections, parasitic diseases, anemia, accidents, and diarrheal diseases.

Health of Adolescents

In 1995, 529 deaths were registered in the age group 10–19 years old. The leading cause of death was external causes, which accounted for 53%, followed by malignant neoplasms, which accounted for a much smaller proportion (6%). Traffic accidents accounted for 23% of the deaths due to external causes. While there are no significant sex differences in mortality in the 10–14 age group, 79% of those who died in the 15–19 age group were males.

In 1995, the primary reasons for medical visits in Ministry of Public Health establishments by persons in the 15–19 age group were acute respiratory infections, anemia, accidents, and parasitic diseases.

Drug addiction, alcoholism, and juvenile delinquency are serious problems among young people. These problems are associated with urbanization and marginalization in urban areas.

Health of Adults

More than half the country's population (53%) is between 15 and 60 years of age and 28% of all deaths occur in this group. The percentage of male deaths in this group is 62% and that of females is 38%.

The leading causes of death among adults, particularly those aged 15–44 years, are accidents, homicides, and some infectious diseases such as tuberculosis and Chagas' disease. Among women aged 15–49, the principal causes of death are malignant neoplasms, accidents, and heart disease.

In 1995, there were 104 registered maternal deaths, 29% due to abortion and 24% to sepsis. Additional significant causes were "other complications of pregnancy, childbirth, and the puerperium," toxemia, and hemorrhage, in that order.

In the 45–64 age group, the leading causes of death in 1995 were cardiovascular diseases and accidents.

In 1995, the most common reasons for medical consultation in this age group were acute respiratory infections, anemia, accidents, and hypertension.

Health of the Elderly

The group (65 years old and older) makes up 5.2% of the total population and accounts for 56% of total deaths. The primary causes of death in this group in 1995 were cardiovascular diseases (ICD-9, 391–398; 410–429; 441–459), which accounted for 28%; cerebrovascular disease (ICD-9, 430–438), which accounted for 18%; malignant neoplasms (ICD-9, 140–239), which accounted for 13%; diabetes (ICD-9, 250), which accounted for 6%; pneumonia and influenza (ICD-9, 480–487), which accounted for 4%; and hypertension (ICD-9, 401–405), which accounted for 3%.

In this age group, the leading reasons for medical visits at Ministry of Public Health establishments were hypertension, acute respiratory infections, anemia, and accidents.

Health of Women

In 1995 the maternal mortality rate was 130.7 per 100,000 live births. In Paraguay, discrimination against women persists and affects all women, but especially those in the lowest economic strata. Of every 10 illiterate persons, 6 are women. More than one-fifth of all households are headed by women. Women have little power in the political sphere, as evidenced by the fact that 94% of the members of the National Congress are men, and only one government minister is a woman. Only 3.2% of the recipients of development loans and grants are women.

The majority of women work in unpaid jobs that are not reflected in official employment statistics (family farming, housekeeping, child care, care of the elderly and disabled). Those who do have paid jobs receive lower wages than their male counterparts who perform similar work. In almost all domestic violence cases, the victims are women and children.

Through the Secretariat for Women's Issues, which was created in 1994 and has ministerial status, the Government implements programs that target gender-related issues (violence against women, reproductive health and family planning, sex education, job training, etc.).

Workers' Health

There is no specific institution responsible for workers' health, and no studies of work-related health risks have been undertaken. Nevertheless, the Ministry of Public Health and Social Welfare, the Ministry of Justice and Labor, and the Social Security Institute (IPS) coordinate activities related to health and safety in the workplace through the Occupational Health and Safety Council.

No reliable data on occupational illnesses are available. There is a shortage of professionals specializing in occupational health and no technical and legal provisions under the health and labor codes regulating conditions in the workplace.

According to data from IPS, which refer only to its beneficiaries, in 1989 there were a total of 2,174 work-related accidents or illnesses, resulting in a rate of 22.1 cases per 1,000 beneficiaries. In 1993, 4,097 cases were registered, which increased the rate to 29.6 per 1,000.

Health of the Disabled

A lack of information, coupled with problems relating to coverage and definitions, make it difficult to adequately assess the situation of this group. According to data from the 1992 census, in Asunción there were 5,335 persons with some kind of disability, while the figure for the entire Central Department was 7,786.

The National Institute for the Protection of Exceptional People (INPRO) was created under Law 780, enacted on 30 November 1979. Since 1985, the Institute has been providing diagnostic, treatment, and rehabilitation services for the disabled. As of 1995, with the goal of extending the coverage of its services, INPRO integrated all governmental and nongovernmental agencies working in the area of disability to which the institute provides technical and financial assistance. That same year, a community-based rehabilitation program was implemented. The program includes extrainstitutional care for the disabled and is being extended to other parts of the country. According to INPRO statistics, there are 22,000 disabled persons nationwide.

Health of Indigenous People

During the last quarter of this century, as a result of migration and occupation and settlement of indigenous lands, the traditional habitat of indigenous peoples has steadily shrunk and deteriorated. Despite efforts of private organizations and the National Institute of Indigenous Peoples (INDI), indigenous communities have deeply deteriorated and disintegrated.

According to data from the 1992 national census, the indigenous population totaled 49,500, of which 43.8% were under 15 years of age and 2.7% were 65 and older. The indigenous population comprises five groups (Tupí Guaraní, Mataco-Mataguayo, Guaicurú, Lengua-Maskoy, and Zemuco) and 17 ethnic subgroups.

The total fertility rate in the indigenous population averages 5.7 children per woman, with differences between ethnic groups ranging from 3.7 for the Lengua group to 7.8 for the Aché ethnic group.

The infant mortality rate—calculated by using the Coale-Trussel variant of the Brass method and based on 1992 census data—was 106.7 per 1,000 live births for the indigenous population as a whole. Interethnic differences ranged from 64 per 1,000 for the Maká to 185 per 1,000 for the Chamacoco.

In addition to having the highest infant mortality rate in the country, the indigenous population has the highest rate of tuberculosis—10 times the national average. Almost 80% of indigenous households are infested with *Triatoma infestans,* a vector of Chagas' disease.

Analysis by Type of Disease

Communicable Diseases

Vector-Borne Diseases. Malaria persists as a health problem, although the number of cases has remained stable over the past three years, never exceeding 1,000. Up to 90% of the cases, all of them due to *Plasmodium vivax,* are concentrated in eight districts within the departments of Alto Paraná, Caaguazú, and Canendiyú.

Since the dengue epidemic of 1988–1989—which was caused by serotype 1 and resulted in more than 40,000 cases—no new cases have been reported, although the vector, *Aedes aegypti,* is present throughout the country.

Chagas' disease is the most serious vector-borne disease in Paraguay and one of the country's important public health problems. Estimates by the Intergovernmental Commission for the Elimination of *Triatoma infestans* and the Commission for the Interruption of Transmission of American Trypanosomiasis by Blood Transfusion indicate that the prevalence of *Trypanosoma cruzi* infection in Paraguay is 11.6%. This percentage is diminishing as a result of control activities. In 1986, 98% of blood used for transfusions was serologically tested, and the prevalence of *Trypanosoma* antibodies in donors' blood was found to be 5.7% and 4.1%, respectively, for 1995 and 1996. A prevalence of 15% was found in a study of 5,042 pregnant women conducted in 1995 in the departments of Paraguarí and Cordillera. Some surveys of the Chaco indigenous population have found up to 80% serologic prevalence.

Cutaneous leishmaniasis is also a serious public health problem. There are approximately 1,000 cases each year, although there is significant underreporting and there is an annual variability that can be explained not by epidemiologic hypotheses but by notification problems. In the past few years, 85% of the cases have occurred in three departments: Canendiyú, Alto Paraná, and San Pedro. The presence of cases and the increase in their number is related to the development and settling of new agricultural lands. Consequently, the most affected population consists of males over the age of 20.

Vaccine-Preventable Diseases. Measles has decreased dramatically in recent years. Up to 1993, epidemics occurred every three years, causing 2,000 cases annually, but between 1993 and 1996 the number of cases dropped from 2,066 to 142 to 69 to 13, respectively, for each year in that period. In May 1997, however, there was an outbreak that mainly affected the department of Alto Paraná, whose most populated cities—Ciudad del Este, Presidente Franco, and Hernandarias—border Brazil. By the end of 1997, more than 300 cases had been reported, 180 of which were confirmed through laboratory analysis or epidemiologic investigation. The last case of poliomyelitis occurred in 1985. In 1995, 23 cases of acute flaccid paralysis were investigated, and between January and October 1996, 19 cases were investigated. Wild poliovirus was ruled out in all cases. During 1992–1995, the numbers of cases of neonatal tetanus were 18, 28, 18, and 16, respectively. As of October 1996, eight cases had been reported. One case of diphtheria was reported in 1995 and none in 1996. Cases of whooping cough totaled 372 in 1992 and

272 in 1993. In 1994, the number dropped to 49, and in 1995 and 1996, only 13 and 16 cases, respectively, were reported.

Cholera and Other Intestinal Diseases. Since the cholera epidemic began in the Americas, Paraguay has reported seven cases: three in 1993 and four in 1996. All cases were laboratory confirmed and all were caused by *Vibrio cholerae* 01, biotype El Tor, serotype Inaba.

Between 1992 and 1996, public health services reported around 40,000 cases of diarrhea per year. Both the number and the proportion of cases in persons under and over the age of 5 years remained about the same during that period (80% of the cases occurred in children under age 5 and 20% in the rest of the population).

Chronic Communicable Diseases. Tuberculosis continues to be a serious public health problem, particularly among indigenous and rural populations. The disease mainly affects adults 15 years old and older. In 1992 and 1993, the annual incidence was 43.3 per 100,000 population; in 1994, it was 38.4; in 1995, 36.1; and in 1996, 37.2. Of these cases, 95% were the pulmonary form; 45% of the cases that occurred in 1995 were confirmed by sputum smear microscopy. Case reporting continues to be incomplete and irregular, especially cases confirmed by bacteriological analysis, and the figures do not reflect the true magnitude of the problem. The most recent cohort studies show cure rates of around 70% and treatment abandonment rates of 17%.

Between 1992 and 1996, the number of new cases of leprosy remained relatively stable; 365, 338, 376, 227, and 386 cases were reported for each year of that period. The national prevalence rate is 2.5 per 10,000, although there are problems with underreporting. The departments with the highest rates are Alto Paraguay, Amambay, and Canendiyú.

Acute Respiratory Infections. Acute respiratory infections continue to be the principal reason for medical consultation. In 1995, they were the leading cause of death in the age group 1–4 years old, and they accounted for 14.5% of all reported deaths of children under 5 years. Between 1991 and 1996, 200,000 cases were reported annually.

Rabies. The incidences of canine rabies in Paraguay increased from 227 cases in 1994 to 572 cases in the period between January and October 1996. In 1992, there were three cases of human rabies; in 1996 there were six cases. In 1995, more than 15,000 people sought medical attention because they were at risk of contracting rabies. Canine rabies occurs most frequently in the central part of the country. The Central, Paraguarí, and Caaguazú departments accounted for 90% of reported cases; the Central Department accounts for 80% of those cases.

AIDS and Other STDs. Between 1986 and December 1996, a total of 253 cases of AIDS were reported in Paraguay, with a case fatality rate of 57%. During the first four years of the epidemic, the annual mean number of cases remained under 10. During the next five years, about 20 cases were reported per year, and during the last four years, the yearly average was 35. The annual incidence rate is 1 per 100,000 population.

The age groups most affected by AIDS are those between 30 and 34, followed by those between 35 and 39. More males than females are affected; the disease is becoming increasingly frequent among women, however. The first female case of AIDS was registered in 1990—five years after the first case was reported nationwide. Since then, there have been approximately 10 new cases of AIDS in women each year.

In 66% of the cases, exposure to the virus has been through sexual contact. Early in the epidemic most cases occurred among homosexuals, but in recent years many heterosexuals have been affected. About 12% of cases acquired the virus through intravenous drug use, 3.8% through blood transfusions, and 2.9% through perinatal transmission.

Available information on HIV infection indicates that persons between the ages of 20 and 24 constitute the group at highest risk. According to data from the National Blood Transfusion Center, the prevalence of HIV infection in blood donors is 0.2%.

The number of cases of syphilis remained relatively constant between 1988, when 763 cases were reported, and 1990, when 765 cases were reported. In 1992 the number of reported cases climbed to 1,022. Rates have not fluctuated much since then. In 1995, the Ministry of Public Health recorded 1,016 cases, of which 263 (26%) were diagnosed in pregnant women, and 56 (5.6%) were cases of congenital syphilis. As of October 1996, 683 cases of syphilis had been reported. The same year, only 66% of blood for transfusions were subjected to serologic testing with the VDRL test. The prevalence of seropositivity among donors was 3.4%.

Noncommunicable Diseases and Other Health-Related Problems

Nutritional Diseases and Diseases of Metabolism. Protein-energy malnutrition is not a serious problem in Paraguay. However, deficiency disorders, such as anemia, endemic goiter, and some vitamin deficiencies, are common, especially in the lowest-income population. According to a 1993 height-for-age survey, the prevalence of malnutrition in schoolchildren was 10.3% nationwide. The rate was twice as high in rural areas, and in public schools the rate was three times that found among students in private schools. The lowest rate (3.7%) was found in Asunción, and the highest

(15.3%) was in the department of Canendiyú. In 1995, 88 deaths due to nutritional diseases, vitamin deficiency, and anemia (ICD-9, 260–269; 280–285) were registered, 33 of which were deaths of children under 5.

Cardiovascular Diseases. In 1991–1992, the Institute for Health Sciences Research at the National University of Asunción conducted a study to analyze the prevalence of certain risk factors for cardiovascular disease. The sample consisted of 1,606 people of both sexes who were between 20 and 70 years of age and lived in Asunción or the surrounding metropolitan area. Results showed that the prevalence of diabetes was 6.1%, while that of glucose intolerance was 11.5%; 11.5% of the study population (9.5% of the men and 12.4% of the women) had high blood pressure and 17.2% of the men and 10.4% of the women had elevated triglyceride levels. Of the total study population, 53.8% were obese (45.8% of the men and 57.4% of the women) and 40% had a sedentary lifestyle, with higher prevalence among women aged 30–49.

In 1995, diseases of the circulatory system (ICD-9, 390–459) accounted for 5,537 deaths. Of these, 2,013 were due to cerebrovascular disease (ICD-9, 430–438), 1,573 to acute myocardial infarction and ischemic heart disease (ICD-9, 410–415), and 319 to hypertensive disease (ICD-9, 401–404). Of the 5,537 deaths due to these causes, 4,535 (82%) occurred in the age group older than 60 years.

Malignant Neoplasms. In 1995, malignant neoplasms (ICD-9, 140–239) accounted for 1,930 deaths, representing 12% of all deaths that year. Mortality from this cause for both sexes was 40 per 100,000 population—46 per 100,000 for females and 33 for males. Among women, the largest numbers of deaths were due to malignant neoplasm of the uterus and uterine cervix (12 per 100,000), breast (5 per 100,000), and stomach (4 per 100,000). For men, the highest death rates were from malignant neoplasm of trachea, bronchus, and lung (7 per 100,000) followed by prostrate and stomach (each at 5 per 100,000).

Among women, cancer of the uterus and uterine cervix, breast, and stomach, and leukemia, in that order, are the four leading causes of death from malignant neoplasms, accounting for 49.7% of all female deaths from that cause. Of the 295 deaths attributed to malignant neoplasm of the uterus and cervix, 120 originated as cervical cancer and 25% occurred in women under 45 years of age.

In men, the four leading causes of death from this cause were cancer of the respiratory system, prostate, and stomach, and leukemia, which together accounted for 59% of all male deaths from malignant neoplasms.

Accidents and Violence. Accidents and violence are an important cause of death and hospitalization. Traffic accidents are the most frequent type of accident and rank ahead of work-related and domestic accidents. In 1995, 58% of deaths due to accidents and violence occurred in the 15–24 age group and 24% were in the 25–44 age group; in 80% of these deaths, the victims were males.

In the first four months of 1995, the number of deaths due to traffic accidents increased by 40% compared with the first four months of 1994. Whereas 93 people died in 1994, in 1995 the number of deaths totaled 130. A total of 461 and 761 accidents were reported in 1994 and 1995, respectively.

In Alto Paraná, accidents are the second leading cause of death and homicide is the third. One of every five homicides in the country takes place in Alto Paraná.

In 1995, 515 deaths due to homicide (ICD-9, 960–969) were recorded, which was 3.2% of all registered deaths; 91% of the homicide victims were males.

Behavioral Disorders. In 1991, a study on mental health and substance use habits was conducted. The study population consisted of persons aged 12–45 years who resided in the 10 most populated cities in the country. The study detected abuse of sedatives, hypnotics, or stimulants in 10.3% of the sample and abuse of amphetamines in 4.6%. One-third (32%) of those surveyed smoked or had smoked; of this proportion, 14% smoked on a regular basis, and 10% smoked more than 10 cigarettes per day. The prevalence of marijuana use was 1.4%; that of cocaine use was 0.3%; and that of use of analgesics for nontherapeutic purposes was 3.0%. Inhaled substances were used by 2.5% of the sample, and 6.6% used sedatives without a medical prescription. The most frequently used substances with the highest potential for addiction were alcohol and pain killers.

In 1995, 121 deaths due to suicide (ICD-9, 950–958) were registered; 70% were males.

Oral Health. A study was carried out in 1995 to determine the DMFT (decayed, missing, filled teeth) index, but the results are not yet available. According to studies conducted in 1989, the most common oral health problem is dental caries, which affects 98% of schoolchildren and 100% of adults.

Hantavirus Pulmonary Syndrome. In November 1995, several clinical cases of respiratory problems, as well as asymptomatic infection with the Sin Nombre strain of Hantavirus, were found in adults living in the city of Filadelfia, located in the center of the Chaco Region. Of 24 possible cases, 23 tested positive for antibodies, as did 4 of 27 contacts and 44 of the 345 residents in the locale. *Calomys laucha* was the most frequently captured rodent as well as the species with the highest rate of antibodies to the Sin Nombre virus.

RESPONSE OF THE HEALTH SYSTEM

National Health Plans and Policies

The National Constitution adopted in 1992 identifies health as a basic right of all citizens and establishes that the National Health System will carry out integrated health actions, with policies that will promote joint formulation and coordination of programs and services by the public and private sectors.

The national health policy seeks to respond to the population's health needs through coordinated actions of public and private sector institutions. It assigns priority to maternal and child health and nutrition; control of vaccine-preventable diseases, communicable diseases, and zoonoses; environmental health; strengthening of health services; interinstitutional coordination; community participation in the health system; and care for marginal populations and indigenous communities.

In December 1996, the Congress adopted Law 1,032, which creates a National Health System. The system basically aims at delivering services to all people in an equitable, timely, and efficient manner—without discrimination of any kind—in the areas of health promotion, recovery, and rehabilitation. The system establishes inter- and intrasectoral links and incorporates all institutions that were created for the specific purpose of participating in health activities.

Health Sector Reform

The National Health System Law is part of the strategy for health sector reform. This law incorporates the principles of equity, quality, efficiency, and social participation. Its implementation began with a process of decentralization at the departmental and regional levels, as well as with the execution of two projects funded by the World Bank and the Inter-American Development Bank (IDB), which sought to strengthen health services in the 11 departments where 71% of the population resides.

The principal strategies of the Ministry of Public Health and Social Welfare are the following: to establish a national health care system that complements and coordinates the entities responsible for developing health activities, with a view to improving care and increasing the coverage of services; to put into action the national government's decentralization policies through ongoing implementation of departmental and district health councils; to strengthen local health systems, which, in turn, will strengthen self-management of the different levels of health care and help optimize the use of available local resources; and to create the National Health Data Center, an agency of the Ministry of Public Health and Social Welfare whose primary purpose will be data collection and processing to facilitate management of

the health sector. The private sector will also be involved in this project.

Organization of the Health Sector

Institutional Organization

The National Health Council is responsible for the coordination of health sector activities. The Council is made up of key health institutions and is headed by the Ministry of Public Health and Social Welfare. By law, it is responsible for coordinating and overseeing the plans, programs, and activities of both public and private health institutions.

Health care is the responsibility of three subsectors. The public subsector comprises the Ministry of Public Health and Social Welfare, the military health services, the police health services, municipal health services, the Sanitation Works Corporation, and the teaching hospital of the National University of Asunción. The semipublic subsector is made up of the IPS, the Paraguayan Red Cross, and the Our Lady of Asunción Catholic University Hospital. The private subsector is composed of multiple private medical centers, pharmaceutical laboratories, and pharmacies, linked together under the Association of Private Hospitals, Sanatoriums, and Private Clinics. The private subsector has grown tremendously in the past 10 years.

It is the Ministry's legal responsibility to ensure care for the population not covered by other institutions, particularly the most vulnerable and the lowest-income groups. Of this population, which makes up between 60% and 65% of the total, 40% has no coverage and is concentrated in rural and periurban areas.

Of the total national population, the Ministry of Public Health covers 63%; private services, 15%; the military health services, around 3%; the police health system, less than 1%; and the teaching hospital at the National University of Asunción, approximately 5%. IPS covers about 13% of the population for risks associated with occupational illnesses, accidents, disability, and old age. Both the Ministry and IPS are organized in a regionalized system with various levels of complexity. Municipal health services are responsible for public health activities such as refuse collection, public sanitation, and others.

Organization of Health Regulatory Activities

Health Code 836/88 recognizes the Ministry of Public Health as the highest public authority in matters of health and social welfare. The Ministry's Department of Health Surveillance is charged with registering and marketing drugs. However, the Department is staffed by few professionals, who are responsible for all administrative processes involved in registering products and licensing health establishments, including all the pharmacies in the country.

The Ministry of Public Health maintains a quality control system under an agreement with the National University of Asunción and its Center for Multidisciplinary Technological Research. This center conducts quality control testing of drugs before they are marketed, as well as post-marketing analysis, if so requested by the Ministry pursuant to a routine inspection or submission of a complaint. Paraguay is currently in the process of implementing the MERCOSUR rules and regulations for quality control of pharmaceutical products and verification of good manufacturing practices.

Reporting of communicable diseases has been mandatory for all public, private, and social security health services since 1915; however, in practice, reporting is limited to public services and, to a certain degree, those of IPS. The Ministry of Public Health, through the Department of Epidemiology, is responsible for compiling disease reports. Weekly reporting is required for 40 diseases and health events. Of these, 16 are under intensified surveillance, and any suspected cases must be reported immediately. HIV/AIDS and Hantavirus pulmonary syndrome are the two diseases most recently incorporated into the system. Epidemiological surveillance results are published in a quarterly epidemiological bulletin. Health inspection of ports, airports, and ground transportation terminals—which is carried out by various agencies of the Ministry of Public Health—is also part of the surveillance system.

The National Food and Nutrition Institute (INAN), an agency of the Ministry, was created in May 1996 and is responsible for food safety and quality control at the national level. The creation of this agency, coupled with coordination of control activities by the National Food Safety Commission (made up of representatives of the ministries of Public Health, Agriculture, and Industry and Commerce) and the integration of Paraguay into MERCOSUR, has substantially enhanced food quality control in Paraguay.

Health Services and Resources

Organization of Services for Care of the Population

Health Promotion. The Ministry carries out health education and communication activities to support the programs on AIDS, cholera, family health, infant survival, prevention of drug and tobacco use, nutrition, and adolescent health. However, the national scope of these programs has not been evaluated.

In March 1997, agreements were signed with 10 *municipios,* including Asunción, for the development of a healthy communities strategy.

Knowledge about how to maintain good health and how to prevent illness and accidents is limited because of lack of information and education. Health education programs do not reach every corner of the country because of shortages of human and financial resources. In addition, at the health services level, little emphasis is placed on health promotion.

Research on health education and communication is limited, and there is little coordination between the social sectors for coordination and implementation of joint programs.

Drinking Water and Sewerage Services. In 1996, 48.3% of the urban population and 18.3% of the rural population had access to drinking water, with an average coverage nationwide of 27.1%. The availability of sewerage systems nationwide is 14.8%. In the interior, only two localities have a sewerage system. Coverage is concentrated in Asunción, where half the population has access to such systems. There are no systems in 11 of the country's departments, and in the remaining 6, coverage is under 10%.

The sewerage system in Asunción discharges wastewater directly into the Paraguay River at a mean rate of approximately 1.5 m^3/sec. The volume of wastewater discharge is not expected to reach a high-risk level of 5.0 m^3/sec until the year 2000. The discharge has an approximate dilution of 1/2,000, which eliminates the need for treatment plants. The same is true of other units that also discharge wastewater into the Paraguay River. Nevertheless, if population growth and industrialization continue at their current pace, the river could become extremely polluted.

Environmental Quality. The situation with regard to the environment and natural resources is characterized by rapid deforestation, loss of biodiversity, and deterioration of the ecosystem, with erosion of the soil in the eastern region and salinization in the western region resulting in the loss of fertile land. Various natural ecosystems and animal and plant species are in danger of extinction. Moreover, this environmental degradation is destroying indigenous habitats, which in turn leads to loss of cultural identity. There is a serious problem with surface- and underground water pollution— the result of poor management of solid, liquid, industrial, and domestic waste—as well as air pollution, which is mainly due to motor vehicle emissions and industrial activities. The most outstanding environmental problems are those linked to development of new agricultural lands, human settlements, and the hydroelectric plants in Itaipú and Yacyretá.

Air pollution is a relatively minor problem, but it is becoming more serious in some cities, especially Asunción, as a result of increased industrialization and motor vehicle traffic.

The country has an Environmental Health Program, in which all the institutions with responsibilities in the area of the environment, water, and sanitation participate. The program's main components are drinking water supply and excreta disposal; pollution control; improvement, monitoring, and control of water quality; and sanitary waste disposal.

The Sanitation Works Corporation, an agency of the Ministry of the Interior, is responsible for providing drinking water, sewerage, and storm drainage services for communities with more than 4,000 inhabitants; communities with 4,000 or fewer inhabitants are served by the National Environmental Sanitation Service.

The Ministry of Agriculture and Livestock regulates the use of water resources. Once a year, analyses of heavy metals and pesticides are conducted, mainly in the Paraguay River, which is the main source of drinking water for the city of Asunción. A special laboratory detects pollution produced by alcohol factories.

Funding for environmental protection activities comes from water and sewerage service fees, taxes on alcoholic and nonalcoholic beverages, real estate taxes, and loans from banks and international organizations.

The National Environmental Sanitation Service plans, establishes standards, develops projects, and constructs works for water supply and excreta disposal systems. The services are administered by local sanitation boards.

Organization and Operation of Personal Health Care Services

Since 1990, the 18 health regions have been strengthened through increased financial and human resources and through decentralization; these improvements have given them greater autonomy and better operating capabilities. Services are structured on four levels. The first, or primary care level, provides for the basic needs of rural, isolated, or remote communities with fewer than 1,000 inhabitants. It consists mainly of health posts staffed by health volunteers, nursing auxiliaries, and birth attendants. The secondary, or basic, level provides care of moderate complexity for rural and periurban communities with populations between 2,000 and 20,000. The second level consists of health centers with a few beds (6–19) and a health care team that includes doctors; dentists; biochemists; pharmacists; nurses; obstetricians; health inspectors; and technical, administrative, and auxiliary personnel. The tertiary, or basic complementary, level is responsible for meeting more complex needs through general medical services and some specialized services. It consists of hospitals and regional health centers. The fourth, or specialized, level provides comprehensive care in specialized areas and serves as a referral center for the network of regional health services. Its principal resources are the National Hospital, the Cancer and Burn Hospital, the Juan Max Boettner Sanatorium, the Urgent Care Hospital, and the Central Laboratory and Institute of Tropical Medicine.

The health sector has no plan for coordinating the development of the operating capacity of its various institutions. Each one functions independently, which leads to duplication of services in the country's principal cities. In 1996, the physical resources of the public, private, and semiprivate sectors consisted of 1,140 establishments, including 47 hospitals, 25 regional hospitals, 197 health centers, 657 health posts or infirmaries, and 214 clinics and sanatoriums. Of the 1,140 establishments, 706 were administered by the Ministry of Health, 100 by IPS, 65 by the military health services, 23 by the police health services, 2 by the National University, 2 by the Catholic University, and 1 by the Red Cross; 241 were private.

The Ministry has 10 specialized hospitals, 15 regional hospitals, 137 health centers, and 477 health posts. IPS maintains 1 central hospital, 7 regional hospitals, 22 health centers, and 70 health posts. The military health services consist of 1 central hospital, 3 division hospitals, 35 health centers, and 26 infirmaries. The police health services include 1 central hospital and 22 infirmaries. The National University of Asunción has a teaching hospital and a neuropsychiatric hospital. The Catholic University has two hospitals—one in Asunción and the other in Villarrica.

The total number of hospital beds is estimated at 6,655, of which 2,905 are in establishments of the Ministry of Health, 1,816 in the private sector, 1,118 in IPS institutions, 539 in the teaching hospital of the National University of Asunción, 187 in the armed services hospital, and 90 in the police hospital.

In 1995, a total of 2,544,482 medical visits and 94,696 hospital discharges were registered in establishments administered by the Ministry of Public Health; 45% of the discharges were of women admitted for childbirth. The bed occupancy rate was 45%. According to data from the Ministry, in 1995 physicians attended 40% of the births that occurred in the Ministry's establishments; another 40% were attended by nurses or midwives, 16% by traditional birth attendants, and 4% by other personnel.

In 1995, there were 311,029 prenatal visits in Ministry of Public Health establishments; 30% were attended by physicians, 38% by nurses or midwives, and 32% by auxiliary personnel.

There are several centers that offer diagnostic imaging services, but it is not known whether they meet safety standards.

Considerable progress has been made in screening blood products and blood used for transfusions, thanks to strengthening of the National Center for Blood Transfusions. By law, all blood must be screened for HIV infection, Chagas' disease, syphilis, and hepatitis B; screening for hepatitis C is currently being undertaken. Through a strategy of providing staff training and a timely supply of reagents, the barriers to effective control of public and private blood banks are being overcome.

There is a shortage of mental health professionals, including psychologists with clinical experience, especially in rural areas.

There is also a lack of postgraduate courses in psychiatry. The scarcity of mental health units and services in general hospitals and health centers makes this one of the least-developed areas.

There are no mechanisms for maintaining up-to-date information on the number and complexity of health establishments and on the equipment they house.

With regard to services for the elderly, there is a national plan under the supervision of Social Welfare. The plan is based on interinstitutional and intersectoral coordination and incorporates social and community programs for older adults, societal motivation and sensitization programs, a program to support and strengthen institutions that provide services for the elderly, and a program to develop and modify related legislation.

Inputs for Health

The national pharmaceutical industry (or pharmaceutical companies located in the country) is in an initial stage of development and is mainly geared toward the formulation, processing, packaging, and other activities related to the final preparation of pharmaceutical products. All the raw materials are imported. The country has no chemical-pharmaceutical industry.

In November 1996, the Senate approved a law for quality control of pharmaceuticals, cosmetics, domestic cleaning products, and similar products. The law is still being reviewed in Congress.

A national list of essential drugs has been developed based on the International Nonproprietary Names and essential drugs list of WHO. This list is used as a guide for the procurement and use of drugs in health services.

Purchases of drugs are currently funded through budget allocations from some local governments. The items are procured through a competitive bidding system coordinated by the Ministry of Public Health. For information and training, there is the National Pharmacopeia, which was adopted in 1943 and has not been updated. However, in practice, the United States Pharmacopeia (USP) is used as a reference.

Community pharmacies have been established in the country with initial funding from the Ministry of Public Health and Social Welfare, which facilitates access to essential drugs at low cost.

Human Resources

According to data from the Ministry, in 1995 the country had 3,730 physicians, 1,279 dentists, 433 professional nurses, 1,547 licensed midwives, 1,875 pharmacists, 892 biochemists, 96 licensed social workers, and 1,561 psychologists.

Of a total of 5,226 people employed in 1995 in services administered by the Ministry of Public Health, 13% were physicians; 3.7%, dentists; 1.2%, biochemists; 9.5%, nurses or midwives; 8%, technical personnel; 37%, nursing auxiliaries; and 25%, administrative or service personnel. The distribution of Ministry personnel by health regions was fairly uniform, although in 5 of the 18 health regions there was a marked shortage of doctors in relation to the size of the population.

Most of the country's oral health professionals are in private practice, including dental assistants and a large number of dental technicians, who make prostheses, crowns, and other dental apparatuses. In the public sector, in 1995 the Ministry of Public Health employed nearly 200 dentists, more than half of whom were in Asunción and the Central Department, where 34% of the population lives. In 8 of the 18 departments there is a serious shortage of oral health personnel.

The Ministry of Public Health has stressed training for personnel in hospital administration, statistics, epidemiology, public health, and maternal and child health as well as training for technical and auxiliary personnel. In addition, a process of redistributing personnel and improving compensation and benefits based on performance and productivity has been implemented. Nevertheless, there are serious flaws in the strategy as well as problems in planning training activities and supervising educational processes.

Research and Technology

With financial backing from international organizations, the National University of Asunción, through the Institute for Health Sciences Research, participates in basic and applied biomedical research.

University programs generally do little to encourage scientific research, and research methodology courses are insufficient. There is no information system through which scientific knowledge is compiled and research is disseminated. Most health studies are merely descriptive.

Scientific and technological research activities are carried out mainly in response to specific events and not as the result of an explicit policy. In addition, there is little financial support, minimal institutional structures, and a marked lack of human resources for such research; consequently, technological production and knowledge are scarce.

Expenditures and Sectoral Financing

Of total health spending, 20% comes from the overall national budget. IPS contributions represent 26%, and direct expenditures by the population account for the remaining 54%.

Public expenditure for health as a percentage of GDP in 1990–1993 was 1.2%. Between 1984 and 1995, the share of the Ministry of Public Health and Social Welfare in the national budget ranged from a low of 4% to a high of 7.5%. Lack of information makes it impossible to accurately estimate the share of private and IPS spending.

In 1996, 64% of the financing for the Ministry's budget came from the Treasury, 14% from revenues of the Itaipú hydroelectric plant, 6% from resources of the Ministry itself, 6% from foreign credit, 5% from special resources, and 5% from other resources.

Income from private prepayment systems totals approximately US$ 26 million annually, which is 13% to 15% of public sector spending.

IPS is financed through the trilateral support of employers, workers, and the State. In addition, IPS receives income from investment of reserve funds, contributions to the special system, contributions of pensioners and retirees, and proceeds from surcharges, penalties, etc. Workers contribute 9% of their earnings, employers contribute 14% of the amount paid to their employees, and the State contributes 1.5% of the taxable wages that firms pay their workers. Under the special system, public- and private-sector teachers, university professors, independent contractors, and domestic workers contribute 8% of their earnings.

External Technical and Financial Cooperation

The Government has negotiated many bilateral and multilateral technical cooperation agreements aimed at extending the coverage of health services and improving health care for the population. Foreign cooperation has been received for development of the regionalized health services system, water supply and sanitation in rural areas, developing and strengthening institutions, maternal and child health, food and nutrition programs, control of leprosy and other specific diseases, prevention of blindness, research into a method for detecting Chagas' disease, the national AIDS program, and programs for immunization, diarrheal disease control, basic sanitation, and rural health.

The Government has also entered into agreements for projects with IDB, the World Bank, and the Japanese International Cooperation Agency (JICA), especially in the area of maternal and child health. These projects will run for approximately five years and will cover 12 departments, where 73% of the population resides. The total amount of project financing is US$ 75 million: 62% from the IDB, 30% from the World Bank, and 8% from JICA.

The country also has projects with the German Development Bank; the international development agencies of Germany, Brazil, France, Japan, and the United States (USAID); UNICEF; the United Nations Population Fund; the Kellogg Foundation; the World Food Program; the United Nations Development Program; the International Development Research Center of Canada; Rotary International; and the United States Peace Corps.

USAID has provided aid for pilot projects to develop or enhance district health councils. UNICEF has provided US$ 1.2 million in support for activities in the areas of maternal and perinatal health, child survival and development, and assistance for children living in precarious conditions. A loan from the German Credit Bank has been invested in infrastructure and equipment in the southern part of the country, and another US$ 2.5 million is expected to be invested in the expansion of maternal and child health services in southern departments.

The Spanish Government has extended a loan for US $32 million for specialized hospital equipment, health establishments in the capital, and health posts throughout country.

PERU

GENERAL SITUATION AND TRENDS

Socioeconomic, Political, and Demographic Overview

Peru is located in the central-western part of South America. It has a surface area of 1,285,216 km² and is divided into three large natural regions: the coast, the mountains, and the jungle. Peru is a multicultural, multilingual, and multiethnic country. The Constitution of 1993 established the department as the main political-administrative unit (the country has 24 departments subdivided into 192 provinces, which, in turn, comprise 1,812 districts, plus one "constitutional province").

State policy is influenced by two main trends: the promotion of economic liberalization and the effort to respond to basic social needs, many of which are unmet. According to the 1993 census, 53.9% of households had at least one unmet basic need. In response, the Government has decided to reform the functions of the State and reorient public spending in order to achieve greater efficiency in the use of resources and ensure that expenditures do not exceed tax revenues. This process implies limiting public functions to those areas that cannot be take over by the private sector for reasons relating to national security, social equity, and market regulation. There are two basic objectives of State reform: (1) to free up financial resources by deregulating the market, privatizing State-run companies, and creating an institutional framework that is favorable to free enterprise; and (2) to restructure the general and specific functions of the State and to find the most effective and efficient use of proceeds. The State reform process is taking place in a context of fiscal and monetary austerity coupled with efforts to pay off foreign debts. Within the context of the restructure of general and specific State functions, alleviation of extreme poverty is a medium-term goal and forms the basis for the Government's social policy. Within this policy, the health sector defines its target population through decentralized strategies.

The Peruvian economy has evolved with considerable ups and downs. The mid-1970s marked the beginning of a prolonged economic crisis that peaked in 1983 and 1989, with reductions in the gross domestic product (GDP) along the order of 12.6% and 11.7%, respectively. The periods of expansion have been short-lived, owing basically to the policy of import substitution that was promoted by the State and applied in combination with a relative price structure that was highly distorted. This policy collapsed in 1988 and generated a serious recession that was accompanied by hyperinflation, social disorder, and violence. Inflation began to be brought under control only in August 1990, when the new Government introduced stabilization measures. That year, the country experienced an unprecedented level of inflation (a 7,650% cumulative increase in prices). Since the fourth quarter of 1990, however, inflation has declined steadily, dropping to 12.5% in 1994 and to 10.4% in 1996.

Between 1987 and 1992, national output decreased 23.5%, and per capita output dropped 28.9%, which exacerbated the already high levels of poverty. Between 1993 and 1995, the gross national product (GNP) showed an upward trend, thanks to which in 1995 it was possible to recover the real levels of production that had prevailed in the country in 1987. This recovery occurred in a framework of stabilization and restructuring of the economy, as well as actions aimed at quelling internal violence and reintegrating the country into the international economic community. The recovery of private investment was supported by the success of anti-inflation measures and an increase in the Government's credibility. Private investment rose in almost all sectors, especially in construction, commerce, agriculture, and manufacturing.

Despite the economic growth of the past several years and the political will that gave rise to poverty alleviation programs, progress in the social sector has been limited. Based on two methods of measuring poverty—the poverty line and unmet basic needs—it is estimated that around one-half of Peruvian families live in poverty. According to the national surveys of living standards (ENNIV) conducted in 1985, 1991, 1994, and 1996, poverty levels declined from 53.6% to 49.6% between 1991 and 1994, and the latter value was maintained in 1996. According to the definition that has been consistently applied in the ENNIV surveys since 1985, poverty is the inability to cover the cost of a basic market basket of food and other goods and services. In 1994, 20% of the national population was living in extreme poverty. The percentage was even higher in rural areas of the coastal, mountain, and jungle regions (66%, 68%, and 70%, respectively). Extreme poverty is defined as the inability to cover the cost of a market basket consisting only of food that meets minimum nutritional requirements. The Lima metropolitan area has the lowest percentages of poor and extremely poor population: 38% and 5%, respectively. According to the 1993 census, 53.9% of Peruvian households had at least one unmet basic need. In rural areas, the proportion was 88.2%, while in urban areas, it was 39.2%. In 16 of the 25 departments, more than 60% of households had at least one unmet basic need. All except one were located in the Andean region or in the jungle. Based on these figures, the National Institute of Statistics and Information Science (INEI) classified the population in five "poverty strata." The provinces in which the poorest strata reside had the highest proportions of young people (under 15 years of age) and the lowest levels of intercensus growth, owing to migration of the population to escape poverty and political violence.

In 1995, the Ministry of Labor and Social Promotion redefined the concept of underemployment, which has altered its time-series data. "Open underemployed" describes workers who work less than 35 hours a week, who want to work more, and who are capable of doing so. "Hidden underemployment" refers to the situation of those who work more than 35 hours a week but earn less than the minimum wage. The minimum wage is based on the cost of a minimum market basket for a family of five with two income earners. According to data from late 1996, 7.1% of the economically active population (people over 15 years of age who are working or are actively seeking employment) was unemployed, 42.4% was underemployed, and only 49.0% had adequate employment. Underemployment based on income (hidden underemployment, 27%) was greater than underemployment based on hours of work (open underemployment, 16%), owing to a shorter work day. Underemployment was higher among females (51%) than males (37%) and among those with only a primary education (50% compared with 29% for those with a university education).

Illiteracy rates decreased from 18.1% to 12.8% in the intercensus period between 1981 and 1993, although notable differences between males and females persist, especially in rural areas. In 1993, the illiteracy rate was 7.1% among males;

among females it was 18.3%. In rural areas the rates were very high: 17.0% of males and 42.9% of females.

According to the IX Population Census and the IV Housing Census conducted in 1993, the total population of Peru was 22,639,443 inhabitants. The average annual population growth rate between 1981 and 1993 was 2.0%, maintaining the downward trend of the past 30 years. On the basis of this intercensus growth rate, it is estimated that the total population of Peru as of 30 June 1996 was 23,946,800. In 1993, 70.1% of the national population was urban (15,870,250 inhabitants). The growing process of urbanization is evident when this figure is compared with the figures for 1972 (59.5%) and 1981 (65.2%). Between 1981 and 1993, the average annual growth rate of the urban population was 2.8%, while that of the rural population was 0.9%. In that same year, females made up 50.3% of the total population, and more than a third of the population (37.0%) was under 15 years of age. The proportion of the population aged 65 and over increased from 4.1% in 1981 to 4.6% in 1993.

The crude birth rate declined from 35 births per 1,000 population in 1980 to 26 per 1,000 in 1996. The total fertility rate, which until the 1960s was more than 6.5 children per woman, declined to 4.0 children per woman in 1991. The total fertility rate varied at the departmental level, ranging from a low of 2.2 children per woman in Callao to highs of 6.5 and 5.9 in Huancavelica and Apurímac, respectively. According to the 1996 Demographic and Family Health Survey (ENDES), the total fertility rate was 3.5 children per woman nationwide (2.8 in urban areas, 5.6 in rural areas, and 2.5 in the Lima metropolitan area). Fertility also varied considerably with the educational level of women: from a total fertility rate of 6.9 among women with no schooling and 5.0 among women with only a primary education to 3.0 and 2.1 for women with secondary schooling and higher education, respectively.

Life expectancy increased from 53.6 to 66.3 years between 1970 and 1993. In 1993, the departmental rates ranged from 54.4 in Huancavelica to 77.1 in Callao; these differences have persisted over time. In the 1993 census, 22.3% of the population (4,921,020 inhabitants) indicated that they had been born in a place different from their place of residence at the time of the census. Most of this internal migration was absorbed by Lima (48.1%) and Callao (7.8%). Other urban centers that received significant proportions of the migrant population were Arequipa (5.1%), La Libertad (4.0%), Lambayeque (3.7%), San Martín (3.6%), and Junín (3.5%). The departments that lost population due to migration were Cajamarca (9.9%), Ancash (7.5%), Ayacucho (6.5%), and Puno (6.1%). In addition to the traditional causes of internal migration, a sizable number of people migrated to escape violence and its attendant problems, although the precise number has not been determined. In the past three years, internal migration has intensified as displaced persons have returned to their places of origin, thanks to successful efforts to stem violence and to the development of new agricultural and mining areas in mountain and jungle regions. International emigration has increased in recent decades. The country registered a net population loss of 36,000 in the 1975–1980 period and 370,000 in the 1990–1995 period.

Mortality Profile

In 1992, underreporting of deaths at the national level was estimated at 50.8%. The departments with the highest levels of underreporting were Ayacucho (99.4%), Amazonas (80.5%), Loreto (79.7%), and Huancavelica (76.9%); the departments with lowest rates were Ica (14.3%), Tacna (19.6%), and Lima (22.6%). For the five poverty strata, the underregistration rates are 27.1%, 36.0%, 53.0%, 74.9%, and 75.1%, respectively. Of all reported deaths, the proportion with death certificates was 70.6% nationwide. The rate at the departmental level ranged from 97.9% in Callao to 24.4% in Apurímac. By poverty stratum, the rates ranged from 90.6% in stratum I to 33.0% in stratum V. The proportion of deaths attributed to ill-defined signs, symptoms, and conditions was 30.6% overall. In poverty stratum I this proportion was 9.9%, and in stratum V it reached 69.8%.

Analysis of proportional mortality by the six major groups of causes showed that at the national level communicable diseases were the leading cause of death, followed by diseases of the circulatory system and malignant neoplasms, which accounted for 27.5%, 19.4%, and 15.2% of all deaths, respectively. In stratum I, diseases of the circulatory system ranked first (22.1%), closely followed by communicable diseases (21.5%) and malignant neoplasms (19.3%). In stratum V, on the other hand, communicable diseases were responsible for 44.0% of all deaths; diseases of the circulatory system for 10.2%; and malignant neoplasms for only 4.6%. The risk of dying from a communicable disease was 6.3 times greater in stratum V than in stratum I (mortality rates of 6.9 and 1.1 per 1,000 population, respectively). Mortality from certain conditions originating in the perinatal period also showed marked differences among strata (43.2 per 1,000 live births in stratum V and 12.6 per 1,000 in stratum I).

With regard to the structure of mortality by age groups, of all the deaths in stratum I, 13.1% and 2.9%, respectively, occurred among children under 1 and children aged 1–4 years; in stratum V these percentages were 29.3% and 11.1%, respectively. The risk of dying was five times higher for children under 1 in stratum V than in stratum I (151.1 and 31.0 per 1,000 children under 1) and seven times higher for children aged 1–4 (13.9 per 1,000 children aged 1–4 in stratum V compared with 1.8 in stratum I).

The 10 leading causes of death were acute respiratory infections (16.3%), intestinal infectious diseases (7.7%), diseases of pulmonary circulation and other forms of heart disease (5.4%), tuberculosis (5.0%), cerebrovascular disease (4.0%), diseases of the urinary system (3.5%), diseases of other parts of the digestive system (3.2%), nutritional deficiencies and anemias (3.2%), ischemic heart disease (3.2%), and hypoxia, birth asphyxia, and other respiratory conditions of the fetus or newborn (3.1%). This analysis, classified by strata, shows enormous variability. While acute respiratory infection was the leading cause of death in all strata, the relative importance of this cause increased with the degree of poverty: from 9.3% in stratum I to 25.2% in stratum V, which means that the risk of dying from this cause was 8.6 times greater in stratum V than in stratum I. The relative risk of dying from intestinal infectious diseases in stratum V was 7.8 times greater; from tuberculosis, 2.6 times greater; from hypoxia, birth asphyxia, and other respiratory conditions of the fetus or newborn, 6.0 times greater; from nutritional deficiencies and anemias, 4.3 times greater; and from appendicitis, hernia of the abdominal cavity, and intestinal obstruction without hernia, 18.5 times greater.

SPECIFIC HEALTH PROBLEMS

Analysis by Population Group

Health of Children

According to the 1993 census, infant mortality was 59.0 per 1,000 live births nationally, and ranged from 22.9 per 1,000 in Callao to 113.9 per 1,000 in Huancavelica. For the period 1995–2000, this indicator was estimated at 45.0 per 1,000 live births. The 1996 ENDES survey revealed a rate of 42.8 per 1,000. Neonatal mortality, according to the same source, was 25.0 per 1,000 live births. In 1992 the leading cause of death in children under 1 year of age was communicable diseases (39.8%), followed by certain conditions originating in the perinatal period (33.9%). Within the group of communicable diseases, acute respiratory infections (26.6%) and intestinal infectious diseases (11.1%) accounted for the largest proportions of deaths. However, these proportions varied significantly among the different poverty strata: communicable diseases and conditions originating in the perinatal period accounted for 29.7% and 39.3%, respectively, of deaths of under-1 children in stratum I and 49.6% and 29.1%, respectively, in stratum V. Among children aged 1–4, communicable diseases were the leading cause of death (66.7% at the national level, 55.2% in stratum I, and 74.7% in stratum V), followed by external causes (7.3%). Among the communicable diseases, respiratory infections caused 28.5% of all deaths and intestinal infectious diseases caused 25.1%.

According to the first national height census of school-children in the first grade of primary school (1993), 48.0% of children aged 6–9 suffered from chronic malnutrition. The situation was more serious in males (54%) and in rural areas (67%). The department that had the highest rate of malnutrition was Huancavelica (72%), while the lowest rates were found in Tacna (18%) and Callao (20%). According to mortality data from 1992, the principal causes of death in this age group were communicable diseases (46.8%) and external causes (20.2%).

Health of Adolescents

According to the 1993 census, adolescents made up 23.0% of the total population. The leading causes of death in the group aged 10–14 years were communicable diseases (40.2%) and external causes (21.7%); these proportions are reversed in the group aged 15–19 years (25% and 39.0%, respectively). The same census revealed that 13.6% of children aged 10–14 years were not attending school. The proportion increased to 26.7% in the group aged 15–17 years. The problem was most pronounced among females in rural areas (23.7%). In the group aged 10–14 years, 5.1% worked. Among those between 15 and 17 years of age, 17.9% worked. It was also found that, in urban areas, 69.0% of adolescents aged 12–14 had consumed alcohol at least once and 17.0% had used tobacco; in the group aged 15–18 years these percentages were 84.0% and 50%, respectively. With regard to the use of other drugs, 7 of every 1,000 children aged 12–14 admitted to having used marijuana at least once.

The fertility rate among adolescents has declined in recent decades, although not in the same proportion as in other age groups. Among women aged 45–49, fertility dropped 67.0% between 1961 and 1993, but in those aged 15–19 years it decreased only 43.0%. In 1993, 1.2% of girls aged 12–14 years and 6.0% of those aged 15–17 years had already had a child or were pregnant for the first time. Among adolescents in rural areas, the latter figure was 10.6%. Although 29.0% of adolescent girls aged 15–19 years who were in a sexual relationship indicated that they used some method of contraception, only 11.0% used a modern method. The vast majority of pregnancies among adolescents are unwanted, and they almost always end in abortion. In 1993, adolescents accounted for 15.0% of all maternal deaths, and an estimated 20.0% of maternal deaths from abortion occurred in this age group.

Health of Women

In 1996, 64.0% of women living with a male partner were using some method of contraception. In urban areas, the per-

centage was 70.0%, and in rural areas it was 51.0%. Seventy-five percent of women with higher education used some type of contraceptive method, while only 38.0% of women with no schooling did so. The most widely used method continues to be the rhythm method (18%), followed by the intrauterine device (12.0%) and female sterilization (10.0%). In 1992 and 1996, 63.9% and 66.2% of pregnant women, respectively, received prenatal care from a health care professional; in rural areas, the proportion was 44.5%, while in the Lima metropolitan area it was 87.4%. In the same two years, 52.5% and 55.1% of women, respectively, received professional care during childbirth. This indicator is lower in rural areas (19.1%) and in the jungle region (34.4%) compared with Lima (93.0%).

The maternal mortality rate is 265.0 per 100,000 live births. It is estimated that around 1,670 women die annually as a consequence of complications of pregnancy, childbirth, and the puerperium. In urban areas, the rate is 200.0 per 100,000 live births, and in rural areas it is 448.0 per 100,000. The maternal mortality rate is 10 times higher among illiterate women than among those with a higher education (448.0 and 49.0 per 100,000 live births, respectively). The leading direct obstetric causes of maternal mortality are hemorrhage (23.0%), abortion (22.0%), infection (18.0%), and toxemia (17.0%); the leading indirect cause is pulmonary tuberculosis.

Health of Adults

In 1992 the leading causes of death in the population aged 15–59 years were infectious diseases (21.9%), external causes (20.8%), and malignant neoplasms (17.6%). The distribution classified by poverty strata I and V was as follows: malignant neoplasms (23.8%), infectious diseases (21.3%), and external causes (11.8%) for stratum I; infectious diseases (32.3%), external causes (18.2%), and malignant neoplasms (6.5%) for stratum V. There were significant differences in the causes of death among men and women. Among men, the leading causes were tuberculosis (10.0%); homicide and intentional injury, injuries due to legal interventions and operations of war (8.4%); other accidents, including after-effects (6.6%); acute respiratory infections (6.4%); and motor vehicle traffic accidents (5.4%). Among women, the leading causes were tuberculosis (9.6%), malignant neoplasms of the uterine cervix (7.0%), acute respiratory infections (6.1%), cerebrovascular disease (4.5%), and malignant neoplasm of the breast (4.0%).

Health of the Elderly

Among the population aged 60 and over, diseases of the circulatory system are the primary cause of death (30.2%), followed by infectious diseases (20.9%) and malignant neoplasms (19.1%). In stratum I, diseases of the circulatory system accounted for 31.7% of all deaths, followed by malignant neoplasms (21.8%) and infectious diseases (17.3%); in stratum V, communicable diseases continued to be the leading cause of death (34.7%), followed by diseases of the circulatory system, which ranked a distant second (18.9%), and malignant neoplasms (5.9%). There are no significant differences according to sex.

Workers' Health

The Peruvian Social Security Institute (IPSS) has an Occupational Health Program, but it covers only 28.0% of the country's economically active population (7,814,809 people). Only 7.8% of wage earners are unionized. Since 1997, the Ministry of Health also has had an Occupational Health Program. According to IPSS, between 1995 and 1996 the occupational accident rate rose from 12.0 to 20.0 per 1,000 workers and fatal accidents increased from 0.7 to 1.9 per 10,000 workers. In part, these figures reflect an improvement in record-keeping, although in the case of fatal accidents the increase is real, because it has been verified on the basis of information provided by unions and by other ministries. Accidents occur mainly as a result of inadequate working conditions, combined with increases in workload. In the mining sector alone, 102 fatal accidents were registered in 1995 (compared with 68 in 1992, 57 in 1993, and 87 in 1994). Data on occupational illnesses are limited, although several studies have suggested that there are serious problems (hearing loss, asbestosis, pneumoconiosis). Another major problem is lack of access to occupational health services for workers in the informal sector (53.9%); the situation of these workers is exacerbated by a higher risk of becoming ill or being injured because of poor and hazardous working conditions and low wages. Based on the 1991 national census, in 1993 the INEI estimated the total number of children aged 6–14 who work at 175,022; the estimate of the Ministry of the Presidency for 1995 was 1,100,000 working children under the age of 18. These children work mainly in mining, agriculture, and in gold ore processing.

Health of Indigenous People

The indigenous population of Peru can be classified according to language and place of residence. Based on native language (Quechua, Aymara, or another indigenous language), a 1993 census identified 4,035,300 indigenous persons, 52% female and 48% male. Of this number, 75.0% resided in mountain areas, 9.0% in the jungle, and 17% in coastal regions, including the Lima metropolitan area. Of the indigenous population over 6 years of age, 22.0% had no schooling; the situation was even more serious in rural areas, especially among women. Forty-two percent of the indigenous population lived in extreme poverty—double the national average. A significant proportion were rural or unskilled workers, with cultural traits that often put them at a disadvantage for finding employment. Those who resided in rural mountainous areas and in the jungle had limited access to education and health services, owing partly to the geographic characteristics of their place of residence and partly to language and cultural barriers. With respect to basic sanitation services, 54% of Quechua speakers and 70% of Spanish-speaking indigenous persons had water service in their homes; the coverage of wastewater systems was 15% and 40%, respectively. Among the Quechua speakers, only 32% of those who reported that they had been sick or injured in the four weeks before the interview had received medical attention, compared with 46% of the Spanish speakers. The average expenditure of a Spanish-speaking person was 65% greater than the average expenditure of a person who spoke some indigenous language. These data suggest that investing in bilingual education that is adapted to indigenous cultural features is an essential strategy for overcoming the poverty that affects this group.

With regard to the indigenous communities living in jungle areas, in 1993 there were 13 linguistic families and 65 ethnic groups. The total population was 299,218 inhabitants (48% female and 52% male). The most populated departments were Loreto, with 83,746 indigenous inhabitants; Junín, with 57,530; Amazonas, with 49,717; and Ucayali, with 40,463. Of the total population surveyed, 49.7% were under 14 years of age, 48.8% were between 15 and 64, and 1.5% were 65 or older. By educational level, 32% had no schooling, 49% had a primary education, 16% had a secondary education, and 2.5% had a higher education. The curricula studied by the indigenous population were the standard curricula used in urban areas and did not take into account indigenous languages or sociocultural characteristics. Seventy-four percent of the indigenous population lived in poverty and more than half lived in extreme poverty; these figures are much higher than the national averages (49.6% and 20.2%, respectively). In the Campa-Ashaninka group, the fertility rate was 8.1 children per woman and infant mortality was 99 per 1,000 live births. Among the Machiguenga of Cuzco and Madre de Dios, the fertility rate was 8.4 children per woman and infant mortality was 100 per 1,000 live births. In the Peruvian jungle, the majority of the population engages in subsistence activities such as farming, hunting and gathering, and fishing. The indigenous population also makes greater use of medicinal plants. These communities have been exposed to political and social strife and to violence associated with drug trafficking, as well as forced migration, abandonment of their environment, and precarious living conditions. The Government has identified priority areas of intervention in health, education, and agriculture, as part of the strategy for poverty alleviation and support for communities in border areas.

Analysis by Type of Disease or Health Impairment

Communicable Diseases

Vector-Borne Diseases. The number of cases of malaria increased from 30,814 in 1989 to 211,561 in 1996, with an incidence rate of 885.0 per 100,000 population. The annual parasite index (API) increased from 2.4 per 1,000 in 1992 to 8.8 per 1,000 in 1996. The proportion of cases due to *Plasmodium falciparum* increased alarmingly from 1.6% in 1992 to 28.3% in 1996. Malaria is associated geographically and environmentally with the tropical and irrigated desert areas of the northern coast and the northeastern mountainous jungle region, the central-southeastern jungle region, and the lowland or Amazon jungle. The seasonal nature of the disease is evident along the northern coast and northwestern region of the country (higher incidence in the first half of the year), but transmission rates remain constant in the Amazon basin. In 1996, the population in high-risk areas numbered 2,382,035 (9.9% of the total population of the country), which reflected a reduction with regard to the at-risk population in 1994 (15.9%). That same year, 77.9% of the reported cases were concentrated in five regions and health subregions (Loreto, Jaén, Luciano Castillo, Junín, and San Martín), and 88.4% of the *P. falciparum* cases were concentrated in the first three. Loreto and Jaén reported 55.2% of all cases. The incidence leveled off in 1996, when a significant decline was observed in some high-risk areas located along the northern coast, but epidemic and unstable behavior persisted in lowland jungle areas, especially the Loreto region (where even the city of Iquitos was affected) and the Jaén subregion. Stratification by API between 1994 and 1996 revealed an increase from 20.7 to 119.1 per 1,000 in Loreto and from 27.7 to 39.8 per 1,000 in Jaén. The proportion of cases due to *P. falciparum* in 1996 was 32.2% in Loreto and 48.2% in Jaén. In the latter year, there were 46 reported malaria deaths, 40 of which occurred in Loreto (87.0%). Of the *P. falciparum* cases, 20% to 26% were resistant to chloroquine and 9.1% were resistant to sulfadoxine/pyrimethamine. Intense internal migration, the development of new irrigation areas for rice and cotton farming, the spread of the vector *Aedes darlingi,* and difficulties in management of the control program in hard-to-reach areas contributed to this epidemiological situation. Since 1994, control efforts have focused on detection, diagnosis, and treatment of cases as well as comprehensive and selective vector control, prevention and control of epidemics, and systematization of the analysis of operational

and epidemiological information. Between 1994 and 1996, coverage of the control program increased from 41.4% to 75.0% in the general health services, and the capacity for the detection, examination, and diagnosis of fever cases increased 472%. The efficiency of the administration of treatment increased during the same period from 63.2% to 83.1% for *Plasmodium vivax* malaria and from 56.7% to 82.6% for chloroquine-resistant *P. falciparum* malaria.

The first epidemic of dengue fever occurred in 1990, when 9,623 cases were reported. Control activities reduced the incidence to 714 cases in 1991 but since then the trend has been upward: 1,905 cases in 1992 and 2,837 in 1996. The serotypes involved in the period 1990–1995 were dengue 1 and, to a lesser extent, dengue 4. Dengue 2 began to circulate in 1995; it was first isolated in Los Órganos (Grau region in the northern part of the country) and in 1996 was detected in other areas of the northeastern region and in the Amazon basin. The most affected geographic areas have been the northern coast (Tumbes and Luciano Castillo) and the northeastern and central jungle region (Loreto, Ucayali, Huánuco, Junín, and San Martín). In 1996 outbreaks were registered in several new localities not considered endemic (Jaén, Bagua, and Juanjui). It was estimated that the population at risk in 1996 totaled 2,750,000 people.

Leishmaniasis is present in 24 health subregions—in particular, the mountain and jungle departments. Between 1960 and 1980 the incidence of the disease remained relatively stable, ranging from 6.5 to 8.4 per 100,000 population. Between 1985 and 1994 an increase in incidence was observed; the rate increased from 12.7 to 40.0 per 100,000 population. In 1995 a total of 7,343 cases were reported (31.9 per 100,000 population). The total for 1996 was 7,756 (32.4 per 100,000 population), which points to a new period of stabilization. In 1996, 86.7% of the cases were the cutaneous form and 13.3% were the mucocutaneous form. The most affected subregions were Madre de Dios (1,071 cases) and Chachapoyas (659 cases). The Andean cutaneous form affects primarily children under 15 and is associated with the increasing use of child labor for brush clearing and preparation of farmlands on mountain slopes of the Andes, as well as with transmission around the home. The mucocutaneous form occurs most frequently in persons over the age of 15 years and is associated with temporary migration or settlement of highland and lowland jungle areas for agricultural and extractive activities (gold mining, logging, oil drilling), as well as with road-building and hunting.

In 1995, jungle yellow fever reached epidemic proportions, with 503 reported cases and a case fatality rate of 38.8%. The disease affected predominantly farmers aged 15–44 years who were of Andean origin and resided in the departments in the central jungle (Pasco, Junín, and Huánuco). The large increases in internal migration beginning in 1994, coupled with the opening up of new agricultural and industrial areas in enzootic areas, were decisive factors in the occurrence of the outbreaks. Intensification of vaccination activities brought about a reduction in the incidence to 86 cases with 34 deaths in 1996. In April 1995, yellow fever vaccination was incorporated into the regular activities of the Expanded Program on Immunization.

In 1996 the total number of cases of Chagas' disease in endemic areas was estimated at 24,170 (1,209 were acute or oligosymptomatic forms and 22,961 were chronic forms). Most cases occurred among people between the ages of 20 and 54. The area where Chagas' disease is most prevalent is located in the country's southern portion (departments of Ica, Arequipa, Moquegua, Tacna, Ayacucho, and Apurímac), where household infestation with *Triatoma infestans* has been detected in 21 provinces and 90 districts. In this geographic area, which represents 9% of the national territory and contains 160,000 dwellings, 473,918 people (2% of the total population) are at risk for the disease. Seroprevalence surveys in these areas have revealed infection rates ranging from 0.7% to 12.0% in the population and from 3.0% to 12.0% in blood banks. In 1996 the country developed national standards and formulated regional control plans.

Between 1945 and 1969, the incidence of bartonellosis declined from 9.6 to 0.25 per 100,000 population and remained stable until 1974, when it began to rise steadily. In 1995, a rate of 3.34 per 100,000 population was registered. Bartonellosis affects the departments of Ancash, La Libertad, Cajamarca, and Amazonas. The exposed population of 1,687,236 people lives mainly in ecological niches located between 1,000 and 3,200 m above sea level. The incidence is highest in children under 15.

Vaccine-Preventable Diseases. Since 1990, vaccination coverage in children under 1 year of age has exceeded 80%. In 1996, coverage levels were 96.9% for the measles vaccine, 99.6% for BCG, and 100% for polio vaccine and DTP. The last measles epidemic in Peru occurred in 1992, when 22,605 cases and 263 deaths were reported (case fatality rate of 1.8%). The measles elimination program was launched in 1995 with surveillance of eruptive febrile illnesses and door-to-door vaccination activities, as a result of which 96.8% of children aged 9 months to 4 years were vaccinated. A total of 224 cases of measles were confirmed in 1995, and only 2 cases were confirmed in 1996. A campaign to eliminate neonatal tetanus as a public health problem was launched in 1991. High-risk districts were identified and all women of childbearing age were vaccinated with tetanus toxoid (TT). In addition, traditional birth attendants and health workers were trained both in how to provide care at delivery and in how to administer vaccines. A total of 128 cases were reported in 1994, 9 in 1995, and 46 in 1996; the majority were

from high-risk districts in the jungle and in marginal urban areas of the coastal region. All cases were in children of mothers who had not received at least two doses of TT, and the mother had given birth in a health institution in only 5% of the cases. According to the 1996 ENDES, 70.1% of the mothers who had given birth to children in the five years before the survey had received at least one dose of TT. The last confirmed case of poliomyelitis in the Americas occurred in Peru in 1991. As of early 1997, the country maintained adequate monitoring of all suspected cases and adhered to international surveillance requirements. Diphtheria is under control; 10 or fewer cases of the diseases were reported between 1992 and 1996, with the exception of 1993, when 31 cases were reported, and most of those (24) occurred during an outbreak in a rural area of the department of Cuzco. Peru ranks among the countries with medium endemicity of the hepatitis B virus. Various seroepidemiological studies have revealed that endemicity in the jungle is medium to high, with prevalence of the surface antigen (HBsAg) ranging from 2.5% in Iquitos to 20.0% among the native population. Along the coast, the prevalence ranges from 1.0% to 3.5%, and in the mountains, from 2.0% to 15.0%. The disease is hyperendemic in Huanta and Abancay, where the prevalence of HBsAg is as high as 54.4% and that of the hepatitis delta virus is 14% in apparently healthy schoolchildren. In these areas, horizontal transmission in children is frequent. In 1996, immunization of children under 1 year with the hepatitis B vaccine was initiated in provinces with high and medium levels of endemicity (25% of the total area of the country).

Cholera and Other Intestinal Infectious Diseases. In 1996, the point prevalence of diarrhea in children under 5, on the 15th day before the survey, was 17.9%, much lower than the figure found in a 1986 survey (31.9%). The prevalence was higher in children aged 6–23 months (29.0%), in rural areas (20.3%), and in jungle areas (25.6%). The seriousness of diarrheal disease, as measured by the proportion of cases with dehydration and serious dehydration, decreased from 34% and 4%, respectively, in 1994 to 25.5% and 1.5%, respectively, in 1996. According to the National Household Survey for the fourth quarter of 1995, 92% of children under 5 with diarrhea received oral rehydration therapy. The proportion of diarrhea cases that received appropriate treatment in the health services of the Ministry of Health increased from 7% in 1993 to 25.4% in 1996.

The appearance of cholera in early 1991 revealed the serious deficiencies in drinking water supply and basic sanitation services. Since then, the disease has shown a downward trend (322,562 suspected cases in 1991, 71,448 cases in 1993, and 4,369 cases in 1996) and has occurred mainly in persons over 15 years of age. The department with the highest rate of cholera in 1996 was Ucayali, which reported 239 cases per 100,000 population. The average case fatality rate has remained at 0.09% since the beginning of the epidemic; however, higher figures have been reported in outbreaks occurring in areas with limited access to health services. National monitoring of *Vibrio cholerae* strains indicates the absence of serotype O139. Cholera is endemic in Peru, and isolated cases of the disease routinely occur between December and March along the coast and between June and October in the jungle.

Chronic Communicable Diseases. Rates of tuberculosis increased between 1985 and 1992, when a steady downward trend began and continued until 1996. Case reporting has improved substantially since 1991. In 1996, 47,498 cases were diagnosed and treated nationwide; the prevalence rate declined from 256.1 per 100,000 population in 1992 to 227.9 in 1995 and 198.4 in 1996. The rate of incidence of the disease dropped from 243.2 per 100,000 population in 1992 to 162.1 in 1996. The most affected age group consisted of individuals between 15 and 44. The proportion of sputum-positive cases detected in children under 15 was 4.8%. The incidence rate of tuberculous meningoencephalitis in children declined from 2.01 per 100,000 population in 1993 to 1.57 in 1995. Mortality decreased slightly from 5.2 to 4.9 per 100,000 population between 1992 and 1995; the reduction occurred in all age groups but was most evident in the youngest groups. The first annual survey of risk of infection was conducted in 1997. A study of tuberculosis drug resistance in Peru in 1995–1996 found that 15.4% of cases were resistant to one drug and 2.4% were multidrug resistant. In 1990 only 25% of the country's health services were carrying out diagnosis and treatment activities, but by 1996 96.0% guaranteed free access to such care. The number of sputum microscopy examinations quintupled between 1990 and 1996 (211,000 and 1,160,000, respectively). In the 1980s, only 50% of diagnosed patients completed treatment, and in 1996 the average cure rate nationwide was 90.9%. An assessment of treatment efficiency through cohort studies revealed that the cure rate increased from 74.1% in 1991 to 90.9% in 1996. The treatment abandonment rate declined from 13.8% in 1991 to 4.2% in 1996.

The prevalence of leprosy in endemic areas of the jungle in 1995 was 0.9 per 10,000 population, and the incidence was 0.35 per 10,000 population. These rates were higher than in 1993 (0.6 and 0.1, respectively), mostly because of better detection of new cases. The most affected departments were Ucayali and Loreto. Of the 240 cases recorded in 1995, 195 were multibacillary (81.3%) and 45 paucibacillary (18.8%). Of the 90 new cases, 14.4% were detected in children under 15, which indicates recent transmission of the disease; 13.3% have second-degree disability, which suggests a late diagnosis. The latter percentage is lower than in 1993 (20.4%).

Acute Respiratory Infections. Acute respiratory infections are the leading cause of mortality in childhood; it is estimated that every year they cause about 12,000 deaths in children under 5 years, of which a high proportion are due to pneumonia. Acute respiratory infections are the leading reason for health service visits, accounting for more than 40% of all such visits and 30% of hospitalizations in this age group. The highest incidence of pneumonia is registered in the mountains (Pasco and Apurímac) and in the jungle (Jaén, Madre de Dios, and Amazonas). Between October and November 1995 a survey on quality of care in health services determined that 39.2% of the cases of acute respiratory infections received appropriate treatment in hospital outpatient clinics, health centers, and health posts.

AIDS. Since its detection in Peru in 1983, AIDS/HIV infection has spread rapidly. The cumulative total of AIDS cases as of August 1997 was 6,443; the estimated number of cases is 10,000 for AIDS and 70,000 for HIV infection. The presence of HIV/AIDS has been confirmed throughout the country, although it is more prevalent in the large cities, particularly in Lima and Callao. Sexual transmission predominates and accounts for 95.4% of the cumulative total of cases; transmission by blood accounts for 2.4% of cases and the trend for this route of transmission is downward; perinatal transmission accounts for 2.2% of cases and the trend is upward. Significant changes in transmission patterns include the rise in heterosexual transmission and the increase in the number of women and young people who are affected. The male/female ratio of cases was 20:1 in 1985 and 3:1 in 1997. In the same period, the median age at the time of AIDS diagnosis dropped from 38 to 29 years, which suggests that HIV infection is occurring at increasingly younger ages. Since 1994 the National Program for the Control of Sexually Transmitted Diseases and AIDS has implemented new control strategies, including marketing of condoms, modification of risk behaviors, and syndromic management of other diseases. In addition, the Ministry of Health has instituted a program that administers AZT free of charge to infected pregnant women and newborns, and it is carrying out activities aimed at eliminating congenital syphilis and ensuring mandatory screening in blood banks. Law 26626, enacted in 1997, and its accompanying regulations establish the legal framework for carrying out these activities and provide explicit protection of the rights of people with HIV/AIDS.

Rabies and Other Zoonoses. During the 1993–1996 quadrennium, 112 deaths from rabies were reported; in 65 of these cases (58%) the source of infection was dogs and in 47 (42%), vampire bats. In marginal areas of the large cities, most cases of human rabies are due to dog bites; males and school-age children are most often affected. Human rabies transmitted by vampire bats has become a serious problem in the Amazon jungle as a result of human intrusion into bat habitat. In the 1993–1996 period, 1,582 cases of canine rabies were reported.

Between 1990 and 1992, Peru had 460 cases of anthrax. The largest number of cases (223) was reported in 1992; in 1993 and 1994 no cases were reported; in 1995, 25 were reported; and in 1996, 12 cases were reported. The departments that periodically report cases of anthrax are Lima and Ica as well as the Constitutional Province of Callao.

Brucellosis is limited to certain regions of the country and is related to consumption of fresh homemade cheese produced with infected goat milk. A total of 3,606 cases were reported between 1993 and 1995. In 1996, 274 cases were reported in Lima alone.

The endemic area for plague is limited to four departments in the northern part of the country: Piura, Cajamarca, Lambayeque, and La Libertad, where periodic outbreaks occur in the inter-Andean valleys. An outbreak of bubonic plague began in October 1992 and eventually spread to 122 localities in 31 districts of the four departments. Between 1994 and 1996, 1,288 cases and 54 deaths were reported, most in the department of Cajamarca. The occurrence of cases is related to the proliferation of wild rodents as a result of deficient environmental sanitation and poor housing conditions in these areas.

Human hydatidosis occurs in the Andean region (Pasco, Huancavelica, Junín, and Puno), where sheep breeding is a major economic activity and herds of sheep live in close contact with dogs infested with the adult parasite. Between 1993 and 1995, 4,829 cases of hydatidosis were diagnosed, mainly the pulmonary and hepatic forms.

Noncommunicable Diseases and Other Health-Related Problems

Nutritional Diseases and Diseases of Metabolism. In 1996, 7.9% of children under 5 had weight-for-age deficits and 1.1% had weight-for-height deficits, figures moderately lower than those registered in 1992 (10.8% and 1.4%, respectively). Low height-for-age affected 25.9% of children under 5 overall, but in those close to their fifth birthday the proportion was 30.5%. The high prevalence of chronic malnutrition can be attributed to inadequate intake, poor use of food, and frequent and prolonged episodes of infection that trigger a vicious cycle of malnutrition and infection. The highest level of chronic malnutrition, 40.6%, is found in rural areas. In the Lima metropolitan area, in contrast, the figure is 10.1%. The prevalence is 17.1% along the coast, 37.9% in the mountains, and 33.3% in the jungle. Also, 50.5% of the children of mothers with no formal education suffer from chronic malnutrition compared with 5.3% of those whose mothers have higher education. There are

no up-to-date statistics on vitamin A and iron deficiency. A study conducted in Piura in 1991 found that 32.8% of children under 6 had serum levels of vitamin A less than 20 μg/dl. In 1987 it was established that iodine deficiency was endemic in most of the mountain and jungle provinces of the country. In 1990, 70% of the salt consumed in the country was iodized. By 1995, according to the National Household Survey for the fourth quarter, 93.9% of the population was consuming iodized salt.

The practice of breast-feeding is prevalent in Peru, but the period of exclusive breast-feeding usually is very short. Supplementation with other liquids and food—usually prepared under poor hygienic conditions—occurs at early ages. In 1996, 38.9% of children under 3 months of age were already receiving food supplements, and among those 4–6 months old, only 32.3% continued to be exclusively breast-fed. The proportion dropped to 5.6% in children aged 7–9 months.

Studies conducted in three coastal areas showed the prevalence of diabetes to be between 7% and 8%. The prevalence of hypercholesterolemia was between 14% and 42% in the same areas.

Cardiovascular Diseases. In recent decades noncommunicable diseases have gained importance in Peru. Proportional mortality from diseases of the circulatory system between 1980 and 1992 ranged from 11.8% to 19.4% of all deaths from defined causes. The estimated mortality rates from these diseases for the 1990–1992 period were 186 and 209 per 100,000 population in men and women, respectively. The prevalence of hypertension in adults was estimated at 17% in coastal regions and at about 5% in mountain and jungle regions, although studies conducted in three areas of the coast showed prevalence rates of 15% to 34%.

Malignant Neoplasms. Data on the incidence and prevalence of malignant neoplasms at the national level are not available, although information is available from two regional reporting systems, one in the Lima metropolitan area and another in the city of Trujillo. In Lima, the incidence was 88.3 per 100,000 population in 1968 and 112.3 in 1990–1991. Mortality from cancer in 1990–1992 was estimated at 113 and 138 per 100,000 population in males and females, respectively. According to the cancer registries of Trujillo (1988–1989) and Lima (1990–1991), the most frequent cancer sites in males are the stomach, prostate, and lung; in women, they are the uterus, breast, and stomach. In men, between 1968 and 1991 the frequency of stomach cancer decreased 37%, while that of prostate cancer increased 48%. In women, cervical cancer decreased 32%, while breast cancer increased 43% in the same period.

Accidents and Violence. Homicides (12 per 100,000 population) and traffic accidents, together with various forms of violence against children, adolescents, and women, constitute a serious public health problem in Peru. In adults, accidents are the most frequent reason for hospitalization and for trips to hospital emergency rooms. Between 1980 and 1995, the National Police registered close to 990,000 traffic accidents, with 320,000 injuries and a case fatality rate of 12.3%.

Oral Health. In 1996, 95% of children aged 3–14 had dental caries, 85% suffered from periodontal disease, and 75% from malocclusion. In children aged 6–14 years, the average number of permanent teeth affected by caries was six, with premature loss of first permanent molars in 45% to 50%. In the same year, the Ministry of Health launched a program to promote topical fluoride application as a part of comprehensive child health services.

Ocular Health. It is estimated that 10% of the country's total population suffers from refractive defects; in the school-age population of some areas of the country this proportion is as high as 15%. The prevalence of blindness in adults over the age of 60 is estimated at 3.4%. Some 300,000 people suffer from a severe visual impairment due to nonoperated cataracts, and 6 of every 10,000 children suffer from blindness due to preventable or curable causes, such as congenital cataracts and glaucoma or premature retinopathy.

Natural Disasters and Industrial Accidents. Because of its location in the Pacific "Ring of Fire," Peru is exposed to earthquakes and volcanic events. Eighty percent of the population is considered to be at risk of suffering injury from earthquakes. Lima, Callao, and the southern border—especially Tacna, Ilo, Cuzco, and the Amazon region—are the most vulnerable sites. The country's mountainous terrain experiences frequent landslides. Human settlements in high-risk areas, indiscriminate logging, and mining operations with inadequate planning increase the risk. The National Civil Defense Institute estimates that 35% of the population is exposed to this threat.

RESPONSE OF THE HEALTH SYSTEM

National Health Plans and Policies

Although the country continues to face serious social problems, it has achieved the necessary political and economic stability to enable it to formulate medium-term social policies in the framework of State reform. The general objective of the medium-term social policy for the year 2000 is targeting of public spending; the operational goal is reduction of extreme poverty by 50%. In this context, the Basic Social Spending Program is carrying out programs in the areas of education, health, food, and justice. In the area of health, the Basic Health-for-All Program, launched in 1994, seeks to increase the response capacity of primary care health facilities, beginning with those located in the areas of greatest poverty. In 1996, the budget of the Program represented 21% of the total budget of the Ministry of Health. In 1995 the Ministry defined the following policy guidelines for the health sector for the period 1995–2000: universal access to public and individual health care services, and ensuring that the poorest segments of the population have access to a basic package of health services is a priority; modernization of the sector in terms of technology, management, information systems, and institutional development; restructuring of the functions of financing, service delivery, and control in order to develop competitiveness and improve accessibility and quality; prevention and control of urgent health problems; and promotion of healthy living conditions and lifestyles through sectoral and multisectoral actions.

The General Health Law, enacted in June 1997, assigns to the State the inalienable responsibility of providing public health services and of promoting conditions that will guarantee adequate coverage of services for the population in terms of safety, timeliness, and quality. It defines the delivery of health services as a matter of public interest, regardless of which institution provides them. In addition, the State is responsible for monitoring, preventing, and treating problems of malnutrition, mental health, and environmental health, as well as health problems of underprivileged children, adolescents, mothers, and disabled and elderly persons. The law also envisions that State financing is to be oriented toward public health activities and the partial or full subsidy of medical care for low-income populations who are not covered by any other public or private health care system. Finally, it expresses the will of the State to promote universal and progressive health insurance for the population.

Health Sector Reform

Since 1995 the global restructuring of the State apparatus has been under way, with the primary aim of promoting efficiency in public operations. In the framework of the aforementioned health policies, as well as the restructuring of public functions deriving from State reform, the Ministry of Health has established the following policies for reform of the public health sector: to improve equity in health care by optimizing the allocation, programming, and utilization of resources through the restructuring of health care financing; to develop a user identification system and a basic package of health services as instruments for targeting health spending; to develop governmental capacity in response to the new environment in the public sector at the central and local levels, as well as the function of regulating the health services market; to improve the administration, management, and quality of public health services through organization of public health facilities in networks at the primary and secondary levels; and to implement a program for modernization of the management of national and regional public hospitals as well as specialized institutions.

While the Ministry of Health will concentrate on the formulation of policies, strategic planning, regulation, and control in the area of health, specialized agencies will be created to oversee the administration of financial resources and of the networks of basic public health care establishments, which will have their own decentralized management. The process of reform has received strong support from international cooperating agencies, especially the projects "Strengthening of Health Services" (IDB), "Peru 2000" (USAID), and "Basic Health and Nutrition" (World Bank).

The Law on Modernization of the Social Security System, enacted in 1997, relaxes the public monopoly on the delivery of medical services to the beneficiaries of IPSS with a view to improving the quality and coverage of services. It also allows beneficiaries the freedom to affiliate themselves with private health care providers, known as health service delivery companies. This process aims to develop the health services market in order to increase coverage for low-income populations, improve the quality of services, and promote efficiency in the allocation of resources.

Organization of the Health Sector

Institutional Organization

The health sector comprises institutions in the public sector (Ministry of Health, IPSS, the armed forces and police health services, and social welfare agencies), private insurance and providers, and nonprofit institutions. According to the second Census of Physical Infrastructure and Resources of the Health Sector, in 1995 the country had 7,304 health facilities, of which 5,931 (81%) were administered by the Ministry of Health; of these, 134 were hospitals, 1,028 were health centers, and 4,762 were health posts. Given that in 1992 there were 4,630 establishments, these figures reflect an overall increase of 63.4% and an increase of 61.1% in primary-level health facilities in only four years. This growth can be attributed to the large-scale investment program that the country is carrying out, mainly through the Basic Health-for-All Program and the Program for Strengthening of Health Services.

Nationwide, there was 1 bed per 767 population in 1995, an increase with respect to 1992, when there was 1 bed per 835 population. In some areas of the country, however, the ratio is 1 bed per 1,680 population, and in others it is 1 per 220 population. In Lima there is 1 bed per 666 population, and in the rest of the country there is 1 bed per 1,250 population.

Between 1992 and 1996, the availability of physicians increased from 7.6 to 9.8 per 10,000 population, that of nursing personnel from 5.2 to 6.2 per 10,000, and that of dentists from 0.7 to 1.1 per 10,000 population. Although these national averages reflect an acceptable availability of resources, one of the health sector's principal problems is the inequitable distribution of its human resources. The departments with the highest poverty levels generally have the fewest health workers. For example, in Huancavelica, Apurímac, and Cajamarca, the rates of physicians per 10,000 population are 2.8, 2.8, and 3.1, respectively, while in Callao, Lima, and Arequipa, the rates are 22.9, 17.3, and 14.5, respectively. To compensate for this uneven distribution, the Government, through the Basic Health-for-All Program, contracts personnel to serve the population in the most impoverished areas of the country. An important development in the organization and management of health services is the creation of local health administration committees, which are made up of community members and personnel from the health centers and posts. The State transfers financial resources to these committees to hire personnel and pay for other expenses associated with operation of the establishments for which they are responsible. In addition, these committees play an important role in local programming, administration and management of resources, evaluation of services, and assessment of the performance of personnel, as a result of which they have become a key element in the process of decentralization.

Of the population covered by the Ministry of Health in 1993, 31.9% used health services and each user had 2.3 visits; in IPSS, the corresponding figures were 35.9% and 4.3 visits in 1994. A problem affecting the Ministry of Health is that of "overlapping benefits," which occurs when its limited resources are used to care for people who have access to other health care systems. For example, in 1994 the Ministry provided care for 20% of the beneficiaries of the Armed Forces Health Service, 13% of the beneficiaries of the IPSS, and 9.8% of the people covered by private insurance. In addition, some programs are still poorly organized. For example, regular preventive maintenance and upkeep programs still have not been implemented in the Ministry, and in IPSS these programs are centralized. The information on production of services is incomplete, as is epidemiological information; moreover, this information is not always timely or totally compatible between providers, and its dissemination is limited.

Utilization and Demand for Health Services

According to the National Household Survey of 1995, 29% of those interviewed indicated that they had experienced some symptom of disease or suffered an accident within the 15 days prior to the survey. Of this proportion, 94% had experienced symptoms of disease and 6% had suffered some accident. The proportion of disease symptoms or accidents was greater in women (55%) and in children and older adults (26%). An association was found between low income and likelihood of suffering symptoms of illness (16% in the highest-income quintile reported symptoms of disease, compared with 28% in the lowest-income quintile), while an inverse correlation was found between educational level and illness or accident (69% of those with a primary education had suffered some illness or accident versus only 10% of those with higher education). Fifty-eight percent of the population that reported having experienced some disease symptom or accident failed to seek medical attention (51% of the urban population and 69% of the rural population); in 65% of these cases, the main reason cited was lack of economic resources. The decision to seek medical care was positively correlated with educational level (54% of those with higher education sought care, compared with 40% of those with primary education) and with level of income (56% in the highest-income quintile compared with 29% in the lowest-income quintile). Income level also influenced the type of health personnel and institution from which care was sought: those with a higher income tended to see private providers, while those with a lower income sought care mainly from establishments of the Ministry of Health, pharmacies, and traditional healers. Nevertheless, consultation of pharmacy personnel was a customary practice at all income levels. According to the 1991 and 1994 ENNIV surveys, the participation of the public sector (Ministry of Health and IPSS) and pharmacies as health service providers increased, while that of private clinics and physicians decreased. This phenomenon can be explained by the economic recession that lasted until 1992 as well as rising levels of poverty, underemployment, and unemployment, as a result of which some of the middle-income group that had been served by the private sector undoubtedly began to turn to the public sector for health services.

Health Services and Resources

Organization of Services for Care of the Population

Health Promotion. In Peru, many individual, family, and community health problems are related to unhealthy practices, habits, and behaviors and to the conditions of poverty in which a large percentage of the population lives. For a long time, health promotion and protection were not considered priorities among sector policies. Since 1995, however, in the framework of the health policy guidelines, the Ministry of Health began to stress the promotion of healthy living condi-

tions and lifestyles as a way to improve the population's quality of life. In 1996 the Ministry of Health launched the "Healthy Communities for Sustainable Human Development" initiative, in which community participation and social communication are the principal strategies. The management of adolescent pregnancy, prevention of violence against children, environmental management, and communicable disease prevention have been among the most important activities carried out.

Epidemiological Surveillance Systems and Public Health Laboratories. The national epidemiological surveillance system comprises 2,690 health facilities (208 hospitals, 924 health centers, 1,504 health posts, and 54 other facilities), 33 epidemiology departments, and a national office of epidemiology, distributed among the three levels of the Ministry of Health: local, subregional, and central. This system monitors and reports weekly on 15 diseases of importance to public health: cholera, plague, yellow fever, *P. falciparum* malaria, dengue, human rabies, meningococcal meningitis, measles, acute flaccid paralysis, neonatal tetanus, tetanus in adults, diphtheria, whooping cough, AIDS, and epidemic typhus. The country's public health laboratory network includes a national reference laboratory (in Lima) and 11 regional reference laboratories (in Piura, Chiclayo, Cajamarca, Iquitos, Tarapoto, Huancayo, Ayacucho, Cuzco, Arequipa, Tacna, and Puno). The basic functions of the regional laboratories are to carry out serological tests using ELISA and bacterial cultures for diagnosis of communicable diseases. The national laboratory, in addition to these functions, isolates viruses and, in its molecular biology department, performs polymerase chain reaction procedures.

In 1995, not all blood was being screened for the various diseases that can be transmitted through transfusion. The coverage of screening was 60% for HIV, HBsAg, and syphilis and 4% for Chagas' disease. The prevalence of infection in blood banks was 0.28% for HIV, 0.70% for HBsAg, 1.21% for syphilis, and 0.03% for Chagas' disease. Law 26454, enacted in 1994, and its accompanying regulations, which were adopted in 1995, established standards and requirements for the acquisition, donation, transfusion, and supply of human blood. The National Hemotherapy and Blood Bank Program was established within the Ministry of Health in 1996.

Food Safety. The country does not have an integrated food safety program. Each sector (agriculture, health, trade, and industry as well as local governments) has food safety standards, which often overlap or leave gaps. In recent years, selling food on the streets has proliferated; there are approximately 60,000 street food vendors in Lima. Many street food stands do not have ready access to sanitary services or a supply of safe drinking water. On average, foodborne diseases accounted for 35% of all communicable diseases reported up to 1990. In 1991, the percentage of foodborne diseases increased to 56.15% because of the cholera outbreak. In 1996 and 1997, several cases of botulism were reported in persons who had consumed canned food that was improperly handled during the canning process.

Environmental Health. Environmental management is divided among several sectors. Law 26410 establishes the National Environmental Board as the national regulatory and policy-making body in this area. The National Environmental Board, which is a decentralized agency under the President of the Cabinet, is designed to plan, coordinate, and monitor activities for safeguarding the environment and the country's natural resources. The General Environmental Health Directorate (DIGESA), a division of the Ministry of Health, is the technical agency at the national level responsible for setting standards, evaluating, and coordinating activities with local governments and other sectors in the areas of environmental protection, basic sanitation, food safety, control of zoonoses, and occupational health. The National Institute of Environmental Protection for Health formulates standards and policies on environmental protection. With specific regard to drinking water and sewerage services, the National Water and Sanitation Authority, under the Ministry of the Presidency, is responsible for ensuring the supply of drinking water services, sewerage, storm drainage, and excreta disposal. The Authority is empowered to develop, monitor, and assess the performance of sanitation service providers throughout the country. In addition, the Special National Program on Drinking Water and Sewerage (PRONAP) centralizes most of the investment in water and sanitation. In rural areas, there is no agency within the Ministry of the Presidency that establishes investment policy or investment amounts for sanitation. The main agencies concerned with environmental health in rural areas are the Ministry of Health, the National Compensation and Social Development Fund, the Repopulation Support Program, and PRONAP. Public sanitation services are handled by the *municipios* themselves, which contract or grant concessions to private companies to provide the services.

Environmental Risks. Deterioration of water quality is a critical problem in some regions of the country, due basically to pollution by effluents from industrial activities, especially metallurgy, and by domestic and agrochemical waste. In Lima and Callao alone, close to 15 m^3/s of untreated wastewater is discharged into the sea. However, studies and projects to clean up the coastal area of Lima are being carried out. In addition, the need to implement a water quality surveillance system at the national level has been acknowledged, as has the need for an integrated approach to the problem in which all productive sectors of the country will be active participants. Work is currently under way to implement this approach in two of the country's river basins (Santa and Rímac). Finally, the Program for Protection of Coastal Areas and Beaches monitors conditions on 70 beaches throughout the country.

Air quality is poor in some areas of the country, including the Lima metropolitan area and industrial areas of Chimbote, Ilo, and Cerro de Pasco. The leading causes of this deterioration are industrial development with inadequate measures to prevent and control pollution and the increase in the size and poor condition of the motor vehicles. Measurements taken throughout 1996 in the center of Lima indicate that the annual average concentration of particulate matter was 270.48 μg/m^3 (allowable limit: 150 μg/m^3), and the annual average concentration of nitrogen dioxide was 142.9 μg/m^3 (allowable limit: 100 μg/m^3). The levels of lead (0.415 μg/m^3) and sulfur dioxide (0.0424 ppm) were within allowable limits (0.5 μg/m^3 and 0.06 ppm, respectively). In Ilo, measurements taken by DIGESA indicate that the concentration of sulfur oxides exceeds the recommended limits set by WHO.

Soil quality also is a problem in several areas of the country. Along the coast, an increase in salinization has occurred as a result of improper use of water and deterioration of forests due to indiscriminate logging and overgrazing by goats. In the mountains, the deterioration in agricultural lands is due to inappropriate farming practices and the consequent destruction of the protective layer of soil on mountain slopes. In the jungle, deforestation is increasing as a result of the clearing for new agricultural lands.

According to the National Household Survey of 1995, 82.4% of the population in extreme poverty occupies dwellings with dirt floors, 56.7% have adobe or mud walls, 31.9% have corrugated metal roofs, and 10% have thatched roofs. In non-poor households, on the other hand, 67.1% of the dwellings have cement, parquet, wood, or tile floor; 51.3% have brick or cement-block walls, and 37% have concrete roofs.

There is no single body charged with monitoring the management of chemical substances from their production to their final disposal; these functions are carried out by various government agencies. However, in 1996 a multisectoral working group was formed to develop a national system for the management of chemical substances. The National Civil Defense System is responsible for organizing emergency response in case of chemical disasters, and the country has a Center for Toxicological Information and a telephone hotline system to ensure continuous availability of information about toxic substances.

Drinking Water and Sewerage Services. The country's drinking water supply systems are severely flawed, and, consequently, water is often supplied under poor conditions and the population is forced to get it from other sources. In urban areas, 66.1% of the population is served by household connections to the public water supply system, 8% by connections to the public system outside their dwellings but within the building, 7.7% by public water tanks, 3.7% by wells, 12.1% by tank trucks, and 2.4% obtain water from watercourses. The supply is intermittent in most of the country. Only 8% of the population has water supply 24 hours a day, 73% receives water for 16 to 20 hours daily, 18% for 6 to 15 hours, and 1% for 0 to 5 hours. Of 9,531 water samples analyzed between 1990 and 1996 in several cities of the country, 7,633 (80.1%) had residual chlorine levels higher than 0.1 ppm; of these samples, 3,069 (32.2%) had residual chlorine levels of more than 0.4 ppm. In rural areas, 13.2% of the population is served by public water tanks, 27.3% by wells, 7.0% by tank trucks, and 52.5% get their water out of watercourses. With regard to sewerage, according to the 1995 fourth-quarter National Household Survey (ENAHO-IV95), 47.4% of the population has sewerage service and 21.95% has latrines. In urban areas, close to 66% of the population is served by sewerage systems and about 20% has latrines, while in rural areas about 9% of the population is served by sewerage systems and 24% has latrines.

Solid Waste Disposal Services. Although limited information is available on these services, averages have been calculated based on several studies. It is estimated that 48% of the paved roadways in the various localities of the country have street-sweeping services and that between 60% and 65% of the population has refuse collection services. Except in the Lima metropolitan area, which has sanitary landfills, and Piura and Trujillo, which also have some kind of landfill (although they have operational problems), in urban areas solid waste is disposed of in open-air dumps or watercourses. The country does not have adequate systems for the treatment of hospital waste, incineration is very limited and inefficient, and there are no landfills where this hazardous waste can be disposed of safely.

Inputs for Health

The General Department of Drugs and Medicinal Products (DIGEMID), an agency of the Ministry of Health, is responsible for regulation and control of drugs in Peru. In 1994, the value of the pharmaceutical market (factory prices) was estimated at US$ 60 million for the public sector and US$ 422 million for the private sector. The process of opening up the market and deregulating prices that has been under way since late 1990 has made a wide range of drugs available. According to DIGEMID, 43% of the 7,447 generic and trademark drugs

on the market in August 1995 were domestic products and 56.7% were foreign products. The Peruvian pharmaceutical industry imports slightly more than 90% of the raw materials for drug manufacturing processes, and the only existing chemical-pharmaceutical company produces two beta-lactam antibiotics that are marketed mainly abroad. In 1992–1993, of 56 laboratories inspected (of 65 registered laboratories), only 25% were complying with good manufacturing practices. Of 312 drugstores and drug importers visited, deficient storage conditions were found in 33%. Street drug sales are a growing problem in the country, and counterfeit and adulterated products sometimes find their way into formal distribution networks.

Peru has been a pioneering country in the implementation of essential drugs programs. The Basic Essential Drugs List was revised most recently in 1992 and is applied today to a limited extent. Since 1994, the country has had a program for shared drug management, which provides a set of 63 low-cost essential drugs to some 1,000 health centers and 4,500 health posts at the primary level of care. The principal strategies of the program are subregional administrative autonomy, administration of revolving funds, and community participation. As of late 1995, the program was operating in all the health subregions, with an approximate coverage of 12 million people and with annual sales amounting to US$ 12.6 million (in Ministry of Health establishments, drugs are provided free of charge only to indigent patients and to those receiving care under the various disease control programs). In addition, IPSS, with an annual budget of US$ 50 million for drugs (1996) and some 6 million beneficiaries, has its own drug supply system based on a list that is differentiated by level of care. The practice of generic substitution in the private and public sectors occurs in 35% and 70% of cases, respectively, according to a rapid assessment of the national pharmaceutical situation conducted between October and December 1996. In Ministry of Health establishments the average number of drugs prescribed is 1.9. The average percentage of drugs prescribed by their generic name is 45.6% and the average percentage prescribed from among the drugs included on the Basic Essential Drugs List is 59.6%. Of patients who receive care in physician's offices, 28.2% receive injectable drugs and 49.2% receive antibiotics. The average percentage of a group of 40 essential drugs available in warehouses, hospitals, health centers, and health posts was 65.5%.

Health Research

The sector does not have a defined research policy, although there is a demand for epidemiological and socioeconomic research in connection with the current process of sectoral restructuring. The principal institutions that conducted research during the period between 1991 and 1996 were non-governmental organizations (58%), public health institutions (30%), universities (5%), the National Institute of Statistics and Information Science (5%), and international cooperating agencies (2%). The fragmentation of research and its limited dissemination, discussion, and application constitute impediments to its use. The Ministry of Health has created a commission that is responsible for proposing research policy within the framework of sectoral reform.

Expenditures and Sectoral Financing

In 1995, total spending on health amounted to 3.6% of the GDP. This percentage has remained stable since 1992. The per capita expenditure on health was US$ 89. Spending by the Ministry of Health, the *municipios,* and the Public Compensation and Social Development Fund is about 1% of GDP (the per capita expenditure was US$ 38), while IPSS spending represented 1.3% of GDP (per capita expenditure of US$ 115). Private expenditure is similar to that of the IPSS: 1.2% of GDP, which is less than in 1992 (1.5%). The health sector's share of public-sector spending rose from 9.9% to 13.1% between 1992 and 1995. The expenditure of the Ministry of Health is slightly greater in the subregions that have the best health indicators, which suggests an inadequate distribution of spending. Although public spending is greater, the proportion of private expenditure is significant. A greater proportion of private spending goes toward the purchase of drugs than toward payment of fees charged by private providers.

The health sector's budgeting and programming procedures are extremely complex, owing to the existence of various sources of financing and budgetary resources for the health subregions. Funding is provided by multiple institutions (various programs and institutions of the Ministry of Health, the Ministry of Economy and Finance, and international cooperating organizations). As a result, the chain of financing is intricate and is not consolidated in overall budgets at the regional level. There is no policy concerning the generation of income by health institutions; rather, criteria differ depending on the type of health facility. This situation engenders inequities, and it hinders the targeting of funds and services to poor populations and the application of cost-effectiveness criteria in rate setting. Several studies have revealed imbalances between the supply and the demand for services, with very low usage rates in many establishments, which suggests the need for restructuring the existing installed capacity.

External Technical and Financial Cooperation

In 1992, based on data from a UNDP report on development cooperation, Peru received foreign aid totaling US$ 875,871,000, which included a concessionary loan of US$ 376 million from the Government of Japan for business sector reform; 20.5% came from multilateral sources, 77.9% from bilateral sources, and 1.6% from international nongovernmental organizations. The principal sources of foreign aid were Japan (US$ 474.6 million), the United States of America (US$ 94.7 million), IDB (US$ 94.3 million), Italy (US$ 42.8 million), Canada (US$ 19.5 million), and the European Union (US$ 3.9 million). The five areas that received the largest amounts were economic management (54.9%), international trade in goods and services (10.8%), regional development (7.2%), transportation (4.8%), and health (3.9%). In the period 1992–1996, bilateral cooperation accounted for 60% of the external resources received, multilateral cooperation accounted for 35%, and nongovernmental organizations accounted for 5%. In 1993, the Office of Financing, Investment, and International Cooperation of the Ministry of Health formulated the National Program of International Technical Cooperation for the Health Sector, which emphasizes three priority areas: development and strengthening of programs and services, human resources development, and Andean cooperation in health.

PUERTO RICO

GENERAL SITUATION AND TRENDS

Socioeconomic, Political, and Demographic Overview

Puerto Rico is a commonwealth associated with the United States of America; as a result, political, social, and economic events that occur in that country have a direct impact on the island. Since 1992, when the newly elected administration began its term in the United States, both Puerto Rico and the United States have developed plans for health reform that have prompted several social and economic changes. In order to adapt the island's social reality to these changes and trends, the Government of Puerto Rico has established a new public policy and strategies relating to health.

The highest rate of real economic growth for the 1990–1995 five-year period was registered in 1995. The gross product that year rose 3.4%, compared to increases of 3.3% in 1993 and 2.5% in 1994. Various factors helped to accelerate the island's economic growth rate in 1995, including increases in consumer spending, government consumption, and gross domestic fixed capital formation. However, the latter investment was partly offset by an increase in the negative balance of net sales of goods and services to the rest of the world.

The Government of Puerto Rico continued to apply its New Economic Development Model, whose economic, social, financial, regulatory, institutional, and human resource strategies were determining factors in the economic recovery. Among the advances achieved were the creation of 40,000 jobs, employment growth in the manufacturing sector (the first such increase since the 1990–1991 period), and an increase in jobs created under the aegis of the Economic Development Administration in the manufacturing sector. In addition, civil servant salaries and wages rose as a part of the wage fairness program. The tourist industry also experienced growth, as evidenced by the fact that both the number of people registered in hotels and their expenditures increased, as did the number of available hotel rooms. The Government

played a significant role in the growth of the construction industry, particularly through investments in infrastructure works such as roads, electricity and telephone lines, and prison facilities.

During fiscal year 1995, financial reforms to reduce tax rates were approved, which was expected to increase the amount of disposable personal income in the next fiscal year. In addition, within the framework of the Government's privatization policy, the sale of the Shipping Authority was finalized and the privatization of hotels and companies such as the Sugar Corporation and Lotus Pineapple Company continued. During the period, Puerto Rico opened trade offices in Chile, Costa Rica, the Dominican Republic, Mexico, and Panama to promote the island's exports.

The real growth in the United States's economic production benefited Puerto Rico, as there was greater demand for manufactured products; this, in turn, led to an 11.1% monetary increase in Puerto Rican exports to the United States. In addition, domestic economic activity and higher income on the island had an effect on imports. Many of these imports (75.6%) were capital goods, raw materials, and intermediate products, which helped to increase Puerto Rico's productive capacity and meet the demand for raw materials for industrial use. In fiscal year 1995, the gross domestic product (GDP), in current prices, rose to US$ 42,363,700, which represented an increase of 7.2% with respect to the previous year.

Owing largely to the economic recovery, personal income increased 5.5% in 1995, surpassing the previous year's figure (4.1%). Total personal income amounted to US$ 27,016,700, compared with US$ 25,609,300 in the previous year, for an absolute increase of US$ 1,407,400. This increase translated into a rise in per capita personal income and in average family income. At current prices, per capita personal income was US$ 7,296 in 1994–1995, higher than the previous year, when it was US$ 7,009.

In fiscal year 1995, the total number of employed persons, according to a Survey of the Department of Labor and

Human Resources, averaged 1,051,000, which reflects an increase of 40,000 jobs with respect to the previous year. The level of employment measured by this survey excludes agricultural workers and self-employed persons, who total 896,000 people. The increase in jobs resulted in a reduction in the number of unemployed people, which was 168,000. That year the unemployment rate was 13.8%.

The U.S. Federal Government participates actively in the island's economy through net disbursements. These consist of net federal transfers to individuals and to the public sector, as well as the net operating expenditures of the federal agencies that are active in Puerto Rico. The net disbursements of the U.S. Federal Government have increased over time. In fiscal year 1995, they totaled US$ 6,367,100, representing an increase of US$ 430.8 million (or 7.3%) with respect to 1993–1994. These disbursements account for 22.4% of the island's gross domestic product. The increase registered in 1994–1995 exceeded the average rate of growth over the 1990–1995 five-year period, which was 5.4%.

The basic unit used to analyze the geographic distribution of the population of Puerto Rico is the *municipio*, or county (the island is divided into 78 *municipios*). Each *municipio* is made up of an urban or semiurban nucleus (city, town, or village) and may include both urban and rural areas.

The population density has been increasing: in 1990 there were 396.9 inhabitants per km^2, but by 1995 this figure had risen to 416.0 inhabitants per km^2; it is estimated that by the year 2000 the population density will be 432.7 inhabitants per km^2. The population of the *municipio* of San Juan, the capital of Puerto Rico, accounted for 12.2% of the island's population in 1995, with a population density of 3,643.7 inhabitants per km^2. The next largest *municipio,* Cataño, had 3,068.8 inhabitants per km^2. Two of the *municipios* with the lowest population density in 1995 were Maricao (50.3 inhabitants per km^2) and the island *municipio* of Culebra (54.7 inhabitants per km^2).

According to preliminary estimates of the Bureau of the Census, an office within the Puerto Rico Planning Board, as of 1 July 1995, the total population of Puerto Rico was 3,720,018, which represents an increase of 34,288 people (0.9%) with respect to July 1994. The cumulative increase over the previous five years was 192,918 persons. The population growth rate was 17.9% (1.7% per year) in the 1970s and 9.9% (1.0% per year) in the 1980s. In the 1990–1995 period, the annual average growth rate was 1.1%.

As of 1 July 1995, the female population totaled 1,918,499, which amounts to an increase of 17,684 (0.9%) with respect to 1994. The male population, which totaled 1,801,519, grew by 16,604 with respect to the previous fiscal year. The total population of Puerto Rico in 1994 was 3,685,730 people.

For many years, migration has been one of the demographic variables that has most affected Puerto Rico's population dynamics. The bulk of the migration is between Puerto Rico and the United States: Puerto Ricans frequently migrate to the mainland and then return to the island, a phenomenon known as return migration. This results in a continuous flow of migrants in both directions, facilitated by the fact that, as United States citizens, Puerto Ricans need no passports or visas to enter the United States.

Net migration in Puerto Rico in fiscal year 1980, was –16,101 persons, whereas in 1994 it was +26,853. According to preliminary data for 1995, a negative net balance of 1,326 people was registered, the lowest since fiscal year 1971, when the figure was –2,525 people.

In 1994, 33,200 marriages were registered, 62 fewer than in 1993. The rate of marriages per 1,000 population aged 15 years or more was 12.3 in 1994, compared with 12.6 in 1993. A total of 13,724 divorces were registered, which represents a rate of 5.1 per 1,000 population aged 15 years or more. In 1993, the divorce rate was 5.4.

The birth rate, which was 24.8 per 1,000 population in 1970, dropped to 18.8 in 1985 and to 17.5 in 1994. With regard to the specific fertility rate, the available data reveal a falling trend during recent decades in all age groups of mothers, except those aged 15–19. In the group aged 20–24 years, for example, the specific fertility rate in 1970 was 187.7 births per 1,000 women, but this rate fell to 138.0 in 1992; in the group aged 25–29 years, the corresponding rates were 179.4 and 122.0, respectively. In the group aged 15–19 years birth rates have fluctuated: the specific fertility rate in this group was 71.9 births per 1,000 women in 1970, 76.3 in 1980, 63.5 in 1985, and 73.3 in 1992.

Morbidity and Mortality Profile

The Ongoing Health Study is a field study of the Evaluation Division of the Office of the Undersecretary for Planning, Evaluation, and Statistics of the Department of Health. It is based on the guidelines of the National Health Interview Survey (NHIS) of the National Center for Health Statistics, a branch of the United States Department of Health and Human Services. The survey gathers statistical data on hospitalization, physician and dentist visits, acute and chronic morbidity, and days of restricted activity. The sample of dwellings used is a subsample of the group of workers of the Statistics Division of the Department of Labor and Human Resources. The population under study consists of noninstitutionalized civilians in Puerto Rico.

Data from the survey reflected a total of 5.5 million chronic disorders in 1992. This figure indicates a rate of 154.4 chronic disorders per 100 population, equivalent to 1.5 disorders per person per year, which means that one person reported suffering one or more chronic disorders in the four weeks immediately prior to the interview. The rate begins to increase at 6 years of age and reaches a peak of 429.4 disorders per 100 people in the group aged 65 years and over.

In 1992, as in previous years, diseases of the circulatory system were the leading cause of morbidity, with rates of 25.6 per 100 population; next, in terms of frequency, were diseases of the respiratory system (20.7), diseases of the musculoskeletal system and connective tissue and endocrine diseases (both with rates of 12.5), and diseases of the digestive system (10.6). The rate of chronic disorders in women was higher than that in men (174.0 per 100 women, compared with 133.6 per 100 men).

In 1992, according to data obtained from a sample of Puerto Rico's noninstitutionalized civilian population of Puerto Rico during two quarters of the year, the estimated incidence of acute morbidity was 4.5 million disorders. Women showed a higher rate (138.9 per 100 women) than men (113.9 per 100 men). The incidence of acute disorders tends to vary with age. Children under 6 had the highest rate of acute illness (229.1 per 100 population per year); the lowest rate was found in the groups aged 45–64 and 25–44 years (99.0 and 129.9 per 100 population per year, respectively). Diseases of the respiratory system accounted for the highest rate of acute illness in 1992 (55.8 per 100 population), followed by infectious and parasitic diseases, injuries, and diseases of the digestive system (25.9, 8.9, and 7.8 per 100 population, respectively).

All births, deaths, marriages, and fetal deaths that occur in Puerto Rico are registered at local offices of the Population Registry located throughout the island. Death registries are very complete, and causes of death are certified by physicians: 52% by family doctors, 37% by physicians who base their certification on the results of autopsies and medical records or other tests, and the remaining 11% by physicians who utilize other sources of information.

Mortality has remained relatively stable: in 1970 the rate was 6.6 per 1,000 population; in 1980, it declined to 6.4 and remained at 6.5 during the first four years of the 1980s; subsequently it rose to 7.0 in 1987 and continued to increase until reaching levels of 7.9 in 1993 and 7.7 in 1994. An important factor that explains the increase in this rate is the natural aging of the population and the rapid growth of older age groups. Another factor in the rise in mortality is the increase in the diseases that are the leading causes of death.

In 1994, 28,444 people died from all the causes (16,707 men and 11,737 women). In that same year, heart disease (rate of 157.7 per 100,000 population) and malignant neoplasms (116.6 per 100,000 population) were the two leading causes of death, together accounting for 35.6% of all deaths.

Diseases of the heart continue to be the leading cause of death. Some 5,814 people died from this group of causes in 1994 (3,169 men and 2,645 women), while 4,298 died from malignant neoplasms (2,516 men and 1,782 women). To-

gether, cardiovascular diseases (including heart disease, cerebrovascular disease, hypertensive disease, and atherosclerosis) were responsible for 8,401 deaths, representing 29.5% of the total.

Among women, there were 1,782 deaths from malignant neoplasms; the most frequent form was breast cancer, which was the leading cause in this group of causes and accounted for 294 deaths (6.8%), followed by colon cancer, which caused 153 deaths (3.6%). Among men, 2,516 deaths from malignant neoplasms occurred; prostate cancer was the most frequent, causing 505 deaths (11.7%), followed by cancer of the trachea, bronchus, and lung, which caused 386 deaths (9.0%).

As in the previous years, diabetes mellitus ranked third as a cause of death, accounting for 1,868 deaths, or 6.6% of all deaths in 1994; of these, 1,028 were women. In 1993 diabetes mellitus caused 1,876 deaths.

The fourth leading cause of death was AIDS. A total of 1,549 deaths from this cause were reported: 1,210 (78.1%) males and 339 (21.9%) females.

Cerebrovascular disease was the fifth leading cause, accounting for 1,428 (5.0%) deaths. This cause ranked fourth in 1993, when it accounted for 1,443 deaths (5.1%).

SPECIFIC HEALTH PROBLEMS

Puerto Rico's social transformation over the last 50 years has brought with it a significant increase in longevity and life expectancy. It is expected that this trend will continue and that by the year 2030 some 15% of the population will be 65 or over. This and other trends, such as the transition from a rural agricultural society to an urban industrial society, have led to changes in the patterns of morbidity and mortality. The epidemiological profile has changed. Chronic degenerative diseases now coexist with acute infectious diseases, and the prevalence of cardiovascular diseases and cancer is high. Alcohol and tobacco use have become more common; the population has grown more sedentary; the diet is often poor, with a high fat and protein content; and illegal drug use is on the rise.

Analysis by Population Group

Health of Children

In 1992, children under age 6 had the highest rates of acute illness (229.1 per 100 population per year), and the incidence was highest among the youngest in this age group. The patterns are similar in males and females. Children under 6 years old also had the highest incidence of common cold and influenza (83.5 per 100 children per year) and other infections of the respiratory system (37.2 per 100 per year). This age group also experienced a greater number of episodes of dysentery and gastroenteritis, with a rate of 24.9 per 100 population. As for diseases of the digestive system, a rate of 3.1 episodes of non-specific gastroenteritis and colitis per 100 children under 6 years of age was reported.

In 1994, there were a total of 738 deaths in this age group, or 11.5 per 1,000 live births (557 neonatal and 181 post-neonatal). The leading causes of infant mortality were conditions related to prematurity and low birthweight (215 deaths), congenital anomalies (142 deaths), respiratory distress syndrome (92 deaths), conditions originating in the perinatal period (24 deaths), and accidents and injuries (ICD-9, E800–949) (18 deaths).

In the under-1 age group, 30 deaths occurred, and the leading cause was accidents (9 deaths). Among 2-year-olds, 16 children died, and the principal cause was heart disease. Among 3-year-olds, 21 children died, and malignant neoplasms were the leading cause, and among 4-year-olds, 9 children died, and the leading cause of death was accidents.

In 1994, 53 children aged 5–9 years old died, for a rate of 16.0 per 100,000. The leading cause of death was accidents (13 deaths, rate of 3.9), followed by AIDS and diseases of the nervous system, which caused a total of 8 deaths each (rate of 2.4). Among males, the leading cause of death was accidents, which accounted for 11 deaths (6.5 per 100,000), followed by diseases of the nervous system and sensory organs, which caused 6 deaths (rate of 3.6). Among females, the leading cause of death was AIDS, which accounted for 5 deaths (rate of 3.1), followed by congenital anomalies, which accounted for 3 deaths (rate of 3.1).

Abuse and neglect of minors are critical issues in Puerto Rico. During the 1994–1995 period, the Department of Family Services reported a total of 48,705 cases of child abuse, 30,388 due to some type of neglect and the other 18,317 to some type of mistreatment (this includes exploitation; institutional, emotional, physical, or multiple types of abuse; and sexual harassment). Of all the cases reported, 11 children died. In 1995, 49,913 cases of neglect and abuse were reported.

Health of Adolescents

In 1994 it was estimated that there were 355,355 adolescents aged 10–14 years and 341,902 aged 15–19 years. For both groups, the principal health problems were accidents, homicide (especially drug-related homicide), and pregnancy. That year, 452 young people in those age groups died. The general death rate was 29.0 per 100,000 in the group aged 10–14 years and 102.1 in the group aged 15–19 years. The two leading causes of death for the younger adolescent group were accidents, which accounted for 37 deaths (rate of 10.4),

and homicide, which accounted for 14 (rate of 3.9). In the group aged 15–19 years, the leading causes of death were also homicide, which accounted for 187 deaths (rate of 54.7), and accidents, which caused 83 deaths (rate of 24.3). The order varies slightly by sex.

According to a risk survey conducted by the Centers for Disease Control and Prevention in public and private schools throughout the island during the first quarter of 1995, sexual activity among adolescents has increased compared to 1992. In that year, 30% of the young people enrolled in grades 9–12 were sexually active, while in 1995 the percentage was found to be 36.35%. In the 1995 survey, 8.4% of those surveyed reported having had four or more sexual partners and only 39.1% had used condoms during their most recent sexual encounter. The exact number of adolescent pregnancies is unknown, but a steady rise in the birth rate among mothers under 20 years of age has been noted since 1988, when 17.2% of all births were reported among adolescents. In 1994, of 64,325 births, 12,779 (19.9%) were to mothers under the age of 20 (444 were to mothers under 15 and 12,335 were to mothers aged 15–19 years). Of these 12,779 births, 8,165 were to unwed mothers (63.9%). Of the children of adolescent mothers, 1,215 (9.5%) had low birthweight (< 2,500 g) and 204 (1.6%) had very low birthweight (< 1,500 g).

Health of Adults

In 1994, 2,195,594 people, or 59% of the population, were between 15 and 59 years of age; 1,050,395 were male and 1,145,199, female.

Of the 64,325 births that occurred in 1994, 63,854 were to mothers between 15 and 49 years of age. Within this group, most births were registered in the subgroup aged 20–24 years (20,469 births and a specific fertility rate of 133.8). During the same period, one out of every four pregnant women did not receive prenatal care until the third trimester. In 1994, 1.2% (764) of women did not receive any prenatal care. This led to higher maternal and infant morbidity and mortality. It is difficult to identify and provide timely treatment for conditions originating as a result of late prenatal care, which may affect both the mother and the child. The maternal mortality rate was 7.8 per 100,000 live births, the lowest since 1990. Three of the five maternal deaths that occurred in 1994 were of women in the 20–24 age group.

The most recent survey of reproductive health was conducted between November 1995 and July 1996. This study, which analyzed a representative sample of 5,944 women aged 15–49, revealed that one in four (22.5%) was not using any contraceptive method. The three most frequently utilized methods were female sterilization (45.2%), oral contraceptives (9.7%), and male condoms (6.4%). The least used were

Norplant (0.1%); vaginal methods, including sponges, jellies, creams, and foams (0.2%); and intrauterine devices (1.0%). The natural family planning method was used by 6.2% of the women interviewed.

Of the 28,444 deaths registered in 1994, 7,981 (28.1%) occurred in the population aged 15–59 years. In the group aged 15–24, there were 862 deaths (729 men and 133 women), which represents 3.0% of total deaths. Of these deaths, 435 (50.5%) were due to homicide and 199 (23.1%) were the result of accidents.

In the subgroup aged 25–49 years, 4,598 people died (16.7% of the total), 3,439 men and 1,159 women. Slight variations were noted between the sexes with regard to the leading causes of death. Among men in the subgroup aged 25–29, the leading causes of death were homicide (156) and AIDS (111), while among women, AIDS (56) was the leading cause, followed by accidents (16). The leading cause of death among men aged 30–39 years was AIDS (507), followed by accidents (195). Among women in that age range, the leading causes were AIDS (156) and malignant neoplasms (53). For the subgroup aged 40–44 years, the leading cause of death among men continued to be AIDS (238), followed by diseases of the digestive system (72), while among women, malignant neoplasms (69) were the leading cause, followed by AIDS (46). The leading causes of death among men aged 45–49 years were AIDS (159) and heart disease (85). Among women in this group, the leading causes were malignant neoplasms (86) and heart disease (48). In the 50–59 age group, 2,521 people died (1,682 men and 839 women), and the two principal causes of death for both sexes were heart disease and malignant neoplasms.

Health of the Elderly

In 1994, according to data from the Planning Board, 13.2% of the population of Puerto Rico was 60 or more years of age. Of the total of 487,381 people aged 60 or more, 224,055 were men and 263,326, women. The health situation of this age group is influenced by normal aging processes, as well as by injuries or diseases. Diseases of the circulatory system, diseases of the musculoskeletal system and connective tissue, endocrine diseases, and diseases of nutrition and metabolism were the chronic disorders that prevailed in this age group in 1992. In that year, a total of 19,493 people died. The leading causes of death were diseases of the heart (ICD-9, 390–398, 402, 404–429), malignant neoplasms (140–208), and diabetes mellitus (250). Other important causes of death included chronic liver disease and cirrhosis (571), hypertensive disease (401, 403), cerebrovascular disease (430–438), and chronic obstructive pulmonary disease and related disorders (490–496).

The Population and Housing Census of 1990 found that 66,187 elderly people lived alone, which is 19.4% of this age group. Analysis by *municipio* indicates that between 14.0% and 24.9% of the elderly lived alone. In almost all the *municipios*, there was a higher percentage of women than men living alone. These data are particularly important for planning health and other services for this population. The principal sources of income for the elderly population are social security, pensions, and public assistance. According to the Department of Family Services, 18,202 elderly people participated in the Economic Assistance Program during fiscal year 1990, and 22,432 participated during fiscal year 1993–1994.

Family Health

The Government of Puerto Rico has launched several assistance programs for needy families, which are administered by various agencies. One is the Department of Family Services, whose mission is to facilitate and promote the development of families who face social, economic, and/or physical disadvantages so that they can contribute to and benefit from the progress of Puerto Rican society. The Office of the Undersecretary for Public Assistance administers programs of the Department of Family Services designed to provide economic assistance to families that lack enough resources to meet their basic needs. This assistance is channeled through programs that provide food and nutritional assistance, economic assistance, and clothes and shoes for schoolchildren, as well as the electricity subsidy program and the energy crisis subprogram. These programs offer services for children, persons with physical and mental disabilities, the elderly, the homeless, and families in general.

According to data from the 1990 census, in that year 435,665 families participated in the program for nutritional assistance; in 1994 the number rose to 490,813. The total value of the assistance provided in 1994 was US$ 995,824,899. That year, 23% of the families served were headed by women.

The Health Department within the Office of the Undersecretary for Health Promotion and Protection has several programs aimed at the maternal and child population, as well as programs for older persons. The Division of Maternal and Child Health prepares manuals to facilitate the implementation of procedures and regulations concerning the various activities of the program: family planning, prenatal and postpartum care, high-risk delivery and neonatal care, health maintenance for children and adolescents, school health, and care for pregnant adolescents. The managers of the divisions of maternal and child and adolescent health participate with other health programs in the preparation of special protocols on topics such as counseling before and after HIV-testing and administration of AZT to pregnant, HIV-positive women and their children. These manuals and protocols are distributed and discussed with regional primary care providers.

Workers' Health

In fiscal year 1994–1995, the State Insurance Fund Corporation, the agency responsible for covering medical care (including hospitalization and supply of drugs) for workers who suffer work-related accidents or illnesses, reported that 75,823 claims were filed out of a total of 1,051,000 employed persons. The public sector reported 31,646 cases and the private sector reported 44,177. The amount of compensation paid totaled US$ 159.5 million. In that fiscal year, 30,077 certificates of disability were issued, 688 (2.3%) for permanent disability.

The injuries that gave rise to the largest number of claims were contusions (13,691), injuries to the back (12,318), and cuts and lacerations (8,047). The number of claims filed by sex was 31,889 for women (42.1%) and 43,934 for men (57.9%).

Health of the Disabled

The Office for the Protection of Persons with Impediments (OPPI) is the government agency responsible for safeguarding the rights of the population with physical, mental, or sensory impairments. This Office attends to problems, needs, and claims of this group through the provision of guidance, referrals, legal advisory services, protection, and intercession. It also intervenes in the fields of education, health, housing, employment, transportation, recreation, and culture.

The State Council on Developmental Deficiencies is concerned with persons aged 5 and older who have serious chronic disorders, such as mental retardation, epilepsy, autism, spina bifida, deafness, blindness, serious emotional disorders, and Down's syndrome. The Council seeks to increase employment opportunities for these people and promote the organization of community activities aimed at preventing, identifying, and treating developmental disorders in children (early intervention).

According to data from the statistical compendium of OPPI (1993), in 1990 there were 704,407 people in Puerto Rico with some type of disability, including some 140,881 with visual impairments and 176,102 with developmental problems. OPPI calculates the total number of people with disabilities by means of an empirical methodology based on a model that uses population data from the census. The definitions of disability used in the 1990 Population and Housing Census focus mainly on the relationship between disability and the capacity to work.

Data obtained through the Maternal and Child Health Program of the Office of the Undersecretary for Health Promotion and Protection from pediatric centers that serve children with special health needs indicate that the number of persons under 21 seen in these centers has increased. In 1993–1994, 15,363 people received care, while in 1994–1995, the number was 21,335. Of the 21,335 children with special needs served in that latter fiscal year, 11,620 were 6 years of age or under, 8,864 were between 6 and 17, and 851 were 18 or over.

According to data from the last census, these pediatric centers cover 1.5% of the children in Puerto Rico and 27% of the children who need services. The most frequent problems treated in the centers are delayed psychomotor development, cerebral palsy, neural tube defects, speech and language disorders, and cleft palate.

Data from the Department of Education reveal that mental retardation and specific learning disorders are the most common conditions diagnosed among persons between 6 and 21 years of age. Hearing impairments account for 2.2% of all the disorders treated and visual impairments, for 1.5%. In 1994, the Department of Special Education served a total of 37,278 children and young people aged 6–21 years.

The Office of the Undersecretary for Family Services within the Department of Family Services administers a program whose purpose is to help blind, disabled, and elderly adults achieve greater well-being and, wherever possible, become self-sufficient and productive members of their families and communities. The Office offers housekeeping services, foster homes, day care, and prosthesis and orthesis services. In 1993–1994, of the 70,261 people served, 3,163 (4.5%) were disabled.

Analysis by Type of Disease or Health Impairment

Communicable Diseases

Vector-Borne Diseases. In 1993, the Dengue Control Program established an active surveillance system that made it possible—through a communication network linking nurse-epidemiologists, physicians in public and private hospitals, and environmental health workers—to immediately investigate any increase in the incidence of suspected cases.

In a 1994 epidemic outbreak of dengue, 24,252 suspected cases were reported and 5,390 cases were laboratory confirmed, 3 of them fatal. The outbreak was due mainly to the widespread use of water storage containers and tanks by large segments of the population, caused by water shortages and rationing during much of 1994. A general state of alert was declared, and mass media campaigns were developed to provide educational information and guidance on the management and maintenance of stored water.

In 1995, 2,046 cases of dengue were confirmed by laboratory testing; in 1996, 1,804 cases were confirmed. The presence of dengue-3 virus has not been detected since 1977. In recent outbreaks, serotypes 1, 2, and 4 have been identified.

Vaccine-Preventable Diseases. In a re-emergence of measles, the highest number of cases was recorded in 1990, when 1,805 cases (51.3 per 100,000 population) and 12 deaths were reported. In 1993, 355 cases were reported (10.1 per 100,000 population), of which 254 (72%) occurred in preschoolers (0–5 years) and 116 (33%) occurred in infants (under 12 months of age). In order to interrupt the transmission of measles by 1996, the Health Department launched a Measles Elimination Program, an island-wide collective effort that included a mass vaccination campaign, increased surveillance, and control of outbreaks. The mass vaccination campaign of 1994 succeeded in covering 77% of the target population (children aged 6 months to 5 years). The strategy adopted was based on PAHO's recommendations for measles elimination. In May of that year, Puerto Rico participated in a national coverage study (estimated population based on 64,336 births), achieving 87% coverage (four doses of the triple vaccine against diphtheria, tetanus, and pertussis [DTP], three doses of oral polio vaccine [OPV], and one of the vaccine against measles, mumps, and rubella [MMR]). In July 1994, the initial phase of the National Immunization Registry was implemented.

In 1994, 2 cases of tetanus were reported, 3 of whooping cough, 2 of mumps, 3 of meningitis (due to *Haemophylus influenzae* type B), 415 of hepatitis B, and 46 of measles. That same year, two deaths from tetanus, both of males, were reported. No deaths from diphtheria, pertussis, or measles were reported.

In 1992, with the adoption of Law 59, which created the Hepatitis B Immunization Program, the hepatitis B vaccine began to be administered to employees in the public and private sectors at high risk from occupational exposure. As of 30 June 1995, 110,224 doses had been administered in the public sector and 17,681 in the private sector.

In 1992, a hepatitis B perinatal growth protocol was established with a view to offering early treatment to infected mothers and vaccination of the children of identified mothers. In 1993 the hepatitis B vaccine was included in the vaccination series for children under age 1, and the age of coverage is to be increased successively every year. The ultimate objective is to cover the entire population aged 0–18 by the year 2000.

Cholera. Puerto Rico has had no reported cases of cholera in the twentieth century.

Chronic Communicable Diseases. The incidence of tuberculosis has shown slight variations over the years: 312 cases were reported in 1992 (rate of 8.9 per 100,000 population), 257 cases in 1993 (7.3 per 100,000), 274 cases in 1994

(7.8 per 100,000), 263 cases in 1995 (7.5 per 100,000), and 222 cases in 1996 (6.3 per 100,000). The distribution by sex was as follows: in 1994, 73.4% of the cases occurred in males and 26.6% in females; in 1995, 65% occurred in males and 35% in females; and in 1996, 72% of the cases were in males and 28% in females. In 1996, 90% of the cases were the pulmonary form of the disease. During that same year, the distribution of cases by age group was as follows: 6.3% in the group aged 0–14 years, 1.4% in the group aged 15–19 years, 39.2% in the group aged 20–44 years, 15.3% in the group aged 45–54 years, and 33.8% in the group aged 55 and over. The age of 4% of tuberculosis patients is unknown. Mortality from tuberculosis was 1.7 per 100,000 population in 1994, 1.6 in 1995, and 1.7 in 1996. The incidence of multidrug resistance in the reported cases was 11 cases in 1994, 8 in 1995, and 4 in 1996.

From 1994 to 1995, an increase was seen in the percentage of tuberculosis cases in people who are also infected with the human immunodeficiency virus (HIV). In 1993, in accordance with the definition of AIDS established that year by the United States Centers for Disease Control and Prevention (CDC), 72 of 257 tuberculosis patients had AIDS (28.0%). In 1994, 81 of 274 tuberculosis patients had AIDS (29.6%); in 1995, 57 of 263 (18.0%); and in 1996, 60 of 222 cases (27.0%).

Acute Respiratory Infections. According to a study conducted by the Basic Sampling Division of the Department of Health on acute disorders, the estimated incidence of acute morbidity in the noninstitutionalized civilian population in 1992 was 4.5 million episodes. The highest incidence was for diseases of the respiratory system, with a rate of 55.8 episodes per 100 population. The most frequent respiratory disorders were the common cold and influenza (39.7 per 100 people), other diseases of the respiratory system (10.7), and acute bronchitis (3.2). Among children under age 6, the most frequent diseases were the common cold and influenza and other diseases of the respiratory system, with rates of 83.5 and 37.2 per 100 children per year, respectively. The rate of common cold and influenza in the population aged 65 and over was 47.7 per 100 population.

A study of the prevalence of chronic disorders found 737,435 episodes of acute respiratory disease (rate of 20.7 per 100 people) in 1992. The most frequent were asthma (309,403 episodes) and respiratory allergies (234,596 episodes). Among males, 362,529 episodes of respiratory disease were registered. The group aged 6–16 had the highest prevalence (108,283 episodes) and asthma was the most common disorder (66,720 episodes). Females suffered 374,906 episodes of respiratory disease and women aged 25–44 were most frequently affected (112,034 episodes); again, asthma was the most frequent disorder (152,125 episodes) and the largest concentration of episodes occurred in the group aged 6–16 (40,601), followed by the group aged 25–44 (35,647). Respiratory allergy was the most frequent disorder in the group aged 25–44 (43,022).

In 1994, as in 1993, pneumonia and influenza (1,187 deaths, 639 in males and 548 in females) and obstructive pulmonary disease (1,186 deaths, 643 in males and 543 in females) were the seventh and eighth leading causes of death, respectively (together accounting for 2,373 deaths).

Rabies and Other Zoonoses. The Office of the Undersecretary for Environmental Health is charged with controlling or eliminating environmental factors that pose a health threat to Puerto Rican residents. One of its programs is the zoonoses program, which seeks to prevent the transmission of animal diseases to man, especially rabies. During fiscal year 1994–1995, 5,908 animals were vaccinated against rabies, a figure that surpassed the number programmed by 11%. In that same period, 211 suspected cases of animal rabies were investigated and 51 animals tested positive, as a result of which rabies treatment was administered to 51 people.

AIDS and Other STDs. In 1994, AIDS was the fourth leading cause of death in Puerto Rico, accounting for 1,549 deaths, with a mortality rate of 42.0 per 100,000 population. Of the 1,549 deaths, 1,210 (78.1%) were of males and 339 (21.9%) were of females. However, AIDS is the leading cause of death for both men and women in the 25–49 age group. As of December 1994, 16,109 cases of AIDS had been confirmed; of that number, 11,400 patients (71%) had died. According to more recent data, as of 30 April 1997 there were 19,625 confirmed cases, with 12,752 (65%) deaths. Of the total number of diagnosed cases, 19,261 occurred in adults and adolescents and 364 occurred in the pediatric population. Forty-five percent of those affected were between 30 and 39 years of age and 23% were between 40 and 49. The primary risk factors were drug use in males (56%) and heterosexual relations with an HIV-infected partner in women (57%). The incidence of AIDS declined 27% from 1993 (89) to 1994 (65). At present, there is no HIV/AIDS registry in Puerto Rico.

The incidence of primary and secondary syphilis declined 34% from 1993 to 1994 (13 and 9 cases per 100,000 population, respectively). The incidence of gonorrhea declined 5% from 1993 to 1994 (15 and 14 cases per 100,000 population, respectively). In contrast, five times more *Chlamydia* infections were reported in women in 1994 than in 1993 (109 and 19 cases per 100,000 population, respectively).

Noncommunicable Diseases and Other Health-Related Problems

Nutritional Diseases and Diseases of Metabolism. Diabetes mellitus is an important cause of morbidity, disability,

and mortality in Puerto Rico. The Vital Statistics Report for 1994 indicates that it is the third leading cause of death, outranked only by heart disease and malignant neoplasms. In 1994, 1,868 people died as a result of diabetes mellitus (1,028 females and 840 males). This disease ranked among the first five causes of death of males in the 55–59 age group, with 60 deaths and a rate of 87.3 per 100,000 population, and it accounted for the greatest number of deaths (139) in the group aged 70–74, with a rate of 329.4 per 100,000 population. Among women, it figured among the first five causes of death in the group aged 45–49 years, accounting for 19 deaths (17.7 per 100,000 population), and its importance is increasing. In the group aged 85 and over, diabetes accounted for 211 deaths, with a rate of 1,060.7 per 100,000 population. In 1983, mortality from diabetes mellitus was 31.0 per 100,000 population; in 1994, the rate was 50.7 per 100,000 population—an increase of 63.5% in 10 years.

According to a study by the Basic Sampling Division on chronic conditions of Puerto Rico's noninstitutionalized civilian population, 5,496,140 suffered from some chronic disorder in 1992. The group of diseases comprising endocrine, nutritional, and metabolic disorders ranked fourth, affecting 443,452 persons. A total of 206,644 people suffered from diabetes mellitus. The most diabetics were found in the group aged 45–64 (91,763), followed by the group aged 65 and over (77,152). Among males, 86,592 had diabetes mellitus, and the highest prevalence was observed in the group aged 45–64 (41,269). Among females, 120,052 were diabetics, and the disease also was most prevalent in the 45–64 age group (50,494 diabetics), followed by the group aged 65 and over (47,882).

Puerto Rico's Department of Health estimates that the prevalence of diabetes, including both diagnosed and undiagnosed cases, in the adult population is 13.98%. According to the National Institute of Diabetes and Digestive and Kidney Diseases, 10.9% of Puerto Ricans who reside in the United States of America have diagnosed or undiagnosed diabetes.

Cardiovascular Diseases. According to data on chronic morbidity from the Basic Sampling Division, diseases of the circulatory system were the most frequent disorders in this category in 1992, affecting a total of 909,409 persons. Of these diseases, hypertensive disease (400,293 cases) and heart disease (160,807 cases) were most prevalent. The group aged 45–64 had the highest number of cases of hypertensive disease (192,103), while the group aged 65 years and over had the greatest number of cases of heart disease (72,188).

Among women, diseases of the circulatory system were most common (569,927 cases), and hypertensive disease was most prevalent (226,863 cases). The group aged 45–64 years was most affected, followed by the group aged 65 years and over. Among men, a total of 339,482 suffered from diseases of the circulatory system, and hypertensive disease was most prevalent (173,430 cases). Again, the group aged 45–64 was most affected (89,053 cases).

In 1994, cardiovascular diseases, including heart disease, cerebrovascular disease, hypertensive disease, and atherosclerosis, caused 8,663 deaths (4,589 males and 4,074 females), which was 30.4% of all deaths in that year, yielding a mortality rate of 235.0 per 100,000 population. Mortality from heart disease was the highest (157.7 per 100,000 population). Of 5,811 deaths from heart disease, 3,169 were of males and 2,642 of females. For both sexes, ischemic heart disease caused the most deaths (3,372–1,895 males and 1,477 females). Among men, heart disease becomes the leading cause of death in the group aged 50–54 and among women, in the group aged 65 and over.

Malignant Neoplasms. According to a study conducted by the Basic Sampling Division, in 1992 a total of 14,982 malignant neoplasms were reported. The most affected age groups were those comprising persons 45 years old and over, for both males and females. Of the 6,652 cases of malignant neoplasms in the male population, 5,425 occurred in the group aged 45 years and older. Among women, 8,330 cases were reported, 7,693 in the group aged 45 years and older.

Malignant neoplasms were the second leading cause of death in Puerto Rico in 1994, accounting for a total of 4,298 deaths. The most frequent cancer sites were the digestive organs and the peritoneum (1,426 deaths in 1994), the genitourinary organs (866), and the respiratory and intrathoracic organs (657). Within the last two categories, malignant neoplasms of the trachea and lung caused 569 deaths (386 male deaths and 183 female deaths), while prostate cancer caused 505 deaths of men. Of the 866 persons who died from malignant neoplasms of the genitourinary organs, 623 were males and 243 were females. The most frequent cancer site in men was the prostate and in women, the placenta and uterus (64 deaths) and the ovaries (54 deaths). Among women aged 35–64, malignant neoplasms were the leading cause of death. After age 65 they dropped to second place, while among men they became the second leading cause of death after 50 years of age.

Accidents and Violence. In 1994, accidents were the sixth leading cause of death, accounting for 1,313 deaths (1,006 males and 307 females). Of all deaths due to accidents, 48.1% are attributed to motor vehicle accidents (631); of these deaths, 144 were of persons aged 15–24 and 117 were of persons aged 25–34 years.

Homicides were the ninth leading cause of death in 1994. A total of 1,017 deaths were attributed to this cause (931 males and 86 females), which yields a mortality rate of 27.6 per 100,000 population. Homicide is among the first three causes of death in group aged 10–14 and in the group aged 35–39. Of the 1,107 homicide victims, 816 (65.6%) were between 10 and 39 years of age and of this group, 759 were males.

Of 355 suicide deaths registered in 1994, 320 were males and 35 were females. Suicide figures among the first five causes of death in men aged 10–39 (141 deaths). In the group aged 40 and over, 202 people committed suicide.

Behavioral Disorders. In 1994, the Program for Treatment of Alcohol Abuse within the Substance Abuse and Mental Health Services Administration (ASSMCA) treated 7,391 people who tended to share several characteristics. In 1995, it was found that the persons treated by the Program generally were single persons between 25 and 54 years of age who were employed full-time and had had some schooling; 59.3% indicated that they had been incarcerated, 61.7% had not been treated previously, 36.0% had received treatment, and 2.3% gave no information in this regard.

In 1994, of all the people treated (7,391), 7,042 were males (95.3%) and 349 were females (4.7%). The largest percentage of males treated fell into the 35–44 age group (32.2%); the next largest percentage were in the group aged 45–54 (24.1%), and the third largest percentage were in the group aged 25–34 (23.0%). These groups account for 83.3% of all the cases treated (79.3% were males and 4.0% were females). In both males and females, the group aged 35–44 was most likely to be treated repeatedly for excessive consumption of alcohol (33.8%), followed by those aged 45–54 (24.9%), and those aged 25–34 years (24.6%).

In 1994, a total of 36,604 people were treated in ASSMCA facilities for drug addiction (87.8% males and 12.2% females). ASSMCA has six specific programs to address this problem, and its facilities range from evaluation and rehabilitation centers to mobile clinics. "Drug-free" programs also have been developed for minors and adults.

The mental health services follow a biopsychosocial approach that takes into account biological and psychological aspects of human behavior, as well as its social dimension, based on the relationship of the individual with his or her immediate environment. Seven mental health institutions and 12 outpatient care centers operate on the island. In 1994, 4,109 more people than in the previous year were treated in the outpatient services, of which 3,658 were treated in mental health centers. Of the total number of patients treated in mental health facilities (102,117), 95.8% received outpatient care. Of these, 54,937 were male (53.8%) and 47,108 were female (46.2%).

According to a study by the Basic Sampling Division on chronic morbidity, 264,798 of the individuals interviewed had suffered some form of mental illness in 1992. Neurosis was the most frequent disorder (193,383 cases). The age group with the largest number of cases of mental illness was the group aged 45–64 (106,255), followed by the group aged

25–44 (77,285). Among men there were 128,481 cases of some type of mental disorder and among women, 136,317. In both sexes, neurosis was the most common disorder and the groups aged 45–64 and 25–44 were most frequently affected.

Oral Health. Although Puerto Rico's legislature was the first in the world to make fluoridation of water mandatory, and despite the fact that fluoridation is the most cost-effective means of preventing dental caries, in recent years the practice has been stopped due to lack of funding. Studies are being conducted with a view to reinstating it.

In 1994, 68 people died from malignant neoplasms of the oral cavity. According to the Ongoing Health Study (Basic Sampling), in Puerto Rico there were 3.5 million dental visits among the noninstitutionalized civilian population in 1992 (1.0 visits per person). This rate was the same as that recorded in 1989. The rate of visits per person per year was 1.2 for the female population and 0.8 for the male population. The group aged 45–64 had the highest rate of dental visits (1.3 per person per year), followed by the group aged 6–24 (1.1 visits per person per year). There is a direct correlation between income level and number of visits per person. The highest rate per person per year (1.5) was registered among persons with an annual income of US$ 20,000 or more, while the lowest rate was found among those earning less than US$ 5,000 per year (0.6).

RESPONSE OF THE HEALTH SYSTEM

National Health Plans and Policies

In recent years, health care costs in Puerto Rico have sky-rocketed, as they have elsewhere in the world. Curbing this increase and ensuring that every Puerto Rican receives good and reasonably priced health care are at the core of current health reforms. The model now in effect also seeks to have the Department of Health delegate responsibility for the delivery of services to the private sector—the aim being to eventually have a single health care system—while maintaining responsibility for ensuring that the population receives appropriate health services. The model emphasizes a preventive approach, including education and promotion of healthy lifestyles, in order to minimize long-term costs for hospitalization and treatment of catastrophic illness.

In order to provide better health services, the Government has made it a top priority to restructure the health regions and their levels of care, as a way to avoid duplication. Its strategies include the establishment of national and regional interdisciplinary working groups to prepare and implement a model for the evaluation of the regions, preparation of normative guidelines that establish which services are to be pro-

vided at each level, streamlining and improvement of the system for referral of patients among health care system levels, and utilization of health facilities at the various levels and community organizations as key instruments for mass health education campaigns.

Health Sector Reform

The new model for health service delivery to the indigent seeks to improve the accessibility and quality of services in a framework of equity and social justice. Once the model has been fully implemented, it is expected to eliminate many of the barriers that hinder access at the various levels of the health care system (primary, secondary, and tertiary).

As of October 1997, 61 of Puerto Rico's 78 *municipios* in Puerto Rico (78%) had been brought into the health sector reform process, and health insurance coverage had been extended to more than 1 million indigent persons. It is expected that another 14 municipios will have been included by the end of fiscal year 1997–1998. Unlike in 1994–1997, when leasing was used to try and privatize health institutions, the current model envisages the sale of health institutions to the private sector.

One of the principal goals of health sector reform is to control the costs associated with the delivery of health services. This goal can be reached by providing universal access to necessary medical care, controlling the costs of care, restructuring the service system, establishing and maintaining a high level of quality in the services provided, developing primary level services with emphasis on disease prevention and health promotion and protection, and ensuring that all beneficiaries pay a reasonable amount for their health care in accordance with their income.

The government insurance plan covers services that are necessary to maintain good physical and mental health, namely, outpatient care, medical and surgical services, hospitalization, dental care, laboratory services, and drugs. Insurance cost and the deductible amounts are determined according to the beneficiaries' ability to pay. Beneficiaries are entitled to select a health care provider from a network of providers in their area of residence.

The incorporation of the new public policies on health into the operations of the Department of Health and its Health Facilities and Services Administration is considered a priority. The strategies for accomplishing this include preparation, organization, and dissemination of information on prevention of the most common diseases; design and implementation of educational programs, emphasizing chronic diseases and lifestyles; and creation of mechanisms to enable Puerto Ricans to actively participate in caring for and maintaining their own health. Among activities under way are the identification of volunteer organizations and their guidance services, and the identification of barriers that impede access to Health Department's services.

Another high priority is the strengthening of technical and administrative capabilities for the delivery of optimal services for the prevention and treatment of AIDS. The strategies envisaged for this purpose include putting in place mechanisms for analyzing, monitoring, and evaluating plans for risk reduction and education, in order to measure their progress; identifying factors that reduce effectiveness or efficiency; determining the need to continue, refine, reduce, reorient, or expand operations; expanding facilities of regional immunology centers; identifying community leaders who could collaborate in AIDS prevention; and identifying the physical and psychosocial needs of HIV-infected women of childbearing age and HIV-infected children and their family members.

Priority also is being assigned to the strengthening of health services in order to ensure that people age 65 and older receive regular health care services. The strategies in this area include analysis of existing community resources that provide specific services to this age group, coordination of these services, and organization of health promotion, health education, and disease prevention activities.

Another priority area involves improving the availability and quality of mental health services at the primary care level. The strategies consist of equipping facilities for the provision of basic mental health services, creating positions and recruiting the necessary personnel for every center that provides such care, and developing a continuous mental health care system in the framework of the Substance Abuse and Mental Health Services Administration.

Organization of the Health Sector

Institutional Organization

Law No. 101, known as the Health Facilities Law, establishes that the Department of Health shall be the sole public authority responsible for planning health services. In order to fulfill this responsibility, the Department of Health designed a regionalization scheme, which it began to implement in 1958. The first region to be designated was the area served by the Bayamón District Hospital, which included the San Juan metropolitan area and 16 *municipios*. In 1960, the rest of island was divided into five regions, each with a population of between 350,000 and 900,000. The three levels of care included in this scheme were the local health centers (primary care), the regional hospitals (secondary and tertiary care), and the Río Piedras Medical Center in the metropolitan area (specialized care).

In 1970, the existing system was restructured and the island was divided into three regions: northeast, south, and west. The medical centers in Río Piedras, Ponce, and Mayagüez were designated as base hospitals for each of these regions, respectively. In 1977, the geographic and functional aspects of the regionalization scheme were again modified. The new system, which remains in effect today, comprises seven regions (Metropolitan Area, Bayamón, Arecibo, Mayagüez, Ponce, Caguas, and Fajardo) and two subregions (Aguadilla, in the region of Mayagüez, and Humacao, in the region of Caguas), which in turn have been subdivided into 16 areas.

Various linked levels of care have been established, which makes it possible for users to receive the care they need as quickly and effectively as possible. The primary level is the gateway into the health system, to which every person has direct access and from which referrals are made to higher levels. The services are accessible to the population and are oriented toward prevention and treatment of the diseases that have a high probability of affecting people at some time during their lives.

The primary level has emergency and ambulatory services, as well as facilities and equipment for the treatment of disease in diagnostic and treatment centers, family health centers, and public health clinics and units. Health promotion and protection and disease prevention activities are stressed. These activities are complemented by health education and combined with treatment and rehabilitation activities.

The secondary level is responsible for treating health problems that occur relatively infrequently in isolated individuals but whose prevalence is significant in population groups of more than 25,000 people. Early detection of disease is emphasized. Medical care is intermittent and patients access this care through referral from the primary level, to which the secondary level offers support services. Secondary level services are provided in subregional and area hospitals, which, in turn, have outpatient and inpatient services in the basic medical specialties (internal medicine, obstetrics and gynecology, and pediatrics). At this level, surgical, ophthalmologic, and other procedures can be performed, and radiology and clinical laboratory services are always available.

The tertiary level concentrates on infrequent diseases, the prevalence of which can only be predicted in populations across several *municipios*. This level requires costly specialized services, complex technology, and highly skilled professionals. The regional specialized and semi-specialized hospitals provide services at this level. The Mayagüez, Ponce, and Río Piedras medical centers and the Cardiovascular Center of Puerto Rico and the Caribbean offer highly specialized services.

The growth of the population in various areas of the island, coupled with extensive use of health services, has affected their accessibility and quality. Under the new model, the regional offices have been maintained but their functions have changed radically in order to focus more on health promotion and protection. Rather than operational functions relating to direct provision of health care to the population, the offices are now carrying out normative functions, and the strategy of healthy communities and "total wellness centers" are being applied as instruments of social participation. The importance of forming alliances among the various levels is also being emphasized.

The Department of Health has implemented several strategies to achieve the integration of administrative components, both at the central and regional levels. Administrative Order 99/104, issued in June 1995, seeks to integrate areas with similar functions and reduce the size of the government apparatus.

Health Legislation

Health sector reform requires changes in the existing legal framework. At the central level, committees have been created expressly to advance decentralization and to eliminate obsolete regulations. The new approach to privatization also has required that the law on privatization of health care facilities be amended, in order to permit the sale of such facilities to the private sector and to incorporate other privatization models.

Organization of Health Regulatory Activities

Health Services Delivery: Facilities and Standards of Care. The Office of the Undersecretary for Regulation and Accreditation of Health Facilities (SARAFS) is the agency within the Department of Health responsible for the regulation and quality control of health services and the operation of health facilities in Puerto Rico. In addition to the Office of the Undersecretary, it includes the Office of Administration, the Division for Certification of Need and Suitability, the Drug and Pharmacy Division, the Laboratory Division, the Division of Health Institutions, the Medicare Coordination Division, and the Division of Medical Emergencies. The Drug Bioequivalence Board also comes under this Office. It monitors the adoption of state and federal laws and standards that regulate health services; provides advice and guidance to the general public on the regulations applicable to health services; and develops and reviews laws, regulations, standards, and related procedures. Among its more specific responsibilities is the enforcement of regulations, procedures, executive orders, and memoranda issued by regulatory and fiscal agencies and entities with the public administration system and the Regional Office of the United States Health Care Financing Administration (HCFA).

The Division for Certification of Need and Suitability evaluates requests for expansion of services, purchase and sale of health facilities, contract extensions, remodeling, capital investment, and acquisition of highly specialized medical equipment. It guides and advises persons who plan to offer a health service on the applicable laws, regulations, and bidding processes. It also investigates complaints relating to possible violations of laws and regulations, and the Division's staff testify as needed in administrative and legal proceedings. Its principal mission is to promote the orderly planning of health services and institutions in order to meet the needs of the population, control the costs of services, and ensure the availability of services where they are needed.

The Drug and Pharmacy Division is responsible for providing guidance and information and granting licenses to establishments where drugs, medications, pharmaceutical products, and chemical products are manufactured, produced, packaged, sold, and distributed. It also carries out inspections in these establishments and maintains the Puerto Rico Drug Registry.

The Laboratory Division carries out yearly inspections, and licenses clinical and pathology laboratories and blood banks. It also monitors the processing of clinical analyses in physician's offices.

The Division of Health Institutions inspects health services. It is responsible for inspecting and licensing the 282 health institutions, including hospitals, diagnostic and treatment centers, convalescent homes, mental health centers, vocational rehabilitation centers, public health units, social rehabilitation centers, and medical institutions for the mentally retarded.

The Medicare Coordination Division carries out inspections and certifies health care facilities that participate in the Medicare Program offered under the Federal Social Security Law of the United States, by means of a contract between the HCFA and the Department of Health.

The Division of Medical Emergencies regulates, inspects, plans, and develops services in the area of emergency medicine. Together with the Public Service Commission, it also regulates the operation of ambulances. All ambulance operators must be licensed by the Public Service Commission after passing a training course offered by the Department of Health.

Certification and Practice of Health Professionals. The Office for Regulation and Certification of Health Professionals is in charge of all regulations relating to the practice of the health professions, administration of professional examinations, licensing and certification, registration of licenses, and license renewal every three years upon fulfillment of the continuing education requirement, as established by law. The Office includes boards of examiners for regulated health professionals and a registry of professionals. It provides the boards with the administrative services they require.

Health Services and Resources

Organization of Services for the Care of the Population

Control of Environmental Quality (Water, Air, Soil, Housing, and Chemical Safety, Including Hazardous Waste). Within the framework of the political relationship between Puerto Rico and the United States of America, various federal and state agencies are responsible for the regulation and control of activities relating to environmental protection. At the federal level, the main agency is the United States Environmental Protection Agency. At the local level, primary responsibility rests with the Environmental Quality Board, an agency under the Office of the Governor. Other public corporations and agencies in Puerto Rico that play an important role in this area are the Department of Health, the Department of Natural and Environmental Resources, the Solid Waste Authority, and the Aqueduct and Sewer Authority.

The Environmental Quality Board was created in 1970. Its functions are to adopt rules and prepare regulations, carry out investigations, impose sanctions, initiate legal and administrative actions, and establish requirements for the issuance of permits related to its programs for the control of ground- and surface water contamination and air, soil, and noise pollution. In addition, it is empowered to take necessary action in environmental emergencies, such as oil and chemical spills; for this purpose it administers the funds provided under the law establishing the Environmental Emergency Fund.

The Solid Waste Authority is a public corporation created in 1978. Among other functions, it is empowered to provide technical and economic assistance to the municipal governments for the management and proper disposal of solid waste. If necessary, it is authorized to operate facilities for the disposal of such waste.

The Department of Natural and Environmental Resources was created in 1972. Among other functions, it is responsible for the enforcement of laws concerning forests, water, mines, caves, caverns and sink holes, sand, stone, and gravel. In addition, it has primary responsibility for the management of coastal resources and wildlife conservation in Puerto Rico. The Monitoring Board within the Department, together with the inspectors of the Environmental Quality Board and the Health Department and members of the Puerto Rican police force, are key resources for the operation of the programs designed to ensure compliance with applicable legal provisions in this area.

The Aqueduct and Sewer Authority is a public corporation that is responsible for drinking water supply to communities and administration of sanitary sewerage systems. In addition, it controls the discharge of water to public treatment systems and, when necessary, requires prior treatment. The Department of Health maintains active monitoring of drinking water quality in public water systems. In 1974, the Congress of the United States approved a law known as the Safe Drinking Water Act, which makes the Environmental Protection Agency responsible for the establishment of minimum national standards on drinking water contaminants. These standards determine the maximum allowable concentrations of radioactive substances, organic and inorganic chemicals, pesticides, herbicides, and bacteria in drinking water. The law applies to all water systems that have at least 15 service connections or that regularly serve at least 25 people.

The Law on Protection of Drinking Water in Puerto Rico was adopted in July 1977. In keeping with the provisions of this law, in December 1977 the Secretary of Health issued Regulation No. 42, which has been amended twice. This Regulation sets allowable levels for drinking water contaminants in all public water systems of Puerto Rico. In coordination with the Environmental Quality Board, the Environmental Protection Agency administers the National System for the Elimination of Contaminant Residues in Puerto Rico, which seeks to control the discharge of contaminants into the island's bodies of water. In addition, the Environmental Protection Agency plays an important role in monitoring the management and disposal of hazardous solid waste, as well as in investigation of sites that are contaminated with hazardous substances and design, planning, and implementation of necessary sanitation activities.

Food Protection. The Department of Health has delegated responsibility for food quality control to the Office of the Undersecretary for Environmental Health. In order to prevent unsafe food from becoming a public health problem, several programs have been put in place, including programs on hygiene in food service establishments, hygiene in the processing and handling of milk products, and hygiene in food factories, warehouses, and meat markets.

Health Promotion. The Department of Health is changing its orientation from basically curative activities toward an approach that stresses health promotion. The Office of the Undersecretary for Health Promotion and Protection has a preventive medicine program that carries out health promotion and disease prevention activities in keeping with the objectives of Health for All by the Year 2000. To foster public interest in these activities, mass media campaigns have been developed and talks, workshops, and health fairs have been organized. In addition, collaborative working groups (coalitions) have been formed and given the necessary organizational, technical, and leadership capacity to enlist support from representatives of public and private agencies, businesses, and the mass media in order to join forces to achieve the goals of the program. The activities are aimed at the general public and are carried out in public places such as shopping centers, primary health care facilities, universities, workplaces, isolated communities, hotels, nursing homes, hospitals, schools, and churches.

Epidemiological Surveillance System and Public Health Laboratories. Reporting of infectious diseases by health professionals to the Epidemiology Program is governed by Law No. 81, enacted in March 1912. The Program offers technical and medical assistance at the three levels of the health care system. Trained nurse-epidemiologists, who work at the primary and secondary care levels in each *municipio,* compile and submit weekly reports in their respective health regions on numbers of cases of communicable diseases. At the regional level, a nurse-epidemiologist and an epidemiologist organize and process the data from the *municipios* and communicate them to the Epidemiology Division at the central level. The Division, in turn, coordinates the collection of all epidemiological information, which is then transmitted by modem from regional computers to be analyzed, interpreted, and redisseminated to each of the lower levels.

The Epidemiology Program collaborates directly with the CDC in the collection, analysis, and dissemination of epidemiological surveillance data and reporting of acute outbreaks of infectious disease. The CDC provides the program with advisory and support services and it establishes standards for the disease prevention and control methods used in Puerto Rico. With the support of the CDC, the program provides advisory services to public and private hospitals in all the health regions of Puerto Rico, conducts epidemiological research, and carries out educational activities and training in disease prevention and control.

During outbreaks, the Epidemiology Division works in coordination with the Environmental Health Program and the Institute of Health Laboratories. In the event of a dengue outbreak, the Epidemiology Program collaborates with the CDC Dengue Laboratory located in San Juan.

The Institute of Health Laboratories has five operational programs: the Program for Proficiency Testing of Clinical Laboratories, Program on Alcohol Toxicology, the Program for Certification of Health Laboratories, the Program for Epidemiological Support Laboratories, and the Program for Environmental Health Laboratories.

Drinking Water and Sewerage Services. The Puerto Rico Aqueduct and Sewer Authority administers 208 water systems that supply approximately 97% of the island's population. The remaining 3% is supplied by other means. Seventy-four percent of the urban population is connected to sewer systems (26% have septic tanks), and 80% of the rural population has basic sanitation services, including latrines. The Aqueduct and Sewer Authority reports all drinking water quality problems to consumers.

Solid Waste Disposal. According to estimates of the Solid Waste Authority, in 1994 some 2 million tons of solid waste were generated on the island. The vast majority of this waste was disposed of in municipal dumps. Only a small proportion (7% of the total) was recovered for recycling.

Food Aid Programs. A strategic priority of the Department of Health is the prevention of nutritional risk factors, especially those associated with chronic degenerative diseases, through preventive services offered to vulnerable groups. Among the measures adopted by the Department during fiscal year 1994–1995 were the adoption of a public policy to promote breast-feeding and the provision of advisory services and execution of surveys on nutritional matters. During that period, enrollment in the Federal Supplemental Nutrition Program for Women, Infants, and Children (WIC), administered by the United States Government, reached 197,663, which represented an increase of 40,000 participants with respect to the previous year. The dissemination of information about the services offered under the program was improved through nutritional guidance campaigns aimed at physicians, hospitals, and pediatric clinics. In coordination with other agencies, the referral processes were facilitated, and the identification of eligible mothers increased 2%. In addition, several shelters and institutions for the homeless were identified and the delivery of services to this segment of the population was coordinated.

The Department of Family Services, through the Office of the Undersecretary for Public Assistance, carries out the Program for Nutritional Assistance. This program was established in July 1982 for the purpose of offering economic assistance to low-income families for food supplements and emergencies. During fiscal year 1993–1994, the program served an average of 490,813 families monthly. The total amount of funds distributed was US$ 1,002,817,928 (US$ 2,043.18 per family).

The Food Distribution Program aims to distribute food donated by the U.S. Department of Agriculture to people with low or no income, in order to provide them with a balanced diet. The food is distributed to the beneficiaries of the Economic Assistance Program, residents of public housing projects, and impoverished communities identified by the Program for Economic and Social Rehabilitation. In 1993–1994, a total of 182,326 families participated in this program.

Organization and Operation of Personal Health Care Services

Outpatient, Hospital, and Emergency Services. The health care delivery system includes public, private, and privatized public institutions. Facilities that provide primary care services must be accredited, in accordance with Law No. 101 and Regulation No. 52. According to data from the Office of the Undersecretary for Regulation and Accreditation of Health Facilities (SARAFS), in 1997 Puerto Rico had 68 hospitals, 24 of them public (including privatized public hospitals) and 44 private hospitals. Of the public hospitals, 16 are general hospitals, 3 are specialized, 4 are psychiatric hospitals, and 1 is a federal hospital. Of the private facilities, 38 are general hospitals, 4 are specialized, and 2 are psychiatric. The 24 public hospitals have a total of 5,464 beds, of which 3,930 are available beds; 3,811 of these are in use. The private hospitals have a total of 6,614 beds, of which 6,239 are available beds and 5,818 are in use.

According to the Annual Report on Institutional Statistics, in fiscal year 1993–1994 the public sector registered, at its three levels of service delivery, a total of 2,952,491 visits to outpatient clinics, 2,093,294 visits to emergency rooms, an average hospital stay of 5.33 days, and a bed occupancy rate of 67.17%. At the tertiary level, the average stay was 5.83 days and the bed occupancy rate was 70.26%.

Human Resources

Professionals who provide health services in public and private institutions must have completed a formal course of study in a school or university recognized by the Government of Puerto Rico and must meet the requirements for continuing education stipulated under Law No. 11.

Of the 6,269 physicians who were practicing in 1989–1992, 3,377 worked in the public sector and 1,283 in the private sector, 1,601 had their own private practices, and 8 worked on a volunteer basis. There were 6,707 general nurses in the public sector and 5,252 in the private sector. Of the 7,394 licensed practical nurses, 4,406 worked in the public sector and 2,807 in the private sector, 175 were self-employed, and 6 worked on a volunteer basis. In 1989–1992, 55% of the general nurses, 59.6% of the licensed practical nurses, and 53.9% of the physicians worked in the public sector, while 43.1% of the general nurses, 38.0% of the licensed practical nurses, and 20.5% of the physicians worked in the private sector.

Training of Health Workers. Health workers receive formal training through educational programs within or outside Puerto Rico. These programs must be recognized by the local regulatory authority. The island currently has schools of medicine, nursing, pharmacy, medical technology, and allied health professions (physical therapy, occupational therapy, speech and language pathology, and others), as well as internships in nutrition and dietetics, a graduate school of public health, and graduate programs in psychology and other areas. In addition, there are intern and residency programs in various medical specialties and technical schools and associate degree programs in other health-related disciplines.

Labor Market for Health Professionals. Traditionally, the public sector has provided most employment opportunities for health professionals, but the reform of the health system has changed this. As it gradually takes over health care delivery to the indigent, the private sector is recruiting more professionals. In addition, the growth of the health insurance market has created new job opportunities for health professionals. As service contracts are being established in the various regions where health reform is being implemented, professionals are beginning to move to new sectors. In addition, the Department of Health, in order to fulfill its core functions, requires professionals skilled in policy analysis and public policy-setting.

Research and Technology

Research and technology activities are carried out by university centers in coordination with the Department of Health. Research projects are conducted under agreements with the CDC and others are subsidized with federal funds from the United States Government, especially in the area of treatment of patients with HIV and AIDS.

Expenditures and Sectoral Financing

Between 1986 and 1995, health care expenditures grew at an annual rate of 6.0%. Although annual growth rates appear to have declined (7.1% in 1992, 5.6% in 1993, 2.9% in 1994, and 5.0% in 1995), health care spending has nevertheless increased at a faster rate than inflation in almost every year of this decade. In 1995–1996 the operating budget of the Department of Health and the Health Facilities and Services Administration totaled US$ 1,035,788,933.

As of December 1996, 1,033,777 people had purchased health insurance plans at a total cost of US$ 608 million.

SAINT KITTS AND NEVIS

GENERAL SITUATION AND TRENDS

Socioeconomic, Political, and Demographic Overview

Saint Kitts and Nevis occupies the northern part of the Leeward Islands chain: Saint Kitts has a surface area of 176.2 km^2 and Nevis spans 93 km^2. The twin-island nation is an independent Commonwealth Caribbean country, having assumed full sovereignty from Great Britain in 1983. The government changed for the first time in 1995, as the Labour Party defeated the People's Action Movement at the polls after 15 years of uninterrupted governance.

Saint Kitts and Nevis is readily accessible by sea and air and boasts a modern international airport, and both islands have an adequate network of roads, a modern telephone system, and an improving transportation system.

Saint Kitts and Nevis functions as a federation: the Federal Parliament, the highest decision-making institution in the country, resides in Saint Kitts, and Nevis operates under a local government, the Island Assembly, which has some degree of autonomy. This arrangement results in virtually parallel public service arrangements in both Saint Kitts and Nevis, with the Prime Minister assuming general control of all aspects of the nation's business, but with the Premier of Nevis having an extensive range of local authority. For example, Saint Kitts and Nevis have separate annual budgetary estimates that are approved by each island's statutory entity and are implemented relatively independently of each other. There are some areas, however—such as access to international assistance and implementation of national projects—in which collaboration is mandatory.

The Ministry of Health is the executive arm of the government responsible for mobilizing resources at all levels to promote the nation's health. The Ministry operates within the framework of the General Orders, which are the laws and regulations governing public service.

Saint Kitts and Nevis does not currently have a published National Development Plan, but clear national policy objectives, goals, and targets are presented annually as part of the budget proposals. The present development strategy, as outlined in the 1995 Annual Budget Address, includes the following key elements: promoting service industries such as tourism, informatics, and offshore financial services; encouraging light manufacturing and food processing with potential for niche marketing; diversifying agriculture, with special emphasis on livestock production; pursuing human resource and technological development through education and training and incentives; and supporting and strengthening the social infrastructure.

The economy of Saint Kitts and Nevis has achieved only moderate levels of growth in recent years. Real economic growth has averaged 4.4% during the 1992–1995 period, which compares unfavorably with the annual average real growth of 6.4% recorded between 1988 and 1991. Thus, the Government acknowledges that one of the country's major challenges is economic revitalization and attaining significantly higher rates of real growth.

The leading contributors to the gross domestic product (GDP) have been government services, wholesale and retail trade, construction, and communications. Tourism also has emerged as one of the stronger economic sectors, and its growth has directly affected several sectors, including hotels and restaurants, transportation, and retail trade. Per capita income in the country has grown in nominal terms, from US$ 3,656 in 1992 to US$ 4,473 in 1995.

Unemployment in Saint Kitts and Nevis is among the lowest in the Caribbean. According to the 1991 Population and Housing Census Report, only 4.9% of the population were unemployed at that time. A 1994 survey of the labor force, conducted jointly by the Organization of American States and the Government, confirmed an unemployment rate of just 4.3%. Thus, the trend suggests not only a healthy employment climate, but also the continuing creation of new jobs.

The leading employment area was the service industry (36.5%), which is heavily dominated by tourism-related activities, followed by professional and technical services (13.6%), agriculture and fishing (12.9%), and construction and manufacturing (12.7%). In 1994, income was approximately US$ 18,500 or more in 9.3% of households; between US$ 13,000 and US$ 18,500 in 8.4%; between US$ 9,300 and US$ 13,000 in 13.6%; between US$ 5,600 and US$ 9,300 in 21.1%; between US$ 3,700 and US$ 5,600 in 15.5%; between US$ 1,900 and US$ 3,700 in 17.9%; and below US$ 1,900 in 14.2% of households. Even though school attendance is not compulsory, in 1991 11,789 students were enrolled in public and private schools, representing 88.5% of the country's total population aged 5 to 19 years old. School enrollment in 1994 was 11,608 (89.2%).

According to the 1991 Population and Housing Census Report, the highest educational level attained by most residents of Saint Kitts and Nevis is secondary school education (39.2%), with an almost equal number reporting having completed primary school or basic level education (38.1%). Just 5.3% of the population had a pre-university education, defined as post-secondary vocational training, or a university education. In 1991, there were 12,056 households, an increase of 3.8% since the previous census count of 11,615 in 1980. A total of 8,921 households (74.0%) were owner-occupied and 2,242 (18.6%) were privately rented. The average number of rooms per household increased marginally from 3.2 in 1980 to 3.4 in 1991, while the average household size decreased from 3.7 persons to 3.5 in the period under review. Significantly, 30.3% of households had two rooms or fewer, an improvement over 1980, when the corresponding figure was 38.2%; 19% of households had three rooms, 23.0% had four rooms, and 12.7% had six or more rooms.

Given the low level of local crop and livestock production and in order to satisfy the needs of a booming tourist industry, the country must import most of its food for consumption. In 1992, livestock and crop production was valued at US$ 3.1 million (1.9% of GDP), while the food import bill for that same year was US$ 16.9 million (10.8% of GDP).

The country experienced a negative population growth of 6.2% during the intercensal period 1980–1991. This decline, from 43,291 in 1980 to 40,618 in 1991, was attributed largely to emigration, a phenomenon that has persisted with an average annual net emigration of 456 between 1992 and 1994.

The Planning Unit in the Ministry of Development and Planning estimated the mid-year population of Saint Kitts and Nevis at 43,530 in 1995, with an almost equal distribution of males and females. Just over 30% of the population was under the age of 15 years, while about 11.9% were in the age group 60 years old and older. A total of 35,510 persons (81.6%) live on Saint Kitts, and 8,020 (18.4%) live on the sister island of Nevis (1995).

Between 1992 and 1994 the "Annual Digest of Statistics, 1994," reported an average annual total fertility rate of 2.4 among women 15 to 49 years old. The crude birth rate declined from 19.7 per 1,000 population in 1992 to 18.3 in 1995, with a rate of 19.6 for the period. There is no underregistration of births.

Mortality and Morbidity Profile

The crude death rate for Saint Kitts and Nevis during the 1992–1995 period was 9.2 per 1,000 population. Between 1992 and 1995, the infant mortality rate fluctuated between a low of 22.4 per 1,000 live births in 1993 to a high of 25.1 per 1,000 in 1995.

According to the "Annual Digest of Statistics, 1994," life expectancy at birth for both sexes was estimated at 68.9 years at the end of 1994; disaggregated figures for that year were 67.4 years for males and 70.4 years for females.

Diseases of the circulatory system were by far the leading cause group of death in Saint Kitts and Nevis between 1992 and 1995, with an annual average of 164 deaths (46.1%) falling into this category. Within this cause group, an annual average of 88 deaths was attributed to cerebrovascular diseases and an average of 71 deaths to diseases of pulmonary circulation and other forms of heart disease. The other important cause groups of death were communicable diseases (14.4%), involving mainly respiratory infections and septicemia, and neoplasms (11.8%).

An annual average of 17 deaths (4.9%) has been attributed to external causes, underscoring the impact of all forms of accidents and violence on the mortality statistics. The other defined group, conditions originating in the perinatal period, accounted for 3.5% of deaths.

It is difficult to present a comprehensive analysis of the country's morbidity data, because data are not always available due to delays in computer data entry and analysis, or because the Nevis component is not compiled. The best estimates suggest that hypertension and diabetes are the main causes of morbidity. In 1995, there were 1,147 hypertensives and 882 diabetics registered at health centers throughout Saint Kitts and Nevis.

Regarding infectious diseases in the 1992–1995 period, gastroenteritis has been the most common, followed by sexually transmitted diseases and dengue fever. It must also be noted that viral hepatitis and leptospirosis have been a consistent feature of the morbidity statistics, although the numbers of cases were mostly quite low. There were 14 cases of AIDS reported.

SPECIFIC HEALTH PROBLEMS

Analysis by Population Group

Health of Children

Infants and young children traditionally have been listed among the priority groups targeted to receive special health care services, including prenatal care throughout pregnancy and the provision of trained nurses and physicians to provide intrapartum care and continuous child health care.

Morbidity reports indicate that gastroenteritis and acute respiratory infections were the main causes of illness among children. For example, in 1995 there were 479 reported episodes of gastroenteritis in children under 5 years old, for a rate of 10,788 per 100,000 population. The main causes for hospital admission among children under 5 years of age have been gastroenteritis, acute respiratory infections, and trauma, both internal and external.

Diseases such as diphtheria, tetanus, whooping cough, and poliomyelitis, for which vaccines are widely available, are now unknown. A surveillance program for flaccid paralysis and rash/fever illness is ongoing. In 1994, there were two suspected cases of measles, but the Caribbean Epidemiology Center (CAREC) confirmed neither.

Children under 1 year old have consistently had 100% coverage against common childhood illnesses since 1992 and, although the coverage dipped slightly to 99% in 1995, the record remains excellent. Immunization against BCG is not included in this analysis, since the vaccine is not administered until age 5 years. The Community Nursing Service reports that 587 BCG vaccines were administered in 1995, covering 63% of 5-year-olds.

Hepatitis B immunization was introduced in 1995, targeting children 0 to 5 years old and health workers. However, the program was aborted, reportedly because of damage to vaccine stocks during a hurricane in that same year; cost considerations have delayed restarting the program.

While severe undernutrition is almost absent (0.1% of children under 5 years old seen in child health clinics), the level of mild to moderate undernutrition remains relatively high, although decreasing. In 1992, 7.5% of children under 5 years old attending health clinics were affected; 7.6% were affected in 1993, 5.9% in 1994, and 4.2% in 1995 (an average of 6.3% for the period). Obesity, on the other hand, may be rising slightly—6.5% of the children under 5 years old attending health clinics in 1992 were obese, 6.4% in 1993, 7.3% in 1994, and 6.7% in 1995 (an average of 6.7% over the four-year period). An annual average of 1,855 children under 5 years old were seen in child health clinics. Nutritional status is measured using height- and weight-for-age criteria set forth in the Caribbean Food and Nutrition Institute Growth Chart.

More than 90% of all newborns weigh more than 2,500 g at birth. During the 1992–1994 period, the percentage of low birthweight babies was 8.1% (74 babies) in 1991, 8.6% (73) in 1992, 9.0% (76) in 1993, and 8.8% (80) in 1994, indicating that this issue deserves attention. The percentage of low birthweight babies gathers even more significance when consideration is given to the link drawn by some experts in the country between prematurity and low birthweight and neonatal death.

Breast-feeding is actively promoted among new mothers; the objective is to achieve exclusive breast-feeding of infants for the first 3 to 4 months of life. Out of a total of 442 assessments completed in 1994, only 142 infants (32%) were fully breast-fed up to 3 months of age, and the number had declined to 23 (5.1%) by age 4 months.

Health of Adolescents

Births to teenage women continue to feature prominently among natality statistics. In 1995, 16.7% of all births were attributed to teenage women, and although that figure represented a drop from the 19.7% figure in 1992, the current situation continues to cause concern. There is no documentation on any other significant health or health-related problem among adolescents.

Health of Adults

Because women have been identified as an at-risk group that requires special attention, specialized programs relating to prenatal and postnatal care and family planning services have become institutionalized.

Primary care services cater specifically to the needs of all pregnant women through weekly prenatal sessions held at all health centers. If prenatal attendance at health centers is assumed to represent total prenatal care for the country as a whole, each woman makes an average of about three visits during her pregnancy, half the minimum of six prenatal visits stipulated by the national maternal and child health manual. It should be kept in mind, however, that an unknown number of pregnant women receive care exclusively from private physicians. All deliveries in the country take place in hospitals.

Hemoglobin levels among prenatal women are nearly perfect: according to the Ministry of Health's 1994 Annual Nutrition Report, 75.8% of women fell in the high category, scoring 11 g and higher; 23.9% were in the median range of 9.0–10.9 g; while a mere 1.3% registered hemoglobin levels under 9 grams; no absolute numbers are provided. Unfortunately, similar data are not available for other forms of nutritional disorders such as iodine and vitamin A deficiencies.

The prevalence rate of contraceptive use is known to be relatively high. In 1992, there were 4,090 women, or 56.7% of women of childbearing age (15 to 49 years old) enrolled at health centers as active family planning users. Although the percentage declined slightly to 51.3% in 1995 (6,164 women registered), the level of contraceptive protection remained within acceptable limits. In 1995, oral contraceptives remained the most popular method of birth control among the women enrolled (51.1%), followed by injectables (13.3%), and the IUD (10.3%); a category listed as "other" accounted for 25.3% of current users.

All active family planning clients are offered cervical cancer screening services as part of their routine health care. The number of Pap test examinations conducted at the J.N. France Hospital has more than doubled since 1992, going from 712 to 1,749 in 1995. Similarly, the number of abnormal smears encountered has increased threefold, from 7 in 1992 to 22 in 1995 (including one invasive carcinoma in 1992 and one in 1995).

There has been one maternal death each in 1992, 1994, and 1995; there were no deaths in 1993. Although these figures are minimal, they still are unacceptably high in terms of zero-maternal-deaths target established for the Caribbean.

Health of the Elderly

In 1995, 5,200 persons in Saint Kitts and Nevis were 60 years of age and older, representing 11.9% of the total population. There are no specialized health services for the elderly, although they are exempt from user charges when using regular health care services. The elderly also are a major focus of diabetic and hypertensive clinics conducted routinely nationwide.

Family Health

Based on the 1991 Housing and Population Census Report, there were 12,056 households in the country, of which 9,350 were in Saint Kitts and 2,686 in Nevis. The 1994 Labour Force Survey showed that 5,672 households, or 47% of the total, were headed by women with dependent children under 15 years old. Among women who headed households, 58.1% were employed, 17.1% were retired, and 12.7% were housewives/homemakers.

All family members have access to primary- and secondary-level health services, including maternal and child health services, diagnostic services, emergency care, and treatment of illnesses and injuries.

Analysis by Type of Disease or Health Impairment

Communicable Diseases

Vector-Borne Diseases. There were 27 confirmed cases of dengue fever (16.2 per 100,000 population) in 1995, a significant increase over 1994 and 1993 figures, when only 7 and 1 cases, respectively, were reported. There were no confirmed cases in 1992. No deaths from the disease were recorded over the period.

An *Aedes aegypti* control program has been in operation for almost two decades. The 6% household index reported in 1995 is higher than the 1% recommended level for dengue control. Control methods involve source reduction and chemical treatment, although use of the latter is decreasing.

Vaccine-Preventable Diseases. There have been no confirmed cases of the childhood diseases preventable by immunization since 1992, except for two suspected cases of measles reported in 1994.

AIDS and Other Sexually Transmitted Diseases. A total of 14 confirmed AIDS cases were reported over the 1992–1995 period. Over the same period, a total of 7,157 persons were tested and 48 (0.7%) were found to be HIV-positive, with the highest number (18) occurring in 1993. Out of an annual average number of 322 blood donors routinely screened, only one was found to be HIV-positive.

Underreporting of sexually transmitted diseases is suspected. The figures show a decline in the number of reported cases of gonorrhea by more than 40%, while the number of cases of syphilis has stabilized. Laboratory data indicate that there was a 2.6% positivity rate for hepatitis B among blood donors.

Other Infectious Diseases. An established system is in place for the reporting and monitoring of infectious diseases, especially notifiable diseases, although data are not always complete and reliable. The Health Information Unit of the Ministry of Health is charged with collating and analyzing the information, but its resources are insufficient to do so.

Numerically, gastroenteritis tops the list of infectious diseases, and viral hepatitis, leptospirosis, and tuberculosis have been reported in all years over the period 1992–1995. In fact, leptospirosis has consistently ranked among morbidity statistics—four cases were recorded in 1995, up from two cases in each of the three preceding years. Most cases have been among agricultural workers employed in the sugarcane industry, which has a high rodent population. An information and education program for agricultural workers is ongoing.

Noncommunicable Diseases and Other Health-Related Problems

Oral Health. Dental services within the public system are delivered through a team that includes dentists, dental auxiliaries, and dental hygienists. Unfortunately, the output has declined significantly since 1992 due to shortages in personnel. Most activities involved extractions, although dental hygienists conducted some preventive work among schoolchildren. In 1992, a total of 8,699 patients were seen; there were 1,547 extractions of deciduous teeth and 2,311 extractions of permanent teeth. In comparison, in 1994 only 4,903 patients were seen and there were 863 extractions of deciduous teeth and 1,290 extractions of permanent teeth.

Malignant Tumors. During the 1992–1995 period, malignant neoplasms accounted for 167 or 11.8% of all deaths from defined conditions, ranking this cause as the third leading cause of mortality in Saint Kitts and Nevis. The digestive organs and peritoneum was the most common site, with 29 deaths, followed by the prostate with 28 deaths, female breast with 14 deaths, and the stomach and cervix with 13 deaths each.

Behavioral Disorders. The number of registered psychiatric patients has remained relatively constant between 1992 and 1995: end-of-year figures were 247 for 1992, and 243, 230, and 358 in each of the following three years, for an annual average of 244. Similarly, the total number of attendances among patients visiting community mental health services has remained stable, at an average of 1,416 annually. Of all visits made to mental health services in 1995, 51% (132 patients) was due to schizophrenia, 25% (67 patients) to alcohol addiction and drug induced psychosis, and 10% (26 patients) depression.

Since 1992, the mental health program has benefited from the services of a national psychiatrist. The program emphasizes the development of an integrated approach that links hospital and community services. There are plans to formulate a National Mental Health Plan to provide the framework for the operation of the services.

Accidents and Violence. Of the 9,484 reports made to the Police in 1994, 337 (3.6%) were offenses defined as grievous bodily harm and wounding; another 14.2% involved thefts, robbery, arson, and predial larceny. A total of 16 deaths attributed to homicide were recorded during the period under review, with two deaths attributed to injury undetermined, whether accidentally or purposely inflicted (ICD-9, E980–E989).

RESPONSE OF THE HEALTH SYSTEM

National Health Plans and Policies

Because Saint Kitts and Nevis does not have a national health sector plan, the following information regarding the sector's plans and policies has been collected from various reports and documents and from discussions with key officials.

The health sector is pursuing several broad objectives for the future. First, the sector's strategic and operational planning capabilities will be strengthened at all levels, so that each subsector can develop its own planning process according to an established national framework. Chronic diseases will be combated through an aggressive health advocacy and health promotion program that will cover all schools, nongovernmental organizations service clubs, and community groups. The hospital infrastructure will be improved: new facilities will replace the structurally compromised J.N. France and Alexandra hospitals, that repeatedly were devastated by hurricanes. The new J. N. France Hospital is estimated to cost US$ 14.8 million, and preparations for its construction are in the final stages. Pogson Hospital also will be substantially refurbished, and services at the main hospitals will be expanded to include as complete a range of secondary care as available resources permit. Alternative funding sources to supplement Government funds will be explored, including direct cost recovery for services provided, private sector contributions and/or donations, and direct payment by the social security scheme for services provided to members. For example, Saint Kitts's fee structure for health services provided is being revised. Human-resource development will be strengthened to a point where in-service training programs for technical staff and management training can be undertaken locally; improving the management capabilities of key health personnel is an important component of this objective. Finally, specialized programs that stress community rather than residential care will be put in place for the elderly and the mentally ill.

As a way to achieve these goals, the Government is committed to provide for the needs of all vulnerable groups in society by strengthening programs targeted at women and children, the urban and rural poor, the elderly, and the disabled; to pursue an aggressive health advocacy and health promotion program; to continue the organizational reform of the health sector, involving key personnel in the decision-making process; to implement programs aimed at reducing the incidence and prevalence of chronic diseases, based on morbidity and mortality patterns; and to actively seek international partnerships in health.

Health Sector Reform

A reorganization of the health services is under way, but up to now reforms have taken place only in Saint Kitts. As part of this process and in order to better allocate resources, program areas for service delivery have been reorganized into five categories—administration, preventive services, hospital services, nursing education, and long-term care. In addition, at least four senior technical and administrative positions have been created in the course of the reforms. The new office of Health Planner is responsible for coordinating health sector planning; at this juncture that office is focusing on organizational reform. The new office of Director of Primary Health Care Services subsumes the functions of the Medical Officer of Health, taking responsibility for the technical development and supervision of all primary care services. The Director of Health Institutions is charged with supervising all health institutions under the purview of the Ministry of Health. Finally, the Director of Health Advocacy and Health Promotion oversees the health education, nutrition, and family planning services.

Organization of the Health Sector

Within the public health sector, the Minister of Health is responsible to the Cabinet for implementing relevant policy decisions, the Permanent Secretary functions as a Chief Administrative Officer, and the Chief Medical Officer coordinates the delivery of health services throughout the country. These positions are federal in scope, covering both Saint Kitts and Nevis. Nevis has considerable autonomy, however, and has its own Minister Responsible for Health and a Chief Secretary who directs administration of local health services. In practice Saint Kitts and Nevis operate two independent systems.

Institutional Organization

Health facilities include J.N. France Hospital (150 beds), Pogson Hospital (18 beds), and Mary Charles Hospital (10 beds). In addition, there is the Cardin Home (50 beds) for chronically ill, disabled, and geriatric cases. Nevis has Alexandra Hospital (54 beds) and a 22-bed infirmary that caters to psychiatric patients and the aged-poor. There also are 17 health centers spread throughout the two islands.

The district level has both primary and secondary care services. The network of health centers constitutes the bedrock for the delivery of primary care services: health centers are managed by full-time district nurses/midwives who are supported by a cadre of trained health personnel, including a medical officer, a family nurse practitioner, and a public health nursing supervisor. Mary Charles, Pogson, and Alexandra hospitals provide the first line of secondary care ands J.N. France Hospital functions as the main referral center.

Health Services and Resources

Organization of Services for Care of the Population

Health Education and Promotion. The newly established Health Advocacy and Health Promotion program area consolidates the efforts of traditional health education, nutrition, and family planning services. Its purview expands beyond public information, education, and training to embrace public policy issues, intersectoral cooperation, the mobilization of community support, and the development of media contacts, all of which are part of the Caribbean Charter on Health Promotion.

Health and family life education have been incorporated into the curriculum of all primary schools, which should exert a powerful influence on the lifestyles of the school-age population. Health promotion is considered to be a major strategy for addressing diseases closely tied to lifestyle, such as diabetes, hypertension, cancer, and sexually transmitted diseases.

Community Participation. Despite the existence of a policy to that effect, the community's involvement in the planning and implementation of health programs has been nonexistent. Moreover, there is no evidence that suggests that the health sector is actively seeking this level of involvement from the community.

This having been said, some outstanding examples of community support for health should be highlighted. For example, it has been reported that the ophthalmic unit at J.N. France Hospital has been fully equipped recently with donations from the private sector.

Environmental Protection. Marine environmental protection and preservation is of key importance to the economy of Saint Kitts and Nevis, given the country's reliance on the tourist industry. A Ministry Responsible for Culture and the Environment was created in 1995, and it is charged with preserving cultural heritage and implementing the Government's environmental protection program. The Environment Division within this Ministry is responsible for enforcing the provisions of the National Conservation and Environmental Protection Act; implementing programs in beach protection and coastal preservation, forestry management, soil conservation, wildlife management, and protection against marine pollution; coordinating all environmental protection efforts; and providing technical support to other Ministries in any environmental matter, including implementation of public sector projects with potential environmental impact.

Water Supply. The 1991 Population and Housing Census Report showed that 7,993 households (66.3%) had their water piped into their premises from the communal system, and an additional 2,749 households (22.8%) had access to public standpipes; these figures confirm that at least 90% of households benefited from a potable water supply. The percentage of households that had water piped from the communal system increased from 39.3% in 1980 to 66.3% in 1991. Conversely, the number of households that accessed their domestic water from standpipes decreased from 40.8% in 1980 to 22.8% in 1991.

The Public Works Department in the Ministry of Communications and Works manages the water supply system. Water is chlorinated routinely to maintain bacteriological quality. The Public Health Department in the Ministry of Health is charged with monitoring the quality of water used for public consumption.

Sewage Disposal. The water closet/septic tank system is the most often used sewage disposal system in the country, which represents a change from the situation that prevailed in 1980, when the pit latrine was dominant. It also should be noted that 85.5% of households have exclusive use of their toilet facilities, while 11.1% share them. In 1995, 3.4% of households had no toilet facilities, but the situation is improving.

Occupational Health and Safety. A National Plan for Workers' Health is being formulated by a group made up of representatives from the Ministries of Health and of Labour, the trade unions, and the Employers' Federation, among others. Apart from injuries, no major occupational hazards have actually been reported. This intersectoral committee has identified the following potential problems: injuries, respiratory disorders, mental and physical stress, skin diseases, strains, and optical and hearing disorders.

The social security scheme, which is equivalent to a national insurance scheme, provides injury benefits to an annual average of about 300 of its members. Every worker is required by law to contribute to the scheme, and benefit claims are paid upon medical certification of injury. The scheme now pays about US$ 800,000 annually in sickness benefits, maternity allowances and grants, and medical expenses for its members. The Labour Department and the Ministry of Health monitor work-related injuries.

During the 1992–1995 period, a total of 1,175 injury claims were paid, distributed as follows by nature of injury: 605 for contusions, abrasions, and cuts; 280 for sprains and/or strains; 69 for fractures; 53 for eye injuries; 41 for burns; 26 for amputations; 22 for infections; 12 for dislocations; 4 for poisoning; 4 for concussions; 3 for electric shocks; 2 for tearing of internal organs; 48 for unspecified skin injury, and 6 for miscellaneous other causes.

Disaster Preparedness. A National Disaster Management Agency has been established to coordinate disaster management efforts throughout the country. This agency has a full-time administrative staff of four and receives directions from a Cabinet-appointed Board of Management. An update of the National Disaster Plan is in progress; the plan covers such aspects as disaster management, crisis management, disaster assessment, relief operations, public information, and liaison with nongovernmental organizations. The Plan's health component deals with such issues as mass casualty management, water supply management, and environmental sanitation; it also includes a section on maintenance of health facilities.

Organization and Operation of Personal Health Care Services

J.N. France Hospital provides inpatient and outpatient care in most major specialties. Mostly as a result of the devastation caused by Hurricane Luis, the Hospital's activity decreased in all areas except emergencies between 1994 and 1995. Total admissions fell by 15%, from 4,004 in 1992 to 3,397 in 1995; surgical operations declined by 10%; radiography examinations dropped by 11%; and the occupancy rate fell by 8%.

The system provides coverage in medical care, emergency care, maternal and child health and family planning, and chronic illness care, but the incompleteness of data makes it difficult to measure activity patterns and output in health services outside of hospitals. Gaps in data are most glaring in the area of clinic visits by number of patients and reasons for visits.

Public health nurses and family nurse practitioners conduct a school health program for primary school students aged 5 to 12 years old. During the 1992–1994 period, there were 443 visits to schools and 8,197 children were seen, for an annual average of 148 school visits and 2,732 children seen per visit. A total of 268 children were referred to the District Medical Officer, for an average of 89 per year. Services included rapid health assessments of children and visual and hearing check-ups.

Inputs for Health

Essential Drugs and Supplies. Saint Kitts and Nevis has actively participated in the Eastern Caribbean Drug Service, a regional pooled procurement scheme for pharmaceuticals and medical supplies. The approved 1995 budget for Saint

Kitts's portion of pharmaceutical purchases through the Service amounted to 6.4% of total health expenditure; figures were not available for Nevis.

A National Formulary establishes the type and range of drugs to be purchased within the government system; a comprehensive list of drugs is available within the private system. The trade in pharmaceuticals and medical supplies is largely unregulated, except for those classified as dangerous drugs and for which specific approval must be sought.

Human Resources

The health services in Saint Kitts and Nevis are administered and operated by a team composed of 21 different categories of workers, ranging from highly skilled technicians in the acute care institutions of J.N. France and Alexandra hospitals to the community outreach workers who provide domiciliary care. Human resources available for health in Saint Kitts and Nevis are difficult to quantify, because of the islands' separate budgetary proposals. Previous analyses have not considered this fact, resulting in underestimates.

In 1995, public sector health workers for both Saint Kitts and Nevis, by category, numbered as follows: 47 medical doctors, 8 dentists, 6 dental auxiliaries, 274 trained nurses, 21 pharmacists, 12 laboratory technologists/technicians, 6 radiographers and technicians, 19 public health inspectors, 4 nutritionists/dietitians, 2 veterinary officers, 11 veterinary assistants.

Expenditures and Sectoral Financing

The Government's recurrent expenditure on health for the entire Federation has averaged 10.6% of total recurrent disbursements over the 1992–1995 period. This ranks health as the third largest recipient of government financial resources, behind finance (26.6%) and education (15.4%). Expenditure on health represents 3.5% of the gross domestic product, somewhat less than the WHO's recommended target of 5%. The per capita expenditure on health was US$ 163 in 1995. Differences in how expenditure items are classified in the budgetary estimates of each island preclude further analysis of financial resources.

External Technical and Financial Cooperation

The European Union is assisting the Government with the health sector's redevelopment, with funds allocated mainly to the rehabilitation of the two largest hospitals. There is little evidence of bilateral international aid for health beyond this initiative.

In its effort to find new ways to develop the health sector, the Government is more actively pursuing regional health initiatives and is working in close collaboration with established international and regional organizations such as PAHO and CARICOM. The Government's support for and involvement in the Caribbean Cooperation in Health Initiative is a good example of the latter.

SAINT LUCIA

GENERAL SITUATION AND TRENDS

Socioeconomic, Political, and Demographic Overview

Saint Lucia is a mountainous island, spanning 238 m²; the Atlantic Ocean is to its east and the Caribbean Sea to its west. The population is concentrated along the coastal areas and the less mountainous areas to the country's north and south. Hurricane season extends from June to November, posing a continuous threat to Saint Lucia's agriculture and physical infrastructure. The official language is English; Saint Lucian French Creole is spoken and understood by more than 70% of the population, mainly in the rural areas.

Saint Lucia became independent from Great Britain in February 1979. The country has a democratic system of government patterned after the Westminster model. The most recent parliamentary elections were held in 1992 and the next elections are scheduled for 1997. Saint Lucia is a member of the Commonwealth of Nations and the Organization of Eastern Caribbean States (OECS).

Saint Lucia's centrally controlled political structure began to be decentralized in the 1980s, in order to make government services better respond to community needs and to involve community members in decision-making. Overall, implementation has moved slowly, with the decentralization of government and/or public services gaining more ground than those in the areas of financial control and decision-making. In the health sector, the administration and delivery of public health services has been decentralized and has led to greater collaboration between staff of the various health departments. Regional health teams were established but have not remained functional. The country has 10 administrative districts.

Saint Lucia has experienced continuous economic growth, averaging 3.9% for 1992–1995 and 3.2% for 1988–1991. The growth rate was 7.1% in 1992 and 4.1% in 1995. The vulnerability of the country's economy to natural disasters was demonstrated during recent floods and damaging winds. The economy has depended mainly on agriculture, especially the banana industry. Despite having been plagued with problems such as input shortages, the global liberalization of trade policies resulting in a reduction in the price of bananas on the European market, and tropical storm Debbie that was estimated to have damaged 58% of the banana crop in 1994, the industry recorded a 13.6% increase in production in 1995. This increase contributed to an estimated growth rate of 9.3% in the agricultural sector for that year.

The role of tourism in the economy has increased, mainly due to a 36.9% increase in visitor arrivals between 1991 and 1995. Hotel occupancy rates have averaged 66% between 1991 and 1995. The hotel and restaurant sector has ranked fifth in the sectoral share of GDP for 1991 and 1995, but the percentage contribution of this sector to GDP rose from 9.3% in 1991 to 11.8% in 1995. Other sectors of the economy have grown more modestly. The construction industry, whose performance is heavily determined by public sector projects, experienced its lowest growth in 1995, as major public sector projects reached completion. The manufacturing sector has shown only moderate improvement, because it has had to compete with regional and international low-cost suppliers, face a decreased demand from its major markets, and cope with the state of the domestic economy. In 1994 the sector contracted by 12%, but it rebounded in 1995 to a 14% growth.

The unemployment rate was 15.3% in December 1995 (compared to 16.7% in November 1992): the rate was 12.3% for males and 19.0% for females; it was highest in the age groups 15–19 years old (53.3%) and 20–24 years old (21.2%) and lowest in age groups 25–34 years old (10.7%), 35–44 years old (8.2%), and 45–54 years old (6.2%). The unemployment rates in the 15–19 age group was 63.4% for females, and 46.6% for males. The leading sectors for employment were agriculture (22%), the public sector (14%), wholesale and retail trade (14%), manufacturing (11%), construction (10%), and hotel and restaurants (10%).

Schooling is compulsory for children aged 5–15 years old. The enrollment rate at the 83 primary schools has averaged

99%, roughly evenly distributed among boys and girls. The percentage of students attending secondary schools rose from 27.5% in 1988 to 37.8% in 1992, and 43.8% in 1994. More girls gain acceptance to secondary schools, with the male-to-female enrollment ratio averaging 1:1.13. There are 15 secondary schools. The number of pupils enrolled in secondary schools increased by 20%, from 9,146 to 11,202 between the academic years 1992–1993 and 1995–1996. Enrollment at the Sir Arthur Lewis Community College was 1,176 in the academic year 1994–1995.

The 1990 literacy survey established the literacy rate as 54.1%, the illiteracy rate as 27.2%, and the functional illiterate rate as 18.7%. Most rural students speak French Creole, which puts them at a disadvantage in the formal education system, which uses English exclusively.

In 1995, Saint Lucia's estimated midyear population was 145,213, representing an increase of 6.8% since 1991. The average annual population growth rate was 1.6% during the 1992–1995 period. In 1995 the population density was 270 persons per km², an increase of 7.6% from 1991.

The age and sex structure of the population has changed little since 1991. In 1995, women still constitute a slight majority, at 51.4% of the total population. The population is relatively young, with 45.8% under the age of 20 years old. The birth rate was 27 births per 1,000 population in 1991 and 25 births per 1,000 in 1995. Women of childbearing age (15 to 49 years old) make up 26% of the population. The economically active population (age group 15–64 years old) comprise 59% of the total. The age dependency ratio was 0.69 in 1995. (See Table 1).

It is estimated that 30% of the population lives in urban areas, which has placed increased demands on housing, water, and social services. There is limited data on migration: the 1991 population census estimated that 25% of the population had moved from their place of birth, and that 30% of them resided in the capital city at the time. According to the 1995 poverty assessment survey, 20% of households reported recent migration, and 53% of them had relocated within the country. The United States and other Caribbean countries were the main destination of migrants.

The above-mentioned survey also found that, based on their reported expenditures on food and nonfood items, 18.7% of households and 25.1% of individuals were poor. In addition, 5.3% of households and 7.1% of the population were indigent, in that their expenditures were inadequate to cover their dietary requirements. The study also revealed that in the poorest groups, food accounted for more than half of all household expenditures.

Mortality Profile

In 1995, life expectancy rates for males and females were 67.5 and 73.3 years, respectively.

TABLE 1
Estimated mid-year population by sex and age groups, Saint Lucia, 1995.

Age group (years)	Number			Percent
	Male	Female	Total	
Total population	70,596	74,617	145,213	100.0
0–4	8,703	8,504	17,207	11.8
5–9	7,983	8,189	16,172	11.1
10–14	8,583	8,632	17,215	11.9
15–19	8,019	7,936	15,955	11.0
20–49	28,516	30,411	58,927	40.6
50–59	3,689	4,107	7,796	5.4
60–64	1,316	1,723	3,039	2.1
65 and over	3,787	5,115	8,902	6.1

Source: Government Statistical Department.

The crude death rate was 6.7 deaths per 1,000 in 1991 and 1995, and averaged 6.8 deaths per 1,000 during 1992–1995; in 1995, the rate was 7.3 per 1,000 for males and 6.0 per 1,000 for females.

The average infant mortality rate was 16.5 deaths per 1,000 live births in 1992–1995. There were 3,839 deaths reported during 1992–1995, an average of 960 deaths per year. Noncommunicable diseases are the major cause of death, particularly diseases of the circulatory system (33%), malignant neoplasms (15%), and diabetes mellitus (11%). The major causes of death reported under "diseases of the circulatory system" were acute myocardial infarction, chronic ischemic heart disease, and chronic/unspecified heart failure. The fact that 66 deaths were labelled "cardiac arrest" underscores the problems with the quality and thoroughness of death certificates. The main sites for cancers among males were the prostate (76 deaths), digestive system, excluding stomach (50 deaths); and stomach (49). In women, the most common sites were the breast (42), cervix (37); digestive system, excluding stomach (60), and stomach (26). Communicable diseases (3%) and external causes of death (5%) are not major causes of death.

SPECIFIC HEALTH PROBLEMS

Analysis by Population Group

Health of Children

The major health problems in this group are acute respiratory infections, diarrheal disease, and accidents.

The perinatal mortality rate in 1992–1995 averaged 25 deaths per 1,000 births. In 1995, the infant mortality rate was estimated as 18.5 per 1,000 live births for males and 14.5 per

1,000 for females. Sixty-two percent of infant deaths during 1992–95 were classified under "conditions originating in the perinatal period," of which prematurity and abnormal fetal growth (48%) and birth asphyxia and respiratory problems (36%) were the major causes. The mortality rate for children under 5 years old was 4.6 per 1,000 population for 1992–1995. Deaths in this age group accounted for 7.9% of all deaths during 1992–1995. Of the 62 deaths in the age group between 1 and 4 years old during 1992–1995, 61.3% were males and the main causes were traffic accidents (5), other accidents (11), infections (10), cancers (4), and pneumonia and influenza (4).

Through cord blood screening for sickle cell anemia that was introduced in 1991, abnormal hemoglobin was detected in 378 specimens tested in 1995, which represented 10.3% of all births for that year. This information is used for early identification of children with the disease, for parent education on the disease and on the prevention and management of crises, and for special immunizations.

There were 27 deaths in the age group 5 to 9 years old during 1992–1995, with the major causes of death being traffic accidents (4), other accidents (5), and anemia (4). Information on the morbidity profile of this age group is not available.

Specific health programs targeted to this population group are limited to immunization and physical assessment upon school entry. There is no organized school health program.

Through a community pediatric program launched in 1993, a pediatrician conducts specialty clinics at selected health centers in each of the eight health regions and trains nursing staff. Physical and developmental screening is performed at birth and at 6 weeks and 8 months of age. A "child health passport"—a home-based record of physical growth, immunizations, and major illnesses—is used to monitor growth in the population under 5 years old, but information on the growth chart is not routinely extracted for reporting and analysis.

Adolescent Health

Health services targeted to adolescent age groups (10–14 and 15–19 years old) do not exist. Immunizations are offered to children at school.

Twenty-seven deaths were reported during 1992–1995 in the age group 10–14 years; 19 males and 8 females. The major causes were traffic accidents (4), other accidents (8), and cancers (5). In the group 15–19 years of age there were 41 deaths during 1992–1995, 25 males and 16 females; the major causes of death were accidents and external causes (15) and cancers (6).

The fertility rate for the age group 15–19 years of age was 104 per 1,000 population in in the age group in 1990, and has

remained above 80 per 1,000 during 1992–1995. The 1988 contraceptive prevalence survey indicated that 16% to 17% of girls in this age group were using a family planning method; the most frequently used methods were contraceptive pills (37.0%), condoms (30.1%), and contraceptive injections (21.9%).

In 1991, the National Population Council in collaboration with the Economic Commission for Latin America and the Caribbean published a comprehensive report on the problems of Saint Lucian teenagers in a changing society, which highlighted lack of education and employment as two of the leading problems. Youth leave the formal school system without the appropriate training to prepare them for the job market. The study's results also have been used to develop strategies at local and regional levels to reduce teenage fertility. A project to prevent adolescent pregnancies aims at modifying behavior and building awareness through communication and education.

Data on drug abuse and sexually transmitted diseases in teenagers is limited. Teenagers accounted for between 1% and 5% of admissions to the drug rehabilitation center between 1993 and 1995. In 1994, a review of clinic records of 143 teenagers who attended an STD clinic revealed that 82% were females. For clients for which information was available (114), the majority reported no drug use (74) and alcohol was the main drug used (39). Condoms were rarely used (5 out of 121 instances of sexual intercourse). Data on prostitution and domestic violence are not available.

Adult Health

During 1992–1995, 864 deaths were reported in this age group (20–59 years old), of which 64.5% were males. Accidents and external causes (195) accounted for 22.6% of all deaths, with the leading causes being traffic accidents (60 deaths), other accidents (60), homicides (41), and suicides (30). Diseases of the cardiovascular and circulatory systems accounted for 20.8% of deaths, with the major causes being cerebrovascular disease (48 deaths), ischemic heart disease (35), and hypertensive disease (23). Other major causes of death were cancers (14.5%), disease of the digestive system (8.7%), and diabetes (7.2%). One maternal death was reported during 1992–1995.

Health services for this age group focus mainly on the needs of adult females. There are no services specially designed for the male population.

Reproductive health care services are available at all health centers and include prenatal, postnatal, family planning, cancer screening, and treatment of medical problems including sexually transmitted diseases. The community health nurse is the main provider of preventive reproductive health services. Specialty clinics in obstetrics/gynecology and sexually transmitted diseases are provided at selected health centers and district hospitals.

An estimated 50% of pregnant women use the public health clinics for prenatal care, and of these, 10%–15% register before 16 weeks. The remaining 50% of pregnant women attend private facilities. As of 1994, pregnant women have been advised to have a routine ultrasound examination at 20–22 weeks gestation. This service is available from either the public or the private sector, but the extent of compliance has not been assessed. Between 95% and 99% of deliveries take place in hospitals. Forty-four percent of women who have delivered go to the public sector for their six-week postnatal examination.

The last contraceptive prevalence survey was conducted in 1988 and showed that 54.8% of fertile, non-pregnant, and in-union women were using a contraceptive method of which the most frequently used were contraceptive pills (39.2%), tubal ligation (16.3%), and contraceptive injections (15.9%). In 1995, the Government took responsibility for purchasing contraceptive supplies through the Eastern Caribbean Drug Service. The Saint Lucia Planned Parenthood Association provides family planning services at a clinic in the capital city, at some work places, and through community-based distribution outlets throughout the island.

Cancer screening is limited to Pap tests and the teaching of breast self examination, both of which are given at all 34 health centers, the clinics run by the Cancer Society and the Saint Lucia Planned Parenthood Association, and at private practitioners' offices.

Health of the Elderly

In 1995, persons 60 years old and older constituted 8.2% of the total population, and women accounted for 57% of this age group.

During 1992–1995, 2,564 deaths were reported in this age group, which represented 66.8% of all deaths. Women accounted for 53% of these deaths, and the most frequent causes were cardiovascular disease (39.8%), cancers (15.4%), and diabetes (10.7%). Of the 1,021 deaths classified as cardiovascular, the major causes were cerebrovascular (40.8%), hypertensive disease (16.5%), and ischemic heart disease (13.9%).

Special health services or programs for the elderly do not exist. There are five homes for the elderly, one operated by the Government, three by religious organizations, and one by a private individual.

Persons over 60 years old who have a yearly income of less than US$ 2,222 are entitled to free medical care from the public sector.

Family Health

During 1990–1995, an annual average of 42 cases of domestic violence and 100 cases of child abuse were reported to the social services department: 38% of cases were for physical abuse and 35% for sexual abuse.

Victims receive support and counseling from the social services department and the crisis center. The Ministry of Women's Affairs has prepared materials giving victims and care providers information on victims' rights and available support services.

Approximately 85% of births occur outside of marriage. Information is not available on the number of these births that occur within a common-law union; 40% of households are headed by single women.

Workers' Health

The Occupational Health and Safety Unit is part of the Department of Labor, and is responsible for monitoring, investigating, and enforcing legislation regarding workers' health. Available data on workers' health is limited to an analysis of injury and sick benefit claims submitted to the National Insurance Scheme (NIS), which covers about 60% of workers. During 1989–1994, 80% of claims due to employment injury (718) were submitted by males, and 80% occurred in workers 20–49 years old of both sexes. In 40% of cases the type of injury was unknown or unspecified, 33% were superficial injuries, and 13% were open wounds. Sixty percent of the sickness claims (12,972) were by female workers, and 65% and 75% of them were in the age group 20–39 years for males and females, respectively. In 36% of sickness claims, the disease was not known or was categorized as "ill defined conditions" or "other." Other reasons for sickness benefits were injury (14%), respiratory illness (10.9%), and infections (9.5%).

Health of the Disabled

The 1991 population census recorded 9,449 persons with disabilities, which represented 6.9% of the population: 58% of disabilities occurred in females, 43% occurred in persons 65 years old and older, and 46% occurred in persons 15–64 years old. Locomotor disabilities system and sight impairments accounted for 70% of all disabilities (Table 2). The cause of the disability was not recorded.

Hearing is assessed in 8-month-old children and on persons referred to either of the two health centers equipped to conduct assessment. Ear, nose, and throat specialist services

TABLE 2
Type of disability by age group, Saint Lucia, 1991.

Type of disability	0–4 years	5–14 years	15–49 years	50–64 years	65+ years	Total by type of disability	
						Number	%
Locomotor	32	147	950	1,013	2,297	4,439	47.0
Sight	22	235	610	379	1,030	2,276	24.1
Mental	36	224	617	87	121	1,085	11.5
Hearing	18	98	151	63	275	605	6.4
Speech	24	98	205	49	76	452	4.8
Other	6	35	119	126	306	592	6.2
Total by age group	138	837	2,652	1,717	4,105	9,449	100.0
%	1.5	8.8	28.1	18.2	43.4	100.0	100.0

Source: Saint Lucia Statistics Department.

are available, but speech therapists and audiologists usually only offer their services on a short-term or volunteer basis.

A team of health professionals conducts a monthly clinic for children with multiple handicaps. Community health aides are responsible for community-based rehabilitation and for a pilot program for early stimulation of disabled children.

Analysis by Type of Disease

Communicable Diseases

Vector-Borne Diseases. No cases of yellow fever were reported during 1988–1991 or 1992–1995. Yellow fever vaccine is administered only to those who request it or persons who require it for travel.

The number of reported cases of malaria, dengue, and schistosomiasis were 3, 9, and 8 during 1992–1995, compared with 0, 12, and 21, respectively, for 1988–1991. The two cases of malaria reported in 1995 were imported. Although the Ministry of Health's statistical unit did not receive reports of dengue cases in 1993, four cases were identified through the measles surveillance system. Information on dengue serotyping and location of cases of vector-borne diseases was not available.

Vaccine-Preventable Diseases. Immunization coverage rates during 1992–1995 ranged between 95% and 99% for BCG and between 92% and 98% for DPT and OPV. The rates for MMR were 72% in 1992 and 92% to 94% for 1993–1995. In 1994, 96% of school girls aged 11–15 years were immunized against rubella. Hepatitis B vaccine was last offered to health workers in 1989–1990, when 69% of the 120 staff members who participated received three doses.

Saint Lucia recorded its last case of poliomyelitis in 1970 and was certified as being free of the transmission of wild poliovirus in 1994. Neonatal tetanus was last reported in 1985; one case of non-neonatal tetanus was reported in 1993. The number of reported cases of suspected measles in children under 15 years old has decreased steadily from 37 in 1992 to 8 in 1995. In the 1992–1995 period, no cases of measles or rubella were confirmed through the surveillance system, nor were any cases of diphtheria or whooping cough reported. During the same period, 11 cases of infectious hepatitis were reported, down from the 30 cases reported in 1988–1991. Reports of infectious hepatitis were not recorded by type of virus. *Haemophilus influenza* is not a reportable disease.

Cholera and Other Intestinal Diseases. Cholera has not been reported, but it is being monitored in the subregion with the assistance of the Caribbean Epidemiology Center (CAREC), so that public education and surveillance can be engaged when required.

Routine reporting from the District Medical Officer clinics demonstrated that diarrheal infection epidemics occur every two years, with children under 5 years old accounting for approximately 50% of cases; causative pathogens were not identified. During the reporting period, 3,994 cases were reported, a drop from the 4,536 cases reported for 1988–1991.

Tuberculosis and Leprosy. Eighty-two cases of tuberculosis were reported during 1992–1995, compared to 98 cases reported during 1988–1991; all were respiratory tuberculosis cases. Available information for the 56 cases reported during 1993–1995 indicates that they were equally distributed between males and females and that they occurred in the age groups 40–59 years old (34%), 60 years old and older (30%), and 20–39 years (29%). Five cases have been reported in persons with AIDS. There were 27 deaths caused by tuberculosis for 1992–1995.

During 1992–1995, 34 new cases of leprosy were reported, all of whom were in persons older than 15 years old. In 1995, 24 cases were being treated and 11 were under surveillance.

Acute Respiratory Infections. Reported cases of acute respiratory infections declined between 1988–1991 and 1992–1995. During the latter period, 78 cases of pneumonia in children under 5 years old and 1,731 cases of influenza were reported, compared to 321 and 2,298 cases, respectively, for 1988–1991.

Pneumonia accounted for 44.2% (99) of all deaths due to respiratory disease. Eight deaths were in children under 5 years of age. There were no deaths due to influenza during 1992–1995.

Rabies and Other Zoonoses. Eight cases of leptospirosis were reported during 1992–1995, and no cases were reported in 1988–1991. Information is not available on the age, sex, occupation or location of these cases. One death due to leptospirosis was reported in 1995, in a 45-year-old male from a rural area.

Leptospirosis has been diagnosed clinically and through serosurveys in cows. Cryptosporidiosis has been identified in cows in one area of the island. A survey in 1994 did not reveal any cases of brucellosis or tuberculosis in cows.

Rabies is not present in Saint Lucia. Animals from endemic areas and areas considered to be at risk are barred from entering the country. Imported domestic animals are quarantined in facilities in the United Kingdom for six months before entry.

AIDS and Other Sexually Transmitted Diseases. The first case of HIV infection was diagnosed in 1985 and the first case of pediatric AIDS was reported in 1990. As of December 1995, there were 140 reported cases of HIV infection and a cumulative total of 81 persons diagnosed with AIDS. The cumulative case fatality rate for AIDS was 88.9%. The male:female ratio for HIV infection is 1.2:1, which points to a primarily heterosexual mode of transmission; 52% of cases were in the age group 30–44 years, and 6 were pediatric cases.

A recent analysis of HIV/AIDS surveillance revealed that HIV infection is diagnosed late, since 80% of cases are reported only at the time of diagnosis of AIDS disease; only 20% of cases are reported more than one year before AIDS symptoms are manifested. Data on the clinical manifestations are poor and the burden of HIV infection and AIDS disease on hospital services has not been analyzed. The total number of HIV tests ranged between 4,000 and 5,000 over the last five years, with 33% having been performed by the blood bank, 38% at STD clinics, 20% by medical practitioners in the public and private sector, and 9% as part of seroprevalence surveys.

In 1994, HIV seroprevalence in the prenatal population was estimated at between 0% and 0.6%; the 1995 HIV seroprevalence on cord bloods was estimated at between 0% and 0.5%; and in 1992, PAHO estimated the HIV seroprevalence for Saint Lucia as 0.63%. Based on these data, the seroprevalence rate of HIV infection for the total population was estimated at 0.5%.

Information on sexually transmitted diseases is limited to reports from three STD clinics in the country's north, south, and west, and reports to the epidemiology unit. During 1992–1995, 670 cases of syphilis and 343 cases of gonorrhea were reported to the epidemiology unit, compared to 689 cases of syphilis and 599 cases of gonorrhea reported during 1988–1991.

Noncommunicable Diseases and Other Health-Related Problems

Nutritional Diseases and Diseases of Metabolism. There are pockets of undernutrition, but the extent of the problem is not known. There were nine cases of undernutrition reported in children under 5 years old in 1992–1995, compared to 23 cases during 1988–1991. Iron deficiency is the only micronutrient deficiency that has been identified, but the extent of the problem, particularly among women and children at-risk groups has not been determined. An analysis of prenatal records in 1990 showed that 20% of pregnant women attending public health clinics had hemoglobin levels of under 10gm/dL.

Problems with the way morbidity data on diabetes mellitus get recorded makes this information unreliable. Diabetes accounted for 8.8% (339) of all deaths during 1992–95; women accounted for 65% and those in persons older than 60 years old, 81%.

Cardiovascular Diseases. During the 1992–1995 period, there were 1,304 deaths due to diseases of the circulatory system, accounting for 33% of all reported deaths and ranking as the main group of causes of death. Within this broad group, derebrovascular (35.9%), hypertensive disease (14.8%), and ischemic heart disease (13.6%) were the major causes of death. Morbidity data are not currently available.

Malignant Tumors. The country has no cancer registry. An analysis of histopathological diagnoses of 2,714 specimens examined at the two main hospitals in 1995 revealed that 8.2% (222) were malignant neoplasms. The main sites affected were the uterine cervix (20.7%), skin (18.9%), female breast (12.2%), and digestive system (10.4%). The sites in 20.7% were not specified.

Malignant neoplasms accounted for 14% of all deaths during 1992–1995. The three most common sites of cancer in males were prostate, stomach, and other sites in the digestive system. Breast, uterine cervix, and the gastrointestinal system were the three most common sites in females.

Accidents and Violence. Accidents and violence accounted for 7.7% of all deaths in 1992–1995. The majority of these deaths occurred in the age group 15 to 44 years old, and 81% were in males. The number of deaths reported was 296, and the main causes were traffic accidents (28.7%), homicides (16.2%), drowning (14.5%), and suicides (11.8%).

Legislation requiring the use of seat belts when riding in automobiles and crash helmets when riding motorcycles was passed in Parliament in 1994. The law was enforced after three years, to give car dealers and individuals time to comply with the law and to reap the benefits of a public education campaign.

Behavioral Disorders. Information is not available on smoking patterns or alcohol consumption. The sale of tobacco and alcohol to minors is prohibited by law.

During the 1993–1995 period, 2,217 persons were admitted to the psychiatric hospital. In 1995, there were 761 admissions, of which 75% were males, and 1,872 persons seen at outpatient clinics, of which 61% were males. The predominant diagnosis was schizophrenia (61%), followed by manic-depressive psychoses (20%).

Natural Disasters and Industrial Accidents. An oil spill occurred at the Hess Oil Terminal in 1995 with no major health consequences reported.

Tropical Storm Debbie caused severe floods in September 1994, which led to landslides and damage to the agricultural sector and to the physical infrastructure. Tropical Storm Debbie resulted in three deaths, and total damage was estimated at US $85 million. The storm's major health threats involved overflowing pit latrines, stagnant water, and interrupted water supplies for prolonged periods. Disease surveillance was strengthened and expanded in the post-disaster period.

RESPONSE OF THE HEALTH SYSTEM

National Health Plans and Policies

The Ministry of Health's main policy mandate is "to maintain and upgrade the present and future stock of human resources." The National Health Policy covers revenue collection, use of appropriate technology, health personnel quality, population growth, vulnerable and at-risk groups, substance abuse, workers' health, and environmental issues. Strategies to address these policies are reflected in the National Ten Year Health Sector Plan, June 1993–July 2003.

The Government will continue to improve the health care system through a primary health care/preventive approach, while also increasing the availability and quality of secondary and tertiary services.

Financial constraints, the rising cost of health care, dwindling external funding, and the public's demand for more sophisticated and expensive health care have led Saint Lucia to review health services management. At the heart of this reassessment is the question of how to organize the health services so as to promote equity, efficiency, sustainability, accessibility, quality, and consumer satisfaction.

Reforms already have resulted in greater collaboration with the country's private health sector and with other countries. The focus on health care financing has resulted in an upward revision of user fees including procedure fees, and plans to implement a national health insurance to cover a greater percentage of the population and to address the issue of equity. Other reform initiatives have focused on mental health and pharmacy services and management reforms for hospitals, including a redefinition of the role of district hospitals.

Organization of the Health Sector

The Ministry of Health's technical directorate and the country's health professional organizations are responsible for leadership in health.

At the central level, heads of departments manage staff and different health development programs; they are supported by national program managers, who manage specific health programs. At the district level, health teams manage the health care administration and services. It should be noted that there are only two teams functioning.

In the public sector, health care is broadly grouped into personal health care services, human resources, and physical resources. Health promotion and prevention, curative, and rehabilitation services are offered and delivered at the primary, secondary, and tertiary levels.

Primary health care services are decentralized and offered at 34 health centers scattered throughout the island. Secondary and specialized services are concentrated in the country's north and south at the two general hospitals and the psychiatric hospital. Clinics for obstetrics/gynecology, pediatrics, surgery, sexually transmitted diseases, and mental health services also are conducted at selected health centers and district hospitals.

Everyone may seek care at any health facility, but the administration and management of health facilities are based on a catchment population within a defined area surrounding a major town or village.

The private health sector is made up of health professionals, nongovernmental organizations, and traditional healers.

Medical and dental practitioners have always operated in the private sector, and many work in both the public and private sector. Nurses more recently have been employed in the hotel industry and in private home nursing care.

The Ministry of Health is responsible for establishing user fees in the public sector, but it has no jurisdiction over the operations of private health insurance companies. Most companies refund the insured while a few pay the service provider. The main types of health insurance are private health insurance for individuals and groups and coverage by National Insurance Scheme (NIS). The last entity makes a yearly lump-sum contribution to the Ministry of Health, which is allocated to inpatient hospital expenses for employees who contribute to NIS. Most private health insurance is awarded through group employment plans, with employers and employees contributing to the plan. Others purchase individual policies for themselves and their families.

At the end of the 1992–1995 period, discussions were under way for implementing a National Health Insurance Scheme (NHIS). This scheme would cover contributors and their families for inpatient and outpatient hospitalization. Membership will include employed persons, pensioners, and socially dependent persons. The socially dependent are identified based on family income.

The medical and nursing councils are responsible for the registration and monitoring of doctors and nurses; the Medical Board is responsible for the registration of dentists, pharmacists, and optometrists. The practice of public health professionals is guided by the Public Health laws. Currently, practitioners need not submit proof of continued medical education or a certificate of physical fitness to practice in order to re-register. Health facilities are not registered or licensed, and there are no monitoring mechanisms in place.

There is no national drug regulatory authority; CARICOM is working to establish a Regional Advisory Body on Drugs and Therapeutics (RABDAT), which will serve as the regional regulation authority for the registration of drugs. Trade licenses are required for the importation of drugs, reagents and other medical supplies. Legislation exists to govern prescription of controlled drugs, and their use is monitored by the Chief Pharmacist.

The Ministry of Planning has responsibility for physical development and the environment. Land use has been zoned for agricultural, industrial, and human settlements. The Ministry has increasingly requested Environmental Impact Assessments for certain development projects.

The Pesticide Control Board is responsible for the registration and licensing of pesticides. Mechanisms are in place for the surveillance and control of biological and chemical contamination of water; however, chemical safety and the quality of the air, soil, and housing are not routinely monitored, and monitoring and enforcement of these measures are inadequate.

Food safety and quality are covered under the 1980 Public Health Regulation No. 70, and the executing agency is the Environmental Health Department's Food Unit. By law, food establishments and food handlers must be registered and in possession of a license.

Several pieces of legislation are under review, including legislation on workers' health, the Emergency Powers Act, and the Pharmacy Act. The Public Health laws and the Registration of Nurses and Midwives Ordinance also are under review.

Health Services and Resources

Organization of Services for Care of the Population

Health Promotion, Health Settings and Environments, Social Communication. Health promotion and education within the Ministry of Health come under the Bureau of Health Education; other Ministry departments, other ministries, and nongovernmental organizations also undertake health promotion activities. Popular theater is increasingly being relied upon for health promotion and education purposes, and Creole is being more widely used to disseminate health news to the public through the media. During 1993–1996, 197 male and 515 female peer counselors received training to provide support and information to youth in the areas of family life, values, human sexuality, and fertility.

Programs of Disease Prevention and Control. Preventive services are provided free of charge, except for yellow fever vaccine, vaccines required for college entry, and contraceptive supplies. Pregnant women are screened for anemia, hemoglobinopathies, and syphilis; iron is routinely administered. Cord blood screening is performed. Immunization is routinely offered to children under 15 years old and pregnant women.

Regarding cancer screening, programs are in place for cervical and breast cancer, and prostatic specific antigen is now available for screening for prostate cancer.

Programs also are in place for the prevention and control of schistosomiasis; foodborne diseases; leprosy; AIDS and HIV; and dengue, including *Aedes aegypti* control. Health education, the reduction of risk factors and early detection, form a major component of disease prevention and control.

Oral Health. Dental services, including dental examinations, prophylaxis, dental sealants, fillings, scaling/root planing, and extractions, are provided at seven dental clinics spread throughout the island. X-ray services are available at three clinics, and one clinic provides treatment exclusively for children; root canal therapy is available only to children. A total of

12,049 patients were treated by the Ministry of Health's dental services in 1995.

In 1994, the school dental program expanded its coverage from 7- to 8-year-old children to include preschoolers and children attending day care centers. Seventy percent of these children participated and were offered fillings, extractions and sealants, cleanings, and fluoride treatment.

Oral fluoride treatment for children was discontinued in 1994 because of inadequate funding and erratic supplies. A 1994 study of all water treatment plants showed that most fluoride levels ranged from 0–0.2mg/dL. A water fluoridation program is not feasible at this time, because water treatment facilities are too few and not sufficiently well maintained.

Epidemiological Surveillance Systems and Public Health Laboratories. Surveillance systems are in place for communicable diseases of international, regional, and national interest. Active surveillance is under way for dengue, diarrheal diseases, poliomyelitis, HIV/AIDS/STD, and measles; the measles surveillance system was put in place in 1991, and surveillance for acute flaccid paralysis began in 1992. Information has been traditionally extracted from reports from District Medical Officer clinic registers.

Throughout 1993–1995, health workers were trained in the diagnosis and surveillance of dengue fever, measles, and poliomyelitis, and mechanisms have been put in place to facilitate the transport of laboratory specimens to the main hospital and to CAREC. The country does not have a public health laboratory. The Ezra Long laboratory at the main general hospital has facilities for the investigation of bacterial, parasitic and certain viral infections. The laboratory investigation of other viral diseases such as dengue, measles, poliovirus, and leptospirosis is conducted at CAREC.

Drinking Water Services and Sewerage. The Water and Sewerage Authority is responsible for monitoring and managing the municipal water supply, and it operates 37 raw water intakes that supply water to 31 water treatment facilities. Tropical Storm Debbie extensively damaged water treatment and storage facilities. The 1991 census indicated that 75% of households were connected to the municipal water supply. The Roseau dam was completed in 1996.

The improper disposal of chemicals by the agriculture and manufacturing sectors and the unrestricted access to raw water sources threatens water quality.

A 1995/1996 study conducted by the Ministry of Health on Saint Lucia's existing piped water supply found that approximately 46% of the population is served by water treatment facilities that lack the basic process of chemical sedimentation.

The 1991 census showed that the pit latrine is the main type of sewerage disposal (49%), with septic tanks being used by 29% of households, and 6% of households being linked to the sewerage system. Eleven percent of households concentrated in rural towns and villages had no excreta disposal facilities. The Government operates about 50 public toilet facilities throughout the island.

Solid Waste Management Services. Solid waste management falls under the combined responsibility of the Ministry of Planning, the Environmental Health Branch of the Ministry of Health, the Castries City Council, and the village councils. Approximately 60% of collection under the responsibility of the Castries City Council is contracted out privately.

Solid waste is not properly stored prior to collection, and is often disposed of inappropriately. Solid waste disposal is handled through open dumps, which are inadequate and not properly maintained. Waste generated by public health care institutions is incinerated on the premises; no assessment has been conducted on the adequacy of this practice nor on the way waste generated in the private health sector is disposed of.

A 1992 study examining solid waste management practices and available resources issued recommendations for managing the country's various types of solid waste. As a result, in 1996 a Solid Waste Management Authority was established under the Solid Waste Management Authority Act, and a Saint Lucian component of an OECS solid waste management project was developed; the latter is funded by the Global Environment Trust Fund, the World Bank, the Caribbean Development Bank, and the Government of Saint Lucia.

Air Pollution Prevention and Control. The Ministry of Planning is responsible for the monitoring and control of air quality. The Government is signatory to several international conventions dealing with air quality and has started intersectoral discussions on ways to reduce substances that deplete ozone. In 1994, all Ministry of Health buildings were officially declared as smoke-free areas, and this policy was extended to all government buildings in 1995. There are standards for air quality available, but no air quality policy has been issued.

Food Protection and Control. The Food Unit of the Environmental Health Department is responsible for handling all aspects of food protection, control, and safety, including the inspection of commercial premises involved in food preparation, inspection of meats and other foods, training and registration of food handlers, and the investigation of foodborne illnesses.

Organization and Operation of Personal Health Care Services

Ambulatory Services, Hospitals, and Emergency Services. Medical and pharmaceutical services are available at least once a week at the 34 health centers throughout the island. Inpatient, outpatient, and accident and emergency services are available at the two general hospitals. The two district hospitals offer primary health care services and limited secondary care and emergency services. Patients move from the public to the private sector and between different levels of care to seek medical attention. The referral system within and from the primary health care system is well developed. The referral system from the secondary and tertiary levels to the community level needs to be strengthened, in order to improve the follow-up of clients by community health staff.

Auxiliary Services for Diagnosis and Blood Banks. Laboratory, colposcopy, and diagnostic radiology services are available in the public and private sector. The National Blood Transfusion Service is based at the main hospital. Donors are screened initially by a questionnaire, and then tested for HIV, HTLV-1, HBsAg, and VDRL.

Specialized Services. Specialized services are available in obstetrics and gynecology, colposcopy, radiology, ophthalmology, ear nose and throat, facio-maxillary surgery, psychiatry, and renal dialysis. Physical rehabilitation services are provided by the physiotherapy departments. Turning Point, an alcohol and drug rehabilitation center, offers inpatient and outpatient care to persons suffering from alcohol and drug abuse.

Inputs for Health

Saint Lucia does not produce drugs, immunobiologicals, reagents, and equipment.

Drugs. Saint Lucia procures some of its drugs and pharmaceuticals through the Eastern Caribbean Drug Service (ECDS). The National Drug Formulary Committee selects drugs and pharmaceuticals for procurement and awards contracts to approved suppliers. In 1994, the committee published the 4th edition of the "Regional Formulary and Therapeutics Manual." A comprehensive quality assurance program exists in collaboration with the Caribbean Drug Testing Laboratory.

Drugs, pharmaceuticals, or other medical supplies that do not qualify for pooled procurement are acquired from known agents or manufacturers by the medical supplies department and individual heads of departments; no formal mechanisms are in place for quality control.

Immunobiologicals. All vaccines used in the public sector are procured through PAHO's Revolving Fund, which awards contracts to suppliers and monitors vaccine quality.

The Ministry of Health provides vaccines to the private sector at a minimal cost.

Hepatitis B and *Haemophilus influenza* B vaccines, and hyperimmune sera used in hospitals are purchased from local or overseas drug agents without any mechanisms for quality control.

Reagents and other supplies used in the public sector are procured from different suppliers by the medical supplies department and individual heads of departments.

Equipment. Biomedical equipment is procured by various persons. The many different brands that are acquired pose problems for the maintenance and the purchasing of spare parts.

Human Resources

Availability by Type of Resource. The number of personnel employed by the public sector increased during the reporting period: in 1995, there were 71 medical doctors, 7 dentists, 401 nurses, 15 pharmacists, 5 health educators, and 280 environmental health staff in all categories working at the Ministry of Health and in Saint Jude Hospital, a semi-private hospital serving the population living in the south of the island. Staff employed in the laboratory and radiology services also increased, but no numbers are available. These increases have resulted from an expansion in the type of service offered, increased workload, and the availability of appropriately trained health professionals.

Education of Health Personnel. The Sir Arthur Lewis Community College is the only local institution that trains health professionals. The college began training of general nurses and midwives in 1988, and in 1994 conducted a Community Nutrition Diploma Course for Field Nutrition Officers. Community health aides are trained by the Community Nursing Department. Training for other categories of health professionals has to be pursued at regional and international institutions, and it is severely constrained by lack of financial resources.

In-service training for all categories of health professionals is regularly organized by the Ministry of Health, the National Drug Formulary Committee, and the Saint Lucia Medical and Dental Association. In addition, short courses on reproductive health and adolescent health have been conducted through the University of the West Indies' distance teaching system.

Labor Markets for Health Personnel. Most health personnel are employed in the public sector. Traditionally, medical and dental practitioners and pharmacists represented most health workers employed in the private sector, but a growing number of private facilities has begun to offer diagnostic services and optical care. There are few opportunities for employment of health professionals in the nongovernmental organizations.

Research and Technology

The Ministry of Health has increased the use of new technologies in several areas. The Environmental Health Department has introduced the use of ultraviolet lights, mist blowers, sensitizer strips, and thermometers in its vector control and food quality and control programs, as well as the use of ventilated improved latrines. Ultrasound and colposcopic services are available in the public and private sector, a computed tomography services in the private sector.

The country has no regulatory policies that address health research and technology, nor are there formal structures to assess and evaluate the impact of health research and technology. Health technology use has not been assessed.

During 1992–1995, the Eastern Caribbean Drug Service conducted a study on rational drug use in hypertension and diabetes. Of concern was the use of sulphonylureas in persons over 60 years, the low use of glucophage, and the prescribing of Bezide 5mg when 2.5mg has been shown to be as effective. Health care providers were informed of the results through drug utilization seminars.

Expenditures and Sectoral Financing

Information on public health expenditure is available for health institutions and specific programs. Information is not available, however, on private health expenditure or on the resources of institutions, corporations, and community and nongovernmental organizations.

The health sector is the second highest recipient of total government resources. The approved health budget averaged 12.5% of total government expenditure over the 1993–1995 period. For the fiscal years 1991/1992 to 1994/1995, recurrent public health expenditure averaged 1.6% of the total government budget for preventative health programs, 5.4% for hospitals (excluding Saint Jude Hospital), and 3.9% for drugs and medical supplies (excluding vaccines). The Government pays for the salaries, wages, and gratuities of the staff at Saint Jude Hospital. The execution of major capital works has relied heavily on international aid.

The major source of funding for government recurrent expenditure comes from income tax, other taxes, and user fees. Because Government revenues from all sources are placed in a consolidated fund, revenue from user fees does not directly benefit the department or Ministry that collected the fees. Saint Jude Hospital is an exception, in that it keeps its user-fee revenue for its expenditures.

Recurrent health expenditure is financed from allocations from the consolidated fund, plus the National Insurance Scheme's annual contribution to the fund to cover inpatient hospital expenses for its members. Prior to fiscal year 1993/1994, only one-third of the approved US$ 1.1 million was received from the National Insurance Scheme (NIS). In fiscal year 1993/1994 the Scheme paid part of the funds owed to the Government, accounting for 70% of the health budget for that year. The NIS contribution accounted for 49% of the total health revenue for the fiscal year 1994/1995.

In 1992, user fees for the public sector were reviewed upward, and as a result, the contribution of user fees to total health revenue increased from 29.5% in 1989/1990 to 49% in 1992/1993.

External Technical and Financial Cooperation

Saint Lucia's health sector receives technical and financial assistance from several agencies. The health sector also benefits indirectly from assistance to other ministries and agencies.

The Pan American Health Organization, the Caribbean Epidemiology Center (CAREC), the United States Agency for International Development, the United Nations Children Fund, the Peace Corps, and the French Government have provided technical assistance and funding for training activities; special programs such as immunization, breastfeeding, and cervical cancer control; and hospital furnishings and equipment. The health sector also receives assistance from CARICOM and the University of the West Indies. During the 1993–1996 period, financial support for capital projects has been received from the following donors: US$ 140,000 from the Basic Needs Trust Fund for the Gros Islet Polyclinic; US$ 11.3 million from the European Union for Victoria Hospital's phase II project; US$ 1.06 million from the Government of France for Victoria Hospital's phase I project; and US$ 1.96 million from the Caribbean Development Bank, US$ 2.45 million from the Global Environmental Trust Fund, and US$ 4.56 million from the World Bank all destined for the solid waste management project.

SAINT VINCENT
AND THE GRENADINES

GENERAL SITUATION AND TRENDS

Socioeconomic, Political, and Demographic Overview

Saint Vincent and the Grenadines is located at the southern end of the Windward Islands, between Saint Lucia and Grenada. The country comprises the island of Saint Vincent and seven smaller inhabited islands and islets that together constitute the Grenadines; altogether, the islands cover 388 km².

Saint Vincent and the Grenadines became independent from Great Britain in 1979. It is a parliamentary democracy with general elections held every five years. The present administration has been in power for the last three terms.

The Medium-Term Development Strategy Paper (1996–1999) sets out the Government's policies and policy implementation arrangements designed to bring sustainable economic growth and social development to the nation. The guiding principles have been defined as equity, the provision of essential services to all citizens, the maintenance of an environment in which all citizens can realize their full potential, and the promotion of employment.

The medium-term strategy emphasizes improving banana production and diversifying agriculture, supporting private sector development, expanding tourism, improving fiscal management and budget reform; making public sector delivery more efficient and effective, pursuing human resources development, and managing environmental problems more intensively.

Real GDP grew at an average annual rate of 3.5% during 1992–1995, with most of the increase occurring in 1992 and 1995. This rate contrasts with that in the 1988–1991 period, when the average annual real growth in GDP was about 7%. The decline in economic performance during 1993 and 1994 has been attributed to disruptions in the banana export market and to a drop in production caused by drought; during these years, tourism gathered importance, and its revenues

exceeded those from bananas. In 1995, crop production represented 9.7% of GDP. Construction activity also grew by an annual average of 8% between 1992 and 1995. Per capita GDP in 1995 was US$ 1,987, representing a recovery from the period of stagnation in the growth of per capita GDP during 1993 and 1994. As part of a package of economic incentives, several corporate and personal income tax reforms were begun in 1993, including the reduction of the corporate tax and the highest marginal tax rates by 5% each. The goal is to ultimately reduce corporate tax to 33% and personal income tax to a maximum of 30%.

The 1996 Poverty Assessment Report for Saint Vincent and the Grenadines examined the nature, extent, geographic concentration, severity, and causes of poverty in 13 selected communities. It concluded that 41.9% of the studied population were poor on the basis of their reported expenditures for food and nonfood items. Moreover, 30.5% of households and 36.2% of the population were considered to be indigent. The Report confirmed that about one-third of the population who lived below the poverty line suffered from an inadequate diet. Poverty was greater among households headed by women (34.1%) than households headed by men (27.9%). The report also established that more than 70% of heads of household were employed, thus concluding that poverty conditions and economic stress were more a function of underemployment rather than unemployment. Three out of every ten workers were engaged in the informal sector where work was irregular and economic returns unstable.

The 1991 Population and Housing Census Report estimated the unemployment rate at 19.8%, an improvement over the 25% figure given in the 1980 census. Just prior to the 1991 Population and Housing Census, 22.8% of the employed population was engaged in the agricultural sector, 15.5% in wholesale and retail trade, 10.8% in construction work, and 8.4% in manufacturing. Unemployment levels were highest among persons engaged in construction (32.2%), wholesale and retail trade (10.9%), and agriculture (10.8%).

Although education is not compulsory, almost all of the population aged 5–15 years old attends school (95.3%). The country has 65 primary schools and 23 secondary schools. Most nationals had not studied beyond the primary or basic school level (66.9%), 18.5% had progressed to the secondary level, and 2.4% had reached post-secondary vocational training and university education; the remainder of the population (about 10%) had no formal education and must be deemed to be functionally illiterate.

The 1991 Population and Housing Census Report showed 27,002 households in the country, compared to 20,090 in 1980, a 34.4% increase during the period. The 1996 Poverty Assessment Report revealed that housing conditions were poor in some communities, but it also showed that most households were privately owned.

The 1991 Population and Housing Census Report returned a final count of 106,499 persons, indicating an average annual growth rate of 0.8% since the previous 1980 census. Since then, mid-year population estimates have been set at 108,965 for 1992 and 110,723 for 1995, representing an average annual growth rate of 0.4% between 1992 and 1995, or about 50% of the rate recorded for the previous decade. One-quarter of the population (25.7%) lives in the capital city of Kingstown and its suburbs and may be considered urban; more than 90% of the population resides on Saint Vincent.

The annual average net emigration between 1992 and 1995 has been established as 947, with the most popular destinations being the British Virgin Islands, Barbados, the United States Virgin Islands, and the U. S. A. and Canada. Figures have changed little from year to year.

The population is relatively young: in 1995, 37.2% of the population was younger than 15 years old. Only 6.5% of the population falls into the age group 65 years old and older. Together, these two groups account for 43% of the population, suggesting a somewhat steep dependency ratio. The sex distribution is even. Life expectancy at birth has been set at 70 years, disaggregated as 65 years for males and 72 years for women.

The crude birth rate has shown only marginal decline in recent years, moving from 24.7 per 1,000 population in 1992 to 23.6 in 1995. No change in the total fertility has been observed, having been reported as 2.8 children per woman in both 1992 and 1995. There is no underregistration of births.

Mortality Profile

The crude death rate for the 1992–1995 period was 6.5 per 1,000 population, with slight variations from year to year. This rate was fairly consistent with that recorded over the previous reporting period.

Infant deaths averaged 42 over the 1992–1995 period, while the infant mortality rate varied slightly from 14 to 18 per 1,000 live births. It is noteworthy that in 1995, 35, or 83% of infant deaths, occurred in infants under 1 day old.

The predominant causes of death relate to those diseases that are grouped under the category "diseases of the circulatory system," and accounted for a cumulative total of 1,058 deaths (38.8% of deaths from defined causes) during the period 1992–1995. Within this cause group, 423 deaths resulted from heart diseases (ICD-9, 410–429), 289 deaths from hypertensive disease (401–405), and 264 deaths from cerebrovascular disease (430–438). The second leading cause of death was neoplasms, with 418 deaths (15.4%); followed by external causes, with 196 (7.2%) deaths; and conditions originating in the perinatal period, with 147 deaths (5.4%). There was a cumulative total of 132 deaths, representing 4.6% of all deaths, that was assigned to "deaths from ill-defined causes" (780–799). Full registration of all deaths is reported.

SPECIFIC HEALTH PROBLEMS

Analysis by Population Group

Health of Children and Adolescents

Children have been listed in the 1991–1995 National Health Sector Plan as one of the country's vulnerable groups deserving special attention. As a result, several specialized programs for young children have become institutionalized within the health care delivery system, including prenatal care of women following set protocols, special child health clinics that provide complete assessment and immunization, ongoing education of parents and guardians, and community follow-up care.

Immunization coverage against common childhood illnesses has neared 100% for many years; as a result, there were no confirmed cases of tetanus, diphtheria, or tuberculosis among the age group under 5 years old between 1992 and 1995. Most of the deaths occurring in children aged 0–9 years old are confined to the first year of life. In 1995, 47 deaths occurred among children under 1 year old. The main causes have been conditions originating in the perinatal period (ICD-9, 760–779) (24 deaths) and congenital anomalies (740–759) (18 deaths). Most newborns weigh at least 2,500 g at birth, but an annual average of 2.1% of newborns exhibit some level of below-normal weight at birth.

Approximately 90% of all children under 5 years old enjoy a satisfactory nutritional status in terms of weight-for-age as set out in the growth chart recommended by the Caribbean Food and Nutrition Institute (CFNI). An annual average of 5.7% suffer from undernutrition, however, with most falling into the category of moderate undernutrition. Although improvements in this index have been observed between 1992 and 1995, the level of undernutrition remains unacceptably high. Moreover, obesity has shown a gradual but steady rise, from 3.8% in 1992 to 4.7% in 1995.

Health of Women

From 1992 to 1995, 22% of all births, on average, occurred in teenage women, while 9% occurred in women 35–49 years of age. Because high-risk pregnancies comprise nearly 30% of all births, a health and family life education program has been put in place in primary and secondary schools and youth guidance centers and skills training programs have been established.

Women of childbearing age (15–44 years old) are one of the priority groups targeted for special attention by the Government. A range of programs providing prenatal and post-natal care, family planning services, and general medical care has been established for women.

The protocol governing the delivery of maternal and child health services stipulates a minimum of six prenatal checks. Records show that 82% of all pregnant women now satisfy this criterion. Virtually all mothers and children receive the minimum of three postnatal checks within the first ten days of delivery. In 1995, 7.0% of all pregnant women making their first prenatal visit displayed hemoglobin levels under 10 g. Identical levels were seen among women at 32 weeks and over their pregnancies on repeat visits. Indeed, anemia in pregnancy has been listed as one of the main concerns among obstetrical patients admitted to the Kingstown General Hospital: 2.0% of 12,290 total admissions to the maternity ward in the 1992–1995 period were seen for this problem. Other major problems were abortion (3.6% of total admissions), premature labor (1.8%), pre-eclampsia (1.5%), and postpartum hemorrhage (1.4%).

The National Health Sector Plan (1991–1995) is committed to increase the number of deliveries occurring at the district level, outside of Kingstown General Hospital. To this end, Barrouallie Health Centre was upgraded to a maternity unit in 1993, as a means of encouraging district deliveries. In 1992, only 20% of total births occurred at the district level, however, and the number barely increased to 23% in 1995.

Records show that in 1995 there were 10,458 women, or 39.4% of women of childbearing age, who were using family planning methods obtained from Government-run clinics; figures for 1992 were 13,625 women or 55.8% of women of childbearing age. The lower 1995 figures are considered to be more accurate, since they were arrived at following a comprehensive review of the record-keeping system. The most popular family planning method remains the contraceptive pill (69.1%), followed by injectables (22.3%).

Four of the seven deaths attributed to maternal causes occurred in 1994, a number that is higher than the target of zero deaths set for the Caribbean.

The 1991 Population and Housing Census Report showed that 9,040 (33.5%) of all single-parent households with one or more children were headed by women. Almost 90% of these women were never married, while 36.3% of them had responsibility for four or more children.

Health of Adults and the Elderly

In 1995, 23.6% of all deaths occurred among the age group 20–59 years old, a level that held throughout the 1992–1995 period. Of the 179 deaths attributed to this age group, the leading causes were neoplasms, endocrine and metabolic diseases, and immune disorders.

In 1995, 8.9% of the population fell into the age group 60 years old and older. Persons in this cohort have been shown to be at greatest risk from chronic noncommunicable diseases. The major causes of illness and death among this age group have been hypertensive diseases, malignant neoplasms, and cerebrovascular accidents.

The Government operates a 120-bed home for the aged that mainly provides general care. Current policy encourages noninstitutional care of the elderly within the community, and a task force has been set up to determine the scope of problems among the elderly, indicate appropriate responses, and adopt holistic approaches to care.

There are no specialized health services for the elderly, although legal provisions have been made to exempt them from user fees. The elderly also are the main beneficiaries of the routine diabetic clinics that are conducted at all health centers.

Everyone has access to health care through the general health services delivery system that includes maternal and child health and diagnostic services at the primary level and any available secondary care services. By law, prenatal, postnatal, and family planning services are provided free of cost, and children under 17 years old are exempt from charges.

Two institutions provide services for the disabled in Saint Vincent and the Grenadines—the School for Children with Special Needs, which has campuses in Kingstown and Georgetown, and the Sunshine School for the Disabled in Bequia. As a way to streamline programs, for the past five years the disabilities of children attending these institutions have been continually assessed according to international criteria. In 1995, of a total enrollment of 94 children, 18 were hearing-impaired, 3 were visually impaired, 32 were mentally retarded, 7 were physically challenged, 6 were autistic, and 28 were learning-disabled. All students attending these institutions must, by law, be fully immunized against common childhood illnesses. Routine medical checks also are provided to all students, in collaboration with the public health service delivery system.

Analysis by Type of Disease or Health Impairment

Communicable Diseases

Infectious diseases have decreased in terms of morbidity and mortality statistics. Infectious diseases ranked eighth among the ten leading causes of death between 1992 and 1995, and only skin infections featured among the main reasons for visits to public sector clinics. Gastroenteritis, once a scourge among young children, accounted for just 1.2% of medical visits 677 in 1995.

Vector-Borne Diseases. Dengue fever and leptospirosis have been the two vector-borne diseases of public health significance. There were 224 reported cases of dengue in 1995, of which 115 were confirmed by laboratory diagnosis, compared to 56 cases (7 laboratory-confirmed) in 1992.

The relatively high prevalence of the *Aedes aegypti* mosquito illustrates the severity of the problem: the household index for the mosquito was reported at 16.5% in 1995, up from 14. 8% in 1992. Moreover, the Breteau Index averaged 27.7 over the 1992–1995 period. Both indices are much higher than the safety zone of 1% infestation that has been established by PAHO/WHO.

Leptospirosis has made a comeback in Saint Vincent and the Grenadines within a very short time. The disease was insignificant at the beginning of the decade, but by 1995 there were 42 suspected cases, with 13 confirmed and 3 deaths. This resurgence is closely associated with a reported increase in rodents that is a result of uncontrolled dumping of solid waste in many communities. Intensive public education programs have been launched, and the upcoming solid waste management project should help reduce the problem.

Tuberculosis. New cases of tuberculosis averaged seven between 1992 and 1995, peaking in 1993 with 13 new diagnosed cases, the highest number of cases recorded in any one year for more than a decade. An annual average of two deaths from this disease were recorded over the period. The incidence of tuberculosis has been highest among those aged 40 to 54 years old.

AIDS and Other Sexually Transmitted Diseases. By the end of 1995, a total of 182 HIV-infected cases had been confirmed by laboratory since the first case in 1984; of these, 73 had developed full-blown AIDS and 71 had died. Sixteen new cases of HIV infection were confirmed in 1992, 27 in 1993, and

26 each in 1994 and 1995. In 1992 there were 7 new AIDS cases, 8 in 1993, 15 in 1994, and 6 in 1995. In Saint Vincent and the Grenadines, the case fatality rate among AIDS patients is 94%; about 75% of infected persons fall into the age group 25–44 years old, with the 25–29-year-old age group being most affected (25.4%); heterosexual transmission (59%) is the main mode of spread, and only 1.9% has been by vertical transmission; and HIV transmission through intravenous drug use and blood transfusion is unknown.

Noncommunicable Diseases and Other Health-Related Problems

Of the total 56,131 visits for medical consultation at all 38 health centers in 1995, the leading noncommunicable disease diagnoses were musculoskeletal problems (11.4%), hypertension (10.5%), arthritis (6.2%), and diabetes (6.0%). Thus, chronic diseases predominate even among the leading causes of morbidity.

Diabetes and Hypertension. Prevalence rates for diabetes and hypertension are unknown. However, records show that in 1995 there were a combined total of 5,863 persons suffering from these conditions who were registered at health centers. Of these, 1,280 (21.8%) were diabetics, 3,589 (61.2%) were hypertensives, and 994 (17%) suffered from both. Special clinics for persons suffering from these conditions are held weekly at all health centers.

Malignant Tumors. Malignant neoplasms are among the leading causes of death in Saint Vincent and the Grenadines, causing 411 deaths in the 1992–1995 period (103 in 1992, 99 in 1993, 103 in 1994, and 106 in 1995). The main cancer sites were the digestive organs and peritoneum (127 deaths in the period); genitourinary organs (114 deaths in the period); lymphatic and hemopoietic tissue (47 deaths); bone, connective tissue, skin, and breast (43 deaths); and respiratory and intrathoracic organs (31 deaths).

Cervical cancer screening services are available to all women in both the public and private sectors. Screening programs seek the early detection and treatment of cervical carcinoma. As a matter of policy, all women who are registered in the Government's family planning program are screened routinely for this condition. A total of 12,612 Pap smears were analyzed during the 1992–1995 period, with the following results: invasive cancer, 15; cancer in-situ III, 48; cancer in-situ II, 84; and cancer in-situ I, 180; the remainder were normal.

Behavioral Disorders. Activity statistics of the Mental Health Centre, the country's only psychiatric hospital that also functions as a residential drug abuse treatment facility, indi-

465

cate that substance abuse (48.9%), drug-induced psychosis (21.3%), and schizophrenia (20.8%) were the main causes of admission between 1992 and 1995, accounting for 91% of the 1,199 admissions during the 1992–1995 period; mental retardation, epilepsy, and manic depression accounted for 2.4%, 2.2%, and 1.3% respectively.

In terms of community mental health, an annual average of 1,040 follow-up home visits were made to outpatients, and attendances at outpatient sessions averaged 3,029 per year; the purpose of the visits was to conduct ongoing psychiatric assessment of all discharges, refill or change medication as necessary, and provide consultation to community-based staff. These community assessments are conducted by a core team on a monthly basis. In 1995, there were 1,241 active patients on the community mental health register.

Mental Health Centre admission records for the 1992–1995 period indicate that of the 587 admissions due to substance abuse, 47.5% were for marijuana, followed by 27.7% for cocaine, and 24.8% for alcohol. About 91% of all admissions for substance abuse were males, while the most vulnerable age group has been shown to be 15–29 years, with 63% of all admissions falling into this category.

Accidents and Violence. There were 196 deaths resulting from external causes (accidents and violence) during 1992–1995: transportation accidents accounted for 30 of them (15.3%), homicide and injury purposefully inflicted by others for 35 (17.8%), suicide and self-inflicted injury for 22 (11.2%), and other violence for 55 (28.1%). The last group includes deaths due to injury unknown whether accidentally or purposely inflicted.

In 1994, a National Committee Against Violence was established to educate the public on all forms of violence, especially domestic violence; provide social and psychological support to victims of violence and their families; and maintain a data base on all aspects of violence.

Oral Health. Government-run oral health services are directed toward providing qualitative and affordable oral health care to the population, particularly school-age children. The number of appointments at the main Kingstown Dental Clinic and the three satellite centers increased 11.9% from 69,124 in 1992 to 77,381 in 1995. On average, 35% of these visits were for extractions, decreasing by 6% over the period, while the number of restorations increased by 8%.

In 1993, a survey on the status of dental health among schoolchildren was completed with PAHO's assistance. The survey revealed that 69% of all schoolchildren (5–15 years old) were affected with dental caries, a known major cause of tooth loss that helps to explain the high demand for extractions. The other major problem was calculus, with 20% of the surveyed population being affected.

The introduction of fluoride treatment at the primary-school level has been achieved. Currently, all children under 16 years of age attending dental clinics are treated with topical fluoride gel. There is no fluoridation of the communal water supply system.

RESPONSE OF THE HEALTH SYSTEM

National Health Plans and Policies

The Government's overall strategy for economic growth, as articulated in the 1991–1995 National Development Plan, centers on increasing output and improving productivity primarily in the agriculture, tourism, education, and health sectors. The Government has acknowledged that economic growth and development are compatible but not synonymous, and that efforts should be made to ensure that the benefits from growth reach all of society.

The Government's social development policy focuses on the need to promote self-sufficiency for disadvantaged groups; for example, by encouraging the community to work together to solve its own problems. In this regard, efforts have been carried out in the agriculture, health, education, housing, and community development sector.

According to the 1991–1995 Health Sector Plan, the Government views access to health care as a basic human right and an integral part of national development and acknowledges that all citizens have the right and duty to participate individually and collectively in the planning, implementation, and evaluation of their health care services at all levels; that health cannot be achieved through the efforts of the health sector alone, but must involve close collaboration with all other sectors; and that the fullest and best use must always be made of national resources to promote health and development. To this end, the Government is committed to provide comprehensive and affordable health care services at primary, secondary, and tertiary levels; facilitate intrasectoral and intersectoral collaboration in providing health care to the population; strengthen links with the community, the private sector, and nongovernmental organizations; institute necessary regulatory mechanisms to ensure the availability of quality health care; and establish dynamic management systems that facilitate the delivery of effective and efficient health care.

The key development areas in health that the Government pursued during the 1991–1995 period were health education and health promotion; disease prevention and control; maternal and child health, including family planning; strengthening of environmental health services; continued development of community and hospital care services; strengthening of pharmaceutical supplies management; drug abuse prevention and control; strengthening of health information systems; and reform of health legislation.

As part of its effort to attain universal access to health care, the Government has identified mothers and children, the poor, and the aged as vulnerable groups requiring special attention. As a result, various services are targeted toward women and children, and the poor, aged, and unemployed are granted concessions in accessing health care services.

Since 1991, the Government has pursued a policy of health sector reforms as a way to increase efficiency in the use of resources and improve cost recovery within the system. Reforms have involved the establishment of new management structures and the streamlining of systems to encourage greater accountability; legislative initiatives also were undertaken to adjust user charges. A review of the health sector's management systems was completed in 1994, leading to changes in organizational structure and functional relationships. The process resulted in the creation of a Senior Management Committee and the adoption of protocols to guide the delivery of services and new forms and schedules for reporting.

Organization of the Health Sector

Health services in Saint Vincent and the Grenadines are basically offered at the primary and secondary levels; at least two major institutions provide social support as well as health care.

At the primary care level, 38 health centers spread over 9 health districts provide services. Each health center is staffed by a full-time district nurse/midwife, a nursing assistant, and a community health aide. Other district health team members such as the district medical officer, pharmacist, and environmental health officers provide support.

On average, each health center covers a population of 2,900 and no one is required to travel more than three miles to access care. Available primary care services include emergency care; medical care; prenatal care and postnatal care; midwifery services; child health services, including immunization; family planning services; and communicable and noncommunicable disease control.

At the secondary level, the 209-bed Kingstown General Hospital is the country's only government acute care referral hospital that provides specialist care in most major areas. Five rural hospitals, with a combined 58-bed capacity, provide a minimum level of secondary care services for which specialist intervention is not indicated. In addition, there are three small, privately owned and operated acute care hospitals with a total capacity of 24 beds. The Government also operates the 120-bed Mental Health Centre, which provides care to acute and chronic psychiatric patients, and the Home for the Aged, which caters to the indigent elderly population and functions as a refuge for abandoned persons with disabilities.

Health Services and Resources

Organization of Services for Care of the Population

Health Promotion and Community Participation. The Health Education Unit has grown into an active unit within the Ministry of Health and the Environment; its main program involves information, education and communication, health promotion, and community outreach activities. To date, there are ongoing training programs in health and family life education for parents, students, out-of-school youth, and community members; daily radio and television programs; and continuous production of a range of audiovisual and graphic materials. The Health Education Unit also coordinates health promotion activities.

There is an ongoing experiment to stimulate community participation in health by promoting the active involvement of community members in the planning, implementation, and evaluation of health programs. Community action is facilitated at the health committee or health center level and at the higher district health team level. It is hoped that this initiative will further involve the community in efforts to modify lifestyles and alleviate health problems. Although some success from this effort has been recorded over time, performance has been spotty.

Environmental Protection. The Government of Saint Vincent and the Grenadines has declared the 1990s as the "Decade of the Environment." To that end, the portfolio of the Ministry of Health was extended to include the environment, and the Ministry became known as the Ministry of Health and the Environment; a new Environmental Services Coordinator post was created in 1995, with responsibility for coordinating all national plans and activities related to environmental protection and preservation; and a National Environmental Advisory Board was appointed by the Cabinet in 1995 to advise the Minister on policies and programs aimed at the environmental protection.

The main environmental issues that have been targeted for attention are the protection of the nation's flora and fauna; the protection of beaches from pollution and sand mining; controlled use of chemicals and pesticides, especially in agriculture; and the proper management of solid and liquid wastes.

Water Supply, Sewerage Systems, and Solid Waste Disposal. The most recent reliable data on the main sources of water supply among households are contained in the 1991 Population and Housing Census Report. The report indicates that almost one-half of all households (47.6%) have water from the communal supply system piped into their premises (yard and house), and an additional 29.4% receive their water from a public standpipe. This means that more than three-quarters of all households (77%) benefit from a reliable potable water supply. It should be noted, however, that 10.8% of households still receive their domestic water supply from suspect sources such as springs, rivers, streams, and communal catchments.

The pit latrine remains the most prevalent means of sewage disposal among households (62.3%), followed by the septic tank (30.1%). It should be noted, however, that the number of households without any approved form of sewage disposal has declined from 8% in 1980 to 3.7% in 1991. Some parts of the capital, Kingstown, are linked by a commercial sewage system that encompasses 3.1% of premises.

In 1995, approximately 64% of all households were provided with a once-weekly refuse collection service, representing a 16% increase in coverage between 1992 and 1995. This service is also augmented by a widespread distribution of community refuse collection bins that are emptied as necessary.

Saint Vincent and the Grenadines is a participant in the Organization of Eastern Caribbean States (OECS)/World Bank Solid Waste Management Project. The project will establish four sanitary landfill sites, two on mainland Saint Vincent and two in the Grenadines, and will extend collection service nationwide.

Food Safety. Broad promotional campaigns have been launched to develop positive attitudes and practices in the handling, preparation, storage, and sale of food that is sold for human consumption. For example, all health districts now routinely conduct clinics for food handlers that provide information and education, demonstrations, medical examination, and, where necessary, treatment. In 1995, there were 2,733 food handling establishments and 3,655 food handlers registered with the public health authority. There are also itinerant vendors, however, who operate without basic sanitary facilities and outside of the reach of public health regulations.

Workers' Health. The Accidents and Occupational Diseases Act No. 24 of 1952 mandates employers to notify the Department of Labour about any accident arising out of and in the course of the employment of any worker that causes loss of life or disability. In 1995, 11 cases of injury on the job were reported. In strict interpretation of and compliance with the law only very serious accidents are reported, and the consensus is that the legislation should be expanded to enforce the notification of all occupational health and safety problems.

Factory Act No. 5 of 1955 regulates employment conditions in factories and other workplaces regarding the health, safety, and welfare of persons employed therein and allows for the inspection of the plant, machinery, and any inputs. This Act is enforced by Environmental Health Officers, who work closely with the Department of Labour, the Trade Union Congress, and the Employers' Federation.

Disaster Preparedness. Saint Vincent and the Grenadines is the home of the La Soufriere Volcano, which last erupted in 1979. The islands also are vulnerable to tropical storms and hurricanes, although no major disasters have occurred recently. However, there is a national consciousness of this vulnerability and the need for continuous disaster preparedness and vigilance.

The Central Disaster Preparedness Committee, which operates under the chairmanship of the Prime Minister, encompasses five subcommittees responsible for disaster management, relief operations, disaster assessment, health conditions, and public information and education. All of these aspects are addressed in the National Disaster Plan. The health component establishes responses in the event of various disasters; the main considerations are mass casualty management, environmental sanitation, food protection, and the potable water supply. The plan also spells out necessary equipment and supplies that must be available at health facilities at the peripheral and central levels in response to disasters.

Organization and Operation of Personal Health Care Services

The occupancy level at the Kingstown General Hospital has averaged 71% per year between 1992 and 1995, a 2% increase over the immediately preceding period. The most active wards have been maternity, surgery, and medicine, in descending order. After a consistent level of activity between 1992 and 1994, hospital admissions fell by 6.2% in 1995. This drop was observed mainly in the maternity ward and may indicate a small measure of success in the efforts to encourage more deliveries at the community level. General hospital utilization is also reflected in the period's average length of stay of 6 days.

All rural hospitals report occupancy levels below 35%, suggesting a high degree of underutilization; reasons given for this low activity include the absence of diagnostic facilities (laboratory and radiography) and of specialist care; the situation is under review. The leading causes of admission to these institutions have been gastroenteritis and maternity cases.

The Mental Health Centre, by contrast, operates at a 120% occupancy level, and the Home for the Aged never falls below maximum capacity. A recent evaluation of the psychiatric services in Saint Vincent and the Grenadines emphasized the need for strengthening the community outreach program as a way to divert the emphasis from institutional care.

Community services are the cornerstone of the health care delivery system. Every year, more than 90,000 visits are made to health centers for the full range of services offered, and almost 48,000 household visits are made by various health staff categories.

Inputs for Health

Essential Drugs and Medications. Saint Vincent and the Grenadines is a founding member of the Eastern Caribbean Drug Service (ECDS), and, as such, benefits from an average 25% savings on the pooled procurement of pharmaceuticals and medical supplies. In recent years, the range of items covered by the service has been expanded to include contraceptive supplies, resulting in even greater economy. About 11.8% of the total recurrent health budget is allocated to the purchase of pharmaceuticals and medical supplies.

The range of drugs available within the public health system is dictated by the National Formulary committee, which is responsible for formulating and updating National Formulary. The National Formulary is closely linked to the Regional Formulary that has been established by ECDS.

A new drug inspector post was created in 1995, designed to monitor the implementation of the legal provisions regarding the dispensing of prescription drugs, drug registration, and drug importation. Relevant legislation is currently being reviewed to facilitate the work of this officer.

Human Resources

All traditional categories of health personnel are available, with nurses, nursing assistants, and doctors representing the highest proportions. There were 574 health personnel posts in 1995, of which 53 were physicians (48 per 100,000 population) and 231 trained nurses of all categories (141 per 100,000 population). As of 1995, upward of 90% of all permanent positions provided for under the budgetary estimates were filled. This is a considerable improvement from 1990, when chronic staff shortages existed in essential categories such as medical doctors, dentists, and nurses. In 1996, there were only limited shortages in the areas of physiotherapy, pharmacy, and medical technology.

Training of Human Resources. Considerable emphasis has been placed on training at the basic technical level and in the area of continuous education. Saint Vincent and the Grenadines has two training institutions for health care professionals: the Government-run School of Nursing and the private offshore Kingstown Medical College, an affiliate of the St. George's Medical School headquartered in Grenada. Health care professionals also receive training at regional and international institutions. Moreover, the emphasis on efficiency and productivity has led to strengthening of managerial and supervisory functions.

Expenditures and Sectoral Financing

From 1992 through 1995, actual Government expenditure on health averaged just under 15% of the total recurrent expenditure. The actual recurrent expenditure on health for the four years was US$ 37.46 million, out of a total recurrent expenditure of US$ 250.90 million, and 4.6% of GDP was spent on health; in the previous four-year period the recurrent expenditure on health averaged 15.4% of total recurrent expenditure. Health now ranks as the third largest consumer of Government's recurrent expenditure, behind the servicing of public debt and education, in that order. Even so, health still attracts 40% of all recurrent expenditure in the social sector.

In 1995, Kingstown General Hospital received 33.7% of all expenditure, and this pattern has held over the period under review. Although the way that the services are organized and the manner in which the budget is presented preclude a precise quantification of expenditure on primary health care, it is known that community health centers and associated services and environmental health services together are allocated 29.2% of the recurrent health budget. Personnel salaries across programs account for 58% of health expenditure.

In January 1995, the Government enacted legislation to revise the user-fee schedule within the public sector, which led to the first revision of the user fee structure in 20 years. This initiative sought to rationalize user charges for hospitalization and diagnostic services, and to introduce charges for dental services and pharmaceuticals, as a way to increase revenue collection from 2% to 6% of actual Government expenditure in the public health sector.

In a related initiative, in 1995 Parliament agreed to introduce a National Insurance Programme. A Cabinet-appointed Steering Committee is currently in the process of undertaking all of the background work required to establish this program. It is hoped that this mechanism will bring greater efficiency to health service delivery and make revenue collection more reliable. Finally, a reform package for the sector seeks to strengthen general and supplies management systems, introduce cost tracking mechanisms, revise admission and billing procedures, and launch a consumer education program.

SURINAME

GENERAL SITUATION AND TRENDS

Socioeconomic, Political, and Demographic Overview

Suriname is located on the northeast coast of South America, and covers 163,820 km². In the north, it borders the Atlantic Ocean, in the east, south, and west it borders French Guiana, Brazil, and Guyana. The country's topography encompasses a narrow coastal plain that extends from east to west, a savanna belt, and a highland tropical rainforest that borders Brazil.

Suriname also is divided into urban, rural, and the Interior areas, in terms of population and economic activity. The urban area comprises the capital city of Paramaribo and parts of Wanica district, and has relatively dense population and an economy based on commerce, services, and industry. The rural area, which includes portions of the coast and the savanna belt, has agriculture, fishing, and bauxite mining as the main economic activities. The Interior, comprising about 80% of the country, is sparsely populated by tribal communities who depend on hunting, fishing, and slash-and-burn agriculture. Forestry, gold mining, and tourism operations also are conducted in the Interior.

The country is divided into 10 administrative districts that are governed through the Ministry of Regional Development, and each district is divided into "ressorts." Each of the country's 62 "ressorts" has its own council. The National Assembly has legislative power in Suriname and consists of 51 members who are elected for a period of five years. The President, who is chosen by the Assembly, has executive power.

The ethnic composition of Suriname's population is 35% Creole, 35% East Indian, 16% Indonesian, 8% Maroon or Bushnegro, 3% Amerindian, 2% Chinese, and 1% European, Lebanese, and others. The main religions are Christianity (42%), Hinduism, (27%), and Islam (20%).

During the 1980s, the country experienced political and economic problems as a result of falling bauxite and alu-minum prices and the suspension of development aid from the Kingdom of the Netherlands. The 1986–1992 period was marked by war in the Interior, with civilian rule being reestablished in 1992. During this period, the population suffered the decay and destruction of the infrastructure. The health sector was affected by a shrinking financial base, lack of investments in and maintenance of facilities and equipment, a scarcity of drugs and reagents, and the departure of trained public health professionals, medical specialists, and registered nurses.

Inflation was 44% in 1992, 143% in 1993, 368% in 1994, and 236% in 1995. The situation improved after the Government instituted structural economic adjustment programs, which resulted in economic and monetary stability and economic growth of 4% in real terms in 1996. The Government had a surplus of cash, made possible by the rise in aluminum prices and the success of a direct tax collection system. The Central Bank intervened, building up currency and gold reserves, and controlling the exchange rate (from a level of Sf 600 to about Sf 400 per U.S. dollar in 1996). The prospects for increased revenue are limited, but a 15% value-added tax was planned for 1997.

Suriname's economy continues to depend on the bauxite sector. Gold mining activities are growing but they also bring about social and public health disruptions such as increased crime and violence, prostitution, drug abuse, and sexually transmitted diseases. Tensions exist between prospectors and villagers, who see creeks turned into mud streams and their access to ancestral lands limited. Development of the timber sector is a source of debate in parliament and the media. Investors applied for timber concessions of 2 million hectares, but environmental concerns delayed decisions.

Suriname was admitted to CARICOM in July 1995, but to participate in the market, it must produce competitive goods. During the country's 15 years of crisis, the deterioration of the infrastructure has hindered attempts to increase production and exports. Rice production, a major source of income, suffers from inadequate infrastructure to limit climatic effects of heavy rainfall and drought. High proportions of domestic goods are imported, and less than 1% of the land is dedicated to food production.

Although the macroeconomic situation has improved, living conditions and the health situation have not. Inflation was accompanied by imbalances in income distribution: 70% of the population was living under the poverty line in 1993. The Government structural adjustment resulted in job losses. Salaried workers, government transfer recipients, and pensioners were the hardest hit. The average real wage fell by 65% between 1990 and 1993. Wages for unskilled jobs decreased to less than US$ 10/month in 1994.

The structural adjustment program was discontinued in 1996, and emphasis placed on "empowerment of the people." Other planned adjustments, however, such as the value-added tax and tariffs for hospitals and utilities that reflect real costs of the services, could affect the majority of the population.

There have been no data on poverty since 1993, and little is known about the informal sector of the economy. The Warwick Institute concluded in 1992 that living standards were still reasonable because of general accessibility of basic services and income sources in the informal sector. Data showed a decrease of jobs in the formal sector in the 1980s that continued during the 1992–1995 period, when they declined by 4%, to 87,282 jobs. The public sector accounted for 40% of formal employment in 1994. Unemployment was estimated at 33% of the economically active population. In 1990–1994, household surveys that considered the informal sectors in Paramaribo and Wanica showed that unemployment declined from 16% in 1990 to 11% in 1994. Between 32% and 35% of the working population (depending on the season) were women. Of those working less than 15 hours per week, between 67% and 81% were female.

Many women started businesses in recent years, and the Ministry of Labor supports them with 22 day-care centers provided through the Foundation for Management of Day-Care Centers. The Government is creating opportunities for their participation in the political process and strengthening their organizations.

It is recognized that one-parent households (usually headed by women) suffer more from poverty. Of 80,000 persons receiving an allowance from the Ministry of Social Affairs and Housing, 60%–65% are women. Groups such as refugees, the elderly, the handicapped, and those in certain urban areas and the Interior are also living under extremely poor circumstances.

About 7,000 refugees returned to the Interior in 1992, but they still lack adequate housing and public services in their tribal lands. Many schools and health centers were rebuilt in 1995 and 1996, but recovery of other infrastructure in the Interior is hampered by logistical and financial problems. Services such as police and vital statistics have not been restored. Armed miners and drug traffickers threaten safety, while malaria and other diseases endanger health. Consequently, many refugees moved to Paramaribo, joining the 13,000 displaced persons already there, and further straining the housing and infrastructure.

Hyperinflation and structural adjustments resulted in decreasing government expenditures in the areas of health care and social protection. While expenses rose from Sf 2.7 million in 1980 to Sf 175 million in 1995, this represents a decline in expenditures from US$ 93 million to US$ 2.2 million.

There are government and nongovernmental programs to strengthen social protection through improvements in health care, welfare services, education, and housing and special subsidies for people living below the poverty line. However, trained personnel to manage these programs are lacking. Of the 39,000 government workers in 1994, 67% had attained only primary education; 33%, secondary education; and only 4% had higher education.

To protect the health status of the population, the Government formulated the Policy Paper 1996, which aims to provide material and social support on a needs basis to individuals and groups in vulnerable socioeconomic situations, and ultimately to enable target groups to become self-sufficient. The Ministry of Social Affairs and Housing provides the existing system of supports, which includes cash transfers to the elderly and to poor families, child allowances (covering 27,659 mothers and 64,000 children in 1994), and free medical care for the poor (about 25% of the population). A system providing subsidized packages of commodities was set up to safeguard the availability of foods and a basic nutritional status, as well as to stabilize prices and ensure equitable distribution of limited goods. Today, there are 130,000 recipients of these packages, including households and institutions. The system will be phased out, providing cash payments amounting to about US$ 37 each, an amount that is insufficient to meet the cost of living of the elderly and the poor.

The operational cost of the Ministry of Social Affairs and Housing was US$ 17 million in 1996 and US$ 51 million in 1997. There is a need for more programs to protect vulnerable groups, but the size and composition of the target groups are not known. Research institutions should be engaged in efforts to improve the availability of statistical information on these groups.

The Vital Statistics Bureau estimated a population of 423,400 in 1996, 70% living in Paramaribo (222,800) and Wanica (72,400) districts on 0.4% of the land. The population increased through 1971; thereafter, growth rates slowed and some years even showed a decrease. Birth rates decreased to their lowest levels of 20.2 per 1,000 in 1994 and 20.7 in 1995. From 1972 to 1996, emigration to the Netherlands was a determinant of population dynamics. However, since 1994, it lost its primary role and growth now depends mostly on the balance between births and deaths. In 1994, 2,836 people emigrated, and 1,716 did in 1995, after rules for traveling to the Netherlands were tightened. Legal immigration, mostly from the Netherlands, Guyana, and the Far East accounted for nearly 2,300 people annually from 1989 to 1991, decreasing to 1,350 in 1994–1995.

Fertility rates declined from 134.8 per 1,000 women aged 15–44 in 1982 to 90.9 in 1991. Factors contributing to this trend are high use of contraceptives, abortion, and emigration. There is also a lack of reliable data from the Interior, where fertility rates are higher.

Mortality and Morbidity Profile

The crude mortality rate fluctuated between 7.3 per 1,000 and 6.2 per 1,000 in the 1986–1996 period. Life expectancy at birth continued to be relatively low, with the latest figures estimated at 68.8 years for males and females combined. Figures on death rates by sex are not available.

In the past 15 years, approximately 85% of deaths were medically certified. This declined to 70% in 1992, 66% in 1993, and 59% in 1994, because of untimely reports made by physicians. The epidemiology unit of the Ministry of Health searched records in the largest hospitals in Paramaribo to find missing certificates, yielding an increase in identified deaths to 85% in 1992, 84% in 1993, and 77% in 1994. Incomplete mortality statistics are also a result of certificates describing the cause of death by vague symptoms or as "unknown." On average, about 15% of medical death certificates are in the category of unspecified diseases, the majority of which cite "unknown" or "old age" as cause of death.

Infant mortality in the 1990–1994 period fluctuated from 19.5 deaths per 1,000 live births in 1993 to 25.1 deaths in 1994. Perinatal mortality ranged from 18.6 in 1990 to 32.9 in 1992, remaining around that level in 1993 and 1994. This increase was attributed to underreporting of stillbirths prior to 1992. The maternal mortality rate was low in 1990 (1.1 per 100,000 live births) and fluctuated over the 1991–1994 period between 6.4 and 12.2. Again, underreporting is considered the main cause of year-to-year variations.

In the 1992–1994 period, the leading causes of death were hypertension and heart disease, accounting for 17% of all deaths (1,167); cerebrovascular accidents, 11% (758 deaths); malignant neoplasms, 9% (601); accidents and trauma, 8% (520); gastroenteritis, 5% (377); conditions originating in the perinatal period, 4% (294); diabetes mellitus, 4% (279); pneumonia and influenza, 3% (177); suicide, 2% (130); and cirrhosis of the liver, 2% (123). The most significant trends were: a decline from 274 suicides in the 1983–1985 period to 130 in the 1992–1994 period (pesticides were the most commonly

used method, followed by hanging); a decrease in deaths due to accidents and trauma from 733 in the 1989–1991 period to 520 in 1992–1994; and an increase in deaths due to gastroenteritis from 280 in 1989–1991 to 377 in 1992–1994.

From 1994 to 1996, the Bureau of Public Health, the Regional Health Service, the Medical Mission, and several hospitals undertook to improve their health information systems. The basis for a national system is in place: morbidity data are collected in all care institutions, but are not analyzed. Standardization of definitions and procedures for comparisons is needed.

An important source of information on morbidity is the registration system for patient visits to Regional Health Service polyclinics. Reasons for visits are not standardized, so comparability is questionable, but data provide ethnic, environmental, or service utilization categories. The system shows percentages of visits to Regional Health Service polyclinics attributed to groups of causes in 1993 in urban and rural areas. Where Creole populations predominated, 9% of visits were related to upper-respiratory infections, 12% to hypertension, and 8% to diabetes mellitus. In contrast, where East Indians and Indonesians were in the majority, 14%–17% of visits were due to upper-respiratory infections, 7%–9% to hypertension, and 4%–6% to diabetes mellitus. Differences in visits for asthma and emphysema by area of influence were noted. Inner-city Regional Health Service polyclinics reported them in 0.1%–0.6% of the visits; in contrast, rural polyclinics reported them in 5% of visits. At the Medical Mission polyclinics in the Interior, 8% of visits were for upper-respiratory infections, 5% for malaria, 3% for diarrhea, 1% for accidents, and 0.2% for urethral discharge among males. In the Academic Hospital, the only facility with a 24-hour emergency medicine department, about 8% of cases were related to traffic accidents, other types of accidents accounted for 39%–44% of cases, and 40% were classified as "drop-ins," or patients with non-emergency complaints. The high percentage in the last category is a result of the unavailability of general practitioners outside normal working hours.

SPECIFIC HEALTH PROBLEMS

Analysis by Population Group

Health of Children

The number of live births per year declined from 9,835 in 1992 to 8,717 in 1995. The Medical Mission, which provides health service in the Interior, recorded 1,179 live births in that region in 1996. About 80% of deliveries take place in hospitals, the rest are attended by midwives and traditional birth attendants in the Interior.

The number of infant deaths increased from 192 in 1992 to 211 in 1994 (rates of 19.5 per 1,000 live births and 25.1, respectively). Data were not computed for the Interior, but before the war, 20% of deaths and 10% of births occurred in the Interior each year. Perinatal mortality remained stable during the 1992–1994 period, with 32.9 deaths per 1,000 births in 1992, 31.0 in 1993, and 29.8 in 1994. An estimate calculated by the Diakonessenhuis Hospital, which cooperates with the Medical Mission in the Interior, indicated that perinatal mortality in 1994 in the Interior was 47.5 per 1,000 births, compared with the national rate of 29.8. This suggests either a higher risk of perinatal mortality in the Interior or an over-representation of high-risk pregnancies.

In the age group under 1 year old, the major causes of death were conditions originating in the perinatal period (284 deaths), gastroenteritis (70 deaths), congenital anomalies (43 deaths), malnutrition (34 deaths), and pneumonia (22 deaths), representing 75% of 604 deaths. In the 1988–1990 period, the annual mean mortality rate due to diarrhea was 5.7 per 1,000 births, compared with 2.6 for 1992–1994.

In 1996, the Diakonessenhuis Hospital reported low birth-weight in 12% of 1,710 live births.

In 1993, the General Statistics Bureau estimated the 1–4-year-old population to be 37,400 (9% of the total), based on the 1980 census data on births, deaths, immigration, and emigration.

There were 149 deaths among 1–4-year-olds in the 1992–1994 period, with 44 in 1992, 58 in 1993, and 47 in 1994, resulting in specific death rates of 1.1 per 1,000 in 1992 and 1.3 in 1993. The leading causes of deaths in the 1992–1994 period were gastroenteritis (40 cases), accidents and trauma (16), malnutrition (10), and pneumonia (10), accounting for 50% of deaths. The annual mean mortality due to gastroenteritis was 23.3 per 100,000 in the 1988–1990 period, and was estimated to be 35.6 for 1992–1994. In the 1992–1994 period, accidents and trauma caused an average yearly mortality rate of 14.3 per 100,000. The yearly mean mortality rates for pneumonia were 20.9 and 8.9 in the 1988–1990 and 1992–1994 periods, respectively.

The 1993 population of 5–14-year-olds was estimated by the General Statistics Bureau to be 89,200, 22.1% of the total. There were 127 deaths in this age group between 1992 and 1994. The leading causes of death were accidents and trauma (54 cases), gastroenteritis (8), and meningitis (5), representing more than 50% of deaths in this group. Four girls in the age group committed suicide. In the 1988–1990 period, annual mean mortality due to accidental trauma was 14.1 per 100,000, with boys outnumbering girls 1.5 to 1. In 1992–1994, the rate was 20.2 per 100,000, with a boy-to-girl ratio of 1.4:1.

Hospitalizations of malnourished children increased from 307 in 1992–1993 to 355 in 1994–1995. This also represents a 3.5-fold increase with respect to 1988–1989. In 1993, most malnutrition-related hospitalizations in s'Lands Hospital affected infants of 6–9 months. In 1994, an increase in hospitalizations involved a majority of 1–2-year-olds. The 1–2-year-olds appeared more vulnerable than infants, who could benefit from breast-feeding. Milk was rationed in this period, with only pregnant women, parents with children under 5 years old, and the elderly allowed to buy a weekly ration of 5 liters at the only milk factory.

A 1994 study on the health status of former refugees in Marowijne district showed that 17% of 278 children aged 0 to 6 years were malnourished (97% chronically), but none of the 0–6-month-old infants were. In 1995, an unpublished study at a clinic for children under 5 years old in a rural village south of Paramaribo (populated mostly by Indonesians and East Indians) found more than 25% of children with a weight-for-age below the third percentile of the United States National Center for Health Statistics (NCHS) standard, while a 1989 study reported 8%.

Acute malnutrition increased during the 1980s in primary school children in Paramaribo. In 1994, a study in Paramaribo among 1,871 schoolchildren aged 4–11 found that 13% of boys had a weight-for-age below the third percentile, twice that of girls (7%). Wasting (weight-for-height below percentile 3 of standard) was the same for boys and girls, with an overall prevalence of 16%. A similar finding was made in 1989 (18%).

Health of Adolescents and Adults

The General Statistics Bureau estimated the 1993 population of 15–44-year-olds to be 199,400 (49% of the total), with 101,200 males and 98,200 females. A total of 1,192 deaths were registered in this age group during 1992–1994. The leading causes of death were accidents and trauma, with 20% of all deaths (233 cases); hypertension and heart disease with 9% (106); and malignant neoplasms with 6% (70). More male (64%) than female deaths were recorded. The pattern of deaths by accidents and trauma and malignant neoplasms differed by sex—24% and 4% for males, and 12% and 10% for females, respectively. An important trend was a decrease in deaths due to accidents, trauma, and suicides among females, from 88 in 1989–1991 to 51 in 1992–1994. There were 21 deaths in this category in the 1986–1988 period, and 34 in 1983–1985. No reasons for this steep decrease in 1989–1991 were readily found.

Between 1981 and 1990, maternal mortality rates fluctuated between 7 and 9 per 10,000 live births. These rates continued to vary from 8.8 in 1991, 12.2 in 1992, 6.4 in 1993, and 8.7 in 1994. Underreporting played an important role in these fluctuations. According to one study, 42 maternal deaths occurred in 1991 and 1992, a maternal mortality rate of 22.4, or 3.5 times higher than the official figures. Postpartum hemorrhage and pregnancy-induced hypertension were the most frequent causes of death, accounting for 29. Lack of transport and blood transfusion facilities were determinants in these unnecessary deaths. A study of pregnant women in 1992 found that half were anemic (hemoglobin < 7 mmol/l).

The total fertility rate fell from 7.3 per woman in the 1950s to 2.9 in 1990. Global fertility rates dropped from 129.4 per 1,000 women aged 15–44 in 1985 to 90.9 in 1991. A national survey indicated differences in global fertility rates by ethnic group; they were 240 for Bushnegroes, 140 for Indonesians, 100 for East Indians, and 90 for Creoles.

In 1988, 1,500 of the 9,094 births (17%) occurred in mothers under 20 years old. The Diakonessenhuis Hospital reported in 1994 that 10% of births were to women under age 20. Between January and August 1994, 622 teenagers visited Stichting Lobi (the family planning foundation) for a pregnancy test, and 15% were pregnant. Figures from s'Lands Hospital showed that out of 262 abortions performed there, 40 (15%) were for women under age 20. It was estimated that trained personnel attended 80% of births in 1994; the average number of prenatal visits per pregnancy was six.

In 1992, a contraceptive prevalence survey done in a sample of women aged 15–44 found that 8% of the women knew nothing about contraceptives, 58% knew four or more methods, and 38% were current contraceptive users. Of the women sampled, 27% were married, 20% were in common-law unions, 25% in visiting partner, and 28% were single. More East Indian (74%) and Indonesian (58%) women were married, while more Creoles (58%) and Bushnegroes (47%) were in visiting unions. The stated order of preference for different contraceptive methods was the pill (54% of women), the condom (23%), tubal ligation (9%, mostly women over age 34), injectable forms (8%), and the IUD (5%, mostly women over age 25). However, the pill was the most frequently used method with 68% of users; followed by tubal ligation with 12%; the condom, 10%; injectable forms, 4%; and the IUD, 3%. Contraceptive use was uneven across social groups, but higher among older women and Indonesians, and lower among adolescents, Bushnegroes, and Amerindians. Bushnegro and Amerindian women were at higher risk than other ethnic groups with respect to age of first intercourse, age of first pregnancy, number of live births, and level of contraceptive use. Seventy percent of women between 15 and 19 years old who had partners did not use a contraceptive method at the time of the survey, and 59% of all adolescents who had been pregnant stated their pregnancies were unplanned.

A survey among students attending a vocational school showed that while 62% of sexually active students did not use contraceptives, most stated they did not want to get pregnant. In 1992, a survey by Stichting Lobi among women of child-bearing age showed that 48% used contraceptives; 36% made the decision to use them on their own, 52% decided with their partner, and in 8% of cases the man made the decision. Another Stichting Lobi survey among 900 female clients of a clinic in 1988–1989 revealed that 34% of the women had had at least one abortion before they registered for family planning. Of those younger than 20 years, 35% had had at least one abortion. Reasons for termination of pregnancy were: "young age" (27%), "wants to finish school" (15%), "spacing" (19%), "just had a child" (14%), "has no job" (10%), "family already complete" (9%), and "other" (6%).

The 1993 population of 45–64-year-olds was estimated at 24,200 males and 26,300 females. A total of 1,661 deaths were recorded in this age group during the 1992–1994 period. As in previous periods, hypertension and heart disease remained the most important causes of death with 382 cases (23% of deaths), followed by malignant neoplasms with 231 deaths (14%), cerebrovascular accidents (226 or 14%), and diabetes mellitus (114 or 7%). In contrast with other age groups, accidents and trauma ranked fifth, with 97 deaths (6%).

In the 1988–1990 period, mortality rates (corrected for undercertification) among this group were 246.5 per 100,000 population for hypertension and heart disease, 113.6 for cancer, 87.9 for accidents and trauma, 81.6 for cerebrovascular accidents, and 55.9 for diabetes mellitus. In the 1992–1994 period, the uncorrected yearly average rates were an estimated 251.9 for hypertension and heart disease, 152.3 for cancer, 64.0 for accidents and trauma, 149.0 for cerebrovascular accidents, and 75.2 for diabetes mellitus. A correction factor for undercertification would increase these figures by about 20%. The increase in the number of deaths due to malignant neoplasms, cerebrovascular accidents, and diabetes may in part be a result of improved case-finding and availability of diagnosis (Pap tests and CT scan).

Health of the Elderly

In 1993, it was estimated that 5% of the total population was in the 65 and older age group. There were 3,188 deaths in the 1992–1994 period, 51% (1,635) among males. The most frequent causes of death were hypertension and heart disease with 606 cases (19%), followed by cerebrovascular accidents (448 deaths, or 14%), malignant neoplasms (269 deaths, or 8%), gastroenteritis (167 deaths, or 5%), and diabetes mellitus with (137 deaths, or 4%). The proportion of deaths by group of causes was similar between males and females, except for cerebrovascular accidents, which were more frequent among females (17% of deaths) than males (12%). In contrast to causes of death in the 1989–1991 period, gastroenteritis appeared among the top five causes of death, while accidents and trauma disappeared from the top five causes.

Health of Refugees and Urban Poor

Two high-risk groups include those in the Interior, especially returning refugees, and those in poor neighborhoods that serve as migrating stations between the Interior and the city.

In 1994, a study on returned refugees in Marowijne found that sanitation and housing were poor and the cost of living high. Although there were three polyclinics (including the Albina Hospital of the Regional Health Service), two auxiliary medical posts, and one private dental clinic in the area, people were largely dependent on Paramaribo for their health care. The study estimated immunization coverage to be 42% among 205 children sampled, lower than the national coverage of 71% in 1994.

Albina, the district's administrative center, had infrastructure problems, particularly with electricity and piped water services. Only Moengo and Albina had piped drinking water. In the surrounding villages, pit latrines either had no lids or were too full. River water was used for drinking, bathing, and other household purposes. Rainwater and well water were also used for drinking. Defecation took place in the woods, rivers, and creeks, and near dwellings, increasing water source contamination. Due to lack or high costs of transportation, outreach health work in the surrounding villages ceased.

Refugees were distinguished as those who returned to their traditional villages and those who settled in the areas of Moengo and Albina. Living conditions in the traditional villages were relatively better for children, since food was guaranteed and small children were always in the company of their mothers. In the semiurban Moengo and Albina areas, mothers were often working away from home, garbage was not collected, and sewage systems did not work. Theft, assault, prostitution, and drug abuse were rampant. Most food came from Paramaribo.

In 1996, the Salvation Army carried out a house survey in the poor neighborhood of Pontbuiten-East (Paramaribo). It has 824 households with a population of about 6,000, 60% under 18 years of age. Of those households participating (73%), 82% reported a monthly income below the poverty level (US$ 100/month). Piped water was available in 75% of households, 17% at all times. In 44% of households, people did not receive at least one daily meal with vegetables and meat or fish. A bed was present in 57% of homes.

A total of 83% of the households surveyed perceived an unsatisfactory health situation, and 86% said medical services were inadequate. Thirty-five percent had state health insurance, 30% were covered by the Ministry of Social Affairs, 20% used private sources, and 8% had company arrangements. Traditional herbal medicines were used in 60% of households. The five leading perceived living condition problems, in descending order, were bad roads, bad sewer systems

and flooding, crime, lack of streetlights, and lack of running water. The lack of a polyclinic and drug abuse ranked eighth and eleventh. A day-care center was regarded as the most needed social service, followed by a market, an old people's home, a police post, and a center for battered women.

Analysis by Type of Disease

Communicable Diseases

Vector-Borne Diseases. In 1993–1994, Suriname had a dengue epidemic, resulting in 201 confirmed cases, 109 hospitalizations, and 10 deaths. Dengue type-4 virus was isolated at that time. In 1996, another epidemic occurred with 182 hospitalizations and 1 death, but only 2 cases were confirmed. This reflects a policy whereby a confirmed diagnosis is not attempted for every suspect.

Malaria is a major public health problem that limits development of the Interior. Due to overlapping diagnostic services of the Medical Mission and the malaria control unit of the Bureau of Public Health, many cases may be counted more than once. In 1996, malaria reached unprecedented levels, with 23% positives out of 68,674 slides examined for malaria. *Plasmodium falciparum* was found in 94% of positive slides, *P. vivax* in 5%, and *P. malariae* in 1%, while mixed infections (*P. falciparum* with *P. vivax* or *P. malariae*) were seen in 15 slides. Almost one-quarter of the reported 11,059 positives seen by the Medical Mission in the Interior were children under 5 years old. In 1996, 14 malaria deaths were reported.

Malaria control activities resumed in 1993, although prewar levels have not been attained. Government policy aims to integrate control with the regular Medical Mission health care programs. In the last quarter of 1996, the Government established a task force with extra funds for malaria control, thus increasing activities. The goal of the task force was to reduce malaria prevalence to "acceptable levels" within three months.

Schistosomiasis transmission is restricted to limited areas in the coastal zone, mainly in the district of Saramacca, 40 km west of the capital city. No recent data are available on its prevalence.

Suspected cases of leptospirosis increased at a rate of around 50% per year, from 50 in 1992 to more than 200 in 1996. However, the number of confirmed cases has remained at around 50 per year since 1991. Because of a lack of laboratory confirmation in all cases, and because some suspected cases turn out to be hepatitis-A or -B, it is not clear how significant the trend is.

Vaccine-Preventable Diseases. The last confirmed case of poliomyelitis was in 1982 and was vaccine-related. Six suspected cases were investigated in 1992, 15 in 1994, 3 in 1995, and 4 in 1996, and in all cases the diagnosis of poliomyelitis was discarded. In the 1988–1992 period no cases of diphtheria were reported, but there were 33 reported cases of suspected pertussis in 1990, indicating the vulnerability left by low coverage. In the 1993–1996 period, no cases of diphtheria were reported, but in 1996 two suspected cases of pertussis were investigated. One case of neonatal tetanus was seen in 1988 and one in 1989, but there were no cases between 1990 and 1996. One case of tetanus was reported in 1994, no cases in 1995, and two in 1996. In 1992 there was an outbreak of rubella, with 17 suspected cases reported from July to December. In 1996, 10 confirmed and 20 suspected cases were seen. In 1994 there were 49 reported cases of mumps; in 1995, 863 cases; and in 1996, 124 cases.

The Expanded Program on Immunization began in Suriname in 1976 with the vaccination of children under 1 year of age against diphtheria, pertussis, tetanus, and poliomyelitis. After a large measles epidemic in 1980–1981, measles vaccination was included in the routine immunization schedule. Girls in the first year of grammar school receive the rubella vaccine. Since 1993 the measles, mumps, and rubella (MMR) vaccine has been given to children at 12 months of age. In 1992, the national vaccination coverage fell to 74%, and in the coastal area, the Regional Health Service achieved only 54% coverage. Reasons for low coverage were lack of DTP and polio vaccines in the country for 3 to 4 months, the breakdown of the public transport system, and the fact that more mothers were working. The immunization program was also hurt by the departure of trained staff members of the Bureau of Public Health and the Regional Health Service, the agencies responsible for EPI supervision and implementation.

In 1993 and 1994, DTP3 and OPV3 coverage rates remained low at 76% and 74%. Coverage was 85% in 1995, but the delivery system was weak, and in 1996 coverage dropped again to 79%. Measles vaccination rates were 62% in 1991 and 68% in 1992. After a special mass campaign, in which 94% of a target population of 46,000 children under age 5 were vaccinated, routine measles vaccination rates returned to the low levels of 61% in 1993, 71% in 1994, 79% in 1995, and 71% in 1996.

AIDS and Other STDs. The first case of AIDS was diagnosed in 1983, and as of 31 December 1996 597 cases of HIV-infection (including AIDS) had been reported. The male-to-female ratio in this group was 1.7:1. From 1992 to 1996 the percentage of new HIV/AIDS cases and of persons tested were: 7% HIV-positives of 685 tested in 1992, 5% of 1,406 in 1993, 5% of 1,394 in 1994, 4% of 1,958 in 1995, and 9% of 1,306 in 1996. Of the 80 who tested HIV-positive in 1995, 46 were men and 34 were women. About 75% of AIDS cases die within three months of diagnosis. Recently, the first AIDS case was reported from an Amerindian village near the Brazilian border.

Reasons given for HIV-testing in 1995 were: unprotected sex (29%), clinical diagnosis (24%), request for insurance or blood transfusion (14%), for prevention prior to marriage or pregnancy (4%), for surveys (3%), HIV-positive contact (2%), perinatal HIV contact (0.5%), other (17%), and unknown (8%). The highest number of positive tests was found in the HIV-contact category (8 of 36) and in the perinatal HIV-contact category (2 of 9). Those tested by request of a third party were positive in 1 out of 274 cases (0.4%), while 1 of 52 (2%) in a survey were positive. Of 563 who tested because of having unprotected sex, 9 were positive (2%).

Syphilis reporting at the Dermatologische Dienst (the national center for the control of sexually transmitted diseases) varied in recent years, from 80 cases in 1988, to 295 in 1992, and 225 in 1995 (or 5% of all STDs). The male-to-female ratio was 0.8:1. At sentinel stations, the trend was similar: from 35 cases in 1991, to 226 in 1992, and 175 in 1996.

In the 1988–1992 period, gonorrhea cases averaged about 1,600 cases per year. In 1995 there were 2,072 cases (42% of all STDs). At sentinel stations there were 450 cases in 1991 and 1,840 in 1995.

Other Communicable Diseases. In February 1992 there was an outbreak of cholera near the border with French Guiana. Twelve cases were reported, of which seven were confirmed, including an 11-year-old girl who died. There was no further transmission of the disease and no cases of cholera reported in the 1993–1996 period.

The prevalence of leprosy decreased during the 1980s from 58.6 per 100,000 in 1981 to 25.8 per 100,000 population in 1989. The decline continued slowly in 1990, 1991, and 1992 with rates of 15.4, 14.1, and 12.4 per 100,000, respectively. In 1996 the rate was 11.0 per 100,000. The goal of eradicating leprosy in the year 2000 is an official policy target of the Ministry of Health.

Since 1990, the Bureau of Public Health reported between 47 and 72 cases of tuberculosis per year, fluctuating from 17.9 per 100,000 in 1990, to 14.9 per 100,000 in 1996. Experts estimated that the incidence could be between 25 and 40 per 100,000 (between 100 and 150 cases per year). An incidence rate of 35 per 100,000 was found among Surinamese in Holland. In 1995, 6 of 72 reported tuberculosis cases were HIV-positive, and in 1996, 14 of 63.

From August 1992 to February 1993 there was a countrywide epidemic of shigellosis, caused by a multiple resistant strain of *Shigella flexneri*, including a total of 107 hospitalized cases and 26 deaths. Deteriorating sanitary conditions and poor nutritional status created opportunities for shigellosis to become endemic. In 1994, 229 cases and 17 deaths were recorded, and in 1995 there were 235 cases and 12 deaths.

After the onset of the war, there was a decline in the number of typhoid fever cases reported. Incidence rates per 100,000 were 5.7, 5.6, and 6.4 in 1984, 1985, and 1986, respectively. In the 1988–1996 period the incidence rates fluctuated between 1.7 and 2.7 per 100,000.

Strongyloidiasis, ascariasis, and other parasitic helminthic infestations are major health problems, especially among young children, that can be attributed to poor excreta disposal practices. Ascariasis and other parasitic helminthic infections affect the population with prevalence rates of about 60% in the 0–14-year age group. Recent surveys in Paramaribo have found prevalence rates of about 60% in the general population. Since 1991, strongyloides have become the leading soil-transmitted helminths. The program for their control examined 5,497 fecal smears in 1995. Of these, 35% were positive for *Strongyloides stercoralis*, 27% for *Ascaris lumbricoides*, 18% for *Trichuris trichura*, and 7% for *Necator americanus*, several of them being mixed infestations.

Noncommunicable Diseases and Other Health-Related Problems

Malignant Tumors. In the review period, early cancer detection and data collection activities were initiated, including the cervical cancer screening program of Stichting Lobi, and the cancer registry project of the Academic Hospital.

A total of 892 malignant neoplasm cases were diagnosed between 1991 and 1993. More than 80% occurred among people 40 years and older, 59% were females, and 48% were Creoles. The predominance of Creoles could not be explained, and needs further analysis.

Cancer of the cervix (140 cases) followed by breast cancer (116 cases) were the most frequently observed malignant neoplasms among females, while prostate cancer (66 cases) and lymphoma (35 cases) were the most frequent among males. Since 1990, 45 cervical cancer cases were reported, on average, each year. Of those cases, 43% were diagnosed in the 25–44-year age group. This reflects, to some extent, the case-finding efforts of Stichting Lobi, women's groups, physicians, and pathologists, among others. Stichting Lobi made 11,532 Pap tests in 1995 and 11,893 in 1996. Between 10 and 25 women die from cervical cancer yearly.

Violence and Crime. According to national figures, there were 49 cases of murder and manslaughter in 1994 and 50 in 1995. There were 568 personal assaults registered in 1994 and 537 in 1995. Because of changes in procedures at the statistics unit of the Ministry of Justice, it is not possible to analyze trends.

In 1993, the Police registered 620 applications for assistance at its Juvenile Affairs Division in Paramaribo. These cases were mainly among youths (70% were boys) between the ages of 12 and 16, who were victims of violence or sexual abuse; were runaways, school dropouts, shoplifters, or juvenile prostitutes; or were considered "unmanageable" by their parents. In 1994, 700 requests for assistance were recorded, 70% linked to children from low socioeconomic classes.

In 1993, a study based on police and hospital data revealed that 54% of police reports involved women. Twenty percent of reports involved women abused by male partners or ex-partners, violence that was often repeated. In 80% of cases of violent abuse against women, the crime took place at home. Academic Hospital emergency unit data showed that 95% of victims of sexual assault were female, and 20% were girls under 10 years of age. A total of 99 rape cases were recorded in 1994, and 108 in 1995.

Little information is available on drug use, including alcohol, but according to the Bureau for Alcohol and the District's Attorney office, illegal substance abuse among youth and drug trafficking were increasing. The police reported an increase in crimes committed to obtain money for drugs. There was anecdotal evidence of increased child prostitution in Paramaribo and the mining areas of the Interior.

Behavioral Disorders. Problems with mental health care are associated with the lack of community-based services for the mentally ill. Ambulatory outreach is very limited and there is only one psychiatric hospital. Care delivery is strictly centralized and mainly oriented toward tranquilizing medication and social constraint of seriously deranged patients. About 60% of inpatients at the psychiatric hospital were over 65 years of age and had been hospitalized for more than 30 years.

Oral Health. The Youth Dental Service Foundation has operated in Suriname since 1968 to improve dental health in the age 0–18-year age group. In 1995, they made a survey of 202 6-year-olds and 214 12-year-old schoolchildren in Paramaribo and Wanica. The 6-year-olds had an average decayed, missing, filled teeth (DMFT) index of 6.05, and 13% had flawless teeth, while the 12-year-olds had an average DMFT of 5.6. These results were consistent with a 1990 survey of the same sample.

Environmental Health. Piped drinking water is provided to 95% of the urban population. About 90% of urban dwellers have house connections and another 5% have easy access (faucets in the yards or on public lands). A program to bring piped water into villages in the rural areas was implemented before the war, and 47 rural systems function in the coastal area. About 70% of the rural population has piped water in the house and 20% near the house. People in the Interior depend on water from rivers and creeks for their supply.

477

Public water supplies use groundwater, but saline intrusion in the coastal area affects its quality. To improve quality in these areas, water from wells is mixed with water piped to Paramaribo from Republiek, 40 km to the south. Although water is not chlorinated, water pumped into the mains exceeds WHO guidelines on quality. However, in many areas piped water is not safe for drinking because of broken mains. Because pressure is often insufficient to supply individual household lines, people break the mains below ground level to secure water.

New buildings are required to install septic tanks for sewage disposal. In Paramaribo there is a functioning sewage treatment plant, and an oxidation pond for sewage disposal at the state prison. About 15% of households in Paramaribo use pit latrines and about 5% have no facilities. A neighborhood of Paramaribo had a sewage treatment system which, due to inadequate maintenance, stopped functioning in 1986–1987. This left sewage spills and, during heavy rainfall, one-third of households experience sewage flooding the house. Plans to provide 1,200 houses with septic tanks are being implemented. In rural districts, pit latrines are the dominant forms of excreta disposal.

The disposal of solid wastes is a major problem, particularly in urban areas. Garbage is dumped in a municipal open site located in a swampy area in northern Paramaribo. Because of the serious economic situation, poor garbage collection services, and lack of awareness, garbage is dumped along roads, city streets, empty lots, canals, and rivers.

The health and environmental effects of agricultural pesticides and fertilizers, hydroelectric power plants, mining, the use of insecticides in the Interior against malaria mosquitoes, and the effect of slash-and-burn cultivation in the Interior are matters of concern. Many of these issues are closely related to issues of economic development. The problem of pesticide use is compounded because aerial spraying leaves pesticide residue on roofs where people collect rainwater.

Other environmental problems receiving attention in the media are the disposal of feces from septic tanks by sanitation trucks into the Suriname river, the open mining of sand for construction, which turns large areas into lakes, and the use of mercury by gold prospectors along rivers in the Interior.

RESPONSE OF THE HEALTH SYSTEM

National Health Plans and Policies

The 1997–2001 Policy Paper of the Ministry of Health identified two core problems in the health care system: financing and the lack of trained personnel. The focus of the Ministry's policies for the 1997–2001 period is to stop the decline of the health care sector. Measures planned to regulate and reorganize the system include institutionalization of a National Health Council; strengthening of management; updating health legislation; continued privatization of government hospitals, the Regional Health Service, and other institutions; and restoration of health care facilities in the Interior.

The Central Office of the Ministry of Health will be reorganized to enable it to function as a center for policy development, supervision, and coordination. The provision of services to the public will stop being a function of the Ministry of Health. Policies aimed at better cooperation among hospitals and the division of specialized functions among hospitals will be continued.

The Policy Paper gives priority to "participation of local communities, mobilization of local resources, and decentralization of health systems management." Women will play a role as catalysts in community participation. Programs aimed at the target groups of women, children, and the working class are diarrhea control, immunization, and cervical cancer screening (conducted by Stichting Lobi). In March 1993, the National Assembly ratified the International Convention of the Rights of the Child. New legislation has been formulated to bring the laws of the land in line with this Convention.

To limit the problems of cost and accessibility of health care services, the Policy Paper states that the Government will implement "a compulsory national health insurance system for the total population, including mechanisms to regulate salaries of service providers, to control prices of drugs and other inputs, and to control the costs of intramural care." Financial policies will focus on stopping open-ended financing of hospitals, budgeting programs, and the gradual elimination of subsidies.

Targets for health care budgeting, including the limit of government expenditure to between 6% and 8% of GNP, are addressed in the Policy Paper. Intramural care should be limited to less than 52% of the health care budget. Budgeting will put a halt to the current "open-ended" approach to financing health services.

Managerial development is a priority, for which development of information systems is an essential component. Health personnel will be strengthened by training professionals (including postgraduate training) and improvements in the remuneration of health workers (especially nurses).

Disease control programs given high priority are those against malaria; dengue; schistosomiasis and soil-transmitted helminthes; sexually transmitted diseases, including HIV-infections; leprosy; and tuberculosis. Priority is also given to the rehabilitation of the Medical Mission facilities in the Interior. The process of privatization of the Regional Health Service is ongoing, as well as changes in its organization that emphasize decentralization of management, strengthening of local health centers, and community participation.

Organization of the Health Sector

Institutional Organization

The Government is responsible for providing access to an integrated health care system. The Ministry of Health supervises health care providers based on norms and standards. The Central Office of the Ministry includes the Medical, Nursing, and Pharmacological Inspectorates; the Legal Department; the Planning Department; and a General Administrative Department. To support the Ministry's leadership and advocacy roles, a National Health Council will be established in the 1997–2001 period. The policy will give the Inspectorates more autonomy in controlling service quality.

Organization of Health Regulatory Activities

Health legislation is outdated and, except for a few changes in laws regulating pharmacies, there have been only ad hoc and minor adaptations. Updating legislation is a priority, especially in the areas of strengthening the control functions of the Ministry of Health, and the establishment of a National Health Council. The Legal Department of the Ministry of Health is charged with coordinating efforts with the Ministry of Justice and the Permanent Commission on Health in the National Assembly to update health legislation and to provide a comprehensive legal framework for health systems development. This will include the formulation of new laws and regulations regarding: licensing and registration of medical and paramedical professionals; reporting communicable diseases, especially AIDS and HIV infections; the role of the Inspectorates; environmental protection; the use, advertising, and sale of alcohol, cigarettes, and other drugs; institutionalization for behavioral disorders; and the importation of drugs, reagents, and medical technologies. A revision of the "Public Morality Act" to permit the promotion of condoms and the regulation of prostitution is also a priority. There is also a need for legislation that protects drinking water resources by regulating mining activities, dumping of waste, the use of surface water, etc.

Registration and certification of physicians, midwives, and pharmacists and their assistants is regulated and supervised by the Ministry of Health. Physicians are licensed by the Ministry and need permission from the Director of Health for clinical practice. Other health professions are not recognized or regulated.

The Pharmaceutical Inspectorate enforces laws on the registration and importation of drugs and vaccines. There are no regulations regarding technologies. The Public Health Laboratory of the Bureau of Public Health is responsible for quality control of food and other products, including drinking water.

The Environmental Inspectorate of the Bureau is responsible for inspection of restaurants, food-handlers, food processing companies, and public as well as private sanitary systems, including the disposal of solid wastes and sewage.

Health Services and Resources

Organization of Services for Care of the Population

Disease Prevention and Control. The Bureau of Public Health is the main organization for health care and includes a health education department, an epidemiology and biostatistics department, and several programs for family health and disease control. The Bureau has about 400 employees, of whom 20 have university degrees.

The Bureau of Public Health provides information on disease distribution through its epidemiology unit, which operates a surveillance system on communicable diseases in cooperation with the Regional Health Service. The system depends on weekly reports of 27 sentinel reporting stations. Other organizations with disease control activities and health promotion are the Dermatologische Dienst of the Ministry of Health, the Veterinary Service of the Ministry of Agriculture, the so-called "Cross Associations" (nongovernmental organizations with well-baby clinics), and foundations such as Stichting Lobi and the Youth Dental Service Foundation.

The Dermatologische Dienst has the following goals: the control of STDs and HIV/AIDS; the elimination of leprosy by the year 2000 (an official policy target of the Ministry of Health); and the control of dermatological conditions such as yaws, leishmaniasis, and other communicable diseases. Services are provided through a central polyclinic in Paramaribo, the district hospital in Nickerie, and the district health center in Wonoredjo.

Each year, the Dermatologische Dienst handles 24,000 patient visits and performs 46,000 laboratory tests. Between 25% and 30% of visits are due to STDs, and only 7% have been related to leprosy. The institution offers syphilis serology for the hospitals (except the Academic Hospital), the blood transfusion service, and the Regional Health Service. It employs 3 dermatologists; 1 general physician; 18 registered nurses; 2 social workers; and 21 administrative, technical, and housekeeping personnel.

Family Planning. The Stichting Lobi foundation promotes family planning and the prevention of cervical cancer deaths. Priority target groups are adolescents, young adults, and inhabitants of the Interior. Stichting Lobi estimates that of 80,000 men and 84,000 women, 45% need family planning services, which would require some 470,000 rounds of the contraceptive pill and 5 million condoms per year. It currently distributes 320,000 rounds of oral contraceptives and 550,000 condoms, or 68% and 11%, respectively, of the estimated needs. Stichting Lobi also screens women for cervical cancer, with 10,000 to 12,000 Pap tests yearly. It is planning to organize a countrywide program allowing women to have free Pap tests during a period of three years. Stichting Lobi aims to expand its services to people covered by the State Health Insurance Fund. Expenditures in 1995 were US$ 489,783, covered by income from grants, sales, client fees, and fundraising.

Oral Health. The Youth Dental Service Foundation promotes dental health by providing free dental care to children 0–17 years of age. In 1996, a total of 207,516 activities were carried out, including 33,738 dental extractions. The Foundation operates a training center and 30 dental clinics in the periphery (10 located in health centers and 20 in schools). In 1996, the Foundation employed 63 dental nurses and 38 dental assistants and had a budget of US$ 340,000, receiving an additional US$ 500,000 from the Ministry of Health.

Water Supply, Sewerage Systems, and Solid Waste Disposal. The Ministry of Public Works is responsible for collection and disposal of solid wastes and construction and certification of sewage systems. The policy is to privatize garbage collection services and to set up a semi-private "Sewage Authority" to take care of sewage systems.

The Suriname Water Company and the Ministry of Natural Resources are responsible for the establishment and operation of piped drinking water networks. The Ministry of Natural Resources operates small local systems in the districts and in the Interior. The company covers Paramaribo and parts of Wanica, Nickerie, and Albina; it also serves a strip of 500 meters on both sides of the 50-km road connecting Paramaribo and the International Airport in Zandery. The provision of drinking water by the company increased to about 22,220,000 liters in 1996. The Paramaribo Water Supply Project, which started in 1994, will provide a sufficient supply of drinking water to every home in Paramaribo. Long-term policy is to have one drinking water system for the entire coastal area. The Suriname Water Company will take over rural areas that are now serviced by the Ministry of Natural Resources, including the Moengo area.

Organization and Operation of Personal Health Care Services

Approximately 89% of households are within 5 km of a polyclinic or health post and 60% use them on a regular basis. Institutions and organizations providing primary care include the Regional Health Service, the Medical Mission, private practices, polyclinics of private companies, the emergency department of the Academic Hospital, the Dermatologische Di-

enst, the Youth Dental Service Foundation, the Bureau of Medical Psychology (a department of the Bureau of Public Health), and the disease control clinics of the Bureau of Public Health.

The Regional Health Service, a semi-private, government-subsidized institution, provides health care for the poor in the coastal areas. It serves 120,000 people covered by the Ministry of Social Affairs and Housing and another 25,000 covered by the State Health Insurance Fund. It offers free service for immunizations, counseling, family planning (in cooperation with Stichting Lobi), and dental services for schools (in cooperation with the Youth Dental Service Foundation). The number of patients covered by the Ministry of Social Affairs and Housing increased from 78,448 in 1991 to 93,124 in 1995. Visits made by these patients more than doubled, from approximately 200,000 per year in the 1991–1994 period to more than 400,000 in 1995. Visits by State Health Insurance patients also doubled from 50,000 visits per year in the 1991–1994 period to more than 100,000 in 1995. It is not clear whether this increase reflects improved administrative procedures or increased utilization of services.

The Regional Health Service operates 11 health centers offering medical, pharmaceutical, and laboratory services, and clinics for children under age 5; 27 polyclinics offering medical and pharmaceutical services and clinics for children under age 5; and 19 auxiliary posts located in villages in the districts and operated by visiting doctors and nurses a few days per month. The Regional Health Service employs 55 doctors, 20 assistant-physicians, 48 nurses, 59 nursing auxiliaries, 28 nursing-assistants, 39 pharmacy assistants, 10 laboratory technicians, 15 trained midwives, and about 250 administrative and support staff. The operational costs were US$ 2.2 million in 1996 and US$ 3.2 million in 1997. Special projects of the Service receive financial and technical assistance from the Dutch Government and PAHO. One such project is the "Global Restructuring Project," which involves restructuring the Regional Health Service, emphasizing decentralization of managerial authority to district health centers, and community participation through local and regional health councils. The project also covers the renovation of 32 polyclinics and personnel housing in the districts. The policy of the Regional Health Service is to reopen all polyclinics and to expand their numbers in the Commewijne River area.

The Medical Mission is a private, nonprofit organization that receives government subsidies and acts as an umbrella organization for missionary foundations. It aims to develop an affordable health care system based on the needs of the community and the promotion of health awareness. The Ministry of Health assigned the Medical Mission with the responsibility for all medical care in the Interior. The target population of the Medical Mission is 48,500 (80% Bushnegroes and 20% Amerindians). With the gold rush in the Interior, many urbanites and foreigners have entered the territory.

The Medical Mission employs 170 persons, including 4 physicians, 6 registered nurses, and 62 "health assistants." After four years of training, the health assistants play a central role in the system; they are able to recognize and treat common health problems, assist in uncomplicated deliveries, and promote disease prevention and healthy lifestyles. The Medical Mission has a coordinating office in Paramaribo and operates 45 health posts, including 6 clinics in the Interior. It maintains a logistical support system with canoes, road vehicles, airlift services provided by the Missionary Aviation Fellowship, and CB radio between clinics and the central office.

There are four general hospitals in Paramaribo and one in Nickerie. There is one psychiatric hospital. In January 1996, there were 3.1 beds per 1,000 population: 387 in Academic Hospital, 304 in s'Lands Hospital, 227 in Diakonessenhuis Hospital, 287 in St. Vincentius Hospital (a Roman Catholic hospital), and 60 in Nickerie District Hospital. In 1989, the combined occupancy rate of the four major hospitals in Paramaribo was 62%, a rate that increased slightly to 67% in 1995. The average length of hospitalization decreased from 11 days in 1989 to 10 in 1995.

The Academic Hospital supports a smaller, "dependent" hospital with 50 beds for chronically ill patients, drawing patients from the coastal area. Patients can be admitted after referral by general practitioners.

Academic Hospital is the only hospital with a department for emergency medicine. In 1994, 33,131 patients were admitted to the emergency unit and in 1996 there were 33,959 admissions. The number of deliveries at the hospital rose from 746 in 1995 to 894 in 1996. The operational costs for the hospital were about US$ 7.4 million in 1996.

The s'Lands Hospital has several special functions. Almost one-half of all babies are delivered in this hospital (4,269 in 1995). The Mother and Child Health Department offers prenatal services and provides women with Pap tests. The hospital also performs renal dialysis (in cooperation with the Kidney Foundation). Of 8,705 patients admitted in 1995, 60% were covered by the Ministry of Social Affairs, and 24% by the State Health Insurance Fund. Operating costs for s'Lands Hospital were US$ 3.2 million in 1996.

Diakonessenhuis Hospital has 100 beds reserved for patients of the Medical Mission; in 1996, there were 559 admissions from the Interior. In 1994, 1,385 babies were delivered at this hospital. The hospital has a policy of linking hospital with primary level services and maintains a general polyclinic that is open to the public until 11 p.m. and on weekends. It has a department for community and home-based care to limit the duration of stay in the hospital. The hospital also established a day-care center on its premises. Diakonessenhuis Hospital operational costs in 1996 were about US$ 2.8 million.

About 1,300 babies were born in St. Vincentius Hospital in 1992. The neonatology unit is a special feature of this hospital. In 1996, 60% of admitted patients were covered by the State Health Insurance Fund, and fewer than 8% by the Ministry of Social Affairs and Housing. The hospital had a budget of US$ 3.7 million in 1996.

Nickerie District Hospital has an operating room, an obstetrics department, an X-ray facility, and a medical laboratory. The hospital was renovated in 1993–1996 with a loan of US$ 8 million from the Inter-American Development Bank. The major problem faced by this hospital is the lack of medical specialists.

The s'Lands Psychiatrische Inrichting, the 300-bed psychiatric hospital, is a division of the Ministry of Health. Its facilities include a ward for crisis intervention (short-stay patients), a ward for forensic psychiatry, and a pavilion for psychogeriatric and chronic patients.

Inputs for Health

The State Pharmaceutical Company is the central importer, producer, and distributor of drugs and medical supplies. It maintains 14 pharmacists and 15 pharmacies, and the Regional Health Service has 32 additional auxiliary pharmacies at its facilities. Some 2,150,000 pharmacy prescriptions were processed in 1990 and 2,525,000 in 1996. The Company sold US$ 3.9 million worth of drugs and US$ 740,000 in other supplies in 1996.

The Cancer Foundation developed a project to set up an orthovoltage radiotherapy unit for cancer patients and submitted it for Dutch Treaty Fund financing. The project for the provision of essential drugs will be expanded to include drugs for chemotherapy. Also on the drawing board is a project to set up a unit for angiograms in the Academic Hospital.

A program for the supply of medical equipment and consumables is being implemented with financing through the Dutch Treaty Funds. As part of the program, quality control and local production of drugs are upgraded, and standard lists are assembled for different categories of supplies. Suriname is following the essential drugs policy advocated by WHO, and has developed a national formulary. Better maintenance of medical equipment was achieved through the establishment in 1993 of a Joint Technical Unit, with the contribution of all hospitals and laboratories. With help from the Belgian Government, the infrastructure of the Joint Technical Unit is being improved.

Currently there is an arrangement for sending patients to the Netherlands for medical procedures not performed in Suriname. The State Health Insurance Foundation has paid an average of US$ 20,000 per case (with assistance from the

Netherlands). The 1996 budget was designed for 200 such cases. The policy is to decrease this need by improving facilities in Paramaribo. Since an argon laser was installed in the Academic Hospital, patients no longer went to the Netherlands for laser treatments. The capacity for open-heart surgery will be established in cooperation with the Academic Hospital of the University of Leiden and visiting Dutch medical teams. Also needed are facilities for a heart catheterization center, the establishment of an oncology team, and decentralization of renal dialysis services.

Human Resources

A 1996 study by the Planning Bureau of the Ministry of Planning and Technical Cooperation found that there are about 500 vacancies for personnel with university degrees at the central offices of Government Ministries (not including vacancies in the field). There were shortages of nurses, medical specialists, pharmacists, dentists, veterinarians, dieticians, nutritionists, physiotherapists, psychologists, pharmacy assistants, laboratory analysts, and environmental health inspectors. According to the Planning Bureau, in the past five years 33% of 567 health care professionals left the sector or the country (primarily senior nurses and medical specialists). Many professionals will retire in the next decade: 64% are 50 years or older. The lack of public health professionals able to make the necessary analyses and reports undermines the functional and leadership capacity of the Ministry of Health.

The health sector employed approximately 5,100 people in 1992, including administrative and other support personnel. About 70% were government employees. In 1996, there were 190 general practitioners, 95 medical specialists, 20 psychologists, 31 dentists, 9 veterinarians, 24 laboratory analysts, 13 physiotherapists, 14 pharmacists, 3 dieticians/nutritionists, and 81 nurses with university degrees. There were also 550 auxiliary nurses, 40 midwives, 95 pharmacy assistants, 27 X-ray technicians, and 63 dental nurses.

In 1993, 9 physicians graduated from the Medical School of the University of Suriname, 15 graduated in 1994, 8 in 1995, and 22 in 1996, after finishing a seven-year curriculum. The Central School of Nursing and the intramural training programs of the Academic Hospital and St. Vincentius Hospital are training nurses and nursing auxiliaries, but the programs cannot keep up with the demand. The duration of courses is four years for registered nurses and three years for auxiliaries. In 1996, 80 enrolled for the registered nurse course and 135 for the nurse auxiliary course. The Nursing School has a new study program for a bachelor's degree in Nursing. There are plans to shift responsibility for the Nursing School from the Ministry of Health to the Ministry of Education. By ending

the requirement that applicants be working in a hospital, the numbers of applicants should increase.

The Youth Dental Service Foundation has a training program for dental nurses. Of the more than 120 dental nurses trained since 1976 (about 80% of all students), only 63 were still working for the Foundation in 1997. After a temporary interruption in 1995–1996, the program admitted 12 new trainees.

The Medical Mission has a special training program for health assistants, and Stichting Lobi has one for midwives. About 10 to 15 registered nursing students are admitted each year. The duration of the course is three years. The Bureau of Public Health also has a training program for environmental inspectors.

The University of Suriname introduced a public health curriculum in 1992–1993 to strengthen the primary health care orientation of medical students. A "skills lab" was started in 1995 to improve teaching methods. The University also initiated a course for physiotherapists in 1996 with 15 students.

Expenditures and Sectoral Financing

In the 1991–1996 period, the Ministry of Health accounted for 4% of government expenditures. In 1996, government expenditures were US$ 210 million. More than one-half of Ministry of Health disbursements were for personnel, while other general costs accounted for 25%. Total national spending on health care (government and private combined) was estimated at US$ 40 million in 1996, 8% of GDP. Of this amount, the Government financed at least 62%. The Ministry of Health (including the Central Office, Bureau of Public Health, Dermatologische Dienst, and the psychiatric hospital) received US$ 8,128,100. Subsidies to the Medical Mission amounted to US$ 985,500; to the Youth Dental Service Foundation, US$ 492,600; and to the Central Nursing School, US$ 123,200. Compensation of financial shortfalls for the Regional Health Service cost US$ 1,283,300; for s'Lands Hospital, US$ 206,900; for Academic Hospital, US$ 194,600; and for Nickerie District Hospital, US$ 51,700. The Ministry of Social Affairs and Housing received US$ 8,620,700 and the Ministry of Finance received US$ 13,546,800 (for the State Health Insurance Fund). Private sector expenditures on health care amounted to US$ 18,472,300.

External Technical and Financial Cooperation

The major international and bilateral partners in the development of the health sector are the Governments of the Netherlands and Belgium, PAHO, United Nations Children's Fund (UNICEF), and IDB.

Some of the most important projects developed through technical and financial cooperation include: (1) reorganization of the Bureau of Public Health, using Dutch Treaty Funds; (2) the Drugs and Medical Supplies Project, financed through Dutch Treaty Funds; (3) restructuring the Regional Health Service, financed through Dutch Treaty Funds and PAHO; (4) the Malaria Control Program financed by Dutch Treaty Funds and PAHO; (5) treatment of patients overseas; (6) the National AIDS Program, a project supported by the European Union and PAHO; (7) the Tuberculosis Control Program, supported by PAHO; (8) the National Immunization Program, supported by PAHO and UNICEF; and (9) the maternal and child health program supported by PAHO and UNICEF.

TRINIDAD AND TOBAGO

GENERAL SITUATION AND TRENDS

Socioeconomic, Political, and Demographic Overview

Trinidad and Tobago is a twin-island State situated at the southern end of the Caribbean chain of islands. Having gained its independence in August 1962, the country is a democratic republic within the British Commonwealth. Tobago is administered separately by the Tobago House of Assembly, which was established in 1980. Trinidad is currently organized into 13 administrative areas or Regional Corporations as set up under the 1981 Regional Corporation Act. Most official data, however, continue to be reported by the original eight Counties and three Municipal Corporations because there have been delays in establishing all of the Regional Corporations.

Since the 1960s, the economy has been characterized by heavy dependence on the production and export of petroleum and gas. Per capita GNP peaked in 1982 at US$ 6,600, followed by sharp contractions until 1988, when the Government implemented an economic reform program. The lowest per capita GNP of US$ 3,160 was recorded in 1989. Since then there has been steady improvement—primarily due to measures of trade and currency liberalization; diversification strategies into agriculture, manufacturing (non-oil), and tourism; and restructuring, divestment, and liquidation of a number of State enterprises. In addition, a tax reform program introduced a 15% value-added tax and reduction of personal and corporate taxes, tighter control of public expenditure and reduction of the fiscal deficit, and increases in public utilities tariffs. In 1994 the GNP was US$ 3,740.

The currency value has remained fairly stable since the floating of the dollar in 1993 (from TT$ 5.40 to TT$ 6.30= US$ 1). There has been, however, slippage of about 10% between mid-1996 and mid-1997. Inflation rates, as measured by the change in the index of retail prices, declined to about 3.2% for 1996. In keeping with this economic recovery, there has been a reversal of the unemployment trends because of in-

creases in the non-oil sectors of tourism and other service industries. The labor force is growing (521,000 in 1995 from 467,700 in 1990), with declining unemployment rates (17% in 1995 from 20% in 1990) and growing participation rates (60% in 1995 from 56% in 1990). Among women, unemployment rates are higher (23% compared with 19% for men), and participation rates are lower (45% for women compared with 75% for men), probably due to lower levels of education, sociocultural factors, and a difficult employment situation. Approximately 22% of households have no employed participant.

Over the period of Trinidad's economic recession (1982–1989), the available data indicate an increase in the levels of poverty—from 3.5% of households in 1981 to 14.8% in 1988. While it is difficult to measure the impact of the Government's structural adjustment program on the welfare of the population, it is likely to have resulted in a decline in living standards and an increase in unemployment. Recent estimates indicate that poverty levels continued to increase from 1988 to current levels of 21%–22% of the population, with a further widening in the distribution of income. About half of these are individuals classified as extremely poor—those unable to afford the cost of a minimum food basket.

Poverty is evenly divided between urban and rural areas, although the severity of poverty is worse in urban areas. Almost one-half of the poor live in Saint George County. In urban areas, the economic pressures of the poor, coupled with high youth unemployment, have contributed to growing problems of crime and drug use—the problem is particularly acute among young males.

There has been a steady and significant improvement in the level of educational attainment in the population. In 1970, approximately 8% of the population had no education and by 1990, this had been reduced to about 3%. Between 1980 and 1990 there was a steady increase in the percentage of both men and women achieving secondary (from 32.7% to 44.4%) and tertiary (from 2.2% to 2.9%) education levels. The adult literacy rates also testify to sustained achievement (94% and

96% for 1970 and 1980, respectively). There is, however, growing concern about functional literacy.

The revised 1995 mid-year population estimate is 1,259,971 based on the 1990 census population of 1,238,800 and an average annual growth rate of 1.1% over the period 1990–1994 (down from 1.27% in the 1985–1989 period). The male-to-female ratio is 101:100. The slowing of population growth is partly due to declines in the total fertility rate (2.4) and crude birth rate (from 19.7 in 1990 to 15.8 in 1995), a stable crude death rate (6.7 in 1990 and 7.1 in 1995), and stabilized emigration between 1980 and 1990 (estimated at 131,918).

These trends are also reflected in a more constrictive-shaped population pyramid: 33.5% of the population is under 15 years of age and 6% are over 65. Based on present trends, however, the expectation is that by 2015 the age group under 15 years old will fall to 23.9%, with the group over age 65 increasing to 7.5% of the total population. Nearly 72% of the population is considered urban.

The ethnic composition of Trinidad and Tobago consists of almost equal proportions of persons of African and East Indian descent—approximately 40% each. The remaining 20% is made up mainly of persons of mixed ethnicity (18.5%) and less than 2% of all other groups (Caucasian, Chinese, and "other" or not stated). There are significant differences by county—persons of African descent are most predominant in Tobago (92%) and in Saint George (50%); persons of Indian descent are predominant in Caroni (67%) and Victoria (62%). Between 1980 and 1990, every ethnic group showed a decline in representation except the mixed ethnic group, which increased from 16.3% in 1980 to 18.5% in 1990—an increase of approximately 13%.

Mortality and Morbidity Profile

Life expectancy at birth continues to increase; in 1990, the figure was 72.7 years for females and 69.3 for males. Between 1980 and 1990, much of the gain in life expectancy at birth was, however, in the under-15 age group, with less than a one-year gain at age 65.

A major reason for the improvement in overall life expectancy over the last 30 years has been the drop in infant mortality from 110 per 1,000 live births in the 1940s to 21.7 per 1,000 in the 1980s, and 18 per 1,000 live births in the 1990s. In addition, the mortality rate for the 1–4-year age group remained fairly stable over the 1985–1995 period, at around 4.8 per 100,000 population.

Mortality by the broad groups of causes is ranked as follows (percentages shown are for 1994 data): diseases of the circulatory system (39.7%), tumors (13.4%), diabetes (12.5%), external causes (7.3%), communicable diseases (5.6%), and certain conditions originating in the perinatal period (1.9%).

Treatment for common diseases is readily available from a network of 101 health centers, 7 hospitals, and approximately 400 private general practitioners. At the point of access, government centers are free, including diagnostic and pharmaceutical supplies. However, two major national surveys, the 1992 Survey of Living Conditions and the 1995 National Health Survey, show that persons seek care in the private sector (45% and 43%, respectively, by survey) or public hospitals (36% and 19%, respectively) significantly more than at the government health centers (9% and 22%, respectively).

The 1995 National Health Survey was conducted as part of the pre-implementation work for the health sector reform program. It was principally designed to fill the data gap about the overall health status of adults and therefore focused on those 15 years old and over. The results are intended for use as baseline information on health needs, morbidity, and patterns of service utilization in conjunction with routine information collected by public sector facilities. The survey contacted 3,240 households and interviewed 6,342 adults, with a response rate of 97.7%. Only persons 35 years and over were questioned about diabetes, hypertension, and heart disease. Responses were based on self-reported disease.

The survey showed that whereas acute symptoms were reported by 38% of the population, chronic conditions affected health status and health behavior to a greater extent. Injury, for example, did not emerge as a major problem until it became a long-standing condition. Chronic or long-standing conditions appear to cause the most burdens in terms of health status. The 1995 survey also showed that the variable that most affected the choice of provider and the cost of health care was a chronic medical condition.

SPECIFIC HEALTH PROBLEMS

Analysis by Population Group

Health of Children

The infant mortality rate in 1994 was 13.8 per 1,000 live births. Problems with underreporting of infant deaths, particularly in the neonatal period, have been identified and plans have been implemented to strengthen the reporting system by: (1) agreement on the procedures for reporting stillbirths and births of gestational age greater than or equal to 28 weeks, and (2) improving the completion of death certificates.

The implementation of "baby friendly" initiatives in the hospitals has improved the prevalence of breast-feeding. In 1995, about 43% of infants attending health centers were totally breast-fed for at least 1 month and 25% for at least 3.

Immunization programs are well organized and continue to have consistently high rates of success and coverage. The programs are also well monitored, and given the high national attendance at primary school level, they benefit from being linked to criteria for admittance to school. Dropouts and missed opportunities are usually picked up at this stage. Polio and DTP immunizations start at 3 months of age, and measles and yellow fever inoculations are given by age 2 years.

Improvements in socioeconomic conditions, environmental conditions, and access to child health services (free in the public sector) have influenced the dramatic fall in both mortality and morbidity in the 1–4-year age group. In 1994, the mortality rate for this age group was 4.8 per 100,000 population. In that year, 16.6% of deaths were due to external causes.

There is low prevalence of satisfactory breast-feeding practices for infants under 1 year old, and areas of malnutrition and poor coverage of routine screening for children between 2 and 5 years old are suspected to be on the rise. Morbidity reports from public sector clinics show no significant change in recent years. Skin complaints (32%) and acute respiratory tract infections (18.8%) are the most common reasons for visits at this age. Diarrhea is reported more often as a recurrent event on the communicable disease surveillance system (15,355 cases in 1994).

First visits to clinics by infants in the first and second years of life amount to about 80% of the target population, but at 2 years of age, coverage is less than 50%. The mean number of visits by infants under 1 year is 4.2, sufficient to produce adequate immunization; 20% of infants are visited at home. On average, each child attends a clinic 1.7 times between the ages of 1 and 4 years.

Deaths from external causes account for approximately 42.8% of male deaths and 22.7% of female deaths in the 5–14-year age group. Neoplasms account for 14.3% of male deaths and 11.4% of female deaths, while communicable diseases account for 6.1% mortality in males and 15.9% in females. Children in this age group make few contacts with the health services, except for illness and immunization.

The school health service has inadequate resources and is currently under review. Programs geared to prevent HIV/STDs and teenage pregnancy, and to promote nutrition and physical activity start at the primary school level. While there are sporadic attempts by the Health Education Department, Ministry of Health, and some NGOs, these programs are not sustained. The Ministry of Education, through its family life programs and other projects such as the "Youth Self-Esteem Project," is doing more in this area.

Health of Adults

The major contributor to mortality in young adults 15–24 years old is external causes, accounting for 64.1% of deaths in males and 32.9% in females. Mortality rates for motor vehicle accidents, drowning, homicide, and suicide contribute equally to male deaths in this age group. Among females, however, homicides and suicides are responsible for 67.8% of these deaths. Neoplasms account for 10.6% of deaths in males and 6.3% in females.

Morbidity reports for this age group are not available. Incomplete data from HIV/STD services indicate that STD rates have not declined. Teenage pregnancy rates are high in urban areas (13.5% of all live and stillbirth deliveries were to teenagers, with an age-specific fertility rate of 45.9%). Data from the National Drug Abuse Unit indicate increasing rates of marijuana and cocaine use in this age group. These data are based on reports of the police and health services.

In 1994, among adults aged 25 to 44 years old, approximately 31.2% of male deaths were due to external causes (motor vehicle accidents, 18.3%; suicide, 24.8%; and homicide, 31.7%). Circulatory diseases caused 14.2% of deaths from defined causes. The leading causes of female deaths were distributed as follows: circulatory diseases (20.1%), communicable diseases (5.6%), cancer (19.1%), and deaths from external causes (13.2%). The 1995 National Health Survey indicated disability prevalence rates of 12.5% in males and 15.2% in females; prevalence of self-reported diabetes and hypertension of 3% and 11%, respectively (in the 35–44-year age group); 13% prevalence of a history of injury in males and 7% in females; and mental illness reported in 4.5% of males and 6% of females.

Circulatory diseases dominated the mortality profile among older adults (45–64 years old) in 1994, accounting for 39.8% of deaths in males and 39.5% in females. Diabetes ranks second for both males and females (17% in males and 21.2% in females). Cancer is also an important cause of death in this age group (20.5% in females, 12.1% in males). Although deaths due to external causes were proportionally less, these accounted for 9.1% of deaths in males and 2.2% in females.

Health of the Elderly

Although the elderly (age 65 and older) currently represent only 6% of the population, the proportion is growing. The principal causes of death in this age group are circulatory diseases (46.8% in men and 51.2% among females), neoplasms (15.4% in men and 11.8% in females), and diabetes (11.7% in men and 14.9% in women).

In the 1995 National Health Survey, 49% of persons over age 65 reported that they had a chronic condition that limited their usual activities. The data show that 12% reported severe pain, 33% were limited in their social activities, 27% had difficulty carrying parcels, 12% had difficulty walking 10 yards, 5% had a problem dressing, 36% had difficulty reading, 19% had a hearing problem, and 23% had a memory or learning disability.

Family Health

The delivery of family planning services is shared mainly by the Ministry of Health—as an integral part of its maternal and child health program in health centers and in postnatal wards and clinics of hospitals—and by the Family Planning Association of Trinidad and Tobago, an NGO. With the collaboration of the Ministry of Education, both agencies carry out targeted public education programs and family life education programs in schools.

Since 1989, clinics of both the Family Planning Association and the Ministry of Health have recorded a decreasing number of new family planning acceptors. This trend has been most marked with regard to adults, among whom the figure for new attendance at health centers and family planning clinics totaled 29,805 in 1995, a decrease of nearly 30% from 1993. The range of contraceptive methods available is limited. The most popular method remains condoms, followed by oral and injectable hormonal methods; the IUD is not widely used. Sterilizations requested at the Family Planning Association are mostly for women, although a few vasectomies are performed. Consistent supplies of contraceptives are a problem in the health centers.

Health of the Disabled

Based on the 1995 survey, 22% of the population 15 years old and over have some disability. Chronic medical conditions contributed to 40% of this disability for the age group under 65 years and 60% for those older than 65 years. Disability has a significant effect on the reporting of health status and a profound one on employment, income, need for care, utilization and many variations of health status. Specific types of disability were also measured. Visual disability affecting reading was high across the whole population (14% in males and 20% in females). Hearing disability affected 6.3% of females and 4.5% of males. As expected, disability as a whole increased to 50% for those over age 65 and increased markedly for each type of disability.

Analysis by Type of Disease or Health Impairment

Communicable Diseases

Communicable diseases are still an important cause of death and morbidity in Trinidad and Tobago, causing 7% of deaths. They are the second most frequent cause of admission to acute-stay hospitals (8%).

Vector-Borne Diseases. Surveillance of mosquito-borne diseases has been stepped up in 1996–1997, particularly as it applies to the control of dengue and dengue hemorrhagic fever. Emphasis has been on community-based interventions rather than insecticide control.

Although dengue is transmitted by vector, the vector's association with water storage is a factor contributing to its endemic aspect. There is poor coverage in terms of potable water supply and efficient wastewater treatment. The Water and Sewerage Authority continues to work with the other agencies to improve this situation but the solutions are largely determined by the necessity to invest large sums of money in the national infrastructure.

Vaccine-Preventable Diseases. Free routine immunization of infants and children is offered in all health centers. In accordance with PAHO protocol, antigens are administered in the first year of life. Coverage for DTP and polio (three completed doses) was 90% in 1995. Yellow fever, measles, mumps, and rubella (MMR) vaccines are given in the second year. In 1995, 89% of the target population received MMR vaccination, while 83% of 1-year-olds received yellow fever vaccines. Booster shots are given according to schedules at all schools. Pregnant women receive tetanus boosters as needed. BCG is not given routinely. A national measles vaccination campaign in 1997 achieved 95% coverage of the target population (children 1–14 years old).

Hepatitis A is endemic, with occasional epidemic outbreaks.

Cholera and Other Intestinal Diseases. Surveillance of diarrheal disease has been stepped up since 1991, when cholera began to reemerge in the Americas. In 1997, the cholera prevention campaign was reactivated after new cases were identified in nearby coastal areas in Venezuela. Trinidad and Tobago has remained cholera-free.

There are relatively few deaths that can be directly attributed to poor environmental sanitation. Outbreaks of communicable diseases, however, still occur from time to time. Although there has been a reduction in mortality from diarrhea, a steady rate of reported cases continues. Both viral and bacterial diarrheas are prevalent.

Acute Respiratory Infections. Influenza and gastroenteritis are the most frequently reported diseases to the National Surveillance Unit. Influenza reports are not laboratory confirmed and may include other types of acute respiratory infections.

Rabies. Surveillance for bat-transmitted rabies continues and involves the veterinary public health unit of the Ministry of Health.

AIDS and Other STDs. The AIDS epidemic continues to cause premature deaths among young (20–35-year-olds), sexually active males and females, and the children of HIV-positives (accounting for 71%, 7%, and 7.2%, respectively, of total AIDS deaths from 1983 to 1995). The pattern of this disease in Trinidad and Tobago is that of heterosexual transmission (51.9% of cases in 1983–1995). Incidence rates are still rising (from 14.0 per 100,000 population in 1990 to 27.2 per 100,000 in 1995) as are the laboratory-reported HIV-positives (from 31.4 per 100,000 in 1990 to 53.4 per 100,000 in 1992), and this trend is expected to continue. Hospital costs are difficult to estimate, as only 1,077 patient days were attributed to AIDS in 1990.

It is important to note that other STDs among adolescents may be on the increase along with HIV incidence, making the efficiency of the STD surveillance system an important factor in controlling AIDS. Unpublished data from the Department of Pediatrics, Port-of-Spain General Hospital, indicate that many women discover they are HIV-positive only after their child is diagnosed as such. The possibility of prenatal testing for women is under consideration.

Data on STDs come from government STD clinics, and they are generally underreported. Crude rates for both syphilis and gonorrhea have declined over the past 10 years. Gonorrhea cases have declined from 311 in 1985 to 160 in 1994 for both sexes. When the rates are disaggregated by age and sex, males in the 15–24-year age group have the highest rates. These figures continue to be a source of concern.

In 1991, there were 1,153 admissions due to pelvic inflammatory disease in acute care hospitals. This disease is not reported under the communicable disease surveillance system.

Noncommunicable Diseases and Other Health-Related Problems

A 1990 study on chronic diseases indicated that tobacco, alcohol, exercise, and nutrition were the risk factors needing most attention. Data from the 1995 National Health Survey indicate that chronic diseases cause the greatest impact on the health sector by increasing health service demand, increasing disability, and curtailing the ability to choose a provider.

Nutritional Diseases and Diseases of Metabolism. The best data available on the nutritional status of children came from a national survey of primary school entrants in 1989–1990. Because these are the results of a single survey, they must be interpreted with caution. It appears that severe malnutrition is uncommon in Trinidad and Tobago, but that selected areas have high rates of moderate stunting and wasting.

The food available to the population is sufficient to meet its basic needs with an excess of energy (30%), protein (60%), and fat (50%). Information is insufficient regarding current consumption patterns. Three surveys have shown that a body-mass index >30 is about 40% for females and 20% for males. The 1995 National Health Survey reports that the poor tend to choose more full-cream milk, fewer green vegetables, and more white flour. Iron deficiency is still too high among women of reproductive age and young children.

A national nutrition policy focusing on the prevention of noncommunicable diseases is being formulated. According to the 1995 National Health Survey, 72% of respondents reported that they always added salt during food preparation and 19.6% said they sometimes did, which makes potential excessive salt intake a matter of concern.

Diabetes mellitus is increasing in prevalence (self-reported diabetes was 11% in the adult population 35 years old and older), with mortality rates increasing from 48.6 per 100,000 population in 1977 to 80.5 in 1990. It is the third-ranking cause of death for males and the second-ranking cause of death for females. The St. James Cardiovascular Study found that East Indian males had higher prevalence rates (1 in 6) than East Indian females and other ethnic groups (1 in 10).

Over 90% of diabetics in Trinidad are non-insulin dependent. While there is a strong genetic influence, research indicates that early obesity is the avoidable risk factor needing mitigation if incidence is to be reduced. Case fatality rates were high according to the St. James study. Almost 50% of diabetic deaths take place before age 65. Despite the high prevalence, hospital and community service clinics appear to have low proportions of diabetics among their attendees, but this may be due to the tendency to code only the main condition for which the patient seeks care.

In the 1995 National Health Survey, 80% of self-reported diabetics reported that they were limited in their activities. Disability was three times more common in diabetics than in non-diabetics. Diabetics were also 3.3 times more likely to have used health services than non-diabetics, and 4.2 times more likely to have received a prescription in the last 12 months.

Cardiovascular Diseases. Heart disease is the highest-ranking cause of death in Trinidad and Tobago, causing over 3,000 deaths per year. High prevalence rates of diabetes and hypertension are contributing factors. Smoking prevalence is lower than it is in North America (30% in males and 7% in females, according to the 1995 National Health Survey), but the number of schoolchildren who experiment with smoking is high.

In addition to high prevalence for hypertension and diabetes, the mean body-mass index is high and regular exercise indicators are low (2% in the 1995 National Health Survey).

According to the 1995 survey, only 64% of respondents aged 35 years and older had had a blood-pressure check in the last 12 months and only 16% had ever had a cholesterol test. There is no coordinated national program aimed at primary prevention, but several NGOs run screening programs aimed at secondary prevention. Except for some funding from international organizations, most of the funding applied to chronic disease goes into treatment.

Malignant Tumors. Cancer has been the second ranking cause of mortality since 1987, with a rate of 94.9 per 100,000 population in 1990. These rates have been increasing since the 1960s. When rates are adjusted for age, the only cancers showing significant increase are prostate, breast, and lung; there is a significant decline in cervical cancer.

Cancer is the leading cause of death before age 65 in females (accounting for 16% of all female deaths under age 65 in 1994) because of the earlier age of onset of cervical and breast cancers. Breast cancer mortality rates have been increasing (17.6 per 100,000 population in 1990 to 19.5 in 1994), while cervical cancer rates have been declining (9.1 in 1990 to 7.3 in 1994). Cervical cancer screening is generally unavailable at government clinics, but NGOs such as the Cancer Society and the Family Planning Association provide services at subsidized rates. According to the 1995 survey, only 43% of female respondents aged 35 and older had ever had a Pap test, one-third in the past year. The National Cancer Registry Report indicates that more breast cancer cases are seen than cervical cancer, although these data are not population-based.

In 1994, the most common cancer sites in males were prostate (34 per 100,000), lung (10 per 100,000), colorectal (7 per 100,000), and stomach (7 per 100,000).

Accidents and Violence. The importance of injury as a cause of death and morbidity cannot be overemphasized. Rates have been increasing since the 1960s, and between 1990 and 1992, all categories of injury showed an increase in rates. Injuries are the major cause of death in all age groups up to 45 years old, but deaths due to injury occur at all ages. Injury is the most important contributor to years of potential life lost (YPLL) in males.

The biggest increase has been in homicide rates, which doubled between 1990 and 1994 for both males and females. In a recent survey of 20 general practices, acute injury was one of the most common reasons given for consultation. Hospital activity statistics indicate that injury is also the most important cause for hospital admissions (20% of discharges and 16.1% of patient days in 1993). Suicide is the second leading cause of injury-related deaths and is a major problem in the 15–24-year age group. Insecticide ingestion is the most common method, and measures to control the availability, storage, and distribution of these toxic chemicals need to be addressed.

Mental Health. A significant proportion of the population of Trinidad and Tobago does not have access to mental health

services, despite efforts to distribute the services throughout the country. Problem areas for mental health services include: psychiatric emergencies; long-standing psychiatric conditions; mental health problems of patients attending primary-care providers, ambulatory services at secondary levels, and inpatient services at acute-care hospitals; and psychiatric and emotional problems of high-risk groups.

Tobacco, Alcohol, and Drug Use. In 1995, 13% of males aged 15–24 years old and 30% of all males over 15 years old reported that they had smoked 100 or more cigarettes in their lifetime. Prevalence was highest in the 35–44-year age group (37.6%) and declined in older age groups. Smoking in females appeared to be much lower: 5.1% in all age groups over age 15, and highest (7.1%) in the 45–54-year age group. Smoking prevalence was significantly higher in households reporting low per capita income and among less educated respondents. Smoking was highly correlated with being male and with drinking 21 or more units of alcohol per week.

The Ministry of Health has established a no-smoking policy in all publicly funded health institutions, discourages its organizations from using funds obtained from tobacco companies for sponsoring health events, and informs all new applicants of the Ministry of Health's no-smoking policy. The Ministry has also taken the initiative for the development of a national no-smoking policy.

Eighty percent of males and 54% of females reported that they had consumed 12 or more alcoholic drinks in their lifetime. Persons with low educational attainment reported a higher prevalence of drinking. Heavy drinking (at least 21 units per week) was reported by 10.5% of males; the percentage rose to 13% in the central region of the country where the sugar industry is based.

Alcohol-control regulations are not effectively enforced. Some education and health promotion efforts take place in schools, workplaces, and in the community, but these are far from adequate.

There are no reliable data on psychoactive substance abuse, although there are indications of an increase in drug-related crimes—a possible proxy indicator of increasing abuse of illegal drugs (in particular, marijuana and cocaine). The Ministry of Health has a substance abuse clinic under the management of Saint Ann's Psychiatric Hospital.

Oral Health. Oral health services are mainly geared to the population under 15 years old. A cadre of dental nurses was trained in the 1970s to deliver dental education to this age group in schools and clinics. Dental clinics in the health offices provide screening and simple treatment on demand. There have been no recent population-based studies on oral health.

Several administrations have considered adding fluoride to the water supply, but this has never been implemented mainly because of the irregularity of the water supply. Instead, the Government has adopted the use of fluoridated salt, but this policy may need to be reviewed when national nutrition policy on noncommunicable disease prevention is being formulated.

Environmental Pollution. Sewerage plants that were built during the oil boom years are now in serious disrepair and are polluting tributaries along the country's northwest corridor, beaches, and inland ecosystems. In addition, the water distribution system is plagued with leakage. In response, the Water and Sewerage Authority has introduced changes in management in preparation for a major infrastructure improvement project. The newly established Environmental Management Authority coordinates the various agencies that play a role in environmental protection.

RESPONSE OF THE HEALTH SYSTEM

National Health Plans and Policies

The Macro-Planning framework and the updated Medium-Term Policy Framework (1996–1998) have remained relatively stable since 1989, despite changes in administration in 1991 and 1995. The Government remains firmly committed to the principles of equity and social solidarity. In keeping with these principles, the Government provides free public education and health services at the point of delivery; carries out social safety net programs targeted at the elderly, female-headed households with children, and persons with disabilities; maintains unemployment relief programs (primarily public works programs); supports the role of the National Insurance System and new programs aimed at helping the "new poor," which include strengthening the capacity of NGOs and the private sectors in poverty alleviation efforts; has developed and implemented housing programs for low- and middle-income groups; has established job training programs for unemployed youths; and provides retraining support for displaced workers and economic support for microenterprise development.

Eight Ministries currently deliver these various components, and efforts are now under way to develop an overall policy framework to establish priorities and streamline service delivery. The Ministry of Social Development has been identified as the lead Government agency, and a program of institutional strengthening has been implemented to support this new role.

Health Sector Reform

The Government has embarked on the first phase of the comprehensive 1996–2002 Health Sector Reform Program

designed to strengthen the health sector's policy-making, planning, and management capacity; separate the provision of services from financing and regulatory responsibilities; shift public expenditure and help steer private expenditures toward high-priority problems and cost-effective solutions; establish new administrative and employment structures that encourage accountability, increased autonomy, and incentives to improve productivity and efficiency; and reduce preventable morbidity and mortality by promoting lifestyle changes and other social interventions.

In order to reach those goals, the program envisions reforming the Ministry of Health in order to make it a policy, planning, sponsorship, and regulatory body; devolving service delivery and management to Regional Health Authorities that will contract with the Ministry of Health to provide cost-effective services, using both public and private providers; developing a human resources strategy, including the establishment of a funded pension plan for RHA staff, to foster an adequate skills mix and appropriate staffing levels; rationalizing the health services and infrastructure to focus activities on cost-effective and high-priority interventions that emphasize health prevention and promotion and strengthen primary care; and developing a comprehensive financing strategy for the sector, including the evaluation of user charges and a national health insurance system as potential financing mechanisms.

Organization of the Health Sector

In 1994, the Regional Health Authorities Act was enacted, establishing five Regional Health Authorities (RHAs)—four in Trinidad and one in Tobago—as independent statutory authorities accountable to the Minister of Health. The RHA territories have been drawn to coincide with those of local governments (the Regional Corporations), to ensure that they effectively coordinate with the latter in providing a range of health services to their catchment populations.

Ownership of publicly financed health facilities has been transferred to the RHAs, and the Act includes provisions for the staff working in public facilities to transfer employment to the RHAs. RHAs will operate according to negotiated annual services agreements aimed at linking expenditure levels to services delivery; agreements will be implemented in 1998.

The Ministry of Health retains responsibility for setting the national framework and priorities, ensuring that public funds effectively meet the population's health needs and improve its health status, and establishing standards and monitoring achievement of these standards by RHAs and other service providers. The national policy framework, or purchasing plan, is being developed on the principles of health gain and health needs assessment. Over time, RHA budgets will shift to a more equitable allocation based on the population's health needs. Health sector reform focuses on the new roles for the Ministry of Health and the RHAs and is consistent with the Government's overall strategy for improving public sector performance, particularly with plans for reorganizing the Ministry of Social Development and strengthening local government initiatives.

Health Services and Resources

Organization of Services for Care of the Population

Food Programs. The Government does not receive food through international food aid programs. Direct and indirect government subsidies for a wide variety of basic food items have been removed. The national school feeding program has been reorganized to include some children in secondary schools and an increased number of primary schools. Voluntary groups also provide food to schoolchildren and the needy. Public assistance grants, old age pensions, and other temporary grants for the destitute and needy provide a minimum cash payment for the purchase of food; these grants are administered by the Ministry of Social Development.

Iodination and fluoridation of salt and the fortification of flour with iron, thiamine, riboflavin, and niacin are carried out to overcome identified deficiencies.

Oral Health. Dental services, which are widely distributed but limited in content, are provided free in about half of the health centers. Dental practitioners (21) provide basic services to schoolchildren and pregnant women, as well as palliative treatment to adults. The service is more focused on extraction than restorative treatment. The dentists are supported by dental nurses, who provide simple dental treatment, restorations, and prophylaxis to children under 12 years old, as well as screening of schoolchildren and dental health education in clinics and schools. Fifty-four health centers, six of them in Tobago, have dental clinics.

Oral and maxillofacial surgery and dental services are available at the two general hospitals. Since it opened in 1991, the Dental Hospital at the Eric Williams Medical Sciences Complex has provided complete dental care on a fee-for-service basis. Two levels of dentistry operate in the private sector: professional dentists and unlicensed dental operatives who practice illegally.

Mental Health Services. The psychiatric services provided by the Ministry of Health are still centered around the only major psychiatric hospital in the country. Decentralized inpatient services for the acutely mentally ill also are provided at the general hospitals, county hospitals, and four extended care centers for the elderly with chronic mental illness. Community psychiatric services are organized by sectors on a geographic basis and are provided free on an outpatient basis at selected health centers.

The community services provide psychiatric, preventive, and therapeutic care for chronic and acutely ill patients, substance abusers, and disturbed children and adolescents; the services also offer follow-up care for persons discharged from hospital. A specialized substance abuse unit is the main center for drug abuse treatment, but there are also several small therapeutic and rehabilitative centers maintained by NGOs. Six or more NGOs organize support groups and offer counseling to prevent acute episodes of mental illness. A child guidance clinic, located at the Eric Williams Medical Sciences Complex, serves the whole country by addressing the needs of children individually and through the education system. Both psychiatrists and psychologists offer private sector care for the mentally ill.

Programs for the Disabled. The Ministry of Social Development has responsibility for the needs of disabled persons. Four major NGOs that provide therapeutic care and education for disabled children receive government subsidies. Services are provided in north and south Trinidad and in Tobago. Special teachers to assist disabled children are posted in very few of the mainstream primary and secondary schools. Some estimates put the number of children on waiting lists for entry to special institutions at triple the number of places.

The blind receive a pension after age 40, and other associated grants are given to disabled adults who have no support. Employment for disabled persons is limited.

Cancer Screening. The Cancer Society, the Family Planning Association, and the Eric Williams Medical Sciences Complex provide screening programs for breast cancer and cervical cancer. Free routine Pap tests are performed in some health centers and in gynecological clinics at government hospitals. The Cancer Society also has a screening program for prostate cancer. In 1996, with the support of the Ministry of Health and the Port-of-Spain Municipal Corporation, the Cancer Society established a national cancer registry.

Environmental Health Services. Environmental services are mainly provided by the Government. The Water and Sewerage Authority, which is heavily subsidized by the Government, has the statutory responsibility to supply potable water to the nation and to collect and dispose of liquid waste. Their services are performed for a fee. Private sector companies play a limited role in the provision of environmental services, and their fees are relatively high.

In urban areas, 87% of the total population has house connections and the remaining 13% have access to standpipes.

All of the water supply in urban areas is chlorinated and meets WHO standards. In rural areas, 87% of the total population has access to safe water, which is either piped or supplied by truck. A 1992 survey found 78.5% of households with running water. Of these, however, 70.6% reported having water from the mains in the last week, and 78.3% reported that they stored water.

The entire urban population has adequate excreta disposal: 30% through house connections and 70% through privies. Almost all (97%) of the rural population has adequate excreta disposal.

Local authorities provide households with free regular collection and disposal services for domestic garbage. This service is unavailable in unauthorized or inaccessible squatter settlements, and garbage is picked up at a collection point. Other forms of refuse are collected by arrangement, for a fee. Private companies remove industrial and commercial waste, but use the local authority's disposal site. Local authorities clean drains and streets.

Arrangements for the disposal of toxic waste are made on an ad hoc basis or the waste is buried at the municipal dump. In both cases, there is risk of seepage that may contaminate soil and underground water supplies.

The insect control division is responsible for insect surveillance, most importantly for *Aedes* and *Anopheles* mosquitoes.

Health Promotion. The Government of Trinidad and Tobago has expressed its support for the strategy of health promotion by endorsing and participating in activities related to the Caribbean Charter of Health Promotion. In 1994, a national meeting on health promotion brought together representatives from the public and private sectors and NGOs, who committed themselves to the goals of the Caribbean Charter and recommended that a National Health Promotion Council be formed to link all the agencies that dealt with health issues. The concept of health promotion and the goals of the Caribbean Charter were presented to a group of community organizations and NGOs. A series of regional workshops followed, where participants chose various projects to work on, such as the Healthy Communities Initiative and a plan for the prevention of noncommunicable diseases. The Healthy Communities Initiative builds on the WHO Healthy Cities Program and will depend on cooperation between the RHA, the Municipal Corporations, and the community. As a part of health reform, the Health Education Division is now linked to health planning in the new Directorate of Policy, Planning, and Health Promotion.

Social and Community Participation. There are ongoing efforts to improve the capacity of NGOs to provide services and to strengthen their relationship with government agencies. It also is hoped that the proposed regionalization will bring about a closer partnership between the community and the health services.

In terms of primary health care, reform proposals being discussed by NGOs and the Ministry of Social Development include the development of a strategy for care of the elderly and the disabled within the community. It is believed that many of those occupying hospital beds have no real need for clinical care and would be better supported by services in community settings. It was agreed that the Government should have one lead agency to set standards and to monitor NGOs, and that the Ministry of Social Development would take on this role, with support of the Ministry of Health.

The RHAs are able to maximize use of community resources since they are free to buy services from outside the public sector. This represents an important tool as the Government pursues a more effective use of existing resources.

The Health Education Division supports the Ministry of Health in the dissemination of information, and there are several activities being carried out in collaboration with the community, such as a cholera awareness program, promotion of breast-feeding, and the "Healthy Communities" initiative. Within the scope of the reform, the Division is considered a key player in health promotion.

Disaster Preparedness. The emergency relief system remains basically unchanged, although certain aspects have been streamlined. The National Emergency Management Agency has a full-time coordinator and committee representing many governmental and nongovernmental agencies and is responsible for the national emergency preparedness and relief plan. Risk maps have been drawn and circulated to many community organizations, and a manual that lists resources that can be accessed during a disaster has been prepared.

The Ministry of Health has its own disaster coordinator, and activities have been undertaken in terms of increasing awareness, training, vulnerability analysis, and preparation of disaster plans for the health sector. Each RHA is being supported in its development of disaster plans. This arrangement has particular significance for the central and southwest RHAs since they include the airport, the Point Lisas Industrial Estate, and petroleum plant sites. Simulation exercises have taken place, and transport and communications were identified as potential problems in the event of a disaster.

Organization and Operation of Personal Health Care Services

Both public and private sectors provide personal health care; NGOs, industrial corporations, and the national security services also provide some services. Public sector care is available at institutions located throughout the country. Secondary and tertiary care are provided at one general hospital in Port-of-Spain and one in San Fernando (1,245 beds), at two county hospitals in Trinidad (111 beds), and at one hospital in Tobago (96 beds). Specialized hospitals and units also provide women's health, psychiatric, chest disease, substance abuse, geriatric, oncology, and physical therapy services, for a total 1,513 additional beds (the psychiatric hospital is the largest, with 1,060 beds). A comprehensive range of diagnostic services is available at the two general hospitals.

Primary health care is provided at 101 health centers, 19 of which are in Tobago. The number of health centers per RHA in Trinidad varies from 16 in the eastern RHA to 30 in the central RHA. The ratio of population to health center ranges from less than 3,000 per center in Tobago to more than 21,000 per center in Saint George West.

Inpatient and ambulatory care are provided free at the publicly funded institutions now administered by the RHAs. Minimum charges are made for certain diagnostic procedures, but at present there is no formal user-charge system, except at the Eric Williams Medical Sciences Complex, which operates on a fee-for-service basis.

Private general practitioners, specialists, diagnostic laboratories, and hospitals are dispersed throughout the two islands, although they are clustered in the cities and larger towns. Of the 33 private hospitals registered with the Private Hospitals Board, 13 have operating theaters and offer some diagnostic services. It is reported that about 45% of the population uses private sector services as a first choice, particularly for ambulatory services; however, private inpatient care is costly, and the range of emergency services is limited.

NGOs provide diagnostic and screening facilities for the early detection and treatment of specific prevalent diseases and disabilities. Charges for services are modest, but since most NGOs are located in the cities (for example, Pap tests are performed at the Family Planning Association), the cost of transportation may discourage utilization by disadvantaged persons who live in remote areas.

Large commercial enterprises provide health services for employees, either directly, through specially contracted services, or through group insurance plans. Dependents are included in the benefits, and one plan includes retired employees. The national security services provide primary care for their officers and staff, and dependents are included in some programs. Secondary or tertiary care for security service officers is initially sought at RHA hospitals. It is estimated that less than 10% of the employed population is covered by health insurance.

Referral systems within the public sector and between the public and private sectors are not well established, and more than 50% of admissions at hospital emergency departments are self-referrals. The Eric Williams Medical Sciences Complex was the first hospital in the country to be administered by a

board responsible to the Minister of Health. Primary (walk-in), secondary, and tertiary health care—both inpatient and ambulatory—are being provided on a limited scale, as the hospital's commissioning is still in progress. Diagnostic services are almost fully operational and the cardiology laboratory, commissioned in 1992, is now in operation. The Ministry of Health provides the hospital with a large subsidy, but the hospital charges the Ministry for patients referred from government institutions. The Complex is now administered by the central RHA. The health sector reform program has projected capital and recurrent resources for its new role as a secondary care hospital for the population of the central RHA and as a national tertiary center. The financing issue will be resolved within the overall financing strategy of the public health sector.

A gradual increase in annual hospital discharges was observed in the 1990–1994 period, peaking in 1994 at both general hospitals: 66,187 at Port-of-Spain and 51,185 at San Fernando. Since then, discharges have decreased, down to 65,580 at Port-of-Spain and 44,767 at San Fernando in 1995, and to 59,350 and 47,873, respectively, in 1996. A similar trend has been seen in Tobago, where discharges averaged 4,822 annually for those years.

The average length of stay at general hospitals is 3–4 days, with average occupancy rates of 63%–70%, except at San Fernando General Hospital, which maintained a bed-occupancy rate above 80% in 1995 and 1996. The occupancy rates for the smaller hospitals varied, but were generally less than 30%, with higher than average lengths of stay (ranging from 7 to 35 days in the medical wards). All of these smaller hospitals, with the exception of Point Fortin Hospital in the southwest RHA, were closed in 1995, pending replacement by new District Health Facilities.

The general hospitals conduct outpatient clinics in major specialties and subspecialties and the three county hospitals provide outpatient clinics in major specialties. In addition, health centers provide general medical consultations on designated days.

Over the 1994–1996 period, the number of first visits and return visits to health centers decreased, with 1996 showing 108,068 for general medical office first visits for the year and 491,681 for total number of visits for all sessions, including child health services. This is consistent with the 1995 National Health Survey data showing that persons prefer the private providers or the hospital emergency department as their first choice in medical care. Figures for private sector outpatient consultations and diagnostic services are not available.

The Eric Williams Medical Sciences Complex, the two general hospitals, the three smaller regional hospitals, and the private sector offer pathology, biochemistry, and hematology laboratory services.

Over 50% of pregnant women attend free prenatal clinics that are provided in the health centers. At each visit a midwife conducts an examination, and at least twice during the pregnancy, a medical officer conducts an examination. This system facilitates the referral of women with complications (about 19% of clients) to specialist clinics at six hospitals. The established protocol for prenatal care at the health centers includes anemia and VDRL tests, screening for diabetes, and tetanus immunization. Iron and folic acid supplements are recommended to pregnant women but are not generally available free at the health centers or the hospital.

About 90% of all deliveries take place in government institutions, which have facilities for cesarean sections, blood transfusions, and acute neonatal care. The other 10% take place in private hospitals and nursing homes (most of which have facilities for cesarean sections), with minimal numbers taking place in homes and "other places." Almost 90% of all deliveries are supervised by midwives, the other 10% by doctors or "other persons." Only about 10% of mothers use postnatal services at health centers.

Inputs for Health

The deterioration of the physical infrastructure, including equipment, is of particular concern to the Ministry of Health and the new RHAs. The lack of ongoing prevention and routine maintenance systems, skills, and budgets are not confined to the Ministry of Health, but exist throughout the public sector.

To address the issue of sustainability of investment in the physical infrastructure, a National Health Services Plan was developed during the design phase of the health sector reform program. The plan will guide investment in infrastructure and, to a large extent, the human resource development required to achieve the new emphasis on primary and preventive care.

According to the National Health Services Plan, essential components of the health services rationalization effort for primary health care services include: reinforcing the network of existing facilities by upgrading selected health centers, constructing new ambulatory facilities and enhanced health centers with some diagnostic and specialist services, and converting the remaining health centers to outreach centers that will offer preventive services.

Also planned is a reduction in the number of acute-care hospitals (from 13 to 5) and hospital bed capacity (reduction of 800 beds by the year 2002); an increase in the ability of hospitals to offer ambulatory and diagnostic services; and improvements in the inpatient facilities in keeping with the rationalization of tertiary services. When the Eric Williams Medical Sciences Complex is commissioned it will include a national cancer treatment center providing radiotherapy and chemotherapy (following the relocation of the National Radiotherapy Center from St. James Medical Complex in 1999). A shift of inpatient care of the elderly and disabled to a private or NGO community-based setting is under review. Finally, an emergency transport system will be introduced to improve access and integration of the rationalized network of health facilities.

Essential Drugs and Blood Transfusion Services. The Ministry of Health has developed national drug policies addressing the provision of safe and effective drugs to those who require them. Efforts to introduce concepts of rational drug prescribing in the public sector were initiated in 1990. These were intended to build on the use of the vital essential and nonessential drugs list to manage the selection and procurement of drugs for the public sector. There are ongoing attempts to develop alternative methods of estimating drug requirements and standardize treatment protocols, starting with the more common diseases and conditions.

In 1992, the procurement, logistics, and distribution of drugs for the public sector were contracted to a statutory body. The outcome has been generally positive, despite the shrinking budget in real terms due to the devaluation of the Trinidad and Tobago currency. Computerized inventory management and drug dispensing systems have been introduced in all major hospitals and the system will be linked to Central Supply in the near future. In 1994, a National Drug Formulary was produced for use in the public sector; it should significantly contribute to awareness of possible options, treatment costs, and perhaps the need for better rational drug-prescribing practices.

Blood transfusion services are centralized, and a fully operational national unit is responsible for setting the standards for collection and distribution of blood products. All blood donations are done on a voluntary basis, and 100% of blood collected is screened for hepatitis B, HTLV I, and HIV.

Human Resources

Reliable and useful human resource data that could be used for manpower planning and projecting are limited, because the Ministry of Health does not maintain data by category of staff or place of work. No reliable data are available for the health professionals in the private sector, or for traditional medicine or nonmedical providers.

There is currently about 1 physician per 1,200 population in Trinidad and Tobago, a figure deemed acceptable by international standards. There still are, however, shortages in the hospital services with respect to the number of junior staff, house officers, and interns. To cope with the problem, nonnationals have been contracted for these posts. It was estimated that in 1993 there were approximately 150 foreign doctors working in the public sector.

A similar situation exists for dentists as for physicians. Current dentist-to-population ratios are satisfactory by international standards. There were 20 graduates from the new Dental School at the Medical Sciences Complex in 1994, and 25 in 1995.

Trinidad and Tobago continues to suffer from a nursing shortage, although the availability of nurses has improved. Nursing training recommended in 1989 and new nurses entered into the system beginning in 1992. Post-basic courses have been strengthened and a significant amount of the training budget has been channeled to specialist nursing training, such as nursing education, administration, intensive care, oncology, and occupational health.

There are many vacancies at the primary care level as a result of constraints in training, recruitment, and qualification. Nursing requirements for the strengthened primary care system call for a significant increase in staffing. Critical shortage areas have been identified in professions allied to medicine, such as dietetics and nutrition, radiology, physiotherapy, occupational therapy, and pharmacology. Each area requires detailed evaluation of current organization and delivery of services to determine what other types of providers can be trained, and to develop and implement training programs.

Training of Health Personnel. Training of health personnel, except for undergraduate and basic nursing training, is centered at the Eric Williams Medical Sciences Complex. There are undergraduate and postgraduate education programs for doctors, dentists, and veterinarians. The newly opened Medical School of the University of the West Indies graduated the first class of doctors in 1994. Most students are Trinidadians, but many are from other Caribbean countries and elsewhere.

The responsibility for nurse training has been transferred from the Ministry of Health to the College of Nursing of the National Institute of Higher Education, Research, Science, and Technology. The College of Health Sciences also offers training programs for radiographers, laboratory technicians, and other allied health professionals, as well as continuing education programs. Training for pharmacists, public health inspectors, and community-based nurses (health visitors and district nurses) is given as part of the University of the West Indies program of continuing studies.

Research and Technology

In accordance with the health sector reform program, the Ministry of Health has undertaken health systems research which has led to an in-depth review of national strategies and policies. Methodologies will be formalized under the Ministry of Health's new Policy, Planning, and Health Promotion Department, which will be responsible for generating the necessary information for identifying priorities and planning services. A research and development function that will include technology assessment also will be developed.

The National Institute for Higher Education, Research, and Technology has the mandate to develop a policy for the introduction of new technology in Trinidad and Tobago. A draft policy was issued in 1996 and a final version is expected by 1997.

The Essential National Health Research Committee was established in 1996 to develop a system for coordinating health research in the country. Its first mandate is to develop an essential national health research policy for ratification. It is integrated by public and private sector professionals and is fully recognized by the Ministry of Health.

Expenditures and Sectoral Financing

There has been a significant reduction in public sector health expenditure over the 1981–1992 period, ranging from a high of TT$ 677 (constant 1985 dollars) in 1982 to a low of TT$ 250 in 1989; it rose to TT$ 256 in 1992. Within the 1981–1986 period, the annual real expenditure per capita, in constant 1985 dollars, was TT$ 528 as compared with TT$ 279 in the 1987–1992 period. It should be noted that structural adjustment measures resulted in the devaluation of the Trinidad and Tobago dollar in 1985, 1988, and 1993.

In terms of recurrent expenditure, whereas approximately TT$ 3.6 billion were spent in the 1981–1986 period, only TT$ 2.3 billion were spent over the 1987–1992 period. The decrease was caused primarily by the overall economic recession, the reduction in public sector compensation packages, and the increase in vacancies within the Ministry of Health, particularly in nursing.

Capital expenditure declined significantly during the 1988–1992 period, with most of the expenditure being directed to the construction of the Eric Williams Medical Sciences Complex (84%). The bulk of the remaining capital expenditure was channeled to other hospitals, with less than 1% directed at community health services.

The pattern of allocation of the recurrent budget shows that the bulk of recurrent expenditure is for personnel (73%) and goods and services (19%). Expenditures on personnel were channeled primarily to hospitals and laboratories (75%), with only 9% going to community or local health services. There are budgetary variations across programs and divisions, with the personnel component accounting for as much as 90% in some areas.

While most of the focus tends to be on public sector spending, National Health Insurance Scheme studies estimate that an almost equal amount is being spent in the private sector. Since less than 10% of the population is covered by health insurance, it is difficult to determine the exact extent of private sector expenditure. These studies, based on a small survey of the insurance claims and extrapolation from qualitative data, indicate that total spending on health care services in Trinidad and Tobago as a percentage of GDP is approximately 4.7%, totaling TT$ 1.1 billion in 1993—2.4% and 2.3% from the public sector and private spending, respectively. Estimates of the private sector outlay were also considered to be conservative.

External Technical and Financial Cooperation

As a middle-income country, Trinidad and Tobago does not qualify for major donor assistance. The major inputs are from PAHO, UNDP, and, in 1993–1995, from the IDB for health sector reform design studies, totaling about US$ 5.2 million. Although the percentage of assistance is small (about 1%–2%), it has significant impact because it is usually provided in a priority area identified by the Government and in the form of technical cooperation or consultant services. The Government of Trinidad and Tobago would be unable to access many of these services because of inflexible national financial regulations. In the future, as this inflexibility is removed by system reform, the Ministry of Health and the RHAs will need to develop new systems of identifying, allocating, and using technical cooperation funds.

TURKS AND CAICOS
ISLANDS

GENERAL SITUATION AND TRENDS

Socioeconomic, Political, and Demographic Overview

The Turks and Caicos Islands, a British dependent territory, is located at the southeastern end of the Bahamas chain. The two island groups—the Turks Islands to the east and the Caicos to the west—extend for approximately 193 mi^2.

The Turks and Caicos Islands received its first constitution in 1976, which gave the territory significant internal autonomy and a ministerial system of government; a new constitution was drafted in 1987. A Governor, who acts as the Queen's representative, shares executive power with an elected House of nine seats that is headed by a Chief Minister. As does the Cabinet in independent Caribbean countries, the Executive Council functions as the supreme executive body; the Governor presides over it.

Tourism earnings outdistanced those from fishing and financial services; the latter two sectors now rank behind tourism in the economy. During the decade of the 1980s and in the early 1990s, most tourism development took place in Providenciales. The fishing industry was endangered by overexploitation, until the Government instituted seasonal harvesting regulations. Export revenues have been slowly increasing, but the trade deficit remains sizable.

The tourism boom in Providenciales brought with it a rapid population growth, which, in turn, has been accompanied by social problems: young people who are drawn by this highly seasonal work are left idle and frustrated for prolonged periods of time. In addition, many illegal immigrants, mainly Haitians and Dominican Republic nationals, also have also been drawn by the economic boom in Providenciales. Both trends have led to an increase in antisocial behavior and other behavioral problems manifested by an increase in accidents, intentional injuries, and other crimes, as well as the

doubling of the prison population between 1990 and 1996. A memorandum of understanding signed between the governments of Haiti and the Turks and Caicos Islands in 1996 agrees to a phased repatriation program.

The total resident population, based on the 1990 census, was 11,465; 50.9% of whom were males. Approximately one-third of the population was under 15 years of age, with another 5% aged 65 years or above, for a dependency ratio of 37.2%. The most populated island was Providenciales, the business hub for the territory; its 4,821 residents accounted for 42% of the total resident population. The administrative seat of the Government is located on Grand Turk, the second most populated island, with 32.2% of the population.

The resident population grew exponentially between 1980 and 1990, exceeding the expected population of 8,913 by an additional 28.6%. An analysis reveals that during this period the only two inhabited islands with positive percentage increases were Providenciales (493%) and Grand Turk (19%). The percentage increase in the population of "belongers" (citizens by parentage, birth, or naturalization) was only 16%, compared to an increase of 494% in the expatriate population.

Given the rapid development in Providenciales, estimates had to be made in order to arrive at realistic population figures for calculating rates for the post-census years. Unfortunately, because there were no universally accepted post-census estimates from the territory, figures from external sources such as the United Nations Population Division and the Caribbean Epidemiology Center (CAREC), in Trinidad, had to suffice. CAREC's figures were somewhat lower than the UN estimates, but the former were used for post-census years, because CAREC gave estimates for various age groups, as well as total population estimates. For censal years, the actual census count of residents was used as a denominator. Because the Turks and Caicos population is so small, data should be interpreted with caution.

Fertility Patterns

The data reported here reflect only those births registered in the territory's Registrar General's Office. It is assumed that these are underestimates, because birth registration has been shown to be incomplete and because residents routinely travel abroad for health care, including for obstetrics and gynecology services.

Data from the 1990 census showed the population of women in childbearing age (16–49 years old) was 3,050, 54.2% of the total female population. This percentage varied greatly across islands, however, from a low of 32.7% in Salt Cay to a high of 64.4% in Providenciales. The high percentage in Providenciales reflects the number of immigrants to that island, who contribute significantly to the fertility rate.

Since the 1970s, the crude birth rate in the Turks and Caicos decreased from 33.3 per 1,000 population in 1970, to 23.5 in 1980, and to 20.9 in 1990. In 1995, there were 234 registered births, for a crude birth rate of 18.6 per 1,000. Although these estimated birth rates may well be underestimates, it is believed that they are indicative of the true birth trend, particularly among "belongers."

The pregnancy rate, particularly among teenagers, has been on the rise. Teenage pregnancies pose potential health risks to both mothers and children, and many of these children become wards of the State or an added burden to the community. The number of abortions also has grown. Hospital admissions data for 1996 show abortions as one of the leading causes of admissions, 5.9% of all admissions for that year. Because of the social stigma and secrecy that surrounds abortion, these figures almost certainly are underestimates; moreover, many women have abortions done abroad in an effort to seek confidentiality.

Estimates of the age distribution of pregnant women are obtained from records of women seeking care at the community health clinics in Providenciales and Grand Turk. During 1996, there were 116 births in Providenciales and 86 in Grand Turk. Five of the births in Providenciales (4.3%) were to teenage mothers between the ages of 15 and 19 years, and 7 (6%) were to mothers older than 35 years old, two age groups at greater risk for complications.

Available data also show an increasing number of pregnant women of other nationalities: 97 of the 116 births in Providenciales in 1996 were to citizens of other nationalities, with 93 (80.2%) to Haitian nationals alone. In Grand Turk, the percentage was not as high (52.3%), but high enough to cause concern. This trend is expected to continue, as it was observed not only among women who gave birth, but also among prenatal care attendees. In Providenciales, there were 283 new prenatal clients, 168 (59.4%) of whom were Haitian nationals, with another 9.1% of other nationalities.

Prenatal services used to be offered for free or at a minimal cost. To offset the burden that this represented on the health budget, Ministry of Health officials revised the payment schedule for prenatal and childbirth services. This change may already have resulted in a reduction in demand, and its overall impact on the health of pregnant women and infants remains to be seen.

Mortality Profile

Cause of death coding in the Turks and Caicos Islands is not systematized. Although all deaths must be certified, many, particularly those that occur on less populated islands, are certified by nurses. Access to and use of diagnostic facilities to confirm clinical diagnosis are limited, and the autopsy rate is not very high.

In an attempt to identify the underlying cause of death, CAREC conducted a detailed review of all registered and unregistered deaths in the Turks and Caicos from 1980 through 1995. Unregistered cases were identified through records kept by the Ministry of Health. Results indicated that from 1990 through 1994, underregistration—estimated by comparing deaths identified in the study with the number of registered events—was 12.1%, a similar figure to that for the 1985–1989 period, which was estimated at 12.2%, and to that for 1990–1994, which was 12%. All mortality data reported here is based on the CAREC study.

Since the 1970s, mortality trends indicate an overall increase in both the number of deaths and the death rates, with periodic decreases. In 1970, there were 47 deaths, which decreased to 30 by 1980. In the 1980s, the number of deaths increased again, peaking in 1985 at 65, before dropping again to 45 in 1990. In 1995, 80 deaths were recorded in the Turks and Caicos Islands, the largest number recorded in recent times. The crude death rate was 636.4 per 100,000 population, up from the 1990 figure of 392.5.

In terms of distribution by gender, most deaths in 1995 were among males (51.3%), in contrast to the previous year, when there were more deaths among women (54.9%). This inconsistent pattern, which was evident throughout the 1980s, may be expected wherever the population is relatively small.

Between 1990 and 1995, the highest age specific death rates were observed in the population aged 65 years old and older, followed by those in the age group under 1 year old. The lowest rates were in the school-age population, children aged 5–14 years.

The number of infant deaths between 1991 and 1995 ranged from a low of 1 in 1991 to a high of 10 in 1995. The highest infant mortality rate for this period was 42.7 infant deaths per 1,000 live births observed in 1995; it is not known whether this increase is indicative of a change in the quality of care. Between 1992 an 1994, the infant mortality rate averaged 23.2 per 1,000 live births. Registered births were used in the calculations.

Between 1993 and 1996, the highest neonatal mortality rate was 34.2 deaths per 1,000 live births; estimates of stillbirth rates were obtained using hospital based statistics. During 1996, the estimated stillbirth rate per 1,000 deliveries was 16.7, compared to 13.5, 14.9, and 33.7 for 1995, 1994, and 1993, respectively. The highest number of stillbirths recorded at the hospital during this period was 6 in 1993.

Among adults, the leading cause of death in 1995 was diseases of the circulatory system, accounting for just over one-quarter (26.3%) of all deaths, followed by deaths due to communicable diseases and external causes, both at 16.3%. Neoplasms accounted for 10% and conditions originating in the perinatal period, for 7.5%.

Of the 362 deaths for the 1990–1995 period, one of every four deaths (27.3%) was due to diseases of circulatory system, most of them resulting from strokes and heart attacks. Communicable diseases ranked second, primarily due to the rise in the number of deaths from AIDS, and accounted for 18%; deaths due to external causes ranked third, accounting for 13%. Of these deaths, 7.5% were the result of neoplasms, and another 5.2% were due to conditions originating in the perinatal period. Deaths due to symptoms, signs, and ill-defined conditions, which is often an indicator of the quality of diagnostic capabilities, accounted for 14.4%.

Morbidity

Reasonably accurate figures on the number of hospital admissions are readily available from ward records. The current system, however, does not allow for an in-depth analysis of these data, and data on admissions and discharge diagnoses are insufficient to allow for an accurate coding according to the principles of the International Classification of Diseases.

In order to determine the main causes of hospital admissions, this report attempts to group available admission diagnosis data for 1996 into selected categories. Data were taken from the general ward that houses both adult and pediatric patients admitted for medical or surgical services. Information from the maternity and geriatric wards was excluded.

During the five-year period ending in 1996, the number of hospital inpatients steadily increased, but bed capacity did not. In 1996, there were 705 admissions to the general ward of Turks and Caicos General Hospital, up 14% from the 619 admissions recorded in 1995. Of these, 58.5% were female and 41.5%, male. Approximately one of every two inpatients (53.1%) admitted that year were between the ages of 15–44 years, one-fifth (20.4%) were patients under the age of 15

years, and 12.7% were 65 years old and older. Whereas approximately 70% of inpatients under the age of 5 years were males, two-thirds of patients 15 years old and older were females.

Based on admissions diagnoses, conditions associated with the gastrointestinal tract accounted for 12.3% of all inpatient stays in 1996; accidents and violence, primarily poisonings, stab wounds, and burns, were responsible for another 10.5%. Other conditions frequently recorded included hypertension (5.4%) and abortions (5.9%). During 1995, there were 402 surgical procedures performed at the hospital and the overall average length of stay was 3.4 days.

The 1,755 outpatients recorded in 1995 represented an increase of 10.2% over the 1,593 visits recorded for 1994, and up 57.4% over the total visits for 1992.

SPECIFIC HEALTH PROBLEMS

Analysis by Population Group

Health of Children

During 1995, 10 deaths in infants (0 to 4 years old) occurred in the Turks and Caicos Islands, and most of them (7 deaths) occurred during the first 7 days of life. Causes of death were listed as prematurity, respiratory distress syndrome, septicemia, acute gastroenteritis, and other conditions originating in the perinatal period. The infant mortality rate for that year was estimated at 42.7 deaths per 1,000 live births, which represents an underestimate given that registered births were used as the denominator.

Prematurity is closely tied to the risk of infant death, and the percentage of deliveries <2,500 g is an indicator of prematurity. The most reliable estimate, based on 1995 data abstracted from the maternity ward book at Grand Turk Hospital, places this figure at 10.8% of deliveries.

Mortality in children between the ages 1–4 years is not a problem in the territory, but acute respiratory infections and diarrheal diseases are. For example, there was only one recorded death resulting from an accident in 1995, but between 1993 and 1996, there were 2,674 acute respiratory infections reported. The 465 cases reported in 1994 represents the lowest annual figure for the period, and the 830 cases reported during 1995, the highest. There were 707 cases of gastroenteritis reported, most of them (209) reported in 1995.

Child health services, in terms of preventive care, immunization, and growth monitoring, as well as curative care are considered priorities. Vaccines are given for DTP, OPV, and MMR, and in 1996 coverage for all neared 100%. Of 552 growth monitoring visits carried out in 1995, 18.3% were considered obese. Based on 1995 data from Grand Turk, the percentage of mothers breast-feeding exclusively at 3 months was below 2%. This figure would improve if mothers were better prepared for breast-feeding after giving birth.

During the 1994–1995 school year, 1,625 primary and 1,058 secondary schoolchildren enrolled in the territory's 10 primary and 4 secondary schools. Grand Turk had the largest proportion of secondary students and Providenciales had the highest number of primary schoolchildren, which reflects the large number of women of childbearing age on the latter island. The school health program offers booster shots, revaccinations, vision and ear screening, and general health education; vision problems are referred to an ophthalmologist.

Data from the Department of Social Welfare indicates a considerable number of orphaned, unsupported, and abandoned children. Many families are single-parent units, and neglect by fathers is common. Drug abuse and AIDS also have affected many families, resulting in even more children being placed on welfare. During 1994–1995, of the 262 persons receiving benefits from the department, 35.4% received such assistance as financial support for the families, placement of children in foster homes or up for adoption, and support for children of delinquent parents. It has been observed recently that school-aged children are being encouraged to work to help supplement household incomes.

The Turks and Caicos Islands currently has no comprehensive program addressing the health of adolescents.

Health of Adults

According to the 1990 census, persons between the ages of 15 and 64 account for approximately 63% of the total population. The percentage of males between 15 and 49 years old is greater than that of females in that age group, but the percentage of females between 50 and 64 years old surpasses that of males in that age group. The unusual preponderance of males between 15 and 64 may very well reflect the gender distribution of the resident migrant population, most of whom are male in the productive age groups.

The leading causes of death to persons in this group are similar to those for the entire population, and include diseases of the heart, cancer, AIDS, accidents, and violence.

The prenatal program aims at having every pregnant woman in for a first visit as early as possible. This is especially important given the many high-risk pregnancies in teenage women and in women aged 35 years old or older. During 1996, only 25.1% of the 283 new prenatal clients in Providenciales made their first visit within the first 16 weeks of gestation and 17% did not make their first visit until after the 28th week. Calculated stillbirth rates of 4.2% and 2.3% in Providenciales and Grand Turk, respectively, only add to the concern.

Observed low hemoglobin levels during pregnancy have raised concern about women's health. Overall, 16.6% of 283 prenatal clients in Providenciales in 1996 were found to have low hemoglobin levels (<10 g) and 24.4% of 98 tests performed in Grand Turk were low. However, not all national groups were equally at risk, as observed in Providenciales—whereas only 4.5% of the Turks and Caicos Islanders were found to have low hemoglobin levels, 23.8% of Haitians and 11.5% of other nationalities had low levels. Similarly, whereas 2 (0.7%) of 89 nationals tested positive for HIV in Providenciales, 9 of 168 (3.1%) Haitians did. HIV-testing with informed consent is conducted on each prenatal client. Nationality specific data from Grand Turk was unavailable.

Health of Women

Data for 1996 from the Female Health Maintenance Clinic in Grand Turk revealed that of 38 Pap tests performed, 30 were on nationals, and 8 (21%) were on non-nationals. The figure for non-nationals is much lower than utilization figures observed for other services; it is known, however, that current health education efforts do not adequately reach this population group. Cervical cancer screening services are available for all women, but women of childbearing age are specifically targeted. Clinics also offer breast examinations.

Family planning services also are offered through the Community Health Clinics. In 1996, 75 new family planning clients were seen at the clinic in Providenciales, 35 for oral contraceptives and 40 for injectibles. Total clients seen for the year was 677, 63.4% of them between the ages of 25–34 years; 13 were under age 20. In 1966, 177 packets of condoms were distributed as a part of the AIDS prevention strategy.

Health of the Elderly

Based on the 1990 census, 574 residents in the Turks and Caicos Islands were aged 65 years old and older, representing 5% of the total population—322 (56.1%) were females and 252 (43.9%) were males.

The Government requires that employees retire at age 55, but National Insurance benefits do not begin until age 65, and noncontributory pensions do not start until age 68. Government services are channeled through the Department of Social Welfare, with welfare benefits provided for most persons starting at age 60.

Over the years, the social and economic burden carried by this age group has increased dramatically, and many of them must provide for themselves and for grandchildren left in their care. The Government, acknowledging that this population groups requires special attention, in 1994 conducted a study on services for the elderly as part of the health sector adjustment project. Study results pointed to the need to better integrate the delivery of health and welfare services to this group.

The geriatric ward at Grand Turk Hospital provides institutional care for the elderly. The ward can only accommodate about 12 patients, all of whom are referred by the welfare department, primarily with diagnoses of senility and fractures. Given the ward's low bed capacity and the absence of any homes for the elderly, social welfare services are provided for elderly persons who live alone, including financial support and payments to home helpers. In the fiscal year 1994–1995, 73 elderly persons received monthly welfare payments. Some churches also provide assistance for their elderly members, as do other, mostly church-affiliated, community groups. Home visits are included as part of the services offered by the staff of the Community Health Department.

Chronic diseases rank as the leading causes of death and hospitalization in this age group.

Analysis By Type of Disease or Health Impairment

Communicable Diseases

Data on communicable diseases are based on case reports that the Community Health Department forwards to CAREC every month. Between 1993 and 1996, the most frequently reported communicable diseases in children under 5 years old were influenza (3,361 cases), acute respiratory infections (2,674), and gastroenteritis (707).

There were no reported cases of vector-borne diseases during this period and very few vaccine-preventable diseases. Seven cases of the mumps were reported in 1993, followed by three in 1994; the last known cases of measles were four cases reported in 1993. After several years with no reported cases of tuberculosis, three cases were reported in 1996.

Sexually transmitted diseases, particularly gonorrhea, continue to be a problem. There were 30 reported cases of gonorrhea between 1993 and 1996, with 16 cases reported in 1996 alone. The number of syphilis cases during the period was 21, with 6 reported in 1996. One case of hepatitis was reported in 1996.

Over this four-year period, 74 cases of foodborne illnesses were reported, with 28 in 1996 alone. Many required hospitalization.

AIDS. AIDS continues to be a major public health problem as a cause of death and as a contributor to years of life lost, as well as in terms of its socioeconomic impact on the community.

From 1985, when HIV testing first began in the Turks and Caicos, through December, 1996, there were a total of 94 AIDS cases diagnosed in the territory—53 (56.4%) of them were males and the predominant mode of transmission was heterosexual contact. Persons aged 20–44 accounted for 63.8% of all cases, with the age group 30–34 years old alone responsible for one-fourth (25.6%). Only three pediatric cases (under 5 years old) were identified. Most of the cases (38.3%) were from Providenciales, followed by those in Grand Turk and South Caicos with 27.7% and 24.5%, respectively. Through December 1996, 75.5% of all cases were known to have died.

The male:female ratio was 1:1 on Providenciales, 1.8:1 on Grand Turk, and 1:1 on South Caicos. Seventy-nine (84%) of all cases were Turks and Caicos Islanders, with persons of other nationalities accounting for the remaining 16%. In Providenciales, which has a higher percentage of immigrants, the percentage of cases among non-nationals was 33.3%; in Grand Turk it was 15.4%; and in the other islands combined it was 3.1%.

Annual HIV-infection tests are performed on applicants for resident and work permits, pregnant women, and blood donors. Because there are no reliable statistics, prevalence estimates must be derived from the testing of prenatal clients on Grand Turk and Providenciales. In 1995, of 101 prenatal clients tested on Grand Turk, 8 (7.9%) tested positive. In 1996, of 283 tests of prenatal clients performed in Providenciales, 11 (3.9%) were found to be HIV-positive.

Statistics show a steady increase in the percentage of non-nationals among new cases of AIDS diagnosed between 1993 and 1996, from 13.3% to 33.3%. These full-blown AIDS cases, however, reflect the infection rate of 5 to 10 years earlier. A more appropriate indicator for the current infection rate would be one based on HIV statistics. Of the 8 HIV-positive cases positive in Grand Turk in 1995 and the 11 in Providenciales in 1996, 87.5% and 81.8%, respectively, were non-nationals. Whether or not this is indicative of a higher prevalence of HIV infection among non-nationals is unknown, although evidence based on prenatal testing in Providenciales tends to suggest this. During 1996, the percentage of national prenatal clients who tested positive was 2.2%, as compared to 4.6% for non-nationals.

Health authorities are actively addressing the AIDS/HIV situation, but gaps remain in prevention efforts. First, a more systematic and data driven approach needs to be taken with regard to the routine testing for HIV and to the collection, analysis, interpretation, and dissemination of this information. Policies must be established that determine who should be tested, so that this effort can become more cost-effective and can be useful for planning. Strategic approaches to the reduction in the numbers of HIV-infected individuals cannot be based exclusively on AIDS statistics. Given the long delay between infection and the onset of symptoms and the fact that in a territory with such a small population such as the Turks and Caicos the epidemiology of the disease may change very rapidly, programs that do not take into account HIV-infection statistics as well as AIDS statistics may be misdirected even before they are put in place. The decision to implement more targeted education campaigns renders the use of HIV statistics even more important. Recent trends in HIV infection—such as rates in pregnant women—indicate a higher prevalence among legal and illegal immigrants who speak a different language and come from a different culture. Since 1995, ODA discontinued its assistance to the AIDS program; currently the program is totally funded through the recurrent national budget, which raises some concern as to whether the program can be sustained at the previous level.

Noncommunicable Diseases and Other Health-Related Problems

Accidents and Violence. External causes have gathered importance as a cause of death. Deaths due to accidents and violence have risen from a single case in 1980 to 2 in 1985, representing 3.1% of all deaths. In the 1990s, the impact of accidents and violence increased further, to 5 cases in 1990 and 13 in 1995, representing 11.1% and 16.3% of all deaths, respectively.

Data for the 1992–1995 period were combined. During this period, there were 36 deaths due to either intentional or unintentional injuries, accounting for 13.7% of all deaths. Twenty-six, or approximately three of every four of these deaths (72.2%), were males. The age group with both the highest actual number of deaths and death rate per 100,000 population was the 25–44-year-old age group, accounting for 13 (36.1%) of the 36 deaths for a rate of 87.8 per 100,000. This was followed by persons aged 15–24 years, with 8 deaths (22.2%) and a death rate of 80/100,000.

The major causes of death due to external causes in the Turks and Caicos Islands are motor vehicle accidents, drowning, and homicides. Between 1992 and 1995, these three causes accounted for two of every three such deaths. Motor vehicle accidents were responsible for 10 deaths, 27.8% of all deaths due to external causes during this period; 7 of the 10 were males. There were 9 drowning deaths; 8 (88.9%) were males. Homicides and injuries purposely inflicted by others accounted for 5 deaths, two of whom were female. Three deaths were the result of accidental falls and two were due to suicide.

Injuries that result from acts of violence or accidents are among the leading causes for hospitalization, accounting for approximately 10.5% of all admissions in 1996. In addition to those causes that result in death, namely motor vehicle accidents, drownings, and acts that result in homicides, other common causes of admission include poisonings and burns; fish poisonings are by far the most common.

Not reflected in the mortality statistics but of increasing public health concern is the escalating incidence of violence against women. Cultural patterns leave many episodes unreported, or, when reported, unpunished. Efforts to curb this trend must be incorporated into the existing family health program.

Malignant Tumors. From 1992 through 1995 there were 23 deaths attributed to malignant neoplasms; 3 in 1992, 9 in 1993, 3 in 1994, and 8 in 1995. Of the total, 13 (56.5%) were male and 10 (43.5%) female. Cancer remained a disease predominantly of the elderly, with 65.2% of all deaths occurring in persons 65 years old and older.

During this same period, 7 deaths (30.4%) were due to cancer of the genitourinary organs, 4 of which were males who died from prostate cancer. Cancers of the digestive organs and the peritoneum were the cause of six (26.1%) deaths, four of them males; stomach cancer accounted for four of these six deaths. In addition, there were two deaths due to cancer of the larynx, two due to leukemia, and two females who died as a result of breast cancer.

Although no detailed data are available on the specific causes, cancer also has been cited as one of the leading of admission to the hospital.

Cardiovascular Diseases. Cardiovascular diseases or diseases of the circulatory system are the leading causes of death in the Turks and Caicos. In 1995, these conditions were responsible for 29% of all deaths, disproportionately affecting females (among whom cardiovascular diseases were responsible for 38.5% of all deaths), compared to males (19.5% of all male deaths). When data for the 1992–1995 period were combined, results were similar, though not as obvious. Of the 263 total deaths occurring during this period, 76 (29%) were due to these conditions, with the percentage in females (33.3%) again greater than that in males (24.4%).

For the 1992–1995 period, leading causes within this group were cerebrovascular diseases (31.6%) and myocardial infarctions (25%). Of the 76 deaths, 58% were female. Mortality rose significantly with age, with persons 65 years old and older exhibiting the highest death rates. Almost 9 of every 10 deaths (87.5%) were to persons 45 years old or older.

Although no reliable hospital data were available, hypertension or conditions resulting from hypertensive diseases are recognized as one of the leading causes of hospital admissions. In 1996, approximately 5% of all persons admitted to the general ward of the hospital in Grand Turk had hypertension specifically recorded as the cause of admission, with considerably more having it mentioned as a contributing factor.

Oral Health. Oral health services in the territory suffer from a serious personnel shortage. A single government dentist, assisted by a dental nurse, works out of Grand Turk's main dental clinic, and there is one private dentist in Providenciales. The government dentist and dental nurse schedule visits to the other islands, but a full-time government dentist is needed in Providenciales, where the bulk of the population resides.

The main clinic on Grand Turk offers most dental services, including radiology, periodontics, endodontics, oral surgery, minor prosthetic services, and restorative dentistry. Dental care elsewhere in the territory depends on facilities available on each island. Preventive care, which is mainly carried out through an active school dental health program, also is a priority. Along with educational lectures provided by the department's professional staff, this program also includes screening schoolchildren every five years for decayed, missing, and filled teeth (DMFT) and to assess periodontal index; administering fluoride treatment to every child; and applying sealants for the children's primary and permanent teeth. In addition, approximately 200 talks on dental hygiene were given by the staff in 1995. During 1995, there were 2,550 patient visits made to the main clinic. The average cost per patient visit was estimated at $ 20.00, but the average fee charged was $ 4.00.

Certain oral health problems have raised concern and will have to be addressed in the future, either through services or education. For example, there is a fair amount of fluorosis, which is thought to be partly due to excessive intake of fluoride that occurs naturally in well water. In addition, residents of Providenciales and Grand Turk, particularly children, are presenting with an increasing number of caries, which is thought to be associated with a dietary shift toward less nutritious foods. Finally, there are far too many extractions performed on foreign nationals, because they wait too long to seek dental care.

Behavioral Disorders. The National Drug Council coordinates efforts to curb the impact of illegal drugs in the Turks and Caicos Islands. Originally established in 1989 as a branch of the Ministry of Health, the Council has now been placed under the portfolio of the Minister for Local Government Affairs. Given the unit's growing role, its transformation into a statutory body with more autonomy is currently under consideration.

Council staff supports such activities as an after-care program, drug support groups on most of the islands, a project with the prison, and an anti-drug program in the schools. The Council also was responsible for the ratification of the 1996–2000 National Drug Strategy Master Plan, which calls for institutional strengthening, data collection, drug-traffic reduction, drug-demand reduction, and the development of legislative and judicial frameworks in the battle against drugs.

Statistics on the scope of the drug problem in the territory are not available, but informed opinion holds that it is relatively serious. During the first half of the 1990s, the prison population in the Turks and Caicos doubled. Estimates based on counseling sessions placed the percentage of prisoners who were involved in drug use at 98%. Many cite boredom and peer pressure as the reason for their drug use, which validates the view that offering more community activities for youth will lower the demand for drugs.

Many addicts have sought help through local support groups who, in turn, appeal to the National Drug Council. With no treatment facilities available in the territory, persons are sent to Sandilands Rehabilitation Center in Nassau, the Bahamas, for treatment. Results for 1996 revealed that three clients had successfully completed the six-month treatment at Sandilands and were now in after-care and two were still under treatment; one former client had relapsed. In addition, four clients were admitted.

As part of the after-care program, all clients returning from Sandilands attend weekly sessions for 18 months. Several high-school students who had used marijuana joined the sessions. Fifteen men with drug abuse problems received treatment as part of the prison rehabilitation program, which will seek to enroll parolees in its after-care.

Disaster Preparedness. As a result of efforts of the National Disaster Committee, disaster preparedness has become better structured. The committee is a comprehensive, multidisciplinary body with representatives from government institutions and nongovernmental organizations whose responsibilities include disasters. A National Disaster Coordinator coordinates all committee and subcommittee activities. Education and training through simulation exercises, the dissemination of information, procurement of equipment and supplies, treatment and referrals, data collection and needs assessment; epidemiological surveillance and the control of communicable diseases, and psychological support are areas that have been emphasized.

Within the National Disaster Management Plan, the Primary Health Care Disaster Management Plan serves as the health sector's blueprint of action following a disaster. It provides clearly defined activities to be undertaken by health personnel and the community throughout a disaster's preparedness, response, and recovery stages. The nine government and two private health centers/clinics located throughout the islands are the focal points for the health response to disasters.

The main threats to the Turks and Caicos Islands are hurricanes, floods, fires, and massive transportation accidents such as airplane crashes. Recently, no hurricane has left any significant damage in the territory. Starting in June when the hurricane season begins, however, every committee is mobilized and on alert. During the summer of 1995, severe floods caused extensive damage and property destruction, particularly on North Caicos and Providenciales. Considerable financial and human resources were used in the clean-up.

RESPONSE OF THE HEALTH SYSTEM

National Health Plans and Policies

The Government, which is the main provider of health care, has long had a policy that holds that health care should be available, accessible, and affordable to all residents of the islands. It also acknowledges that nongovernmental organizations and individuals must share in this responsibility if optimal health for the majority is to be a reality. The medical and the dental departments aim to provide efficient, high-quality preventive and curative care to all sectors of the population, working with the community and with private and overseas health care providers. The Environmental Health Department ensures that hotels, restaurants, shops, and private homes adhere to sanitation and health standards as established by law.

Health Sector Reform

In 1989, the Government of the United Kingdom financed a comprehensive health sector adjustment program in order to identify and address the many shortcomings in the health care industry in all British dependent territories in the Caribbean. The program targeted the following five areas for improvements: management structures and processes, planning approaches, financial strategies, quality of care, and health outcomes. Now in its second phase, the program has established operational plans for the Turks and Caicos through the year 2000.

Recommendations from the adjustment program have led to several changes. For example, the fee schedule for medical and dental services has been revised, and an improved financial management system, including a system for revenue collection, will soon be put in place. In addition, the large number of referrals abroad and the need for in-country follow-up care are being examined and the feasibility of establishing a national health insurance system is being explored.

The new management structure established by the health sector adjustment project led to the appointment of a Health Services Manager charged with the administrative aspect of the health services, an area traditionally under the responsibility of the Chief Medical Officer. A Primary Health Care Manager position also was created. Duties from existing posts have been reallocated as a way to fill the new positions.

Policies continue to address infrastructure and personnel deficits that must be dealt with if the quality of services is to improve, as well as the control over health care costs. Priorities are human resource development; access to financial resources; development of an effective health information system that will lead to better program planning and monitoring; improvement to the health infrastructure, particularly at Grand Turk Hospital; the consolidation of ties with nongovernmental organizations; environmental health; drug procurement; health promotion; nutrition; prevention and control of noncommunicable diseases; and the control of HIV and AIDS.

A legislative package also is being explored as part of the health sector adjustment project, which includes provisions for recovery of charges and accident reduction legislation, such as laws on drunk driving or the mandatory use of seatbelts and helmets. A comprehensive review of environmental legislation was completed in 1992.

Because practices such as dietary patterns and food choices play important roles in the etiology of many noncommunicable diseases, a National Nutrition Policy was developed in conjunction with the Caribbean Food and Nutrition Institute (CFNI) and PAHO's nutrition consultant in the Bahamas. The plan will become an important element in the fight against such diet-related conditions as obesity, heart disease, diabetes, and various forms of cancer, which are among the leading causes of morbidity and mortality in adults.

Organization of the Health Sector

Institutional Organization

Health services in the Turks and Caicos Islands comes under the aegis of the Ministry of Health, Education, Youth, and Sports. The services are under the direct responsibility of the Permanent Secretary for Health Services, who is responsible to the Minister. There is some degree of decentralization, and services are categorized into three general areas—medical, dental, and environmental—each with its own budget.

Medical services are further divided into hospital services and community health services. The Chief Medical Officer, who also functions as the medical director of the Turks and Caicos's single hospital located in Grand Turk, is the chief technical officer responsible for all medical and health services. Each section head is administratively responsible to the Permanent Secretary.

The hospital located in Grand Turk is a 36-bed secondary care institution that serves as a referral center for all of the islands; it has a maternity ward; a geriatrics ward; and a general ward that handles all other inpatients. In 1995, the hospital added a hemodialysis unit that can treat up to three patients simultaneously. Before hemodialysis was available, patients had to be transferred abroad for the procedure, at a very high cost.

There are nine community health clinics on six islands: a maternal and child health complex, offering maternal and child health services, female health maintenance, family planning; and school health services on Grand Turk; a general clinic, offering preventive, curative, and rehabilitation services to all age groups, also on Grand Turk; a 10-bed government clinic, providing 24-hour service for general and maternal and child health care on Providenciales; two clinics each on Middle Caicos and North Caicos; and one each on South Caicos and Salt Cay. Depending on demand, clinics are staffed with public health nurses, registered nurse midwives, clinical nurses, and/or community health aides; physicians make scheduled visits.

Maternal and child health services offered by government clinics generally include prenatal and postnatal care, family planning, and child health services.

There are two private clinics located on Providenciales. Many Turks and Caicos residents also regularly travel abroad to the Bahamas or elsewhere for medical care. Private insurance companies offer coverage for medical care to those who can pay. Because the cost for this insurance tends to be exorbitant, the Government is exploring ways of extending locally available services through an arrangement with a visiting specialist. Private physicians also have proposed an arrangement to jointly use and manage the secondary care facility in Providenciales; their proposal is being carefully considered.

Organization of Health Regulatory Activities

The certification and practice of health professionals in Turks and Caicos is governed by the 1978 Health Practitioners Ordinance, which has established a Health Practitioners Board chaired by the Minister responsible for health or his delegate.

The 1992 Public and Environmental Health Ordinance governs the work of the Department of Environmental Health, which is responsible for safeguarding environmental quality—including the preservation of water, air, and soil; housing quality; and chemical safety—and for food protection and safety.

Health Services and Resources

Organization of Services for Care of the Population

Health Promotion. Acknowledging the importance of health promotion to the attainment of health for all, the Gov-

ernment of the Turks and Caicos Islands has embraced the Caribbean Health Promotion Charter and is working to incorporate health promotion activities throughout its programs. The Community Health Department is directly responsible for implementing these programs and activities, many conducted in collaboration with the education and communications sectors. There is, however, a recognized need for a more comprehensive health promotion strategy.

External assistance provides funds for several ongoing health promotion programs, most of them targeting AIDS and drug abuse. Much more can be achieve, however, by developing programs and avctivities aimed at the reduction of other priority health problems such as accidents and violence.

Disease Prevention and Control Programs. Most communicable diseases are reportable by law, and with most of the population routinely attending government clinics, reporting coverage is believed to be quite good. The Community Health Department is responsible for disease prevention, including epidemiological surveillance. Programs such as immunization for mothers, infants, and children; health education activities; cancer screening for adults; screening of schoolchildren; and health education activities are the cornerstones of the Department's prevention activities. The Department's frequent collaboration with other departments, particularly the Environmental Health Department, is essential for the success of such programs as vector control and efforts to control waterborne diseases, foodborne diseases, and diseases that result from biological or chemical contamination.

The integrated vector control project is noteworthy for its efforts to engage the community in the control of mosquitoes and mosquito-borne diseases, especially *Aedes aegypti* and dengue fever. Initially sponsored by the Government of Italy and subsequently funded by the Government of the United Kingdom, the project led to significant reductions in the household index for all mosquitoes, including *Aedes aegypti,* and it was particularly important to those islands near Haiti, where dengue fever is endemic.

Water Supply, Sewerage Systems, and Solid Waste Disposal. Potable water in the Turks and Caicos Islands is mainly obtained through reverse osmosis process, then is distributed from public issue points or via trucks, and finally is stored in water tanks. The public water supply is chlorinated and regularly checked for chemical and bacterial contamination. Many households also rely on well water, a practice that can only be encouraged if the supply is properly treated against bacterial contamination. The current Planning Ordinance requires all new construction to provide for water supply, but many households remain without water storage tanks.

The availability of wastewater and sewage treatment facilities is mandatory. Based on the 1990 census, most households

(52.6%) use septic tank systems, but many (43.6%) still use pit latrines. Large facilities such as hotels have mechanical treatment plants. Because the islands face a chronic water shortage, many hotels, government buildings, and private dwellings use saltwater for flushing systems.

The Environmental Health Department is responsible for the collection and disposal of all waste in the territory. It handled approximately 1,500 tons of solid waste in 1996. On some islands, residential and business collection is handled by private contractors for a small fee. Independent private haulers also provide the service for a fee. Waste is disposed in landfills.

Food Protection and Safety. Food protection and control is important for consumer health and for the economy of the Turks and Caicos Islands, particularly because of the reliance on tourism and fishing. Department of Environmental Health officers trained in food inspection methodologies periodically inspect food preparation, food service, and food dispensing facilities for compliance with sanitation and safety policies and procedures. The Department also is responsible for educating the public on food protection and safety.

Human Resources

Because many health sector areas have shortages of qualified health professionals, the Government must continually recruit foreign nationals. Many of them are hired through short-term contracts, which severely hinders long-term planning efforts.

Recent data indicate that the Ministry of Health employs 5 doctors, 1 dentist, and 34 nurses at various levels; 22 of the nurses had received training as registered nurses or higher. In addition, an allied health staff comprised of eight community health aides, eight geriatric aides, two laboratory technicians, five environmental health officers, and nine vector control officers form part of the public health sector. As of December 1996, only one doctor was a Turks and Caicos national, and almost 50% of nurses, which constitute the largest cadre of

health workers, were foreign nationals; similar situations exist in the support services and environmental health sectors.

The Chief Nursing Officer is responsible for providing leadership to the nursing profession throughout the territory. The Officer also manages nurses and nursing support staff at the hospital and offers educational programs and guidance on career development to all nursing staff. The Chief Nursing Officer reports to the Chief Medical Officer on all technical matters. To assist this professional, a consultant was commissioned to undertake a study analyzing the skill-mix and human resource allocation of nurses; the study's report is under review.

Expenditures and Sectoral Financing

The Government's recurrent expenditure for the 1991–1996 period reveals the rising cost of health care in the Turks and Caicos. The actual cost of health care services to the Government for the 1995–1996 period was 42.3% higher than that for the 1991–1992 period. Health infrastructure development in Providenciales, particularly the new health center that became operational in 1994, is largely responsible for the increase. During the 1995–1996 period, the total amount of the budget allocated to health care was US$ 4,340,652, almost $US 1 million over the 1994–1995 figure and representing 14.3% of the total Government expenditure. For the same period, total revenue was $US 179,100, 72% of which came from medical fees and charges.

In terms of operational expenses, most funds were allocated for medical care services, including the hospital and all clinic services, followed by environmental health. With the cost of services provided at the health center in Providenciales included, the operational budget for medical services for 1995–1996 was $US 1,619,674, a 27% increase over that for 1994–1995. Again, this was due mainly to the increase allocated to the health center in Providenciales, whose range of services were expanded. For the same fiscal year, the operational budget for environmental health services was $US 323,543, 21.6% over that of the previous year.

UNITED STATES OF AMERICA

GENERAL SITUATION AND TRENDS

Socioeconomic, Political, and Demographic Overview

The health situation of United States residents has improved in the last 10 years. Between 1990 and 1995, overall life expectancy at birth increased from 75.4 years to 75.8 years. By 1995, a person who had reached the age of 60 years could expect to live an average of 21.1 more years, for a total of 81.1 years. A person reaching the age of 65 could expect to live an average of 17.4 more years, to 82.4 years. Life expectancy at birth was much higher for white males (73.4) than for African-American males (65.4); the gap is shrinking, however. Increases in life expectancy in the 1990s were 0.7 years for white males and 0.9 years for African-American males. The difference in life expectancy at birth for white and African-American females was 5.6 years. The 1990–1994 data are final, but 1995 data are preliminary and therefore subject to change. Preliminary data are available for whites, African-Americans, and Hispanic populations, but are not available for other racial and ethnic groups.

An estimated 36 million people were living in poverty in 1995. The national poverty rate was 13.8% in 1995, compared with 15.1% in 1993. The poverty rate among African-Americans, the largest minority group, was 29.3%—nearly triple the rate among the white population.

The poverty rate for female-headed households with children declined sharply, from 47.1% in 1991 to 41.5% in 1995, and the poverty rate among children decreased from 21.8% to 20.8%. In 1995, the percentage of African-American children living in poverty (42%) was about 2.5 times that of white children (16%). Poverty levels among Hispanic children (40%) were similar to the levels seen among African-American children.

The resident population of the United States totaled 263 million in 1995, a 6% increase over the 1990 population. Between 1990 and 1995, the population 75–84 years of age grew by 11% to 11 million, and the population 85 years and older grew by 20% to 3.6 million. The African-American population increased by 8%, to 33 million, and the Hispanic population increased by 20%, to 27 million. The Asian and Pacific Islander population grew by 24%, reaching 9 million persons.

Mortality Profile

In 1995, an estimated 2,312,180 deaths were registered in the United States, a rate of 880.0 deaths per 100,000 population. This was 0.5% above the rate of 875.4 per 100,000 in 1994 and the same as the rate in 1993. The age-adjusted death rate, which eliminates the effects of aging of the population, was at a record low of 503.7 per 100,000 population, 0.7% below the 1994 rate of 507.4, and 1.9% below the 1993 rate of 513.3. For most of the 10-year age groups for females and all of the age groups for males, death rates declined between 1994 and 1995 for all races combined. However, death rates increased for females 85 years and older. The most important contributing factor in lower death rates for the white population and African-Americans in the 15–24-year age group was the decrease in homicides.

The age-adjusted death rate in 1995 for all causes combined was about 70% higher for males than for females. For each of the 15 leading causes of death, male mortality was also higher. The greatest differential between genders was seen for HIV infection, where the age-adjusted rate for males was 5.1 times that for females. The smallest sex differential was for diabetes mellitus, with a male-to-female ratio of 1:1.

During the 1990s there were major declines in rates for three of the leading causes of death: heart disease, stroke, and unintentional injuries. Much of the decrease can be attributed to the reduction in risk factors that cause illness. Accompanying these trends are increased public awareness of the risks posed by such activities as tobacco use and driving while under the influence of alcohol.

Between 1990 and 1995, the age-adjusted death rate for heart disease, the leading cause of death, declined 9.1%. This dramatic reduction reflects increased high blood pressure screening and control, a decline in cigarette smoking, and increased awareness of the role of dietary fat in production of cholesterol. The decline in heart disease mortality since 1990 was 10.8% for white men, 7.5% for white women, and 9.7% for African-American men and women. In 1995, heart disease mortality for white men was almost double that for white women; it was more than 64% higher among African-American men than African-American women. In 1993, the age-adjusted death rate for heart disease among males of Asian descent aged 45 years and over (107.6 deaths per 100,000 population) was about 17% lower than the rate for Hispanics, 3.8% lower than the rate for American Indians, 77% lower than for whites, and 149% lower than the rate for African-Americans.

Deaths among white women due to lung cancer showed a 5.8% increase between 1990 and 1995. Death rates from this disease decreased for African-American men by 14.5% and for white men by 8.7%. In 1995, age-adjusted lung cancer death rates for African-American men and white men (73.7 and 51.7 deaths per 100,000, respectively) were two to three times those for African-American women and white women (26.1 and 27.4, respectively).

In 1993, the age-adjusted death rates for all cancers for American Indians, Asians, and Hispanic males aged 45 years and older were similar (92.9, 99.9, and 97.4 deaths per 100,000, respectively); these rates were considerably lower than the rates for whites or African-Americans (156.4 and 238.9 deaths per 100,000, respectively). The most recent available data are from 1993 for certain race groups, including Asians and American Indians.

The age-adjusted death rate from stroke, the third leading cause of death, declined by 3.6% between 1990 and 1995, continuing the downward trend of the 1980s. Declines in stroke mortality since 1980 ranged from 34.1% for African-American men to 36.8% for white men. In 1995, age-adjusted death rates due to stroke were almost twice as high for African-American men as for white men, and 69.4% higher for African-American women than for white women.

Cancer has surpassed heart disease as the leading cause of death for people 45–64 years of age since 1984. In 1995, cancer resulted in 252.5 deaths per 100,000 persons in this age group. Breast cancer rates remain high despite the attention paid to early detection and treatment. Cancer accounts for about one of every four deaths in the United States each year, and, in 1995 it claimed the lives of 537,969 people. Overall, cancer mortality rates have changed little since 1950.

SPECIFIC HEALTH PROBLEMS

Analysis by Population Group

Health of Infants

The infant mortality rate in 1995 was 7.5 deaths per 1,000 live births. Between 1990 and 1995, the infant mortality rate for white infants declined by 17.1%, from 7.6 to 6.3 deaths per 1,000 live births; for African-American infants, it declined by 17.2%, from 18.0 to 14.8. These declines resulted in record low infant mortality rates in the U.S.

In 1994, almost 32,000 infants—about 0.75% of those born—died before reaching 1 year of age. The five leading causes of death in 1995 were congenital anomalies, disorders relating to short gestation and unspecified low birthweight, sudden infant death syndrome, respiratory distress syndrome, and maternal complications of pregnancy.

The overall percentage of live-born infants weighing less than 2,500 g was 7.3% in 1994, up from 7.2% in 1993. The proportion of infants weighing less that 1,500 g at birth (those at greatest risk of death and disability) was stable at 1.3%. In 1994, the percentage of African-American infants weighing less than 1,500 g was three times that of white infants (3.0% as compared with 1.0%). Maternal cigarette smoking has been identified as a risk factor for low birthweight babies in the United States. Other major problems associated with low birthweight include lack of prenatal care, young age of the mother, and alcohol and drug use.

The spread of HIV/AIDS among women and heterosexual men has resulted in increasing numbers of seropositive newborns. Infants born with HIV infection require more intensive health care services throughout their lives. Through June 1996, AIDS was reported in more than 6,900 children under 13 years old.

Health of Children and Adolescents

The coverage rates for DPT, polio, and measles immunizations given between 19 months and 35 months of age were 90%, 79%, and 90%, respectively, in 1994. This represents some improvement over 1992, when the coverage rates were 83% for DPT, 72% for polio, and 83% for measles. Nonetheless, the 1994 level of immunization coverage is lower than in many other countries, including many developing countries.

Outbreaks of communicable diseases still occur throughout the United States, indicating that vaccination programs have not adequately reached many children, especially in rural and inner city areas. Nevertheless, other than an increase in the number of measles cases between 1989 and 1990, especially among preschoolers, there have been no major outbreaks or epidemics of vaccine-preventable diseases in recent years.

Over 42% of all childhood deaths are due to unintentional injuries, and about 30% of these occur as a result of motor vehicle accidents. The number of deaths due to automobile accidents has declined as a result of increased compliance with laws in all 50 states that require the use of car safety restraints for young children.

Among teenagers, the three leading causes of death are unintentional injuries, homicide, and suicide. While motor vehicle deaths involving alcohol are the greatest risk to white males in the 15–24-year age group, homicide is the leading killer among African-American males in the same age group. The death rate from motor vehicle accidents for young white men was 42.4 per 100,000 in 1995.

The suicide rate for American Indian males 15–24 years of age (31.6 deaths per 100,000 population in 1993) was one-third higher than the rate for white youths, 57% higher than the rate for African-American youth, 74% higher than for Hispanic youth, and 150% higher than the rate for Asian youth.

Studies indicate that in the United States, the average age at first sexual intercourse is 16 years, putting high school students at risk for acquiring HIV infection. Through June 1996, there were 2,463 reported cases of AIDS among adolescents (13–19 years of age); and 94,414 among 20–29 year olds. Because the time from infection with HIV to development of AIDS can be 10 years or more, many people with AIDS who are in their twenties were infected as teenagers. The proportion of adolescent AIDS cases diagnosed among females peaked in 1994 (43%) and declined to 40% in 1995.

Mental retardation, learning disabilities, and emotional and behavioral problems are other threats to child health. These conditions seem to be more prevalent among children living in poverty than among children in higher socioeconomic situations.

Health of Adults

In 1994, the fertility rate was 66.7 live births per 1,000 women 15–44 years of age, 1% lower than the rate of 67.6 in 1993, and 6% lower than in 1990 (70.9). There were 3,952,767 babies born in 1994, 1% fewer than in 1993. Preliminary data for 1995 indicate births continued to decline by about 1%.

Between 1993 and 1994, birth rates by age of mother fell 1% for women 15–29 years old. Rates for women in their 30s rose 1% to 2%, while the rate for women aged 40–44 years increased 5%. Rates for the youngest teenagers, 10–14 years, and for women aged 45–49 years were unchanged. The birth rate for 15–17-year-olds dropped to 37.6, and the rate for 18–19-year-olds to 91.5 per 1,000 births, both declines of 1%.

Preliminary data for 1995 suggest that teen birth rates continued to decline.

Fertility rates for women of Hispanic origin declined 1% in 1994 to 105.6 per 1,000. Preliminary data indicate that the 1995 rate (103.7) is the lowest since national data on Hispanic fertility became available in 1989. Despite the decline, Hispanic women in 1994 continued to have much higher fertility than non-Hispanic white women at all ages. For example, the birth rate for Hispanic teenagers was 107.7, compared with 40.4 for non-Hispanic white teenagers. Among Hispanic groups, the fertility of Mexican American women was highest (115.4 in 1994), followed by Puerto Rican women (81.9) and Cuban women (55.9). For Hispanic women not belonging to those three groups the fertility rate was 97.7.

AIDS is the third leading cause of death among women aged 2–44 years. The number of AIDS cases due to heterosexual transmission of the virus to women increased by 165% between 1992 and 1993, partly because of the inclusion of gynecological conditions as markers in the AIDS case definition in 1993; from 1993 to 1995 the number of cases due to heterosexual transmission declined by 14%. Although African-American and Hispanic women make up only 22% of the female population, 74% of the women diagnosed with AIDS since 1981 belong to these ethnic groups.

In 1995, 64.2% of women between 15 and 44 years of age were using some form of contraceptive. New contraceptive choices such as the Norplant implant and the "female condom" are currently available; however, the implant is costly and the extent to which it will be available to low-income women is uncertain. While the female condom has the potential to greatly reduce the incidence of STDs among women who use it, its acceptability in populations at greatest risk for these infections and unwanted pregnancies from its use are still unknown. Data for 1994 show that the abortion rate was 321 abortions per 1,000 live births, down from 345 in 1990. The abortion rate is 21 per 1,000 women in the age group 15–44. This rate remained stable from 1980–1991, and has recorded moderate but consistent annual declines since 1991.

Health of the Elderly

The aging of the population is one of the greatest challenges facing the health care system in the United States. By the year 2000, it is projected that the number of people 65 years and over will rise to 35 million, accounting for 13% of the population. That proportion is expected to climb as high as 23% by the year 2040. Most significant, however, is the rapid growth of the population 85 years of age and over, whose numbers are expected to rise 52%, to 4.6 million by the year 2000. As a result, a considerable increase will be seen in such disabling conditions as hip fractures and Alzheimer's disease.

Heart disease, cancer, stroke, pneumonia/influenza, chronic obstructive pulmonary disease, and diabetes are the major causes of death among persons aged 65 and older. Because pneumococcal disease is three times more prevalent among those older than 65, immunization for older adults is considered a priority preventive service.

Problems such as arthritis, visual and hearing impairments, osteoporosis, incontinence, and dementia also have significant impact on the lives of seniors. Health promotion offers major benefits toward maintaining the health of the elderly. Physical activity and proper diet can increase bone mineral content, reduce the risk for osteoporotic fractures, and help maintain appropriate body weight.

Health of Special Populations

Growth has been much faster among racial/ethnic minority populations than the majority white population over the past two decades, a trend that is expected to continue for at least the next 30 years. It is projected that the African-American population will increase 35% from 1990 to the year 2020, while the population of other minority groups (mostly Asians and Pacific Islanders, but also American Indian/Alaska Natives) will more than double. The Hispanic population is expected to rise by 84%. The projected increase in the white population during this period is only 11%.

While chronic disease conditions are the leading causes of death for both minority and nonminority persons over 45 years of age, minority populations (African-Americans, Hispanics, Native Americans, and Asian American/Pacific Islanders) incur a disproportionate share of death, illness, disability, and adverse health conditions. Commonly used health indicators such as life expectancy at birth and infant mortality rates show continued widening of the health gap between minority and majority populations. Poverty is a major contributing factor to the disparities in health status.

African-Americans. African-Americans are the largest minority group, comprising 12% of the nation's population. Although African-Americans live in all parts of the country and occupy every socioeconomic level, one-half of their population lives in urban areas that are typified by poverty, poor schools, and inadequate housing, and one-third of the population lives in poverty—a rate three times that of whites.

Death rates among African-Americans exceed those of the white population by 58.8%. Rates are also higher for most of the leading causes of death. Homicide continues to be responsible for the greatest rate differential between the races. The age-adjusted death rate due to homicide in the African-American population in 1995 was about six times higher than in the white population, and it was the leading cause of death in

1995 among African-Americans 15–24 years of age. Age-adjusted death rates for chronic diseases are one-third to nearly three times higher in the African-American population than in the white population. The death rates for colorectal, respiratory, and breast cancer among the African-American population have decreased in the 1990s, as they have among the white population. The three leading causes of death for which rates were lower among African-Americans than among whites were chronic obstructive pulmonary diseases and allied conditions, suicide, and Alzheimer's disease.

Hispanics. The Hispanic population is the second largest and fastest growing minority group. Hispanic subgroups, including Mexican Americans, Puerto Ricans, Cuban Americans, and Central and South American immigrants, comprised about 10% of the total population in 1995. The birth rate among Hispanics was 25.5 births per 1,000 population in 1994, while that of the total population was 15.2 births per 1,000.

Tobacco use poses a substantial risk to the health of Hispanics, since 43% of Hispanic men currently smoke and teenagers of both sexes smoke more than African-American or white teenagers. Hispanic teenagers also report more frequent use of alcohol than African-Americans and whites.

Asians and Pacific Islanders. Speaking more than 30 different languages and representing many cultural groups, Asians and Pacific Islanders are the nation's third largest minority. Asians who have been established in the United States for generations are virtually indistinguishable socioeconomically from the majority population, and their median income is higher than that of the overall population.

Local studies have identified certain diseases that pose special health risks for Asian Americans and Pacific Islanders. The lung cancer rate is 18% greater for Southeast Asian men than for white men. Higher rates of high blood pressure have been documented among Filipino men ages 50 and older living in California than among the total California population. Tuberculosis and hepatitis B are of particular concern in immigrant communities. Rates for these conditions among Southeast Asian immigrants are 40 times higher than those in the total population.

Native Americans. The Native American Indian and Alaska Natives form the smallest minority group, numbering 2.1 million. About 50% live in urban areas, while many of the rest live on reservations. Health care for this native population is provided by the federal government through the Indian Health Service.

This population is relatively youthful, because large proportions of Native Americans die before 45 years of age and because of a relatively high level of fertility. Age-adjusted death rates for diabetes, liver disease, and tuberculosis are two to three times higher among Native Americans than comparable rates for the total U.S. population.

The major cause of death among Native Americans under the age of 45 is unintentional injuries, which most often follow alcohol use (75%). The injury death rate for American Indians 15–24 years of age is two to three times higher than the rate for any other group. More than half (54%) of the motor vehicle accidents in this population have been attributed to the effects of alcohol.

Alcoholism is the leading health and social problem of the American Indian and Alaska Native people. The 1992 age-adjusted death rate for alcohol-induced causes among American Indians and Alaska Natives was 38.4 deaths per 100,000 population—5.6 times the rate for the total population (6.8 deaths per 100,000). Smoking and other tobacco use are also significant health problems.

Refugees. In 1995, approximately 131,300 refugees were admitted to the United States. Of these, 34% came from Eastern Europe and the former Soviet Union, 28% from East Asia, 3% from the Near East, 30% from Latin America and the Caribbean, and 3% from Africa. The number of refugees entering the United States in fiscal year 1995 represents a decrease of 9% from the number who entered the country in 1992. The number of refugees and entrants from Latin America and the Caribbean increased by 131% in the same period.

Upon arrival in this country, refugee reception and initial placement is the responsibility of 12 nonprofit organizations that operate through federally funded cooperative agreements with the Department of State. Thereafter, the refugees receive assistance from state programs funded by the Department of Health and Human Services.

Because refugees often have health problems that stem from the conditions in their countries of origin, health care services are offered in first-asylum camps located in refugee processing centers. At ports of entry, refugees and their medical records are inspected by quarantine officers who also notify the appropriate state and local health departments of their arrival. Health services are provided by the Refugee Resettlement Program for all refugees who meet a means test.

The Government provided close to US$ 412 million in 1995 to support refugee activities both overseas and domestically. Grant program funds are awarded to state and local health offices for post-arrival health assessments to help identify health problems that might impair effective resettlement, employability, and self-sufficiency of newly arriving refugees.

People with Disabilities. In the United States, more than 49 million people have physical and mental disabilities. For these individuals, disability affects all aspects of their well-being, and has emotional, social, and financial consequences.

In 1994–1995, the National Center for Health Statistics conducted the first-ever comprehensive national disability survey in this country. The survey found that the prevalence of disabilities is disproportionately higher among minority, elderly, poor, and rural populations.

In fiscal year 1997, the Department of Health and Human Services devoted over US$ 62 billion to programs for people with disabilities. Not only do disabilities entail high costs for individuals, but also for states and for the nation as a whole. In 1997, estimated economic losses due to disability, including the increased cost of health care and reduced productivity, was over US$ 350 billion.

Health care is an essential component to helping people with disabilities lead independent lives, and the Department of Health and Human Services is helping to ensure that people with disabilities have access to quality health care throughout their lives. Medicare and Medicaid, the Government's largest public financing programs, in 1997 provided health insurance to about 12 million individuals considered to be disabled based on federal criteria. Spending during fiscal year 1997 is estimated at US$ 21 billion for health care and services under Medicare, and the Government is expected to make US$ 33 billion in Medicaid payments. The budget for FY 1998 includes proposals to help people with disabilities lead more independent lives.

As the Health Care Financing Administration (HCFA), a division of the Department of Health and Human Services, implements the Health Insurance Portability and Accountability Act of 1996, special care is being taken to protect the insurability of individuals with preexisting conditions. The HCFA also continues to support community-based, long-term care for the elderly and people with developmental or physical disabilities.

The Department of Health and Human Services supports and conducts a wide array of research activities on service organization and delivery, quality, and financing of health and long-term care for people with disabilities. In particular, the Agency for Health Care Policy Research helps policymakers plan for meeting the health needs of people with disabilities by examining their access to and use of health services, as well as their views of how the health care system works.

The lack of knowledge about the health needs of women with disabilities resulting from chronic physical impairments prompted the National Institutes of Health Office of Research on Women's Health to sponsor development of health promotion activities. These programs are identifying barriers to health promotion and are developing effective, well-defined interventions that will lead to improved health for women with disabilities.

Other Special Groups. A government-sponsored program known as Health Care for the Homeless (HCH) intends to improve access by homeless individuals to primary health care services and substance abuse treatment. In 1997, 123 HCH programs were supported in 48 states, the District of Columbia, and Puerto Rico. Fiscal year 1997 funding for the HCH program totals US$ 69 million.

Residents of public housing projects have also been targeted for assistance with federal funds to help overcome barriers to health services such as lack of transportation, language difficulties, and lack of financial resources. In 1997, a total of US$ 9 million was awarded to 21 grantees to improve access to health care for people who reside in public housing.

Analysis by Type of Disease or Health Impairment

Communicable Diseases

Vaccine-Preventable Diseases. Among vaccine-preventable diseases, diphtheria, tetanus, pertussis, and polio either decreased or remained at a constant low level between 1988 and 1995. However, a major measles outbreak occurred in 1989–1990, after almost 10 years of relatively few reported cases. The number of measles cases in 1989 was higher than the median number reported annually during the preceding eight years, and in 1990, 27,786 cases were reported. In 1995, only 281 cases of measles were reported.

While the measles outbreak affected all age groups, the most notable increases in incidence occurred in preschool-aged children and adults over 20 years old. In several cities, data indicated that measles vaccination coverage was only 40%–65% in kindergarten children, and low coverage significantly contributed to the spread of the disease. Measles outbreaks also occurred among school-aged children with high coverage rates, prompting 21 states to require that students receive a second measles vaccination upon entering kindergarten, first grade, or middle school.

AIDS and Other STDs. The number of persons infected with HIV in the United States was estimated at between 635,000 and 900,000 in 1992. As of June 1996, 530,397 AIDS cases in adults, adolescents, and children had been reported. The number of AIDS cases more than doubled between 1992 and 1993, partly because of the expansion of the AIDS surveillance case definition in 1993, as mentioned previously. Between 1993 and 1995, the annual number of cases declined by 30%, to 71,300 in 1995.

HIV infection continues to be a major health problem, with racial/ethnic minorities bearing a disproportionate share of the burden. However, annual numbers of AIDS cases among African-Americans and Hispanics decreased 23% and 25%, respectively, between 1993 and 1995, to rates of 91 per 100,000 population in African-Americans and 42 per 100,000 in Hispanics, compared to 15 per 100,000 in whites.

In the 1993–1995 period, there was a larger proportionate decrease in reported cases among men (33%) than among women (18%). For women, 1995 rates were higher among African-Americans and Hispanics (46 and 17 per 100,000 population, respectively) than among whites (3 per 100,000). In 1995, African-American children accounted for 66% of all reported pediatric AIDS cases.

The primary exposure categories for reported AIDS cases in the United States are homosexual males (44%) and injecting drug users (26%). A growing number of people have been infected through heterosexual contact (11%). In 1995, the number of women infected with HIV through heterosexual contact exceeded the number infected through injection drug use.

Prevention programs, directed toward changing behaviors, continue to be the main strategy in the control of HIV/AIDS. Massive education and prevention programs have been undertaken to reduce injection drug use, decrease high-risk sexual behaviors, and increase the use of condoms. Efforts to develop creative preventive programs, improve care of AIDS patients, and conduct research on care have been initiated throughout the country.

Because many AIDS patients do not have medical insurance and others have depleted their private insurance and personal resources to pay for costly treatment, much of the cost for treating HIV/AIDS is borne by local and state programs as well as by Medicaid, a public health financing program.

Women in the United States are at substantial risk for sexually transmitted diseases (STDs). In 1995, rates for syphilis and gonorrhea among women were 6 and 140 per 100,000, respectively; both rates have declined during the 1990s. Once infected, women are less likely than men to have symptoms, less likely to seek care, and less likely to be diagnosed correctly after seeking care. Since STDs in women pose far more serious complications than in men (including infertility, ectopic pregnancy, and cervical cancer), it is important for women to be knowledgeable about the prevention, diagnosis, and implications of STDs.

Tuberculosis. The incidence of tuberculosis rose in the United States in the early 1990s after decades of decline. A total of 26,673 new cases were reported in 1992, a 20% increase over 1985. Since 1992, the annual number of new cases of tuberculosis has declined to about the level of 1985 (22,860 cases reported in 1995). The increase in the early 1990s was due to many factors, including the HIV epidemic, deterioration in the local public health care infrastructure, and increases in the number of cases among immigrants.

The occurrence of resistant and multi-drug–resistant tuberculosis has caused great concern regarding recent outbreaks. A national task force, created to expand the 1989 Strategic Plan for the Elimination of Tuberculosis, developed a national action plan to control multi-drug–resistant tuberculosis. The plan defines steps that must be taken to bring current outbreaks under control, prevent new ones, and work toward the ultimate elimination of the disease.

Foodborne Illnesses. Foodborne illnesses remain a major health problem in the U.S. It is estimated that as many as 9,000 deaths and from 6.5 to 33 million illnesses are food-related. Hospitalization costs alone for these illnesses are estimated at over US$ 3 billion a year and costs for lost productivity for seven specific pathogens have been estimated to range between US$ 6 billion and US$ 9 billion.

Between 1988 and 1992, 2,423 foodborne outbreaks were reported in the United States. Bacterial pathogens were responsible for causing 79% of the 1,001 outbreaks and 90% of the cases for which an etiology was determined. Outbreaks caused by *Salmonella enteritidis* continued to cause significant morbidity and mortality, but decreased by 35% between 1989 (77 outbreaks) and 1996 (50 outbreaks). In addition to bacteria such as *Campylobacter jejuni, Escherichia coli* O157:H7, and *Listeria monocytogenes,* parasites (including *Cryptosporidium parvum* and *Cyclospora cayetanensis*) are emerging as important foodborne pathogens. Multi-state outbreaks of foodborne illness caused by contaminated produce are of epidemiological importance.

While about 400 outbreaks are reported each year in the U.S., most foodborne diseases occur as sporadic, individual cases. In the past, passive surveillance for specific infections was conducted by local, state, and national health authorities to provide a sketch of those diseases. Beginning in 1996, an active surveillance program in five sentinel sites (FoodNet) was initiated to provide more detailed data on sporadic cases of diagnosed infections.

Noncommunicable Diseases and Other Health-Related Problems

Malignant Tumors. It is estimated that 180,200 new cases of breast cancer will be diagnosed in women in 1997, making it the second leading cause of cancer deaths among women. One in 10 women is projected to develop breast cancer in their lifetime. Although African-American women have an 18% lower incidence of breast cancer than white women, their survival rates are significantly lower, probably a result of earlier diagnosis of the disease in white women. The incidence rate of lung cancer in men began to decline in 1984, but the rate among women continues to rise.

Although incidence rates for colorectal cancer have increased since 1973, they seem to have peaked among white males and females. In recent years there have been significant declines in incidence in both sexes in the white population, a modest decline in African-American females, and stability in African-American males. Mortality rates for colorectal cancer have risen somewhat among African-American males; however, for African-American females the mortality rate has been stable in recent years.

Accidents and Violence. In 1995, nearly 151,000 Americans died from injuries sustained from motor vehicle accidents, falls, burns, drowning, poisoning, homicide, and suicide. This translates into more than 400 people who die from injuries each day; at least 58 of these are children. Costs due to injury including direct medical care and rehabilitation as well as lost income and productivity in 1995 are estimated at more than US$ 224 billion. This represents an increase of 42% over the last decade. Accidental injuries kill more people between the ages of 1 and 34 in the United States than any other cause. Many measures for preventing unintentional injury are available, such as safety belts and child safety seats to prevent traffic fatalities, smoke detectors to warn residents of fire, and fencing around swimming pools to prevent drowning, but people do not use them consistently.

Traffic fatalities have decreased remarkably over the past 30 years. Even so, more than 1.2 million people died on the roads during that period, and traffic accidents remain the leading cause of death from unintentional injury. At present, motor vehicle crashes account for nearly one-third of all injury fatalities, and they are the leading cause of death for persons 5–24 years of age. Alcohol is involved in over 40% of all traffic deaths, and is a factor in about 1.2 million crash-related injuries each year. In 1993 alone, there were over 1.5 million arrests for driving while under the influence of alcohol or narcotics. It is estimated that about two in every five persons in the U.S. will be in a traffic accident involving alcohol at some time in their lives.

Every year, nearly 900 people die from injuries sustained while cycling. Another 550,000 injured bicyclists are treated in emergency departments, 33% of these for head injuries. Head injuries are involved in 62% of bicycle-related deaths. Studies have shown that bicycle helmets reduce the risk of head injury by 80%.

The United States currently has the highest overall fire death rate of all industrialized countries. Residential fires are the major cause of overall fire-related mortality. In 1995, 414,000 residential fires claimed the lives of 3,640 individuals and injured another 18,650 people. Direct property damage exceeded US$ 4.2 billion; fire death and injury costs totaled US$ 16 billion. Persons living in residences equipped with functional smoke detectors are half as likely to die in a house fire. About one-quarter of U.S. households lack a working smoke detector.

On an average day, 70 people die from homicide in the United States, 87 people commit suicide, as many as 3,000 attempt suicide, and a minimum of 18,000 survive assaults. Between 1990 and 1995, the age-adjusted homicide rate decreased by 8.9% to 9.2 deaths per 100,000 population, and among males aged 25–44, the rate decreased by 20.4%. However, there were large disparities in homicide rates in 1995 among males aged 15–24. African-American males had rates 18 times higher, and Hispanic males had rates 8.7 times higher than white males. Homicide is the second leading cause of death for young people aged 15–24 and the leading cause for African-Americans in that age group.

In 1994, almost 5,000 women in the United States were murdered. In those cases in which it was known whether or not the perpetrator and the victim knew each other, only 13% were killed by a stranger. Of the women murdered by someone they knew, approximately half were murdered by a spouse or someone with whom they had been intimate. The great majority of assaults on women do not result in death, but in physical injury and severe emotional distress. In 1985, the most recent year for which there are data, an estimated 1.8 million women were physically assaulted by male partners.

From 1980 to 1995, the suicide rate for the U.S. population rose only slightly. Still, suicide was the ninth leading cause of death in 1995. Each year, suicide claims more than 30,000 lives; about 80% of those who die are males. Mortality data compiled for the 1990–1995 period show that the rate of suicide among children under 15 years of age in the United States was double the average suicide rate among that age group in other highly industrialized countries. From 1952 through 1995, suicide rates among adolescents and young adults more than tripled. From 1980 to 1995, the rate of suicide among people aged 15–19 increased by 23%, and among those aged 10–14, the increase was 118%. For African-American males aged 15–19, the rate increased by 146% in this period.

Suicide rates continue to be highest among people aged 65 and older. The 1980–1990 period was the first decade since the 1940s in which the suicide rate for older people rose instead of declined. In 1995, persons aged 65 and older accounted for 13% of the population but almost one-fifth of all suicides. Because this is the fastest growing age group in the United States, it is likely that the number of suicides in this age group will continue to increase.

Behavioral Disorders. In 1994, there were 5,932 mental health facilities in operation in the United States. Nearly 60% (3,216) were operated and/or funded in whole or in part by a state mental health agency. State and county mental hospitals numbered 260 (5%); private psychiatric hospitals, 430 (8%); residential treatment centers for emotionally disturbed children, 459 (9%); general hospitals with separate psychiatric services, 1,612 (30%); Veterans Administration psychiatric

organizations, 161 (3%); and all other mental health organizations, 2,470 (46%).

Mental health facilities received US$ 37.4 billion in funding in 1994. Of this amount, facilities funded in whole or part by state mental health agencies received US$ 23.2 billion, and US$ 7.4 billion of these funds went to state and county mental hospitals. The Medicaid program provided 20.4% (US$ 7.7 billion) of total funds received by all mental health facilities in 1994, and 21.9% (US$ 5.1 billion) of funds received by mental health facilities operated and/or funded by state mental health agencies. Managed care organizations provided funds to 2,662 (46%) of all mental health facilities.

In 1992 (the latest year for which data are available), the one-year prevalence of mental disorders other than substance abuse was 16% among non-institutionalized, non-rural adults between the ages of 18 and 54. Of these adults, 11.1% had a depressive (affective) disorder, and 34.2% obtained treatment. The prevalence of depressive disorders was higher among women (34.2%) than among men (13.1%).

Substance Abuse. Approximately 11% of preventable deaths in the United States are related to alcohol and illicit drug use. Alcohol is associated with motor vehicle crashes and fatal intentional injuries such as suicides and homicides: in 1994, 19,470 deaths were attributed to alcohol-induced causes. Heavy alcohol use, defined as five or more drinks in a row at least once in the prior two-week period, has increased in the past several years. In 1995, the rate of heavy use among high school seniors was reported as 28%; among college students, the rate was 41%.

In 1992, the prevalence of marijuana use among high school seniors began to increase. Of related concern is the continued decline in the proportion of high school seniors who perceive social disapproval of occasional use of marijuana and physical and psychological harm from regular marijuana use. The rate of use among young adults (18–25 years) remained about the same in 1994 and 1995.

The Secretary of Health and Human Services has named the Youth Substance Abuse Prevention Initiative as one the Department's six key initiatives. Consistent with the objectives of the Office of National Drug Abuse Policy, the initiative aims to educate the country's youth and enable them to reject illegal drugs, as well as alcohol and tobacco. Its primary goal is to reverse the upward trend in marijuana use and to reduce by 25% the rate of use among youth aged 12–17.

Oral Health. Dental and oral diseases, including dental caries and periodontal diseases, may be the most prevalent and preventable conditions in the United States, especially among lower socioeconomic groups. Although oral health status has been improving on average, especially among children, expenditures for dental services totaled US$ 45.8 billion in 1995, about 5.2% of all expenditures for personal health care. Of that total, 95.6% was paid either "out-of-pocket" by consumers or through private dental insurance. It is important to note, however, that less than one-half the U.S. population has such insurance.

A nationwide survey conducted between 1988 and 1994 found that more than 60% of children under the age of 10 had a caries-free primary dentition, as had 55% of children and adolescents aged 5–17. While caries in permanent teeth continue to decline among school-aged children, 45% of them still suffer from this preventable disease. Tooth decay is nearly universal among American adults. The survey found that 94% of people aged 18 and older had either untreated decay or fillings in the crowns of their teeth. Women had more caries than men, but they also had slightly less untreated decay. Whites had approximately twice as many coronal caries as African-Americans and Mexican Americans, but these two groups had more tooth surfaces in need of treatment than did whites. Women had better periodontal health than did men, and whites had fewer periodontal problems than did African-Americans or Mexican Americans.

Oral cancer primarily affects adults over age 60 and results in over 8,000 deaths annually. Treatment of oral cancer is costly and frequently results in significant disfigurement and loss of function. The most common risk factors for oral cancers are tobacco and alcohol use and excessive exposure to sun. Early detection and treatment can reduce both morbidity and costs. Workplace or community-based strategies to eliminate use of tobacco could prevent many of the 30,000 new cases of oral cancer that occur each year.

RESPONSE OF THE HEALTH SYSTEM

National Health Plans and Policies

The most comprehensive U.S. policy to improve health and prevent adverse health conditions is called Healthy People 2000. The central goal is to increase the number of people who live long, healthy, and disability-free lives. The second goal of the plan calls for the elimination of disparities in health among population groups. The third goal of the strategy is to achieve access to clinical preventive services for all people.

As overall coordinator of Healthy People 2000, the Office of Disease Prevention and Health Promotion, a program office in the Department of Health and Human Services, works with Public Health Service agencies, other federal agencies and departments, and members of the Healthy People Consortium. The Consortium consists of 345 national membership organizations representing professional, voluntary, and corporate interests and 271 state agencies that collaborate to support

the prevention agenda and achieve the year 2000 goals. The Consortium members have worked on revising and adding to the year 2000 objectives and many have participated in periodic progress reviews chaired by the Assistant Secretary for Health.

In 1994, the Public Health Service undertook a midcourse review of the Healthy People 2000 objectives. The resulting review document showed that of the 300 objectives, 50% were moving toward the target, 18% were moving away from the target, 3% showed no change, and 29% had insufficient data to measure progress. As of 1997, 44 states, the District of Columbia, and Guam had published Healthy People 2000 plans of their own. By 1993, 70% of local health departments were using Healthy People objectives.

At the 1996 meeting of the Healthy People Consortium, at which WHO and PAHO were represented, the foundation was laid for the third generation of these objectives, Healthy People 2010, which will be released in January 2000. Consortium members and federal, state, and local agencies are collaborating to develop a set of objectives that will reflect current prevention science and the most important health promotion and disease prevention issues. Healthy People 2010 is the United States response to the World Health Organization's Renewing the Health for All strategy.

Health Services and Resources

Organization of Services for Care of the Population

Food and Nutrition. Diet plays a critical role in the prevention of diseases such as coronary heart disease, cancers, strokes, and diabetes mellitus, which are leading causes of death and disability in the United States. Improvement of maternal and child nutrition is especially critical to improving national health.

Objectives in improving nutrition nationwide relate to obesity, relationships between diet and disease, the application of the "Dietary Guidelines for Americans" to food service operations, dietary counseling, food labeling, nutrition education in schools, maternal and infant nutrition, and feeding of older people. Strategies to achieve these objectives focus on the following: labeling foods in a way that facilitates consumers' application of the dietary guidelines; ensuring that the dietary guidelines are followed in institutional meal preparation, such as in schools and day-care centers; and nutrition education, particularly for school-aged children, low-income populations, and medical professionals.

The strategy for food safety involves four components: regulatory measures to increase food safety; technical support for states and territories for regulation of food operations; surveillance systems to track the incidence of foodborne pathogens; and communication with consumers about safe food-handling practices.

Environmental Health. Addressing environmental health concerns requires the participation of federal agencies including the Department of Health and Human Services, the Environmental Protection Agency, the Department of Agriculture, and the Department of Transportation, as well as state and local agencies, the private sector and community groups. The wide range of priority areas reflects the broad nature of the problems. Some of the priorities include environmental health education, risk assessment programs for state health agencies, emergency response programs, and water/sanitation projects among migrant and rural people.

In its ongoing efforts in disease prevention, the U.S. Public Health Service recognizes that environmental risks are underlying factors contributing to the disease process. Among the numerous diseases and dysfunctions that have a known or suspected environmental component are cancer, reproductive disorders such as infertility and low birthweight, neurological and immune system impairments, and respiratory conditions such as asthma. Exposure to environmental hazards covers a broad range of factors such as pesticides, toxic chemicals, and radiation. The environmental component of a particular disease or health outcome is frequently the result of repeated and cumulative exposures.

The magnitude of the threat posed by environmental hazards on the health of the nation is evident in the following examples. In 1995, one-third of the United States population lived in an area where the air was too polluted to meet health standards. One in four United States residents lived within four miles of a so-called "Superfund site," which denotes areas assigned highest priority by the Environmental Protection Area for accelerated clean-up of hazardous wastes. Aquifers from which much of the country draws its drinking water are shrinking faster than they can be replenished, and as this happens, they become increasingly vulnerable to toxic contamination.

Family Planning Services. Public funds to provide family planning services come from several programs. The largest source of funds is the federal-state Medicaid program, which focuses on low-income women. In fiscal year 1997, Medicaid reimbursed health care providers an estimated US$ 475 million for their provision of family planning services.

The only federal program dedicated solely to funding family planning services is Title X of the Public Health Service Act, "Population Research and Voluntary Family Planning Programs." Funded agencies provide a variety of contraceptive options, along with education and counseling to low-income women, especially those who do not qualify for Medicaid and lack private insurance. With a fiscal year 1997 budget of US$ 198 million, the Title X program serves 5 million women through a network of 5,000 clinics nationwide. Family planning services are also partially supported in most states with federal funds from the Maternal and Child Health Block Grant and the Social Services Block grant program. In addition, some family planning clinics receive support from state and local sources.

The Adolescent Family Life Program has a fiscal year 1997 budget of US$ 14.2 million for programs to control the number of teen pregnancies. With these funds, it supports community-based demonstration projects focusing on issues of adolescent sexuality, pregnancy, and parenting. Prevention projects encourage adolescents to abstain from early sexual activity. Parental consent is required for receipt of these services.

Research and Technology

Research. Biomedical and behavioral research and training are conducted through a vast network of extramural programs involving the country's major universities, medical schools, and research centers. The federal government supports nearly 40% of all biomedical research and development in the country through the National Institutes of Health (NIH). The highest funding priority at NIH is basic research. This research investment has led to many achievements: new knowledge about the body, from the level of the gene to organ systems; research and clinical technologies; new diagnostic techniques; new drugs to fight illnesses; and new vaccines to prevent disease. Through its training programs, NIH ensures a steady flow of young researchers into the biomedical research community.

The total NIH budget for fiscal year 1998 is approximately US$ 13.6 billion, which includes US$ 1.6 billion for AIDS research. Approximately 79% of the budget supports extramural research and training in the United States and abroad and about 11% of the budget supports intramural research conducted at NIH's own laboratories. Although international cooperation accounts for only about 1.5% of the total NIH budget, it is an important component of the NIH research portfolio. Interaction on a global scale among biomedical and behavioral researchers, technicians, and laboratories increases the opportunity to capitalize on scientific opportunities and new technologies for the diagnosis, prevention, and treatment of disease.

Technology Transfer. Technology transfer has gained increased importance in the United States. It involves the dissemination of research results; collaboration between public, academic, and industrial organizations on research and development projects; licensing of intellectual property rights; and introduction to the marketplace of new devices, vaccines, diagnostic and therapeutic drugs, etc. Effective partnerships between these entities increase the capacity to conduct laboratory and clinical research, facilitate the movement of scientific discoveries into public health advances, and contribute to economic growth. NIH is considered the preeminent government technology transfer entity in the United States, since it accounts for over 80% of the royalty income generated by the entire Government.

While technology transfer activity has increased, there have been numerous issues and concerns regarding its administration, such as how academic and industrial collaborations and agreements affect NIH-funded activities. Another area of concern is how public investments in research are reflected in the price of health care products. NIH has addressed this issue by using careful selection procedures for its partners, constructive negotiation techniques, aggressive monitoring of licensee's timely achievement of established benchmarks, and ensuring that discoveries move as rapidly as possible into the marketplace to improve public health.

The management of intellectual property, such as human genome research discoveries, is a new area requiring careful consideration. At issue is whether intellectual property derived from government-funded research should be patented or made available to the public.

Health Services Research. Increased emphasis is being placed on research to improve delivery of health services, patient outcomes, and assessment of health care technology. The Agency for Health Care Policy and Research (AHCPR), a part of the Public Health Service, is the lead agency charged with supporting research designed to improve the quality of health care, reduce its cost, and broaden access to essential services. The fiscal year 1997 budget for AHCPR was US$ 143.5 million. These funds support research to test assumptions on which current health policies and practices are based; to examine new ways to organize, finance, and deliver health services; and to improve health care technology assessment methods.

Surveillance and Data Systems

Health information is vital to understanding the health status of the population and the planning, implementation, description, and evaluation of public health programs designed to control and prevent adverse health events. Data must be accurate, timely, and available in a usable form to allow the successful tracking of the status of public health objectives. The foundation for planning and evaluating the Healthy People 2000 objectives for the nation is information and its analysis.

The Public Health Service has established national surveillance and data system objectives in order to improve the coverage and effectiveness of public health data systems. Important activities at the national level include the direct collection and compilation of data collected by other agencies; analysis and dissemination of health information about progress toward achieving the Healthy People 2000 objectives by other federal, state, and local agencies; assistance to state and local agencies in conducting public health surveillance and evaluation of data; and coordination of a federal, state, and local surveillance network for diseases of public health importance.

Expenditures and Sectoral Financing

National health expenditures in 1995 were US$ 988.5 billion, up from US$ 937.1 billion in 1994. Growth in health spending in 1995 was slightly higher than the 5.1% increase registered in 1994, while spending rose by US$ 156 per person from US$ 3,465 in 1994. Growth in the nation's health care spending decelerated steadily from annual double-digit and near double-digit increases in the 1980s and early 1990s to 6.9% in 1993. The growth rates for 1994 and 1995 are the slowest in more than 30 years. National health expenditures represented 13.6% of the gross domestic product in 1995.

The health care system in the United States relies heavily on the provision of payment for medical care through private insurance. Private insurance provided by employers or purchased individually covers about three-quarters of the population; 14% of the population has no medical coverage at all.

Medicare and Medicaid funded about 36% of all spending for personal health care in 1995 and accounted for 80.9% of the public share of health care financing. These two programs financed 47% of hospital care and about 26.9% of physician services.

Medicare, created in 1965, was designed to protect people 65 and older from the high costs of medical care. In 1972, it was expanded to cover other populations such as disabled workers and people with end-stage renal disease. Unlike other federal health programs, Medicare is not financed solely from the general revenue. In 1995, 85.4% of the hospital insurance portion of the program came from a 1.45% payroll tax levied on both employers and employees. The Supplemental Medical Insurance portion of Medicare that covers physician services is financed through monthly premiums paid by the 35.7 million beneficiaries.

Spending has grown faster for Medicare than the private sector, primarily because the private sector has garnered greater savings from managed care. Medicare must base its managed care payments on a formula related to Medicare fee-for-service costs. Therefore, under current law, Medicare may not benefit from discounts and other factors that generate savings for the private sector. This is a primary reason why private sector spending grew at a rate of 2.9% in 1995 while public sector spending grew by 8.7% in that year.

Managed care is characterized by its emphasis on preventive care, elimination of unnecessary services, negotiated price discounts, and smaller copayments and deductibles. More than half of the U.S. population was enrolled in managed care in 1995.

Medicaid, also initiated in 1965, is a combined state-federal program intended to provide services to the poor. The federal government determines broad eligibility guidelines and mandatory services. Individual states have the option of expanding the basic coverage package by offering additional services. In 1995, Medicaid provided services to 36.3 million people and had actual expenditures of US$ 328.9 billion.

Medicaid expenditures are mostly institutional, with 39.1% spent on hospital care and 27.2% spent on nursing home care. It is the largest third-party payer of long-term care expenditures, and financed 46.5% of nursing home care in 1995. One-fourth of program benefits went to poor Medicaid recipients, while the blind and disabled, who account for only one-third of the Medicaid population, used three-fourths of the benefits.

External Technical and Financial Cooperation

The United States provides technical assistance in health to other countries primarily through the U.S. Agency for International Development (USAID). In fiscal year 1996, the Center for Population, Health, and Nutrition obligated approximately US$ 916 million for such assistance. The Department of Health and Human Services works with countries directly or in partnership with USAID on technical cooperation health activities of mutual benefit.

Global public health issues have an increasing effect on the health of the population of the United States. Trends such as emerging and reemerging infectious diseases, food and pharmaceutical harmonization, global disease surveillance mechanisms, and the increasing importance of chronic diseases all are serious concerns. The United States is an active participant in multilateral and bilateral efforts to address the growing importance of these issues.

There is ongoing international collaboration on several fronts. Programs under the supervision of the Office of International and Refugee Health, Department of Health and Human Services, include: the Health Committee of the Gore-Chernomyrdin Binational Commission; the promotion of enhanced cooperation with Mexico, with special emphasis on the border; the U.S./Mexico Binational Commission; the development of a new program with USAID in Egypt, focusing on health policy and decision-making; support for the Gore-Mbeki Commission, a bilateral agreement with South Africa; cooperation with Israel, the Netherlands, Japan, and China on health policy and related issues; provisions of departmental support for global programs with WHO, UNAIDS, UNICEF, and PAHO; and ongoing cooperation with the Office of Refugee Resettlement and USAID on refugee health issues and emergency response capacity.

The United States is using the lessons learned from Healthy People 2000 to develop Healthy People 2010. The country is seeking to share its own experience and learn from other countries to improve the next generation of health for all.

URUGUAY

GENERAL SITUATION AND TRENDS

Socioeconomic, Political, and Demographic Overview

Uruguay, known officially as the Eastern Republic of Uruguay, has the smallest land area (176,215 km^2) of any country in South America. The country's economy is based on agriculture, especially livestock. There are no appreciable mining resources, and industry is based on the processing of farming and livestock products. Since the creation of the Southern Common Market (MERCOSUR), the tertiary (service) sector has gained importance. Uruguay has a population of slightly more than 3 million people, 51.6% of them women. Of the total population, 89.1% reside in urban areas and 42.2% in Montevideo Department.

Uruguay is a representative democracy, with voting for national and municipal authorities in elections every five years. The Executive Branch is made up of a president and 12 ministers, and the Legislative Branch consists of 30 senators, the Vice President of the Republic, and 99 representatives. The Judicial Branch's highest body is the Supreme Court of Justice. Administratively, the country is divided into 19 departments. Departmental and municipal governments have little autonomy from the central government but can levy or eliminate certain types of taxes and do have responsibilities in health care. The department with the smallest area is Montevideo, but it has the most inhabitants. Uruguay is not divided into regions. When departmental data are analyzed, the tendency is to consider, on the one hand data from Montevideo, and on the other hand, data on the "interior," that is, the 18 other departments. The most notable recent political event was approval of a reform of the National Constitution through a plebiscite in December 1996.

The reform of the social security system, approved by law at the end of 1995, allows private companies to operate in the pensions and retirement market. These companies are called Pension Fund Administrators.

In 1995, the Government initiated earnest efforts toward educational reform, aimed at strengthening the public education system—but not the private system—in all four of its areas: primary, secondary, technical, and professional education, as well as teacher training and upgrading. One of the main objectives is to extend preschool education to all children aged 4 and 5, which began in 1997.

In 1995, some 700,000 students were enrolled in public and private primary, secondary, and technical and professional schools (excluding universities). Of these, 166,500 were secondary and technical/professional students in the public system.

Economic and Social Situation

The most noteworthy economic event was the creation of MERCOSUR in mid-1993, fully implementing the agreement signed between Argentina, Brazil, Paraguay, and Uruguay. MERCOSUR permits the free movement of goods and services among these countries and equalizes the tariffs on various products for third-party countries.

The growth in the gross domestic product (GDP) was 6.8% in 1994; 2.4% in 1995, and 4.9% in 1996. For 1997, an increase in the GDP of 3% was expected. Between 1985 and 1990 inflation ranged from 60% to 80% per year. In 1991, it reached 82%, then fell to 24% in 1996. The Economics Institute of the University of the Republic estimated that inflation would be 20% in 1997, and the Government expected that it would range from 14% to 17%. The budget deficit was 1.7% of the GDP in 1996. Up to 1991, the balance of trade was positive but became negative in 1992. In 1996, the negative balance was US$ 925.6 million.

Between 1984 and 1996, the purchasing power of wages grew at an annual rate of 2.3% (3.2% in the private sector and 1.3% in the public sector), while the purchasing power of retirees and pensioners grew at an annual rate of 5.5%. From

1992 to March 1997 the national minimum wage (in current dollars) did not vary significantly. It was US$ 89.6 per month in 1992, US$ 87.7 in 1994, US$ 92.4 in 1996, and US$ 90.5 in March 1997. In 1990, 8.5% of the economically active population was unemployed. In 1995 the figure was 10.3% and in 1996, 11.9%. It was estimated that unemployment in 1997 would be around 11%.

In *Social Panorama of Latin America 1996,* the Economic Commission for Latin America and the Caribbean points out that economic growth and lower inflation played a significant role in reducing urban poverty in Uruguay, which fell from 12% in 1991 to 6% in 1994.

The overall reduction in unmet basic needs throughout the country in the 1984–1994 period was approximately 40%. This reduction may be related to housing programs, expansion of the drinking water supply, and development of the health services in the urban areas of the interior. Among the residents of Montevideo, the percentage of people with unmet basic needs decreased from 14.7% in 1984 to 9.1% in 1994. In urban areas of the interior it fell from 28.9% in 1984 to 17.3% in 1994. A breakdown of unmet basic needs by age indicates that children under 15 have the highest rate of unmet basic needs.

In the urban areas of the interior, 3.5% of the dwellings are not supplied with drinking water, and 2.2% have no adequate waste disposal system. In 1996, in Montevideo, 98.8% of all dwellings had piped drinking water.

Population

According to the May 1996 National Census, Uruguay had a population of 3,163,763. The census showed a decrease in the rural population, continuing the trend found in previous censuses. The average annual population growth rate during the 1985–1996 period was 0.6%. The crude birth rate during 1990–1995 was 17.6 live births per 1,000 population. In the same period, the general fertility rate was 70.6 live births for every 1,000 women aged 15 to 49 years. The total fertility rate was 2.33 children per woman. The crude net reproduction rate was 1.14 daughters for every woman aged 15 to 49 years.

In 1995, the crude death rate was 10.0 per 1,000 population, and life expectancy at birth was 73.3 years overall, 69.3 years for men and 77.4 years for women. The population is clearly aging, with a large proportion in the advanced age group and low, declining percentages in the infant and juvenile populations. In 1996, 25.1% of the inhabitants were under 15 years of age, 62.1% were aged 15 to 64, and 12.8% were 65 or older. The annual growth rate of the group aged 65 and older is four times higher than the average for the country.

The literacy rate in 1996 was 95.7%. There has been a steady increase in the average years of schooling among the adult population aged 15 and older. There are nine years of compulsory education—six years of primary school and three years of secondary school.

Mortality and Morbidity

In Uruguay, 100% of deaths are recorded, and all death certificates are completed by a physician. In 1995, there were 31,700 deaths in the country. Of that total, 4% were children under 5 and 70.6% were people 65 and older.

Of the total deaths in 1996, 6.8% were "ill-defined symptoms, signs, and conditions." The total death rate of 8 per 1,000 in the 1950s has risen slowly since then, reaching 9.9 per 1,000 in 1995. The trend in proportional mortality by age has gone down in all groups except those aged 65 and older. Proportional mortality in this group increased by 70.6% between 1980 and 1995.

The infant mortality rate for the entire country was 19.6 per 1,000 in 1995 and 17.5 per 1,000 in 1996. Almost all births (99%) occur in a hospital, and 100% are certified by a physician or university-trained midwife. Underreporting of births is very low, 2.3%. Unreported births tend to be detected later through various mechanisms.

There are no reliable data on morbidity from the most prevalent diseases. However, the Ministry of Public Health routinely collects certain morbidity data, almost exclusively from outpatient visits and only for the population using the Ministry's services. There is underreporting of this information and the data that are collected are not processed on a regular basis. With the exception of the mandatory disease reporting system, the country has no information system for collecting morbidity data from all its various institutions.

In 1996, the Ministry of Public Health, in collaboration with the IDB, conducted a study of losses from disability-adjusted life years (DALY) attributable to different causes. The results were consistent with what was already known, that is, that noncommunicable diseases are much more significant in Uruguay and produce the greatest loss of DALY, far ahead of communicable diseases and external causes (homicides and accidental injuries).

SPECIFIC HEALTH PROBLEMS

Analysis by Population Group

Infant Health (under Age 5)

In 1996, there were 58,928 births in Uruguay, and 1,033 children under the age of 1 died, for an infant mortality rate of 17.5 per 1,000 live births. Neonatal mortality was 9.6 per 1,000 and postneonatal mortality, 7.9 per 1,000. Of total deaths in children under 1 year, 48% occurred in public health services, 31% in private facilities, and 17% at home.

In 1996, the leading causes of death in children under 1 year were birth defects (3.3 per 1,000 live births), hyaline membrane disease (1.8 per 1,000), acute respiratory infections and pneumonias (1.4 per 1,000), and prematurity, neonatal sepsis, and meconial aspiration syndrome (each with a mortality of 1.1 per 1,000).

The leading causes of hospitalization for children under 1 year in the hospitals of the Ministry of Public Health in the interior of the country were acute respiratory infections (28%) and intestinal infections (17%). There is no information on the private sector, although it is thought that the situation is similar. In the infant population aged 1 to 4 years, the three leading causes of death in 1995 were accidents and injuries (16.1 per 100,000 live births), malignant neoplasms (10.2 per 100,000), and birth defects (6.3 per 100,000).

Health of Primary-School Children (Ages 5 to 9)

In 1995, 41% of the deaths in children aged 5 to 9 came from three causes: accidents (with mortality of 12.8 per 100,000), malignant neoplasms (3.5 per 100,000), and birth defects (2.7 per 100,000). In the group from 5 to 14 years, injuries in general were the leading cause of hospitalization (15%), and acute respiratory infections were the second cause (10%).

Health of Adolescents (Ages 10 to 14)

In 1995, accidents remained the leading cause of mortality in the group from 10 to 14 years. In fact, 60.5% of all deaths from accidents of all types among all age groups occurred in the 10–14 age group. Malignant neoplasms were the second cause of mortality in the 10–14 age group, and diseases of the circulatory system were third.

Health of Adults (Ages 15 to 64)

Of the 31,700 deaths that occurred in Uruguay in 1995, 23.0% were in the group aged 25 to 64. As with the 10–14 age group, the leading causes of death of those between 15 and 34 were accidents and injuries. Between the ages of 35 and 64, malignant neoplasms (breast cancer in women and lung cancer in men) were the leading cause of death, followed by cardiovascular disease.

The maternal mortality rate was 2.1 per 10,000 in 1994, when 12 maternal deaths were reported in the entire country. It is believed that there is significant underreporting of maternal mortality, but the true extent is unknown.

In the adult population, 34% of the hospitalizations in Ministry of Public Health facilities are for normal childbirths. Other major reasons for hospitalization are complications during pregnancy, childbirth, and puerperium (16%); injuries and poisonings (7%); and mental disorders (3%).

Health of the Elderly (Age 65 and Older)

The proportion of deaths that occur at age 65 or older is rising, particularly among women. The leading cause of mortality is cardiovascular diseases, and the second is tumors. Among cardiovascular diseases, ischemic heart disease ranks first in the group aged 65 to 79, and cerebrovascular disease among those 80 and older. The second cause of death in this group is malignant neoplasms, most frequently of the trachea, bronchia, and lungs among people aged 65 to 79, and of the rectum and colon for persons 80 and older.

One problem that the Ministry of Public Health considers a priority among the elderly is social isolation, particularly among women who live alone.

Analysis by Type of Disease or Health Impairment

Communicable Diseases

Vector-Borne Diseases. Cases of malaria, dengue, plague, schistosomiasis, and yellow fever do not occur in the country. *Aedes aegypti* was eradicated from Uruguay in 1958. However, in 1997 uninfected larvae of this mosquito were found in areas bordering on Argentina. There is evidence that the spread of Chagas' disease was halted in Uruguay in 1997.

Vaccine-Preventable Diseases. Cases of poliomyelitis, neonatal tetanus, and diphtheria have not been reported for more than 15 years. Eleven cases of whooping cough were reported in 1994, 69 cases in 1995, and 17 cases in 1996. Twelve measles cases were reported in 1994, 5 in 1995, and only 1 in 1996. There were two cases of nonneonatal tetanus in 1994, two cases in 1995, and one case in 1996.

In 1996, vaccination coverage for tuberculosis prevention with BCG in children under 1 year was 98%. Coverage for diphtheria, whooping cough, and tetanus with three doses of DTP vaccine was 89%; for poliomyelitis, with three doses of live oral polio vaccine was 89%; and for measles, mumps, and rubella with the MMR vaccine was 85%.

Cholera and Other Intestinal Infectious Diseases. The cholera epidemic that began in 1991 in the Americas did not spread to Uruguay, where no cases have been recorded during this decade. As a cause of mortality in children under 1 year, acute diarrhea ranked eighth in 1995, with a rate of 0.4 per 100,000 live births. In 1996, 3,565 cases of viral hepatitis and one case of typhoid fever were reported.

Chronic Communicable Diseases. Mortality from tuberculosis was 2.8 per 100,000 in 1986 and 2.2 in 1995. The incidence of tuberculosis in all its forms was 19.3 per 100,000 in 1995. Continuing to decrease, leprosy has ceased to be a priority health problem. Prevalence in 1996 was 3.8 per 100,000 population.

Acute Respiratory Infections. Acute respiratory infections ranked sixth as a cause of mortality in children under 1 year in 1995, with a rate of 5.6 per 100,000 live births.

Rabies and Other Zoonoses. In the past 10 years, there have been no reports of human or canine rabies. The rate of surgical prevalence of hydatidosis (the number of people undergoing surgery for hydatid cyst in relation to the total population) was 12.4 per 100,000 population in 1993, falling to 10.5 in 1994 and 9.4 in 1995.

AIDS and Syphilis. From 1983 through 31 January 1997, 851 cases of AIDS were reported. In 1993, 103 cases were reported, 119 in 1994, 127 in 1995, and 156 in 1996. In January 1997, 11 cases were reported. The fatality rate has been 56% for the 851 reported AIDS cases. Approximately 60% of the HIV-positive and AIDS patients use Ministry of Public Health facilities. From 1983 to 31 January 1997, 2,153 people were reported with HIV-positive serology. In 1993, 239 seropositives were reported, 242 in 1994, 257 in 1995, and 309 in 1996. During the month of January 1997, 23 cases were reported. The last sentinel study of HIV, conducted in late 1996, showed a prevalence of 0.2% in the general population, which means that there are about 6,300 people infected in the country. A 1995 study had found an estimated prevalence of 0.24%.

AIDS continues to occur primarily among men; in 1996 there were 4.6 male patients for every woman. Sexual transmission predominates (68.7%), far outranking blood-borne transmission through intravenous drug abuse (26.9%). There are no seropositive cases attributable to blood transfusion. Mother-to-child transmission, however, is rising, moving from 2.6% of the total cumulative cases as of 1992 to 4.3% of the total cases as of 31 January 1997.

In 1996, 879 cases of syphilis were reported.

Noncommunicable Diseases and Other Health-Related Problems.

Nutritional Diseases and Diseases of Metabolism. Fat consumption has always been very high in Uruguay. An FAO/WHO report indicated that in 1993 fats accounted for 32% of total caloric intake.

The 1994–1995 Household Spending and Income Survey confirmed that as earnings increase, so does the percentage of calories consumed in the form of fats. In the poorest households, 24% of the total calories consumed come from fats, while in the wealthiest households the percentage is 34%. Daily dietary cholesterol intake is also very high and also increases with income. Fish consumption is very low and also increases with income, but is very limited at all income levels.

Fruit and vegetable consumption is limited but rising. According to the Household Spending and Income Survey, average daily consumption of fiber is 23 g in the interior and 24 g in Montevideo. The poorest 10% of the households in Montevideo consume a daily average of 18.7 g of fiber, while the wealthiest 10% of households consume an average of 28 g.

There is a high prevalence of obesity in some sectors of society. For example, 9% of the children treated in the private-sector collective health care institutions were obese, while the percentage was only 3% for children treated by the public sector. In a representative sample of 4,000 adults in the city of Montevideo, overweight or obesity—defined by the body mass index—was found in 47% of men and 58% of women. There was a strong statistical correlation between obesity and low socioeconomic status in women. In men, however, the correlation was inverse and less pronounced.

According to a ministerial report submitted in 1997, 28% of the 5,543 children under 5 cared for in Ministry of Public Health facilities between 1994 and 1997 showed retarded growth, as determined by their height-for-age.

Endemic goiter and blindness due to vitamin A deficiency are not public health problems in Uruguay. Table salt has been iodized since 1963.

The prevalence of diabetes in the country is estimated at 7.6% in men over 18 years of age and 10.0% in women in the same age group. Diabetes ranks fifth as the cause of death, with a rate of 20.2 per 100,000 population.

According to a study conducted in October 1996, 50.5% of children under 1 month of age are not exclusively breast-fed. The rate of exclusive breast-feeding is 37.5% in infants under 4 months. For children aged 6 to 9 months the rate of appropriate supplementary feeding is 30%.

Cardiovascular Diseases. For 40 years, cardiovascular diseases have been the leading causes of death in Uruguay, accounting for 30% of total deaths in 1996. Mortality from cardiovascular diseases, at 357 per 100,000 in 1995, has remained relatively stable in recent years. Each year some 400 deaths are attributed to hypertension, about 3,700 to ischemic heart disease, and 3,500 to cerebrovascular disease. Of the total deaths from cardiovascular disease, 80% occur in people aged 60 and older. Ischemic heart disease and cerebrovascular disease together account for more than 63% of deaths from cardiovascular diseases.

In recent studies (1991–1993, 1995), hypertension was among the primary causes for medical visits. In a survey conducted in Montevideo, hypertension was found in 20% of the adult population. Among the general population in the cities of Rivera and Tacuarembó, the prevalence of hypertension was 24%, with a 15% prevalence for borderline hypertension. In two research studies on workers being issued health cards in Montevideo and San José, the percentages of hypertensives were 7% and 10%, respectively.

Malignant Neoplasms. In 1995, 7,029 people in Uruguay died from tumors of all types. The mortality was 221.9 per 100,000 population, and higher in men (263.7 per 100,000) than in women (182.2 per 100,000). Cancer ranked second as a cause of mortality, accounting for 22.3% of deaths. As in previous years, in 1995 lung cancer was the leading cause of cancer death in males, followed by cancer of the prostate, rectum and colon, stomach, and esophagus. In women, breast cancer continued to rank first, followed by cancer of the rectum and colon, stomach, uterus and cervix, and pancreas.

Accidents and Violence. In 1995, accidents and injuries together were the third leading cause of death, with 7.1% of all deaths. The corresponding mortality was 70.3 per 100,000, which indicates an increase in recent years (in 1991 the figure was 45.2 per 100,000). A possible reason for this increase is the growth in the number of automobiles in the country, which almost tripled between 1991 and 1996.

Accidents in general and traffic accidents in particular are the leading cause of death in people under 30. Accidents account for 28% of deaths in children aged 1 to 4 and 50% of deaths in the 15 to 19 group.

Reporting of all traffic accidents that cause some type of physical injury and require taking the injured to an emergency service began in November 1995. In December 1996, the Registry of Injured Persons, part of the Ministry of Public Health, was operating in most of the country's departments. According to the data from the Registry, 56% of those injured in traffic accidents were between the ages of 15 and 39.

In March 1997, Breathalyzer tests for alcohol and blood alcohol tests began to be administered to drivers in Montevideo and along various national highways. By law, those who refuse to submit to a Breathalyzer test are regarded as probably intoxicated and are sent to the appropriate court. Maximum tolerance levels are 0.8 mg of ethanol per 100 ml for drivers in general and 0 mg for those who work as drivers.

Behavioral Disorders. In a survey conducted in 1995 to study the prevalence of smoking in Uruguay, almost 22% of a representative sample of people over the age of 13 in urban areas throughout the country admitted to being regular smokers. The prevalence of smoking was higher in Montevideo (23.6%) than in the interior (20.2%), and higher among men (2.2 male smokers for every woman), with most smokers belonging to the group aged 30 to 39. Male smokers differ significantly from female smokers. Most men who smoke have a basic level of education, do manual labor, receive low pay, and work long hours. Among women, smokers more frequently have an average or higher level of education, are engaged in intellectual pursuits, and have high incomes.

There are no good data on alcoholism. Mortality from cirrhosis of the liver rose from 8.5 per 100,000 in the 1986–1991 period to 11.0 per 100,000 in 1995, and affects men much more than women.

Mortality from mental disorders increased significantly between 1984 and 1995, from 7.2 to 24.8 per 100,000.

Oral Health. There was a countrywide decline in the DMFT (decayed, missing, filled teeth) Index from 4.1 in 1991 to 2.5 in 1996 among children under age 12. The sale of fluoridated salt began in 1991. Of the salt sold for household use in 1996, 60% was fluoridated.

Emerging and Re-emerging Diseases. In February 1997, the first case of hantavirus was diagnosed in Uruguay. It was confirmed by laboratory tests, and the patient survived. In 1996, 382 cases of meningitis were reported in the country.

RESPONSE OF THE HEALTH SYSTEM

National Health Plans and Policies

The Constitution of the Republic establishes that the State will legislate on all issues related to health and public hygiene, seeking the physical, moral, and social betterment of all the country's inhabitants. All residents have the duty to protect their own health, as well as to seek care when ill. The Constitution also says that the State will provide measures for prevention and will give care free of cost only to the indigent or those who lack sufficient resources. In 1934, the Organic Public Health Law created the Ministry of Public Health and established its commitments to public health, health care, monitoring health, and the setting of standards.

The Ministry of Public Health is the agency responsible for setting standards and regulating the health sector, developing preventive programs, and administering its healthcare services. In recent years, there has been a continuity in Ministry policies concerning the decentralization of services—begun in 1987 and accelerated in 1995—the targeting of actions to priority problems, and the maintenance of moderate state control over the private sector.

The Government is engaged in the reform of social policy, with the goal of improving public administration, increasing productivity, readjusting services, and refining spending. Reform of the public sector to gradually phase out nonessential state services is considered a priority. This has been reflected in a Ministry policy of increasing its effectiveness and efficiency, while still ensuring universal and equitable access to health services of acceptable quality and efficiency. A gradual reduction in its activities in the direct delivery of services is proposed through the transfer to third parties of all functions considered nonessential and by redistributing responsibilities and resources through a decentralized model for the administration of the health services.

In 1995 the Government signed two loans, one with the World Bank to finance the Project for Institutional Strengthening of the Health Sector, and the other with the IDB to finance the Strengthening the Social Area project.

As part of the first project and based on a legislative strategy approved by the World Bank, two draft decrees have been prepared. One would create a legal framework to operate public hospitals with decentralized management, and the other would implement a Single Registry of Formal Healthcare Coverage, under the General Health Bureau of the Ministry of Public Health. This registry would make it possible to gather the necessary information on medical coverage for all residents of the country, thus detecting cases of dual coverage—very frequent in Uruguay—and identifying where this harms the State Health Services Administration (ASSE) if the bill for services received is not paid by the appropriate institution.

In recent years, there has been a tendency to separate two normative roles in health care administration, that of regulation and that of oversight. Beginning in 1987 with the creation of ASSE as an autonomous agency within the Ministry of Public Health, the two functions began to be differentiated. The project transforming ASSE into a decentralized service is moving in the same direction. Also, departmental health directors were created beginning in 1995; they have functions similar to those of the Director-General of Health, but they work only in their own departments.

Created in 1979, the Public Resources Fund (PRF) is a public entity, not a Government one. Its aims are to collect and administer the resources necessary to pay for the services of highly specialized medical facilities. It pays for highly complex and costly procedures, and the country's entire population is covered. The PRF finances heart surgery, pacemaker insertion, hip prostheses, chronic hemodialysis, transplants, the treatment of serious burns and, as of 1992, chronic peritoneal dialysis on an outpatient basis, knee prostheses, and lithotresis. The list of treatments covered by the PRF can be expanded, reduced, or modified through a resolution of an Honorary Administrative Commission. The sources to finance the PRF are varied, but its basic sources are contribu-

tions from the State to care for users of Ministry services and contributions from the private-sector collective health care institutions to cover care for their members, who are generally people with average or high incomes.

Health Sector Reform

The strategy for carrying out health sector reform is based on the reassessment of primary care, improved coordination between the public and private sectors, modernization of the health information system, strengthening of the central ministerial level, and decentralization of Ministry of Public Health hospitals.

Now under study is the creation of a national health sector information system. Its development requires the selection of data, the production of information appropriate to the new model of care, and the implementation of a communications network linking all public and private institutions in the health sector.

Strengthening the central ministerial level means improving the government's capabilities in managing the system; formulating health plans and programs; setting technical, administrative, and financing standards; coordinating the activities of public and private agencies; and supervising, auditing, and evaluating compliance with policies and plans.

Decentralization of the management of Ministry hospitals began in 1987 with the creation of ASSE, the public agency responsible for administering Ministry hospital facilities.

In 1995 the Government sent to Parliament a draft proposal for a five-year budget, one of whose articles provided for the decentralization of ASSE. The article was not approved, perhaps due to pressure from the private sector in the country's interior, which perceived the ASSE as a potential competitor.

The Ministry has continued to promote decentralization, especially with the proposal to create public hospitals with decentralized management. The goals of that project—financed by the World Bank—are to improve the management and administration of health facilities, increase efficiency in the allocation and management of sectoral resources, promote functional coordination with the private sector, and effectively use the existing hospital infrastructure.

The creation of public hospitals with decentralized management is intended to improve the response capability of the health services, ensuring recognized levels of quality management, and to formulate a new management model for public hospitals, based on measurement of their processes and outcomes, and centered on the costs and quality of services. Each hospital should prepare a budget defining the hospital product, its management processes, and costs, thus making it possible to evaluate the services provided in terms of efficiency and technical effectiveness. The goal is also to map out a specific legal framework for managing the hospitals and to introduce the concepts of managerial and administrative responsibility in the utilization of resources and the attainment of results.

In the process of transforming the public hospital into a decentralized management hospital, the State must guarantee the population's access to health services and assume the role of regulating the system. This implies the establishment of alternative intervention modalities in the market to help ensure more equitable access to health services for the population, with a resulting redistribution of income.

The health sector reform strategy includes the Medical Center Project. The general objective of this project—financed by an IDB loan for US$ 80 million—is "to help adapt the health system to the specific situation of the country." The specific objectives of the Project include upgrading training and redefining the role of the University Hospital in the national network of health institutions.

Significant among the obstacles to sectoral reform and decentralization is the country's centralist culture and the vested interests of powerful groups.

Organization of the Health Sector

Institutional Organization

The public health system consists of services under the Ministry, provided through ASSE; the University of the Republic, through the teaching hospital (*Hospital de Clínicas*); the health care services of the municipal governments; the armed forces health services; the police health services; and the medical services of other public and autonomous entities. The ASSE provides health services to lower-income persons. It has 65 health facilities throughout the country, with 8,553 beds located in hospitals for patients with acute or chronic conditions (some 2,300 for chronic patients). The university teaching hospital has 700 beds and provides tertiary care to users of Ministry services for free and to the rest of the population for a fee.

The armed forces health services cover approximately 220,000 people and have a 447-bed hospital. Police health services have a 70-bed hospital and cover some 120,000 people.

The Social Welfare Fund covers care for pregnancy and childbirth for pregnant workers or workers' spouses, as well as pediatric care up to age 6. It has its own hospital and several maternal and child centers in Montevideo and in Canelones Department. In the interior, the Fund contracts for services with the Ministry of Public Health or the private-sector collective health care institutions.

The State Insurance Fund has a 160-bed hospital in Montevideo and contracts for services with third parties in the interior. It covers occupational diseases and work-related accidents for workers covered by the Department of Social Health Insurance.

The country's municipal governments provide outpatient health services to the general population.

The autonomous entities and decentralized services are state and semipublic agencies. They offer highly diverse medical services, from hospitalization to payment of private insurance premiums, at the beneficiary's option.

The private health sector consists of 53 collective health care institutions (CHCI), 68 partial-insurance health plans, several highly specialized medical institutes, private physician's offices that charge fees for services, private nursing homes, and some foreign insurance companies.

Of all the public and private health institutions, the most important in terms of coverage are the CHCIs. They serve approximately 55% of the population. Public coverage through ASSE is approximately 28%, and military and police health insurance cover approximately 10%. Although the precise figure is unknown, it is estimated that the partial-insurance plans cover a significant portion of the population. It is estimated that insurance plans registered with the Ministry of Public Health provide coverage to some 800,000 people. These plans cover certain types of medical, surgical, emergency, and dental care.

The CHCIs are private nonprofit organizations that provide services through prepaid health insurance. There are three types: mutual assistance associations, which are based on the principles of cooperation and use a system of mutual insurance to provide medical care to their members; professional cooperatives providing medical care to their members and associates, in which corporate capital is contributed by the respective professionals; and health services created and financed by private companies or quasi-governmental entities to provide nonprofit medical care to personnel and family members.

The CHCIs are independent institutions that compete with each other. The State exercises some legal and technical control over them, but they have a high degree of autonomy. In 1983, it was decreed that each CHCI must have at least 10,000 members; the largest one has 280,000 members. There are three types of affiliation with a CHCI: collective state affiliation through the social security system, collective affiliation paid for by private companies, and individual affiliation, generally for relatives of persons affiliated in one of those first two ways.

Some 35 CHCIs are physicians' cooperatives located in the country's interior and affiliated with each other through an association called the Medical Federation of the Interior.

Workers in private companies subscribe to a compulsory health plan through the Department of Social Health Insurance. The plan affiliates them with the CHCI of their choice and provides total health coverage for themselves, but none for their dependents. In the event of unemployment, the health insurance plan covers the period in which the worker is covered by unemployment insurance, up to six months.

There are four national honorary commissions. They are public, not state, entities and are financed with percentages of different taxes (on alcohol, tobacco, etc.) and rates. They are made up of representatives from public and private institutions, including trade associations and nongovernmental organizations. The primary duty of the Honorary Commission to Combat Tuberculosis and Prevalent Illnesses is to deal with tuberculosis throughout the country and to be responsible for all vaccination activities in the country and the selective detection of congenital hypothyroidism. The three other honorary commissions deal with cardiovascular health, the struggle against cancer, and the struggle against hydatidosis.

Health Legislation

In 1987, the State Health Services Administration (ASSE) was created by law as an autonomous agency of the Ministry of Public Health. ASSE has the authority to transfer the administration or use of health facilities to the departmental governments and may reach agreement with the CHCIs to use their facilities some of the time.

The National Resources Fund was created in 1979 and became fully operational in 1981. It is directed by an Administrative Honorary Commission advised by several technical commissions.

A law regulating the creation of the CHCIs was promulgated in 1981, and the decree regulating investments in CHCI health services was issued in 1983. In 1989, an ordinance established the regulations governing partial-insurance health plans.

When the 1967 Constitution was adopted, the Social Welfare Fund was created and given the task of "coordinating state social welfare services and organizing social security." The Fund centralizes the administration of disability insurance and also administers old-age pensions.

In 1979, maximum centralization in the administration of social security was reached when a General Social Security Administration was created as an agency of the Ministry of Labor and Social Security. It absorbed the activities of the Social Welfare Fund and incorporated into its operations the administration of health insurance plans, family insurance, and maternity and unemployment insurance. In 1986, the General Social Security Administration was eliminated and its functions were taken over by the Fund, which was reestablished.

The State reform currently under way reaffirms two essential duties for the Ministry of Public Health. One is prevention programs and free care to the indigent and other poor persons. The other is health promotion through the control and reduction of risk factors for disease, together with improvements in the quality, timeliness, effectiveness, and efficiency of health care for the entire population.

Health Services and Resources

Organization of Services for Care of the Population

Disease Prevention and Control. For a number of years, the Ministry of Public Health has given top priority to the following problems: morbidity and mortality from traffic accidents; cardiovascular diseases; substance abuse and addictions; infant mortality and poorly monitored pregnancy and childbirth; AIDS; breast cancer; lung cancer; oral health; social isolation of the elderly; Chagas' disease; hydatidosis; violence, especially domestic violence; and disabilities stemming from eye diseases (amblyopia in children and cataracts in the elderly) and from hearing disorders.

In 1995, the Ministry created the Health Promotion Bureau, which includes the Department of Health Education. There is also a National Drug Board, which reports directly to the Office of the President and includes several public agencies.

Uruguay is not subject to major natural disasters except for some flooding in winter and fires in summer. For special situations like these, the National Emergency Committee meets. The Committee is comprised of several public agencies and reports directly to the Office of the President.

Epidemiological Surveillance Systems. Uruguay has a single epidemiological surveillance system, which is directed and coordinated by the Epidemiological Monitoring Department of the Ministry of Public Health. Its objective is to make timely recommendations to the authorities on short-, medium-, and long-term measures to prevent or control diseases subject to surveillance or other unusual or epidemic health situations.

The regular reporting sources are persons who are required to report, basically physicians or the technical administrators of health institutions. Sentinel posts are voluntary reporting services specifically selected because they have a large number of users and a ready willingness to report. Reportable diseases include foodborne diseases.

The National Blood Bank, an agency of the Ministry, regulates, supervises, and controls all the country's blood banks. Donation is voluntary and uncompensated. A strict preliminary screening of donors is performed, through questioning and then serology for HIV, syphilis, hepatitis B, and Chagas' disease. Transfusions must be requested by a physician, who is in most cases a specialist in hemotherapy.

Drinking Water and Sanitation Services. According to the 1985 census, 7.4% of the population was not supplied with drinking water, and the percentage of the population with critical sanitation deficiencies was 8.5%. There are no recent data available, but according to reports from the State Sanitation Works the drinking water system has been extended in recent years in both Montevideo and the interior.

The water in the network has good sanitary treatment controls, and its supply is the exclusive responsibility of Sanitation Works, which is also in charge of controlling surface waters and beaches and informing the population about the level of *Escherichia coli* contamination.

Public sewerage services reach 43% of the country's population and 51% of the urban population. In Montevideo, coverage is close to 80%. When the expansion of this service is completed—financed with an IDB loan—more than 95% of households will be reached.

Solid Waste Management Services. Households in Uruguay generate an estimated 2,000 tons of solid waste per day, and treatment varies from department to department. Generally speaking, there is a notable lack of an effective methodology for final disposal. Also, there are shortcomings in their handling and disposal of hospital, pathogenic, and toxic waste.

Prevention and Control of Air Pollution. The country's favorable atmospheric conditions significantly reduce the amount of air pollution. This is indicated by data from measurements of suspended particulates and sulfur dioxide. Air pollution sometimes occurs in industrialized urban areas as a result of petroleum refining, cement manufacturing, and the burning of fossil fuels.

Food Safety and Control. From 1993 through May 1997, 26 outbreaks of food poisoning reported to the Epidemiological Monitoring Department of the Ministry of Public Health have been laboratory-confirmed. Bacterial agents were the most frequent cause (89%), with foods of animal origin the most implicated (73%) and homes the most frequent location of the outbreak (46%).

Food Assistance Programs. For over 20 years, the Ministry of Public Health has had a supplementary food program to combat malnutrition and low birthweight in the population covered by ASSE, specifically at-risk children and pregnant women. This program has been strengthened by other food assistance programs that are operated by other agencies linked to the Government and by nongovernmental organizations and that are intended not only for pregnant women and children but for older adults as well.

Organization and Operation of Personal Health Care Services

Basically, the physical infrastructure in both the public and private health sectors has not changed significantly in recent decades, although facilities have been remodeled and expanded. In Canelones and Las Piedras—both in metropolitan Montevideo—two new hospitals have been built and will soon start operating.

As part of World Bank and IDB technical cooperation projects, the resizing of the health care network is being studied. In Montevideo, there are a large number of hospital beds, with a high occupancy rate and a high average hospitalization rates. In the interior, hospitalization levels are adequate, but the occupancy rate is about 50%. If the average hospitalization period in the private sector were applied to the number of hospitalizations done by the public sector, half the current number of beds would be enough. This indicates the need to reconsider not only the number of facilities, but basically the operations within each facility.

The private sector requires authorization from the Ministry of Public Health to build new hospitals and import equipment valued at over US$ 20,000. In the mid-1980s, the Ministry opened a Medical Technology Unit that analyzed private sector requests to import technology. The Technology Unit considered not just the technical standpoint, but also the technology's effectiveness and the country's needs. However, once equipment was authorized, since there was no regulation of the fee being charged to use it, monopoly or oligopoly situations were created that were hard to manage. This led interest groups to exert pressure and evade regulation, importing equipment and reducing prices as a result of competition. However, the control only affected the private sector. In the public sector, equipment was acquired with nothing more than a request from the director of an institution, depending on the availability of funds, without planning based on the population's needs or on establishing levels of care. Currently, the budget and infrastructure are inadequate and there is no maintenance program. The country has no national inventory of public or private equipment. There are no data on the availability of replacement parts or staff training.

It is estimated that the private health sector, consisting of the CHCIs and the private sanatoriums, has some 3,500 beds for the hospitalization of acute patients throughout the country. The CHCIs administer a total of 2,800 beds, 1,800 of which are in Montevideo. The private sanatoriums—5 in Montevideo and 34 in the interior—have some 700 beds.

According to 1996 data, CHCI members annually average 5.5 medical consultations, 1.21 hospital stays, and 4.95 days of hospitalization. The average hospital stay is 4.2 days, and 37% of births are by cesarean section. Members receive an average of 10.9 prescriptions per year and 1.9 prescriptions per visit. Of all CHCI members, 16% are over 64 years of age.

Inputs for Health

The supply of drugs in the country is adequate, in both the public and private sectors. Since 1971, the Ministry of Public

Health has periodically published a list of essential drugs (the latest in 1996), with their international generic names.

Pharmaceutical spending accounts for 15% to 20% of all health sector spending. Purchasing is done through public bidding or negotiation with laboratories. The drugs that are marketed must be registered with the Ministry's Office for the Control of Drugs and Related Products, which assesses quality and other characteristics, under the supervision of the Ministry's Quality Control Laboratory.

Drugs are provided at no cost to those with a health care card from the Ministry.

Vaccinations are administered through the Ministry's Expanded Program on Immunization (EPI), in both public and private sector vaccination units. The management of the EPI is the responsibility of the Ministry's Epidemiology Department. In both the public and private vaccination units, vaccines are free, and all people receive care. The vaccines included in the EPI (for tuberculosis, diphtheria, tetanus, whooping cough, poliomyelitis, measles, rubella, and mumps) are required by law. In addition, vaccination is provided against *Haemophilus influenzae* B. Health workers at risk from contact with patients and patients undergoing chronic dialysis are vaccinated against hepatitis B.

Human Resources

The number of physicians, dentists, pharmacists, and nursing assistants is adequate for the population. There are 11,928 physicians (3.7 per 1,000 population) and 4,069 dentists (1.3 per 1,000 population). In contrast, there are not enough professional nurses, as there are only 2,230 (0.7 per 1,000 population).

Health sector education is not planned. Admission to health training is open to anyone who meets the requirements, without admissions quotas. However, in recent decades concern in this area has been growing, and medical associations are promoting the regulation of admissions to the School of Medicine. The number of physicians and their distribution by specialty is being considered. It is believed that there is overspecialization based on technology, and a lack of health services managers and administrators, as well as such public health specialists as epidemiologists and health economists.

Research and Technology

In Uruguay, very little research is conducted, especially in the area of health systems and technology. Epidemiological research, however, is somewhat more developed and its findings do guide policies to resolve specific problems. In other areas, there is only an awareness of the problem and specific research on some subjects. In addition, the training of health professionals in research concepts and methodology is inadequate. In this respect, the education of health workers is very heterogeneous. In the area of technology, research is not conducted before technology is incorporated nor is there any subsequent evaluation of the results of technologies. The limitations are basically the lack of training and an absence of firm policies requiring research findings for decision-making.

Expenditures and Sectoral Financing

Health expenditures in 1995 were US$ 1,781 million, or US$ 564 per person. As a percentage of GDP, total health expenditures have been growing. The share was 6.2% in 1982, 8.3% in 1992, and 10.0% in 1995.

Of total health expenditures in 1995, 28.6% were in the public sector and 71.4% were in the private sector. For some time, spending by the public sector has remained at about 30%, but moving downward, while the private sector has accounted for slightly more than 70% of spending, with that proportion increasing.

The largest portion of spending in 1995 was for the CHCIs, with 49.6%. The State Health Services Administration accounted for 15.1%; spending in pharmacies outside of hospitals was 6.4%; partial health insurance plans accounted for 5.9%, and the contribution from CHCIs (through a surcharge on the fees prepaid by their members) to the Public Resources Fund was 3.9%. The share of spending in the other health entities was small, just 1% to 2% each.

The expenditures for the four public Honorary Commissions (to Combat Cancer, for Cardiovascular Health, to Combat Hydatidosis, and the Tuberculosis Campaign) represented only 0.5% of health expenditures in 1995, amounting to about US$ 9 million.

Of all expenditures, in both the public and private sectors, 45.7% went to pay for personnel costs, 24.9% to materials and other items, 16.7% to drugs, 9.5% to contract third parties, and 3.2% to investment.

In 1995, considering the public and private sectors together, 42.1% of health funding came from the monthly fees paid by CHCI members, 25.4% from direct payments by users, 23.3% from general taxes, 3% from withholdings on employee compensation is allocated to health insurance and other social security agencies, 0.8% from extrabudgetary resources of institutions in the public sector, and 5.5% from insurance premiums such as those for mobile emergency medical services and from direct private spending.

In the public sector, financing for health sector expenditures in 1995 came basically from taxes, which financed 81.1% of spending; 9.1% from withholding on wages; 6.7%

from the sale of services; and 2.9% from the extrabudgetary resources of institutions in the public sector.

In the private sector, 59% of financing came from mutual fees, 33% from income from the sale of services, 0.5% from withholding on wages, and 7.5% from such other sources as partial-insurance health plans, exclusive private care, and nursing homes for the elderly.

External Technical and Financial Cooperation

In 1995, a joint IDB/Government of Uruguay project was announced under the program known as Strengthening the Social Sector. With a budget of US$ 42.5 million—US$ 12.5 million contributed by the Government and US$ 30 million financed by an IDB loan—it will carry out infrastructure and reform projects in education, health, labor, justice, nutrition, and social information. The health objectives include initiating public sector reform, improving institutional efficiency, adapting the supply of health services to the epidemiological profile and needs of the population, expanding coverage, and improving the quality of basic services.

There is another project to strengthen the decentralized management of hospitals, financed by the World Bank.

According to studies conducted by the Economics and Health Commission of the Medical Union of Uruguay, the amount of international assistance received comes to approximately 0.1% of health expenditures.

VENEZUELA

GENERAL SITUATION AND TRENDS

Socioeconomic, Political, and Demographic Overview

The Republic of Venezuela has a land area of 916,445 km². It is comprised of 22 states, a Federal District, and federal dependencies (a group of islands in the Caribbean Sea). The states and the Federal District are divided into 330 *municipios,* which are the basic autonomous political units within the national system. The *municipios,* in turn, are divided into parishes and capital *municipios.* In December 1995 the third election by direct and secret ballot was held for governors, mayors, aldermen of the municipal councils, and members of the parish boards. Representatives of the state legislative assemblies were also elected, and the democratic process and political and administrative decentralization moved ahead.

In the 1993–1996 period, the country experienced uneven economic growth. GDP grew in 1993 (0.4%) and 1995 (2.2%) and fell in 1994 (−2.8%) and 1996 (−1.6%). Inflation was 38.1% in 1993, and in 1996 reached its highest level ever, 103.2%. Per capita GDP was US$ 2,862 in 1993, $2,370.70 in 1994, $3,470.20 in 1995, and $2,804 in 1996. In 1996, the Government launched a fiscal, monetary, and foreign exchange plan of action to lower inflation, balance the budget, restructure and strengthen the financial system, establish a new social security model, transfer resources to the most vulnerable sectors, and transform the structure of the economy and of the framework of legal institutions.

The estimated population in 1996 was 21,377,426, and the population density was 23.84 persons per km². The Federal District has the highest population density, with 1,181.20 inhabitants per km². The states with more than 200 inhabitants per km² are located along the coast (Carabobo, Miranda, Aragua, and Nueva Esparta). The border states (Apure, Amazonas, Bolívar, and Delta Amacuro) have population densities of less than five inhabitants per km². In 1996, 85.4% of the country's inhabitants lived in urban areas; of this urban population, 72% resided in cities of more than 50,000 inhabitants.

The indigenous census of 1992 found 38 indigenous ethnic groups, who together constituted 1.5% of the country's population. Of the 38 groups, 28 resided in the border states of Zulia, Amazonas, and Bolívar. Some 34% of the indigenous population belonged to the Wayuu group, 12.9% to the Warao, and 10.5% to the Pemón.

The total population growth rate was 2.3% in 1992, 2.1% in 1993 and 1994, and 2.0% in 1995. The birth rate declined gradually from 27.4 per 1,000 population in 1992 to 23.8 per 1,000 in 1995. The total fertility rate fell from 3.3 children per 1,000 women in 1992 to 2.9 in 1995. Women between the ages of 20 and 29 have the highest fertility rate. Migration has varied somewhat. In 1992 there was a negative balance of −11,752. The figure grew in 1994 to −90,670, but there was a positive balance in 1995 (6,961).

The Venezuelan population is young: 12.6% are under 4 years of age; 23.6% are from 5 to 14 years, and 55.5% are under 25. Only 4.1% of the population is 65 or older, but this group is growing faster than the general population. Life expectancy at birth in 1995 was 72.2 years (69.3 for men and 75.1 for women).

Poverty estimates that have been elaborated by the Household Survey of the Central Office of Statistics and Information (OCEI) indicate that as of 30 June 1994, 27.3% of the Venezuelan population had unmet basic needs and 21.6% lived in extreme poverty. The states with the most people living in extreme poverty were Apure, Delta Amacuro, Amazonas, and Portuguesa.

The annual cost of the adjusted basic food basket was US$ 157 in 1993, $153 in 1994, $195 in 1995, and $156 in 1996. With the 1996 minimum wage, civil servants could buy 63% of this basket, private sector workers, 95.4%; and rural workers, 57%. The unemployed made up 7.1% of the population in 1992, 10.2% in 1995, and 12.4% in 1996.

In 1995 the illiteracy rate was 7.2% (6.5% for men and 8.0% for women). Among persons between 10 and 24 years of age, illiteracy among males was 3.5%, and the rate for females was half that. Illiteracy in the indigenous population over 10 years of age was 41%.

Morbidity and Mortality Profile

The crude mortality rate has varied little in recent years. It was 4.4 per 1,000 population in 1992 and 4.2 per 1,000 population in 1995. There are no studies on underreporting, but the Latin American Demographic Center estimates it at 13.2%. That would make the actual mortality rate 5.4 per 1,000 population for the period 1990–1995.

In 1995, according to mortality rates for five major groups of causes, diseases of the circulatory system ranked first (142.1 per 100,000 population), followed by accidents and other external causes (69.9), tumors (60.9), communicable diseases (46.1), and certain conditions originating in the perinatal period (25.8). In comparison with 1989, cardiovascular diseases remained in first place, with a 7.0% increase. External causes moved to second place, with a 43.8% increase, edging tumors, which experienced a 0.3% reduction, to third place. Communicable diseases were in fourth place and had a 17.5% reduction. Certain conditions originating in the perinatal period remained in fifth place, despite a 32.9% reduction. Ill-defined symptoms and conditions represented 1.49% of the total deaths recorded in 1995, similar to the 1992 percentage (1.63%).

In 1995, deaths from external causes were five times more frequent in males (115.2 per 100,000 population) than in females. Accidents led external causes (74%), followed by homicides (19%) and suicides (7%). In 1992, 13 men died as a result of homicide for every woman, a number that rose to 16 men for each woman in 1995.

Mortality rates by age group in 1995 are similar to those for 1989. The infant mortality rate remained at 23.1 per 1,000 live births. If an underreporting of 13.2% for deaths and 4% for births is factored in, the rate comes to 27.4 per 1,000 live births.

An analysis of mortality by years of potential life lost (YPLL) for 1995 gives first place to certain conditions originating in the perinatal period and second place to enteritis and other diarrheal diseases, which represented 8.2% of the total YPLL. Traffic accidents ranked third and tumors fourth. Excluding deaths in children under 1 year, traffic accidents account for the greatest number of YPLL. The breakdown of YPLL by sex shows traffic accidents and homicides in second and third place for men, while cancer is second for women and enteritis and other diarrheal diseases is third for them.

SPECIFIC HEALTH PROBLEMS

Analysis by Population Group

Child Health

The infant mortality rate from 1992 to 1995 was stable, with values around 23.5 per 1,000 live births. There are differences among the states. In 1995, Bolívar, Amazonas, Zulia, and Trujillo had rates of 31.1 to 36.1 per 1,000 live births. In Anzoátegui and Sucre the rates were 7.5 and 10.4 per 1,000, respectively, although these states are believed to have significant underreporting of births and deaths. Some 59% of infant mortality is neonatal mortality, which had a rate of 13.4 per 1,000 live births in 1995.

The leading causes of death in children under 1 year of age are hypoxia, asphyxiation, and other respiratory disorders (31.1%), enteritis and other diarrheal diseases (17.9%), and birth defects (11.7%).

No national data are available on low birthweight, but reports from the Concepción Palacios Maternity Hospital, the largest maternity hospital in the country and the referral center for the highest-risk cases, indicate that the percentage of children with a birthweight under 2,500 g fell from 16.0 to 12.1 between 1990 and 1994.

Between 1992 and 1995 the mortality rate in the 1–4 age group remained stable, with figures of close to 1.2 per 1,000 population of that age. In this group, enteritis and other diarrheal diseases ranked second behind accidents as a cause of death.

Health of Primary-School Children and Adolescents

In 1994, the leading causes of death in primary-school children were accidents (32%), followed by malignant tumors (14.8%) and birth defects (12.0%). In that same year, the most frequent causes of death in the group from 10 to 14 years were also accidents and malignant neoplasms. Among those 15 to 19 years old, homicide was the second leading cause of death. Analysis of mortality by sex shows that the leading cause of death in males was homicide, and in females, accidents.

Health of Adults

The total fertility rate has been declining gradually. The highest rate was recorded in the 20–24 age group, followed by the 25–29 age group. However, the states of Barinas, Monagas, Apure, Cojedes, Guárico, Sucre, Portuguesa, and Yaracuy showed comparatively high fertility rates among adolescents.

Studies conducted in the country found that illiterate women who live in rural areas have an average of 8 children, while women with university educations average 2.1. According to figures furnished by the Ministry of Health and Social Welfare, 95.3% of all deliveries in 1994 were attended by physicians.

Mortality from complications related to pregnancy in the group aged 15 to 49 constituted 6.8% of the deaths in the 1993–1995 period, with rates of 6.2 per 10,000 live births in 1993, 6.9 in 1994, and 6.5 in 1995. Over this period, the leading causes of death were hypertension complicating pregnancy, childbirth, and puerperium (28.5%); prepartum hemorrhage, abruptio placentae, and placenta previa (14.2%); and unspecified abortion (13.6%).

Health of the Elderly

According to OCEI data, in 1990 the population aged 65 and older totaled 717,774, representing 3.7% of the population. In 1994 the percentage of persons in this age group was 4.0%, and in 1995, 4.8%.

In 1990, 26.5% of older adults said they were employed; 41.3% practiced some trade or profession in the home; 68% of this population helped their families through various activities. Some 73.5% were economically dependent on others. Households with older adults, and in particular those headed by older adults, had lower per capita incomes. The lack of up-to-date information for recent years makes it impossible to assess changes in income due to inflation.

In 1994, the leading causes of mortality among those 65 and older were heart disease (42.5%), cancer (18.6%), cerebrovascular disease (15.5%), and diabetes mellitus (6.7%). There is a higher mortality rate among older men than among older women. The National Institute of Geriatrics and Gerontology indicated that in 1996 the four leading causes of morbidity, by reason for medical consultation, were hypertension (7.3%), arthritis (6.4%), influenza (3.3%), and diabetes mellitus (2.1%).

Workers' Health

According to OCEI data, in 1994, 7,903,400 people (5,390,600 men and 2,512,800 women) were economically active, and the unemployment rate was 8.6%. The percentage of women over 15 years of age in the labor force has grown since the 1960s, but in recent years, growth has been most pronounced in the group aged 25 to 44.

A series of regulations limit the length of the workday for minors. By law, children under 14 may not work. Those between the ages of 14 and 16 need special authorization, may not perform night work or piecework, and may not work more than six and a half hours per day. According to the School of Social Management of the Ministry of the Family, there is an increase in working minors. Between 1981 and 1991 the percentage of people from 15 to 19 years of age in the labor market rose from 7.7 to 12.8, and the percentage of people from 10 to 14 years of age rose from 0.8 to 1.2. There is an increase in working minors.

Health of the Disabled

The Program for Care of the Disabled of the Ministry of Health and Social Welfare estimates that 10% of the population has some type of disability. It is believed that this percentage is increasing due to the aging of the population, accidents of all types, and degenerative diseases.

The National Health System includes a system of Physical Medicine and Rehabilitation Services that serves an estimated 2% of the disabled population. To date, it has focused on diagnostic and therapeutic activities. Statistical record-keeping problems have been noted, and an information system has been put in place to better understand the actual conditions of this segment of the population.

Health of the Indigenous Population, Border Populations, and Other Special Groups

Venezuela has a richly diverse and complex Amerindian culture even though indigenous persons account for just 1.5% of the country's total population. Indigenous groups are widespread in a number of the border states. In Zulia, Páez *municipio* has an indigenous population of 88.9%, and Mara, 32%. In Delta Amacuro, Antonio Díaz *municipio* has an indigenous population of 82.9%, and Pedernales, 40.5%. In Amazonas, with the exception of Atures, all the *municipios* have indigenous populations. The rest of the indigenous groups are located in the states of Monagas and Anzoátegui, on the coast.

Critical regional and indigenous population problems include the migration from rural and jungle regions to urban areas; illegal mining, which is destroying the ecosystem; economic strangulation; aggressive evangelization; harassment; physical assaults; and health problems. The health problems that have been studied include gastroenteritis and dysentery, malaria, hepatitis B, and onchocerciasis, all of which are serious endemic diseases affecting the indigenous populations in Amazonas. To deal with these problems, health care programs have been launched in Amazonas and Zulia. Malaria is endemic throughout most of the states of Amazonas and Bolívar and constitutes the number-one recorded cause of death (40.1%) among the Yanomamis of Amazonas.

Studies conducted by the Simón Bolívar Amazon Center for Tropical Disease Research and Control on hepatitis B in the Yanomamis of Amazonas (in the communities of Parima and Mavaca) show that some 58.3% to 84.0% of the population is infected at some time during their lives. Hepatitis B is the third leading recorded cause of death after malaria and malnutrition.

In the Mavaca area, gastroenteritis, amoebic dysenteries, and helminthiasis constitute the leading cause for medical consultations and the fourth leading cause of recorded deaths. The situation is worse in the areas that do not have medical care.

Onchocerciasis is found in the Orinoco River basin and extends toward Bolívar State and Brazil. The level of endemicity ranges from 4% to 76%, and it is hyperendemic in the High Orinoco. The most seriously affected ethnic group is the Yanomami. Studies show a strong correlation between altitude and endemicity due to the increase in the variety of vector species and bite rate at higher altitudes.

Medical services in Amazonas State (1 hospital with 65 beds, 7 rural outpatient dispensaries, and 40 dispensaries without physicians) offer little coverage for such an extensive territory (177,617 km² with a density of 0.53 inhabitants per km²); in addition, access to services is difficult for some communities. Independently of these centers, activities are carried out within the framework of the programs for Dermatological Health (control of onchocerciasis and leishmaniasis), for Malariology (control of malaria and parasitic disease), of the Yellow Fever and Plague Division of the Ministry of Health and Social Welfare, the Institute of Biomedicine, and the Research Center of the Central University of Venezuela.

In Zulia State, the hepatitis B control program continued during 1992–1995. Vaccination of 56 indigenous communities moved forward, with the administration of 7,141 doses to 3,500 people of the Yucpa and Baré groups.

In 1992, the rate of new tuberculosis cases in Zulia State was 27.7 per 100,000 population in the nonindigenous population and 167.9 in the indigenous population. In the 1–4 age group the rate was 11.5 per 100,000 population in the nonindigenous population and 116.6 in the indigenous population. The figures emphasize the high transmission rate of the disease among the indigenous groups, a situation worsened by a high percentage of patients (18%) who fail to complete treatment.

The National Border Council is responsible for policies related to the indigenous population. Under draft legislation on Indigenous Communities, Peoples, and Cultures, the Council proposed implementation of a system of bilingual intercultural education and a plan to grant land to indigenous communities, as well as the inclusion and management of resources for the sustainable development of these communities in regional plans, projects, and programs.

Analysis by Type of Disease or Health Impairment

Communicable Diseases

Vector-Borne Diseases. The transmission area for malaria covers 23% of the land area of the country with an elevation of less than 600 m, and has 713,394 inhabitants at risk. The area where malaria has been eradicated or is in the maintenance phase covers 460,397 km² (76.8% of the original area), affecting 16,914,622 inhabitants. The regions in the attack phase include the states of Apure, Barinas, Táchira, and Zulia, where the principal vector is *Aedes nuñeztovari,* whose behavior is exophilic, as well as the states of Apure, Bolívar, and Amazonas, which are inhabited by indigenous groups and mine and timber workers and where the principal vector is *A. darlingi.* The case detection system takes an average of 198,000 blood samples annually. Of all infections, 91% were by *Plasmodium vivax,* 8.4% by *P. falciparum,* 0.2% by *P. malariae,* and 0.4% were mixed. In the first six months of 1997, there were 14,610 cases of malaria, an increase of 19.1% over the same period in 1996.

Some three million inhabitants are at risk from Chagas' disease. Between September and December 1995, in the 20,902 dwellings checked, the triatomine infection rate was 3.1%, and the *Trypanosoma cruzi* infection rate was 15.8%. Between January and August 1996, the rate of infestation found in 18,747 dwellings examined was 0.8%, and the rate of infection by *T. cruzi* was 13.6%. From September to December 1995, the rate of human seropositivity was 6.2% and in 1996, 4.3%. Estimates put the total number of infected people at 800,000.

There were no cases of yellow fever between 1992 and 1997. Between 1994 and 1996 vaccination coverage increased by 350%. In 1996, 1,470,742 doses were administered in the Federal District and the states of Apure, Barinas, Cojedes, Delta Amacuro, Táchira, Portuguesa, Guanare, and Mérida.

In the 1990–1996 period, no cases of human plague were recorded, and the only existing focus at present, located in Aragua State, is inactive.

In 1989 and 1990 there was an upswing in the number of dengue cases, and since then the disease has been endemic. In the five years between 1991 and 1995 this disease, in both its classical and hemorrhagic forms, was on the rise. The most cases occurred in 1995, the 32,280 cases were more than double the number in 1994. Some 5,380 (16.6%) were hemorrhagic, with 43 deaths, and 25 cases were laboratory-confirmed. The case-fatality rate was 0.13%. Serotype 4 predominated, which was a departure from previous years, when the predominant serotypes were 1 and 2. Serotype 3 was not identified in the samples that were processed. In 1996, some 9,180 cases of dengue were reported; 18% were of the hemorrhagic type, with 13 deaths. The States with the highest morbidity were Barinas, Amazonas, Aragua, Mérida, and Lara.

In recent years, schistosomiasis transmission has been limited to isolated foci, and prevalence remained below 2%. Between 1990 and 1996, 2,731 cases were confirmed through serological testing.

There are three large endemic foci of onchocerciasis: the northeastern region, which includes the states of Sucre, Anzoátegui, and Monagas, where 61% of the country's cases were recorded; the north-central region, encompassing the states of Aragua, Carabobo, part of Guárico, Yaracuy, Cojedes, and the Federal District, with 39% of the cases; and the southern region, which includes the southern part of the states of Amazonas and Bolívar and affects mainly the Yanomami, Piaroa, and Makiritare peoples. It is estimated that in 1995 there were at least 70,000 active cases of onchocerciasis.

Vaccine-Preventable Diseases. The last confirmed case of poliomyelitis was recorded on 21 March 1989, and the last compatible case was in 1993. In 1995, 104 cases of acute flaccid paralysis were reported, but none were confirmed. This represents a reduction of 5.45% over 1994, when 110 cases were reported, all of which were ruled out.

The last case of diphtheria was reported in Zulia State in 1992.

The Measles Elimination Plan, which was launched in 1994 with a National Vaccination Campaign for children from 9 months to 14 years of age and achieved a 98% coverage, substantially decreased the number of confirmed cases. In 1995 the reduction was 96%; 652 cases were recorded, with 1 death, and 172 were confirmed. In 1996, 65 of 681 suspected cases were confirmed.

In the past three years, the number of cases of and deaths from whooping cough decreased. In 1994, there were 808 cases and 21 deaths; in 1995, 510 cases and 25 deaths; and in 1996, 384 cases and 7 deaths.

The intervention strategy to reduce neonatal tetanus, especially in the parishes with substandard living conditions, resulted in a decrease from 37 cases in 1991 to 17 cases and 7 deaths in 1995. The states of Apure and Zulia reported cases every year between 1989 and 1994.

With vaccinations, the dropout rates between the first and third doses of the polio and triple (DTP) vaccines are generally above 20%.

Cholera. In June 1996, cholera reappeared in the country. The first cases occurred among the indigenous Wayuus in Zulia State. The epidemic spread, primarily affecting the inhabitants of the areas with the worst living conditions in the states of Delta Amacuro, Mérida, Aragua, Monagas, and Miranda, and in the Federal District. As of 12 July 1997, 1,972

cases had been reported, with 50 deaths (a case-fatality rate of 2.5%).

Chronic Communicable Diseases. The annual risk of infection with tuberculosis is estimated at between 0.2% and 0.4%, and new reported cases of pulmonary tuberculosis have increased by 14% since 1993. The number of cases in children under 15 has not increased. In the 5–24 age group, the increase is in the bacteriologically unconfirmed pulmonary forms. An increase in diagnoses of new bacteriologically confirmed cases was noted in the 25–44 age group. In 1995, 3,056 cases were recorded, and 2,765 were treated. After treatment, 75% of the patients had negative smears. In 1996 there were 3,195 new pulmonary cases and 726 extrapulmonary cases, with 212 relapses. The Tuberculosis Control Program systematically utilizes bacilloscopy to diagnose tuberculosis in patients with respiratory symptoms. Short-term conventional chemotherapy (less than nine months) is administered to all patients with positive sputum. The recording and reporting system recommended by WHO is utilized, and the results for the treatment of new cases are assessed.

Some 3,954 cases of leprosy were recorded in 1995. Of these, more than 65% were expected to be discharged between 1996 and 1997. In 1996, 564 new cases were reported, an increase of 12.3% over the 504 new cases detected in 1995. This is considered a positive development, since it contributes to the reduction of hidden morbidity, calculated at 500 cases. It was expected that the elimination phase would be declared in 1997, in keeping with the goal proposed by WHO of a prevalence of less than one case per 10,000 population.

Acute Respiratory Infections. These diseases are the fifth leading cause of death in children under 1 year and the third in the 1–4 age group. The mortality rate in these age groups was stable between 1989 and 1995. The states with the highest risk of death from this cause in the population under 5 are Delta Amacuro, Zulia, and Trujillo. It is estimated that there are from seven to nine episodes per child annually in urban areas and two to four in rural areas. Acute respiratory infections are the reason for 40% of the outpatient consultations and 40% of the pediatric hospitalizations.

Rabies. In 1994 no cases of human rabies were reported. In 1995 an epidemic began in Zulia State, and five cases were reported. In 1996 there were four reported cases, all from canine bites.

AIDS and Other STDs. The number of newly reported AIDS cases was 966 in 1993; 1,003 in 1994, 746 in 1995, and 226 in 1996, for a cumulative total of 2,941. The annual incidence rate per 1,000,000 inhabitants was 46.2 in 1993, 46.9 in 1994, and 34.1 in 1995. The incidence rate for men was 4.6

per 1,000,000. In 1993, 7.9 in 1994, and 18.4 in 1995, and for women, it was 0.8 in 1993, 1.1 in 1994, and 20.0 in 1995. The male/female ratio for reported cases of AIDS was 6.0 in 1993, 7.1 in 1994, and 9.2 in 1995. Persons 20 to 49 years old have the highest risk. The highest number of cases was reported in the Federal District, including the Sucre *municipio* in Miranda State; next, descending in order of frequency, were the states of Nueva Esparta, Aragua, Mérida, and Bolívar.

According to figures provided by the Ministry of Health and Social Welfare, in the three years from 1993 through 1995, the gonorrhea rate was 72.8 per 100,000. In 1996 the rate fell to 54.1 per 100,000. The syphilis rate in the 1993–1995 period was 40 per 100,000 and declined in 1996 to 24.1 per 100,000. It is believed that the decline in 1996 was due to underreporting.

Emerging and Re-emerging Diseases. Morbidity from meningitis in the 1990–1995 period was erratic. It increased from 6.7 per 100,000 population in 1990 to 10.5 in 1993; in 1994 it declined; and in 1995 it was 11.4 per 100,000 population. An improvement in case reporting has been noted. The states with the highest risk were Mérida, Monagas, and Lara, with average rates of 24.4, 22.0, and 20.8 per 100,000, respectively. In 1995 and 1996, almost 80% of the cases occurred in children under 15. In this group those at greatest risk are children under 5, particularly children under 1 year of age. In 1995 a rate of 3.4 per 100,000 live newborns was recorded. The two circulating serotypes are B and C, representing 18.5% and 37.0%, respectively, of the serotypes identified in 1995.

In August 1995 the first equine encephalitis epidemic in 20 years began, with an incidence higher than that reported in previous outbreaks. Some 12,317 cases were registered, with 24 deaths and a case-fatality rate of just 0.2%. The states of Zulia, Lara, Falcón, Yaracuy, Carabobo, and Trujillo were affected. Zulia had 90.8% of the cases and 62.5% of the deaths, and the Wayuu population was the most seriously affected. The first case observed in horses was reported at the end of April (week 14 of the year) in Yaracuy State. In week 20 the presence of the disease in horses was confirmed in Falcón State, and in week 24, the first human cases were confirmed. Of the recorded cases, 59% were found among individuals between 5 and 24 years of age. At the time of the epidemic, vaccination coverage in horses was very low.

In 1994, 4 cases of Venezuelan hemorrhagic fever were reported; in 1995, there were 8, and in 1996, there were 40 cases and 12 deaths. The 1996 case-fatality rate of 30% was higher than in previous years. In 1996 there was considerable agricultural activity in the affected areas. Most severely impacted was the group aged 15 to 45; they had 70% of the cases in 1996. Preliminary research findings on potential reservoirs point to the rodent *Zygodontomys brevicauda*.

The incidence of the cutaneous form of leishmaniasis has remained stable over the past three years, with a national incidence rate above 1 per 10,000 population. In 1996, 1,409 cases were reported, with an estimated total of 2,234. It is thought that for each reported case there are one or more unrecorded cases. The states with the highest rates were Trujillo, Mérida, Lara, Táchira, Sucre, and Anzoátegui. Up through October of 1996, 33 cases of visceral leishmaniasis (kala-azar) were recorded. Almost half the cases in the country were recorded in Anzoátegui State, followed by Nueva Esparta.

Noncommunicable Diseases and Other Health-Related Problems

Nutritional Diseases and Diseases of Metabolism. The Food and Nutrition Surveillance System (FNSS), which operates in the medical facilities of the Ministry of Health and Social Welfare, is in charge of collecting information on nutrition throughout the country. The diagnostic criterion for "general malnutrition" utilized in the FNSS is weight—2 standard deviations below the reference mean (U.S. National Center for Health Statistics) for the chronological age (weight-for-age). In the population under 15, the proportion of low weight-for-age children declined from 16.2% in 1990 to 11.6% in 1995. Differences among states are found, with the highest percentages found in Portuguesa (20.8%), Delta Amacuro (16.6%), Apure (15.6%), Miranda (14.2%), and Cojedes (13.5%). The percentages of children under 2 with low weight declined, from 16.8% in 1990 to 11.9% in 1995. It also went down for children between the ages of 2 and 6; for this group, the percentage was 29.9% in 1990, 23.7% in 1995, and 20.9% in the first quarter of 1996. In Barinas a rate of 34.56% was recorded; in Apure, 32.73%; in Delta Amacuro, 29.73%; in Amazonas, 26.46%; and in Cojedes, 25.78%. These data should be viewed with caution, since they take into account only the children seen at the health services of the Ministry of Health and Social Welfare.

Death from nutritional deficiencies in children under 15 increased from the 1991–1992 period to 1993; most affected were children under 1 year of age. The states with the highest mortality rates from nutritional deficiencies were Delta Amacuro (20.6 per 100,000 population), Amazonas (17.4 per 100,000 population), and Monagas (8.3 per 100,000 population). All three states have high percentages of unmet basic needs.

In 1994 the prevalence of overweight (defined as weight-for-height above the 90th percentile) reported by the FNSS was higher than in 1988 for all age groups. In children from 2 to 6 years of age, the prevalence increased from 9.0% in 1988 to 11.3% in 1994, and in those from 7 to 14 years of age, from 10.5% to 14%. An analysis of living conditions by the National Foundation for Study of the Growth and Development of the Venezuelan Population showed an increase in overweight 1-year-old children in the high-income strata from 10.7% in 1991 to 17.3% in 1994.

According to OCEI data, consumption of food high in vitamin A declined in the 1990–1993 period. In 1995 in Nirgua, in Yaracuy State, a survey of food consumption conducted by the National Nutrition Institute revealed that 25.7% of the population studied ($n = 165$) aged from 6 months to 6 years suffered from vitamin A deficiency, especially in the 1–3 age group. The rural population was the most seriously affected.

In 1992, according to National Foundation studies, the prevalence of iron deficiency, determined by ferritin serum levels in schoolchildren aged 7, 11, and 15 ($n = 653$) in low-income groups (IV and V), using the Graffar-Méndez method, averaged 36%, with variations of between 30.2% and 47.1% in the different age groups and sexes. In 1993, the government made it mandatory to fortify corn flour (50 mg/kg) and wheat flour (20 mg/kg) with iron (ferrous fumarate). A comparative study of the prevalence of anemia and iron deficiency in Caracas schoolchildren aged 7, 11, and 15 living in critical and extreme poverty showed that one year after fortification of the flours, the prevalence of both iron deficiency (20.4%) and anemia (9.3%) was half the 1992 levels of 42.9% for iron deficiency and 19.0% for anemia. Per capita iron consumption among strata IV children rose from 14.3 mg per day in 1989 to 18 mg per day in 1994. It also improved among strata V children, going from 13 to 16.9 mg per day over that same five-year period.

Iodine deficiency disorders constitute a public health problem, and the Venezuelan Andean region is considered an endemic area for goiter. Through the National Program for Control and Elimination of Iodine Deficiency, the National Nutrition Institute studied these disorders in the Andean region—in Mérida in 1993, in Trujillo in 1994, and in Táchira in 1995—based on a sample of 14,074 schoolchildren between 7 and 14 years of age. The Institute found a 63.5% prevalence of goiter (grade Ia goiter, 40.1%; grade Ib goiter, 20.7%; and grade II goiter, 2.7%). The prevalence of goiter was 62.4% in urban areas and 65.4% in rural areas.

An evaluation of urinary excretion of iodine in 9,592 schoolchildren in 59 urban and 94 rural localities of the three Andean states showed a median urinary iodine excretion of below 10 µg/dl in 43.6% of the rural localities and in 13.5% of the urban localities. This indicates that the risk exposure remains high in rural areas. In 1966, salt iodization was made mandatory. The National Nutrition Institute, through the FNSS and the Division of Food Research, conducts surveillance by collecting samples monthly in the three Andean states and in Zulia State, where the majority of salt producers are found. Sample collection is semiannual in the rest of the country.

The results of salt iodization for the 1993–1996 period varied. In 1993, 67% of samples were adequately iodized; in 1995, 85%; and in 1996, 64%. This is related to competition from the clandestine mills and problems in surveillance and control encountered by the health authorities.

In 1996, the National Nutrition Institute, through the Nutrition Unit of Mérida State, conducted a field study on knowledge, attitudes, and practices related to breast-feeding in the Tovar *municipio* of that state. The results showed that exclusive breast-feeding up through the fourth month was more widely practiced in urban areas (16.7%) than in rural areas (7.7%), while continuous breast-feeding for one year was more prevalent in rural areas (40.3%) than in urban areas (27.1%). It is worth noting that the percentage of mothers who did not work outside the home was 80% in rural areas and 62.4% in urban areas.

Diabetes mellitus is one of the 10 leading causes of death. According to Ministry of Health and Social Welfare morbidity data, its prevalence is estimated at 1% to 6%. It especially affects the 45–65 age group and females, and has a significant economic impact due to the high cost of medical care and loss of productivity. A prevention and control program has been implemented in 33 health services in 18 states and in the Federal District.

Cardiovascular Diseases. These are the leading cause of death. Notable among this group are ischemic heart disease and hypertension. Even with underreporting, morbidity from cardiovascular diseases is significant. According to information provided by the Ministry of Health and Social Welfare, the prevalence of hypertension in adults is 20% to 30%. A high prevalence of risk factors is noted in the population, including smoking, hypertriglyceridemia, diabetes mellitus, obesity, sedentary lifestyles, and alcoholism.

Malignant Neoplasms. Malignant neoplasms constitute one of the leading causes of mortality. In 1995 they ranked second, after heart disease. For both men and women, stomach cancer declined up through 1995. Lung cancer is rising steadily, with the trend becoming more pronounced in recent years and more marked in men than women. Prostate cancer is also increasing. Cervical cancer had been decreasing until 1985, when the trend reversed. Breast cancer has also been on the rise in recent years.

Accidents and Violence. Since 1996, Venezuela has had a surveillance system in metropolitan Caracas for fatal and nonfatal injuries resulting from violence. The Central University of Venezuela and the General Division of Forensic Medicine of the Judicial Police's Technical Corps work together on this system, with support from the National Science and Technology Research Council. Since 1997, a quarterly newsletter with data on deaths from violent causes in metropolitan Caracas has been published. Up through June 1997, homicides were the most frequent cause of violent death (69.8%), followed by accidents (23.6%) and suicides (6.5%). Homicides are on the rise, and the persons at highest risk are males from 10 to 49 years of age. The Federal District is the most affected area.

Smoking. Smoking was treated as a program area in the Division of Chronic Noncommunicable Diseases until 1995, when it became a program under the Ministry of Health and Social Welfare. Smoking control activities are interinstitutional and interprogrammatic, and are aimed at prevention among secondary school students. Protection for nonsmokers is sought through strategies to increase smoke-free spaces, mainly in the work environment. Smokers are helped through consciousness raising and training by health professionals, who offer individual assistance and also develop group strategies. Cigarette consumption has been on the decline since 1983, when all radio and television advertising was banned and a vigorous public education campaign was carried out. Annual per capita consumption has dropped from 1,950 in 1990–1992 to 900 in 1994–1996.

Oral Health. The National Directorate of Oral Health of the Ministry of Health and Social Welfare, utilizing the DMFT (decayed, missing, filled teeth) Index has noted the high prevalence of this health problem. In the 7–14 age group, 8 out of every 10 children have dental damage, and in the over-35 group, the figure is 9 out of every 10. An analysis conducted in December 1995 by the Directorate revealed that this situation had not changed.

The Salt Fluoridation Program was established in 1993. It was expanded in 1994 and 1995 with resolutions that established standards, techniques, and procedures to carry out the program and to repackage and market edible salt. The National Fluorine Commission is comprised of representatives from business, government, trade associations, and research institutes. In 1994 the country's five most important salt mines began fluoridating salt for human consumption, ensuring 85% national coverage.

Natural Disasters and Industrial Accidents. Earthquakes are the greatest natural hazard in Venezuela, since approximately three-quarters of the nation's territory is in seismic areas. On 9 July 1997, an earthquake of medium intensity rocked the eastern part of the country and, to a lesser extent, the central region. Its greatest impact was felt in the areas of Cariaco, Casanay, and Cumaná in the Sucre State. There were a total of 67 dead and 511 injured, and damage to infrastructure was estimated at US$ 25 million. The national authorities in the Ministries of Health and So-

cial Welfare and of Internal Relations, through Civil Defense, carried out the Humanitarian Supply Management (SUMA) System for disasters. Storms have also caused considerable damage, but with very few human deaths. Industrial accidents are on the rise, largely because of growth in the petroleum and petrochemical industries. In the 1981–1995 period, more than 15 major accidents occurred. Legal tools and technology have been developed with a view to reducing these numbers.

RESPONSE OF THE HEALTH SYSTEM

National Health Plans and Policies

The institutional basis, objectives, and guidelines for Venezuela's health policies are contained in the Ninth National Plan, a national economic and social development plan from which the priorities for the Executive Branch's five-year work plan are derived.

The principal elements of the health policy are:

• to reaffirm the right to health and equity and to combat inequalities and social inequities with regard to health, disease, death, and access to goods and services
• to improve the efficiency and effectiveness of the health services system and to give outpatient-services units the authority to make decisions
• to assign special priority to activities for health promotion and damage and risk prevention, thus strengthening primary care and the outpatient network
• to reaffirm the role of the State in developing health services and to democratize the health structure, with broad societal participation
• to ensure the guidance role for the Ministry of Health and Social Welfare in determining policies; managing, coordinating, and regulating the health sector; and establishing appropriate regulations.

The Ministry of Health and Social Welfare shares operational coordination and the fulfillment of medical care, social welfare, and environmental sanitation programs with 23 federal entities, as well as mayors' offices, *municipios,* and civil society, in order to jointly implement conceptual management and financing models based on individual and collective needs in the field of health.

Health Sector Reform

The 1993–1996 period was marked by a State reform process that moved ahead in decentralizing the different national sectors, especially the health sector. What drove the reform was the commitment of all of society, the promotion of health education, and social organization for active participation in the movement toward change. It is hoped that the reform will generate new management models capable of ensuring access to the health services. Its principal strategies are the restructuring and decentralization of activities. Restructuring involves restoring one of the basic attributes of the Ministry of Health and Social Welfare, that is, its guidance role in the management of the health sector. Decentralization, on the other hand, includes three essential elements: environmental health, coverage in the health care subsystems, and the organized municipalization process. The intent is for the guiding actions of the State to reach society through a system organized into mayoralties and *municipios,* conceived as links between the State and the community.

Decentralization is a sociopolitical process that seeks to link State actions with individuals, sharing management responsibilities with civil organizations under new legal arrangements. The Ministry of Health and Social Welfare becomes an agency responsible for generating policies, standards, and techniques and ceases to perform operational functions, which are now transferred to the state or municipal level or to society itself. Some of the difficulties associated with decentralization have to do with instability in ministerial management, operational conflicts (macro- and microcorporate), resistance to change, financial constraints, lack of trained staff, and the long time required to implement decentralization.

The restructuring of the Ministry of Health and Social Welfare is being carried out on three levels: managerial, strategic, and tactical. It exercises the guidance role and is responsible for insurance, subsidiary action, cooperation, management, financing, and regulation. The goal is thus to simplify functions, levels of management, upper management, and cooperation for health.

In order to restructure it is necessary to reorganize the outpatient network, strengthen organized community participation, train health personnel, improve health programs, and develop financing models with an adequate public budget. It is expected that 10% of the national budget will be allocated to health, which, together with the contributions from other sources, will make it possible to create a collective fund for the benefit of population segments that do not have the ability to pay or access to financial intermediaries.

A Restructuring Committee has been created, presided over by the Minister of Health and comprised of a Director General and sectoral directors general, in charge of managing and monitoring the reorganization of the Ministry of Health and Social Welfare.

The sources of financing for the sector are:

• the central government, through budgetary transfers from sector agencies and from the constitutional allocation of funds to the state governments, insurance companies, and private groups
• national resources from the National Health Fund; these funds will not be a permanent payment but will go to the states based on population, socioepidemiological and geographical situation, and level of poverty and rurality
• the state governments, through agreements and contracts with the municipal governments and health service centers and with financing modalities such as the Social Development Research Fund and the National Health Fund or State Health Funds, which pool resources from different sources and redistribute them on the basis of established criteria

The Comprehensive Health Service Plan, intended to provide health care for citizens, will be financed with national and state contributions to the system. Other services not included in the Comprehensive Plan will have a fee-for-services system and will be paid for by private or group insurance, direct user payments, or public funds when the decision is made to exempt beneficiaries from payment.

The centers providing hospital services will be autonomous establishments that will receive public funds based on the volume and quality of services provided and will be responsible to the individual organizations of every state.

Organization of the Health Sector

Institutional Organization

The health sector is made up of the public, private, and mixed (social security) sectors. Its most important institutions are the Ministry of Health and Social Welfare, the Venezuelan Social Security Institute, the Social Welfare Institute of the Ministry of Education, the Institute of Social Welfare of the Armed Forces, the Government of the Federal District, and the Municipal Council of Sucre, Miranda State. The private sector has grown without any planning or control, and many of its services are inefficient and costly, which increases inequity in health care.

The health facilities network provides different levels of care and is distributed throughout the entire country, but the care model and the financing and human resources policies do not guarantee accessibility, effectiveness, and quality of medical services. In general, the outpatient centers are short on supplies and proper equipment and lack health professionals. Even well-equipped hospitals and outpatient centers may not have made organizational changes. The labor situation, with its poor collective bargaining conditions, low pay, and inadequate incentives, has an adverse impact on the performance of professionals. That led to a medical strike in December 1996 that paralyzed emergency services in all the public hospitals of the country.

In March 1997 the Draft Legislation for the Comprehensive Social Security System was prepared, covering everything from medical care and the use of free time to pensions for retired persons. The project is guided by such principles as management unity, solidarity as a social obligation, the efficiency and effectiveness of the service, the participation of public and private societal players, universal protection for the inhabitants of the Republic, and financing to guarantee the delivery of services.

The Ministry of Health and Social Welfare is charged with health research and surveillance, as well as the promotion, provision, and operation of health services. Since 1996 it has been performing these functions in a dispersed manner in 10 states. In the remaining 13 federal entities, the provision and operation of the services has been transferred to the state governments.

Organization of Health Regulatory Activities

Drugs. One of the health problems confronting the country is access to drugs. Some experts believe this crisis has been accentuated by the lack of development and enforcement of a pharmacological policy backed by legislation to ensure its execution. Congress is currently studying a provisional draft of a Drug Law that governs drug production, registration, control, supply, and prices.

Drug regulations are based on legislation such as the Pharmacy Practices Law and its Regulations (1937–1993), the Organic Law of the National Health System (1987), the regulations of the decree creating the National Institute of Hygiene (1993), the standards of the Pharmaceutical Products Review Board, and the Standards for Good Manufacturing Practices of the Pharmaceutical Industry.

At present, the country has a modern registration system, mechanisms for inspecting pharmaceutical establishments, official quality control laboratories, a National Drug Control Center, a Drug Review Commission, and advisory groups that ensure the marketing of effective, safe, high-quality drugs. The operations of this system are carried out by the Ministry of Health and Social Welfare, the National Institute of Hygiene, and the states, based on the standards contained in the aforementioned laws and regulations.

Medical Supplies. With regard to paramedical products (diagnostic kits, equipment, and materials used to prevent, diagnose, and treat disease, excluding drugs), the sanitary control system has an office in charge of the registration and control of imports and the establishments that distribute them. Quality control of these products is performed in various institutions, including universities, health institutes, and private laboratories accredited for that purpose. Since January 1977, all products entering the country have had to be registered in advance.

Environmental Quality. The Ministry of the Environment and Renewable Natural Resources, together with the Ministry of Health and Social Welfare, have programs that address the quality of the environment. There are 125 drinking water treatment plants that guarantee the level of water treatment in urban areas. In the rural areas, water supply is still inadequate, and, in some cases, there are no plants to treat the water that is supplied. A sectoral analysis of drinking water and sanitation carried out in 1997 found that 80% of urban communities have drinking water service through direct connections. The remaining 20%, located in lower-income areas, receive drinking water by means of tank trucks or public spigots.

There are programs to monitor and evaluate the air in metropolitan and industrial areas, with 14 national sampling stations. The country participates in the Program for Global Information on the Environment.

The National Government has developed programs to reduce the lead content of the gasolines used in the automotive sector. In addition, programs to use natural gas have been developed, mainly in the public sector.

Soil contamination from the inappropriate use of pesticides and the presence of solid and liquid wastes has been studied, and there are standards and regulations to correct or prevent it, in addition to the Criminal Law of the Environment (1992).

The country has a significant housing shortage. The principal cities have chaotic makeshift settlements, with the impoverished segment of the population occupying high-risk areas with inadequate services. The National Government promotes housing development policies (Housing Policy Law) and has formalized projects to grant parcels of land with services in order to alleviate this problem.

Health Technology Assessment. The Ministry of Health and Social Welfare regulates the technology in the services according to guidelines that take into account the complexity of the establishments and their geographical and population coverage. In the private sector, state-of-the-art technology has been applied in the most highly developed geographical, population, and social centers. Equipment maintenance problems are becoming worse due to disorganized services, poor supervision and control, inadequate technical information, and the lack of training for personnel.

There is a scientific and technical infrastructure in the country's research centers for technology development. Ex-

539

amples of this are the progress in bioengineering made at Simón Bolívar University, the quality of the manufacturing of drugs and biologicals, the plans to link developments in science and technology with community participation that are being promoted by the National Board of Science and Technology and the activities of regional foundations such as ASCARDIO, which in 10 years has created a technical support service for the production of equipment to meet needs in Lara State. The need to identify areas for work in technology is recognized, incorporating players from civil society.

Health Services and Resources

Organization of Services for Care of the Population

Health Promotion. The Ministry of Health and Social Welfare is promoting the implementation of a new model that makes it possible to increase the autonomy and managerial capacity of the *municipios* in order to meet the most urgent needs of the population. Along these lines, the Healthy *Municipios* Strategy was adopted as one of the activities for health promotion. Begun in January 1994, the Strategy contained a proposal to promote health, foster sustainable development, improve the environment, and increase solidarity and equity in health. The process promotes health at the *municipio* and parish levels and encourages citizen participation and an intersectoral approach under the leadership of the mayoralties. As of June 1997, 15 activities were implemented in 14 federal entities; including 13 community projects. Of the community projects, 35% involved basic sanitation; 32%, social problems; 10%, program development; 8%, community organization; 6%, problems concerning morbidity and mortality; 4%, training; and 3%, information systems.

The specific programs dealing with family health are:

• Family grants program. This program provides an allowance of US$ 10 a month per student on a bimonthly basis to low-income families with a maximum of three children. Its goal is to protect the income of the family groups that are most vulnerable socioeconomically. In 1996 the program covered 3.05 million children.
• School snack program. The goal is to protect the nutritional health of children between the ages of 2 and 14, both in and out of institutions, by providing from 15% to 20% of their protein and energy needs. In 1996 the program covered 1,206,194 children.
• School food program. This attempts to improve the nutritional health of institutionalized children in preschool or grades one through six or in special education programs in government and private educational establishments. It guarantees them a daily balanced meal containing no less than 30% of their total nutritional requirements. In 1996, the program served 729,291 children.
• Maternal and child food program. The objective is to help decrease the mortality and morbidity rates for pregnant women, nursing infants, and children from 6 months to 6 years of age, by providing them with nutritional supplements. In 1996 the program covered 500,000 households.
• Multi-home program. This program provides comprehensive care for poor children under the age of 6 who are not registered in school. In 1996 the program served 350,000 children.

Programs and Health Care Policies for the Over-60 Population. Since 1978, the National Institute of Geriatrics and Gerontology, by law, has been responsible for the policies on health care for people aged 60 and over. The Institute has 29 geriatric units throughout the country—2 of them psychiatric—and offers services to 3,500 elderly people. It provides residential care with medical, social, rehabilitation, and nutrition services. In addition, it offers outpatient consultations for preventive, curative, and odontological care, in 11 metropolitan areas and in 6 states in the interior of the country. There are 4 day-care centers with a capacity for 50 elderly people. They offer all services, without separating the elderly person from his or her family circle. In metropolitan Caracas, a count taken by the National Institute of Geriatrics and Gerontology found 62 private geriatric units sheltering 2,500 elderly people.

Disease Prevention and Control. The General Sectoral Bureau of Malariology and Environmental Health is responsible for programs to eradicate malaria and to control Chagas' disease, ancylostomiasis and other intestinal parasitic diseases, schistosomiasis, other vector-borne diseases, and *Aedes aegypti.*

The Institute of Biomedicine is the organization within the Ministry of Health and Social Welfare responsible for programs to control leprosy, leishmaniasis, onchocerciasis, and other dermatoses. In Amazonas State, responsibility for these programs belongs to the Simón Bolívar Amazon Center for Tropical Disease Research and Control.

The objective of the Endemic Disease Control Project of the Government of Venezuela and the World Bank is to reduce the incidence of communicable diseases by strengthening the institutional capacity of the implementing units.

The Technical Directorate of Programs coordinates activities to prevent and control tuberculosis, cardiovascular diseases, diabetes mellitus, mental disorders, and AIDS and other sexually transmitted diseases.

Epidemiological Surveillance Systems and Public Health Laboratories. Suspected cases of diseases subject to surveillance are reported weekly to the regional or state epidemiology service by telephone or telegram. In the event of an epidemic, reporting is done daily. Every week the states send the epidemiological information to the Epidemiology Department headquarters, where the data are processed and analyzed, and where a weekly bulletin, *ALERTA,* is published for distribution throughout the country. The epidemiological information on suspected cases is also included in the monthly reporting system. Using technology developed in the Ministry of Health and Social Welfare in November 1996 the National Epidemiological Information System began operations, permitting electronic data transmission from the state level to the national level.

The virology laboratory of the Rafael Rangel National Hygiene Institute operates as a national reference center. It performs virological and serological diagnosis of infectious diseases and also manufactures biologicals (vaccines and serums).

Each laboratory in the network is equipped with an ELISA-test reader and a washer. Five laboratories are in operation, in the states of Aragua, Barinas, Falcón, Lara, and Zulia. The Aragua laboratory serves the states of Guárico, Apure, Carabobo, and Cojedes.

Drinking Water and Sanitation Services. Official figures show that drinking water supplied by direct connection reaches 80% of the people in urban areas and 65% of those in rural areas. Regarding sewer sanitation, service coverage of 69% is reported in urban areas, with the remaining 31% using septic tanks or latrines. The percentage of wastewater treated does not exceed 5% of the amount distributed.

Solid Waste Disposal, including Hospital Waste. The Municipal Waste Collection and Disposal Service has been decentralized. The mayoralties are responsible for this service, and many of them have opened the business to private operators. The major metropolitan areas receive adequate collection and transportation service. Deficiencies are noted at the final disposal sites, which are usually dumps and not sanitary landfills. The State, through the Venezuela Social Investment Fund, the Decentralization Fund, and the Municipal Development Foundation, is spending funds to improve the final disposal sites for municipal waste.

Decree 2,218 (Standards for the Classification and Management of Waste in Health Facilities) governs hospital waste. This regulation is being implemented around the country and its enforcement is considered of the utmost importance, since not all health facilities have incinerators to dispose of waste properly.

Prevention and Control of Air Pollution. There are pollution prevention programs backed by specific guidelines and regulations. Decree 2,215 establishes standards to control the use of substances that damage the ozone layer. There are projects to control industrial pollution, and other petroleum and petrochemical industry projects. One project, the Corporate Project of the Venezuelan Corporation of Guayana, made possible the installation of a network of air quality monitoring stations for Ciudad Guayana. The Project for the Elimination of Lead in Gasolines is also under way, with a timetable for its adaptation by industry. Lead levels in the atmosphere in the metropolitan areas under surveillance are below those called for internationally, except in the El Silencio area of Caracas, where the established limits were exceeded in 1993, 1994, and 1995.

Organization and Operation of Personal Health Care Services

Health Care Network. In 1995, the network of public establishments consisted of 583 hospitals and 4,027 outpatient centers (662 in the urban areas and 3,365 in the rural areas). The private sector had 344 hospitals. The average number of beds was 2.4 per 1,000 population. The public sector hospitals are type I, II, III, and IV, based on a scale of increasing complexity. Type III and IV hospitals also carry out university and postgraduate training.

Private health services are concentrated in the large population centers and serve higher-income persons. There is a trend toward emergency care, in both the hospitals and outpatient centers. There are more emergency surgeries than elective ones, and preventive consultations are infrequent. One explanation for this behavior is that elective interventions and preventive consultations have been affected by the actions of the various trade and union groups.

In recent years the physical infrastructure of the health network has deteriorated. This is seen not only in the poor physical condition of the facilities, but also in the lack of basic services, such as water and electricity, which is associated with the low rate of investment in the construction of public patient care facilities and with the lack of a maintenance policy.

Blood Banks. These facilities conduct tests to detect AIDS, hepatitis B and C, *Trypanosoma cruzi,* and syphilis. The serological reagents used to screen for these diseases are evaluated at the National Institute of Hygiene before their distribution to the blood banks.

In 1994, full coverage for these diseases, except for hepatitis C (31.6%), was provided to 202,247 donors. The results showed a 6.8% prevalence for hepatitis B, 1.3% for *T. cruzi,* 1.1% for syphilis, 0.9% for hepatitis C, and 2% for HIV. In 1995, the highest prevalence found from the screening of 202,515 donors was again for hepatitis B, with 5.9%. For syphilis, the figure was 1.1%; for hepatitis C, 0.8% (screening coverage was 57%); for *T. cruzi,* 0.8%; and for HIV, 0.4%.

Specialized Rehabilitation Services. The National Rehabilitation Program estimates the coverage of care for the disabled at between 1% and 2%. The social welfare benefits are limited to the population covered by the social security system; the rest of the disabled depend on nongovernmental organizations and some official entities. In order to increase the care available, community-based rehabilitation activities have been launched, specifically in outpatient centers.

Inputs for Health

Drugs. During 1996 and the first half of 1997, 50% of the drugs that were marketed in the country were produced domestically. That amount was 45% less than in 1990. This can be attributed to the globalization of the pharmaceutical industry and to the country's economic and financial crisis. Domestic production of pharmaceutical products and preparations is broad, and the vast majority of the essential drugs are made in the country.

Drug imports are limited to the products that have been registered in the country, except for "orphan drugs" used to treat rare disorders. Narcotics and psychotropics are subject to strict control, and their imports must be reported lot by lot.

The Pharmaceutical Products Review Board establishes guidelines that regulate the production and marketing of drugs. Advertising must follow ethical and health criteria so as to contribute to the rational use of drugs, must be compatible with national health policy, and must follow national regulations. There are different criteria for marketing depending on whether the product requires a doctor's prescription or may be sold over the counter in pharmacies.

Marketing is carried out through the laboratory/drug-store/pharmacy chain. Pharmacies dispense the products to patients. There are other marketing modalities for certain types of products, such as anti-cancer drugs or hormones. Patients receive these drugs through nonprofit foundations or institutions, for example, the Antineoplastic Drug Bank or the Endocrine Drugs Support Unit. This procedure has increased the availability of drugs for all levels of the population. The value of the Venezuelan drug market is US$ 518,628,000. Of that, $487,043,550 (93.91%) is in the private sector and $31,584,450 (6.09%) is in the public sector.

Since 1986, the producing laboratories have been subject to inspection for good manufacturing practices. The 62 producing laboratories are evaluated at least once every two years. Quality control is conducted at the government and private levels. For the government, the National Institute of Hygiene conducts surveillance through periodic planned inspections,

inspections resulting from complaints, and the checking of the first production lots. At the private levels, every manufacturing laboratory conducts surveillance, since each is required to have a quality control department in its production facilities.

Immunobiologicals. The legal base for immunobiologicals is the same as the one governing the registration and control of drugs. Domestic production is carried out by the National Institute of Hygiene, an agency that produces a portion of the vaccines utilized in the Expanded Program on Immunization of the Ministry of Health and Social Welfare. The immunobiologicals produced there are the DTP vaccine (diphtheria, tetanus, pertussis), the tetanus toxoid, and the human and canine rabies vaccine. There is a production plant and a project under way to produce blood derivatives on an industrial scale. The Institute of Biotechnology of the School of Pharmacy of the Central University of Venezuela produces polyvalent anti-venom immune serum for the treatment of snake bite and serum for the treatment of scorpion stings in quantities sufficient to meet Venezuela's needs.

Leaving out some exceptions, the importing laboratory handles importing and marketing using the same ethical and technical guidelines that govern drugs. Distribution is done directly to private entities or to the Ministry of Health and Social Welfare, which utilizes these products for its immunization programs. For certain types of products (for example, blood derivatives) the importing laboratory distributes directly to the public. Quality control is conducted at the National Institute of Hygiene by means of the Office for National Control of Biologicals.

Staff at the headquarters of the Ministry of Health and Social Welfare or the National Control of Biologicals inspect for good manufacturing practices. Venezuela participates in the Regional Network of Laboratories for Quality Control of Biologicals sponsored by the PAHO Special Program on Vaccines and Immunization and the Regional System for Vaccines.

Reagents. Until July 1997, there was no sanitary control of reagents. A proposal is being drafted to regulate their importation, marketing, and use. Domestic production is virtually nil, with the exception of a minimal amount produced in the Physics Center of the Venezuelan Institute for Scientific Research. These substances are controlled by the Ministry of Energy and Mines.

Human Resources

Some 14,676 professional nurses, 53,818 physicians, 8,571 pharmacists, and 13,000 dentists are registered in the General Sectoral Bureau for Sanitary Control of the Ministry of Health and Social Welfare. There are 31,629 nurse's aides who work for the Ministry of Health and Social Welfare.

In the health sciences, there are 12 medical schools, 7 dentistry schools, and 3 pharmacy colleges, as well as 7 nursing schools with degree programs. All are public institutions, except for two dentistry schools (Santa María University and Nor Oriental Gran Mariscal de Ayacucho University), and one pharmacy school (Santa María University).

Health sector reform changed the concept of training, viewing it as part of the work process and geared toward changing the health situation. Training is conducted in work teams and not individually, and is supported by a process that is reflexive, problem-based, democratic, and participatory.

Financing for training comes from the Ministry of Health and Social Welfare, with approximately US$ 4.5 million from the regular funds of the Ministry itself, and funds from the Social Development Project (financed by the World Bank) and Project Health (carried out jointly by the World Bank and the Inter-American Development Bank).

The Ministry of Health and Social Welfare continues to be the principal employer of the different categories of health professionals. In 1997 implementation of the Plan for the Restructuring and Transformation of Labor began in this Ministry. Within the country, the agencies empowered under the law to license, control, and regulate professional practice in the medical specialties are the associations of physicians and the Venezuelan Medical Federation. The associations of physicians are professional public corporations with legal recognition, their own assets, and all the rights and functions provided by law.

The Law on the Practice of Medicine states that there should be an association of physicians in the Federal District and in each state of the Republic, with headquarters in the respective capital. The Venezuelan Medical Federation is comprised of the medical associations of the Republic; it has professional, commercial, and union characteristics. Like the College of Physicians, it has legal recognition and its own assets, and its headquarters is located in Caracas.

Expenditures and Sectoral Financing

Public funding resources for the health sector, including contributions to social security, amounted to US$ 1,253,055,403.18 in 1993 and $1,206,713,320.46 in 1996.

Health expenditures represented 10.4% of total expenditures in 1993, 9.6% in 1994, and 9.4% in 1995 and 1996. During that same period, health expenditures as a percentage of gross domestic product decreased from 2.09% in 1993 to 1.92% in 1996. Per capita health expenditures were US$ 59.90 in 1993, $58.60 in 1994, $69.42 in 1995, and $54.10 in 1996. The Ministry of Health and Social Welfare and the Venezuelan

Social Security Institute account for 76% of public spending on health, a percentage that climbs to 93% when the state governments are included.

The distribution of the Ministry of Health and Social Welfare budget to the decentralized states and entities reveals differences. The states with the highest indices of extreme poverty are Apure, Delta Amacuro, Portuguesa, Amazonas, Barinas, Guárico, and Zulia. The states with the lowest population density—an indicator of rurality—are Amazonas, Delta Amacuro, Barinas, Portuguesa, Guárico, and Cojedes. The states characterized by both rurality and extreme poverty are Amazonas, Delta Amacuro, Portuguesa, Barinas, and Guárico. However, the budgetary allocation does not give preference to these states.

Systematized official information about private health sector financing and expenditures is not available. As a result, private health expenditures must be inferred from households' expenditures for final consumption of goods and services. The expenditures for health and education were US$ 1,308,721,887 in 1993 and $1,350,026,991 in 1994. This represented 9.4% and 10.1% of final consumption of services in 1993 and 1994, respectively. The consumer price index rose 66% between 1993 and 1994, and 55.1% between 1994 and 1995.

The financial resources allocated to the science and technology sector increased from US$ 313,090,071.31 in 1993 to $362,107,428.57 in 1995. These numbers represent 0.52% of the GDP for 1993 and 0.47% for 1995. The budget allocation for research, experimentation, and services in science and technology for institutions attached to public agencies or receiving contributions from the State rose from 11.9% in 1993 to 54% in 1995.

The financing granted by the central government through the National Science and Technology Council to promote research and technological innovation, by administrative region, decreased from US$ 1,617,195.5 in 1992 to $627,428.6 in 1995. In 1995, the central region received 40% of that financing, followed by Zulia with 21%, the Capital with 19%, the northeastern region with 12%, and the Andes with 9%.

External Technical and Financial Cooperation

The economic, political, and social crisis became acute in the early 1980s, resulting in the need to request financial cooperation to support the reform of the different national sectors. The IDB provided approximately 90% of the total funding.

The Official Development Assistance funds, understood as the net disbursements of subsidies and loans granted to the country by the Development Assistance Committee, with the basic objective of promoting economic development and well-being, decreased from US$ 81 million in 1990 to $49 million in 1993 and $31 million in 1994. Cooperation provided by the European Economic Community in 1991 and 1992 was part of this component. Official assistance totaled approximately $22.8 million. The "health and population" component received $668,366 as a donation, which was 3% of the total assistance, distributed among 15 projects.

IDB. The Ministry of Health and Social Welfare is implementing the Project for Modernizing and Strengthening the Health Sector, at a cost of US$ 300 million (of which the IDB contributes 50%). The objective of the project is to improve the coverage, efficiency, and quality of the health service networks through more appropriate and efficient spending in the sector, and to develop and strengthen the institutions responsible for coordinating the delivery of public health services. Financing from the Andean Development Corporation was also received in two subcomponents, the Program for Promotion and Prevention in Health and the Program for Strengthening and Modernizing the Ministry of Health and Social Welfare.

The Social Investment Fund of Venezuela and the Ministry of the Family are carrying out the Local Social Investment Program, involving US$ 140 million, of which the IDB contributes 60%. The objective of the program is to target resources toward social infrastructure works that improve social services for low-income groups.

The World Bank. The Ministry of Health and Social Welfare is carrying out the Health Sector Reform Program, for a total of US$ 108 million, 50% of which is financed by the World Bank. The project supports the design, implementation, and development of the comprehensive health system reform process and the policies that govern it.

The Ministry of the Family is responsible for the Social Development Program, which is part of the strategy to support decision-making to steer social sector expenditures toward targeted, efficient programs. The World Bank contributes 28%, and the total cost of the project is US$ 355 million.

The Foundation for Community Development and Municipal Promotion conducts the Program for Neighborhood Urban Improvement, totaling US$ 85 million, 47% of which is contributed by the World Bank. The stated goal is to improve the standard of living of neighborhood residents, to train the *municipios* so that they can plan, administer, and efficiently carry out investment projects, and to strengthen the Foundation in its capacity to provide technical assistance to the *municipios*.